THE TRAU
TRAUMA
CARE SUR

Fourth Edition

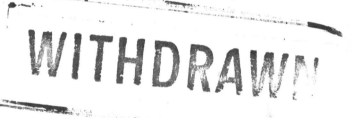

WITHDRAWN

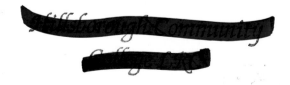

THE TRAUMA MANUAL: TRAUMA AND ACUTE CARE SURGERY

Fourth Edition

Editors

Andrew B. Peitzman, MD
Mark M. Ravitch Professor
Chief, Trauma and General Surgery
Department of Surgery
University of Pittsburgh School of Medicine
Pittsburgh, PA

Donald M. Yealy, MD
Professor and Chair of Emergency Medicine
University of Pittsburgh/University of Pittsburgh Physicians
Pittsburgh, PA

Timothy C. Fabian, MD
Harwell Wilson Alumni Professor and Chairman
Department of Surgery
University of Tennessee Health Science Center
Memphis, TN

Michael Rhodes, MD
Professor of Surgery
Thomas Jefferson University
Chair, Department of Surgery
Christiana Care Health Systems
Wilmington, DE

C. William Schwab, MD
Professor of Surgery
Department of Surgery
Perelman School of Medicine
University of Pennsylvania
Division of Traumatology, Surgical Critical Care & Emergency Surgery
Hospital of the University of Pennsylvania
Philadelphia, PA

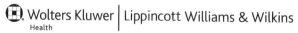
Wolters Kluwer | Lippincott Williams & Wilkins
Health

Philadelphia · Baltimore · New York · London
Buenos Aires · Hong Kong · Sydney · Tokyo

Acquisitions Editor: Brian Brown
Product Manager: Brendan Huffman
Production Manager: Bridgett Dougherty
Senior Manufacturing Manager: Benjamin Rivera
Marketing Manager: Lisa Lawrence
Design Coordinator: Teresa Mallon
Production Service: Aptara, Inc.

©2013 by LIPPINCOTT WILLIAMS & WILKINS, a WOLTERS KLUWER business
Two Commerce Square
2001 Market Street
Philadelphia, PA 19103 USA
LWW.com

Printed in the United States of America

Library of Congress Cataloging-in-Publication Data available upon request
ISBN-13: 978-1-4511-1679-3
ISBN-10: 1-4511-1679-3

To purchase additional copies of this book, call our customer service department at (800)
638-3030 or fax orders to (301) 223-2320. International customers should call (301) 223-
2300.

Visit Lippincott Williams & Wilkins on the Internet: at LWW.com. Lippincott Williams &
Wilkins customer service representatives are available from 8:30 am to 6 pm, EST.

10 9 8 7 6 5 4

This book is dedicated to those who have given their lives, and those who daily risk their lives, in the care of the injured.

Contributors

Michel B. Aboutanos, MD, MPH, FACS
Professor of Surgery
Director, International Trauma System
  Development Program
Division of Trauma, Critical Care &
  Emergency Surgery
Department of Surgery
Virginia Commonwealth University
  Medical Center
Richmond, VA

Syed M. Faisal Alam, MD
Vascular Surgery Fellow
Division of Vascular and Endovascular
  Surgery
Department of Surgery
The University of Tennessee Health Science
  Center
Memphis, TN

Louis H. Alarcon, MD
Medical Director, Trauma Surgery
Associate Professor of Surgery and Critical
  Care Medicine
University of Pittsburgh School of Medicine
Pittsburgh, PA

Darwin Ang, MD, PhD, MPH
Associate Professor of Surgery
Trauma Medical Director, Ocala Regional
Director of Research USF/HCA Trauma
  Network
University of South Florida
Tampa, FL

Derek C. Angus, MD, MPH, FRCP
Chair, Department of Critical Care
  Medicine
The Mitchell P. Fink Endowed Chair in
  Critical Care Medicine
Professor of Critical Care Medicine
University of Pittsburgh School of Medicine
Pittsburgh, PA

Juan A. Asensio, MD, FACS, FCCM, FRCS
Professor of Surgery
Department of Surgery
University of Miami Miller School of
  Medicine
Director, Trauma Clinical Research,
  Training and Community Affairs
Department of Surgery
University of Miami Miller School of
  Medicine
Miami, FL

Vishal Bansal, MD, FACS
Assistant Professor of Surgery
Division of Trauma, Burns and Surgical
  Critical Care
University of California San Diego Health
  Sciences
San Diego, CA

Philip S. Barie, MD, MBA, FIDSA, FCCM, FACS
Professor
Departments of Surgery and Public Health
Weill Cornell Medical College
Chief
Preston A. (Pep) Wade Acute Care Surgery
  Service
New York-Presbyterian Hospital/Weill
  Cornell Medical Center
New York, NY

Tiffany K. Bee, MD
Associate Professor of Surgery
The University of Tennessee Health Science
  Center
Memphis, TN

Matthew V. Benns, MD
Assistant Professor of Surgery
School of Medicine
University of Louisville
Louisville, KY

Timothy R. Billiar, MD, FACS
George Vance Foster Professor and
  Chairman
Department of Surgery
University of Pittsburgh School of Medicine
Pittsburgh, PA

Thane A. Blinman, MD
Associate Director of Trauma
Division of General, Thoracic and
  Fetal Surgery
The Children's Hospital of Philadelphia
Philadelphia, PA

Deanna M. Blisard, MD
Department of Critical Care Medicine and
  Surgery
University of Pittsburgh Medical Center
Pittsburgh, PA

Amir Blumenfeld, MD, MHA
Former Chief, Trauma Branch
Israeli Defense Forces
Israel

Charles C. Branas, PhD
Professor of Epidemiology
Perelman School of Medicine
University of Pennsylvania
Philadelphia, PA

Benjamin Braslow, MD, FACS
Associate Professor of Surgery
Division of Trauma, Emergency General
    Surgery & Surgical Critical Care
Section Chief of Emergency General
    Surgery
Department of Surgery
Perelman School of Medicine
University of Pennsylvania
Philadelphia, PA

Susan Miller Briggs, MD, MPH
Associate Professor of Surgery
Harvard Medical School
Director, International Trauma and
    Disaster Institute
Massachusetts General Hospital
Boston, MA

**L.D. Britt, MD, MPH, FACS, FCCM, FRCSEng
(Hon), FRCSEd (Hon), FWACS (Hon),
FRCSI (Hon), FCS(SA) (Hon)**
Brickhouse Professor and Chairman
Eastern Virginia Medical School
Department of Surgery
Norfolk, VA

Joshua B. Brown, MD
General Surgery Resident
Department of Surgery
University of Pittsburgh Medical
    Center
Pittsburgh, PA

Jodie A. Bryk, MD
Chief Internal Medicine Resident
University of Pittsburgh School of
    Medicine
Pittsburgh, PA

Christopher H. Byrne, MD
Assistant Professor of Surgery
Department of Surgery
The University of Tennessee Health Science
    Center
Memphis, TN

Asim F. Choudhri, MD
Assistant Professor of Radiology and
    Neurosurgery
The University of Tennessee Health Science
    Center
Memphis, TN
Director of Neuroradiology
Le Bonheur Neuroscience Institute
Le Bonheur Children's Hospital
Memphis, TN

William L. Chung, DDS, MD
Associate Professor
Department of Oral & Maxillofacial
    Surgery
University of Pittsburgh Medical Center
Pittsburgh, PA

Mark Cipolle, MD, PhD
Medical Director, Trauma Program
Christiana Care Health System
Wilmington, DE

Mitchell J. Cohen, MD
Associate Professor of Surgery
Division of General Surgery
Director of Acute Care Research
San Francisco Injury Center
University of California
San Francisco, CA

Raul Coimbra, MD, PhD, FACS
The Monroe E. Trout Professor of Surgery
Executive Vice-Chairman, Department of
    Surgery
Chief Division of Trauma, Surgical Critical
    Care, and Burns
UC San Diego Health System
San Diego, CA

David C. Cone, MD
Professor and EMS Section Chief
Department of Emergency Medicine
Yale University School of Medicine
New Haven, CT

Michael W. Cripps, MD
Assistant Professor of Surgery
UT Southwestern Medical Center
Dallas, TX

Martin A. Croce, MD
Professor of Surgery
Chief, Trauma and Surgical Critical Care
The University of Tennessee Health Science
    Center
Memphis, TN

Frederick J. Denstman, MD
Section, Colon and Rectal Surgery
Christiana Care Health System
Wilmington, DE

Jennifer M. DiCocco, MD
General Surgery Chief Resident
Department of Surgery
The University of Tennessee Health Science
  Center
Memphis, TN

Soumitra R. Eachempati, MD, FACS, FCCM
Professor of Surgery and Public Health
Weill Cornell Medical College
Chief, Trauma Services and Surgical
  Intensive Care Unit
New York-Presbyterian Hospital
New York Weill Cornell Center
New York, NY

Philip A. Efron, MD
Assistant Professor of Surgery and
  Anesthesiology
Co-director, Laboratory of Inflammation
  Biology and Surgical Science
Associate Director, Trauma ICU
Program Director, Surgical Critical Care
  Residency
Department of Surgery, Division of Acute
  Care Surgery and Surgical Critical Care
College of Medicine
University of Florida
Gainesville, FL

Timothy C. Fabian, MD
Harwell Wilson Alumni Professor and
  Chairman
Department of Surgery
University of Tennessee Health Science
  Center
Memphis, TN

David V. Feliciano, MD
Professor
Department of Surgery
Emory University School of Medicine
Surgeon-in-Chief
Department of Surgery
Grady Memorial Hospital
Atlanta, GA

John Fildes, MD, FACS, FCCM
Professor and Vice Chair
Department of Surgery
Chief, Division of Acute Care Surgery
University of Nevada School of Medicine
Las Vegas, NV

Abe Fingerhut, MD
Hippokration Hospital and Medical School
Athens, Greece

Gerard Fulda, MD, FACS, FCCM
Director, Surgical Critical Care and
  Surgical Research
Christiana Care Health Systems
Associate Professor of Surgery
Jefferson Medical College
Newark, DE

Gary N. Galang, MD
Vice Chairman for Operations
UPMC Rehabilitation Institute
UPMC Mercy Hospital
Pittsburgh, PA

Frederick Giberson, MD, MS
Assistant Professor of Surgery
Jefferson Medical College
Program Director, General Surgery
Christiana Care Health Services
Newark, DE

Steven P. Goldberg, MD
Assistant Professor of Surgery
Division of Pediatric Cardiothoracic
  Surgery
The University of Tennessee Health Science
  Center
Le Bonheur Children's Hospital
Memphis, TN

Daniel J. Grabo, MD
Division of Traumatology, Surgical Critical
  Care and Emergency Surgery
Perelman School of Medicine
University of Pennsylvania
Philadelphia, PA

Vicente H. Gracias, MD
Professor of Surgery
Department of Surgery Chief
Trauma, Emergency Surgery, Surgical
  Critical Care
UMDNJ-Robert Wood Johnson Medical
  School
New Brunswick, NJ

Francis X. Guyette, MD, MPH
Assistant Professor, Department of
  Emergency Medicine
Medical Director, STAT MedEvac
Pittsburgh, PA

Amy N. Hildreth, MD
Assistant Professor
Department of Surgery
Wake Forest School of Medicine
Winston-Salem, NC

William S. Hoff, MD, FACS
Clinical Professor of Surgery
Temple University School of Medicine
Trauma Program Medical Director
St. Luke's University Health Network
Bethlehem, PA

Daniel N. Holena, MD
Assistant Professor of Surgery
Division of Traumatology, Surgical Critical
   Care, and Emergency Surgery
Perelman School of Medicine
University of Pennsylvania
Philadelphia, PA

James H. Holmes IV, MD, FACS
Director, WFBMC Burn Center
Associate Professor of Surgery
Department of General Surgery
Wake Forest University School of Medicine
Medical Center Blvd
Winston-Salem, NC

John A. Horton, III, MD
Assistant Professor
Department of Physical Medicine and
   Rehabilitation
University of Pittsburgh School of Medicine
Pittsburgh, PA

Rao R. Ivatury, MD
Professor of Surgery
Chair, Division of Trauma, Critical Care
   and Emergency Surgery
Virginia Commonwealth University
Richmond, VA

Steven A. Johnson, MD, FACS
Assistant Professor of Surgery
Jefferson Medical College
Director, Surgery and Surgical Critical Care
Capital Health, Hopewell Medical Center
Pennington, NJ

Gregory J. Jurkovich, MD
Chief of Surgery
Denver Health and Hospital Authority
Bruce M. Rockwell Distinguished Professor
   and Vice Chairman
Department of Surgery
University of Colorado School of Medicine
Denver, CO

Michael Kalina, DO, FACOS
Assistant Professor of Surgery
Jefferson Medical College
Thomas Jefferson University
Associate Medical Director of
   Trauma
Surgical Critical Care Associates
Christiana Care Health System
Newark, DE

John A. Kellum, MD
Professor and Vice Chair
Department of Critical Care
   Medicine
University of Pittsburgh
Pittsburgh, PA

Mousa Khoursheed, MD, FRCS
Department of Surgery
University of Kuwait
Mubarak Al-Kabeer Hospital
Safat, Kuwait

Patrick K. Kim, MD
Assistant Professor of Surgery
Division of Traumatology, Surgical Critical
   Care and Emergency Surgery
Department of Surgery
Perelman School of Medicine
University of Pennsylvania
Philadelphia, PA

Edward Kwon, MD
Trauma and Critical Care
Department of Surgery
University of Nevada School of
   Medicine
Las Vegas, NV

Peter D. Le Roux, MD, FACS
Department of Neurosurgery
Perelman School of Medicine
University of Pennsylvania
Philadelphia, PA

Luke P.H. Leenen, MD, PhD, FACS
Professor of Trauma
Department of Surgery
University Medical Center Utrecht
Utrecht, The Netherlands

Ari K. Leppäniemi, MD, PhD
Chief of Emergency Surgery
Department of Abdominal Surgery
Helsinki University Hospital,
   Meilahti
Helsinki, Finland

L. Scott Levin, MD, FACS
Paul B. Magnuson Professor of Bone and
Joint Surgery
Chairman, Department of Orthopaedic
Surgery
Perelman School of Medicine
University of Pennsylvania
Philadelphia, PA

Ryan M. Levy, MD
Assistant Professor of Thoracic Surgery
Department of Cardiothoracic Surgery
University of Pittsburgh Medical Center
Pittsburgh, PA

James D. Luketich, MD
Professor of Surgery
Chair, Department of Cardiothoracic
Surgery
Director, Heart Lung Esophageal Surgery
Institute
Chief, Division of Thoracic and Foregut
Surgery
Co-director, Minimally Invasive Surgery
Center
University of Pittsburgh Medical Center
Pittsburgh, PA

Robert C. Mackersie, MD, FACS
Professor of Surgery
University of California
San Francisco, CA
Director, Trauma Services
San Francisco General Hospital
San Francisco, CA

Louis J. Magnotti, MD
Associate Professor of Surgery
The University of Tennessee Health Science
Center
Memphis, TN

Neil R. Malhotra, MD
Assistant Professor
Department of Neurological Surgery
University of Pennsylvania
Philadelphia, PA

R. Shayn Martin, MD
Assistant Professor of Surgery
Department of Surgery
Wake Forest School of Medicine
Director, Surgical Critical Care
Wake Forest Baptist Medical Center
Winston-Salem, NC

Federico N. Mazzini, MD
Attending Surgeon
Trauma & Emergency Surgery
General Surgery Department
Hospital Italiano de Buenos Aires
Buenos Aires, Argentina

Samir Mehta, MD
Assistant Professor, Department of
Orthopaedic Surgery
Perelman School of Medicine
University of Pennsylvania
Chief, Orthopaedic Trauma & Fracture
Service
Hospital of the University of Pennsylvania
Philadelphia, PA

Ali Y. Mejaddam, MD
Division of Trauma, Emergency Surgery,
and Surgical Critical Care
Massachusetts General Hospital and
Harvard Medical School
Boston, MA

J. Wayne Meredith, MD, FACS
Richard T. Myers Professor and Chair,
Department of Surgery
Director, Division of Surgical Sciences
Wake Forest School of Medicine
Winston-Salem, NC

Lyle L. Moldawer, PhD
Professor and Vice Chairman
Department of Surgery
College of Medicine
University of Florida
Gainesville, FL

Frederick A. Moore, MD
Professor
Department of Surgery
Head, Division of Surgical Critical Care &
Acute Care Surgery
Department of Surgery
University of Florida
Gainesville, FL

David Morris, MD
Senior Associate Consultant
Trauma, Critical Care, General Surgery
Department of Surgery
Mayo Clinic
Rochester, MN

A. James Moser, MD
Division of Surgical Oncology
Beth Israel Hospital
Boston, MA

Alan Murdock (Dr.) Col, USAF, MC
Chief, Acute Care Surgery
Department of Trauma and General
   Surgery
UPMC PUH
Pittsburgh, PA

Michael L. Nance, MD
Director, Pediatric Trauma Program
The Children's Hospital of Philadelphia
Templeton Professor of Surgery
Perelman School of Medicine
University of Pennsylvania
Philadelphia, PA

Lena M. Napolitano, MD, FACS, FCCP, FCCM
Professor of Surgery and Associate Chair
   Division Chief
Acute Care Surgery (Trauma, Burn, Critical
   Care, Emergency Surgery)
Department of Surgery
University of Michigan
Ann Arbor, MI

Mayur Narayan, MD, MPH, MBA
Assistant Professor, Department of Surgery
Trauma/Critical Care/Acute Care &
   Emergency General Surgery
Director, Center for Injury Prevention &
   Policy
R Adams Cowley Shock Trauma Center
University of Maryland School of Medicine
Baltimore, MD

Matthew D. Neal, MD
Resident
Department of Surgery
University of Pittsburgh School of Medicine
Pittsburgh, PA

Juan B. Ochoa, MD, FACS
Professor of Surgery and Critical Care
University of Pittsburgh
Pittsburgh, PA
Medical and Scientific Director
Nestle Health Care Nutrition/Nestle
   Health Science
North America

Mark W. Ochs, DMD, MD
Professor and Chair
Department of Oral and Maxillofacial
   Surgery
University of Pittsburgh School of Dental
   Medicine
Pittsburgh, PA

Andrew B. Peitzman, MD
Mark M. Ravitch Professor
Chief, Trauma and General Surgery
Department of Surgery
University of Pittsburgh School of Medicine
Pittsburgh, PA

Jean-Francois Pittet, MD
Professor and Vice Chair, Department of
   Anesthesiology
Director, Division of Critical Care
   Anesthesiology
University of Alabama School of Medicine
Birmingham, AL

Patrick M. Reilly, MD
Professor of Surgery
Chief Division of Traumatology, Surgical
   Critical Care and Emergency Surgery
Department of Surgery
Perelman School of Medicine
University of Pennsylvania
Philadelphia, PA

Michael Rhodes, MD
Professor of Surgery
Thomas Jefferson University
Chair, Department of Surgery
Christiana Care Health Systems
Wilmington, DE

Matthew R. Rosengart, MD, MPH
Associate Professor
Department of Surgery
University of Pittsburgh
Pittsburgh, PA

Ronald N. Roth, MD, FACEP
Professor, Department of Emergency
   Medicine
Chief, Division of EMS
University of Pittsburgh School of Medicine
Pittsburgh, PA

Michael F. Rotondo, MD, FACS
Professor and Chairman, Department of
   Surgery
The Brody School of Medicine, East
   Carolina University
Greenville, NC
Chief of Surgery, Director of the Center of
   Excellence for Trauma and Surgical
   Critical Care
Vidant Medical Center, Vidant Health
   System

Grace S. Rozycki, MD, MBA
Professor of Surgery
Emory University School of Medicine
Grady Memorial Hospital
Atlanta, GA

James M. Russavage, MD
Assistant Professor of Plastic Surgery
University of Pittsburgh
Pittsburgh, PA

Matthew Sanborn, MD
Assistant Professor
Department of Neurological Surgery
University of Pennsylvania
Philadelphia, PA

Babak Sarani, MD
Associate Professor of Surgery
Chief, Trauma and Acute Care Surgery
The George Washington University
Washington, DC

Thomas M. Scalea, MD
Physician in Chief, Shock Trauma Center
Francis X Kelly Professor of Trauma and
    Director Program in Trauma
University of Maryland School of Medicine
Baltimore, MD

Vaishali D. Schuchert, MD
Clinical Assistant Professor of Surgery and
    Critical Care
Associate Director of Acute Care Surgery
University of Pittsburgh School of
    Medicine
Pittsburgh, PA

C. William Schwab, MD
Professor of Surgery
Department of Surgery
Perelman School of Medicine
University of Pennslyvania
Division of Traumatology, Surgical Critical
    Care & Emergency Surgery
Hospital of the University of Pennsylvania
Philadelphia, PA

Ayan Sen, MD, MSc
Critical Care Fellow
Department of Critical Care Medicine
University of Pittsburgh Medical Center
Pittsburgh, PA

John P. Sharpe, MD, MS
General Surgery Resident
The University of Tennessee Health Science
    Center
Memphis, TN

Lachlan J. Smith, PhD
Research Associate
Department of Orthopaedic Surgery
Perelman School of Medicine
University of Pennsylvania
Philadelphia, PA

Jason L. Sperry, MD, MPH
Assistant Professor of Surgery and Critical
    Care Medicine
Division of Trauma and General Surgery
University of Pittsburgh School of Medicine
Pittsburgh, PA

S. Tonya Stefko, MD
Assistant Professor of Ophthalmology,
    Otolaryngology, and Neurological
    Surgery
University of Pittsburgh School of Medicine
Pittsburgh, PA

Glen Tinkoff, MD
Associate Vice Chair of Surgery
Christiana Care Health System
Newark, DE

Meredith S. Tinti, MD
Assistant Professor of Surgery
Associate Medical Director, Surgical
    Intensive Care
UMDNJ-Robert Wood Johnson Medical
    School
New Brunswick, NJ

Samuel A. Tisherman, MD
Professor
Departments of Critical Care Medicine and
    Surgery
University of Pittsburgh
Pittsburgh, PA

Glenn Updike, MD, MMM
Medical Director
Magee-Womens Hospital Outpatient Clinic
Assistant Professor
Department of Obstetrics, Gynecology, and
    Reproductive Sciences
University of Pittsburgh Magee-Womens
    Hospital
Pittsburgh, PA

Cory J. Vatsaas, MD
Division of Acute Care Surgery
Department of Surgery
University of Michigan
Ann Arbor, MI

George C. Velmahos, MD, PhD, MSEd
John F. Burke Professor of Surgery
Harvard Medical School
Chief, Division of Trauma, Emergency
  Surgery, and Surgical Critical Care
Massachusetts General Hospital
Boston, MA

Thai Vu, MD
Assistant Professor
Trauma and Surgical Critical Care
Penn State Hershey Medical Center and
  Penn State College of Medicine
Hershey, PA

Brett H. Waibel, MD
Assistant Professor of Surgery
Trauma and Surgical Critical Care
The Brody School of Medicine at East
  Carolina University
Greenville, NC

Henry E. Wang, MD, MS
Associate Professor and Vice Chair for
  Research
Department of Emergency Medicine
The University of Alabama at
  Birmingham
Birmingham, AL

Gregory A. Watson, MD, FACS
Assistant Professor of Surgery & Critical
  Care
University of Pittsburgh School of
  Medicine
Pittsburgh, PA

Hunter Wessells, MD, FACS
Professor and Nelson Chair
Department of Urology
University of Washington School of
  Medicine
Seattle, WA
Harborview Injury Prevention and
  Research Center
Seattle, WA

James F. Whelan, MD
Assistant Professor of Surgery
Division of Trauma, Critical Care, and
  Emergency Surgery
Department of Surgery
Virginia Commonwealth University
Richmond, VA

Sean P. Whelan, MD
Chief Resident in Surgery
University of Pittsburgh Medical Center
Pittsburgh, PA

J. Scott Williams, MD, PhD
Associate Professor of Radiology
Case Western Reserve University
Cleveland, OH

Donald M. Yealy, MD
Professor and Chair of Emergency
  Medicine
University of Pittsburgh/University of
  Pittsburgh Physicians
Pittsburgh, PA

Kent Zettel, MD
Chief Resident in Surgery
University of Pittsburgh Medical Center
Pittsburgh, PA

Feihu Zhou, MD, PhD
The Clinical Research, Investigation, and
  Systems Modeling of Acute Illness
  (CRISMA) Center
Department of Critical Care Medicine
University of Pittsburgh School of Medicine
Pittsburgh, PA
Department of Critical Care Medicine
Chinese PLA General Hospital
Beijing, People's Republic of China

Brian S. Zuckerbraun, MD
Associate Professor of Surgery
University of Pittsburgh School of Medicine
Attending Surgeon, University of
  Pittsburgh Medical Center and VA
  Pittsburgh Healthcare System
Pittsburgh, PA

Preface

The 4th edition of *The Trauma Manual* reflects the maturation and evolution of the field. Common to the patients for whom we provide care is their urgent presentation and often time-dependent illness, whether from injury or non-trauma critical disease. The 4th edition of *The Trauma Manual* has expanded its coverage of all components of the field: trauma, critical care, and emergency surgery. The chapters are organized by disease processes and based on the chronology of patient care. The emergency department and the trauma/acute care surgery services at many hospitals are essentially the "safety nets" for the inpatients and the critically ill outpatients. *The Trauma Manual* incorporates the diverse disease processes and care that we deliver every day.

We have built upon the success of the first three editions of this book by expanding the authorship of the chapters to more international and national experts. The chapters on trauma care have been updated and revised. New chapters on critical care have been added to this edition. Chapters on emergency general surgery have been expanded and reorganized.

As with the first editions, these chapters are written by experts in these fields. The recommendations made are backed by the extensive clinical experience of the authors. Rather than listing every option in a clinical situation, a consensus recommendation is generally presented. We have attempted to keep the content of *The Trauma Manual* practical and direct.

The goal of *The Trauma Manual* remains to serve as a ready pocket reference for all who provide care for the patient with acute surgical diseases. The format of the book is that of a user-friendly pocket manual rather than a comprehensive textbook. With that said, this book contains a great deal of information covering all phases of trauma and acute care surgery.

Contents

1 Introduction to Trauma Care

Amy N. Hildreth, R. Shayn Martin and J. Wayne Meredith

I. **INTRODUCTION.** Trauma is mechanical damage to the body caused by an external force. The trauma patient has been defined as "an injured person who requires timely diagnosis and treatment of actual or potential injuries by a multidisciplinary team of health care professionals, supported by the appropriate resources, to diminish or eliminate the risk of death or permanent disability." This chapter describes the current impact of injury on society, the structure of modern trauma systems, and the way injuries are measured and quantified as well as common patterns of injury seen with blunt, penetrating, and blast injury mechanisms.

II. **EPIDEMIOLOGY**
- **A.** Overall, trauma is the fifth leading cause of death in the United States and is the leading source of mortality for patients between 1 and 44 years of age. In 2007, 182,479 people died secondary to injury, representing 60 deaths per 100,000 population. Of these, 123,706 were unintentional in nature while 53,371 were caused by violence. A fatal injury occurs approximately every 5 minutes.
- **B.** Mortality after trauma can be characterized by three time periods during which the majority of deaths occur. As seen in Figure 1-1, approximately 50% of deaths occur immediately and are usually secondary to severe neurologic injuries or exsanguination from major blood vessel injuries. These deaths can only be avoided through injury prevention. The second peak of approximately 30% of deaths occurs during the initial hours post-injury, and preventing these deaths is the goal of modern trauma. Finally, 20% of deaths occur late (1 to 2 weeks from injury) and are secondary to sepsis and multiple organ failure. It is believed that improved early management of injury and associated shock may prevent these late complications.
- **C.** In 2009, there were over 36 million medically attended, non-fatal injuries in the United States. Data from 2007 reveal an estimated 42.4 million injury-related emergency departments and 80 million office-based visits. Injury represents the greatest cause of years of potential life lost (YPLL) before age 65, totaling over 2.4 million years or 20.1% of all YPLL. The total cost for injuries occurring in 2005 including medical expenses and lost wages was estimated to be 355.3 billion dollars.
- **D. Specific injury patterns and mechanism**
  - **1. Age.** While people 44 years old and younger account for the majority of fatal and non-fatal injuries, the impact of trauma on the elderly is far more severe. The death rate for injuries among patients 0 to 44 years old is approximately 45 per 100,000 population, whereas this rate is 113 per 100,000 for people over 65 years old and 169 per 100,000 for people over 75 years old.
  - **2. Gender.** Sixty-nine percent of all injury-related deaths occur in males, accounting for twice the number of female deaths.
  - **3. Mechanism**
    - **a. Motor vehicle crashes** (MVC) are the leading cause of injury-related death, accounting for 42,031 deaths in 2007 or 13.8 deaths per 100,000 population. Over 2.6 million people sustained non-fatal injuries secondary to MVC in 2009. Despite this, the death rate per vehicle miles traveled (VMT) has declined steadily throughout the century.
    - **b. Firearm-related injury** resulted in 31,224 deaths in 2007 and was the third leading cause of injury-related mortality for all ages. Fifty-six percent were a

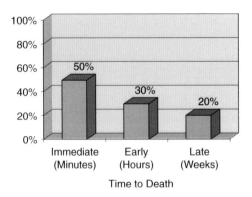

Figure 1-1. Distribution of death after injury. Adapted from: Trunkey DD. Trauma. Accidental and intentional injuries account for more years of life lost in the U.S. than cancer and heart disease. Among the prescribed remedies are improved preventive efforts, speedier surgery and further research. *Sci Am* 1983;249(2):28–35 .

result of suicide while 41% were homicide-related. Non-fatal gunshot wounds were identified in 66,769 patients in 2009. Predominately, fatal shootings involve young males; the number of deaths in the 15- to 34-year-old age range is over seven times the number of female deaths. Firearm-related injuries peak at 19 years of age.

- c. **Falls** are the leading cause of non-fatal injury, resulting in approximately 8.8 million injuries and 23,443 deaths throughout all age groups. Falls are most common among the young and the elderly with both groups demonstrating injury rates of greater than 4,000 injuries per 100,000 population. Despite this similarity, falls are the leading cause of death in patients 65 years or older while death in children is uncommon. The death rate due to falls in elderly patients is more than 170 times that of children less than 10 years old. The peak incidence occurs at age 85.
- d. Other common mechanisms contributing to trauma mortality include poisoning, suffocation, drowning, cutting/piercing, and burns.

III. TRAUMA SYSTEMS
A. Overview
1. As defined by the Trauma System Agenda for the Future, "A trauma system is an organized, coordinated effort in a defined geographic area that delivers the full range of care to all injured patients and is integrated with the local public health system."

Historical perspective. The systematic care of trauma changed significantly with the publication of, "Accidental Death and Disability: The Neglected Disease of Modern Society" in 1966. This document revealed the deficiencies in injury management and initiated the development of systems to improve trauma care. The Emergency Medical Services Systems Act was passed in 1973 to support the development of regionalized Emergency Medical Services (EMS systems. In 1976, the American College of Surgeons (ACS) Committee on Trauma (COT) published, "Optimal Hospital Resources for the Care of the Seriously Injured" which established criteria that identified hospitals as trauma centers. This document has been revised as knowledge about trauma systems has evolved. More recently, the Model Trauma Care System Plan created by the Health Resources Services Administration (HRSA) was published to further define and guide trauma system development.

2. **Function.** Trauma systems have been designed to be *inclusive* in nature and use all available resources to provide appropriate care to all injured patients.
3. **Designation and verification.** Facilities within a trauma system require identification of injury management capabilities so that resource assessments can be achieved. A government group designates a hospital as a trauma center after evaluating the facility's resources and the ability to provide a specific level of care.

B. Fundamental components
1. **Injury prevention** has become an essential focus for all trauma systems in order to proactively reduce the impact of injury.
2. **Prehospital care** includes community access and communication systems as well as EMS systems and triage protocols. Universal access to emergency care (i.e., 911) is essential to allow efficient activation of the system. A robust communication system provides coordination of prehospital resources as well as proper transfer of information to receiving facilities. Standardized curricula for training EMS personnel provide a more consistent knowledge base and skills set. Developed trauma systems have insured more efficient emergency response through improved geographical placement of EMS providers versus only facility-based responders.
3. **Acute care facilities** provide a range of injury management from initial stabilization and transfer to all-inclusive definitive care. On the basis of available resources, facilities are characterized by injury management capabilities and many are designated as trauma centers using a scale of 1 to 4, with Level 1 centers providing the most comprehensive level of care.
4. **Post-hospital care** is an important part of reducing disability and improving an injured patient's long-term outcome.

C. Trauma system infrastructure elements
1. **Leadership.** A lead agency should be established to coordinate trauma system development and provide necessary administration.
2. **Professional resources.** Successful trauma systems rely on competent and energetic health care providers to insure optimal injury care.
3. **Education/Advocacy.** Trauma systems must endeavor to improve public awareness about trauma as a disease state and the ability of injury prevention to reduce the societal impact of trauma.
4. **Information Management.** Trauma data registries at the local and national levels provide an invaluable resource for performance improvement, research, and trauma system management. Ideally, trauma data should be consistently captured and incorporated into regional and national databases to provide the most accurate depiction of the status of injury care.
5. **Finances.** Adequate financial support is essential for both trauma system development and the continued provision of trauma care. Increased public and political awareness of the magnitude of the problem is required to improve governmental funding.
6. **Research.** To continue improving the care of the injured, research endeavors must be encouraged and efforts to increase financial support for trauma research are crucial.
7. **Technology.** The potential of novel and developing technologies must be adopted and applied to the field of trauma care.
8. **Disaster preparedness and response.** Trauma systems are charged with the task of being prepared to respond to potential disasters by developing a systematic and organized approach that can be implemented if the need arises.

IV. INJURY SCORING
A. Principles
1. **Purpose.** Injury scoring systems have been developed to accurately and consistently quantify the magnitude of injury from an anatomic, physiologic, or a combined standpoint. Scoring systems are used in triage decision making, quality improvement and benchmarking initiatives, prevention program analyses, and research endeavors.
2. **Database use.** Scoring systems are commonly included in trauma databases to provide a quantifiable means of patient comparison. (See Chapter 20.)
3. **Correct use of scoring.** Systems used for triage decision making must be easy to calculate from rapidly available information. Scoring is commonly used in the research setting and in this case, should be able to identify patients with comparable injuries. Evaluation of responses to therapy may benefit from applying

a physiologic scoring system. The combined scores are valuable when assessing outcome after injury.

  4. Limitations. Since each injured patient is unique, there is no single scoring system that can provide a perfect description.

B. Scoring Systems (see Chapter 60)

  1. Anatomic scores

   a. Abbreviated Injury Score (AIS), Injury Severity Score (ISS), New Injury Severity Score (NISS)

   b. American Association for the Surgery of Trauma (AAST), Organ Injury Scale (OIS)

   c. Survival Risk Ratios (SRR)/ICD-based Injury Severity Score (ICISS)

   d. Anatomic Profile (AP)

   e. Penetrating Abdominal Trauma Index (PATI). PATI is a scoring system designed to quantify the effects of penetrating abdominal injury. Each organ has a predetermined risk factor score (1 to 5) and injured organs are assigned a severity score (1 to 5) based on published criteria. The severity score is multiplied by the risk factor score and the sum of all of these results are the PATI.

  2. Physiologic scores

   a. Glasgow Coma Score (GCS)

    i. A GCS of 8 or less is usually indicative of severe brain injury and may be suggestive of required intervention (e.g., intubation).

    ii. The motor component of the GCS has been found to correlate well with the entire GCS and be the most predictive of outcome.

    iii. Revised Trauma Score (RTS)

    iv. Systemic Inflammatory Response Syndrome Score (SIRS Score)

   b. Trauma Score (TS)

  3. Combined Scores

   a. Trauma and Injury Severity Score (TRISS)

   b. A Severity Characterization of Trauma (ASCOT)

C. Validation of scoring systems

  1. After the development of a scoring system, a process of validation is required to confirm its accuracy and predictive nature. This can often be accomplished by challenging the scoring system against a large, well-constructed trauma database such as a state trauma registry, governmental database, or the NTDB.

V. MECHANISMS OF INJURY

A. Principles. Trauma can result from multiple mechanisms of injury, including blunt injury, penetrating injury, thermal injury (discussed in a later chapter), or some combination of these three. These mechanisms often result in discrete injury patterns; recognition of injury patterns common with each mechanism is essential to prompt diagnosis and treatment of associated injuries. Knowledge of injury mechanism provides guidance in determining the proper approach to an injured patient.

B. Blunt injury

  1. Types

   a. Motor vehicle collision

    i. Determinants of injury

     a) Magnitude of force/energy of collision

     b) Direction of force

     c) Location of occupant in vehicle

     d) Use of restraint device

     e) Type of vehicle(s) involved in collision

    ii. Injury patterns

     a) Front. Injuries in this type of collision tend to follow one of two injury patterns—either an "up and over" or a "down and under" pattern. The former occurs when the chest and abdomen strike the steering wheel and the head impacts the windshield. In this case, the cervical spine takes much of the load of the collision. Common injuries may include rib fractures as well as pulmonary and myocardial contusion from chest wall—steering wheel impact. Shear forces may contribute to injuries to the aorta or liver. Brain injury is common due to direct compression, and acute neck flexion or hyperextension may lead to cervical spine injury. In the latter pattern of injury, the occupant is pushed under the steering column, often striking the knees on the dashboard. In this case, the upper leg absorbs much of the impact. Commonly noted injuries include knee dislocation, femur fractures, and posterior hip dislocation with acetabular fracture.

b) **Lateral.** If energy is transferred to the vehicle directly and the vehicle stops, this mechanism results in an injury pattern compatible with a lateral crushing injury to the spine, torso, and pelvis. Common injuries include flail chest, pulmonary contusion, liver injuries, and splenic injuries. Brain injury is also common in this scenario. However, if motion is imparted to the vehicle, the torso is often pushed laterally as the head remains in its original position, resulting in lateral flexion and rotation of the cervical spine, leading to fractures and ligamentous injuries.

c) **Rear.** Injury patterns with this mechanism will depend upon the presence or absence of subsequent impact after the initial collision as it is common to strike another object ahead of the vehicle as a result of the collision. The most common injury seen is cervical spine hyperextension and resultant injury during forward acceleration following impact.

d) **Rotational.** In these collisions, injury patterns are commonly a combination of front and lateral impact patterns.

e) **Rollover.** Rollover collisions are highly unpredictable in terms of injury patterns, as there may be trauma to the vehicle occupant from a multiplicity of directions.

f) **Ejection.** Those vehicle occupants who are ejected during a collision have the greatest potential for injury. In a collision, some protection is afforded to the occupant by the vehicle. Those who are ejected do not have this protection, and they have the velocity of the vehicle as they are ejected, resulting in the potential for serious injury. Ejected occupants have been found to be four times as likely to require admission to an intensive care unit and five times more likely to die following injury.

iii. **Role of restraints**

a) **Injury prevention.** Three-point seat belt restraints were first introduced in 1967 by Bohlin, resulting in significant decreases in mortality when compared to unbelted occupants during collisions. Recently, the National Highway Traffic Safety Administration (NHTSA) has reported these belts to be 43% to 50% effective in reducing traffic fatalities and to have decreased serious injury by 45% to 55%. NHTSA data indicate that air bag use alone decreases mortality by 13%; used in combination with restraints, the mortality reduction increases to 50%. However, air bags are most effective in frontal collisions. Side air bags when available are more useful in lateral collisions and rollovers.

b) **Associated injuries.** Although restraint systems and air bags have significantly decreased morbidity and mortality from collisions in recent years, their deployment has also been associated with specific injury patterns. If lap belts are applied above the iliac crests, they contribute to what is known as the *seat belt syndrome.* Bowel and other intraabdominal injuries may occur. Increased intraabdominal pressure can cause diaphragmatic rupture, and lumbar spine injuries are seen. Injuries attributable to the shoulder strap include rib fractures, clavicle fractures, and blunt cerebrovascular injury. Improper positioning of seat belt restraints increases the likelihood of these associated injuries. Air bag deployment also has the potential to cause injury. Trauma to the eyes, face, cervical spine, chest, abdomen, and upper extremities has been reported. However, 96% of all airbag-associated injuries have been reported to be minor.

b. Motorcycle collision. As with motor vehicle collisions, injury pattern in motorcycle collisions is dependent on the type of collision. Common motorcycle collision types are listed below.

i. Frontal. In this type of collision, the motorcycle tips forward, and the rider is thrown over the handlebars. Head, thoracic, and abdominal injuries are common. If the rider's feet are in contact with the pegs when collision occurs, femur fractures may occur.

ii. Angular. Crush injuries to the lower extremities are common following angular impacts.

iii. Ejection. If the rider is ejected from the motorcycle, as with motor vehicle collisions, there is a significant potential for serious injury. Specific injuries are unpredictable, given multiple directions of force.

iv. Rear. Injuries from rear impact result from rapid acceleration followed by hyperextension and subsequent crush from impact or from the colliding vehicle.

c. Pedestrian–auto collision. The injury pattern caused by these collisions is dependent upon both the size of the pedestrian and the size of the automobile causing injury.

i. Adult. When an adult is struck by a motor vehicle, the car bumper may first impact the lower leg, resulting in tibia and fibula fractures. Subsequently, the pedestrian is thrown onto the hood. The femur and pelvis will often make the first hood impact, followed by the thorax, abdomen, and craniofacial area. A third impact results from the pedestrian striking the ground, causing further injury. The classic triad of injuries includes fracture of the tibia and fibula, injury to the trunk, and injury to the brain (Waddell's triad).

ii. Child. In contrast, a child who is struck by a motor vehicle usually receives the initial impact of the bumper at the level of the pelvis or femur. The hood usually strikes the thorax, and the child is often dragged under the vehicle, often resulting in severe multisystem trauma.

d. Falls. Falls may result in multiple impacts; the height of the fall typically determines the severity of injury. The landing surface is also of importance. Landing on the feet after an approximately vertical fall may result in a common injury pattern of bilateral calcaneus fractures, vertical sheer injury to the pelvis and thoracic and lumbar spine fractures due to axial loading.

e. Assault. Head and facial injuries are the most common injuries with this mechanism. Defensive posturing may result in upper and lower extremity injuries. However, torso injuries may also be present as a result of kicking or stomping.

C. Penetrating injury (see Chapter 23)

1. Types

a. Gunshot wounds. A basic knowledge of ballistics is necessary for the surgeon providing care to a patient injured by a gunshot wound. Ballistics refers to the study of the flight, behavior, and mechanics of projectiles. When describing a projectile and its motion, three categories of ballistics apply: Internal, external, and terminal ballistics.

i. Internal ballistics. The effects of bullet and weapon design and material within the weapon are known as internal ballistics.

a) Bullet characteristics. Characteristics of the path down the weapon are imparted by the bullet's material. Bullets are often manufactured of lead, but lead bullets leave significant deposits along the barrel of a weapon at high velocities. Therefore, these lead bullets are often coated with a harder metal to prevent deformity, known as a jacket, usually of copper. If the bullet is completely surrounded by the jacket, the covering is termed a *full metal jacket*. Partially encased bullets are *semi-jacketed*; these bullets have exposed lead at the tip and are referred to as *soft-point bullets*. Soft-point bullets are meant to deform on contact. Bullets called

| TABLE 1-1 | Ballistic Data for Handguns | | | |

Caliber (in.)	Weapon type	Bullet weight (grains)	Muzzle velocity (ft./s)	Kinetic energy (ft–lbs)
0.22	22 short	29	1,000	72
0.25	25 automatic	50	810	73
0.38	38 special	158	870	263
0.354	9 mm Luger	115	1,155	341
0.357	357 magnum	158	1,410	696
0.44	44 magnum	240	1,470	1,150

hollow-point bullets may also have an open cavity at the tip which also predisposes to deformation.

b) Weapon characteristics. Modern guns with the exception of shotguns, discussed later, have a series of spiraling ridges (referred to as lands) and grooves lining the interior of the barrel in order to impart spin to the bullet along its longitudinal axis. These lands and grooves are termed rifling. The spin of the bullet lends stability after it leaves the weapon (Tables 1-1 and 1-2). Guns with rifled barrels are referred to as being of a certain "caliber," which refers to the approximate internal diameter of the barrel of the weapon, usually expressed in hundredths or thousandths of an inch.

ii. External ballistics. The main forces acting on a bullet that affect its behavior after leaving the barrel of the weapon are gravity and drag.

a) Gravity. All projectiles have the same rate of acceleration toward the ground due to gravity. However, faster projectiles will travel farther than slower projectiles prior to hitting the ground.

b) Drag. Drag is the force produced by the resistance to air or fluid as the bullet passes through. Drag increases exponentially with velocity; sectional density (mass divided by cross-sectional area) decreases drag. Therefore, drag has the least effect on a heavy, narrow projectile.

c) Stability. The stability of a projectile in flight is also subject to variation. Bullets may develop a slight wobble upon leaving the barrel due to imperfections in the bullet, pressure differences in the barrel, and slight movement of the barrel. This wobble is called *precession* and is a rotation around the center of mass of the bullet. Bullets may also develop *yaw*, a rotation of the nose of the projectile away from the line of flight and measured by the angle between the long axis of the bullet and its flight path. *Nutation* is a smaller circular movement at the tip of the bullet. Any of these movements increase drag and decrease velocity.

| TABLE 1-2 | Ballistic Data for Rifles | | | |

Caliber (in.)	Weapon type	Bullet weight (grains)	Muzzle velocity (ft/s)	Kinetic energy (ft–lbs)
0.22	Remington 22	40	1,180	124
0.223	M-16	55	3,200	1,248
0.30	AK-47	123	3,500	1,725
0.270	270 Winchester	150	2,900	2,810
0.308	30–0	150	2,910	2,820

iii. Terminal ballistics. Terminal ballistics describes the behavior of a projectile in tissue.

  a) Kinetic energy. Kinetic energy (KE) of a missile is proportionate to the mass (m) of the missile times its velocity (v) squared.

$$KE = 1/2\,mv^2$$

  Therefore, the amount of kinetic energy of a bullet is highly dependent upon its velocity. Modern bullets have been designed to maximize the amount of kinetic energy dissipation into the tissue.

  b) Cavitation

  1) Permanent. The size of the permanent cavity caused by the bullet's path through the tissue is usually relatively small, especially if there is minimal yaw. As yaw increases, the amount of tissue crushed and thereby the permanent cavity increases. This cavity's size may also be increased by the use of soft-point and hollow-point bullets. These often deform into a mushroom shape, increasing surface area and wound severity. Bullet fragmentation increases the size of the permanent cavity as well.

  2) Temporary. When a bullet passes through tissue, a temporary cavity is formed in addition to the permanent cavity. This cavity is a result of the waves created by the bullet which are perpendicular to the direction of the bullet's travel, which compress adjacent tissues. High-energy projectiles tend to cause a larger temporary cavity. The type of tissue the bullet passes through also determines the effect of the temporary cavity. In solid organs, the effect of the temporary cavity is greater than in air-filled organs. Tumbling and fragmentation may also affect the size of the temporary cavity.

b. Shotgun wounds. In contrast to the barrel of a handgun or rifle, the inside of a shotgun barrel is smooth. A shotgun fires multiple metal spheres at a high velocity. These pellets decelerate rapidly because of their unfavorable aerodynamics, and have greatest wounding capacity at a relatively close range (4 to 5 m). Shotguns are generally referred to in terms of "gauge." This term originally described the quantity of lead shot capable of fitting in the diameter of the barrel. Smaller pellets fired from a shotgun are traditionally known as "bird shot"; larger pellets are known as "buck shot." Within a shotgun shell, the pellets are separated from the powder by plastic or cardboard wadding. Search for wadding when a patient is wounded by a shotgun, as it is not identifiable radiographically. Take care to serially examine these wounds, as the greatest extent of tissue destruction may not be immediately apparent.

c. Stab wounds. In contrast to gunshot wounds, stab wounds are low-energy wounds caused by "hand-driven" weapons. The most commonly used weapon is a knife, but other sharp objects of various types may be used to cause stab wounds as well. History of weapon type and length is poorly predictive of actual injury.

D. Combined injury

1. Blast injury. In addition to the current military experience, there were a reported mean of 1327 bombing incidents per year between 1989 and 2002 in the United States. Familiarity with associated injury patterns is essential for any practicing trauma surgeon.

  a. Primary blast injury. Primary blast injury is caused by pressure differentials. The most vulnerable tissues are the tympanic membrane, the lungs, the bowel, and the brain. If the tympanic membrane is uninjured, injury to other organs from primary blast injury is much less likely.

  b. Secondary blast injury. When debris from the explosive device is picked up by the blast wave and accelerated toward the victim, this results in secondary blast injury. These injuries are more common than primary blast injuries, and may cause significant blunt and penetrating wounds. It must be noted that as the explosion occurs, debris is scattered widely, so be careful to assess for wounds distant from the site of most obvious injury. Significant bony injury is also common.

c. **Tertiary blast injury.** Tertiary injury occurs after a blast when there is structural collapse and subsequent entrapment. Injury pattern is highly dependent upon the type of blast and structure, but compartment syndromes and crush syndrome resulting in rhabdomyolysis may occur.

d. **Quaternary injury.** Thermal and other environmental exposures contribute to quaternary injuries. These injuries may include burns or inhalation injuries.

Suggested Readings

Baker SP, O'Neill B, Haddon W Jr, et al. The injury severity score: a method for describing patients with multiple injuries and evaluating emergency care. *J Trauma* 1974;14(3):187–196.

Carter PR, Maker VK. Changing paradigms of seat belt and air bag injuries: what we have learned in the past 3 decades. *J Am Coll Surg* 2010;210(2):240–252.

Champion HR, Copes WS, Sacco WJ, et al. A new characterization of injury severity. *J Trauma* 1990; 30(5):539–545; discussion 545–546.

Champion HR, Sacco WJ, Copes WS, et al. A revision of the Trauma Score. *J Trauma* 1989;29(5):623–629.

Fast stats A to Z. U.S. Department of Health and Human Services Web Site. http://www.cdc.gov/nchs/fastats/Default.htm. Accessed August 17, 2011.

Hoyt DB, Coimbra R. General considerations in trauma. In: Mulholland MW, Lillemoe KD, Doherty GM, Maier RV, Upchurch GR, eds. *Greenfield's Surgery: Scientific Principles and Practice*. 4th ed. Philadelphia, PA: Lippincott Williams & Wilkins; 2006.

Hunt JP, Weintraub SL, Marr AB. Kinematics of trauma. In: Feliciano DV, Mattox KL, Moore EE, eds. *Trauma*. 6th ed. New York, NY: McGraw Hill Medical; 2008.

Maiden N. Ballistics reviews: mechanisms of bullet wound trauma. *Forensic Sci Med Pathol* 2009;5(3): 204–209.

Malone DL, Kuhls D, Napolitano LM, et al. Back to basics: validation of the admission systemic inflammatory response syndrome score in predicting outcome in trauma. *J Trauma* 2001;51(3):458–463.

Meredith JW, Evans G, Kilgo PD, et al. A comparison of the abilities of nine scoring algorithms in predicting mortality. *J Trauma* 2002;53(4):621–628; discussion 628–629.

Rutledge R, Osler T, Emery S, et al. The end of the Injury Severity Score (ISS) and the Trauma and Injury Severity Score (TRISS): ICISS, an International Classification of Diseases, ninth revision-based prediction model, outperforms both ISS and TRISS as predictors of trauma patient survival, hospital charges, and hospital length of stay. *J Trauma* 1998;44(1):41–49.

Trunkey DD. Trauma. Accidental and intentional injuries account for more years of life lost in the U.S. than cancer and heart disease. Among the prescribed remedies are improved preventive efforts, speedier surgery and further research. *Sci Am* 1983;249(2):28–35.

Volgas DA, Stannard JP, Alonso JE. Ballistics: a primer for the surgeon. *Injury* 2005;36(3):373–379.

WISQARS. CDC Web Site. http://www.cdc.gov/injury/wisqars/index.html. Accessed August 1, 2011.

2 Physiologic Response to Injury

Luke P.H. Leenen

I. Multiple changes occur in an organism following injury. The initial responses are protective, followed by compensation for the changes experienced and attempts to restore integrity and homeostasis. After the initial physiologic mechanisms to compensate, processes are initiated to prepare the organism to repair and ultimately heal. The response to injury is composed of a local response, tissue level reaction, and a general, systemic, response. After the first hit and the initial response, an individually determined response is evoked by the organism on a systemic level, depending on the extent of the injury.

A. Immediate changes experienced after injury (Table 2-1):
  1. Tissue injury, disrupting the integrity of the tissues
  2. Hemorrhage, followed by:
   a. Hypovolemia
   b. Hypercarbia
   c. Hypoxia
   d. Acidosis
   e. Coagulopathy
  3. Tissue edema and volume shifts

B. The immediate changes are followed by a fight or flight response, which is an adrenocortical response to stress and leads to increased production of corticosteroids and catecholamines. This redistributes the blood flow to essential organs such as the heart and brain. The hypothalamic–pituitary (ACTH, endorphins, ADH)–adrenal (corticosteroids, epinephrine) axis is activated, as well as kidney response (renin) and sympathetic response (catecholamines). These activations lead to a hormonally driven homeostatic response, composed of:
  1. Increase in heart rate
  2. Increase in respiratory rate
  3. Fever
  4. Leukocytosis
   This immediate response is supported by:
   a. Excitation of the sympathetic nervous system, because of the pain elicited by the trauma. This leads to hypertension, a high pulse rate and cortisol release.
   b. Stimulation of baroreceptors, atrial as well arterial, leads to vasoconstriction and increased hormonal activity.
   c. Specific changes in the blood composition lead to stimulation of chemoreceptors, which elicit compensatory changes.

C. After the immediate response, several other processes ensue:
  1. Hemostasis
  2. Volume shifts
  3. Local and systemic immune response
  4. Initiation of tissue repair through local tissue reaction involving (Fig. 2-1):
   a. Complement. Based on ischemia and endothelial injury; invading microorganisms also may activate plasma proteins
   b. Oxygen radicals
    i. Produced by leukocytes and parenchymal cells
    ii. Consist of toxic products, such as hydrogen peroxide, superoxide, and hydroxyl radicals

TABLE 2-1	Organ System Response
Organ system	**Physiologic response**
Cardiovascular	Tachycardia
	Blood pressure
	Cardiac output higher
Renal	Lower output
Adrenal	Higher cortisol release
Pulmonary	Increased minute volume:
	By higher frequency and tidal volume
CNS	Altered mental state (direct or indirect)
Splanchnic	Decreased blood flow
	Disintegrated barrier function
General	Edema:
	■ Higher body salt
	■ Interstitial fluid
	■ Capillary permeability
	■ Hyponatremia
	■ Local cytokines
	Hypermetabolism
	Leukocytosis/platelets

    c. Cytokines. Responses by local tissues, but also by systemic organs such as the liver

    d. Eicosanoids. Prostaglandins, leukotrienes, and thromboxanes

    e. Nitrogen oxide. From endothelial cells as a homeostatic factor for the immediate regulation of the blood pressure. Increased by inflammation and may contribute to profound hypotension and decompensated hemorrhagic shock.

    f. Others. Release of several growth factors such as platelet-derived growth factor and endothelial-derived growth factor

II. HEMOSTASIS: THE EFFECT OF TRAUMA ON COAGULATION

    A. Coagulation is a complex process which attempts to maintain integrity of the vascular system. Important in this respect, is the process of thrombocyte aggregation to plug the gap with thrombus formation. Coagulation abnormalities have long been thought to be only secondary to hemodilution from resuscitation and hypothermia. We now understand that tissue injury directly influences coagulation (acute traumatic coagulopathy). As mentioned above, the coagulation system is influenced by our treatment, as following factors influence coagulation:

      1. Dilution

      2. Hypothermia

      3. Hypoxia

      4. Acidosis

    Currently, however, trauma and, more importantly, tissue hypoxia are seen as important, independent factors in the development of coagulation disorders after trauma.

      Trauma-induced coagulopathy (TIC) and its component acute traumatic coagulopathy lead to endogenous coagulopathy, which is present in up to 25% of trauma patients entering the emergency department. It is induced by a combination of tissue injury and shock and related to tissue hypoperfusion. The driver seems to be the systemic activation of the protein C pathway (Fig. 2-2), resulting in:

      a. Coagulation inhibition. Thrombomodulin is presented by the damaged endothelium and forms the Thrombomodulin complex which can no longer cleave fibrinogen

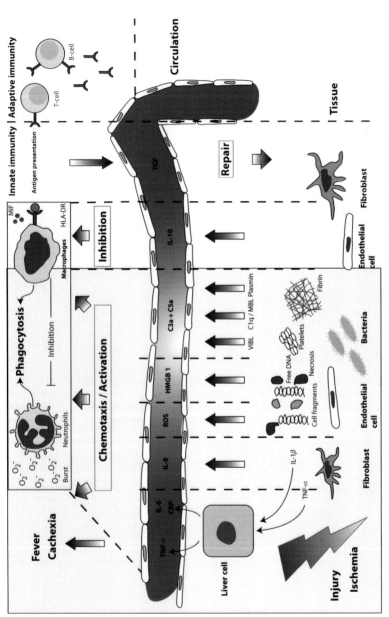

Figure 2-1. Cascade of processes after injury (left lower corner). Role of various cells and cytokines and their actions. Redrawn after Hietbrink et al. *WJES* 1:15.

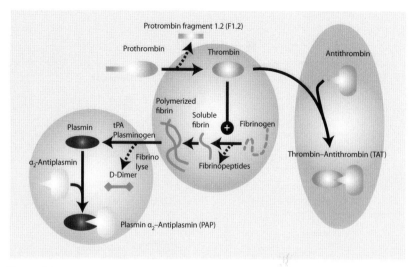

Figure 2-2. Trauma induced coagulopathy driven by activation of the Protien C pathway.

    b. Decreased fibrinogen utilization
    c. Increased fibrinolysis. Tissue plasminogen activator (tPA) is presented by the endothelium by injury and hypoperfusion. tPA cleaves plasminogen to initiate fibrinolysis. Moreover, a potent inhibitor of tPA, plasminogen activator inhibitor-1 (PAI-1) is consumed leading to hyperfibrinolysis.
  B. Elevated admission INR is an independent predictor of poor outcome in trauma patients. Currently, thromboelastography (TEG) is utilized to further clarify the coagulopathy of trauma.

III. CONTINUED VOLUME SHIFTS

  A. Hypoxemia at the tissue level and the effects of microparticles released after tissue damage compromise the integrity of the endothelial lining and the natural barrier is lost, resulting in a rapid redistribution of the fluids over the compartments (Fig. 2-3).
  B. Three phases of volume shifts after trauma:
    1. Phase I: Shock and active hemorrhage
    This phase controls bleeding and lasts from admission to the end of operation for hemostasis. Pre-capillary vasoconstriction reduces the hydrostatic efflux of fluid, electrolytes, and protein into the interstitium. The interstitial matrix and plasma volume are contracted as electrolytes and proteins are mobilized into the circulation.
    2. Phase II: Obligatory extravascular fluid sequestration
    To restitute fluid in the interstitium, volume shifts into the interstitial and intercellular spaces, leading to oliguria, if insufficient fluid is given. An obligatory sequestration phase follows. This sequestration gives a modest rise in the volume of the intercellular fluid compartment and a marked expansion of the interstitial space. This leads to a reduction in plasma volume and plasma proteins and albumin relocation into the interstitial space.
    3. Phase III: Fluid mobilization and diuresis
    In this phase, fluid again is mobilized from the interstitial spaces, resulting in an acute increase in plasma volume sometimes resulting in volume overload, hypertension, and pulmonary dysfunction.

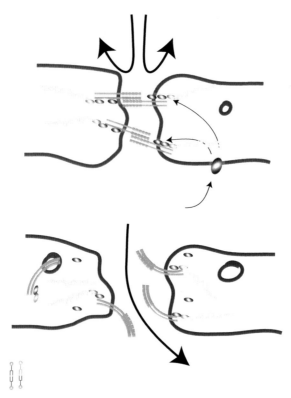

Figure 2-3. The integrity of the endothelial lining is compromised resulting in loss of barrier function and subsequent fluid loss to the interstitium. Redrawn after Le and Slutsky. *NEJM* 2010;363:689.

IV. THE IMMUNE RESPONSE

The immune system plays a pivotal role in defense and repair after external and internal threats.

A. Local versus systemic

At a local level after the bleeding ceases, the damaged tissues attract (Fig. 2-1) leukocytes that start to remove the debris and counteract the invading microorganisms. Local vasoconstriction further attenuates bleeding and a mesh of fibrin is woven in which the invading cells can reside.

At a systemic level, after trauma or infection, the organism is at a heightened state of alertness. This is reflected by fever, tachycardia, tachypnea, a complex of symptoms known as the systemic inflammatory response syndrome (SIRS). This SIRS state can be further elevated by secondary insults such as operation or superimposed infections, often termed the *second hit*. This hyper-vigilant state is counteracted by anti-inflammatory agents, resulting in the compensatory anti-inflammatory response syndrome (CARS), a weakened vigilance, sometimes resulting in infection and/or sepsis (Fig. 2-4). These are thought to be processes following each other in time; however, currently it is thought that this anti-inflammatory response with immune paralysis is in place early post-injury. This makes the organism susceptible for infection and sepsis.

B. The immune response can be divided into the adaptive and the innate immune reaction (Fig. 2-1).

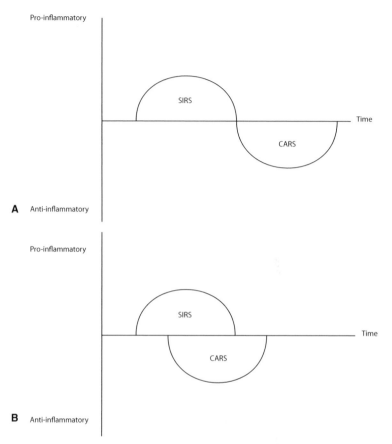

Figure 2-4. A: Classic hypothesis of systemic inflammatory response syndrome and the subsequent Compensatory anti-inflammatory response syndrome, which would follow up each other in time. **B:** New theories indicate that possibly already at the moment of a severe inflammatory response a less vigilant immune system results, resulting in an early immune compromised host.

1. Innate immune system:
   a. Activation of immune cells
   b. Cytokine secretion
   c. Complement activation
   d. Activation of the coagulation cascade
2. Adaptive immune system that adapts to the specific stimulus and attempts to counteract the invader built specific plasma cells and cytotoxic T-cells to eradicate microbes and other non-autologous materials.
3. The end effector organ is the leukocyte, which attempts to locate the threat and react to it. The leukocyte is influenced by many systems, both locally and systemically (Fig. 2-1), as will be elucidated further in this chapter. Just recently it has been hypothesized that trauma related, damage associated molecular patterns (DAMPs), act on the same pathway as the pathogen associated molecular patterns (PAMPs) related to pathogens such as microbes (Fig. 2-5). Thus, explaining why both trauma and infection elicit similar reactions of the body, with differentiation between both genesis of an inflammatory reaction, is difficult.

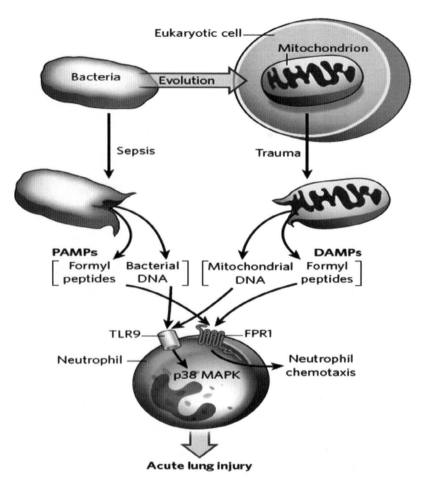

Figure 2-5. Current hypothesis of a common pathway of PAMPs and DAMPs (see text) resulting in a comparable expression and function of leukocytes.

C. Early immune response (Fig. 2-1):
   1. Local activation at the site of the insult:
      a. Activation of immune cells
      b. Local secretion of mediators
      c. Counteraction of anti-inflammatory cytokines to limit the response
   2. With the goal of:
      a. Hemostasis
      b. Prevention of invasion of microorganisms
      c. Start of tissue repair
      d. Wound healing
   3. In patients or injuries where:
      a. The local response is overwhelmed
      b. The host is more vulnerable for the insult
   4. Mediators are released in the circulation leading to a systemic response with release of pro- and anti-inflammatory cytokines, leading to release of leukocytes and invasion of immune cells into the site of injury. In an even higher stimulation of the immune system, for example, in severe trauma or a vulnerable host,

dysregulation leads to an overwhelming immune response (SIRS) with ultimately an immune paralysis (CARS). This overwhelming immunologic reaction with leukocyte infiltration in the tissues leads to:
- **a.** Increased endothelial permeability
- **b.** Endothelial damage
- **c.** Bacterial and endotoxemic translocation
- **d.** Dysfunctional microcirculation
- **e.** Tissue damage
- **f.** Organ failure (lung, kidney, liver, brain, nervous tissue)
- **g.** Because of the depletion of potent leukocytes, the host is more susceptible to microbiologic invasion and subsequent sepsis

V. NEUTROPHILS

A. Tissue damage and reperfusion result in the production of reactive oxygen species (ROS). The local inflammatory mediator production provides homing signals for neutrophils, mainly leukocytes. On the basis of these homing signals from the injured tissues (provided, e.g., by IL-8 and ROS), neutrophils are attracted to these tissues. They leave the circulation and enter the tissues by diapedesis through the blood vessel walls (Fig. 2-5). In the tissues, they exert their action to clear the unwanted material and bacteria. However, in certain situations these actions can act against the host itself resulting in tissue damage, e.g., adult respiratory distress syndrome or multiple organ failure.

B. Neutrophils excrete injurious products:
- **1.** ROS
- **2.** Proteases:
  - **a.** Collagenase
  - **b.** Elastase
    These products result in increased permeability, by elastase mediated endothelial injury (Fig. 2-3). This process is only possible with close contact between neutrophils and the endothelium. After stimulation with bacterial products such as fMLP and endotoxin or complement (C5) the leukocytes adhere to the endothelium to cause vascular injury, governed by molecules expressed on the surfaces of both cell types.

C. The normal function of the leukocyte (Fig. 2-5)
After production in the bone marrow, the leukocyte circulates in the bloodstream. A subset of the leukocytes, the neutrophil, is the most active part of the cell line. After specific messages, the neutrophil changes its membrane properties and expresses selectins. These selectins (L-selectin, P-selectin, and M-selectin) interact with the endothelium, whereafter the leukocyte adheres to the endothelium and starts rolling along the surface of the vessel. The integrins then set in and cause firm adherence to the endothelium, so the leukocyte comes to a stop. The neutrophil transmigrates through the vessel wall into the interstitium, where it acts by phagocytosis of debris or microbes and the release of active substances, influencing the local surroundings in a paracrine way, attracting new leukocytes for further action. In support of the leukocytes, mast cells release serotonin, histamine, and bradykinin.

VI. MACROPHAGES

A. Primary function: Wound healing
B. Are generated from monocytes, attracted to the tissues by cytokines and bacterial products
C. Secrete active substances, for example, growth factors
D. Phagocytose bacteria
E. Mediate antigen presentation to lymphocytes
F. Less activity (or over use) is correlated with infectious complications
G. Inhibited by macrophage inhibiting factor

VII. CYTOKINES (see Figs. 2-1 and 2-6)

A. Pro-inflammatory (TNF, IL-1b, IL-6, IL-8)
- **1.** Lead to upregulation encoding genes for phospholipase A2, COX-2, NO synthase

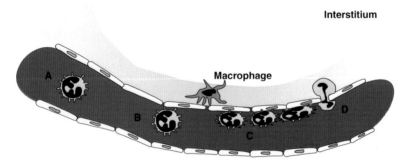

Figure 2-6. Normal function of the leukocyte A. Free floating in the bloodstream B. Rolling along the endothelial wall C. Adherence to the endothelium D. Diapedesis through the vascular wall into the tissues to ensue their lethal function.

  2. Initiate neutrophil action
     a. Function as chemoattractants
     b. Lead to upregulation of leukocyte–endothelial adhesion
     c. Initiate neutrophil degranulation
  3. Trigger clotting cascade
B. Anti-inflammatory (IL-10)
C. Proinflammatory cytokines
  Proinflammatory cytokines are produced by monocytes, macrophages, immune, and endothelial cells initiated by trauma, ischemia, LPS (gram negative bacteria), or infection.
  IL-1β
  1. This cytokine is produced early in the inflammatory reaction and only detectable for a short period of time after the injury.
  2. Initiates the production of TNF-α and IL-6 by hepatic cells
  3. Plays an important role in the development of ARDS, inducing inflammation in the pulmonary compartment
  TNF-α
  Effects:
  Low concentrations
  1. Higher expression of selectins and integrins, causing leukocyte adherence
  2. Up-regulation of endothelial IL-8 production causing higher leukocyte attraction
  3. Promotes apoptosis of certain cells
  High concentrations
  1. Fever
  2. Acute phase protein synthesis
  3. Cachexia
  4. Myocardial depression
  5. Disseminated intravascular coagulation
  6. Hypoglycemia
  IL-6
  1. Produced by liver cells and seen as a general acute phase factor.
  2. One of the factors best correlated to injury severity. However, its role in the inflammatory process is still to be determined.
  3. Frequently used as a monitor of the inflammatory reaction of the host.
  IL-8
  1. Produced at the site of injury

2. Leads to leukocyte recruitment
3. Attracts leukocytes to site of injury
HMGB1
1. High mobility group box-1 is a nuclear DNA binding protein acting as a DNA transcripting regulator
2. Produced by immune cells
3. Signals cell necrosis
4. Results in endothelial barrier disruption leading to vascular leakage and tissue hypoperfusion

D. Anti-inflammatory cytokines
IL-10
1. Produced from the onset of the inflammatory process on, however, peaks hours after the event
2. Forms negative feedback to TNF-α, IL-6 and IL-8
3. Suppresses monocyte function

Reactive oxygen species
In the normal oxidation processes in the mitochondria, oxygen is processed to deliver fuel for intracellular processes. However, in a small percentage of cells this process is incomplete and highly ROS are formed as a result. After ischemia/reperfusion injury, this process is enhanced producing high levels of these toxic products. The damaging effects on remaining normal tissue are:
1. Lipid peroxidation
2. Protein denaturation
3. Nucleic acid denaturation
4. Cell matrix injury
5. Apoptosis

Complement
Complement has heat-labile components that complement the lytic function of antibodies. These are proteins that interfere with several aspects of the inflammatory response. They are formed by two distinct processes as depicted in Figures 2-7 (A) and (B). The functions are:
1. Osmotic cell lysis
2. Opsonization of foreign particles or organisms to facilitate binding to macrophages and leukocytes, to enhance phagocytosis
3. Stimulation of the inflammatory process by stimulation of degranulation and oxidative burst
4. Clearance of immune complexes in the circulation
The active components C3a and C5a are the result of the classical (IgG or IgM related) and alternative (foreign particle related) pathway and result in:
  a. Vasodilatation
  b. Increased vascular permeability
  c. Neutrophil related action:
    i. Chemotaxis
    ii. Diapedesis
    iii. Degranulation
    iv. Free radical production
    v. Emergence of complement receptors on the leukocyte membrane
Complement activation is also related to ischemia reperfusion injury, by forming a C3–IgM complex.

Eicosanoids
Eicosanoids are vasoactive and immunomodulatory remnants of membrane fatty acids which are produced by many cells in response to several stimuli. They are:
  a. Prostaglandins, with effects on:
    i. Vasculature. Vasodilation and thrombocyte aggregation
    ii. Nervous system. Temperature elevation related to inflammation
    iii. Renal system. Increase in glomerular filtration rate and blood flow
    iv. Gastrointestinal tract. Contraction of GI muscle
    v. Respiratory tract. Relaxing respiratory smooth muscle

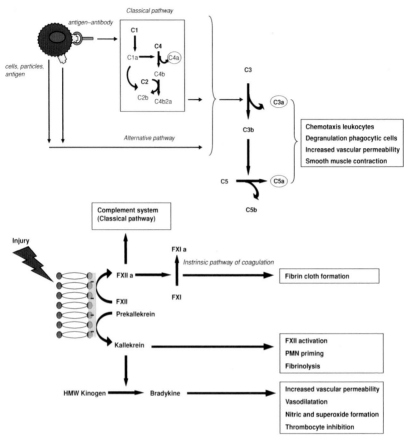

Figure 2-7. Complement system in classic **(A)** and alternative **(B)** pathways. For specific function see text.

    b. Leukotrienes:
        i. Neutrophil chemotaxis and activation
        ii. Bronchoconstriction
        iii. Increasing vascular permeability
    c. Thromboxanes. Active in vasoconstriction and thrombocyte aggregation
        i. Vasoconstriction
        ii. Bronchoconstriction
        iii. Enhanced platelet aggregation
        iv. Increased membrane permeability
        v. Neutrophil activation
          These agents are primarily active only locally because of their relative short half-life.

AXIOMS

■ The reaction to trauma is multifactorial and consists of both a local and a systemic response.
■ Both humoral and cellular body systems react to changes in the homeostasis.

■ The degree of the systemic response depends on the extent of the trauma, level of resulting hypoxia, and specific host factors.

Suggested Readings

Ledgerwood AM, Lucas CE. A review of the effects of hemorrhagic shock and resuscitation on the coagulation profile. *J Trauma* 2003;54:S68–S74.

Park MS, Martini WZ, Dubick MA, et al. Thromboelastography as a better indicator of hypercoagulable state after injury than prothrombin time or activated partial thromboplastin time. *J Trauma* 2009;67:266–275.

Tieu BH, Holcomb JB, Schreiber MA. Coagulopathy: its pathophysiology and treatment in the injured patient. *World J Surg* 2007;31:1055–1064.

3 Airway Management and Anesthesia

Henry E. Wang, Jean-Francois Pittet and Donald M. Yealy

I. **GENERAL CONSIDERATIONS.** Ensuring adequate oxygenation, ventilation, and protection from aspiration are the first priorities when treating an injured patient. Trauma patients have physiologic and anatomic challenges that magnify the complexity of airway management. For patients requiring acute surgical intervention, these challenges may complicate the provision of anesthesia. This chapter provides an overview of the basic principles of adult trauma airway management and anesthesia.

A. Airway management consists of both basic (e.g., bag-valve-mask [BVM] ventilation) and advanced (e.g., endotracheal intubation [ETI]) airway interventions. **Basic airway interventions are more important than advanced interventions.**

B. **Airway management must follow a clear, deliberate, systematic plan, including the anticipation of failure and having alternative/rescue interventions.**

C. **Assume all trauma patients have a cervical spine injury, head injury, and hypovolemia.** All airway management interventions must be performed with cervical immobilization and avoid hypoxemia (which can worsen any neurologic injury).

D. **Most trauma patients require the use of pharmacologic agents to facilitate ETI.** Only properly trained and experienced personnel should use deep sedatives and neuromuscular blocking agents (NMB; paralytics) to facilitate ETI.

E. **Airway procedures should be performed by the most experienced person available and without distraction.** No other procedures should occur during intubation or other airway management efforts.

F. **Airway management of the trauma patient is a team effort.** Communication between the airway manager and the trauma team leader is essential. The ultimate decision to perform ETI or other advanced airway procedures should rest with the trauma team leader.

G. **Resuscitation of the major trauma patient begins in the field and Emergency Department (ED), continues during surgery, and is ongoing in the intensive care unit.** Anesthesia and surgical intervention may exacerbate fluid and blood losses. Trauma teams must work together and bridge resuscitative efforts across these three areas.

II. **ANATOMY.** The key structures that are visualized during ETI include the epiglottis, vallecula, vocal cords, and aryepiglottic folds (Fig. 3-1). A cross-sectional view of airway structures during orotracheal intubation is depicted in Figure 3-2. Anatomical landmarks for cricothyroidotomy are depicted in Figure 3-3.

III. **BASIC AIRWAY INTERVENTIONS.** All patients should receive basic airway interventions. All interventions must be performed with inline cervical immobilization. Two or three operators may be needed to maintain basic airway control.

A. **In alert and spontaneously breathing patients,** apply a **non-rebreather mask** with 100% oxygen (10 to 15 L/min).

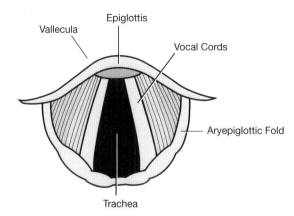

Figure 3-1. Pertinent laryngeal anatomy.

B. In semi-conscious or obtunded patients:

1. If possible, insert an **oropharyngeal** or **nasopharyngeal airway.** (Use extreme caution when inserting a nasopharyngeal airway in a patient with a suspected midface or basilar skull fracture.)
2. Use the **jaw-thrust** maneuver to open the airway. Do not use head tilt/chin lift on trauma patients because of the risk of cervical spine injury.
3. If the patient is spontaneously breathing, use a non-rebreather mask with 100% oxygen.
4. If the patient is not breathing spontaneously, if respiratory effort is inadequate, or if oxygen saturation cannot be maintained >95%, use **BVM ventilation.**
    a. BVM of the trauma patient requires at least two operators: One to perform a jaw thrust and seal the mask, and one to squeeze the bag.
5. Use large-bore suction to keep the airway clear of blood and secretions.

IV. ADVANCED AIRWAY INTERVENTIONS—ETI (OROTRACHEAL).
If basic airway interventions fail or will not sustain adequate oxygenation and ventilation, advanced airway management may be considered. ETI is the most common method of advanced airway management. ETI may protect the airway from aspiration and facilitate controlled ventilation. Orotracheal intubation is the most common and the preferred method of ETI in trauma patients. Alternate/rescue and surgical airway techniques are described in Sections VII and VIII.

A. General considerations

1. ETI of the trauma patient is best approached as a "difficult airway" at all times, and ETI should be attempted by the most qualified operator available. There is high potential for ETI failure in trauma patients and alternative strategies must be planned.
2. Perform ETI with manual inline cervical immobilization, cervical collar removed. Flexion and extension of the head should never be used to facilitate ETI in trauma patients. Likewise, the sniffing position is contraindicated in trauma patients.
3. ETI requires the coordination of multiple tasks. It is best done with three rescuers.
4. Most trauma patients will require pharmacologic agents (deep sedation or rapid-sequence intubation [RSI]) to facilitate ETI (Section VI).
5. In the event of serious facial injury distorting oral or airway structures, it may be necessary to proceed directly to another advanced intervention (e.g., a supraglottic or surgical airway).

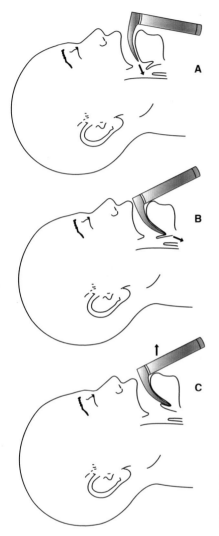

Figure 3-2. Laryngoscopy technique for orotracheal intubation of the trauma patient. Note that the cervical spine must be maintained inline—flexion and extension of the head are contraindicated.

B. Indications for ETI. These are general indications and do not encompass all possible clinical scenarios.
1. Apnea or near apnea
2. Airway obstruction or respiratory compromise unrelieved with basic interventions
3. Depressed consciousness from head trauma or any other cause
4. Combativeness unresolved with oxygen
5. Respiratory distress (severe tachypnea, increased work of breathing, cyanosis, hypoxemia, etc.)
6. Facial or neck injury with potential airway compromise
7. Chest wall injury or dysfunction with respiratory compromise
8. Persistent or refractory hypotension

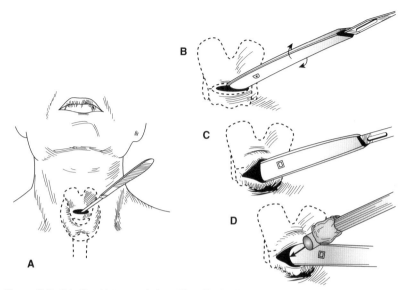

Figure 3-3. Cricothyroidotomy technique. (From Trunkey DD, Guernsey JM. Cervicothoracic trauma. In: Blaisdell FM, Trunkey DD, eds. *Surgical Procedures in Trauma Management.* New York, NY: Thieme Inc; 1986:303, with permission.)

    9. Need for diagnostic or therapeutic procedures in patients at risk for deterioration (e.g., computed tomography in somnolent patient, etc.)

C. Technique for orotracheal intubation

    1. Prepare and test all intubation equipment *prior* to patient arrival.

        a. For a typical 50 to 80 kg adult, use a **curved (Macintosh no. 3 or 4)** or **straight (Miller no. 3) blade.** Test the light.

        b. Use a no. 7.0 to 7.5 endotracheal tube on average-sized adult females and a no. 7.5 to 8.0 tube on males. Children under 8 years require smaller uncuffed tubes (Chapter 46). Insert a stylet, then test the cuff.

        c. Prepare and test large-bore suction.

        d. Prepare pharmacologic agents (Section VI).

        e. Prepare an alternate/rescue airway plan (Sections VII and VIII).

    2. Oral intubation requires at least three rescuers (Fig. 3-4).

        a. Rescuer 1: The most experienced provider; performs laryngoscopy and placement of endotracheal tube.

        b. Rescuer 2: Performs manual cervical immobilization and applies cricoid pressure.

        c. Rescuer 3: Provides oxygenation, assists rescuer 1 with laryngoscopy (handing equipment to intubator, etc.), facilitates verification of tube placement, and performs postintubation ventilation.

    3. Most patients will be supine—if not, lay the patient flat and adjust the bed height to ease laryngoscopy. **Rescuer 2 maintains manual cervical immobilization.** We recommend that rescuer 2 stand to the patient's side, facing the intubator—this gives the intubator more room while making it easier to use both hands to support the neck and jaw.

    4. Rescuer 3 should oxygenate the patient using a non-rebreather mask or BVM ventilation (Section III). Use 100% O_2 (10 to 15 L/min); if possible, optimize oxygenation and ventilation (spontaneous breathing or assisted) for 3 to 4 minutes; this technique maximizes pulmonary oxygen reserves. If possible, oxygenate to SaO_2 of 100%.

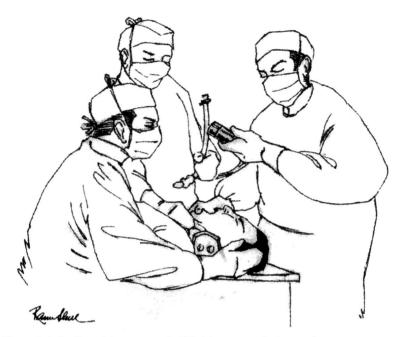

Figure 3-4. Positions of three rescuers for ETI of the trauma patient.

5. **Ensure a functioning intravenous catheter for drug administration.**
6. When directed, **rescuer 2 unfastens the cervical collar while maintaining cervical stabilization.** Apply firm cricoid pressure only when requested by the intubator—the maneuver does not universally aid or prevent harm.
7. **Give sedative and/or paralytic drugs** (Section V).
8. **Perform laryngoscopy** (insert the laryngoscope blade and expose the vocal cords) (Fig. 3-2).
    a. With a **curved (Macintosh) blade,** insert the blade in the right side of the patient's mouth and sweep the tongue to the left. Insert the tip of the blade in the vallecula (the space between the tongue and the epiglottis)—pressure placed on the hyoepiglottic ligament will lift the epiglottis and expose the vocal cords. With a **straight (Miller) blade,** similarly insert the blade in the right side of the patient's mouth, but directly lift the epiglottis with the tip of the blade.
    b. Maintain inline stabilization of the cervical spine. **Head tilt/extension, neck flexion, and "sniffing position" should never be used in trauma patients.** Cricoid pressure may improve laryngoscopic view but again is done at request only.
    c. **Limit the duration of each laryngoscopy attempt to 30 seconds. Stop earlier if SaO$_2$ drops $\leq$90%.** (Caution: Oxygen desaturation may be precipitous in trauma patients.)
    d. No other procedures should be performed while the laryngoscopy is being attempted.
9. **Insert the endotracheal tube.**
    a. Place the tip of the tube just past the vocal cords. In a typical 70 kg patient, the tube should be placed to a **depth of 21 to 22 cm for adult women and 22 to 23 cm for adult men** (denoted by depth markers on the tube) measured at the patient's teeth.

b. If encountering difficulty passing the endotracheal tube through the vocal cord opening, consider using a gum elastic bougie. This is a semi-rigid stylet and can be more easily inserted when glottic view is limited. The endotracheal tube can then be passed over the bougie and through the vocal cords.

c. Hold the tube manually—**do not release the tube until placement is confirmed and the assistant is prepared to secure the tube. Similarly, do not release cricoid pressure until proper tube position is confirmed.**

d. Inflate the cuff with 10 mL of air, remove the stylet, and attach the bag-valve device.

e. If tube placement fails, stop and reventilate with BVM. Then, re-attempt ETI with improved positioning. If unsuccessful after a total of three ETI attempts or if hypoxemia occurs despite BVM use, go directly to alternate/rescue airway techniques. Proceed to an alternate/rescue airway sooner if clear intubating barriers are encountered during initial ETI attempts.

10. Confirm correct tube placement. Unrecognized tube misplacement (esophageal or hypopharyngeal) can be rapidly fatal. No singular method of monitoring or tube confirmation is infallible. Use a combination of focused examination and adjunct devices to confirm tube placement.

  a. Directed physical examination. Auscultate the epigastrium—it should be quiet. Auscultate the apices and bases of both lungs; breath sounds should be present and equal, and the chest should rise normally. Each of these findings can be misleading or difficult to appreciate, particularly under resuscitation conditions.

  b. End-tidal carbon dioxide detection. If the tube is correctly placed, carbon dioxide will be present in the endotracheal tube. This is the most accurate method for confirming tube placement but not infallible. Note that these devices may be inaccurate in cardiac arrest or severe shock.

  i. The presence of expired CO_2 suggests correct tracheal placement (although rarely, hypopharyngeal placement will allow CO_2 detection). The absence of expired CO_2 means either incorrect placement (i.e., esophageal) or poor perfusion.

  ii. Colorimetric carbon dioxide detectors turn from purple to yellow in the presence of carbon dioxide. They are inaccurate when wet or exposed to air for extended periods.

  iii. Digital capnometers or **waveform capnographers** are preferable because they are not susceptible to moisture and provide continuous information.

  c. If any uncertainty exists, perform laryngoscopy (direct revisualization) to visually confirm the tube passing through the vocal cords. **(Caution: This technique may be inaccurate, especially when airway structures are distorted from injury.) If still uncertain, remove the tube, try BVM ventilation, or move to the failure option.**

  d. Methods that should not be relied upon for confirming tube placement: Tube fogging (gastric contents can fog the tube), chest x-ray (identifies vertical position only, not intratracheal placement), and oxygen saturation (desaturation may not occur for several minutes after tube misplacement).

11. Secure the tube using adhesive tape, umbilical tape, or a commercial tube holder.

12. Release any cricoid pressure and replace the cervical immobilization collar.

13. Place a nasogastric tube (oral if facial trauma is present) unless contraindicated.

D. Features suggesting difficult ETI. While the difficulty of an ETI is often relative to the experience of the operator, the following features are associated with ETI difficulty. The presence of multiple factors should lower the threshold for proceeding to alternate/rescue airway interventions. Note that this is not a comprehensive list of potential factors. In general, all trauma patients should be considered potentially difficult intubations.

1. **Anatomic features associated with ETI difficulty**
   a. Obesity
   b. Short neck
   c. Small mouth
   d. Overbite or underbite
   e. Limited neck mobility
   f. Airway trauma or injury
2. **Clinical scenarios associated with ETI difficulty**
   a. Head/face/neck trauma or other major injury
   b. Hypotension
   c. Intoxicated or combative patient

E. Managing failed ETI efforts. A common mistake is failing to recognize futile intubation attempts and delaying alternate/rescue airway interventions.

1. ***Assume all attempts at intubation will fail.*** Establish a clear alternate/rescue airway plan prior to the first ETI attempt.
2. **Reassess, oxygenate, and ventilate prior to each successive attempt.**
3. **Change the ETI equipment, technique, or operator with each intubation effort**—avoid repeating the same unsuccessful approach.
4. **Perform no more than three total laryngoscopy attempts** (regardless of the number of operators). If unsuccessful after three attempts, go directly to an alternate/rescue airway plan.

V. PHARMACOLOGIC ASSISTANCE DURING INTUBATION
A. General considerations

1. While deeply comatose or cardiac arrest patients can be intubated without drugs, **most trauma patients are awake, combative, or unrelaxed and must receive sedative and NMB to facilitate safe and rapid ETI.** A secondary purpose of pharmacologic assistance is to minimize autonomic response (e.g., blood pressure and intracranial pressure) to ETI, which can be stressful on a patient who is already in physiologic compromise from injury.
2. When choosing a drug regimen for the trauma patient, it is best to **assume that both hypovolemia and traumatic brain injury exist.** This approach allows for a greater margin of safety because either condition can be difficult to exclude in the first minutes after patient arrival. Short-acting agents should be used to facilitate rapid recovery if ETI efforts fail.
3. The use of NMB as a part of RSI is a helpful advanced technique but contains potential risks. A pharmacologically paralyzed patient has no airway tone or respiratory effort; if ETI cannot be readily accomplished, this condition can rapidly lead to death. **NMB agents should be used only by the most advanced and properly trained personnel.**

B. Preferred regimen in acute trauma—etomidate + succinylcholine. The combination of short-acting sedative/inductive and NMB is preferred for injured patients. This will optimize intubation conditions while allowing for rapid recovery if ETI failure occurs. **Based on this consideration, while there are many potential drug regimens, we recommend the drug combination etomidate + succinylcholine.** Give both agents consecutively and in rapid sequence (IV over 3 to 5 seconds for each drug). See Table 3-1 for summary of other sedative/induction and NMB.

C. Pretreatment with other drug agents is often suggested in RSI protocols but has unproven value.

1. Intravenous lidocaine may blunt physiologic and intracranial response to ETI, but the benefit of this technique in trauma patients is uncertain and dwarfed if prolonged attempts occur.
2. Pretreatment with a nondepolarizing NMB may prevent succinylcholine fasciculations but offers little practical benefit.
3. Atropine can help offset succinylcholine-associated bradycardia in pediatric patients (Chapter 46).

TABLE 3-1	Drugs Commonly Used to Facilitate Endotracheal Intubation	
Drug	**Dosage**	**Notes**
Sedation/induction		
Etomidate	0.2–0.3 mg/kg IV; 15–20 mg in a 70 kg adult. Onset: 30–60 s. Duration: 10 min.	May cause hypotension. May cause adrenosuppresion (clinical relevance unclear)
Ketamine	1–2 mg/kg IV; 70–140 mg in a 70 kg adult. Onset: 30–60 s. Duration: 5–10 min.	Raises intracranial pressure— avoid with head injury
Fentanyl	2–5 mcg/kg IV; 150–350 mg in a 70 kg adult.	Less likely to cause hypotension than other opioids. No amnestic effect
Propofol	1–2 mg/kg IV; 70–140 mg in a 70 kg adult. Onset: <1 min.	Causes hypotension
Thiopental	3–5 mg/kg IV; 210–350 mg in a 70 kg adult	Causes hypotension
Methohexital	1–3 mg/kg IV; 70–210 mg in a 70 kg adult	Causes hypotension
Neuromuscular blocking agents		
Succinylcholine	1–2 mg/kg IV; 70–140 mg in a 70 kg adult. Onset: 1 min. Duration: 5–7 min.	Causes fasciculations. May cause hyperkalemia. Relative contraindications: Burns >24 h old, >1 wk of paresis or motor dysfunction, globe/eye injury, impending cerebral herniation
Vecuronium	0.08–0.10 mg/kg IV; 5–7 mg in a 70 kg adult. Onset 2–3 min. Duration: 30–35 min.	
Rocuronium	0.6–1.2 mg/kg IV; 45–85 mg in a 70 kg adult. Onset 1.0–1.5 min. Duration: 20–30 min.	

D. Postintubation paralysis and sedation

    1. Maintenance of paralysis may be required after intubation. We recommend an initial dose of vecuronium (0.04 to 0.075 mg/kg IV; 3 to 5 mg in a 70 kg adult) that will provide 30 to 35 minutes of paralysis. Repeating lower doses (0.01 to 0.02 mg/kg IV; 0.7 to 1.4 mg in a 70 kg adult) will provide an additional 12 to 15 minutes of paralysis. **(Caution: The effects of NMB are often cumulative, and repetitive dosages may cause prolonged paralysis).**

    2. Provide concurrent sedation with a benzodiazepine such as **lorazepam** (0.025 to 0.05 mg/kg IV; 2 to 4 mg in a 70 kg adult) or **diazepam** (5 to 10 mg IV). **Propofol** (5 to 50 mg/kg/min constant infusion, adjusted as needed) may also be used.

E. Discouraged techniques

    1. Except for patients who are comatose, obtunded, or in cardiac arrest, we discourage intubation of trauma patients without drugs. Not only is this cruel, but it is technically difficult, is less likely to result in successful intubation, and may be hemodynamically stressful on a patient who is already in a tenuous condition. We discourage the sole use of topical anesthetics (e.g., lidocaine, tetracaine, cetacaine) for the same reasons.

    2. We also discourage "light sedation" alone to facilitate ETI, usually attempted with benzodiazepines (midazolam, lorazepam, or diazepam) or opioids (morphine, meperidine, hydromorphone). At conventional sedative doses, these agents have a slow and unpredictable onset and often do not provide adequate intubating conditions.

3. **It is important to recognize the airway management difficulty and the likelihood of intubation failure.** Examples are spontaneously breathing patients with major facial injuries and/or patients with significant bleeding into the airway. **RSI in this setting, making a spontaneously breathing patient an apneic patient, converts a difficult situation to a catastrophe.** In these situations, NMB are contraindicated (e.g., anticipated very difficult intubation, or the absence of personnel experienced with RSI), and we recommend the cautious use of deep sedation alone using etomidate (0.15 to 0.3 mg/kg IV; 10 to 20 mg in a 70 kg adult). Intubation must be by the team member with the most experience with difficult airways. The patient must be prepped and instrument trays open for immediate surgical airway if this fails. We discourage the routine use of this technique in trauma patients. However, patients who present with such tenuous airways must be recognized and managed appropriately.

VI. **ALTERNATIVES TO OROTRACHEAL INTUBATION (ALTERNATE/RESCUE AIRWAYS).** In the event of failed or non-feasible ETI efforts, alternate or rescue airway techniques are needed. Surgical airways are alternate/rescue airways and are described in Section VIII.

A. **Laryngeal Mask Airway (LMA), Combitube and King Laryngeal Tube (King LT) are supraglottic airways** commonly used as alternatives to ETI. These devices are relatively easy to insert and are believed to ventilate almost as well as an endotracheal tube. Both devices may provide an adequate "bridge" airway until the execution of alternate ETI techniques or placement of a surgical airway. Prehospital EMS personnel may use supraglottic airways on major trauma patients. (These alternatives are discussed in detail in Chapter 8.)

B. Whether inserted in the prehospital or ED setting, **resist the temptation to immediately remove and replace the supraglottic airway.** It is best to assume that conventional laryngoscopy will be very difficult in these patients. While there are several strategies for converting a supraglottic airway to an endotracheal tube, we recommend using a fiberoptic bronchoscope and a hollow flexible intubating stylet (Aintree catheter). Alternatively, in the setting of severe facial trauma or the anticipated need for prolonged ventilation, early tracheostomy may be prudent. If the supraglottic airway is functioning adequately, the conversion to an endotracheal tube or tracheostomy may occur on a less urgent basis.

C. We discourage nasotracheal (nasal) intubation in major trauma patients. **Nasotracheal intubation** is usually performed in a "blind" fashion in patients who are spontaneously breathing. Nasotracheal intubation is technically more difficult than orotracheal intubation, can cause significant airway trauma, and offers little advantage over oral intubation. Nasotracheal intubation is contraindicated in apneic patients or those with midface, nasal, or basilar skull fractures. A nasotracheal tube may cause significant sinusitis after 48 hours. Nasotracheal intubation requires the use of smaller diameter endotracheal tubes which may complicate ventilator management. Conversion of a nasotracheal tube to an orotracheal tube should be considered after 24 hours if the patient is stabilized; this may require a careful plan and bedside team of experts.

D. **Other ETI techniques.** There are a variety of alternate approaches to ETI; for example, tactile **(digital)** ETI, and **lighted-stylet** (transillumination) ETI. These approaches require specialized equipment or skill and may not be practical in the injured patient. Intubation over a flexible bronchoscope **(fiberoptic intubation)** requires special equipment and skill and is best left to specially trained operators (anesthesiologists who are facile with this technique). This technique is rarely appropriate in the trauma resuscitation area.

VII. **SURGICAL AIRWAYS.** Surgical airways are required when basic interventions and ETI efforts are not likely to succeed or have failed. The equipment for these techniques is specialized and should be readily available in the resuscitation suite. Landmarks for these techniques are depicted in Figure 3-3.

A. Cricothyroidotomy ("open cric") is preferred to jet insufflation because of the simpler equipment and the ability to provide optimal protection from aspiration and to place a large-bore airway for suctioning. Most clinicians are more familiar with this technique.

  1. Technique (Fig. 3-3)

  a. Palpate the thyroid cartilage—identify the depressed cricothyroid membrane immediately caudad.

  b. Make a 3 cm midline, longitudinal incision over the membrane. In a thin neck with clear landmarks, it is acceptable to perform a transverse skin incision.

  c. Spread the skin with fingers or retractors and identify key landmarks by palpation (thyroid cartilage, cricothyroid membrane). This procedure is performed by palpation, not visualization.

  d. Make a transverse incision (1.5 to 2.0 cm) through the cricoid membrane. The procedure is essentially performed using tactile input; if the membrane cannot be seen, incise where the soft membrane is palpated. **Do not fracture the cricoid cartilage during the procedure.** Gain access through transverse spreading, not vertical.

  e. Insert a no. 5 or 6 Shiley tracheostomy tube or a no. 5.5 or 6 endotracheal tube and inflate the cuff.

  f. Attach a bag-valve device and confirm tube placement.

  2. Complications include hemorrhage (avoid by limiting the size of incision and controlling bleeding with local pressure), misplacement, hypoxia secondary to prolonged procedure time, esophageal perforation, laryngeal fracture, and subcutaneous emphysema. Stenosis is often a problem if left in place for extended periods because of the narrow and contained diameter of the cricoid area; a cricothyroidotomy should be converted to a tracheostomy after the patient is stabilized.

  3. Relative contraindications to cricothyroidotomy include laryngeal trauma or pediatric patients (age less than 10 years). Only needle techniques (jet ventilation) should be used on pediatric patients because the cricoid membrane is delicate and can be easily transected.

  4. Percutaneous dilator-based cricothyroidotomy kits are available. These kits use a Seldinger guidewire technique with a series of dilators. These kits may be easier to insert by less experienced operators. However, familiarity with any technique is essential prior to the need to urgently attempt it.

B. Tracheostomy is generally reserved for nonemergent situations. A possible exception is the presence of laryngeal fracture or where the cricoid membrane integrity is compromised.

C. Percutaneous translaryngeal catheter insufflation ("needle cric" or "jet ventilation")

  1. Technique

  a. The trachea is used as a passive port for exhalation. Thus, the only absolute contraindication to jet ventilation is complete airway obstruction. Using the special jet ventilation device, tidal volumes of 700 to 1,000 mL can be achieved.

  b. Contrary to popular misconceptions, correct jet ventilation can be used for unlimited periods of time, if used with the proper high-pressure source (40 to 50 psi) at an inspiration: Expiration rate of 1:3 seconds.

  c. Complications of jet ventilation include barotrauma, local hemorrhage, hypotension from overventilation and decreased venous return, inadvertent placement with resulting subcutaneous or mediastinal emphysema, hypoxia, hypercarbia, and dysrhythmias from prolonged attempts.

  2. A transtracheal catheter can be easily converted to a conventional cricothyroidotomy. We recommend leaving the catheter in place and using it as a guide for identifying the cricoid membrane. A Seldinger-type guidewire can also be passed through the catheter to provide similar guidance.

VIII. ANESTHESIA FOR THE MAJOR TRAUMA PATIENT
A. General Considerations
   1. Resuscitation of the major trauma patient begins in the ED but continues during surgery in the operating room and after surgery in the intensive care unit. Anesthesia and surgical intervention may exacerbate fluid and blood losses. It is essential to anticipate and proactively treat fluid and blood losses before, during and after the surgical intervention. The anesthesiologist plays an important role in bridging resuscitation care between the ED, operating room and intensive care unit.
   2. As most anesthetics are direct vasodilators and negative inotropes, these agents should be given in reduced doses during the early phase of resuscitation when the trauma patient is hemodynamically unstable.

B. Vascular Access
Early vascular access is essential in the major trauma patient. Once draped for emergent surgical intervention, access to the patient may prove difficult. Therefore, early anticipation for and placement of vascular catheters are advisable.
   1. Peripheral venous catheters
   a. Two large-bore intravenous catheters should be placed into peripheral veins of severely traumatized patients (14 to 16 gauge catheters). For rapid transfusions of large amounts of resuscitation fluid or blood products, a 7 to 7.5 French introducer may be placed in a large vein of the upper extremity.
   b. Site of insertion should be the upper extremity unless there is the possibility of major venous injury in the arm, upper chest, or ipsilateral neck that will interfere with the flow of fluids into the central circulation.
   c. Placement of a large-bore intravenous catheter in the upper extremity is critical if an injury to one of the iliac veins or the vena cava inferior is suspected as the fluid administered via a femoral vein catheter may not reach the central circulation.
   d. In difficult situations, cutdowns may be required. Cutdowns are usually placed at the level of the antecubital crease into the basilic or cephalic vein or at the level of the ankle into the greater saphenous vein.
   e. Intraosseous access is an alternative when intravenous access is difficult or not possible. The preferred site of access is the anteromedial surface of the tibial tuberosity. Other reported sites for intraosseous access are sternum, distal femur, lateral or medial malleoli, iliac crest, and possibly distal radius.
   2. Central venous catheters
   a. Central catheters are frequently inserted in subclavian, internal jugular, or femoral veins in severely traumatized patients using the Seldinger technique.
   b. These procedures require expertise because of the risk of serious complications (pneumothorax, hemothorax, infection, ventricular arrhythmias, arterial puncture). If time permits, use an ultrasound to guide vessel identification and catheter placement.
   3. Arterial catheters
   a. Placement of an arterial catheter is critical for the continuous monitoring of the systemic arterial pressure and frequent measurement of arterial blood gases.
   b. The preferred access site is the radial artery using a Seldinger technique. Alternative access sites are the ulnar, brachial, or femoral arteries.

C. Fluid Resuscitation
Principles of fluid resuscitation are covered in detail in Chapter XX. General considerations include:
   1. Monitoring and assessment of volume status is essential in the major trauma patient and can be accomplished by both invasive and non-invasive means.
   2. Fluid resuscitation starts in the ED but continues through the operating room phase. Fluid resuscitation in the operating room must account for fluids and blood products previously given in the ED. Some clinicians use a strategy of "permissive hypotension" for severely bleeding patients limiting fluid administration to a maximum of 20 mL/kg and targeting a MAP of 60 mm Hg.

3. Isotonic crystalloid solutions such as normal saline or Lactated Ringer's solution are typically used for fluid resuscitation in trauma. Large amounts of normal saline solution should be avoided because of the potential for hyperchloremic metabolic acidosis. Colloid solutions including albumin, hydroxyl ethyl starch and dextran have been used for the treatment of uncontrolled hemorrhage.

4. Patients who are bleeding should receive **red blood cell transfusions** as soon as possible. **Plasma** and **platelets** should be given with red cells whenever more than 3 to 4 units are needed. Many centers use massive transfusion bundles of 6 units of RBC, 4 units of plasma FFP, and 1 unit ("4 or 6 pack") of platelets.

5. Vasoactive drugs (catecholamines, vasopressin) can be used in severe uncontrolled hemorrhagic shock to restore tissue perfusion. Vasoactive agents should not be used instead of fluid resuscitation, but as additional transient therapy to maintain organ perfusion pressure.

D. Anesthetics

1. General anesthesia

   a. Patients with severe trauma are usually intubated at the scene of injury or shortly after admission to the hospital. If the trauma patient is intubated in the operating room, the principles summarized in the previous paragraphs of this chapter should be applied.

   b. After induction, general anesthesia is generally maintained with a combination of volatile anesthetics and narcotics. As most anesthetics are direct vasodilators and negative inotropes, these agents should be given in reduced doses during the early phase of resuscitation when the trauma patient is hemodynamically unstable.

   c. If there is concern about awareness during the initial phase of emergency surgery for severe trauma (e.g., because of the intolerance to anesthetics), small doses of benzodiazepines can provide adequate amnesia for the perioperative period.

   d. Trauma patients should be paralyzed intraoperatively to optimize ventilation and decrease oxygen consumption. Monitoring of the neuromuscular function is critical as liver and renal function may be abnormal after severe trauma.

   e. Trauma patients should be ventilated with volume-controlled ventilation with a tidal volume of 6 to 8 mL/kg ideal body weight and with a small amount of PEEP (4 to 6 cm H_2O). $PaCO_2$ should be maintained between 30 and 35 mm Hg by adjusting the respiratory rate, not the tidal volume. Patients should be ventilated with 100% O_2 or a mixture of oxygen and air. There is no real advantage in adding nitrous oxide to the gases delivered by the ventilator.

   f. Body temperature should be continuously monitored to target a core temperature close to the physiologic value except for traumatic brain injury patients or post-cardiac arrest (where controlled, moderate hypothermia is desirable.)

   g. Urine output should be monitored during the anesthesia, seeking at least 0.5 to 1.0 mL/kg/h.

2. Regional anesthesia

   a. Regional anesthesia can be used for isolated trauma of the extremities if the patient is hemodynamically stable and has no coagulopathy or other contraindication to this approach. Regional anesthesia is not appropriate for thoracic, abdominal, pelvic, or neurosurgical procedures, nor for patients with signs of hemodynamic compromise.

   b. Advantages of regional anesthesia include an attenuation of the stress response, decreased risk for blood loss or venous thrombosis, improved outcome with microvascular surgery, and better pain management.

   c. Disadvantages of regional anesthesia include the inability to correct impaired oxygenation or ventilation, the risk of epidural abscess or hematoma after neuraxial anesthesia, damage to peripheral nerves after conduction blocks, sympathectomy, and possibly nerve damage.

d. Regional anesthesia can be used as the method of analgesia in trauma patients if the specific contraindications for this technique are respected. Thoracic or lumbar epidural analgesia may provide excellent analgesia for patients with severe thoracic or abdominal trauma.

AXIOMS

- Basic airway interventions (e.g., BVM ventilation) are more important than advanced interventions (e.g., ETI).
- Airway management must follow a clear, deliberate, systematic plan, including the anticipating failure and having alternative/rescue interventions.
- Assume all trauma patients have a cervical spine injury, head injury, and hypovolemia. All airway management interventions must be performed with cervical immobilization until that injury is excluded.
- Most trauma patients require the use of pharmacologic agents to facilitate ETI. Only experienced personnel should use NMB (paralytics) to facilitate ETI.
- Airway procedures should be performed by the most experienced person available. No other procedures should occur during intubation or other airway management efforts.
- The ultimate decision to perform ETI or other advanced airway procedures should rest with the trauma team leader and the most experienced person is best suited to perform this procedure.
- Use caution when administering anesthetic agents as the usual body mass dosing may be too high because of the hypovolemia associated with severe trauma.

Suggested Readings

Bolliger D, Gorlinger K, Tanaka KA. Pathophysiology and treatment of coagulopathy in massive hemorrhage and hemodilution. *Anesthesiology* 2010;113:1205–2019.

Fouche Y, Sikorski R, Dutton RP. Changing paradigms in surgical resuscitation. *Crit Care Med* 2010;38:S411–S420.

McCunn M, Gordon EK, Scott TH. Anesthetic concerns in trauma victims requiring operative intervention: The patient too sick to anesthetize. *Anesthesiol Clin* 2010;28:97–116.

Roberts JR, Hedges JR, Chanmugam AS. *Clinical Procedures in Emergency Medicine.* 4th ed. Philadelphia, PA: WB Saunders; 2004.

4 Initial Assessment and Resuscitation*

Michael Rhodes and Michael Kalina

I. INTRODUCTION

A. Resuscitation of the adult patient is an intense period of medical care in which initial and continuous patient assessment guides concurrent diagnostic and therapeutic procedures. As a dynamic period, resuscitation requires the trauma team to rapidly develop a differential diagnosis based on effectiveness of treatment and results of available diagnostic studies. When possible, the surgeon and emergency physician should direct this crucial activity. The supervising physician must ensure that the optimal resuscitation space, personnel, and equipment are present.

B. Resuscitation of the trauma patient requires an organized, systematic approach utilizing a well-rehearsed protocol. Advanced Trauma Life Support (ATLS) is a single-physician resuscitation course of the American College of Surgeons that prescribes an initial approach to an unstable patient with life-threatening injury (Table 4-1). The principles of ATLS resuscitation are also applicable to the Trauma Center environment and should be supplemented by a **team approach** to the trauma patient. The approach of a trauma team should be multispecialty and pro-tocol driven based on patient **"stability"** and **mechanism of injury** (blunt vs. penetrating) (Fig. 4-1). This chapter presents a team-oriented approach for initial assessment and resuscitation.

II. PATIENT STABILITY

A. The term **"unstable"** has classically referred to physiologic parameters such as vital signs (pulse, blood pressure, and respiratory rate). Patients with abnormalities of these vital signs are usually sending out a clear distress signal. However, in the context of trauma resuscitation, the definition of unstable can be expanded to include patients who are considered **metastable** (the capacity to change at any time). These patients exhibit subjective, objective, or anatomical findings that may predict need for specialized trauma care in the Trauma Center. These expanded criteria for instability (and metastability) are liberal and refer to the potential need for operative intervention or the intensive care unit (ICU) (Table 4-2). Patients who meet these expanded criteria usually have injuries that are life- or limb-threatening. A subcategory of unstable patients, those who present **in extremis** (sometimes referred to as "agonal"), requires a tailored approach.

B. Blood pressure **response to initial fluid challenge** is also a measure of stability. Hypotensive patients who sustain a normotensive response to the first 1 to 2 L of fluid are responders and considered stable. **Transient responders** and **non-responders** are **unstable** (generally from ongoing bleeding) and should be treated accordingly.

C. **Significant injury may also be suspected** from interpretation of key phrases verbalized by patients.
- "I'm choking"—airway dysfunction
- "I can't swallow"—airway dysfunction
- "I can't breathe"—ventilatory dysfunction
- "Let me sit up"—ventilatory dysfunction, hypoxia, cardiac tamponade
- "Please help me"—blood loss, hypoxemia

---

*(see Chapter 21 for Special Populations)

TABLE 4-1	Phases of Initial Assessment

Primary survey (15 s)
- **A**irway with C-spine control
    - → Voice, air exchange, patency, cervical immobilization
- **B**reathing
    - → Breath sounds, chest wall, neck veins
- **C**irculation
    - → Mentation, skin color, pulse, blood pressure, neck veins, external bleeding
- **D**isability (neurologic)
    - → Pupils, extremity movement (site and type), voice
- **E**xpose the patient

Resuscitation
- Generic—ECG leads, pulse oximetry, IV, draw labs
- Concurrent with life-threatening injuries identified on primary survey
- Include gastric and urethral catheters, or perform with secondary survey

Secondary survey
- Head-to-toe examination (including spine)
- AMPLE history (A, allergies; M, medications currently taken; P, past illness; · L, last meal; E, events related to injury)
- Imaging
- Second survey may be delayed until after operating room in unstable patient or patient *in extremis*

Definitive care
- Surgery (may be in resuscitation phase)
- Splinting
- Medications (3 As): Analgesics, antibiotics, anti-tetanus
- Consultants
- Transfer

Tertiary survey
- Repeat primary and secondary surveys within 24 h for occult or missed injuries
- Creation of injury "problem" list with specific identification of physician handling each one

Modified from American College of Surgeons Committee on Trauma: *Advanced Trauma Life Support Manual*. Chicago: American College of Surgeons, 2008.

- "I'm going to die"—blood loss, hypoxemia
- "I'm thirsty"—blood loss
- "My belly hurts"—peritoneal irritation
- "I need to have a bowel movement"—hemoperitoneum
- "I can't move my legs"—spinal cord injury

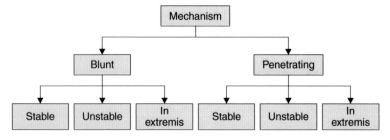

Figure 4-1. Initial emergency department triage.

TABLE 4-2	Criteria for Adult Unstable (or Metastable) Trauma Patient[a] (Blunt or Penetrating Trauma)

Altered physiology
- Glasgow Coma Scale (GCS) score $\leq$14
- Pulse <60 or >120 beats/min
- Blood pressure <90 mm Hg after 2 L fluid challenge
- Blood pressure >190 mm Hg systolic
- Respiratory rate <12 or >24 breaths/min
- Poor gas exchange (e.g., SaO_2 <90%)
- Temperature <92°F (33°C)

Altered physical findings
- Paralysis
- Hoarseness/inability to talk
- Labored respirations
- Severe pain
- External hemorrhage site(s)
- Combative

Altered anatomic findings
- Severe deformity(ies): Spine, neck, chest, extremities
- Penetrating wound from head to popliteal fossa

[a]**Increased index of suspicion:**
- Age >55 y
- Coronary artery disease
- Obstructive lung disease
- Liver disease
- Insulin-dependent diabetes mellitus
- Anticoagulation or history of coagulopathy
- History of mental illness
- Pregnancy

- "Please do something for my pain"—significant injury
- "Where am I?"—head injury, hypoxia, hypercarbia

III. *STABLE* ADULT WITH BLUNT TRAUMA

A. Assess for airway, breathing, circulation, and neurologic disability.

B. Immobilize cervical spine.

C. Administer O_2 nasally or by mask.

D. Insert at least one peripheral intravenous (IV) (18 gauge or larger).

E. Perform "stable patient" laboratory studies.

F. Splint deformed extremities.

G. Assess for occult injury.
   1. Head, neck, chest, abdomen, pelvis, spine, and extremities.
   2. Selective rectal and pelvic examinations.

H. Consider Insertion of a nasogastric tube (unnecessary in most stable patients).

I. Insert urinary catheter (if patient unable to void or pelvic fracture).

J. Limit IV fluid (e.g., 1 L in first 30 minutes).

K. Perform **Select** radiologic studies as indicated by mechanism of injury and physical examination.
   1. Chest x-ray (usually routine).
   2. C-spine—no x-ray if no symptoms or signs and not intoxicated (see Chapter 25).
   3. Pelvis—no x-ray if no symptoms or signs.
   4. CT of head with any alteration in consciousness, amnesia, headache, or history of anticoagulation.

5. CT of abdomen—if tenderness, macroscopic hematuria or microscopic hematuria with signs and symptoms (see Chapter 30).
6. Ultrasound of abdomen (selective)—if abdominal tenderness.
7. CT chest (with CTA) if history of acceleration/deceleration injury (e.g., MVC >25 mph, fall >10 ft
8. CTA neck if seatbelt sign to neck.
9. Spine and extremity films (selective)—if tenderness.

IV. *UNSTABLE* ADULT WITH BLUNT TRAUMA
A. Assess airway (with C-spine immobilization).
1. Patency, voice, stridor, foreign body, tongue, lacerations, O_2 saturation
2. Treatment **options** (see Chapter 3 for specific indications)
   a. Administration of $100\%O_2$ (by mask)
   b. Suction
   c. Chin lift
   d. Oral airway (if obtunded)
   e. Nasopharyngeal airway
   f. Laryngeal mask airway (LMA)—very selective
   g. Endotracheal intubation
   h. Surgical airway
B. Assess breathing.
1. Facial expression (distress, anguish, flat), depth and quality of respiration (shallow or labored), skin pallor or cyanosis, use of accessory muscles (neck and abdomen)
2. Trachea (midline, crepitus), neck veins (flat or distended), breath sounds (diminished or absent), chest symmetry (look for anterior or lateral flail, or splinting), respiratory rate, central cyanosis, O_2 saturation (pulse oximetry)
3. Treatment **options** (see Chapter 28 for specific indications)
   a. Endotracheal tube
   b. Needle decompression of chest, unilateral or bilateral
   c. Chest tube(s), unilateral or bilateral
   d. Ventilator (manual or mechanical)
   e. Analgesia (systemic titrated opioids, inhalational opioids, intercostal block, paravertebral blocks, epidural)
   f. Thoracotomy
C. Assess circulation.
1. Skin color, mentation, palpable pulse
2. Quality of pulse, blood pressure, capillary refill, peripheral cyanosis, skin temperature, external hemorrhage, agitation, ECG monitoring, O_2 saturation
3. Treatment **options** (see Chapters 5)
   a. Two large-bore peripheral IVs, draw "unstable patient" labs
   b. Central line if peripheral access unavailable—subclavian or femoral
   c. If no IV access, consider adult IO (intraosseous) or cutdown at ankle or groin; IO in children.
   d. 1 to 2 L of warmed Ringer's lactate IV as fast as possible (monitor response)
   e. With profound or persistent hypotension, early blood transfusion
   f. If signs of persistent hypovolemia (e.g., thirst, base deficit, tachycardia, or hypotension), check for occult blood loss in one of six areas
      i. **External.** (Look under dressings), back, buttocks, occiput, axillae
      ii. **Thoracic cavity.** Trachea, neck veins, auscultation/percussion, early chest x-ray, chest tube
      iii. **Abdominal cavity.** Palpation, ultrasound, diagnostic peritoneal lavage (DPL) (selective), exploratory laparotomy
      iv. **Pelvis.** Physical examination, perineal laceration, unstable pelvic ring, pelvic binder, pelvic x-ray, arteriogram, or external fixation
      v. **Extremities.** Fractures, particularly if bilateral or femoral
      vi. **Spine.** Extensive fractures with hemorrhage (lumbar)

4. If the search for bleeding is unrevealing, other **causes** of **hypotension** include the following:
   a. Tension pneumothorax
   b. Cardiac rupture or tamponade
   c. Neurogenic shock (spinal cord injury)
   d. Severe blunt cardiac injury with acute heart failure (very uncommon)

D. Neurologic disability
   1. Perform and document focused neurologic examination (see Chapters 23 and 25) **before** patient is **intubated** and paralyzed: Glasgow Coma Score (GCS), pupils, movement, and gross sensation of **all** extremities.
   2. Palpate head and spine (log roll).
   3. Treatment **options**
      a. Administration of O_2
      b. Intubation
      c. Mannitol
      d. Emergency imaging of brain and/or spine
      e. Intracranial pressure monitoring
      f. Ventriculostomy
      g. Craniotomy

E. Extremities
   1. Palpate extremities and joints.
   2. Palpate pulses (Doppler).
   3. Perform focused motor and sensory examination.
   4. Treatment **options** (see Chapter 31 for specific indications)
      a. Cover open wounds with sterile dressing.
      b. Apply direct pressure to control hemorrhage.
      c. Consider hemostatic composite pack for large bleeding wounds
         i. Realign gross deformities
         ii. Splint
         iii. Apply traction (femur fractures)

F. Place **nasogastric or orogastric tube** and **urinary catheter** at earliest opportunity **if not contraindicated** or **interfering** with assessment or stabilization of airway, breathing, circulation, or neurologic dysfunction.

G. Imaging in the **unstable blunt trauma patient**
   1. Suggested as time and clinical situation permit (in resuscitation area)
      a. Chest x-ray: Camera at maximal distance (lower resuscitation litter); inspiratory-hold
      b. Cervical spine: If time permits, perform lateral (to rule out gross deformity only), delay full C-spine until patient is stable
      c. Pelvis: Anteroposterior (AP) to rule out site of occult hemorrhage.
   2. Selective (based on assessment)
      a. Extremities
      b. Thoracic and lumbar spine
   3. In general, imaging should be delayed until airway, breathing, and circulatory dysfunction have been stabilized. Exceptions occur when chest x-ray or pelvic x-ray are needed to identify "occult" blood loss (see above). CT done in an unstable patient can be dangerous. Studies in the trauma patient should be done only in CT units with full monitoring capability, easy full patient body viewing, and a nurse-physician team capable of performing any and all life saving procedures (e.g., cricothyroidotomy, chest decompression, decision to operate). Newer rapid helical or spiral scanners can image the head, chest, and abdomen rapidly allowing studies to be performed in select transient responders to fluid challenge when supported by clinical judgment and logistics.
      a. Head: If GCS <15
      b. Chest: If suspected contusion or mediastinal anatomy uncertainty
      c. Abdomen and pelvis: If signs or symptoms or unable to examine
      d. Spine: If suspected by plain films or physical examination

V. *STABLE* ADULT WITH PENETRATING TRAUMA

A. Assess patient for airway, breathing, circulatory, and neurologic dysfunction.

B. Document **number** and **sites** of penetrating wounds.

C. Determine trajectory—this is vital in determination of anatomic structures at risk from missiles.

D. Treatment **options**
   1. Administer O_2
   2. Secure at least one peripheral IV (select so that a potential vascular injury is not between the IV site and the heart)
   3. Selective placement of nasogastric tube and urinary catheter (e.g., penetrating torso wound)
   4. "Stable patient" **lab** studies

E. Assess the patient for significant injury, depending on injury sites: Physical examination and x-ray; both plain film and CT are complementary to accurately determine precise trajectory. Diagnostic **options** include:
   1. **Head:** CT without contrast.
   2. **Neck:** CT with IV and oral contrast, AP and lateral x-rays, contrast swallow study, endoscopy, arteriogram, neck exploration. **(Caution: Check airway repeatedly during diagnostic evaluations with low threshold for intubation.)**
   3. **Chest:** Chest x-ray; if transmediastinal, CT with IV and oral contrast, or angiography, bronchoscopy, esophageal contrast, cardiac window, echocardiography.
   4. **Abdomen, back, or flank:** Local wound exploration, DPL, ultrasound, CT with IV and oral contrast (including rectal), laparoscopy, laparotomy.
   5. **Extremities:** Pulses, motor and sensory examination, ankle brachial index, Duplex ultrasound, CTA, arteriogram, operative exploration.

VI. *UNSTABLE* ADULT WITH PENETRATING TRAUMA

A. Assess patient for airway, adequate gas exchange, circulatory or neurologic dysfunction.

B. Assess number and sites of penetrating wounds.

C. Determine trajectory—this is vital in determination of anatomic structures at risk from missiles.

D. Treatment options
   1. **Airway**
      a. Administer $100\%O_2$
      b. Suction
      c. Chin lift
      d. Oral airway (if obtunded)
      e. Nasopharyngeal airway
      f. Endotracheal intubation
      g. Surgical airway (i.e., for shotgun wounds to face)
   2. **Breathing**
      a. Needle decompression of chest, unilateral or bilateral
      b. Chest tube(s), unilateral or bilateral
      c. Ventilator (manual or mechanical)
      d. Thoracotomy or sternotomy
   3. **Circulatory**
      a. Insert two large-bore IVs, draw **unstable** patient **laboratory studies,** consider large-bore central line, 1 to 2 L of warmed Ringer's lactate IV, blood transfusion with profound or persistent hypotension. **In general, a target BP of 90 mm Hg should not be exceeded until definitive control of the injury in the operating room.**
      b. IV **above** and **below** diaphragm in penetrating **torso** trauma
      c. Avoid IV placement such that the bullet wound is between the IV site and the heart.
      d. If signs of hypovolemia occur (e.g., thirst, base deficit, tachycardia, or hypotension), search for sites of blood loss.

    i. Thoracic cavity. Tracheal deviation, neck veins, bilateral equal breath sounds, chest x-ray, chest tubes (bilateral if precise trajectory not known).

    ii. Abdominal cavity. Exploratory laparotomy, ultrasound, or DPL (stab wounds).

    iii. If hypotension continues, look for cardiac tamponade, tension pneumothorax.

    iv. Occult spinal cord injury.

  4. Place nasogastric or orogastric tube and urinary catheter at earliest convenience.

E. Hemodynamically **unstable patient** with a **penetrating** wound to the **chest** may require chest tube(s) and thoracotomy in emergency department or operating room.

  1. Chest tube may be diagnostic or therapeutic.

  2. If patient is hemodynamically unstable after chest tubes, perform thoracotomy in emergency department or OR.

  3. If stable after chest tubes and mediastinal or transmediastinal trajectory (see Chapter 28), then perform the following.

    a. Repeat ultrasound or pericardial window

    b. Echocardiogram (transthoracic or transesophageal)

    c. Aortogram

    d. Bronchoscopy

    e. Esophageal contrast study

    f. CT with contrast in selected patients

F. The hemodynamically **unstable** patient with a **penetrating** wound to the **neck, abdomen,** or **extremity** requires control of hemorrhage in the **OR.**

VII. PATIENT *IN EXTREMIS*

A. The patient *in extremis* presents with anatomic or physiologic findings that will result in **death within minutes** if not immediately corrected. These patients usually have signs of life such as reactive pupils, spontaneous respiratory efforts, spontaneous movement, or a palpable pulse, but otherwise present with profound shock or respiratory failure. This requires a **treat, then diagnose** approach **(operating room NOW!!)**.

B. If not intubated, **intubate.**

  1. If unable to intubate**, obtain a surgical airway.**

C. Penetrating injury, patient *in extremis* (Fig. 4-2)

  1. Neck

    a. Direct digital pressure if expanding hematoma or active bleeding

    b. IV fluid and blood

    c. Operating room

  2. Chest

    a. Bilateral chest tubes

    b. IV fluid and blood

    c. Left thoracotomy or bilateral thoracotomy

    d. Operating room

  3. Abdomen

    a. IV fluid and blood, avoid systolic blood pressure >80 mm Hg until in the OR.

    b. Move to OR immediately.

      i. Left thoracotomy for aortic control within the chest if abdomen is expanding and blood pressure remains low despite volume resuscitation. Some prefer control of the aorta through a high midline abdominal incision.

  4. Groin and extremities

    a. Apply pressure if expanding hematoma or active bleeding.

    b. IV fluid and blood

    c. Operating room

  5. Multiple penetrating wounds

    a. Apply pressure to sites of active bleeding.

    b. Bilateral chest tubes

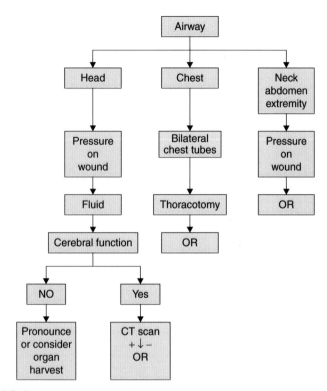

Figure 4-2. Penetrating trauma patient *in extremis.*

    c. IV fluid and blood
    d. Operating room
    e. Left thoracotomy (see Abdomen above)
D. Blunt injury, patient *in extremis* (Fig. 4-3)
    1. Apply pressure to external hemorrhage (consider hemostatic composite pack for large wounds)
    2. IV fluid and blood
    3. Bilateral chest tubes
       a. If ongoing hemorrhage or >1,500 mL on initial insertion of chest tubes, do OR or resuscitative thoracotomy.
    4. Ultrasound (US) or DPL of abdomen
       a. If grossly positive, move to OR.
       b. If negative DPL aspirate or US minimal or if no fluid, **x-ray pelvis.**
    5. X-ray of pelvis. Must identify the exsanguinating patient with pelvic fracture. (A small proportion of patients with major associated vascular injury must be taken to the OR.)
       a. If positive, place pelvic binder, move to angiography (consider aortography after pelvis).
       b. External fixation not usually appropriate for patient *in extremis.*
    6. Priorities with multiple injuries
       a. First → active thoracic hemorrhage or tamponade
       b. Second → abdominal hemorrhage
       c. Third → pelvic hemorrhage
       d. Fourth → extremity hemorrhage

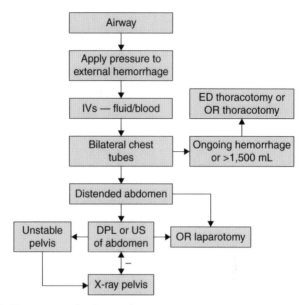

Figure 4-3. Blunt trauma patient *in extremis.*

       e. Fifth → intracranial injury
       f. Sixth → spinal cord injury

VIII. LABORATORY STUDIES
   A. Recent data have suggested a more selective and cost-effective approach to laboratory studies in both blunt and penetrating trauma.
      1. Stable patient
        a. Hemoglobin (Hb) and hematocrit (Hct)
        b. Blood ethanol (ETOH) (depending on hospital protocol)
        c. Urine dipstick for blood, human chorionic gonadotropin (hCG) in women of childbearing age (urine or blood)
        d. Blood screening without cross match unless condition changes
        e. Other studies as indicated by disease history
      2. Unstable patient:
        a. Required
          i. Blood type and cross match
          ii. Arterial blood gas and serum lactate
          iii. Hemoglobin/hematocrit
          iv. Prothrombin time, partial thromboplastin time, platelet count
          v. Urine dipstick for blood, hCG for women of childbearing age
          vi. ECG
         b. Selective (based on hospital protocol)
          i. Na, K, CO_2, Cl, blood urea nitrogen (BUN), creatinine, Ca^{++}, Mg^{++}
          ii. Serum amylase or lipase
          iii. Serum ETOH
         c. Point of care testing is available in many trauma centers

IX. MULTIPLE VICTIMS
   A. When several trauma victims arrive in the resuscitation area simultaneously, priority should be given to the unstable trauma victims.

B. Trauma team leader (most senior physician) should assign physicians and nurses to specific areas, and designees should not cover several areas simultaneously.

C. The trauma team leader should rotate from patient to patient to oversee management, prioritize care, and supervise actions of individual trauma teams.

D. The team leader should decide the need for backup assistance or calling a disaster plan when demand outstrips immediate resources. The team leader should err on the side of calling for additional assistance.

AXIOMS

- The **unstable trauma patient** can be defined by potential requirement for surgery or the ICU as well as cardiopulmonary dysfunction.
- DPL has a selective use in diagnosis of intraabdominal injury.
- Permissive hypotension (systolic BP of 90 mm Hg) is a useful approach in patients presenting with penetrating trauma until definitive control is obtained in the OR.
- The trauma patient who remains unstable after initial resuscitation usually requires operative intervention.
- The trauma patient *in extremis* may require treatment before diagnosis.

Suggested Readings

American College of Surgeons Committee on Trauma. *Advanced Trauma Life Support Manual.* Chicago: American College of Surgeons; 2008.

Moore FA, Moore EE. Initial Management of Life Threatening Trauma. In ACS Surgery, Principles and Practice. Section 7, Trauma and Thermal Injury. March 2010, acssurgery.com

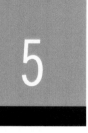

5 Shock

Joshua Brown, Jason L. Sperry and Timothy R. Billiar

Shock is defined as inadequate delivery of oxygen and nutrients to tissues to maintain normal cellular metabolic function.

I. CLASSIFICATION

A. **Hypovolemic and hemorrhagic.** The most common cause of shock in the injured patient is hypovolemia from hemorrhage. This etiology is assumed and treated until proven otherwise for all trauma patients in shock.

B. **Traumatic shock** is a separate entity in injured patients, but includes elements of other forms of shock. Traumatic shock evolves from acute blood loss/hypovolemia and release of pro-inflammatory mediators as a result of direct tissue injury that decreases peripheral vasomotor tone. Acute blood loss itself, irrespective of volume, can also promote pro-inflammatory effects. The combination of these insults results in global hypoperfusion, whereas each component in isolation may not.

C. **Cardiogenic shock** results from inadequate pumping function of the heart. Contractility is impaired and cardiac output falls with resultant hypoperfusion. In the injured patient, cardiogenic shock often is due to direct injury to the heart, most often blunt cardiac injury. Secondarily, intrinsic heart disease becomes more common among trauma patients and may lead to impaired heart pump action associated with the stress of injury on pre-existing cardiac disease.

D. **Vasogenic shock** occurs when vascular resistance is lowered sufficiently to reduce perfusion pressure in peripheral tissue beds. Underlying etiologies include anaphylaxis, adrenal crisis, sepsis, and neurogenic shock, with the latter two forms seen most commonly in trauma patients.

1. **Septic shock** results from infection, often later in the course of injured patients. Shock arises when the local pro-inflammatory response of the body designed to enhance microbe killing becomes systemic with profound vasodilation. There is also a component of capillary leak and loss of intravascular volume.

2. **Neurogenic shock** occurs with loss of sympathetic tone following spinal cord injury in the cervical or upper thoracic region. Loss of sympathetic tone increases vascular capacitance and decreases cardiac output.

E. **Obstructive shock** occurs when preload to the heart is impeded as a result of obstructed venous filling or direct compression of the heart. In trauma, this occurs in the setting of cardiac tamponade or tension pneumothorax, both of which require prompt diagnosis and treatment during the primary survey.

II. PHYSIOLOGIC RESPONSE.
The body mounts a complex physiologic response in the face of hypoperfusion to maintain homeostasis and perfusion to the most important tissues (i.e., brain, heart). This response is adapted in the setting of different types of shock.

A. **Afferent signaling.** The central nervous system integrates several afferent signals in the setting of hypoperfusion and impaired oxygen delivery. Baroreceptors in the carotid bodies and aortic arch, volume receptors in the atria, and chemoreceptors for oxygen tension, CO_2, and PO_2 all sense changes that signal hypoperfusion and act through the hypothalamic–pituitary–adrenal (HPA) axis and autonomic nervous system (ANS) to initiate compensatory mechanisms.

B. **Cardiovascular.** The cardiovascular system has three major responses to hypoperfusion, mediated through neuroendocrine pathways. Activation of the ANS results in an increased heart rate (HR) and contractility through beta-1 receptors, both augmenting cardiac output. Loss of sympathetic input in the setting of neurogenic shock blocks this increase in HR and is classic – albeit not common – for neurogenic shock. Intrinsic pump dysfunction in cardiogenic shock will not be overcome by the increased sympathetic activation. Alpha-1 receptor activation by the ANS and adrenergic hormones result in vascular smooth muscle contraction and increased vascular resistance. The degree of vasomotor tone increase is dependent on the regional tissue bed, with selective shunting of blood from less vital organs (i.e., skin, gut, kidney) to maintain perfusion to the brain and heart during the immediate threat of hypoperfusion. Recent evidence points to decreased HR variability as a poor prognostic indicator in patients with shock, as these highly integrated compensatory relationships become uncoupled and decompensation occurs.

C. Neuroendocrine. Epinephrine and norepinephrine are released from adrenal medulla to produce vasomotor effects. The renin–angiotensin–aldosterone system is activated in addition to the release of antidiuretic hormone to promote water reabsorption in the kidney and further modulation of regional vascular beds. Cortisol and glucagon release contribute to a catabolic state to increase available energy substrates for cells.

D. Immunologic and inflammatory. Although a profound inflammatory and immune response is typified in the setting of septic shock, all forms of shock promote a pro-inflammatory state as local tissue injury can become systemic. Important mediators of this reaction include cytokines, complement, oxygen radicals, eicosanoids, and nitric oxide. Important cytokines that have early effects on the systemic pro-inflammatory response include TNF-alpha, IL-1, IL-2, and IL-6. Many of the eicosanoids have strong vasoactive properties. Nitric oxide is recognized as having an increasingly important role in hypoperfusion modulation.

E. Cellular effects. As oxygen delivery to the cell declines, oxidative phosphorylation and ATP production slow down and the cell shunts substrates into anaerobic metabolism, producing lactate. As the ATP supply is depleted, a variety of energy-dependent cellular functions begin to fail including enzyme synthesis, DNA repair and expression, and signal transduction. Further, the membrane Na^+/K^+ ATPase becomes unable to maintain the cell membrane electrochemical gradient with resultant influx of sodium followed by water, causing cell swelling and lysis. Accumulation of metabolism byproducts and radical species are directly toxic to cells. Local and systemic acidosis ensues leading to alteration in enzyme activity and intracellular calcium signaling. Alterations in the local microcirculation are influenced by many metabolic byproducts and can aggravate oxygen debt in the tissue as well as promote further pro-inflammatory damage as a result of neutrophil trapping and activation.

III. SHOCK MANIFESTATIONS. The findings in a patient with shock are markers of hypoperfusion and the body's attempt to compensate. Signs of early shock may be subtle and must be carefully sought to prevent the cascading events. It is imperative to underscore patently abnormal vital signs as a late finding in shock, particularly hypotension. Patients with a normal/near normal blood pressure may still have profound hypoperfusion; failure to recognize this will lead to increased mortality and morbidity. Findings may vary between the forms of shock and can provide clues as to the underlying etiology.

A. Clinical findings

1. Hypovolemic shock. Depending upon the degree of volume loss, early signs include peripheral vasoconstriction, tachycardia, anxiety, or confusion. Patients on beta-blocking medications may not manifest a tachycardia. As hypovolemia and hemorrhage continues, extremities become cold and clammy, urine output declines (less useful in the acute phase), and mental status deteriorates. Patients may become combative or unresponsive. Hypotension often becomes evident only when 30% or more of the blood volume is lost. Central venous pressure declines with volume loss, but absolute thresholds that identify shock are indistinct—e.g., a "normal" CVP of 8 does not preclude volume depletion.

2. **Cardiogenic shock.** Patients will also show peripheral vasoconstriction and depressed mental status. Tachycardia or other dysrhythmias may be present and new ECG changes such as bundle block or T wave abnormalities may suggest cardiac injury or failure. Often a history of pre-existing cardiac disease or evidence of chest trauma (i.e., sternal fracture) may be obtained. Heart failure on examination or chest radiograph may be evident depending on the acuity of onset and time course. Echocardiography is the test of choice to confirm this diagnosis.
3. **Vasogenic shock.** Patients are marked by a hyperdynamic response, noted by increased cardiac output with tachycardia. Hypotension may be present. In vasogenic shock, vasodilation leads to warm, seemingly well-perfused extremities. Fever and leukocytosis are common particularly in sepsis, which may or may not be accompanied by an obvious source of infection.
4. **Neurogenic shock.** Patients will have similar manifestations as vasogenic shock including warm extremities and hypotension; because of the loss of sympathetic feedback to the cardiovascular system, cardiac output will be decreased. Patients are classically bradycardic, although a normal or fast HR may be present. Patients will have sensory and/or motor defects consistent with a spinal cord injury in the appropriate distribution. Hypovolemia is frequently coexistent, so volume infusion is a key first step.
5. **Obstructive shock.** Patients with tension pneumothorax frequently have rapid progression of severe shock and decompensation. They will develop tachycardia, hypotension, and cool extremities. Breath sounds will be decreased or absent on the affected side. Jugular venous distension is not reliably present. Tracheal deviation is generally a late finding or may be obscured by a cervical collar. Diagnosis and therapy should be performed simultaneously as described below. Cardiac tamponade classically presents with Beck's triad of hypotension, distended jugular veins, and muffled or distant heart sounds, although commonly one finding or more is absent. The electrocardiogram may show low or varying QRS voltage or tachycardia. The degree of clinical derangement is related to the acuity in the development of tamponade rather than volume of hemopericardium. Focused ultrasonography is the key in rapid detection.

B. **Coagulopathy of trauma**
1. **Acquired coagulopathy.** Part of the "lethal triad" of hypothermia, acidosis, and coagulopathy; patients develop impaired coagulation during resuscitation due to hemodilution of circulating clotting factors and functional derangements in clotting cascade enzymes from hypothermia. This phenomenon underscores the importance of using warmed fluids and has led to the concept of hemostatic resuscitation. Massive transfusion protocols in the hemorrhaging patient utilize plasma to blood ratios of at least 1:2 to combat the development of acquired coagulopathy associated with large volume resuscitation.
2. **Acute traumatic coagulopathy.** Now recognized as a separate entity, severe injury and hypoperfusion lead to an endogenous coagulopathy in the immediate post-injury period prior to hemodilution from resuscitation and onset of hypothermia. This traumatic coagulopathy is associated with systemic activation of the protein C anticoagulant system and hyperfibrinolysis. An independent risk of mortality and organ failure has been associated with acute traumatic coagulopathy, and understanding of the complex coagulation response following injury is in its infancy.

C. **Quantification of hypoperfusion**
1. **Oxygen debt.** When oxygen delivery declines, oxygen demand of cells outstrips oxygen delivery resulting in oxygen debt. The degree of oxygen debt correlates directly with the degree and duration of hypoperfusion as well as survival in hemorrhage models. Measurement of oxygen debt directly is difficult, necessitating surrogate measures of ongoing hypoperfusion.
2. **Lactate and base deficit.** Lactate levels and arterial base deficit are better indicators of oxygen debt compared with blood pressure, cardiac output, and volume loss in shock. These two tools are best used to trend debt and therapy rather than defining debt in a singular moment.

IV. MANAGEMENT. Shock requires simultaneous diagnosis and treatment; initial treatment is often empiric. The injured patient in shock frequently has elements from several types of shock and should always be assumed to have underlying hypovolemic shock until proven otherwise.

A. ABCs. The initial approach to shock includes securing an airway in patients with altered mental status and ensuring adequate ventilation for oxygen delivery. Early intravenous access is mandatory with two large bore peripheral lines preferably or central access if necessary. Any external hemorrhage should be halted with direct pressure as a temporizing maneuver. Fluids should be warmed and external warming undertaken to prevent hypothermia and subsequent coagulopathy.

B. Hypovolemic and hemorrhagic shock. Trauma patients should receive an initial 1 to 2 L crystalloid bolus. If profound shock is recognized immediately in a patient with large volume or ongoing hemorrhage, start blood transfusion (uncrossmatched) quickly. Moreover, fluid or blood product resuscitation should never delay operative hemorrhage intervention; any delay to operative control of bleeding will increase mortality in the hypotensive patient. Particularly in penetrating trauma, limited volume resuscitation may be beneficial until surgical control of hemorrhage is attained.

  1. Conceptually hemorrhagic shock patients are classified as responders, transient responders, and non-responders to initial fluid resuscitation. The latter two categories are patients that have ongoing sources of hemorrhage and either deteriorate after early improvement or continue to have ongoing signs of hypoperfusion despite resuscitation. These patients have surgical bleeding and require prompt operative or endovascular intervention to stop hemorrhage.

  2. Chest. Hemorrhage from lung parenchyma, great vessels of the chest, or cardiac wounds can result in significant blood loss. If suspected in deteriorating patients, bilateral chest tubes should be placed. Brisk hemorrhage (>1,500 mL blood returned immediately or >200 mL for more than 3 hours) should prompt operative intervention. In patients in extremis, consideration should be given to resuscitative thoracotomy in the appropriate setting in a patient with signs of life present.

  3. Abdomen. Patients with abdominal pain, peritonitis, or distension in conjunction with shock have evidence for intra-abdominal hemorrhage. Focused abdominal sonography or diagnostic peritoneal lavage can identify hemoperitoneum in patients without obvious examination findings. In patients with evidence of abdominal trauma and deteriorating perfusion absent, another cause should be promptly explored in the operating room

  4. Retroperitoneum/pelvis. Patients with open book or distracted pelvic fractures can lose significant amounts of blood into the retroperitoneum. A pelvic binder should be immediately placed once recognized. If no other source of hemorrhage is found and there is evidence of ongoing blood loss, angiography with embolization can stop bleeding. Pelvic packing may be considered in the persistently unstable patient with pelvic fracture.

  5. Long bones. Patients with femur fractures can lose large amounts of blood. Reduction and splinting can reduce hemorrhage and pain, followed by definitive orthopedic management.

  6. External. Soft tissue injuries can result in external blood loss and are usually easy to identify on examination and from field reports. These are initially controlled with direct pressure until definitive control can be achieved. Figure of eight or running locking sutures may be rapidly placed for persistent hemorrhage such as large scalp wounds if necessary.

C. Traumatic shock. In addition to treating elements of hemorrhagic shock as above, measures to limit secondary and ongoing tissue damage and resultant proinflammatory state should be undertaken. This includes early and frequent debridement of devitalized tissue, stabilization of orthopedic injuries, and meticulous care of soft tissue wounds.

D. Cardiogenic shock. After exclusion of hypovolemia as the cause of shock, fluid administration should be carefully monitored. Patients with known cardiogenic shock benefit from invasive hemodynamic monitoring such as central venous and arterial line placement. There are a variety of both invasive and noninvasive methods to closely monitor cardiac output and other hemodynamic parameters that can guide the use of inotropic support such as dobutamine. In states of refractory shock, an aortic balloon pump may aid. The goal of therapy in cardiogenic shock is supportive until the heart recovers from the insult. If needed, coronary revascularization can improve the function where vessel-based disease complicates acute trauma.

E. Vasogenic shock

1. Septic shock. Fluid resuscitation is the first step in sepsis care. In the trauma patient, sepsis becomes prevalent later in the course or in patients with delayed presentation. Patients who remain hypotensive may require vasopressor support. Norepinephrine and vasopressin are common choices. Patients should also be evaluated for underlying cardiac dysfunction as the pro-inflammatory state can also impair pump function.

  a. Treatment of the underlying infection is paramount. Broad spectrum empiric therapy should be immediately instituted concomitantly with a search for the source of infection. **Source control is essential** and any purulent collections must be drained, devitalized tissue debrided, and infected foreign bodies removed.

  b. Antibiotics should be narrowed to cover likely pathogens as a source is discovered and guided ultimately by culture data and institutional susceptibilities. If no source is found after a comprehensive evaluation, empiric antibiotic therapy should be stopped and the clinical course followed closely.

  c. Immunomodulatory therapies remain experimental at this point. The use of activated protein C has shown promise in sepsis but in patients with lower risk of death may precipitate bleeding and should be used with caution in the trauma patient. Adrenal insufficiency may coexist in the septic patients and should be considered in patients who have evidence of ongoing shock. No consensus on corticosteroid replacement in the trauma patient outside of adrenal insufficiency has been reached.

2. Neurogenic shock. Fluid administration is the initial treatment of choice. Once hypovolemia is corrected or ruled out as a cause of shock, persistently hypotensive patients may require vasopressor support. Phenylephrine is a common choice for its pure alpha agonist activity. The duration of required support is usually less than 48 hours as the body compensates. Invasive monitoring with an arterial line eases vasopressor titration.

F. Obstructive shock. As noted above, obstructive shock should be diagnosed and treated in rapid succession or simultaneously to avoid deterioration and death. For tension pneumothorax, needle thoracostomy followed by tube insertion should be undertaken expediently. In cardiac tamponade, emergent thoracotomy can be performed for patients in extremis. Patients with a more stable course should be taken to the operating room for pericardial window. Percutaneous drainage attempts are usually futile in acute tamponade.

V. ENDPOINTS OF RESUSCITATION. Therapy for shock is successful when oxygen debt and acidosis are eliminated and aerobic metabolism restored; it is difficult to reliably measure when this has been achieved. Although the need for continued resuscitation is clear with abnormal vital signs, normalization of blood pressure, HR, and urine output may occur in the face of ongoing hypoperfusion as measured by lactate levels or base deficit.

A. Lactate and base deficit. Just as markers of acid–base status have proved to be useful in quantifying shock initially, reversal of abnormal acid–base has been shown to predict outcome and guide resuscitation efforts. An inability to clear lactate within 48 hours of injury is associated with increased mortality. Persistently elevated base deficit (up to 96 hours) is a marker for ongoing resuscitation requirements and can be found despite normal vital signs and urine output. As a caution, both measures may be altered in the face of alcohol or drug use.

B. Gastric tonometry. This technology takes advantage of the body's selective shunting of blood during shock, whereby gut blood supply is diminished in favor of other critical organs. Subclinical reduction in gastric blood supply results in regional pH depression; CO_2 from this can be measured through diffusion techniques. Normalization of gastric pH correlates with mortality; however, the cumbersome evaluation of this as well as the need for gastric acid suppression and withholding gastric feeding has limited clinical application.

C. Near-infrared spectroscopy. This emerging technology has growing evidence showing the tissue oxygen saturation (StO_2) $\leq 75\%$ helps identify patients in persistent shock and is associated with poorer outcomes in trauma patients. StO_2 devices used on the thenar eminence are now commercially available for clinical use.

D. Tissue pH, oxygen, and carbon dioxide. Transcutaneous, subcutaneous, or sublingual measurement of regional acid–base status works on the same principles as gastric tonometry but is more clinically accessible. To date, the clinical utility remains uncertain.

E. Right ventricular end-diastolic volume index (RVEDI). Obtained from invasive hemodynamic monitoring, RVEDI correlates best with cardiac preload. Preliminary evidence shows that interventions to increase RVEDI resulted in reversal of subclinical gut ischemia and less organ failure in trauma patients.

AXIOMS

- Shock represents a state of hypoperfusion, which is not precluded by normal vital signs.
- Trauma patients are in hypovolemic shock from hemorrhage until proven otherwise.
- Resuscitation occurs concomitantly with evaluation for the patient in shock.
- Operative intervention for hemorrhage must not be delayed by diagnostic or other therapeutic maneuvers.
- The ultimate goal of resuscitation is restoration of aerobic metabolism to tissues, which can be guided by a variety of measures.

Suggested Readings

Beekley AC, Martin MJ, Nelson T, et al. Continuous noninvasive tissue oximetry in the early evaluation of the combat casualty: A prospective study. *J Trauma* 2010;69:S14–S25.

Blackbourne LH, Baer DG, Cestero RF, et al. Exsanguination shock: The next frontier in prevention of battlefield mortality. *J Trauma* 2011;71:S1–S3.

Cohen MJ, West M. Acute traumatic coagulopathy: From endogenous acute coagulopathy to systemic acquired coagulopathy and back. *J Trauma* 2011;70:S47–S49.

Davis JW. The relationship of base deficit to lactate in porcine hemorrhagic shock and resuscitation. *J Trauma* 1994;36:168–172.

Harbrecht BG, Forsythe RM, Peitzman AB. Management of shock. In: Feliciano DV, Mattox KL, Moore EE, eds. *Trauma.* 6th ed. New York, NY: McGraw Hill Co Inc; 2008:213–234.

Mikulaschek A, Henry SM, Donovan R, et al. Serum lactate is not predicted by anion gap or base excess after resuscitation. *J Trauma* 1996;40:218–224.

Morris JA, Norris PR, Ozdas A, et al. Reduced heart rate variability: An indicator of cardiac uncoupling and diminished physiologic reserve in 1,425 trauma patients. *J Trauma* 2006;60:1165–1174.

Neff LP, Chang MC. Hemodynamic management and shock. In: Flint L, Meredith JW, Schwab CW, et al., eds. *Trauma: Contemporary Principles and Therapy.* Philadelphia, PA: Lippincott Williams and Wilkins; 2008:675–683.

Zuckerbraun BS, Peitzman AB, Billiar TR. Shock. In: Brunicardi FC, ed. *Schwartz's Principles of Surgery.* 9th ed. New York, NY: McGraw Hill Co Inc; 2010:89–112.

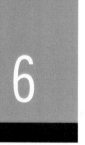

6

Damage Control Surgery

Brett H. Waibel and Michael F. Rotondo

I. HISTORY AND EVOLUTION OF DAMAGE CONTROL. The foundation of **damage control surgery (DCS)** focuses on exsanguinating truncal trauma. The underpinning for damage control is that a traditional operative approach risks physiologic exhaustion, and an abbreviated initial operation controlling only hemorrhage and contamination and allow aggressive resuscitation in the intensive care unit (ICU) is better. Once the trauma cascade of hypothermia, coagulopathy and acidosis is resolved, repair of all injuries begins.
   A. Due to its success, the clinical application of "damage control" has expanded into other areas, such as the septic abdomen and orthopedics, and underlies many triage and planned surgical responses to mass casualties for both military and civilian surgeons.

II. DAMAGE CONTROL INDICATIONS. The patient's physiology will drive the decision to perform DCS. Multiple variables interact to prevent absolute determinants for instituting DCS. *The operative needs must be balanced with the condition and response to the injuries or insult sustained (i.e., fecal peritonitis). Thus, the patient must constantly be reevaluated to identify those who would benefit from an abbreviated approach versus definitive repair.*
   A. Critical physiologic factors
      1. Hypothermia (temperature below 35°C)
      2. Acidosis (pH below 7.2 or base deficit exceeding 8)
      3. Coagulopathy defined as non-mechanical bleeding within or without the surgical field, increase in prothrombin (PT) and/or partial thromboplastin time (PTT), thrombocytopenia, hypofibrinogenemia, or massive transfusion requirements (greater than 10 units packed red blood cells [pRBC] or blood volume replaced)
      4. Prohibitive operative time required to repair injuries (greater than 90 minutes)
      5. Hemodynamic instability or profound hypoperfusion
   B. Injury complexes generally leading to development of instability
      1. High-energy blunt torso trauma
      2. Multiple penetrating torso injuries
      3. Multiple visceral injuries with major vascular trauma
      4. Multiple injuries across body cavities, especially those with competing priority for treatment, such as closed head injury, major vascular injury, and pelvic trauma.
   C. Other considerations
      1. Presence of injuries that may be better treated with nonsurgical adjuncts, such as angiographic embolization: Hepatic or pelvic injuries, deep large muscular bleeding, endovascular stenting, etc.
      2. Limitations in physiologic reserve, often seen in the elderly and those with multiple medical comorbidities.
      3. Complex surgical procedure(s) beyond the scope and training of the initial surgeon or resources of the facility.

III. DAMAGE CONTROL SEQUENCE. The DCS sequence was initially described in three phases. The initial abbreviated laparotomy (DC I) is followed by ICU resuscitation

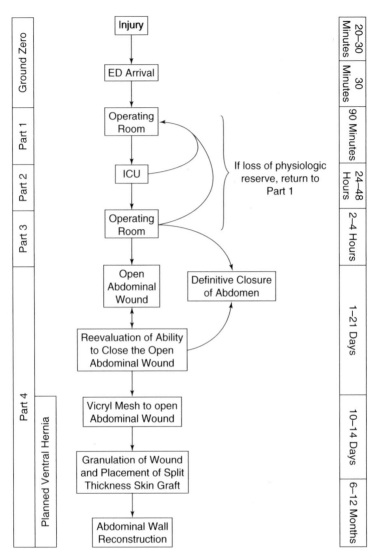

Figure 6-1. Damage control sequence (times are approximations and vary according to patient's injury and condition).

(DC II) then definitive repair of injuries at a subsequent laparotomy (DC III). Definitive closure of the abdominal wall (DC IV) and the initial presentation and resuscitation (DC ground zero) were later added. Damage control is best seen as a series of tactical phases linked by the need to progress the patient from near death to reconstruction and recovery (Fig. 6-1).

A. Ground zero (initial resuscitation)
   1. Prehospital care—see Chapter 9
   2. Initial hospital resuscitation

a. In patients entering the damage control pathway, simultaneous resuscitation, diagnosis, and concurrent onset of definitive care are necessary to hasten the onset of operation. The use of permissive hypotension (targeting systolic BP of 90 mm Hg) is begun in the prehospital setting and continued during the initial resuscitation until surgical control of the bleeding can be obtained. The clinical picture of the patient is generally someone with critical injury, either single or multiple, and profoundly abnormal vital signs as a manifestation of exsanguinations and severe hypovolemia. If Class IV shock exists – hypotension and bradycardia are present and herald a profound under-perfusion of the heart – most of these patients will fail to respond to blood administration and can only benefit from the immediate identification and surgical control of bleeding.

b. Adjuncts – Focused Abdominal Sonography in Trauma [FAST], diagnostic peritoneal lavage, tube thoracostomy, and radiographic imaging of the chest and pelvis – allow rapid localization of hemorrhage sites, but are not infallible. In general, fluid in the peritoneal cavity with hypotension indicates need for celiotomy, while large initial volume evacuation or ongoing drainage from tube thoracostomy (>1,500 mL initial, >200 mL/h over 3 to 4 hours) indicates the need for thoracotomy.

c. Damage control resuscitation (DCR), the aggressive transfusion policy of 1:1:1 (pRBC:FFP:platelets), made popular by the military experience in Iraq has become prevalent for civilian trauma patients. The current opinion favors the combined approach of limited crystalloid infusion, early Type O blood administration, permissive hypotension, and balanced ratio type specific or type and crossmatched blood product resuscitation.

d. While the optimal transfusion ratios have not been proven, most favor equal numbers of packed cells and plasma with early platelet administration. The volume of crystalloid is limited to that which allows organ perfusion and function, but does not return hydrostatic pressures to normal (permissive hypotension). Blood component products provide both volume expansion and function, such as clotting factors and oxygen carrying capacity. Most civilian reports show similar improvements (to the military experience) in mortality with the DCR approach.

e. Massive transfusion programs require protocols to assure the availability of large volumes of blood components quickly. These programs have been shown to lower mortality and not be wasteful of blood products.

B. **Damage control I (initial abbreviated laparotomy).** The goals of the initial celiotomy are to obtain control of hemorrhage and ongoing contamination. Definitive repair of injuries is deferred until subsequent operations to allow a further resuscitation period in the ICU.

1. The peritoneal cavity is opened and packed to obtain initial control, especially for hepatic, retroperitoneal, and pelvic structures. Abbreviated maneuvers are used to control vessel bleeding and perforated or lacerated viscera are temporary packed to limit leakage.

2. Once all injuries are identified, a plan is set to provide minimal acceptable care of all injuries to allow the patient time to reverse the physiologic insult. Shed blood can be collected for autotransfusion, but is effectively devoid of clotting factors and platelets and if heavily contaminated best not re-infused. *The guiding principle at this stage is that the more severe the injury(ies) and the more altered physiology, the less definitive repair during the initial laparotomy.*

3. **Positioning and packing**

a. While positioning for obvious isolated abdominal or thoracic injuries is straightforward, combined thoracoabdominal injuries are less so as neither the supine nor lateral decubitus position will allow simultaneous access to both cavities. The taxicab hailing position will often allow for practical exploration of both cavities, as well as sternotomy. The patient is placed in supine position with the chest laterally rotated about 30 degrees off the coronal plane using folded blankets. The arm is abducted, elbow flexed, and arm rotated above the head to allow exposure to the chest wall.

b. Preparation of a wide area is preferable. The preparation should be from neck to knees bilaterally. Patient warming can be difficult given the extent of exposure, but warming of the environment and intravenous fluids and placement of appropriate warming devices underneath the patient can minimize further heat loss and aid in reversing hypothermia.

c. Upon entry into the abdominal cavity, the four quadrants should be packed to tamponade bleeding. If effective, this allows a period to further resuscitate the patient and communicate important physiologic and lab parameters (pH, temperature, BP, etc.). This pause is used to set the surgical tactics and plan. Packs should be initially removed from areas without active bleeding to develop working space. *It is possible to overpack the peritoneal cavity producing decreased venous return via compression of inferior vena cava and inhibiting pulmonary excursion; continual communication with the anesthesia team is critical.*

4. **Hemorrhage control**

a. Hemorrhage control is a continuum across the multiple body cavities/regions. The surgeon should begin with the most compelling source of bleeding and then proceed to other areas quickly as circumstances evolve. Important in this concept is that some bleeding sites may not be present in the exposed surgical field. For most injuries, control can be achieved with combinations of manual tamponade, vascular clamps, and suture ligation of nonessential vessels.

b. Most major vascular injuries do not need definitive repair at time of DC I. Surgical shunts in major arteries and veins can be used as conduits in the interim in preference to undertaking a complex repair and the time they required. Shunts also avoid ligation of critical vessels (e.g., external iliac artery, SMA, subclavian artery, etc.).

c. Solid organ injuries have approaches that are organ dependent. Some organs, such as spleen and isolated kidney, may be best sacrificed if unsalvageable or to expedite control. Hepatic injuries are generally amenable to packing followed by further definitive control using angio-embolization.

   i. Avoid attempts to do more complex hepatorrhaphies or dissections, unless obvious large vessel bleeding in or around the liver is present.

   ii. Use angiography in any complex injury that is not controlled directly, such as complex renal, pelvic, or soft tissue injuries.

d. Ongoing arterial bleeding, whether in a viscera or cavity, will **not** be controlled with packing alone. Proximal control is needed, or the use of interventional radiology (ideally in the operating room) for these difficult injuries.

e. The operation should not end if ONGOING BLEEDING IS PRESENT, even though the patient remains hypothermic, acidotic, and coagulopathic. LEAVING AN ABDOMEN WITH ONGOING SURGICAL BLEEDING IS DESTINED TO FAILURE AND DEATH.

5. **Contamination control**

a. Hollow viscus injuries predominate and are straightforward in their treatment. Simple suturing or stapling techniques can control defects or rapidly removed injured segments to gain contamination control. Avoid definitive repair of these injuries, reestablishing intestinal continuity, stoma formation, or feeding ostomies at this time.

b. Biliary injuries can be temporized with external drainage, avoiding complex repairs.

c. Pancreatic injuries can be complex to manage. *Packing alone is inadequate for control of pancreatic secretions.* Wide area, closed suction drainage (multiple drains) of these injuries is required for control of the activated digestive enzymes to prevent secondary injury to the surrounding tissues. Definitive treatment and duct evaluation occur later.

6. **Temporary abdominal closure (TAC).** During the initial operation, a TAC is generally chosen. Preferably, the dressing should contain the visceral structures while helping to evacuate contamination. Skin integrity should be well

maintained by effluent control. Minimize tension to reduce the chance of abdominal compartment syndrome.

a. Preserve fascia for later definitive closure. A multitude of procedures exist that provide variable achievements of these goals. Towel clip closures, silo formation (Bogota bag), and suture closure of fascia or skin are used less often than previously. At present, either a commercial vacuum assisted closure system or "vac-pack" style temporary abdominal dressing is generally used. For a vac-pack style closure, a perforated plastic membrane (x-ray cassette cover or bowel bag) or sterile soft cloth towel covered with an adhesive dressing is placed between the visceral block and abdominal wall. Kerlix gauze with embedded closed suction drains is placed in the wound to provide drainage to the abdominal cavity. An adhesive dressing (such as an Ioban^{TM} dressing) is placed to provide closure of the system and maintain skin integrity.

b. Continuous suction applied to the embedded drains will maintain a seal and provide evacuation of peritoneal fluids. The commercial systems have the same basic design, but may be more efficacious in removal of intraperitoneal fluids and medialization of the fascia, helping to preserve domain for later use.

C. Damage control II (intensive care unit resuscitation). Resuscitation is continued in the ICU to reestablish the physiologic reserve in anticipation of definitive repair at the next laparotomy. Central to this goal is reversal of hypothermia, coagulopathy, and acidosis. In addition, control of other metabolic derangements and identification of all injuries must be performed during this period.

1. Hemodynamics and correction of acidosis

a. The goal of damage control management for hemodynamics during DC II is to restore adequate tissue perfusion to reverse the metabolic acidosis associated with trauma. Monitoring of preload and arterial pressure is commonly needed in the unstable patient to optimize preload and cardiac output to provide adequate perfusion of the tissue beds. Multiple endpoints of resuscitation can be used, but no single one alone is ideal. Vital signs are poor indicators alone, as even after their normalization, many patients will demonstrate evidence of inadequate tissue perfusion. Base deficit and lactate levels are often collinear and correlate with outcomes; however, brain injury or hepatic dysfunction may delay lactate clearance despite acceptable reestablishment of tissue perfusion. *Therefore, resuscitation should continue until multiple methods of evaluation indicate that the shock state has resolved.* These include, but are not limited to, normalization of temperature and other vital signs, declining base deficit/lactate levels, improved urine output, and normalization of oxygen saturation, pulmonary hemodynamics, and arterial pulse contour analysis.

b. *Failure to obtain improvement in base deficit/lactate levels or other endpoints of resuscitation should prompt reevaluation of the resuscitation strategy and search for ongoing hemorrhage or contamination which requires return to the operating room or interventional suit for further control or search for missed injury.*

c. No evidence supports one fluid type over another for resuscitation within the ICU. However, fluid choice can have significant effects. The better outcomes seen recently may be due to changes in resuscitation strategy over the last decade and the continuation of DCR into the ICU phase. The blood component resuscitation-limited crystalloid approach results in overall volumes being reduced compared to the very large crystalloid volume resuscitations performed in the past. Better and careful monitoring of the end points of resuscitation (see above) allows constant adjustment to assure organ perfusion and function without volume overload.

2. Core rewarming

a. *Coagulopathy and hypoperfusion cannot be adequately corrected until normothermia is reestablished.* Severe hypothermia is associated with both cardiovascular collapse/malignant dysrhythmias and disruption of coagulation pathway and platelet function. In addition, hypothermia inhibits oxygen dissociation from hemoglobin, impairing tissue oxygenation. Furthermore, increased infectious complications are seen in hypothermic patients.

b. The rewarming process can usually be achieved with removal of wet bedding, increase in ambient room temperature; place convection or insulating blankets/pads, and warm intravenous fluids and ventilator gases. More invasive procedures, such as intravenous heat exchange catheters, cardiopulmonary or extracorporeal venovenous/arteriovenous bypass, and body cavity lavage, are generally not necessary. *The inability to warm the patient suggests continued hemorrhage.*

3. Coagulopathy correction

a. Loss and dilution of coagulation factors and platelets by bleeding, replacement with intravenous fluids or only packed RBCs, the effects of hypothermia and acidosis, and binding of calcium (clotting factor 4) by citrate found in component blood products all interact to produce an acquired coagulopathy. In addition, intracranial, pulmonary, and massive soft tissue injury can release tissue thromboplastin and other factors that contribute to this coagulopathy; a component of the coagulopathy is a direct result of the injury. Thrombocytopenia is the first and most common abnormality to occur.

b. To correct this coagulopathy requires control of hemorrhage, rewarming, and replacement of factors and platelets. Any *clinical* evidence of coagulopathy should prompt replacement of platelets and factors before measurement. Serial evaluation of PT, PTT, platelet counts, and fibrinogen can guide further replacement. Where possible, have some quantity of plasma thawed for emergent use.

c. Recombinant Factor VIIa (rFVIIa) is another adjunct to correct an acquired coagulopathy. However, the CONTROL trial, a recent multi-center randomized controlled trial to evaluate the efficacy of rFVIIa in trauma, was closed before completion due to futility.

4. Ventilator management. Most patients will require mechanical ventilation and optimization of oxygenation during DC II. Given the extent of inflammation induced in severe trauma, patients are at high risk to develop acute lung injury or acute respiratory distress syndrome (ARDS). The goal should be to maintain oxygenation and adequate ventilation while minimizing ventilator induced pulmonary injury from large tidal volumes and pressures (see Chapter 38 – Acute Respiratory Failure and Mechanical Ventilation).

5. Sedation/neuromuscular blockade. Sedation and analgesia are commonly needed to achieve good synchrony between the patient and ventilator; prolonged neuromuscular blockade is rarely needed. The damage control patient with an open abdomen is best treated with continuous infusions of both sedatives and opioid analgesics.

6. Nutritional support. Hold enteral feeding until hemodynamic stability exists to avoid the risk of intestinal ischemia. Placement of enteral catheters is best accomplished early at DC I or DC III, with a nasojejunal tube preferred for feeding or decompression. **Start enteral feeds after restoration of normal physiology and assurance of normal gut perfusion and resumption of gut motility.** TPN has no role in the early phases of damage control; later, TPN is a potential bridge intervention when there is complex or multiple pancreatic, biliary, or foregut injuries.

7. Complete injury identification. Complete injury identification is sought during this period, which includes a tertiary examination and review of radiographic imaging. Again, complete imaging obviated by DC I as soon as physiology is restored and transport (if necessary) from the ICU is safe.

D. Damage control III (subsequent laparotomy/definitive repair). The patient is returned to the operating room for definitive care of their injuries, often 24 to 48 hours from injury. Premature return to the operating room can lead to resumption of the shock state and need to repeat DC I. However, delayed return is associated with increased infectious risks, especially if significant contamination and packing is present.

1. Upon return, packing should be carefully removed in a stepwise fashion, especially from solid organs. This allows an organized control of recurrent or errant bleeding points. After unpacking, fully examine the peritoneal cavity in a structured fashion to ensure identification of all injuries. Inspect prior gastrointestinal repairs/anastomoses. At this time, reestablish gastrointestinal continuity and make other repairs if possible. Any anastomosis performed should be tucked under the fascial edges or covered with omentum to reduce risk of breakdown. Then, do a thorough abdomen washout. If needed, closed suction drainage is preferable, especially for bilious drainage and pancreatic injuries, and these tubes should be brought out as lateral and posterior as possible.

2. While tube enterostomies and stomas are possible, they have increased complication rates and should be avoided. If needed, the stoma should be lateralized, as this will move more anteriorly as abdominal wall geometry returns to normal. Place or reposition nasojejunal tubes at this opportunity. If a colostomy is necessary, these are best done laterally and brought through the musculature between the anterior and midaxillary lines. This avoids large defects in the rectus muscle and preserves components that may be necessary for abdominal wall closure in the future. It also avoids placing a stoma over an open abdomen wound and direct soilage.

3. Some injuries are more commonly missed, especially diaphragm and retroperitoneal structures (duodenum, rectum, bladder, ureters, pancreas, retroperitoneal colon, posterior gastric wall, gastroesophageal junction, mesenteric intestinal border). Look carefully for these in each patient.

4. Definitive closure of the abdominal cavity should *never* be forced or performed prematurely. Such a closure depends upon the swelling of the viscera, need for further abdominal surgery, and ongoing resuscitation. Those with markedly distended viscera (protruding "abdominal block") or needing further resuscitation should undergo repeated placement of a TAC. The risk of developing abdominal compartment syndrome (ACS) should guide the need for a TAC versus definitive abdominal wall closure. During fascial closure, changes in airway pressure may be used to guide capacity for safe closure.

5. *In patients undergoing fascial closure, a radiographic evaluation of the abdomen for retained packing or instruments is recommended at time of definitive closure.* Given the circumstances of the initial laparotomy, closing counts cannot be trusted and imaging provides a permanent record of operating room sponges used and their removal. It must include all areas of the abdomen and pelvis.

E. Damage control IV (abdominal wall closure). Primary fascial closure at DC III cannot be performed in approximately 40% to 70% of patients. A multitude of TACs are present with variable advantages/disadvantages and success rates.

1. In general, if an abdomen cannot be closed in 7 to 8 days, further attempts at closure are usually futile and preceding with some form of mesh closure with eventual split thickness skin graft (STSG) and delayed abdominal wall closure (6 to 12 months) is recommended. Approximately two-thirds of patients are closed by the seventh or eighth day post injury.

2. The dynamic properties of the vacuum assisted dressing are superior and preferred to the early TAC devices (vac-pack – see above).

3. For those requiring more intermediate closures while awaiting resolution of visceral edema for fascial closure, more options are available. Interpositional mesh closures and vacuum assisted abdominal dressings are both options. Sequential closure of the fascia may be performed with these TAC techniques.

    a. Absorbable meshes such as polyglactic acid (Vicryl) or polyglycolic acid (Dexon) have lower tensile strength, and elicit little inflammation. They are the preferred coverage mesh products. Polypropylene meshes have higher tensile strengths, but induce an inflammatory reaction and higher infectious complications; polytetrafluoroethylene is easily colonized and shelters bacteria from the immune system. These nonabsorbable meshes should not be used.

    b. *Avoid complex closures involving permanent meshes, fascial releases, or extensive skin flaps, as they lead to the increased wound complications and infectious* *risks. Furthermore, these techniques can prevent or complicate abdominal wall reconstruction later.*

4. When fascial closure is not achievable, use of a planned ventral hernia is another option. Our first preference is to attempt a skin only closure. If this cannot be achieved, an absorbable mesh is placed and followed by a STSG when granulation tissue integrates with the mesh (usually 10 to 14 days). Abdominal wall reconstruction is performed when the skin graft separates from the underlying viscera (usually 6 to 12 months). Often, this technique requires component separation and/or mesh placement, usually in an underlay position (either subfascial or retrorectus), as lateral retraction of the abdominal wall muscles leads to increasing defect size (Chapter 56).

IV. **MORTALITY/MORBIDITY OF DAMAGE CONTROL SURGERY.** Damage control can improve the chance of survival, but comes at the cost of increased morbidity. Approximately a third of patients will experience a major abdominal complication, such as intraabdominal abscess, anastomotic leak, enterocutaneous or enteroatmospheric fistula, prolonged ileus or obstruction, and abdominal wall dehiscence. Furthermore, damage control patients commonly experience other complications such as abdominal compartment syndrome, ARDS/acute lung injury, renal failure, pneumonia, or multisystem organ failure.

A. **Mortality.** Damage control laparotomy has a survival benefit when compared to similar patients with severe injury treated in more traditional ways. Damage control techniques have survival rates around 60% overall and some series report higher survivals with penetrating injuries. Duchesne has recently reported improved outcomes with layering damage resuscitation into damage control laparotomy (74%).

B. **Abdominal compartment syndrome (ACS) (Chapter 39)**
   1. ACS, the clinical entity marked by hypotension, increased ventilatory pressures, and oliguria in the presence of intraabdominal hypertension, is associated with increased mortality. ACS has global effects beyond the aforementioned symptoms. Decompression of the peritoneal cavity will improve organ perfusion and function.
   2. Risk factors for ACS development include severe hemorrhagic shock, elevated penetrating abdominal trauma index, and large fluid resuscitation (greater than 10 L intravenous fluid or massive transfusion). As such, damage control patients are at high risk for ACS development, especially if fascial closure is performed. *The use of TACs, reducing ACS incidence but does not prevent it.*
   3. Clinical examination and measurement of the abdominal circumference do not correlate with intraabdominal pressure. *Monitoring of intraabdominal pressures with interval bladder pressure measurement is necessary and allows the early detection of intraabdominal hypertension.* The World Society of Abdominal Compartment Syndrome (WSACS) defines ACS as sustained intraabdominal pressures above 20 mm Hg associated with new organ dysfunction or failure.

C. **Intraabdominal abscess (IAA).** Intraabdominal abscess rates vary from 10% to 70%, but appear related to the duration of intraabdominal packing and degree of contamination. Infection rates appear to increase at 72 hours of pack retention. CT imaging aids detection of abscesses in patients with persistent fever or leukocytosis. Once defined they are best handled with radiographically guided percutaneous drainage.

D. **Enterocutaneous fistula (Chapter 39).** Multiple factors, such as extent of bowel injury, anastomoses, length of time of the open abdomen, manipulations, and abdominal closure technique, affect fistula formation. Reports vary, but generally the frequency is between 1% and 15%. Unfortunately, the fistulae seen with open abdomens tend to be the aggressive enteroatmospheric type, where the fistula opens within the granulating wound bed either through the visceral block or laterally in the dead space between viscera and abdominal wall.
   1. Closure rates without surgery tend to be around 25%. Effluent control can be difficult to obtain given the fistula location and several methods to gain effluent control have been described. No single technique can be applied to all situations nor is superior to another.

2. Once effluent control can be obtained, the open abdominal wound can undergo skin grafting and eventually the fistula treated like an ostomy.
3. As recovery occurs, sepsis is controlled, and nutrition improves, abdominal opening contracture and scar maturation should be allowed until the patient has gained considerable weight and well-being. Abdominal wall reconstruction and fistula reversal can be performed in 9 to 12 months.

V. DAMAGE CONTROL IN OTHER AREAS. Damage control identifies those patients with exhausted physiology or high risk of such and seeks to improve survival at the cost of increased morbidity. It is used in other surgical emergencies with similar hemodynamic instability including emergent vascular and gynecologic procedures, as well as complicated pancreatitis. However, orthopedics and the septic abdomen are two domains with emerging experiences with this paradigm.

A. Damage control orthopedics. Before 1950s, surgical stabilization of fractures was not routinely performed. While over the next few decades, the benefits of skeletal stabilization began to become apparent, the prevailing belief remained that patients were too sick to acutely be operated upon and fractures would heal faster if surgery were delayed for 2 weeks. By late 1980s, it was clear that morbidity, postoperative complications, and length of stay improved with a damage control approach after immediate surgical stabilization. This decreased complications and hospital time, although some pulmonary complications and multisystem organ failure occurred. Over the next two decades, this has been refined to minimizing the initial operation (external fixation only) and delaying definitive repair in the multiply injured patient until the inflammatory state resolved. The term damage control orthopedics was coined in 1999 by Scalea and Pollak to describe this sequence.

B. Septic abdomen. The techniques employed in damage control for trauma can easily be adapted to the septic abdomen. The TACs utilized allow for rapid entry and egress from the abdomen, improved peritoneal toilet, and control of effluent. In addition, they allow for reduced incidence of abdominal compartment syndrome, common in this clinical entity. Unfortunately, studies to date have been small with mixed populations preventing a true determination of the efficacy of damage control techniques in this population.

1. The damage control sequence is adjusted for the septic abdomen. The initial resuscitation phase, while only a few hours, is longer than that seen for trauma. The goal of the abbreviated laparotomy is source control, which includes wide drainage of the septic process. A temporary abdominal dressing is used for the described indications. Further resuscitation is performed in the ICU, followed by needed subsequent laparotomies. This sequence can also easily incorporate the surviving sepsis guidelines.

AXIOMS

- DCS is a well-defined five-part approach to the severely injured trauma patient which can be modified to other surgical emergencies.
- Damage control improves the chance of survival with increased morbidity; it should be reserved for those who truly need it.
- Damage control requires complete injury identification and management of all injuries after the initial temporizing period.
- Failure to control hemorrhage or contamination will cause a continuous strain upon the physiologic reserve of the patient, ultimately leading to patient death.
- Packing alone will not control arterial bleeding within a cavity or solid organ. Failure to improve acidosis, reverse hypothermia, or correct the acquired coagulopathy of trauma should prompt reevaluation of the resuscitation strategy and a search for ongoing bleeding.

Suggested Readings

Campbell A, Chang M, Fabian T, et al. Management of the open abdomen: from initial operation to definitive closure. *Am Surg* 2009;75:S1–S22.

Cheatham ML, Safcsak K. Is the evolving management of intra-abdominal hypertension and abdominal compartment syndrome improving survival? *Crit Care Med* 2010;38:402–407.

Damage Control Management in the Polytrauma Patient, Pape HC, Peitzman AP, Schwab CW, Giannoudis PV, eds. New York, NY: Springer; 2010.

Duchesne JC, Kimonis K, Marr AB, et al. Damage control resuscitation in combination with damage control laparotomy: A survival advantage. *J Trauma* 2010;69:46–52.

Giannoudis PV. Surgical priorities in damage control in polytrauma. *J Bone Joint Surg Br* 2003;85:478–483.

Johnson JW, Gracias VH, Schwab CW, et al. Evolution in damage control for exsanguinating penetrating abdominal injury. *J Trauma* 2001;51:261–269.

Miller RS, Morris JA Jr, Diaz JJ Jr, et al. Complications after 344 damage-control open celiotomies. *J Trauma* 2005;59:1365–1371.

Pape HC, Giannoudis P, Krettek C. The timing of fracture treatment in polytrauma patients: relevance of damage control orthopedic surgery. *Am J Surg* 2002;183:622–629.

Perel P, Roberts I. Colloids versus crystalloids for fluid resuscitation in critically ill patients. *Cochrane Database Syst Rev* 2007;(3):CD000567.

Ramirez OMMD, Ruas EMD, Dellon ALMD. "Components separation" method for closure of abdominal-wall defects: an anatomic and clinical study. *Plast Reconstr Surg* 1990;86:519–526.

Rasmussen TE, Clouse WD, Jenkins DH, et al. The use of temporary vascular shunts as a damage control adjunct in the management of wartime vascular injury. *J Trauma* 2006;61:8–12.

Reilly PM, Rotondo MF, Carpenter JP, et al. Temporary vascular continuity during damage control: intraluminal shunting for proximal superior mesenteric artery injury. *J Trauma* 1995;39:757–760.

Rotondo MF, Schwab CW, McGonigal MD, et al. 'Damage control': an approach for improved survival in exsanguinating penetrating abdominal injury. *J Trauma* 1993;35:375–382.

Rotondo MF, Zonies DH. The damage control sequence and underlying logic. *Surg Clin North Am* 1997;77:761–777.

Shapiro MB, Jenkins DH, Schwab CW, et al. Damage control: collective review. *J Trauma* 2000;49:969–978.

Stawicki SP, Brooks A, Bilski T, et al. The concept of damage control: extending the paradigm to emergency general surgery. *Injury* 2008;39:93–101.

7 Blood and Transfusion

Michael W. Cripps, Mitchell J. Cohen and Robert C. Mackersie

I. INTRODUCTION

A. The transfusion of blood and blood products is a key component in reversal of hemorrhagic shock. Blood product transfusions expand volume, improve oxygen carrying capacity, and restore coagulation homeostasis. While it is clear that blood product transfusion saves lives and reduces morbidity, they have associated risks. This chapter will focus on the transfusion management of severely injured trauma patients.

II. EPIDEMIOLOGY

A. Approximately 30 million units of blood are transfused every year in the United States, with 10% to 15% of all RBC units used to treat injured patients. Twenty five percent of trauma patients admitted receive at least a unit of packed red blood cells (pRBCs) and of those, 25% receive a massive transfusion (defined below); this latter group is the most severely injured (and therefore largest potentially preventable mortality) with a death rate of 40% to 70%.

B. Hemorrhage remains a leading cause of preventable death in trauma patients, with approximately 16% of preventable deaths attributed to truncal hemorrhage. Hemorrhage as the cause of death usually occurs within the first 6 hours of admission.

C. It is the failure to control hemorrhage that underlies the cause of many of these possibly preventable deaths. This failure is typically related to either an inability to rapidly control "surgical" hemorrhage (bleeding requiring suture/staple/ligation), or persistent "non-surgical" hemorrhage (bleeding normally expected to stop spontaneously), and an inability to reestablish relatively normal coagulation.

D. While exsanguination from massive (non-surgically repairable) injury is responsible for a large number of deaths, many patients with preventable mortality suffer from coagulopathy and bleeding. Up to one-third of all trauma patients who present to the hospital already have a coagulopathy.

    1. Trauma patients are vulnerable to development of the so-called "bloody vicious cycle" or "Triad of Death," which is comprised of coagulopathy, hypothermia, and acidosis. Each of these variables worsens the other and if not reversed, will lead to death.

    2. Historically, the coagulopathy seen in trauma was thought to be solely the result of dilution and loss of coagulation factors following large volume resuscitation with crystalloids or unbalanced blood component transfusions (dilutional coagulopathy). More recently, a coagulopathy that develops in severe injury through an impairment of hemostasis and activation of fibrinolysis that occurs independent of the development of acidosis, hypothermia, or hemodilution has been described. It has been referred to by many terms including the "Early Trauma Induced Coagulopathy," "Trauma Associated Coagulopathy," and as the "Acute Traumatic Coagulopathy." For the purposes of this chapter, we will refer to this coagulopathy as the acute traumatic coagulopathy (ATC).

    3. Observations from recent armed conflicts refined the concept of hemostatic resuscitation **(see later).** This includes limiting the early administration of crystalloid fluids, advocating the use of tourniquets and hemostatic agents for direct bleeding control, and resuscitation goals directed toward the preservation of physiologic and coagulation homeostasis rather than restoring normal or supranormal vital signs.

4. Conventional resuscitation involves the use of large volumes of isotonic crystalloid solutions to restore normal blood pressure, followed by pRBCs to increase oxygen carrying capacity with fresh frozen plasma (FFP) and platelets administered later to counteract the effects of hemodilution.

5. *Hemostatic resuscitation* aims to maintain intravascular volume, oxygen carrying capacity, and normal coagulation through the preemptive administration of blood and blood products that approximates ongoing losses. While the optimal ratios of pRBCs, FFP, and platelets are uncertain, a strategy of administering a ratio 1 unit of pRBCs to 1 unit of FFP to 1 unit of platelets (1:1:1 ratios) is common now when treating the severely injured.

III. PATHOPHYSIOLOGY

A. Normal coagulation.

Normal coagulation following tissue injury involves subendothelial tissue factor exposure resulting in a series of protease activations (the coagulation cascade), thrombin production, thrombin burst, and the conversion of fibrinogen to fibrin which is crosslinked and combines with platelets to form a plug. These procoagulant actions are balanced by natural anticoagulants (activated protein C, TFPI, and antithrombin) and fibrinolysis which serve to break down clot when no longer needed and prevent an overly thrombogenic milieu. Hence normal coagulation is a balance between hemostatic and fibrinolytic processes, thereby allowing for tissue-specific clot formation in an injured area without resultant systemic thrombosis.

B. Coagulopathy

The inability to control major hemorrhage can be due to "non-surgical bleeding," defined as bleeding that continues despite the surgical control of identifiable bleeding sources. This often manifests clinically as diffuse microvascular hemorrhage. The principal causes are hemodilution resulting from excessive crystalloid administration relative to the administration of blood and blood products (FFP, platelets), and a non-dilutional ATC.

C. Dilutional coagulopathy

Dilutional coagulopathy occurs with hemodilution resulting from the transfusion of large volumes of intravenous crystalloid and/or from an imbalance in blood component resuscitation. The dilutional loss of clotting factors and platelets limits the extent of the fibrin/platelet plug that can be formed at the site of injury. Transfusion solely with pRBCs, containing no platelets or clotting factors, further exacerbates the coagulopathy.

D. Acute traumatic coagulopathy (ATC)

Up to 33% of major trauma patients present initially with a coagulopathy that is neither disseminated intravascular coagulation (DIC) nor dilutional and is associated with major tissue injury and hypoperfusion (shock). Abnormal coagulation that occurs in this setting is often referred to as the ATC.

ATC is characterized by both impaired clot formation and enhanced fibrinolysis. Recent work suggests that activation of the protein C system is a primary cause of ATC.

E. Other causes of coagulopathy

The combination of hypothermia, acidosis, and coagulopathy left untreated is lethal. Each of these problems worsens the other.

1. **Acidosis.** Metabolic acidosis is usually related to inadequate tissue perfusion (shock) leading to an accumulation of lactate. This acidosis can be further exacerbated by administration of large volumes of normal saline which, as a consequence of the high chloride concentration in normal saline (154 mEq/L), can lead to a hyperchloremic acidosis. Acidosis inhibits thrombin and factors VIIa, Xa, and Va. Coagulation factor complex activity necessary for normal coagulation is disrupted by acidosis.

2. **Hypothermia.** Nearly two-thirds of trauma patients have a temperature of $36°C$ or below on presentation; 9% have a temperature $\leq 33°C$. Acidosis and

hypothermia produce a synergistic effect with greater mortality. Hypothermia can be graded as mild (36 to 34°C), moderate (34 to 32°C), and severe (<32°C). The hypothermia of the injured patient is covered in Chapter 42.

a. Hypothermia directly affects the coagulation cascade by inhibiting tissue factor activity, platelet aggregation, platelet adhesion, and increasing the time it takes for thrombin formation. Enzymatic inhibition of the coagulation cascade generally begins at temperatures less than 33°C.

b. Measures to prevent hypothermia include the administration of warm fluids (crystalloid and blood products), use of blankets, warming devices, and increasing the ambient temperature.

c. The contribution of hypothermia alone to overall coagulation disorders is relatively small compared to ATC and dilutional coagulopathy.

3. Hypocalcemia. Calcium is a coagulation cofactor (Factor IV), required at several points in the coagulation cascade. pRBCs are preserved in citrate which binds calcium. While there are no definitive studies that show improved outcomes with reversal of hypocalcemia, intravenous calcium is often used in patients receiving massive transfusions.

4. DIC. DIC is a systemic process of consumptive coagulopathy in concert with diffuse microvascular thrombosis. In trauma patients, there are several mechanisms that can lead to DIC:

a. Tissue factor exposure is induced at the site of tissue injury which leads to activation of the coagulation cascade that in turn, leads to diffuse intravascular thrombin generation.

b. Systemic embolism of tissue-specific thromboplastins from sites of injury (including bone marrow lipid material, amniotic fluid, and brain phospholipids) can also lead to widespread generation of thrombin.

DIC is characterized by simultaneous systemic thrombosis and hemorrhage, and typically occurs in the setting of large amounts of tissue factor exposure in the blood in a short period of time. There may be some clinical overlap between DIC and ATC, but the latter occurs in the absence of the low platelet and fibrinogen levels typically seen in DIC.

IV. LABORATORY MONITORING OF TRANSFUSION AND COAGULATION

The goal of laboratory studies is to provide an ongoing, timely evaluation of coagulation and oxygen carrying capacity. The currently available laboratory studies for transfusion initiation and monitoring includes:

A. Blood type, screening and cross matching. Send this early to prepare for transfusion. Seek cross matching when transfusion is likely.

B. Complete blood count (CBC). The CBC is used primarily for the hemoglobin concentration (to assess oxygen carrying capacity) and the platelet count.

C. Coagulation panel—prothrombin time (PT), partial thromboplastin time (PTT), and international normalized ratio (INR). These tests are used to determine coagulation status.

1. PT. Used to assess the extrinsic pathway of coagulation (Factors I, II, V, VII, and X).

2. PTT. Functional measure of the intrinsic pathway of coagulation (VIII, IX, XI, and XII).

3. INR. The results of the PT may vary among institutions depending on the type of analytical system used. The INR was devised to standardize the results by utilizing an international sensitivity index (ISI) that is specific to each analytical system. The INR is calculated by $(PT_{test}/PT_{normal})^{ISI}$.

However, these tests are problematic in trauma patients for multiple reasons:

1. The coagulopathic state in trauma patients is in constant flux as they are continuously receiving large volumes of blood, plasma, and platelets.

2. The standard coagulation lab examinations take time to analyze, so the result reported does not necessarily reflect the patient's coagulation state when the results are returned.

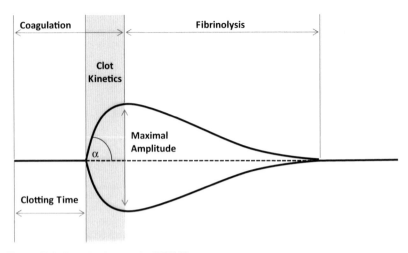

Figure 7-1. Thromboelastography (TEG) Measurement.

3. For the PT/PTT analysis, the patient's blood sample is warmed to 37°C and mixed with platelet-poor plasma, which may not represent the true coagulation state in a hypothermic trauma patient.

A PT greater than 1.5 times normal following severe injury is often a diagnostic criterion for ATC. While the prevalence of prolonged PT is higher, prolongation of the PTT is more specific with more robust predictive value for mortality.

Newer alternatives to traditional coagulation testing such as thromboelastography, may offer a more accurate assessment of actual *in vivo* coagulation. (See Section "Thromboelastography" below).

D. Fibrinogen and D-dimer. Fibrinogen is a soluble plasma glycoprotein that is converted by thrombin into fibrin during blood coagulation. The D-dimer is the fibrin degradation product that is found after clot dissolution.
   1. Low levels of fibrinogen and elevated D-dimer can act as surrogate markers of clotting factor consumption and hyperfibrinolysis, respectively.
   2. The D-dimer is elevated in almost all trauma patients, leaving its absolute clinical value in question.
   3. Recent data indicates that there is a benefit from increased fibrinogen levels, suggesting a role for more frequent fibrinogen level measurements during resuscitation of severely injured patients.

E. Thromboelastography. Thromboelastography (TEG) is an assessment of the viscoelastic properties of clot formation in fresh or citrated whole blood in real time. This test synthesizes information from standardized tests (PT, PTT, thrombin time, fibrinogen level, and platelet count) into a single dynamic readout providing simultaneous information regarding time to clot initiation, clot strength, and fibrinolysis. This allows immediate analysis and goal directed therapy of the coagulation disorder.
   1. The TEG (Fig. 7-1) is measured on a small aliquot of warmed whole blood and measures the clotting time (R value), clot formation (alpha angle), clot strength (MA, maximal amplitude), and clot lysis (LY 30).
   2. Several standardized coagulation parameters can be derived from the TEG, and are calculated in real time by the TEG software:
      a. SP (split point) (or activation with an exogenous procoagulant) until the earliest detectable resistance. Depending on the nature of the activator, this roughly corresponds to the results of the standard PT/INR and PTT coagulation tests.

b. R (reaction time). The time from sample placement or activation until the tracing amplitude reaches 2 mm, corresponding to the initiation phase of clotting. Both SP- and R-times are prolonged in the presence of clotting factor deficiencies, anticoagulants, and hypofibrinogenemia, and may be shortened in hypercoagulable states.

c. K (clot formation time). Time elapsed between the R-time and the point where the tracing amplitude reaches 20 mm, a measure of the amount of time required for a standardized degree of viscoelasticity to be reached once clotting is initiated; this corresponds to the potentiation phase of clot formation during which thrombin begins to cleave soluble fibrinogen. The K-time is prolonged by depletion of clotting factors, fibrinogen, or platelets.

d. Alpha (angle). The angle formed by a line tangent from the R-time to the 20 mm amplitude reached at the K-time, corresponding to a standardized slope of fibrin polymerization and clot strengthening. Reduced alpha angles are seen in clotting factor depletion, hypofibrinogenemia, thrombocytopenia, or platelet dysfunction.

e. Maximal amplitude (MA). The maximal amplitude reached after clot initiation. This corresponds to the maximal clot strength via GP IIb/IIIa–mediated platelet–fibrin interactions. The MA is reduced in the setting of hypofibrinogenemia, thrombocytopenia, or platelet dysfunction.

f. G. A calculated measure of total clot strength based on amplitude. It has been suggested that the G value is a more reliable measure of overall clot strength than MA alone.

V. TRANSFUSION MANAGEMENT IN TRAUMA PATIENTS

The resuscitation of severely injured trauma patients requires specific knowledge about the products available for transfusion and treatment. Each product has its own unique properties and associated limitations. In addition to the blood component therapy that is available for transfusion, there are procoagulant factors that can also be utilized in patients with severe coagulopathy as result of trauma.

A. Packed red blood cells (pRBCs). A typical pRBC unit has a volume of 225 to 350 mL, a hematocrit of 65% to 80% and should raise the hemoglobin by 1 g/dL after transfusion

1. Collection. Units are collected from donors as either allogeneic or autologous units. Autologous units may not be screened if units are drawn and transfused at the same facility.

2. Screening. All allogeneic units are screened for infectious diseases and then grouped according to surface antigen (ABO and Rh) factors. The transfusion of pRBCs in trauma patients should be done as quickly as possible; it could take 15 minutes to get type-specific blood to the patient, so it may not be ready for the patient in early need. Therefore, initial transfusions consist of uncrossmatched type O blood. Women of child-bearing ages should receive type O, Rh-blood, although the exact rate of sensitizing to the Rh antigen when Rh+ uncrossmatched blood used is not known. All others should receive O+ blood if needed before type-specific or crossmatched is available.

3. The amount of type O blood available is limited, so once a blood type is known, type-specific blood should be used.

4. Patients who require further blood transfusions after their emergency type O transfusions should receive crossmatched blood. There is no current data regarding the limit of type O blood that can be transfused before switching to type-specific, but it is suggested that after 8 to 10 units of type O blood, type O should be continued until a re-crossmatch can be obtained.

5. Leukocyte reduction. During unfiltered separation from whole blood, some leukocytes will remain with the unit of pRBCs. These leukocytes are often cited as causal agents in a number of complications associated with transfusions, including nonhemolytic transfusion reactions, immune suppression, and increased post-operative infection. Although slightly more costly, the advantages of leukoreduction are such that most of the blood used in the United States is leuko-reduced.

B. Plasma. Plasma is the fluid component of whole blood once the cellular components have been removed, then frozen immediately after separation and then thawed directly before transfusion, i.e., FFP. Each unit must be ABO compatible, and on average, contains 200 to 250 mL of plasma, but apheris derived units may contain 400 to 600 mL. Plasma contains approximately 250 mg/dL of fibrinogen, as well as all the coagulation factors, including the labile factors V and VIII. In addition to fibrinogen and clotting factors, FFP also contains albumin, fibrinolytic proteins, immunoglobulins, and other proteins.

  1. FFP can be transfused up to 5 days after thawing, and the levels of most elements of FFP will remain stable except for the labile factors which can decrease by as much as 40% after 5 days. Factor VIII is the most significantly affected, with Factors V, VII, X decreased to a lesser degree.

C. Cryoprecipitate. Cryoprecipitate is a protein solution derived from FFP through centrifugation that contains virtually the same total amount of fibrinogen, von Willebrand factor, and factors VIII and XIII as a unit of FFP, but in a much smaller volume (~15 mL). Each unit of cryoprecipitate can be expected to raise the fibrinogen level by about 5 mg/dL. Although there is no clearly defined level at which fibrinogen should be replaced, most transfusion guidelines call for the administration of fibrinogen for levels less than 100 mg/dL. However, recent data suggests that fibrinogen levels decrease early in trauma and that higher fibrinogen levels of as much as 150 to 200 mg/dL may still be associated with increased perioperative bleeding.

D. Platelets. Most platelet units used currently are derived from a single donor through platelet apheresis. This replaces the older method of using a pooled donor platelet "6-packs," and reduces risk due to exposure to multiple donors. One unit of platelets under the pooled method contains about 5.5×10^{10} platelets suspended in 40 to 70 mL of plasma. A unit of apheresis platelets contains $\geq 3 \times 10^{11}$ platelets and is the therapeutic equivalent of to a "6-pack" of pooled platelets. The platelets are taken from the plasma component and stored at room temperature with a shelf life of 5 to 7 days. Each single-donor apheresis unit or pooled 4- to 8-donor "6-pack" can be expected to increase the platelet count by 30,000 to 50,000/μL. Admission platelet counts are inversely correlated with 24-hour survival. Although the platelet count does not give any information regarding the platelet activity, platelet counts less than 100,000/μL are often insufficient in the setting of massive transfusion and ongoing hemorrhage.

E. Procoagulant agents. In addition to repletion of coagulation factors by transfusion, several pharmaceutical hemostatic agents are available for the treatment of severe coagulopathy in the injured patient.

  1. **Recombinant factor VIIa.** Recombinant factor VIIa (rFVIIa) is a serine protease that augments hemostasis through the activation of factor X and inducing a thrombin burst on activated platelets. It was developed and approved for the treatment of hemophilia and congenital factor deficiencies, and subsequently used to reverse the effects of anticoagulants (Coumadin). While once a promising agent in the management of refractory coagulopathy in the setting of massive transfusion, recent data suggest that while the use of rFVIIa reduces blood product consumption, it does not appear to have a clear survival benefit in the trauma population.

  2. **Prothrombin complex concentrate.** Prothrombin complex concentrate (PCC) is a factor concentrate enriched for factors II, VII, IX, and X originally developed for hemorrhagic complications of hemophilia B. While not yet widely available in the US, PCC can rapid reverse warfarin-induced coagulopathy, particularly in brain-injured patients. It is easier to use and less volume than FFP, and PCC will likely become the agent of choice for warfarin reversal in a variety of settings. The utility of PCC in the treatment of other trauma-induced coagulopathy is unknown.

  3. **Antifibrinolytic therapy.** Recent data from clinical studies suggest that *tranexamic acid (TXA)*, an antifibrinolytic that binds the lysine binding pocket of plasminogen, reduces the incidence of all-cause and hemorrhage-related mortality in trauma patients. The low-risk profile of TXA coupled with recent data of an

increased survival benefit in trauma patients suggests that incorporating early administration of TXA into civilian massive transfusion protocols (MTP) may be of benefit.

  a. Aminocaproic acid, a similar lysine-based plasminogen binding inhibitor, reduces perioperative blood loss during elective surgery, but has not been evaluated in the trauma population.

4. Desmopressin. Desmopressin, a synthetic form of vasopressin, was developed for the treatment of inherited bleeding diatheses and to counteract uremic bleeding. Desmopressin acts by inducing endothelial cell release of von Willebrand factor multimers triggering stabilization of plasma factor VIII and leading to enhanced hemostasis. It is used commonly to reverse the anti-platelet effect of aspirin and renal failure. DDAVP has no defined role in trauma-induced coagulopathy.

VI. INDICATIONS FOR TRANSFUSION. Patients who are otherwise hemodynamically normal should not receive blood transfusions for hemoglobins >7 g/dL as they had increased morbidity and mortality, leading to a more conservative approach to transfusions.

In trauma patients with active coronary ischemia, transfusion at hemoglobin levels of <10 g/dL is useful. *Those patients with active large-volume bleeding or any signs of hemorrhagic shock should be transfused irrespective of the hemoglobin level.*

The use of recombinant erythropoietin (EPO) has been touted as a possible solution to decrease the number of blood units transfused in critically ill patients. In a large, randomized study in critically ill patients admitted to the ICU for greater than 48 hours, trauma patients who received EPO had a decreased mortality despite no difference in blood transfusion rates.

VII. HEMODYNAMIC RESPONSE

Patients with severe hypotension (BP <70 to 80 mm Hg) *attributable to hemorrhage* should receive blood immediately. Those with higher systolic blood pressures may be given a fluid challenge to determine their response. Those who respond only transiently before becoming hypotensive and those who do not respond at *all* should receive blood. Those who do respond to the fluid challenge and those who arrive with normal blood pressure do not need blood initially.

VIII. LABORATORY INDICATORS

  A. Base deficit/lactate. Base deficit and lactate both correspond to decreased systemic perfusion. An elevated BD <−6 mmol/L, lactate level >6 mmol/L on hospital admission, and increasing time to normal lactate level <2 mmol/L until ICU admission, are risk factors for early mortality and trigger considering transfusion.

  B. Hematocrit. A single, early normal initial hematocrit cannot refute large hemorrhage. Serial hematocrits may reflect ongoing slow bleeding, but may remain normal with significant hemorrhage.

IX. MASSIVE TRANSFUSION PROTOCOLS (MTP) AND HEMOSTATIC RESUSCITATION. The most commonly used definition for massive transfusion is that requiring ≥10 units pRBCs/24 hours. However, there is an even more critically injured subset of patients for who even a brief interruption in the supply of blood and blood products may mean the difference between life and death. Patients in this category typically require more than 20 to 30 units of pRBCs and a corresponding amount of FFP/platelets in the first 6 to 8 hours.

  A. The coordination required in the procurement and administration of large volumes of blood and blood products in the setting of critical injury requires an MTP and team.

  B. These protocols provide guidance to blood bank and treating physicians, improving survival and coagulopathy. MTP continue to evolve and typically contain the following elements:

Sample MTP:

1. Indications for MTP activation
   a. Transfusion of 3 or greater uncrossmatched blood units in the ED/Trauma Bay with anticipated ongoing transfusion needs
   b. Severely injured patient with elevated base deficit (> -6), hypotensive, tachycardic, with no clinical response to fluid or 2 units of blood
   c. Experienced clinician judgment of severe injury with likelihood of significant resuscitation needs.
2. Personnel authorized to activate MTP
   a. Trauma attending
   b. Emergency medicine attending
   c. Anesthesia attending
   d. Other physicians and senior residents of trauma services in coordination with trauma, emergency medicine, or anesthesia
3. Blood bank response to MTP activation
   a. Immediate release of uncrossmatched type O blood (4 units) to the Trauma Bay
   b. Patient blood sample drawn and sent for type and crossmatch to be used for future blood product units
4. Blood bank begins release of MTP packs containing type-specific units of :
   a. 4 units of pRBCs
   b. 4 units of FFP
   c. 1 unit of platelet (apheresis unit) = 6 pack of platelets
5. MTP pack released every 20 minutes until stopped by treatment team
6. Laboratory draws and ABGs during resuscitation (see MTP targets below)
   a. Done every 30 minutes or at discretion of MTP leader
7. Fibrinogen and/or cryoprecipitate released after 2 MTP packs on the basis of laboratory values
   a. Consider ordering Factor VII at this time if pH >7.2, platelets $>50,000$, fibrinogen >100, and no other contraindications—see Procoagulant agents
8. MTP strategy (e.g., 1:1:1)
   a. The goal is to aim for a 1:1:1 transfusion ratio. One unit of platelet pheresis is roughly equivalent to the number of platelets that would be seen in the same volume of 6 units of blood and FFP. Therefore, 1 platelet pheresis is transfused after 6 units of blood and FFP, making a 1 (blood):1 (FFP):1 (platelet) ratio that most mimics whole blood.
9. MTP monitoring and target values. These include:
   a. CBC, PT/PTT, fibrinogen, ABGs, calcium, metabolic panel
   b. There are no exact criteria which dictate how much blood product should be given for each value, but suggested responses include:
      i. INR >1.4--Give 4 units of FFP
      ii. Platelets $<100,000$--Give 1 apheresis platelets
      iii. Fibrinogen <100 mg/dL—Give 1 unit FFP or cryoprecipitate
   c. The goal of these transfusions typically proceed with a goal of achieving the following MTP targets
      i. Hemoglobin >8 g/dL
      ii. INR <2
      iii. Platelets $>100,000$
      iv. Fibrinogen >100 mg/dL
10. Protocolized transfusion triggers for patients with dilutional coagulopathy or ATC, based upon TEG clotting time, clot formation time, amplitude, and clot lysis index have been suggested for standard and rotational thromboelastography based on single center experience, but have yet to be prospectively validated. Johansson et al. used the following algorithm for transfusion based on TEG analysis (Table 7-1)
11. Indications for termination of MTP
    a. Normalized laboratory values AND/OR no evidence of ongoing bleeding

TABLE 7-1	Proposed Transfusion Algorithm Based on TEG Analysis

TEG parameter	Treatment
R = 11–14 min	2 × FFP or 10 mL/kg
R >14 min	4 × FFP or 20 mL/kg
MA = 46–50 mm	1 platelet concentrate
MA <46 mm	2 platelet concentrate
Angle <52	2 × FFP or fibrinogen
Ly30 > 8%	Antifibrinolytics

Current data suggest that a resuscitation protocol involving high ratios of FFP:RBCs:PLT given early and aggressively while limiting crystalloid improves outcome. This concept has taken hold and largely displaced the previous practice of administering high volumes of crystalloid followed by pRBCs, usually with minimum plasma and platelets.

Current studies suffer from the problem of survival bias—those patients who receive 1:1:1 may survive not because of the actual plasma and platelets, but because they were bleeding less rapidly and survived to receive the plasma and platelets in the prescribed ratios. Many clinicians believe that the benefits of 1:1:1 are real, but that the 'target' population for these high ratios has not been well defined as yet. Because of these concerns, patients **without** the need for massive transfusion are treated in response to specific laboratory deficits.

X. RISKS AND COMPLICATIONS

While necessary to maintain intravascular volume, oxygen carrying capacity and normal coagulation, blood transfusions carry specific risks (discussed below), and have been found in some reports to correlate with increased mortality or multiple organ failure.

A. Metabolic changes in older stored blood. pRBC units can be stored at 4°C for 21 to 42 days, depending on the storage media used. The average age of a transfused pRBC unit is 13 to 37 days depending on the ABO/Rh group and storage media, with older red cell units frequently allocated to high use facilities such as trauma centers. Older banked RBCs may develop what is referred to as a "storage lesion," which is a combination of metabolic and structural changes of the RBC. The morphologic changes can be seen in the cells' shape change, membrane loss of carbohydrates, and changes in membrane lipids that lead to increased cell removal from circulation.

During storage, multiple changes to the unit can occur, including:

1. Potassium concentration. Increase in storage duration leads to an increase in potassium concentrations within the unit.

2. Acidosis. A decreases in pH of the unit can result in acidosis when large volumes of pRBCs are transfused.

3. Oxygen carrying capacity . Decreased levels of 2,3 DPG shift the oxygen dissociation curve to the left, increasing oxygen affinity and decrease oxygen offloading.

4. Pro-inflammatory changes. The physiologic consequence of increased storage time of pRBCs and their clinical significance is debated, but may have deleterious effects including increased incidence of multiorgan failure (MOF) and mortality. The full mechanism causing the increase in MOF and mortality is yet to be elucidated, but several mechanisms including increased levels of cytokines and retained leukocytes have been identified as potential culprits.

B. Infectious disease risks. Each unit of stored blood is screened for possible transmissible diseases. Despite this screening, there is still a chance for a contaminated unit to be transfused into a patient. Although this risk is very small, each patient should be advised of this risk if possible. Emergent transfusions to save the patient's life are an exception.

Estimated risk of transfusion per unit transfused:
1. Human immunodeficiency virus (HIV)—1:2,000,000
2. Hepatitis B—1:205,000
3. Hepatitis C—1:2,000,000

C. **Non-hemolytic transfusion reactions.** Most units of stored RBCs contain leukocytes that were not removed during component separation. A nonhemolytic febrile transfusion reaction is the result of cytokine release from these remaining leukocytes upon activation in the transfusion recipient. This leads to clinical symptoms of fever, chills, or rigors that usually require only supportive treatment.

D. **Hemolytic transfusion reaction.** Hemolytic transfusion reactions can be characterized by immune and non-immune hemolytic reactions.

1. **Non-immune.** When stored RBCs are damaged prior to transfusion, a resulting hemoglobinemia and hemoglobinuria can occur from the immediate destruction of the red cells after transfusion. This non-immune hemolytic transfusion reaction usually has no significant clinical symptoms.

2. **Immune.** An acute hemolytic transfusion reaction is usually the result of transfusing ABO incompatible blood. Antigens on the transfused RBC interact with recipient antibodies resulting in red cell hemolysis. The antibodies involved include immunoglobulin M (IgM) anti-A, anti-B, or anti-A, B. The result of the activation of these antibodies can result in severe, potentially fatal complement-mediated intravascular hemolysis, hemoglobinemia, hemoglobinuria, disseminated intravascular coagulation (DIC), renal failure, and complement-mediated cardiovascular collapse. The incidence of these transfusion reactions and alloimmunization is lower in trauma patients receiving blood than non-trauma patients. This is thought to be related to the immunosuppression associated with hemorrhagic shock.

3. Treatment and work-up of either immune or non-immune hemolytic anemia may include:
   a. Stop the transfusion immediately
   b. Saline as needed to keep urine output at 0.5 mL/kg
   c. Notify the transfusion service
   d. Rule out clerical error by rechecking the unit, transfusion tag and patient identification.
   e. Send new blood samples for lab tests including:
      i. Direct antiglobulin test (DAT) on posttransfusion sample
      ii. CBC
      iii. Bilirubin
   f. Defer future transfusions until workup complete

E. **TRALI—Transfusion related acute lung injury** is a potentially lethal transfusion event that causes hypoxemia and non-cardiogenic pulmonary edema within 6 hours of transfusion. The incidence of TRALI is higher in those patients who have received plasma or platelet transfusions rather than pRBCs. The pathophysiology of TRALI is varied, with both antibody-mediated and antibody independent pathways. Common to both pathways is a susceptible recipient—a patient who has activated granulocytes or pulmonary endothelium. The end result of TRALI is pulmonary edema and alveolar damage. The National Heart, Lung, and Blood Institute (NHLBI) TRALI definition is (1) ALI that occurs within 6 hours of transfusion, (2) no ALI prior to transfusion, and (3) no temporal relationship to an alternative risk factor for ALI.

F. The increased units of FFP utilized in current resuscitations pose some risk for the development of TRALI. TRALI risk reduction strategies (including male-predominant plasma, plasma from parous or transfused females tested for HLA antibodies, and nulliparous females) reduce the incidence of TRALI. Currently, there is little data regarding the true incidence of TRALI in trauma patients.

G. Transfusion associated circulatory overload (TACO). TACO is a condition that is thought to occur as a result of an increase in central venous pressure and pulmonary blood volume immediately following a transfusion. This increase in hydrostatic pressure leads to fluid extravasation into the alveolar space. This condition may be difficult to distinguish between other transfusion reactions, especially TRALI. Patients with TACO typically exhibit many similar characteristics including respiratory distress and interstitial infiltrates on chest x-ray as well as orthopnea, cyanosis, and tachycardia. The distinguishing features that may set TACO apart from other reactions include hypertension, rales, and jugular venous distension, but not all patients with TACO will have these abnormalities.

1. The incidence of TACO is highest on the extremes of age (<3 and >60 years old) and those with underlying cardiac dysfunction. It is estimated to occur in approximately 0.03% to 8% of blood transfusions, but may be as high as 23%. There is no well defined treatment therapy, so it is largely supportive with continued respiratory support, discontinuation of transfusions, and consideration of the use of diuretics. As in TRALI, the ability to accurately diagnose TACO in acute trauma patients as a sole pathologic entity is extremely difficult and there is little data regarding its relevance or incidence in the trauma population.

H. Hypercoagulable risks. Procoagulant agents that augment or accelerate coagulation may increase the risks of post-injury thrombo-embolic events (VTEs). Early concerns surrounding the use of rFVIIa were triggered by observations of otherwise unexpected VTEs in previously healthy combat soldiers. The use of PCC initially noted an increased thrombotic risk with in older studies, but more recent studies using a reformulated product suggest minimal additional thrombotic risk associated with the use of these agents.

1. The use of TXA was not associated with an increase risk of in the rate of VTE when compared to placebo.

2. While these aggregate data suggest that the additional risk of VTE is not enhanced through the use of procoagulants, the risk profile of trauma patients for VTE is high, with recent evidence pointing to the development of a more general hypercoagulable state following major trauma. Prophylaxis and monitoring for VTE remain essential elements in post-resuscitation care.

AXIOMS

- Send blood for type and screen or crossmatch *early* in patients with evidence of blood loss.
- In actively bleeding patients with any findings of shock, give blood (type O if needed) early and begin preparing for massive transfusion in case needed.
- Seek balance in transfusions of pRBC, platelets, and plasma when large volumes are needed, using clotting studies to aid tailoring.
- Avoid the combination of crystalloid dilution, acidosis, and hypothermia in the bleeding trauma patient.
- Reverse warfarin coagulation early with plasma or PCC if any head bleed or ongoing other site losses exist.

Suggested Readings

Arinsburg SA, Skerrett DL, Karp JK, et al. Conversion to low transfusion-related acute lung injury (TRALI)-risk plasma significantly reduces TRALI. *Transfusion* 2012;52(5):946–952.

Brown LM, Call MS, Margaret Knudson M, et al. A normal platelet count may not be enough: the impact of admission platelet count on mortality and transfusion in severely injured trauma patients. *J Trauma* 2011;71:S337–S342.

Dente CJ, Shaz BH, Nicholas JM, et al. Improvements in early mortality and coagulopathy are sustained better in patients with blunt trauma after institution of a massive transfusion protocol in a civilian level I trauma center. *J Trauma* 2009;66:1616–1624.

Differding JA, Underwood SJ, Van PY, et al. Trauma induces a hypercoagulable state that is resistant to hypothermia as measured by thrombelastogram. *Am J Surg* 2011;201:587–591.

Dutton RP, Shih D, Edelman BB, et al. Safety of uncrossmatched type-O red cells for resuscitation from hemorrhagic shock. *J Trauma* 2005;59:1445–1449.

Hebert PC, Wells G, Blajchman MA, et al. A multicenter, randomized, controlled clinical trial of transfusion requirements in critical care. Transfusion Requirements in Critical Care Investigators, Canadian Critical Care Trials Group. *N Engl J Med* 1999;340:409–417.

Hess JR, Brohi K, Dutton RP, et al. The coagulopathy of trauma: a review of mechanisms. *J Trauma* 2008;65:748–754.

Johansson PI, Stensballe J. Hemostatic resuscitation for massive bleeding: the paradigm of plasma and platelets – a review of the current literature. *Transfusion* 2010;50:701–710.

Levi M, Levy JH, Andersen HF, et al. Safety of recombinant activated factor VII in randomized clinical trials. *N Engl J Med* 2010;363:1791–1800.

Lier H, Krep H, Schroeder S, et al. Preconditions of hemostasis in trauma: a review. The influence of acidosis, hypocalcemia, anemia, and hypothermia on functional hemostasis in trauma. *J Trauma* 2008;65:951–960.

Shakur H, Roberts I, Bautista R, et al. Effects of tranexamic acid on death, vascular occlusive events, and blood transfusion in trauma patients with significant haemorrhage (CRASH-2): a randomised, placebo-controlled trial. *Lancet* 2010;376:23–32.

Zink KA, Sambasivan CN, Holcomb JB, et al. A high ratio of plasma and platelets to packed red blood cells in the first 6 hours of massive transfusion improves outcomes in a large multicenter study. *Am J Surg* 2009;197:565–570; discussion 570.

8

Nutritional Intervention

Jodie A. Bryk and Juan B. Ochoa

I. **INTRODUCTION.** Nutrition intervention (NI) is integral to the care of the surgical patient and is comparable to any other form of medical intervention. The biologic beneficial effects of NI are translated into better outcomes including decreased infection, improved healing of surgical and traumatic wounds, while decreasing cost and minimizing waste of health care resources. Similar to any therapy, NI has contraindications, risks and side effects, which need to be carefully prevented or promptly identified and managed. Knowledge of NI is progressing at a rapid pace and requires the surgeon maintain continuing education in this area.

A. Progress in both basic sciences and process-improvement applications are significant and have clarified the therapeutic role of NI, the metabolic effects of specific nutrients as well as the timing, route, and volume that NI should be delivered. **Nutrition intervention in trauma and major abdominal surgery provides unique challenges.**

The traditional goal of NI has focused on minimizing nitrogen loss and achieving a positive nitrogen balance (Fig. 8-1). In the past few years, investigators have moved beyond these goals realizing that:

1. Positive nitrogen balance can only be achieved through a better understanding and regulation of the immune response to injury or critical illness. Catabolism seen in trauma, sepsis, and stress cannot be curtailed by exceeding caloric requirements.

2. Higher than normal amounts of protein are necessary after injury. This may require modular additions of protein to existing enteral nutrition formulas (Table 8-1).

3. Enteral nutrition (EN) is clearly the preferred route of NI with limited roles for the use of TPN. EN provides benefits that are distinct from that of meeting caloric goals including preservation of gastrointestinal integrity and function and preservation of immunity. Starting EN early (as soon as the patient achieves hemodynamic stability) improves outcomes including gastrointestinal tolerance and may reduce mortality.

4. Prolonged starvation (particularly during the first week) builds a "caloric deficit" and may be detrimental. Total parenteral nutrition (TPN) supplementing EN is being tested as a means to overcome the caloric deficit and improve outcomes; the results of these trials are eagerly awaited. Attempts at minimizing starvation are essential for good outcomes.

5. The requirements of macro- and micronutrients such as certain amino acids, lipids, and vitamins are different in trauma and burn patients when compared to normal human beings or even to other critically ill patients including patients with sepsis.

6. The immune system plays an active role in the regulation of the availability of certain nutrients through active destruction or sequestration.

II. **METABOLIC DEMANDS OF TRAUMA AND BURNS.** The trauma patient exhibits significant metabolic changes that profoundly affect the adaptive response to starvation. Trauma patients become catabolic; the degree of catabolism is proportional to the degree of injury. Burn patients exhibit the highest degree of metabolic alterations among injured patients. Changes in burn and trauma may be unique; because of this, the principles that guide NI in other diseases may be unsuitable for the trauma patient.

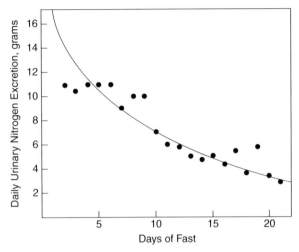

Figure 8-1. Daily urinary nitrogen excretion during prolonged fast. (From Freund E, Freund O. Beitrage zum Stoffwechsel im Hungerzustand. *Med Klin* 1901;15:69.)

A. **Increased protein breakdown.** Protein loss is augmented due to increased catabolism and loss through wounds following injury. Loss of protein can be high: Up to 15% of the lean body mass can be lost in 10 days. Severe protein malnutrition occurs when 25% to 30% of the lean body weight is lost. Thus, protein depletion (not calorie depletion) can become a life-threatening condition in severe trauma. The high catabolic rate is resistant to the provision of calories. However, protein synthetic rate does increase with amino acid infusions. Traditionally, traumatized patients should be offered 1.5 to 2 g/kg/day of protein.

TABLE 8-1	Examples of Different Types of Enteral Nutrition Formulas. Nutrient (Expressed as % calories) From Two Different Companies in the United States			
Name	**Protein**	**CHO**	**Lipid**	**Comments**
Compleat®	18%	48%	34%	Formulated from intact food
Jevity 1 Cal®	17%	54%	29%	Standard polymeric diet with fiber
Isosource HN®	18%	53%	29%	Standard polymeric formula
Nutren® Replete®	25%	45%	30%	High-protein complete formula
Promote®	25%	52%	23%	High-protein complete formula
Peptamen 1®	16%	51%	33%	Hydrolyzed whey protein formula
Bariatric®	37%	31%	33%	For acutely ill obese patient
Vital 1.0®	16%	51%	33%	Peptide-based elemental formula
Impact®	22%	53%	25%	Immune formula
Pivot 1.5 Cal®	25%	45%	30%	Immune formula

Note: The trade name formulas in the table are available as a "family" of products with different characteristics including higher protein or caloric concentrations and the presence of fiber. This allows finding a formula that meets the special needs of the patient. Please refer to the following websites for additional information on these products.
http://abbottnutrition.com/our-products/brands.aspx
http://www.nestle-nutrition.com/Products/Default.aspx

TABLE 8-2	Formulas to Calculate Energy Expenditure

Harris–Benedict equation

EEE (males) $= 66 + 13.7$(wt in kg) $+ 5$(ht in cm) $- 6.8$(age in y)

EEE (females) $= 665 + 9.6$(wt in kg) $+ 1.8$(ht in cm) $- 4.7$(age in y)

Where EEE is estimated energy expenditure, wt is weight, and ht is height.

B. **Hyperglycemia and resistance to insulin.** Hyperglycemia is an independent predictor of poor prognosis with increased risk of infection, multiple organ dysfunction, and death. Hyperglycemia may be present in patients with no evidence of pre-existing diabetes. Hyperglycemia is due to complex factors related to stress. It is attributable primarily to excess hepatic gluconeogenesis due to the liver's increased avidity for gluconeogenic substrates (i.e., lactate, pyruvate, and alanine). Hyperglycemia is also attributable to decreased glucose storage, increased circulating steroids, increased catecholamines, and increased glucagon.
   1. Insulin release is suppressed within a few hours after trauma and restored in the later phase. However, hyperglycemia persists since insulin resistance is also characteristic of severe trauma.
   2. Severe hyperglycemia is associated with decreased neutrophil chemotaxis, phagocytosis, oxidative burst, and superoxide production. Hyperglycemia can be worsened by inappropriate provision of glucose, a situation that can more easily occur with the provision of TPN or an attempt to deliver caloric goals beyond those needed by the patient.
C. **Lipid mobilization.** Mobilization of lipid stores (lipolysis) occurs after trauma. This is a result of the activation of triglyceride lipases by elevation in the levels of catecholamines, thyroid hormones, cortisol, adrenocorticotropic hormone (ACTH), glucagon, and growth hormones. Lipids remain the main energy source during recovery from trauma.
D. Resting energy expenditure (Table 8-2) is increased after trauma and is proportional to the degree of severity of injury. Observations of increased metabolic rates led to the misconception that provision of nutrients should be increased to meet metabolic demands (beyond that of 25 kcal/kg/day) and were traditionally known as "stress factors." There is however, no evidence that increasing provision of nutrients beyond that of basic metabolic demands improves outcome, and indeed may worsen outcomes.
E. **Vitamin deficiencies.** There are no specific guidelines for the replacement of deficient vitamins beyond those advocated for normal individuals.
F. **Immune-mediated amino acid destruction.** Recent observations demonstrate that immune activation during trauma induces the release of arginase 1 contained in neutrophils and the accumulation of myeloid cells expressing this same enzyme occurs within hours of injury in immune tissues such as the spleen. Arginase 1 actively metabolizes arginine to ornithine and urea and can deplete this amino acid locally and systemically. Arginase 1 can also be released from injured hepatocytes and erythrocytes and is significantly abundant in packed red blood cells. Arginine is an essential amino acid for normal T lymphocyte function and nitric oxide production. Arginine depletion is now known to be associated with T lymphocyte dysfunction and decreased nitric oxide production in disease states associated with elevated arginase and may be a relevant problem in trauma.

III. **PUTTING IT ALL TOGETHER.** Nutrition intervention is best done using published guidelines. Clinical management guidelines linked to performance-improvement processes are useful to prevent errors, initiate nutrition interventions, and guide safe therapy. Periodic updates of all protocols should be performed. Utilizing specialized nutrition teams and a registered dietitian skilled in NI are recommended.

Specific NI includes the following categories:
1. Oral intake at will
2. Controlled starvation
3. Enteral nutrition
4. Parenteral nutrition
5. Oral nutrition supplements

Inevitably, NI will fall into one or more of these categories. The option chosen will depend on a careful evaluation of the benefits and risks of a given choice, as well as a comparison with alternative interventional options. The physician should consider the following factors in determining how to make this decision.

A. **Oral intake at will.** Most adult human beings are able to maintain adequate nutrition intake, constantly meeting demands of water, electrolytes, vitamins, micro and macronutrients through volitional intake, and physiologic cues of thirst and hunger. Oral intake is the simplest and most natural way to provide adequate nutrition.

Trauma and critical illness dramatically interfere with the capacity of the patient to maintain normal oral intake. Critically ill and injured patients with altered mental status may be at risk of vomiting and aspiration, have poor splanchnic perfusion or recent GI surgery putting them at risk for complications if allowed oral intake. In addition, disease frequently causes a significant degree of anorexia. Furthermore, access to food may be limited in the hospital. These problems obligate the surgeon to intervene. Careful evaluation of the nutritional history on arrival of the patient, followed by adequate monitoring of caloric/protein intake and a well-constructed plan of NI, is essential.

Oral intake at will should be allowed if possible and daily assessment of intake is desirable. Incorporating the patient and family into discussions of NI is often feasible and may be beneficial for the psychological well-being of the patient; empowering the patient to maintain some degree of control of his/her own care may bring significant benefits.

B. **Controlled starvation.** The decision to prevent oral intake occurs frequently in hospitalized patients. Virtually any member of the health care team can stop or prevent a patient from obtaining adequate oral intake. Orders for "NPO" or "clear fluids" are frequently inappropriate or unnecessary and may be detrimental for patient care.

Short-term "starvation" in the hospital is allowable on otherwise healthy human beings as it can be tolerated for short periods with no apparent ill effects. During starvation, complex biologic mechanisms are induced that allow protection and sparing of resources and stores. For example, increased utilization of lipid occurs when glycogen stores are depleted, protein turnover is significantly decreased, and energy expenditure is significantly reduced. As a result of these metabolic adaptive changes, healthy individuals can maintain normal organ function for weeks or even months at a time. Eventually, these protective mechanisms fail if starvation is prolonged and malnutrition with organ dysfunction occurs.

In critical illness, protective mechanisms observed during starvation become ineffective and malnutrition occurs faster. Increased gut permeability and dysmotility in the traumatized patient can occur with starvation beyond 24 hours. Caloric and protein deficits build rapidly increasing morbidity and mortality. Every effort should be made to minimize starvation in the trauma patient.

C. **Enteral nutrition (EN).** Most trauma patients are able to tolerate oral or enteral intake within the first 24 hours following the injury. **The most important limiting factor for early EN is the presence of shock and poor gut perfusion.** Early EN is associated with easier tolerance to a diet and decreased infection rates. Enteral nutrition increases wound healing and decreases length of stay. Early enteral nutrition may decrease mortality and has become the standard of nutrition interventions in the critically ill and trauma patient.

1. Although it is clear that early EN is beneficial, the amount that needs to be delivered early is still debated. Proponents of early aggressive EN to meet caloric goals (increasing volume of delivery), suggest that mortality is proportional to the "caloric debt" accumulated early in the course of disease; opponents refute

these observations and suggest that the risks of aggressive EN outweighs the benefits. Yet others suggest starting early EN along with supplemental use of TPN. In view of this controversy, the guidelines published by the Society of Critical Care Medicine and the American Society of Parenteral and Enteral Nutrition (SCCM/ASPEN) compromise by stating that a reasonable goal is to provide 50% and 65% of caloric goals by the end of the first week in the intensive care unit.

2. Enteral nutrition does have complications, including those stemming from the placement of a feeding tube, gastrostomy, or jejunostomy. Diarrhea occurs in up to 30% of patients and enteral feeding may also lead to vomiting and aspiration.

A major, although rare complication of EN, is that of bowel necrosis, which is observed when aggressive volumes of EN are delivered, especially in the presence of poor bowel perfusion and shock. Careful evaluation of the risks and benefits of early EN, along with increased supervision of the patient are necessary in the hemodynamically unstable patient.

3. Tube placement and confirmation is important. The tip of the nasoenteral feeding tube can be left in the stomach or advanced into the duodenum or jejunum. Nasojejunal tube feeds appear better tolerated than nasogastric tube feeds and may be associated with less aspiration. In a recent report, up to 2% of the nasoenteral feeding tubes were misplaced within the tracheobronchial tree. Confirmation of a correct position within the stomach by using an abdominal x-ray or chest x-ray is highly recommended before usage. "Tube migration" into the small bowel from the stomach usually occurs quickly, can be enhanced with bedside fluoroscopic manipulation.

D. Total parenteral nutrition (TPN). The advent of TPN in 1968 allowed the provision of complete nutritional support delivered by a central venous catheter. TPN has undoubtedly saved innumerable patients from a certain death when the gastrointestinal tract is not available. TPN indications include:

1. Severely malnourished patient who cannot eat and will be undergoing elective surgery. In this patient population, TPN decreases complications.

2. Patients with short gut syndrome.

3. Patients where enteral nutrition has failed for at least 1 week.

TPN is not indicated when the gastrointestinal tract is functional or during short periods of starvation. Recent work performed by Casear and others, in over 4,000 patients, demonstrated that "supplemental TPN" in patients who were starved or in patients where enteral nutrition failed to meet caloric goals during the first week, showed that supplemental TPN was associated with poor outcomes including increased days on ventilator, increased incidence of infections, increased days on dialysis, and a trend toward decreased mortality. Blood sugars were also moderately elevated in the TPN group.

TPN requires close attention for ordering (composition, additives, rate) line placement, and monitoring. Nutrition teams should work with the primary surgical and critical care team in all cases and standardized guidelines for insertion site care and laboratory monitoring are available. In addition, this nutritional support team and pharmacists skilled in the use of parental nutrition should tailor the macro- and micronutrients delivered based on the patient's goals and needs. Careful monitoring for side effects, complications, and efficacy is required.

E. Oral nutrition supplements. There is a growing variety of nutritional supplements, which can be categorized into three basic categories:

1. Nutritionally complete oral nutritional supplements (ONS). These supplements are intended to provide all the nutrients necessary for an otherwise normal individual. Complete ONS can come with higher protein concentrations and are advocated for the trauma patient with significant wounds. Data suggests a possible beneficial effect including decreased infections with the use of high-protein ONS in patients undergoing surgery for hip fractures.

2. Fortified nutritional supplements. These supplements supply specific nutrients and are given for specific conditions in a patient who may otherwise have a normal dietary intake. These supplements are not to be used as the sole source of nutrition.

An example is improved wound healing with the use of supplemental arginine, vitamin C, or vitamin E in patients with chronic wounds.

3. Specialized ONS. These supplements are considered ONS and are designed to be used for patients with special needs. Examples of specialized ONS include those prescribed for patients with diabetes or chronic renal failure.

F. **Immunonutrition** refers to evidence that some nutrients may be essential for normal immune function. These immunonutrients include certain amino acids (arginine and glutamine), lipids (omega-3 fatty acids), and other components including nucleotides and vitamin C. Supraphysiologic quantities of some of these nutrients to enteral diets or ONS have been added and have been classified as immune-enhancing diets. Of these, the best tested diet contains arginine, omega-3 fatty acids, and nucleotides. Its use in the elective surgery patient is associated with clear benefit that includes a significant risk reduction in postoperative infection, a decrease in other surgical complications, decreased length of stay and cost. Trauma patients may also benefit from the combination of the nutrients described above; however, the number of trauma patients studied to date is limited.

IV. NUTRIENT REQUIREMENTS

A. **Meeting caloric goals.** Traditional nutrition support guidelines for caloric requirements minimize protein breakdown and loss of lean body mass. Multiple formulas have been designed to guide initiation and generally follow a recommendation that a critically ill patient should receive 20 to 25 kcal/kg/day.

1. As discussed above, the exact time to begin NI is variable and depends on the patient's overall condition, severity of injury, extent of burn, and co-morbid conditions.

2. Overfeeding is detrimental and should be avoided. Overfeeding increases length of stay on the ventilator and is associated with increased incidence of sepsis (Table 8-3). Overfeeding occurs in up to one-third of patients when caloric requirements are calculated with the use of conventional formulas (Harris–Benedict equation). Indirect calorimetry, although a more elaborate and expensive approach, allows more careful determination of energy requirements and may be necessary when no demonstrable results are seen with NI.

B. **Carbohydrate requirements.** Several types of carbohydrates are commercially available and are classified according to their complexity. Complexity (the size of the individual carbohydrate polymers) determines the need for digestion prior to absorption. The complexity of carbohydrates is measured in dextrose equivalent (DE) units. The DE of dextrose is 100 and is readily absorbed. In contrast, unaltered cornstarch has a DE value of 1. Intermediate values are given for maltodextrin, corn syrup, and modified cornstarch.

C. **Protein requirements.** The provision of proteins to trauma patients is essential and may minimize loss of lean body mass. Protein intake should be 1.5 to 2.0 g/kg/day or 20% to 30% of the total caloric nutrient intake. Higher *protein intakes have been advocated for the morbidly obese patient.*

1. Several types of protein are available commercially and are classified depending on their source. Sources of protein include casein, soy, and whey protein. To our knowledge, there are no data comparing the effect of the different type of protein on clinical outcome.

2. Predigested protein presentations in the form of simple peptides or individual amino acids are also available. Peptide-based or amino acid–based diets are used in the disease states where there may be impaired digestion and absorption and

TABLE 8-3	Ireton–Jones Equation: Sepsis

$EEE = -1000 + 100(V_E) + 1.3(Hb) + 300(sepsis)$
Where V_E is expired minute ventilation and sepsis is 1 for yes and 0 for no.

may facilitate tolerance to enteral nutrition. Increased plasma amino acid levels are observed in patients receiving predigested whey protein but the beneficial effects on clinical outcomes are unknown.

D. Lipid requirements. Lipids provide the most concentrated energy source of all macronutrients. Lipids are essential in the formation of cell membranes and provide the substrate for production of prostaglandins and leukotrienes.

  1. Traditionally, 30% of the calories delivered to a patient come from lipids. However, this percentage may vary significantly depending on the diet, ranging from 15% to 70% of the caloric goals.

  2. A diet free of lipids will result in fatty acid deficiency (linoleic and linolenic acid) within a few weeks. Thus, the minimum amount of fat provided in the diet should be approximately 2% to 4% of the caloric goals to prevent essential fatty acid deficiency.

  3. The amount and type of lipid provided in the diet may play distinct physiologic roles affecting specific organ function, a fact that is being explored in different specialized diets.

  a. Long-chain fatty acids such as those provided in corn oil (omega-6 fatty acids) are traditional sources of lipids provided in many diets for critically ill patients. Intravenous lipid presentations in the United States are exclusively omega-6 fatty acids.

  b. Omega-3 fatty acids are contained in fish oil and are provided in significant concentrations in specialized enteral diets. Omega-3 fatty acids affect the inflammatory milieu through several mechanisms including changes in the types of prostaglandins generated (PGE3 over PGE2), the production of resolvins and activation of PPAR (peroxisome-proliferator activated receptors) among others. Dietary intake of omega-3 fatty acids is low in the normal population, potentially negatively impacting health. Physiologic intake of omega-3 fatty acids is necessary (http://ods.od.nih.gov/factsheets/omega3fattyacidsandhealth/). The effect of supraphysiologic intake of omega-3 fatty acids in an effort to regulate inflammation in critical illness is less clear. Omega-3 fatty acids may have a significant role in preventing liver damage observed with chronic use of TPN.

  c. Medium-chain triglycerides (containing 14 carbons) are absorbed directly into the bloodstream and can be used as energy sources in the absence of carnitine, which becomes deficient during critical illness. Carnitine is required for transport of long-chain triglycerides into the mitochondria.

  d. Short-chain fatty acids provide a main energy source for the colonic mucosa. Short-chain fatty acids are produced of broken-down digestible fibers.

E. Micronutrients. Little is known of dietary supplementation of micronutrients (vitamins and minerals) in trauma and critical illness. Therefore, under most circumstances micronutrients are provided in quantities sufficient to meet recommended dietary allowance (RDA). It is known that levels of vitamin C drop significantly after trauma or hemorrhagic shock. Preliminary trials suggest that the administration of supraphysiologic quantities of vitamin C as part of the resuscitation protocol may have a significant effect on overall outcome. Definitive trials are pending. Supplemental zinc, selenium, and vitamin C are traditionally used in patients with large wounds and decubitus ulcers.

V. SPECIAL PATIENT POPULATIONS

A. Burn patients. Nutritional needs for burn patients are far different from those observed in other populations. Most severe burn patients are cared for in units where specialized nutritional support is available. Burn patients exhibit high metabolic rates, the need for provision of calories (in the form of carbohydrates) at significant rates, the need for provision of protein, and increased requirements for micronutrients such as zinc, vitamin C, and selenium. (See Table 8-4 and Chapter 33.)

B. Obese patients. An increase in the number of obese patients has been observed in the last 10 years. Obese patients have specific requirements for their care. Obese patients may exhibit occult but significant nutritional deficiencies. Accumulating evidence suggests that obese patients may benefit from the use of hypocaloric and

TABLE 8-4	Ireton–Jones Equation for Ventilated Patients: Burn Patients

EEE = 1925 − 10(age in y) + 5(wt in kg) + 281(sex) + 292(trauma) + 851(burn)
Where sex is 0 for females and 1 for males, trauma is 1 for yes and 0 for no, and burn is 1 for yes and 0 for no.

high-protein diets. Higher protein intake helps achieve positive nitrogen balance even in the presence of lower amounts of calories.

C. Elderly patients. Elderly patients have increased metabolic problems providing significant challenges in nutritional intervention. They may be malnourished prior to injury, and may also have chronic underlying diseases such as renal insufficiency or diabetes. Hyperglycemia after trauma is common in these patients. (See Table 8-5.)

VI. CLINICAL GUIDELINES. The Eastern Association for the Surgery of Trauma (EAST) has created guidelines to assist clinicians in the formulation of NI in trauma. More recently, SCCM and ASPEN have provided updated guidelines for the critically ill patient including trauma patients.

Consider the following:

A. All patients need nutrition. Starvation should be minimized. Orders to keep the patient NPO should be discussed daily. Equally the use of orders for "clear fluids" should be avoided. Oral intake and a regular diet should be encouraged whenever possible.

B. Nutrition intervention is indicated in patients who cannot eat for reasons stated above.

C. TPN should only be started in patients who have clearly failed to tolerate enteral nutrition generally after 7 days of admission. Specialized nutrition teams should be consulted to help in the prescription and monitoring of TPN.

TABLE 8-5	Guidelines for SGA Ranking

Well nourished
No physical signs of muscle wasting
No or minimal subcutaneous fat loss
Dietary intake adequate or marginally inadequate for <2 wks

Mild malnutrition
Mild muscle wasting
Mild subcutaneous fat loss
Inadequate dietary intake of 2–3 wks
Functional capacity: Working suboptimally

Moderate malnutrition
Moderate muscle wasting
Significant subcutaneous fat loss
Inadequate dietary intake 3–5 wks
Functional capacity: Semiambulatory, requiring assistance with activities of daily living

Severe malnutrition
Severe muscle wasting
Severe subcutaneous fat loss
Inadequate dietary intake >5 wks
Functional capacity: Minimally ambulatory, or bedridden

(From Pikul J. Degree of preoperative malnutrition is predictive of preoperative morbidity and mortality in liver transplant recipients. *Transplantation* 1994;57(3):469.)

D. Surgical manipulation of the gastrointestinal tract, including that of bowel resection, should not prevent the clinician from ordering enteral nutrition. Clinical examination alone (i.e., listening to bowel sounds) is not a sensitive mechanism to determine tolerance to enteral nutrition.

E. Enteral nutrition should be started early, ideally within the 24 to 36 hours after the injury. The role of meeting caloric goals early is unclear and will need further research. Increase volume of enteral nutrition to meet 50% to 65% of caloric goals within 7 days. **Feeding the gut when the patient is in shock (either related to resuscitation or sepsis), especially at high-volume rates, may be associated with bowel ischemia and necrosis.**

F. Do not overfeed critically ill trauma patients. Overfeeding is associated with significant morbidity and possibly increased mortality.

G. Consider using a hypocaloric–hyperproteic diet under some circumstances. This is especially significant in obese patients and during sepsis.

H. Monitor nutritional interventions carefully. Avoid hyperglycemia and hyperlipidemia. A low albumin and prealbumin in trauma and critical illness is non-specific and may reflect an inflammatory state rather than malnutrition. Overfeeding patients with low levels of albumin or prealbumin will not hasten the patient's recovery, especially if the patient has a septic focus or significant amounts of necrotic tissue.

I. The use of peptide-based enteral nutrition may improve tolerance and facilitate meeting nutritional goals. Tolerance is increased if a concerted attempt is made early in the course of the disease. The use of prokinetic agents may also facilitate tolerance.

J. Use of immune-enhancing diets should be considered in the trauma patient, particularly with open wounds.

AXIOMS

- Trauma patients are catabolic; the degree of catabolism is proportional to the degree of injury.
- TPN is not indicated when the gastrointestinal tract is functional or during short periods of starvation.
- A critically ill patient should receive 20 to 25 kcal/kg/day as a caloric goal.
- Protein intake should be 1.5 to 2.0 g/kg/day or 20% to 30% of the total caloric nutrient intake.
- Feeding the gut when the patient is in shock, especially at high-volume rates, may be associated with bowel ischemia and necrosis.
- Avoid hyperglycemia and hyperlipidemia when feeding your patient.

WEBSITES

http://www.nutritioncare.org/Library.aspx—ASPEN guidelines for Nutrition in critically ill patients.

http://www.criticalcarenutrition.com/—Excellent resource and critical evaluation of guidelines for nutrition in critical care.

Suggested Readings

Brown R, Hunt H, Mowatt-Larssen C, et al. Comparison of specialized and standard enteral formulas in trauma patients. *Pharmacotherapy* 1994;14:314.

Cresci GA. Nutrition support in trauma. In: Gottschlich MM, ed. *The Science and Practice of Nutrition Support: A Case-Based Core Curriculum.* Dubuque, IA: Kendall/Hunt Publishing Co; 2001:445.

Dickerson RN, Boschert KJ, Kudsk KA, et al. Hypocaloric enteral tube feeding in critically ill obese patients. *Nutrition* 2002;18:241.

Ireton-Jones CS. Equations for estimating energy expenditure in burn patients with special reference to ventilatory status. *J Burn Care Rehabil* 1992;13(3):330–333.

Keys A. Basal metabolism. In: *The Biology of Human Starvation.* St. Paul, MN: North Central Publishing Co; 1950:303.

Kudsk KA, Minard G, Croce MA, et al. A randomized trial of isonitrogenous enteral diets after severe trauma. An immune-enhancing diet reduces septic complications. *Ann Surg* 1996;224:531.

Lin E, Calvano SE, Lowry SF. Systemic response to injury and metabolic support. In: Brunicardi FC, Andersen DK, Billiar TR, Dunn DL, Hunter JG, and Pollock RE, eds. *Schwartz's Principles of Surgery.* New York, NY: McGraw-Hill Medical Publishing Div; 2005:3.

Marderstein EL, Simmons RL, Ochoa JB. Patient safety: effect of institutional protocols on adverse events related to feeding tube placement in the critically ill. *J Am Coll Surg* 2004;199:39.

Moore FA, Moore EE, Kudsk KA. Clinical benefits of an immune enhancing diet for early postinjury enteral feeding. *J Trauma* 1994;37:607.

Sandstrom R, Drott C, Hyltander A, et al. The effect of postoperative intravenous feeding (TPN) on outcome following major surgery evaluated in a randomized study. *Ann Surg* 1993;217:185.

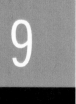

9 Prehospital and Air Medical Care

Francis X. Guyette and David C. Cone

I. TRAUMA TRIAGE. Trauma triage sorts patients on the basis of the **severity of their injuries** and the **availability of resources**. Generally, there are different types of prehospital trauma triage.

A. Field triage involves determining, prior to transport, if a trauma patient requires the services of a trauma center. Field triage uses an estimation of the severity of injury. Trauma triage criteria are used in single-patient events and events with small numbers of patients that do not exceed the capabilities of the local trauma system.

  1. Field triage guidelines. Knowledge of injury, mechanism, and existing comorbid factors are keys to optimal trauma triage. Unfortunately, no single factor will guarantee triage success. The following have been developed by the Centers for Disease Control and Prevention (Table 9-1):

    a. Patient assessment. The initial patient survey identifies and treats immediately life-threatening injuries.

      i. Abnormal vital/physiologic signs suggest the need for rapid treatment and transport to the highest level of care within a trauma system.

      ii. Anatomic locations and types of injuries can predict the need for emergent surgical or specialty care.

    b. Mechanism of injury. Mechanistic criteria enhance the sensitivity of the guidelines by considering the forces involved at the scene and the kinetic energy transferred during the event. **The** mechanism is not as strong a predictor of need for emergent operation or intensive care compared to the anatomic and physiologic criteria. Prehospital personnel should review the case with the direct medical oversight (DMO) physician by phone or radio to choose a destination.

    c. Premorbid conditions. No formal system exists for assessing or ranking premorbid conditions; yet these are often included in decision-making. Some such as pregnancy, age, and anticoagulation may alter the disposition of the patient to a specialty center. As with mechanism of injury criteria, discussion with the DMO physician may be helpful.

  2. Field triage scoring. Several trauma-scoring techniques determine the severity of injury of trauma victims both in the hospital and in the field. Examples include the Trauma Score, CRAMS Scale, Prehospital Index, and Trauma Triage Rule. Accurate trauma scoring is dependent on diagnostic skills and the availability of adjunctive testing, and is limited by field conditions, patient intoxication, and compensatory physiologic mechanisms masking major injuries. Trauma-scoring systems typically look at combinations of the following:

    a. Cardiovascular system
    b. Respiratory system
    c. Central nervous system
    d. Type and location of injury
    e. Abdominal examination

  3. Prehospital triage for air medical transport

    a. The transport of trauma patients directly from the scene should be supported by DMO or pre-approved protocols on the basis of the factors of time, distance, geography, patient stability, and local resources. Air medical transport may reduce blunt trauma mortality rates compared with ground transport. Undue

TABLE 9-1 2011 Guidelines for Field Triage of Injured Patients

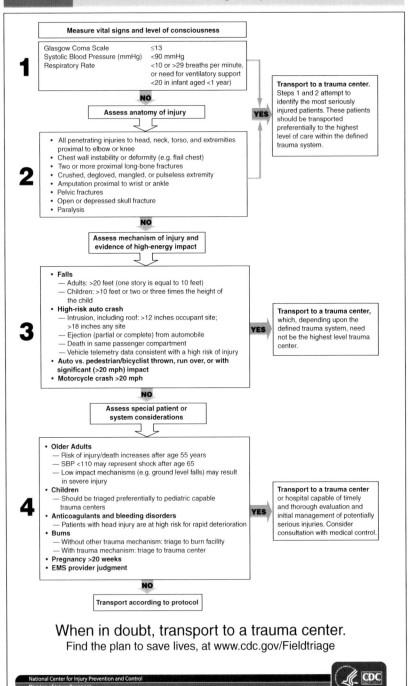

Measure vital signs and level of consciousness

Glasgow Coma Scale	≤13
Systolic Blood Pressure (mmHg)	<90 mmHg
Respiratory Rate	<10 or >29 breaths per minute, or need for ventilatory support <20 in infant aged <1 year)

1

NO

Assess anatomy of injury

YES → **Transport to a trauma center.** Steps 1 and 2 attempt to identify the most seriously injured patients. These patients should be transported preferentially to the highest level of care within the defined trauma system.

2
- All penetrating injuries to head, neck, torso, and extremities proximal to elbow or knee
- Chest wall instability or deformity (e.g. flail chest)
- Two or more proximal long-bone fractures
- Crushed, degloved, mangled, or pulseless extremity
- Amputation proximal to wrist or ankle
- Pelvic fractures
- Open or depressed skull fracture
- Paralysis

NO

Assess mechanism of injury and evidence of high-energy impact

3
- Falls
  — Adults: >20 feet (one story is equal to 10 feet)
  — Children: >10 feet or two or three times the height of the child
- **High-risk auto crash**
  — Intrusion, including roof: >12 inches occupant site; >18 inches any site
  — Ejection (partial or complete) from automobile
  — Death in same passenger compartment
  — Vehicle telemetry data consistent with a high risk of injury
- **Auto vs. pedestrian/bicyclist thrown, run over, or with significant (>20 mph) impact**
- Motorcycle crash >20 mph

YES → **Transport to a trauma center,** which, depending upon the defined trauma system, need not be the highest level trauma center.

NO

Assess special patient or system considerations

4
- Older Adults
  — Risk of injury/death increases after age 55 years
  — SBP <110 may represent shock after age 65
  — Low impact mechanisms (e.g. ground level falls) may result in severe injury
- Children
  — Should be triaged preferentially to pediatric capable trauma centers
- Anticoagulants and bleeding disorders
  — Patients with head injury are at high risk for rapid deterioration
- Bums
  — Without other trauma mechanism: triage to burn facility
  — With trauma mechanism: triage to trauma center
- Pregnancy >20 weeks
- EMS provider judgment

YES → **Transport to a trauma center** or hospital capable of timely and thorough evaluation and initial management of potentially serious injuries. Consider consultation with medical control.

NO

Transport according to protocol

When in doubt, transport to a trauma center.
Find the plan to save lives, at www.cdc.gov/Fieldtriage

National Center for Injury Prevention and Control
Division of Injury Response

CDC

84

Questions that can assist in determining appropriate transport mode are as follows:

- Does the patient's clinical condition require minimization of time spent out of the hospital environment during the transport?
- Does the patient require specific or time-sensitive evaluation or treatment that is not available at the referring facility?
- Is the patient located in an area that is inaccessible to ground transport?
- What are the current and predicted weather situations along the transport route?
- Is the weight of the patient (plus the weight of required equipment and transport personnel) within allowable ranges for air transport?
- For interhospital transports, is there a helipad and/or airport near the referring hospital?
- Does the patient require critical care life support (e.g., monitoring personnel, specific medications, specific equipment) during transport, which is not available with ground transport options?
- Would the use of local ground transport leave the local area without adequate emergency medical services coverage?
- If local ground transport is not an option, can the needs of the patient (and the system) be met by an available regional ground critical care transport service (i.e., specialized surface transport systems operated by hospitals and/or air medical programs)?

Figure 9-1. ACEP/NAEMSP guidelines for air medical dispatch.

delay of transport from the scene to the closest hospital while waiting for a helicopter should be avoided. Rendezvous at the hospital's helipad (helistop) allows for a more efficient use of time and provides additional options should the patient decompensate.

    i. The National Association of EMS Physicians (NAEMSP) and the American College of Emergency Physicians (ACEP) have recommended triage guidelines for air medical dispatch (Fig. 9-1).

  b. Interhospital transport of trauma patients usually involves moving a patient to a facility with a higher level of care.

  c. Weather, geography, logistics, or other factors determine flight suitability. **The final decision to accept the mission rests solely with the pilot, however any member of the crew should have the right to abort the mission. Crew safety is paramount.**

B. Mass casualty triage involves prioritizing patients when needs exceed available resources. The goal is to provide the most benefit to the greatest number of patients. This requires identifying potentially salvageable patients with life-threatening conditions who require immediate treatment and transport.

  1. The first EMS personnel to arrive on scene initiate mass casualty triage. Providers first ensure scene safety and relay basic information regarding the incident to dispatchers, so additional resources can be mobilized and hazards mitigated. The responsibility for patient triage is assigned to more experienced personnel when they arrive. Field triage works best when victims are limited to a small geographic area. Large disaster sites (such as earthquakes and floods) or disasters with geographically distinct areas (such as either side of a train crash, when mobility between and access to the two sides is limited by the wreckage) can require multiple triage sites.

  2. Principles. While it is generally taught that the most critically injured patients are transported first, empiric data are lacking to support this principle. Triage is a continuous process, with frequent reassessment of patient status and resources. Patients are typically re-triaged on arrival at the hospital.

  3. Simple triage and rapid treatment (START) is the most commonly used mass casualty triage system in the United States. Patients who are ambulatory are first removed from the area. Next, patients are classified as "expectant" if obviously dead or if not breathing after one attempt to reposition the airway. Remaining patients are categorized as "immediate" or "delayed," on the basis of the evaluation of respiratory rate, perfusion, and mental status. An abnormality

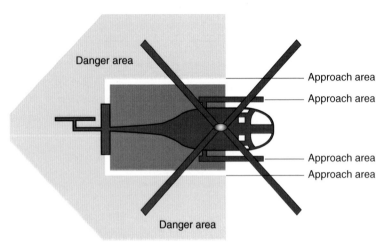

A

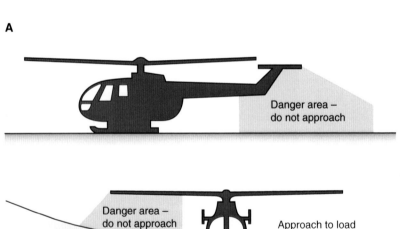

B

Figure 9-2. The same safety standards should be practiced whether the helicopter's engines are running or shut down.

- Do not approach the helicopter unless signaled to do so by a flight team member.
- Remain clear of the helicopter at all times unless accompanied by a flight team member.
- When approaching the helicopter, always approach from the front of the aircraft and move away in the same direction (Panel A).
- When approaching the helicopter on a slope, **never** approach from the uphill side. Always approach from the downhill side because the main rotor to the ground clearance is much greater. Always be aware of the blade clearance.
- **Never** walk around the tail rotor area (Panel B).
- No unauthorized personnel are allowed within 100 ft of the aircraft.
- No IV devices or other objects should be carried above the head, and long objects should be carried parallel to the ground.

TABLE 9-2	**START Triage Guidelines**

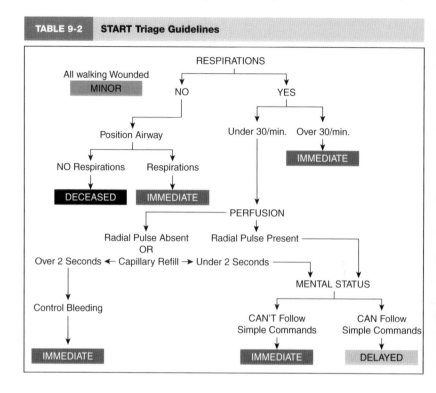

in any one parameter places the victim in the "immediate" category (Table 9-2).

4. **Triage tags** are often used to identify needs in both large and small multi-victim incidents.

   a. **Problems** that can occur with triage tags include:

      i. Separation of the tag from the victim

      ii. Contamination by blood or body fluids

      iii. Limited space for documentation

      iv. Inability to "upgrade" a patient's triage category, since many tags use color-coded strips that are torn off (leaving the patient's categorization attached) and cannot be reattached if a patient's status worsens

   b. **Color codes** are traditionally used to identify patient categorization by injury severity and need for transport:

      i. **Red "immediate"** or the most critically injured. This includes patients with major injuries to the head, thorax, and abdomen for which immediate surgical or specialty care is required.

      ii. **Yellow "delayed"** or less critically injured. This includes patients who are less seriously injured, who still likely require in-hospital treatment, but whose clinical condition permits a delay of several hours without endangering life.

      iii. **Green "ambulatory"** with no life- or limb-threatening injury identified. Ideally, medical personnel will reassess all of the ambulatory patients who are initially moved away from the disaster scene, to identify injuries.

      iv. **Black "expectant"** or dead. Patients who would be triaged to "red" under certain circumstances might be triaged to "black" when resources are limited.

C. **Limitations to triage.** Patient injuries and conditions are dynamic and assessment is limited, making perfect triage difficult to achieve. In both field triage and mass casualty events, over- and under-triage may occur.

1. **Over-triage** (false positives) occurs when a patient who does not require a trauma center or high level of immediate care is assigned to and transported to a trauma center. When resources are not constrained, this results in some degree of wasted resources if activation of the trauma team occurs unnecessarily. In a mass casualty situation, over-triage may limit the ability of a trauma center to provide optimal care for those who need it.

2. **Under-triage** (false negatives) occurs when a patient who may benefit from trauma center/higher level of care is transported to a setting with fewer resources. This can affect ultimate outcomes; in a mass casualty incident, under-triage may be unavoidable as trauma centers become saturated.

3. While it is commonly stated that 50% over-triage is acceptable to achieve 10% under-triage, there are no outcome data to support this supposition.

II. **TRAUMATIC ARREST.** The term "traumatic arrest" refers to the end result of a variety of pathologic processes in response to injury and is not a single clinical entity.

A. **Etiology.** EMS personnel should be trained to recognize the **most common treatable causes of traumatic cardiopulmonary collapse in the prehospital setting: Airway obstruction, hypoventilation or hypoxemia, tension pneumothorax, and uncontrolled hemorrhage. These etiologies are well covered elsewhere. Airway loss or failure remains the most common reversible cause, followed by hemorrhage/volume loss.**

B. **Determination of viability**

1. **Likelihood of survival.** The research on this topic often includes a mixture of clinical conditions, making interpretation difficult. A few general guidelines can be gleaned from the available data.

   a. **Victims of penetrating trauma** have a greater likelihood of survival from cardiac arrest than victims of blunt trauma.

      i. Survival from arrest is more likely after stab wounds than after gunshot wounds.

      ii. Arrest before EMS arrival decreases the likelihood of survival, particularly if transport times are long.

      iii. Presence of recognized *and* quickly treated tension pneumothorax or pericardial tamponade is a positive prognostic factor, but this is usually not done in the field.

   b. **Victims of blunt trauma** who suffer cardiopulmonary arrest have an extremely low likelihood of survival, approaching zero (unless witnessed and treated in the emergency department).

      i. Those found by prehospital personnel to be in arrest with no signs of life (absence of spontaneous movement or respirations, and absence of reflexes including pupillary) and no electrical activity on the electrocardiogram have a negligible chance of survival. Prehospital resuscitation is **not** indicated for these patients.

      ii. The presence of some life sign (eye movement, pupil reaction, corneal reflex, organized cardiac rhythm) in pulseless, nonbreathing patients confers a low likelihood of survival. Because aggressive interventions (e.g., intubation, ventilation, release of tension pneumothorax, and volume resuscitation) result in occasional long-term survival, resuscitation is attempted. Persistence of pulselessness on hospital arrival is uniformly fatal and further resuscitation is not warranted.

      iii. Deterioration into cardiac arrest after EMS arrival but before hospital arrival also has dismal prognosis, but full resuscitative efforts should generally be undertaken. Most data suggest no benefit to emergency department thoracotomy for prehospital blunt traumatic arrest.

C. **Criteria for attempting resuscitation.** Resuscitation should be attempted on patients in arrest caused by major blunt or penetrating trauma, **unless** one or more of the following criteria are met:

1. Injury obviously incompatible with life (e.g., decapitation, incineration)
2. Absent signs of life (no respiratory effort, no pupillary response or eye movement, no response to deep pain) and ECG rhythm of asystole
3. Documented, untreated pulselessness and apnea for 15 minutes (e.g., prolonged entrapment, hazardous scene) in a normothermic patient
4. Rigor mortis or dependent lividity
5. Transport time to an ED or trauma center of more than 15 minutes after the onset of cardiopulmonary arrest

D. Special conditions
   1. Electrical shocks **or lightning.** Since arrest is usually caused by a cardiac dysrhythmia and may be reversible, aggressive resuscitation should be attempted. In cases of multiple casualties from an electrical incident, defibrillation of those in ventricular fibrillation or pulseless ventricular tachycardia arrest should be given first priority.
   2. **Drowning or hanging.** Arrest is usually caused by asphyxia in these situations. Although appropriate trauma care, such as spinal immobilization, should be instituted, the decision to resuscitate can be based on criteria for "medical" arrests. Hypothermia should be considered in drowning victims.
   3. **Hypothermia.** The presence of hypothermia (core temperature below 35°C) can result from or lead to a traumatic event. Hypothermia can make it difficult to detect signs of life. Patients who are severely hypothermic should generally undergo active core rewarming before cessation of resuscitative efforts unless injuries are clearly incompatible with life. Refer to Chapter 43 for more details on this illness and treatment.
   4. **Arrest secondary to medical cause.** It can be a challenge to recognize patients who may have suffered trauma or cardiac arrest because of a medical condition, such as the driver of an automobile who develops ventricular fibrillation with a resultant crash. Unless evidence suggests a fatal injury, a patient whose mechanism of injury does not correlate with the clinical condition should typically undergo resuscitative efforts similar to any other non-traumatic arrest patient. Following return of spontaneous circulation, these patients should undergo a complete trauma evaluation to exclude further injury followed by treatment of the medical condition that precipitated the arrest.

E. Management of traumatic arrest
   1. **At the scene.** Time on scene (excluding extrication) should be as short as possible—often targeted for 10 minutes maximum, absent extrication concerns or other operational delays.
      a. **Ensure scene safety before entry,** particularly in cases involving assaults, fire, hazardous materials, confined spaces, and vehicular traffic. Law enforcement or fire service assistance may be needed to secure the scene prior to EMS operations. Field personnel should not put themselves at risk for a patient with a negligible chance of survival.
      b. **Recognize cardiac arrest**
         i. Determine whether to initiate resuscitation (see Section B).
         ii. Assess for the presence of special conditions such as hypothermia or a primary medical cause that might influence decision or course of resuscitation.
      c. **Start manual and device-based spinal immobilization**
      d. **Perform chest compressions at a rate of 100/minute**
      e. **Open airway using jaw thrust without head tilt.** Inspect oral cavity, and suction or manually remove debris (blood, teeth, etc.).
      f. **Ventilate patient** with basic techniques (e.g., bag-valve-mask) at a rate of 10 to 12 breaths/minute. Use supplemental oxygen to maintain oxygen saturations >95%.
      g. **Control severe external hemorrhage**
      h. **Determine ECG rhythm** (note that above steps may be carried out while assessing rhythm to decide whether to proceed with resuscitation):
         i. Defibrillate for ventricular fibrillation or pulseless ventricular tachycardia.
         ii. An organized rhythm (pulseless electrical activity) confers a greater likelihood of a reversible condition.

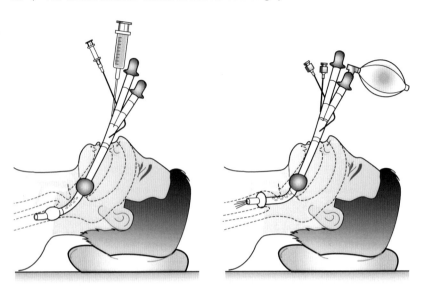

Figure 9-3. Supraglottic Airway; Esophagotracheal Combitube (ETC). (Modified from the Sheridan Catheter Corporation, Argyle, NY, with permission.)

   i. Manage the airway (refer to Chapter 11); this starts with supplemental oxygen in all.
      i. If able to intubate or place a supraglottic airway (Fig. 9-3), confirm proper tube position and carefully secure tube.
      ii. Do not delay compressions, treatment of reversible causes of arrest, or transport to perform endotracheal intubation.
      iii. If unable to perform intubation or place a supraglottic rescue airway device, determine effectiveness of ventilation using basic techniques:
         a) If able to ventilate adequately (chest rise and fall), continue ventilation with basic maneuvers (Fig. 9-4).
         b) If unable to ventilate adequately with a mask device, and *if* the rescuer is properly trained and qualified, perform surgical cricothyroidotomy; otherwise (as is often the case in most EMS situations), initiate rapid transport and continue to attempt ventilation with basic maneuvers.
   j. Assess patient for tension pneumothorax.
      i. Signs: Unilateral (or bilateral) decreased breath sounds, poor or worsening lung compliance (especially with positive pressure ventilation), tracheal deviation, subcutaneous emphysema.
      ii. If pneumothorax is suspected, perform needle decompression (described elsewhere).
   k. Immobilize the patient's spine on a long backboard with straps, rigid cervical collar, and head immobilization device.
   l. Transfer the patient rapidly to the vehicle, and initiate transport.
 2. En route to the hospital.
   a. Ensure ongoing optimal ventilation (using means above, ensuring tube position if present).
   b. Reassess for tension pneumothorax.
   c. Contact DMO and/or receiving facility, based on local protocol.
   d. Initiate intravenous (IV) access, or intraosseous (IO) access if IV access cannot be obtained and the rescuer is qualified.

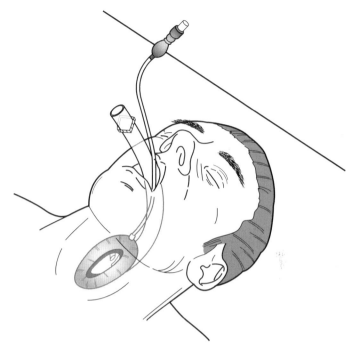

Figure 9-4. Laryngeal mask airway (LMA). (Modified from The laryngeal mask airway: Its uses in anesthesiology. *Anesthesiology* 1993;79:144–183, with permission.)

    i. Two large-bore IV lines (≥16 gauge) are optimal.

    ii. The role of fluid resuscitation is controversial. A pragmatic approach is to guide EMS providers to control any external hemorrhage first, then give isotonic crystalloid fluid to help approach normal circulating volume but not to seek "normal" vital signs until hemorrhage is controlled. In many cases, the latter cannot occur until after hospital arrival.

3. Advanced interventions for **physicians and other advanced providers** may be indicated in some situations, especially when scene or transport time is long.

    a. Surgical airway

        i. Open **cricothyroidotomy**

        ii. Percutaneous cricothyroidotomy

    b. Venous access

        i. Central vein access

        ii. Cutdown of saphenous vein at groin or ankle

    c. Tube thoracostomy. Needle decompression can produce inadequate or only temporary decompression of pneumothorax and is inadequate for drainage of hemothorax.

4. Termination of efforts. Termination of resuscitation efforts should be considered for traumatic arrest patients with 15 minutes of unsuccessful resuscitation efforts and cardiopulmonary resuscitation (CPR).

III. NONARREST PREHOSPITAL TRAUMA MANAGEMENT

A. Airway management.

    1. Introduction. While it has traditionally been taught that airway management is the most important skill to be mastered by EMS personnel, "endotracheal intubation" may delay critical interventions and increase the risk of secondary insult from hypoxia, hypotension, and hypoventilation. Effective airway management with a supraglottic airway device or BVM ventilation may be preferable depending on transport time, patient condition, and provider skill or experience. Regardless, conditions and circumstances encountered by EMS personnel contribute to the challenge of establishing an airway. These include adverse environmental conditions (rain, snow, darkness), limited patient access (entrapment), limited numbers of personnel (often only two providers, only one of whom is trained in advanced airway management techniques), concern for cervical spine injury (precluding or complicating certain airway maneuvers), and patients with full stomachs, head injury, or acute intoxication (each of which can increase complication rates).

2. **Patient assessment.** The airway is assessed by simultaneous evaluation of several simple clinical features. These include level of consciousness, physical findings, and vital signs.

   a. **Level of consciousness.** The patient's general condition of wakefulness is the best predictor of the ability to protect the airway from aspiration or occlusion. Specific simple features are commonly sought using the AVPU scale: Is the patient **awake,** eyes open, and conversing? Is the patient reacting to **verbal** stimuli? Is the patient arousable only to **painful** or noxious stimuli? Is the patient **unresponsive**? Abnormalities of mental status can be caused by hypoventilation, hypoxemia, hypoperfusion, hypoglycemia, drug or alcohol intoxication, or head injury. If the patient's ability to maintain adequate oxygenation, ventilation, or airway patency is impaired, airway interventions are required.

   b. **Physical findings.** Search for findings indicative of poor oxygen delivery to tissues: Pale, cool, moist skin; delayed capillary refill (greater than 2 seconds); noisy or labored respirations (too fast or too slow). Other physical findings more specific to a pure respiratory abnormality include asymmetric or shallow chest excursion, crepitus, thoracic ecchymosis, nasal flaring, accessory muscle use, abdominal breathing, or subcostal retraction.

   c. **Vital signs.** Abnormal vital signs (including pulse oximetry and end-tidal carbon dioxide ($EtCO_2$)) must be addressed and appropriate therapy instituted. Normal vital signs do not guarantee airway protection.

3. **Airway resuscitation** encompasses positioning and clearing the airway, delivering supplemental oxygen, using adjuncts or assist devices, and implementing supraglottic or tracheal intubation techniques. **The steps of airway management are detailed in Chapter 3;** these apply here but are constrained by the providers' training and skill. Field providers should have ongoing training in basic airway management – bag-valve-mask use, airway suctioning and positioning, oral and nasal airways, endotracheal intubation, and alternate supraglottic airway device use – but not be expected to master all options. The key is having the simple steps mastered and two advanced methods well honed.

B. **Other procedures and therapies**
   1. **IV access and fluid therapy**
      a. **IV access** allows the administration of crystalloids, blood products, and medications. Venous catheterization of trauma patients by paramedics is done routinely, even though outcome data supporting this practice are lacking. Currently, pragmatism suggests that IV access should be attempted but without delaying transport or other interventions (especially airway management and hemorrhage control). To limit the on-scene interval, attempts at IV placement should be made during extrication, while awaiting transport resources, or during transport to the hospital. Large-bore (16 gauge) peripheral IV lines are preferred for major trauma patients. If IV access is not readily available consider IO access.
      b. **Failures.** A small number of trauma patients will arrive at the hospital without IV/IO access because of short transport times, uncooperative patients, or

other more pressing priorities (e.g., airway management, spine protection, or hemorrhage control).

c. **Fluid therapy in the field.** Significant controversy exists regarding the composition, amount, and ultimate clinical goals of fluid therapy in trauma patients. No specific heart rate or blood pressure targets exist to guide the amount of fluid; rather, controlled or limited fluid resuscitation (sometimes referred to as "permissive hypotension") appears beneficial, although the endpoint and fluid makeup are still uncertain. Recent data suggest that resuscitation to a palpable pressure or SBP >70 mm Hg is sufficient for penetrating trauma, while recommendations for blunt trauma range from an SBP of 90 to 110 mm Hg.

2. Rapid chest decompression/needle thoracostomy

　a. **Indications.** Needle thoracostomy should be performed when a tension pneumothorax exists or is suspected. **Any trauma patient with severe respiratory distress should be evaluated immediately for tension pneumothorax.** In the field, the diagnosis is critical and must be treated before arrival at the hospital. Tension pneumothorax should be suspected in the trauma patient who is short of breath or hypotensive and with **any** of the following features:

　　i. Decreased breath sounds

　　ii. Tracheal deviation (away from the involved side)

　　iii. Distended neck veins (this may not be seen in the patient who is hypovolemic)

　　iv. Hyperresonance to percussion of the chest (on the involved side)—difficult to assess in the field environment

　　v. If the patient is intubated, increasing difficulty in bag-valve ventilation can be the earliest or sole indication of a developing tension pneumothorax

　　vi. Respiratory distress

　b. **Procedure.** Treatment should proceed rapidly once the diagnosis is suspected; if incorrect, the only harm is creating the need for a formal tube thoracostomy in the receiving facility, whereas failing to recognize and treat can lead to death. Decompress the affected side of the chest by inserting a large-bore IV catheter (12 or 14 gauge) perpendicular to the skin at the second or third intercostal space in the midclavicular line, or the third or fourth interspace in the anterior axillary line (Fig. 9-5). Advance the catheter until a rush of air occurs from the open distal end, or until the hub reaches the skin. Common errors include placing the needle either too close to the sternum or cephalad to the second intercostal space (making heart or great vessel puncture possible), or placing the needle under instead of over a rib (making puncture of the neurovascular bundle, which runs in a groove under each rib, possible). After placement, withdraw the needle, but leave the catheter in place to prevent reaccumulation of pleural gas. If the patient's condition worsens, suspect occlusion of the first catheter and place a second needle.

　　i. **Bilateral decompression.** Occasionally, especially in the patient on positive pressure ventilation or with severe obstructive lung disease, bilateral tension pneumothorax can develop. The asymmetry described above with respect to tracheal and chest findings may not be present. If uncertain, both hemithoraces should be decompressed.

　　ii. **Therapy after needle thoracostomy.** At the receiving facility, a chest tube is usually placed for definitive treatment once needle decompression is performed (whether or not clinical success occurred with the latter). Once the chest tube is in place, the catheter(s) can be withdrawn.

3. Tourniquets. If pressure fails to control hemorrhage from an extremity injury, a tourniquet should be applied. Controversy over tourniquet use began with reports of amputation or fasciotomies when the devices were left in place too long. Tourniquets used during this period were improvised with rubber tubing, rifle slings, and belts, and were often inappropriately narrow resulting in further tissue injury at the necessary tension to stop arterial bleeding.

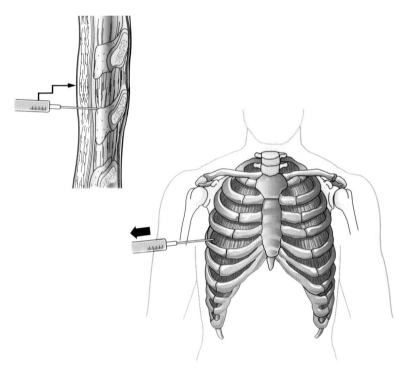

Figure 9-5. Technique for needle thoracostomy. (Modified from Champion HR, Robbs JV, Trunkey DD. Trauma surgery. In: Rob and Smith's Operative Surgery. *London: Butterworth*, 1989:57, with permission.)

Several recent case series and case reports have shown that tourniquet use on the battlefield has resulted in neither limb loss nor permanent disability, even among those who had tourniquets applied that in retrospect were not required. Civilian prehospital studies evaluating the safety and effectiveness of tourniquets are lacking. If direct pressure fails, a tourniquet should be applied. Tourniquets may also be needed in MCIs related to explosive blasts, terrorism, or criminal violence. In these cases there will often be more casualties than skilled providers, and evacuation from the scene may be delayed due to tactical concerns during a criminal or terrorist attack, or because of collapsed and unstable structures in the event of an explosion.

4. **Splinting**
   a. **Indications.** The purposes of splinting are to prevent further injury, decrease blood loss, and limit the amount of pain the patient will have with movement of that extremity during extrication and transport. An injured extremity should be splinted in anatomic position *if possible*, with the splint extending to the joints above and below the fracture site for stabilization. If the patient refuses, or if resistance to straightening exists, splint in a position of comfort. Dressings should be applied to any open wounds before splinting.
   b. **Splint types.** A large variety of splint designs will appear on patients brought to the emergency department. They can be as simple as a rolled-up newspaper, or as complex as a vacuum or traction splint.
      i. Cardboard splints, with or without foam padding, are intended for single use.

    ii. Board splints are common and durable, made of straight pieces of wood, metal, or plastic cut to various lengths.

    iii. Air splints, which encircle the injured extremity, are inflated with air to impart stiffness. They are usually clear to allow visualization of the underlying structures. Over inflation can cause neurovascular compromise.

    iv. Vacuum splints incompletely encircle the injured limb. Instead of air being blown into them, air is withdrawn and a vacuum is produced, which stiffens the splint.

    v. Traction splints are used for femur fractures. Thomas half-ring splints and Hare traction splints are those most commonly used. Specific training is required for proper placement.

    vi. Ladder splints are made from heavy gauge wire in a ladder shape. They are useful for splinting extremities that cannot be straightened because they are bendable and can be shaped to match the extremity. The SAM Splint, with a flexible aluminum alloy core covered with closed-cell foam, is similarly flexible.

    vii. Pelvic binders and compression devices may be made out of bed sheets or commercial devices with compound pulley systems and Velcro to close a disrupted pelvis.

  c. Complications. Although splinting is safe and effective in most patients, complications can develop, including:

    i. Neurovascular compromise. Whichever splint is used, distal neurovascular status must be checked before and after application of the splint. Also, if any patient movement has occurred, the patient reports more pain, or the extremity is noted to be cyanotic or edematous distal to the splint, reexamine the extremity and splint. It is also advisable to periodically check the neurovascular status, even if none of the above occurs. When impaired neurovascular status is seen distal to an injury, the splint should be loosened or adjusted, and the neurovascular status rechecked.

    ii. Pain. When the patient reports pain, search for neurovascular compromise or malpositioning. Gentle repositioning should resolve this condition.

5. Axial spine immobilization

  a. Prehospital indications. Despite the lack of supporting literature, the entire axial spine is immobilized by prehospital personnel whenever the mechanism of injury, injury pattern, or physical examination indicates the possibility of any spinal injury. Patients with obvious physical findings (e.g., bony crepitation, palpable step-offs) or those with neurologic findings (e.g., paresthesia, weakness, paralysis) consistent with spine or cord injury should always receive cervical immobilization before transport.

  b. Clinical assessment of the spine often cannot be performed by field personnel because of time, space, distracting injury, altered consciousness, and other concerns (e.g., airway, bleeding control, vascular access) that can preclude adequate in-field evaluation to rule out spinal injury. The rule in prehospital care is to maintain a high index of suspicion for such injuries with liberal application of spinal immobilization.

  c. The need for spinal immobilization occurs at the injury scene and continues through extrication, transportation, and stabilization in the ED. Immobilization is accomplished with the least possible neck movement, and ends only when physical and/or radiographic findings definitively rule out injury.

  d. Types of immobilization devices. No single method or combinations of methods of immobilization consistently place the spine in neutral position or prevent all motion in the axial spine.

    i. Cervical collars (c-collars). These rigid one- or two-piece devices encircle the cervical spine and soft tissues of the neck, providing (when properly fitted) a snug fit between the tip, the chin, and the suprasternal notch of the anterior chest, and between the occiput and the suprascapular region of the back. These collars limit movement of the head in the coronal and transverse planes, minimizing lateral and rotary motion. They do not, however, provide adequate immobilization in the sagittal plane (flexion–extension motion). For this reason, **a rigid cervical collar alone is inadequate for effective spinal immobilization** and is always used in conjunction with a cervical immobilization device (CID) and a spine board (short or long). Soft neck collars (foam supports covered with loose-weave material) are ineffective at limiting motion of the head and are not intended for use in spinal immobilization.

ii. CIDs are made of plastic, cardboard, or foam. They act to limit both lateral and rotary motion, and they possess restraining straps that are positioned over the patient's forehead and chin. The CID affixes the patient's head and c-collar to a rigid spine board, limiting the head movements of flexion and extension. A CID can be fashioned from blanket rolls, blocks, or sandbags placed alongside the head, with fixation to the spine board via a wide (2 to 3 in) adhesive tape placed over the forehead and chin.

iii. Spine boards have not been demonstrated to benefit patients with spinal injury and have been associated with respiratory compromise, patient agitation, and pressure ulcers. Use of spine boards should be limited to the transfer of the patient to the EMS stretcher and the time on the board should be minimized. Spine boards are termed "short" or "long," depending on the most distal portion of the patient immobilized. Short boards limit flexion and extension from the head to the hips, minimizing movement in all portions of the spine (cervical, thoracic, lumbar). Short boards are primarily used if patient access is limited (e.g., entrapment in a vehicle, or confined space extrication) and stability in the axial spine is needed before and during the extrication process. Once extrication is performed and complete access to the patient is achieved, the patient should be log rolled onto the EMS stretcher and kept supine. Straps provide fixation points at the thorax, hips, and lower extremities (above the knees). Padding between the lower extremities and under the knees enhances both stabilization and patient comfort.

a) Secondary pain after immobilization. With any of these devices, immobilization itself can produce symptoms of discomfort (e.g., occipital headache; neck, back, head, mandible pain). Padding behind the occiput and in the areas of lordosis and kyphosis make intuitive sense, and may be especially important in the pediatric and elderly population, given their anatomy. Once patients arrive at the hospital, prompt removal after appropriate assessment will limit pain and skin breakdown.

IV. AIR MEDICAL TRANSPORT

On the basis of the experience of the Korean and Vietnam Wars, air medical transport has grown to become an integral part of trauma care in the United States. Over 800 private, hospital-based, public service, and military air medical helicopters transport more than 300,000 patients annually. Two-thirds of the transports are interhospital, with the remaining one-third transported directly from the scene.

A. Equipment

1. Most air medical transport today is accomplished with helicopters specifically configured for medical missions. Some flight programs fly instrument flight rules (IFR) missions, allowing transport of trauma patients in weather conditions that previously prevented rotorcraft transport. Most aircrafts with reconfiguration can transport two patients, in addition to two flight crew members and the pilot. The practical transport range for helicopter transfer is generally 150 miles. For longer distance transports or in poor weather conditions, fixed-wing aircrafts are utilized.

2. The flight environment is austere. Noise, vibration, and limited space make simple procedures such as auscultation of blood pressure and breath sounds difficult or impossible. Therefore, non–audible-dependent monitoring is used. Most flight

crews rely on noninvasive blood pressure monitoring, ECG, $EtCO_2$, and pulse oximetry to monitor patients in flight. Rotorcrafts rarely fly at altitudes above 2,000 ft above ground level. At these altitudes, pressure changes have only a minor effect on the volume of air-filled spaces. However, fixed-wing aircrafts are typically pressurized to 8,000 ft, resulting in a decreased partial pressure of oxygen and a roughly 25% expansion of confined gasses.

3. The flight crew communicate with each other and the patient through headsets or helmets connected to internal communication systems. The crew must be able to communicate with the receiving hospital. Advance notification of patient assessment and changes in patient condition are transmitted to the receiving trauma center by radio, cellular, or satellite phone.

B. Flight crew

1. More than 70% of the medical flight crews consist of a nurse–paramedic team. Approximately 20% of programs use two nurses, and only 3% of programs use a flight physician. Respiratory therapists are also combined with nurses in a small percentage of programs when specialty care is required for children or neonates.

2. Mid-level providers including certified registered nurse anesthetists (CRNAs), registered nurse practitioners (RNPs), and physician's assistants (PAs) have a limited role in adding specialty skills and a broader scope of practice to some critical care transport teams.

C. Interventions

1. Transport crews should be experienced in the care of critically ill patients. Crew members should be highly trained in airway management using rapid sequence intubation, as well as resuscitation, vascular access, and control of hemorrhage. These interventions should be initiated prior to lift-off.

2. IV analgesia, sedation, and chemical paralysis, as well as administration of vasoactive substances and blood products, can be done in flight. These interventions must be performed under strict DMO, or predetermined approved protocols.

D. Helipad access team

1. A helipad team trained in helicopter safety is designated to assist the flight crew in unloading and transporting the patient from the helicopter to the emergency department. Helipads should be in close proximity to the resuscitation area, limiting the need for therapeutic interventions on the helipad.

2. When helipads are remote from the resuscitation area (e.g., rooftop with elevator and corridor transport), therapeutic interventions may be required on the helipad. Only a limited number of resuscitative procedures should be performed on the helipad. Focus should be on identifying the need for immediate lifesaving procedures, establishing an airway, decompressing a tension pneumothorax, applying direct pressure to an open bleeding wound, or administering resuscitative drugs and defibrillation for dysrhythmias. Other interventions (IV catheter placement for volume resuscitation or thoracotomy) are best performed in the emergency department.

E. Safety

1. The leading causes of accidents are weather, collision with an object or terrain, and loss of control of the aircraft. Pressure on pilots to fly and failure to observe minimum weather standards are contributing components to accidents. The pilot's decision to complete a mission should be based on aviation factors alone and not influenced by patient criteria. Whenever possible, programs should employ technology to prevent collisions and accidents in adverse weather including collision avoidance systems, weather radar, and night vision systems.

2. In general, a 500 ft ceiling and 1 mile visibility are required for daytime visual flight rules (VFR) operation. This may be geography-specific, depending on the presence of mountains and pockets of fog. Day-local is defined as 25 nautical miles from departure point to destination point, with generally the same terrain elevation.

3. Comprehensive safety orientation programs for local ground EMS personnel that include instruction covering helicopter communication, set-up of landing zones,

patient preparation, and conduct around the aircraft are an essential part of any EMS air medical program. Guidelines for safe operations around a helicopter are provided in Figure 9.2.

V. INTERHOSPITAL TRANSPORT

A. Introduction. Emergent interhospital transport occurs after initial stabilization of the trauma patient at the referring facility. There is evidence demonstrating that trauma outcomes are improved if critically injured patients are cared for in dedicated trauma centers. A trauma center should have a referral and communications center to facilitate transfers, outreach teams to provide referring facilities with continuing education, and public education programs about trauma systems and injury prevention. Transfer of the trauma patient occurs with the expectation that care will continue en route to the receiving facility and that changes in patient status will be identified and treated. These goals require specialized personnel and equipment. Coordination between referring and receiving institutions and medical oversight during transport are fundamental to guarantee continuity of care.

B. Before transport. It is the responsibility of the **referring physician** to decide the best mode of transportation (air vs. ground) and to ensure that the transporting personnel have the necessary expertise and equipment to deal with the patient's condition and possible complications. For example, some non–hospital-based personnel may not be trained in the use of certain hospital equipment (IV pumps, ventilators, or other devices); this should be recognized and addressed before transport. Some transport systems employ **physician medical directors** who are expert in transport medicine and may function as a consultant to the referring physician to aid the delivery of appropriate resources to ensure optimal patient care.

1. The transporting crew can be any combination of paramedics, nurses, or physicians, depending on the patient condition and local policies. A physician, with expertise in prehospital and transport medicine, should provide medical oversight including crew protocols, policies, training, and total quality management. If the referring physician is to provide medical oversight during transport, transfer orders should be discussed before departure.

2. Documentation of key patient care records must be sent with the patient. This includes results of all therapeutic and diagnostic interventions, copies of all imaging studies performed, and patient consent for transfer. Tele-radiology and integrated electronic medical records each allow trauma center personnel to see all records before and after arrival. This also allows the center to help referring facilities manage patients who do not require transfer to a trauma center.

3. It is essential that the transport team establish direct communication with both referring and accepting physicians. Communication with the referring physician must detail the following information:
   a. **Identification** of the patient and medical history
   b. **Mechanism of injury** and circumstances about the incident
   c. **Prehospital management** before arrival to the emergency department
   d. **Interventions** performed during initial stabilization and patient's response
   e. **Pertinent physical examination findings**
   f. **Ongoing therapy**
   g. **Potential complications** that may occur during transport

4. The transport team should then perform its own directed evaluation, equivalent to a primary survey, without delaying transport. This evaluation should include, but not be limited to, the following.
   a. **Airway**
      i. **Recheck the airway** or assess adequate position of the endotracheal tube with appropriate methods that can include direct visualization, $EtCO_2$, auscultation, esophageal detector device, or chest x-ray.
   b. **Respiratory**
      i. **Document respiratory status** before initiation of transport.
      ii. **Check for appropriate functioning of ventilatory equipment.**

      iii. Check or place nasogastric tube to prevent aspiration in obtunded or intubated patients.

      iv. Check position of any tube or device (e.g., thoracostomy). Chest tubes ideally should have pleural drainage devices attached and placed on suction for transport.

    c. Cardiovascular

      i. Document heart rate, pulse, pulse oximetry, and blood pressure before initiation of transport.

      ii. Control external bleeding and reevaluate bandages applied for bleeding control. Consider the use of tourniquets, splints and hemostatic dressings when appropriate.

      iii. Secure two large-bore IV catheters.

      iv. Secure adequate supply of blood products for transfer.

      v. Connect invasive lines (e.g., arterial lines, central venous pressure [CVP] lines, and pulmonary artery catheters) to the transport monitor to allow continued hemodynamic monitoring during the transport.

      vi. Connect the patient to electrocardiograph monitor.

    d. Central nervous system

      i. Document neurologic examination and Glasgow Coma Scale (GCS) score before initiation of transport or administration of paralytic or sedative agents.

      ii. Secure head, cervical, thoracic, and lumbar spine with immobilization devices as needed.

C. During transport. The transport team must know before transport which physician is to be responsible for DMO. Responsibility for medical oversight will vary, based on local practices and the policies of the transport service. The receiving physician, however, must always be made aware of changes in the patient's condition en route.

  1. Once the patient has been stabilized, the transport should be completed without delay. It is expected that care during transport be at the same level as received at the referring institution, within the obvious limitations of the out-of-hospital environment. A provider capable of appropriate medical interventions should accompany unstable patients; this may require a physician.

  2. The transporting unit must have the capability to continue cardiorespiratory support and blood volume replacement. Constant hemodynamic monitoring is essential. Communication via radio, cellular telephone, or satellite phone should occur to obtain medical oversight and to provide updates to the receiving facility.

  3. When standing orders or protocols (the essential component of indirect medical oversight) are given to the transport team, the referring physician must be sure that the orders match the team's capabilities and that the appropriate medications and equipment are present.

D. After transport. On arrival at the receiving facility, the transport team must give a complete report to the receiving trauma team. This should include a brief summary of the initial history and treatments, followed by an update of any changes en route and any interventions. In addition, all documentation from the referring institution must be delivered to the receiving team leader. If the patient was transferred for diagnostic procedures and is to be transferred back to the original institution, the same transfer regulations apply now to the receiving hospital. If diagnostic procedures reveal new evidence of present or potential instability, the patient cannot be transferred back without appropriate stabilization.

VI. LEGAL CONSIDERATIONS. The transfer of patients from one institution to another is regulated by federal statute. The legislation that created the patient stabilization and transfer requirements for hospitals and physicians is the **Consolidated Omnibus Budget Reconciliation Act (COBRA) of 1985,** also known as the "antidumping law." This is the current legal standard. One of the main objectives of this resolution is to guarantee equal access to emergency treatment to all citizens regardless of their ability to pay.

A. COBRA attributes responsibility for the patient's transfer to the referring hospital and physician.

1. Violations can result in termination of Medicare privileges for the physician and hospital.
2. A hospital can be fined between $25,000 and $50,000 per violation.
3. A physician can be fined $50,000 per violation.
4. A patient can sue the hospital for personal injury in civil court.

B. The **Emergency Medical Treatment and Labor Act (EMTALA)** established by COBRA legislation governs how patients can be transferred from one hospital to another. Hospitals cannot transfer patients unless the transfer is "appropriate," the patient consents to transfer after being informed of the risks of transfer, and the referring physician certifies that the medical benefits expected from the transfer outweigh the risks. Appropriate transfers must meet the following criteria:
1. The transferring hospital must provide care and stabilization within its ability.
2. Copies of medical records and imaging studies must accompany the patient.
3. The receiving facility must have available space and qualified personnel and agree to accept the transfer.
4. The interhospital transport must be made by qualified personnel with the necessary equipment.

AXIOMS

- Recognizing trauma severity, assisting breathing in the simplest effective manner, controlling any bleeding, and rapidly transporting to an appropriate hospital are keys to good care.
- Most field trauma patients can be managed with basic life support skills, such as bag-valve-mask ventilation, splinting and spine immobilization, and hemorrhage control. There are no convincing data to support advanced life support interventions in trauma patients.
- The differences between field triage (for individual trauma patients) and mass casualty triage (for multipatient events) must be understood by both field and hospital personnel, and EMS systems must account for these two different types of triage when establishing or refining policies and procedures.
- Safety of patient and EMS crew is paramount during transport; never approach a helicopter without the assistance of the flight crew.
- The medical benefits anticipated from the provision of specialized trauma care at the receiving facility should outweigh the risks of transfer.

Suggested Readings

Accreditation Standards of the Commission on Accreditation of Air Medical Services. 8th ed. Sandy Springs, SC: Commission on Accreditation of Air Medical Services 2009.

Ahn H, Singh J, Nathens A, et al. Prehospital care management of a potential spinal cord injured patient: a systematic review of the literature and evidence-based guidelines. *J Neurotrauma* 2011;28:1341–1361.

American College of Emergency Physicians. *Appropriate Utilization of Air Medical Transport in the Out-of-Hospital Setting.* Dallas, TX: American College of Emergency Physicians; 2008.

Brown JB, Stassen NA, Bankey PE, et al. Helicopters and the civilian trauma system: national utilization patterns demonstrate improved outcomes after traumatic injury. *J Trauma* 2010;69(5):1030–1036.

Davis DP, Hoyt DB, Ochs M, et al. The effect of paramedic rapid sequence intubation on outcome in patients with severe traumatic brain injury. *J Trauma* 2003;54(3):444–453.

Emergency Medical Treatment and Active Labor Act of 1986: Consolidated Omnibus Budget Reconciliation of 1986, §9121, 42USC, §1395dd.

Hopson LR, Hirsh E, Delgado J, et al. Guidelines for withholding or termination of resuscitation in prehospital traumatic cardiopulmonary arrest: A joint position paper from the National Association of EMS Physicians Standards and Clinical Practice Committee and the American College of Surgeons Committee on Trauma. *Prehosp Emerg Care* 2003;7(1):141–146.

Lerner EB, Shah MN, Cushman JT, et al. Does mechanism of injury predict trauma center need? *Prehosp Emerg Care* 2011;15:518–525.

Nathens AB, Jurkovich GJ, Cummings P, et al. The effect of organized system of trauma care on motor vehicle crash mortality. *JAMA* 2000;283(15):1990–1994.

Sasser SM, Hunt RC, Faul M, et al. Guidelines for field triage of injured patients recommendations of the National Expert Panel on Field Triage. *MMWR Recomm Rep* 2012;61(RR-1):1–20.

10 Team Activation and Organization

William S. Hoff

I. **THE TRAUMA RESPONSE.** The response to an injured patient arriving at a health care institution is determined by (1) the manner in which the patient is triaged in the prehospital phase and (2) the type of facility to which the patient is being transported.

A. Institutional capability. The resources available to manage trauma patients are institution-specific. The American College of Surgeons Committee on Trauma has designated trauma centers as follows:

1. *Level I.* Provides a 24-hour, in-house trauma team with the ability to fully resuscitate injured patients and provide definitive surgical care for the most complex injuries. The trauma team is usually led by an attending trauma surgeon, emergency physician or senior-level surgical resident. Level I centers are typically located in population-dense areas. Level I trauma centers also distinguish themselves through research, training, and prevention and outreach programs.

2. *Level II.* Clinical capabilities are similar to Level I centers. However, more specialized resources (e.g., cardiac surgery, microvascular surgery) are not required. An in-house trauma surgeon is not required, but must be available to meet the patient on arrival. Level II centers are frequently located in suburban areas.

3. *Level III.* These centers typically serve rural areas not easily accessible to Level I or II trauma centers. A surgeon must be available in a timely fashion, but certain subspecialties (e.g., neurosurgery) are not required. Complex patients are routinely transferred to level I or II trauma centers.

4. *Level IV.* Provide initial evaluation and assessment of injured patients; typically located in small hospitals or clinics serving the more remote areas. Surgical coverage is not mandatory and most patients will require transfer to higher levels of care.

5. *Non-designated.* The majority of hospitals in the United States carry no specific trauma center designation. Each hospital should be aware of the resources available for management of trauma patients with clearly delineated plans for transfer of patients that exceed the "resource threshold."

B. Levels of response. All hospitals should have some established response to injured patients. In non-designated hospitals, where a full trauma team is not available, an organized procedure (e.g., personnel, tasks, etc.) will facilitate resuscitation and optimize patient outcome. Trauma centers use pre-determined tiered levels of response based on regionally established triage criteria. The composition of the trauma team varies based on the level of trauma response:

1. Full response (e.g., "trauma code," "code red"). Highest level of response designed for patients with physiologic instability, severe traumatic brain injury or who present with obvious life-threatening injuries (e.g., abdominal gunshot wound).

2. Modified response (e.g., "level II trauma," "trauma alert"). Response typically intended for physiologically stable and neurologically normal patients with the potential for serious injury based on injury mechanism or anatomic findings. Composition of the trauma team will vary with the trauma center; emergency medicine physicians frequently assume the leadership role.

3. Trauma consultation. In most trauma centers, this response is reserved for low-energy or single system injuries in stable patients. Patients are fully evaluated by an emergency medicine physician prior to consultation with a trauma surgeon.

II. TRAUMA RESUSCITATION AREA

A. Physical plant

1. A dedicated trauma resuscitation area (TRA) is required for any Level I or II trauma center and should be considered in any hospital emergency department that receives a significant volume of injured patients or where an injured patient may arrive without prior notification.

2. The TRA should be secure, with limited access to non-medical personnel.

3. Convenient access to the operating room, radiology suite, intensive care unit, and staff call rooms are other important considerations in TRA design.

4. The TRA must be sufficiently large to accommodate all members of the trauma team (i.e., 5 to 10 people). Ample space must be provided to allow free movement of prehospital providers into and out of the area, complete resuscitation, basic radiographic evaluation, orthopedic stabilization, and required emergency surgical procedures:

   a. Airway intubation

   b. Cricothyroidotomy

   c. Insertion of central venous catheters

   d. Tube thoracostomy

   e. Placement of urinary catheters and naso/orogastric tubes

   f. Emergency department thoracotomy

   g. Focused abdominal sonography for trauma (FAST)

   h. Diagnostic peritoneal lavage (DPL)

   i. Splinting of fractures

   j. Wound irrigation and suturing

5. Other TRA considerations include:

   a. Lighting should be sufficient and must allow free access to the patient and easy movement of personnel and equipment through the workspace.

   b. Hypothermia must be actively prevented during trauma resuscitation. Specific measures to prevent hypothermia include individual TRA thermostats and overhead heat lamps.

   c. A mechanism should exist to supply the TRA with uncrossmatched packed red blood cells (O-neg), especially for hospitals in which the blood bank is located a significant distance from the emergency department. Ideally, the laboratory or blood bank, as part of the trauma response, can deliver O-neg blood in a cooler to the TRA. Level I and II trauma centers should have a massive transfusion plan designed to supply large volumes of packed red blood cells, thawed plasma and platelets.

   d. Each institution must have guidelines for resuscitation of multiple trauma patients within the confines of the defined TRA or emergency department. A pre-determined plan for temporary expansion into alternate patient care areas is essential to optimal mass casualty triage and disaster management. A plan for mobilization of additional personnel should also be established.

B. Protective garments

1. Any bodily fluid should be considered a potential source of transmissible disease and, thus, barrier precautions should be mandated for all members of the trauma team. Specifically, non-sterile gloves, an impervious gown, surgical mask, protective eyewear, and shoe covers are required for all team members likely to come in contact with a patient.

2. It is not uncommon for radiographic studies to be performed concomitant with the trauma resuscitation. Appropriate protective gear (e.g., lead vests, lead aprons) should be worn by trauma team members who may be working close to the patient while radiographs are being performed. Having these garments available obviates the need to interrupt the resuscitation during x-rays.

3. Protective garments should be available in a designated area adjacent to the TRA in full view of those who may enter the area. The trauma team leader or recorder should monitor and enforce compliance with barrier precautions and radiographic protective gear.

TABLE 10-1	Immediately Accessible Equipment and Supplies

Head of stretcher Equipment for airway management, including multiple endotracheal tubes, oxygen, suction devices, oral/nasal airways, Ambu bags, and laryngoscopes
Tray #1 Equipment for intravenous access, intravenous tubing, phlebotomy, arterial blood gases
Trays #2 and #3 Thoracostomy trays, chest tubes (36 F, 40 F), appropriate suture material
Tray #4[a] Diagnostic peritoneal lavage equipment
Foot of stretcher Chest drainage system (e.g., Pleurovac)
Left side Manual blood pressure cuff, electrocardiogram wires, pulse oximetry monitor

[a]Ultrasound machine.

4. Inevitably, patients will arrive without notification. In these cases, guidelines should be developed for relieving personnel who, by necessity, have entered the TRA without barrier precautions. Protected team members should provide rapid relief for those who have not had the opportunity to don protective equipment. The ultimate goal is to minimize the total number of unprotected individuals during a given resuscitation.

5. Appropriate and visible receptacles available for disposal of used protective gear must be available within the confines of the TRA. Personnel should be discouraged from leaving the TRA with soiled gown, gloves, etc.

C. Equipment. The minimal amount of equipment and supplies necessary to effectively resuscitate should be stored in the TRA. While frequent restocking may be necessary, eliminating superfluous inventory optimizes resuscitation space and facilitates standardization of care.

1. Carts or trays may be utilized to store the most frequently used equipment (e.g., airway cart, thoracotomy tray). Equipment trays should contain only those instruments and materials absolutely necessary to perform a given procedure. Trays should be easily accessible, openly displayed, and clearly labeled for easy identification. One logical approach is to stock supplies in a head-to-toe configuration, with airway equipment and cervical collars stored near the head of the stretcher, thoracostomy trays near the midportion of the stretcher, and splinting materials near the foot of the stretcher.

2. Equipment necessary to manage immediately life-threatening conditions should be stocked close to the stretcher, in proximity to the trauma member most likely to use it (Table 10-1; Fig. 10-1).

3. Additional equipment and materials listed below can be stored along the walls of the resuscitation workspace. Large, portable equipment must be easily visible and accessible. Smaller items can be stored on shelves and counters or in designated trays or bins. Cabinets are not recommended, as closed doors impede rapid identification and ease of access.
   a. Mechanical ventilator
   b. Rapid infusion/warming device
   c. Central venous catheter, pulmonary artery catheter kits
   d. Instrument trays (e.g., basic surgical trays, plastic surgery trays)
   e. Portable monitors
   f. Suture cart
   g. Traction devices
   h. Preformed extremity splints
   i. X-ray view boxes/monitors
   j. Computers

4. A modest inventory of equipment and supplies to replace items used from other areas (e.g., angiocatheters, intravenous tubing) should be readily available.

5. Equipment and supplies should be stocked in a portable carrier that can be transported with the patient outside of the TRA. Suggested contents include:

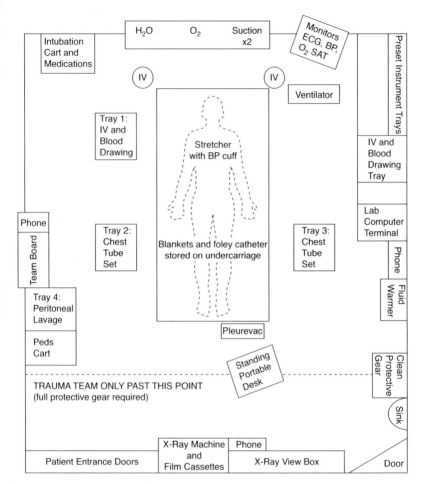

Figure 10-1. Layout of the TRA.

- **a.** Nasal and oral airways
- **b.** Cricothyroidotomy set
- **c.** Suction equipment and tubing
- **d.** Pulse oximetry probe
- **e.** Manual blood pressure cuff
- **f.** Angiocatheters (14, 16, and 18 gauge)
- **g.** Intravenous tubing and adapters
- **h.** Syringes (3, 5, and 10 mL)
- **i.** Phlebotomy supplies
- **j.** ABG syringes
- **k.** Irrigating syringe (60 mL)
- **l.** Dressings, gauze, tape
- **m.** Medications (see II.D. below)
- **n.** Additional forms for documentation
- **o.** Telephone and pager lists

6. Equipment and medications specific for pediatric resuscitation should be stored on a separate cart. The cart should be equipped with a Broselow tape for rapid calculation of medication dosages and selection of appropriately sized equipment.

7. A resuscitation stretcher should be oriented in the center of the resuscitation workspace. Several items should be ideally stored under the stretcher:
   a. Patient gowns
   b. Blankets
   c. Small oxygen tank
   d. Nasogastric/orogastric tubes
   e. Irrigation tray
   f. Automatic blood pressure cuff
   g. ECG leads
   h. Pulse oximetry leads

D. Medications in the TRA. In addition to standard medications stocked on the code cart, a small inventory of medications should be stocked in the TRA. Institutions that utilize computerized drug storage systems (e.g., Pyxis®) in the TRA or emergency department must develop a method to facilitate access for immediately required drugs.

1. Immediately available drugs include those for acute airway management: Etomidate, succinylcholine, rocuronium. Ideally, these agents should be stored in labeled syringes for instant administration.

2. Easily available agents include sedatives, analgesics, long-term paralytics, and antimicrobials: Lorazepam, morphine sulfate, fentanyl, naloxone, vecuronium, tetanus toxoid, cefazolin, and an aminoglycoside.

3. Medications that should be readily available include diphenylhydantoin, 50% dextrose, methylprednisolone, mannitol, thiamine, magnesium, and calcium.

E. Communication. Reliable communication among members of the trauma team and to areas outside of the TRA is essential. Communication in the TRA can be facilitated by the following:

1. Communication with prehospital providers prior to patient arrival facilitates preparation of the trauma team. In extreme conditions (e.g., trauma code, penetrating thoracic trauma, arrival of multiple patients), having this information allows the trauma team leader to brief the members of the trauma team and assure that each member understands their role and to anticipate potential contingencies. Direct report from the medical command physician is the simplest method to provide this information.
   a. A podium provides space to document resuscitation events and serves as an area from which the flow of activity in the TRA may be observed.
   b. Marker board can be useful to record history, physical findings, test results, and to display pertinent pager numbers of on-call consultants and ancillary personnel.
   c. Efficient communication throughout the hospital is essential. Dedicated extensions to the OR, computed tomography suite, blood bank, and the ICU should be available and use of these extensions should be limited to the trauma team. In high-volume trauma centers a laboratory computer terminal and digital radiology station should be considered.
   d. Communication between the trauma team and the OR staff is facilitated by a patient classification system. Such a system allows the OR and blood bank staff to organize resources and allocate personnel. The trauma patient classification system described in Table 10-2 provides an example. Early in the resuscitation, a single individual should be responsible for communicating the OR classification to responsible OR staff.

III. TRAUMA TEAM
A. Definition. The trauma team is an organized group of professionals who perform initial assessment and resuscitation of critically injured patients. Team composition, level of response, and responsibilities of each member are institution-specific.

TABLE 10-2	Trauma Patient Classification System

Class A Unstable patient: Requires immediate surgical intervention; no further injury evaluation (e.g., x-ray or laboratory studies) required.
Immediate access to the operating room is necessary.
Initiate massive transfusion protocol for blood and blood products (e.g., fresh frozen plasma, platelets).

Class B Unstable patient: High probability of surgical intervention within 15–30 min.
Some injury evaluation in progress.
Massive transfusion likely.

Class C Stable patient: Probability of surgical intervention within 2 h.
Complete injury evaluation (e.g., CT scan) in progress.
Crossmatched blood or type and screen sufficient.

Class D Stable patient: Minimal probability of surgical intervention (minor injuries).

Pre-defined roles and placement during the trauma resuscitation are vital to an organized resuscitative effort. Specific personnel include:

1. Trauma surgeon. A general surgeon with demonstrated training and interest in trauma care. In designated trauma centers, the trauma surgeon typically functions as the trauma team leader.
2. Emergency medicine physician. In many hospitals, the emergency medicine physician functions as the trauma team leader depending on the perceived severity of injuries. Ideally, these physicians have advanced trauma life support (ATLS) certification.
3. Anesthesiologist. A physician with special skills in airway management, sedation, and analgesia. In some trauma centers, this role may be fulfilled by a certified registered nurse anesthetist (CRNA).
4. Trauma nurses. Emergency department nurses with specialized training and demonstrated interest in trauma care.
5. Resident physicians. Residents in emergency medicine or surgery and trauma fellows may assume active roles in the trauma team. In Level I and II trauma centers, senior surgical residents and trauma fellows may function as trauma team leaders.
6. Respiratory therapist. Therapist available to assist in the evaluation and management of the patient's respiratory status as well as setting up and managing the mechanical ventilator when necessary.
7. Radiology technicians. Technicians available to obtain x-rays as indicated by the initial assessment and secondary survey.
8. Surgical subspecialists. Although not typically involved in the initial assessment, surgical consultants (e.g., orthopedic surgeons, neurosurgeons) are vital members of the trauma team.
9. Other personnel. The trauma team may also include OR nurses, laboratory technicians, ECG technicians, chaplains, social workers, transport personnel, and case managers.

B. During periods of high-volume or high-acuity (e.g., multiple victims), some internal mechanism should be available to mobilize additional personnel. In addition, appropriate on-call personnel must be available.
C. Roles and responsibilities. With adequate pre-notification, the trauma team can be organized and positioned prior to arrival of the patient. A generic positioning scheme is illustrated in Figure 10-2. Specific responsibilities of respective trauma team members are outlined in Table 10-3.
D. Multiple patient scenario
   1. All hospitals must be prepared for the arrival of multiple trauma patients, a situation that can overwhelm the resources of the best-prepared trauma center.

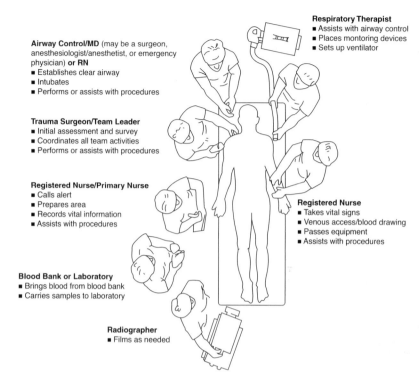

Respiratory Therapist
- Assists with airway control
- Places montoring devices
- Sets up ventilator

Airway Control/MD (may be a surgeon, anesthesiologist/anesthetist, or emergency physician) **or RN**
- Establishes clear airway
- Intubates
- Performs or assists with procedures

Trauma Surgeon/Team Leader
- Initial assessment and survey
- Coordinates all team activities
- Performs or assists with procedures

Registered Nurse/Primary Nurse
- Calls alert
- Prepares area
- Records vital information
- Assists with procedures

Registered Nurse
- Takes vital signs
- Venous access/blood drawing
- Passes equipment
- Assists with procedures

Blood Bank or Laboratory
- Brings blood from blood bank
- Carries samples to laboratory

Radiographer
- Films as needed

Figure 10-2. Positions and roles of the trauma team members.

The definition of "multiple patients" is institution-specific, based largely on the depth of personnel and the availability of resources.

2. The trauma team leader is responsible for assigning available personnel to assure safe and effective resuscitation of each patient.

3. A triage plan for positioning patients and allocating resources should be formulated based on the prehospital report and early clinical findings, for example:

   a. Position patients based on perceived needs—e.g., patients with severe head injury should be positioned near the mechanical ventilator.

   b. Assign a primary resuscitator for each patient under the direct supervision of a trauma team leader. Personnel caring for each patient must be aware of who is functioning as team leader for their respective patient. Effective communication between these individuals is of utmost importance.

   c. Recruit additional personnel. Properly trained nursing staff, prehospital providers, and technicians are potential sources of immediate in-house assistance. On-call personnel (e.g., orthopedic surgeons) may also be mobilized to assist in the resuscitative phase.

   d. Reallocate personnel and resources based on results of each patient's primary survey.

   e. Move stable patients out of the TRA to other areas of the emergency department based on clinical assessment.

IV. TRANSFER OF PATIENT TO THE TRAUMA TEAM

A. A formal report at the time of patient arrival signifies the transition of care from pre-hospital providers to the trauma team. Assuming adequate pre-notification, the

TABLE 10-3	Trauma Team Roles and Responsibilities

Trauma team leader Primarily responsible for directing individual trauma team members, coordinating events of the resuscitation, and formulating the plans for definitive management. In larger centers, especially those with training programs, the trauma team leader may be an attending trauma surgeon, emergency physician, trauma fellow, or senior or chief surgical resident (i.e., command physician).

Primary resuscitator A surgeon or emergency medicine physician responsible for the initial assessment and performance of surgical procedures, as necessary. In smaller hospitals, this individual also assumes the role of team leader.

Airway manager Anesthesiologist, CRNA, emergency physician, or surgeon primarily responsible for assessment and management of the airway. Required procedures can include endotracheal intubation, insertion of nasogastric or orogastric tubes, and assistance with cervical spine immobilization. Also expected to manage paralytics, sedatives, and analgesics relative to intubation and assist with medical management during code situations.

Assistant The assistant is responsible for exposing the patient, placing electrocardiographic leads and pulse oximeter, and assisting with patient transfers. In addition, may be asked to assist with any necessary procedures. Depending on the institution, the assistant may be a physician (e.g., surgical resident) or, in nonteaching hospitals, a trauma nurse or emergency medicine technician.

Trauma nurse Prepares the TRA for arrival of the patient. Serves as the patient's primary nurse during the resuscitative phase of care. Responsible for monitoring vital signs and performing select procedures (e.g., intravenous access, phlebotomy, urinary catheters). Assists with patient transfers, accompanies patient outside of TRA and reports to the receiving unit.

Recorder Should be a nurse with extensive experience in trauma resuscitation. Responsible for documenting events of the resuscitation on an appropriate flowsheet. Facilitates communication and mobilization of additional resources (e.g., blood bank, operating room, consultants). May also assist in coordinating events of the resuscitation.

Respiratory technician Responsible for assessment of the airway and breathing and placement of appropriate monitoring devices (e.g., pulse oximeter). Assists airway manager with intubation and ventilator setup.

Radiology technologist Performs necessary radiographic studies. Assists with positioning the patient for the required studies. Processes films and returns completed radiographs to the TRA.

Laboratory technician Draws blood samples and transports samples to the laboratory for processing. Delivers blood to the TRA before arrival of the patient. Transports additional blood and blood products to the patient as necessary.

Chaplain/social worker/case manager Assists with patient identification. Communicates between trauma team and patient's family.

trauma team can assemble prior to arrival of the patient to receive the prehospital report.

B. With few exceptions (e.g., airway compromise), patients should be maintained on the transport stretcher until the prehospital report is completed. Once the patient has been moved to the resuscitation stretcher, the trauma team may not devote full attention to the report.

C. The prehospital report should be a concise (30 to 45 seconds) summary given by a single prehospital provider and directed to the entire trauma team. The pneumonic *MIVT* offers a concise method for prehospital reporting: M = Mechanism of injury, pertinent associated factors; I = Injuries identified on prehospital survey; V = Vital signs; T = Treatment provided in the prehospital phase.

D. Following the report and transfer of the patient, a designated member of the trauma team should attempt to get a more detailed history from the prehospital providers.

AXIOMS

- Prior notification of patient arrival facilitates an organized response and offers the team leader the opportunity to adjust roles and responsibilities as necessary.
- Barrier precautions should be utilized by all trauma team members who may come in direct contact with the patient.
- The personnel placement scheme for the TRA should be routine. Equipment and supplies should be standardized, easily accessible, and stored in a clinically logical sequence.
- Minimize verbal communication among trauma team members during resuscitation.
- The presence of an identified trauma team leader promotes efficiency and facilitates formulation of a definitive plan.
- The trauma team leader should attempt to maintain a panoramic view of the resuscitation.

Suggested Readings

American College of Surgeons Committee on Trauma. *Resources for the Optimal Care of the Injured Patient*. Chicago, IL: American College of Surgeons; 2006.

Barach P, Weinger MB. Trauma team performance. In: Wilson WC, Grande CM, Hoyt DB, eds. *Trauma: Emergency Resuscitation, Perioperative Anesthesia, Surgical Management, Volume I*. New York, NY: Informa Healthcare USA, Inc.; 2007.

Center for Disease Control. Recommendations for prevention of HIV transmission in health-care settings. *MMWR Morb Mortal Wkly Rep* 1987;36(Suppl 2S):15–185.

Chhangani SV, Papadakos PJ, Wilson WC, et al. Resuscitation suite and operating room readiness. In: Wilson WC, Grande CM, Hoyt DB, eds. *Trauma: Emergency Resuscitation, Perioperative Anesthesia, Surgical Management, Volume I*. New York, NY: Informa Healthcare USA, Inc.; 2007.

Christensen EF, Deaken CD, Vilke GM, et al. Prehospital care and trauma systems. In: Wilson WC, Grande CM, Hoyt DB, eds. *Trauma: Emergency Resuscitation, Perioperative Anesthesia, Surgical Management, Volume I*. New York, NY: Informa Healthcare USA, Inc.; 2007.

DiGiacomo JC, Hoff WS. Universal barrier precautions in the emergency department. *Hosp Physician* 1997;33:11.

Driscoll PA, Vincent CA. Organizing an efficient trauma team. *Injury* 1992;23:107.

Fernandez L, McKenney MG, McKenney KL, et al. Ultrasound in blunt abdominal trauma. *J Trauma* 1998;45:841.

Gunnels D, Gunnels M. The Critical Response Nurse role: an innovative solution for providing skilled trauma nurses. *Int J Trauma Nurs* 2001;7:3.

Hoff WS, Reilly PM, Rotondo MF, et al. The importance of the command-physician in trauma resuscitation. *J Trauma* 1997;43:772.

Maull KI, Rhodes M. Trauma center design. In: Feliciano DB, Moore EE, eds. *Trauma*. Norwalk, CT: Appleton & Lange; 1996.

Moore EE. Resuscitation and evaluation of the injured patients. In: Zuidema GD, Rutherford RB, Ballinger WF, eds. *The Management of Trauma*. Philadelphia, PA: WB Saunders; 1985.

Morgan T, Berger P, Land S, et al. Trauma center design and the OR. *AORN J* 1986;44:416.

O'Brien J, Fothergill-Bourbonnais F. The experience of trauma resuscitation in the emergency department: themes from seven patients. *J Emerg Nurs* 2004;30:216.

TeamSTEPPS®: Strategies and Tools to Enhance Performance and Patient Safety. Agency for Healthcare Research and Quality. Rockville, MD. http://www.ahrq.gov/qual/teamstepps

11 Imaging of Trauma Patients

Asim F. Choudhri

I. **INTRODUCTION.** Medical imaging provides a noninvasive assessment of bone and soft tissue injuries. The most appropriate imaging modality depends upon factors including the location and availability of equipment, stability of the patient, and local expertise and care pathways. The goal of imaging is to provide the maximum information to the trauma team as quickly as possible while minimizing risk to the patient.

Imaging modalities

A. **Conventional radiography** ("x-rays") provides a quick method of evaluating patients; these are well suited for evaluating bony architecture and for screening in chest injuries. The immediate evaluation of the trauma patient starts with anterior–posterior (AP) chest and pelvis radiographs. These studies can be performed using the portable technique, without moving the patient from the trauma resuscitation room. Further radiography, such as of the long bones, is typically deferred until after initial resuscitation and CT scans are performed. However, x-rays can selectively be performed as a part of the primary survey as needed. Spine radiographs have a limited role for the primary detection of fractures in adults, however, remain an important part of the spine evaluation in children.

Initial chest x-ray studies are usually performed in the supine position. After the initial stabilization of the patient, an upright film may be obtained to better assess for aortic injury, pneumothorax, or pleural effusion.

B. **Computed tomography (CT)** has become the standard modality used in the early diagnosis of head, spine, thoracoabdominal, and pelvic injury, often in one combined study. CT provides a comprehensive evaluation of chest injuries and maxillofacial fractures and allows for specific diagnosis of injury to the organs of the abdomen and retroperitoneum. The increasing availability of multislice helical CT in or near the emergency department expanded the role of CT in the trauma setting.

C. **Magnetic resonance imaging (MRI)** has several advantages over CT scan, particularly in the evaluation of soft tissues. MRI offers the ability to obtain images in sagittal, coronal, and oblique planes, and can be used to define shear injuries to the brain, injuries to the spinal column and cord, or vascular abnormalities that are not apparent on other films. However, MRI is time-consuming and allows minimal access to the patient during the procedure; together, these factors limit the application in the initial evaluation of the trauma patient. Currently, MRI is used after stabilization, often to detect neurologic injuries or occult fractures.

D. **Ultrasonography (US)** is a valuable tool for the management of trauma patients. The focused abdominal sonography for trauma (FAST) has largely replaced the diagnostic peritoneal lavage (DPL) in unstable patients. A rapid diagnosis of hemoperitoneum can be made noninvasively in the trauma patient with a sensitivity of approximately 85%. US is quite accurate for the diagnosis of pericardial tamponade, allowing for decreased need for diagnostic pericardial window. US can also be used to assess for peripheral vascular injury.

E. **Angiography.** Standard two-dimensional angiography has been largely replaced by CT angiography in the diagnosis of vascular traumatic injury. If said scans are equivocal or negative in the face of a high index of suspicion, angiography is a dynamic study with a very high spatial resolution, allowing detection vascular extravasation. In addition, its therapeutic role in such injuries has expanded.

Angiography with embolization is the procedure of choice for difficult-to-access injuries (e.g., those to the vertebral artery, pelvic vessels, retroperitoneum) and selected vessels of the chest, abdomen, and large muscle masses.

II. SKULL AND BRAIN TRAUMA

A. Plain-film skull radiography is only used for penetrating injuries of the skull to determine the course, location, or number of gunshots or foreign-body fragments as well as possible depressed skull fragments.

B. Patients with a head injury, history of loss of consciousness (LOC), or postconcussive sequelae require evaluation by non-contrast CT scan. CT scan of the brain should be the initial screening tool for patients with symptoms indicating moderate to high risk of closed head injury. The CT scan images should be displayed with three windows: Brain (shows edema, gray–white interface, ventricles, and cisterns), bone (outlines fractures, bony fragments), and blood (mass lesions, hemorrhage). Contrast enhancement is used selectively after non-contrast if occult extra-axial fluid collections, abscess, tumor, or venous sinus obstruction is sought.

1. **Common CT findings of brain injury**
   a. **Basilar skull fractures** can occur in 20% of craniofacial injuries, and CT is essential for complete evaluation. However, a negative CT scan does not exclude basilar skull fracture, especially with positive physical findings or unexplained pneumocephalus. Basilar skull fractures can be accompanied by cerebrospinal fluid (CSF) leak, damage to the internal carotid artery, and cranial nerve injury. Multislice CT with multi-planar reconstruction of thin sections greatly improves the ease and accuracy of diagnosing basilar skull fractures. CT cisternography, which is high resolution skull base imaging after the injection of intrathecal iodinated contrast, can help localize a CSF leak from an occult skull base fracture; this technique is not typically performed in the acute setting.
   b. **Epidural hematomas** result from the rupture of arteries and large venous sinuses resulting in an accumulation of blood that strips the dura off the inner table of the skull. The temporal region of the skull is most commonly injured, resulting in a tear of the middle meningeal artery. The characteristic appearance of an epidural hematoma is a biconvex (lentiform) fluid collection that does not cross intact skull suture lines but can cross the midline if venous sinuses are ruptured.
   c. **Subdural hematomas** result from the dissection of blood from ruptured veins that bridge through the subdural space. These hematomas are generally located between the dura and the arachnoid membrane. The typical subdural hematoma is a crescent-shaped fluid collection that conforms to the calvarium and underlying cerebral cortex. Recognition of atypical subdural hematomas is sometimes aided by coronal CT scan or repeat CT scan with enhancement. Subdural hematomas often are accompanied by nearby parenchymal contusion.
   d. **Subarachnoid hemorrhage** is seen commonly in the basilar cisterns of patients following head trauma. Non–contrast-enhanced CT detects about 90% of subarachnoid bleeding within the first 24 hours, regardless of cause, as the higher density of blood replaces the water density of CSF in the cistern and sulci. Like non-traumatic subarachnoid hemorrhage, vascular evaluation with angiography is important if the degree of hemorrhage is out of proportion to the mechanism of trauma.
   e. **Shear injury or diffuse axonal injury (DAI).** Most brain parenchymal injuries are caused by shear-strain lesions; multiple and bilateral injuries are common. Linear and rotational acceleration–deceleration mechanisms cause shearing along interfaces of tissue of different densities, such as CSF and brain as well as gray–white junctions with the brain and meninges. Unenhanced CT scan may show multiple small focal hemorrhagic lesions with minimal mass effect, but it is an insensitive test. In a patient who is severely depressed

neurologically with a relatively normal CT study, the possibility of diffuse brain injury (or cerebrovascular injury) should be considered. MRI is more accurate in diagnosing diffuse axonal brain injury, in particular susceptibility weighted imaging (SWI). If SWI is not available, a hemosiderin sensitive gradient imaging (GRE) should be performed in all trauma patients. Areas of hemorrhage will appear as focal dark spots. Multiple petechial hemorrhages, predominantly at the gray–white interface and within the corpus callosum, is characteristic of DAI.

f. **Cerebral contusions and parenchymal hematomas** are relatively common findings seen on brain CT after injury. Such injuries can coalesce or enlarge. Routine follow-up CT is recommended in these patients within 24 to 48 hours, or sooner if there are changes in the neurologic examination. MR of the brain with SWI/GRE can be helpful evaluating the extent of injury which may be underestimated by CT.

III. **FACIAL TRAUMA.** Facial injuries are seldom directly life threatening, but often are associated with airway obstruction, head or cervical spine injury, or globe injury. Occasionally, hemorrhage into the nose, nasopharynx, or mouth requires immediate attention.

A. **CT is preferred to evaluate facial fractures;** plain films often miss injuries and are challenging to interpret due to bony overlap.

B. **CT scans of the face** can be obtained at the time of head CT scan if patient condition permits. Helically acquired CT imaging can be reformatted into thin section axial and coronal bone algorithm datasets. Three-dimensional (3D) reconstructions from the volumetric dataset provide optimal delineation of midfacial fractures and the spatial relationship of the fragments.

IV. **SPINE INJURIES.** Every patient with an appropriate mechanism of injury (MOI) must be considered to have a spine injury until ruled out with imaging or by clinical features.

A. **Cervical spine. An alert, communicative adult trauma victim without distracting injury who denies symptoms, such as neck pain, without drugs or alcohol on board, and has no signs, such as neck tenderness, may be "cleared" on the basis of clinical examination.** Patients with head injury often have accompanying cervical spine (C-spine) injuries, and radiographic evaluation of the C-spine is essential. The unconscious, intoxicated, noncommunicative, or multi-injured patient needs radiographic clearance. The cervical collar must not be removed until the C-spine has been evaluated and cleared.

1. **Techniques for obtaining adequate plain-film radiographs for C-spine clearance**

a. The plain-film lateral view of the C-spine is not adequate unless C1 through the top of T1 are visualized. If the shoulders obscure the lower cervical and upper thoracic spine, caudal traction of the arms must be applied during filming, unless contraindicated on clinical grounds. Useful techniques to further define the C-spine include the "swimmer's view" or left and right oblique views. Failure to adequately visualize the cervicothoracic junction or the craniocervical junction will necessitate CT scan.

b. **Technically adequate lateral, AP, and open-mouth odontoid C-spine films are the minimal views necessary to evaluate the C-spine radiographically.** A very small percentage of patients with C-spine injury have isolated ligamentous injury and grossly normal static plain radiographs. Other studies, such as flexion–extension views, left and right oblique views, CT scan, or MRI, may delineate these injuries or investigate areas that are not well visualized on plain films.

i. Active flexion–extension views are done voluntarily by the alert and cooperative patient only to the limit of pain tolerance. Recent practice tends to use flexion–extension views less often and rely on CT with reformatting and MRI when needed.

    c. The purpose of the radiographic evaluation is to identify potential C-spine bony injury that has not caused a neurologic deficit. In the hemodynamically unstable patient, protect and immobilize the spine, treat the condition causing instability, and clear the spine when the patient's condition permits. **Do not spend time attempting to clear the C-spine in a hemodynamically unstable patient.**

    d. The availability of a CT scan within or near the emergency department facilitates emergent evaluation of C-spine trauma. In particular, **MDCT offers the opportunity to obtain definitive and easily interpretable imaging of the C-spine quickly.** These scanners also offer greater flexibility in 3D image reconstructing. Reliable coronal and sagittal reformations are easily obtained from the initial scan without the need for reimaging. CT scan is the imaging modality of choice for suspected fractures and fracture–dislocations of the spine in which plain films are not diagnostic. These scans are usually performed on an axial plane with thin (1 mm) cuts.

    e. MRI is the imaging procedure of choice for evaluation of injuries to the spinal cord, ligaments, and discs. While MRI is very sensitive to detect marrow edema from fractures or bone contusions; it is best used as a complementary technique to CT and does not replace it. In patients with myelopathy, MRI can establish the location, extent, and nature of the cord injury, as well as demonstrate the location and nature of nerve root injury in patients with radiculopathy. Blood products within a cord contusion (hematomyelia) predict subsequent functional deficits. An MRI should be obtained to evaluate the spinal cord or suspected ligamentous injury, such as disruption of the posterior ligament complex due to anterior subluxation (whiplash).

B. Thoracic and lumbar spine. Plain films of the thoracic and lumbar spine are an initial screening option signs; symptoms of MOI suggest a spine injury. **If head and thoraco-abdominal CT is planned, spine reformats are easily obtained and offer better detail, obviate the need for plain films, and result in no additional radiation exposure.** In the patient with distracting injuries (e.g., chest or pelvic fractures) or a concomitant C-spine injury, a complete thoracic and lumbar (T&L) spine series is necessary. Certain mechanisms of injury warrant radiographic evaluation of the T&L spine: Automobile–pedestrian collisions, rollovers, ejections from a vehicle, collisions involving unrestrained automobile passengers, motorcycle crashes, or falls from a height.

    1. Plain radiographs must include two views of the area of concern: Usually AP and lateral. Oblique views can be helpful, but CT scan directed to the suspected area of injury is preferred. Portable studies are often impractical because of patient size, and the osseous detail required to exclude a fracture. In this circumstance, the patient should have done these films in the radiology department, with proper monitoring and trauma team presence. MDCT also offers the ability to reliably review areas of concern by reformatting images obtained from scans of the chest, abdomen, and pelvis. Some institutions routinely generate 3D reconstruction of the CT thoracolumbar spine images as part of the chest/abdomen/pelvis CT.

V. CHEST TRAUMA

A. The chest x-ray is the fundamental and primary examination in chest trauma. A frontal AP chest radiograph should be obtained in all major trauma cases. Ideally, an erect chest film is obtained because the anatomic alterations caused by the supine position can simulate disease (e.g., a widened mediastinum or interstitial lung disease) and mask pleural effusions or pneumothorax. However, the upright position is usually not possible. To decrease magnification artifacts, the distance from the x-ray tube (camera) to the film should be maximized to approximately 60 to 72 in. (5 to 6 ft) in either the supine or reverse Trendelenberg position.

    1. Acute aortic injury should be suspected in any patient who suffers a significant deceleration injury. The most common type and site of aortic injury is an incomplete tear through the intima and media of the descending thoracic aorta, just distal to the left subclavian artery. Mediastinal hemorrhage is present in most patients with aortic injury. However, 7% to 10% of patients with thoracic aortic injury have a normal admission chest x-ray study. In addition, only 10% to 20% of patients with plain chest film findings of mediastinal widening prove to have an aortic laceration.

  a. A patient who has radiographic evidence of mediastinal bleeding may be clinically stable enough to allow definitive imaging evaluation of the aorta. There are common radiographic findings on plain chest film that are associated with blunt thoracic aortic injury, including a widened mediastinum (>8 cm), obliteration of the aortic knob, aortopulmonary window opacification, left apical pleural cap, deviation of the trachea to the right, depression of the left main stem bronchus, widened paraspinous stripe, and a left pleural effusion. Any of these findings alert the physician to the possibility of aortic injury. Due to limitations of plain-film radiography in the trauma setting, **any adult patient with significant blunt MOI should undergo CT angiography of the thorax.**

  2. **CT scan is now the imaging modality of choice for the definitive diagnosis of aortic injury.** Scanners using spiral and multislice technology are more accurate than earlier generation CT in the evaluation of the thoracic aorta and have been shown to accurately detect aortic injury. A complete scan of the chest plus the abdomen and pelvis can now be obtained without any increase in contrast exposure or time. CT findings of suspected aortic injury should be considered as representing:

  a. Normal (no mediastinal blood, normal aortic contour)
  b. Positive (mediastinal hemorrhage plus abnormal aortic contour)
  c. Equivocal (mediastinal hemorrhage without an apparent aortic or arterial abnormality)

  Any uncertainty regarding aortic or major vascular injury requires catheter angiography, if the patient is hemodynamically stable. If injuries to aortic branch vessels is suspected, angiography is required as these injuries may not be detected on CT.

  3. The diagnosis of **diaphragmatic rupture** is difficult to make on plain film. Apparent elevation and distortion of the hemidiaphragm (usually the left) can be evident along with ancillary findings such as pleural effusion or rib fractures. Disruption of the diaphragm, the presence of abdominal contents outside the contour of the diaphragm (i.e., abdominal organs lying in a dependent position near the ribs), nasogastric tube in the chest, and the "pinched" appearance of a herniated bowel are reliable signs. CT scan using sagittal and coronal reformations can be useful in appreciating the altered contour of the diaphragm, but even with CT scan, this diagnosis can be difficult.

  a. The optimal imaging procedure for diagnosis of equivocal diaphragmatic rupture is MRI in the sagittal and coronal planes. This can only be employed after the patient has been stabilized. In the acute setting, with an unstable or marginal trauma patient, helical CT is the diagnostic procedure of choice.

  4. **Most clinically important lung parenchymal and pleural space abnormalities** are well seen on plain radiograph examinations. CT scan can reveal unsuspected pneumothorax or hemothorax, commonly seen on the upper cuts of an abdominal CT scan.

VI. ABDOMINAL TRAUMA

  A. **Penetrating trauma** from gunshot wounds (GSWs) to the abdomen constitutes a special problem in preoperative evaluation. Chest and abdominal plain films can aid in determining trajectory and localization of opaque foreign bodies and to identify injury in the stable patient. Large radiographs are used with radiographic markers placed over each skin penetration site. Two films are usually necessary, one under the chest and the second overlapping the chest slightly but covering the abdomen and pelvis. There are two important caveats. First, low-velocity missiles do not always go in straight lines. They often strike solid tissue, including bones, the abdominal wall and organs, and then change direction. Second, x-rays are best deferred in the unstable patient with clear intra-abdominal injury.

1. In hemodynamically stable patients with GSWs, some have advocated a "one-shot intravenous pyelogram (IVP)" to evaluate potential renal or ureteral injuries. In addition to demonstrating injuries, it can prove the presence and function of the contralateral kidney. The yield is very low in the patient without hematuria. **We recommend the excretory phase CT,** which involves repeating the pertinent cuts after contrast has reached the collecting system. This accurate evaluation of the renal collecting system adds only a few minutes to the standard abdominal CT, and may also be valuable in evaluating blunt renal injury.

2. **Technique for a plainfilm IVP**
   a. Large-bore intravenous (IV) catheters are used to inject contrast material.
   b. 100 mL of 60% contrast is infused rapidly.
   c. A 2 minute post-injection film is obtained to show a bilateral nephrogram.
   d. Contrast material should be visualized in the renal collecting system and ureters on a 10 minute film.
   e. This study is contraindicated in patients with a severe allergy to iodinated contrast.

3. **Findings include**
   a. Delayed function and visualization can be seen in renal contusion and minor parenchymal fractures.
   b. Nonvisualization of a portion of the kidney usually indicates injury to that specific area and requires additional studies (i.e., CT scan or angiography).
   c. Nonvisualization on one side is typical of major vascular injury such as renal artery injury, thrombosis, or renal pedicle avulsion. Unilateral nonvisualization prompts immediate arteriography or surgery to establish diagnosis.
   Some centers prefer plain-film evaluation and surgical exploration with on-table IVP. This is best used when clinical need for rapid exploration of the abdomen already exists and avoids unnecessary delays.

4. **Stable** patients with stab wounds to the back or flank can be evaluated by **triple-contrast–enhanced CT scan.** GSWs that are thought to be tangential or extraperitoneal also can be evaluated with this study. Contrast material is administered orally, intravenously, and rectally prior to imaging.

B. **Blunt trauma.** In selecting the various diagnostic methods to evaluate blunt abdominal trauma, many factors are considered: Clinical status of the patient, accuracy of the results, experience and expertise of those performing and interpreting the examination, cost, safety, and availability of the procedure.

1. **Plain radiography is not helpful for identification of significant abdominal injuries following blunt abdominal trauma.**

2. **CT scan has replaced DPL** as the method for screening blunt abdominal trauma in **stable** patients. (**FAST** has replaced DPL as the screening tool for abdominal injury in **unstable** patients.) The major time factor in CT evaluation lies in the transport and positioning of the patient. Actual scanning and reconstruction of the images are done quickly. CT is accurate in identifying and quantifying hemoperitoneum, as well as identifying the site and extent of solid-organ injury; CT diagnosis of bowel injury is more challenging. A patient who remains hemodynamically unstable following resuscitation is not a candidate for CT scan or other potentially time-consuming diagnostic imaging studies. In these patients, US or DPL is recommended.
   a. CT provides valuable information regarding the depth and extent of abdominal visceral injuries, the extent of hemorrhage, and other criteria that correlate with the American Association for the Surgery of Trauma (AAST) grade of injury and prognosis. A properly performed and interpreted CT scan reliably demonstrates active bleeding (extravasation), which usually indicates a need for surgery or transcatheter angiographic embolization.
   b. The technique for abdominal CT scan is
      i. Intravenous contrast with or without oral contrast media. No IV contrast material should be given until the head scan is completed. The IV contrast (100 to 150 mL of 60% contrast) must be administered at a rate of

2.5 to 3.0 mL/s. In those with contrast allergy or renal failure not on dialysis should not receive IV contrast.

ii. The oral contrast material is a dilute solution (2%) of aqueous iodinated contrast medium (e.g., gastrografin or gastroview). Alert patients can drink the solution, whereas patients with altered sensorium have the solution administered through a nasogastric or orogastric tube after evacuation of stomach contents. Although the safety of oral contrast has been demonstrated, there is still much debate about its utility in the trauma setting, notably aspiration risk and real added value in detecting injury. We recommend using this selectively rather than routine, deploying it when hollow viscus injury is suspected in a stable patient. Again, CT absent oral contrast is a good tool in initial care.

iii. If used, give oral contrast as early as possible prior to the scan in order to facilitate bowel opacification and to minimize delays within the CT scan suite. Any delays in obtaining the scan in order to allow gastrointestinal passage of contrast material are not recommended.

c. Routine scans are done with slices taken at 5 mm intervals from the nipple line (upper heart) to the upper thigh (lesser trochanter). Helical CT scanners allow faster acquisition of higher resolution scans. MDCT scanners may acquire contiguous 1.0 to 2.5 mm thick sections. These are usually viewed as 5 mm thick sections, while the thinner sections are utilized to construct high-resolution, sagittal, coronal, and 3D images.

3. **Ultrasonography (FAST)** is useful in the diagnosis of hemoperitoneum. US is less accurate than CT in the diagnosis of injuries to solid abdominal viscera and does not depict bowel injuries nor the source of hemorrhage. **FAST** examination is used concomitantly with early resuscitation to rapidly determine hemoperitoneum, hemopericardium, or hemothorax. Due to the potential for false negative examinations, stable patients with appropriate MOI should undergo abdominal CT.

4. The diagnosis of hollow viscous injury is probably the most challenging aspect of the radiographic evaluation of the trauma patient. CT findings indicative of bowel injuries include extraluminal air or oral contrast, and suggestive findings include bowel wall or mesenteric thickening, and free intraperitoneal fluid. CT has been proven to be highly accurate when there is a positive finding or in the setting of a completely negative scan. But, sensitivity of CT for hollow viscus injury has been reported to be 70% to 90%. **If the CT is equivocal or there is a high clinical suspicion of bowel injury, close clinical monitoring with serial examinations is mandatory. Patients without intact neurologic status are especially problematic, and diagnosis is often delayed.**

VII. PELVIC TRAUMA

A. **The plain AP pelvic film is the key to the early diagnosis of pelvic fracture.** If the alert and communicative patient is asymptomatic without distracting injuries, this x-ray study is not essential. This radiographic examination requires a frontal pelvic view that includes the iliac crests, both hip joints, and the proximal portion of both femurs. This can be supplemented by angled projections of the pelvis of the caudal ("inlet") and cephalad ("outlet") because these provide a more accurate delineation of the extent and relationship of pelvic fractures and joint disruptions.

B. **Traditionally, CT scan has had a minimal role** in the immediate evaluation of the acutely injured pelvis. However, helical CT is now an easy and fast way to accurately identify active hemorrhage associated with pelvic fractures. CT scan is also the most accurate method for assessing the need for operation. Computer-generated 3D images from the axial CT sections of the pelvis assist in preoperative display and reconstruction of complex pelvic fractures. No second scan is necessary; therefore using 3D reconstructions will not delay any operative intervention. Pelvic CT scan is essential in determining:

1. Pelvic ring disruptions
2. The spatial orientation and relationship of complex or displaced pelvic ring fragments
3. The presence of joint instability
4. Intra-articular fragments
5. Fractures of the articular surface of the acetabulum or femoral head

C. Immediate pelvic angiography is best in patients with hemodynamic instability from pelvic fracture, allowing identification of pelvic arterial bleeding sites and transcatheter embolization. Between 6% and 18% of patients with unstable pelvic ring disruption have pelvic arterial injuries that warrant embolization. When pelvic arterial bleeding is found at angiography, embolization successfully occludes the bleeding artery in 80% to 90% of cases. Completion arteriography is required to ensure control of hemorrhage after therapeutic embolization. If the patient has a torn venous plexus or cancellous bone fragments are bleeding, angiographic embolization may not succeed and immediate operative intervention may be required.

D. **Retrograde urethrography (RUG)** is essential in the evaluation of urethral injuries. Rupture of the bladder or urethral laceration occurs in approximately 20% of patients with pelvic ring disruptions. RUG is indicated for any male patient who has blood at the urethral meatus or a scrotal or perineal hematoma. When any of these findings are present, a RUG should be performed prior to insertion of a Foley catheter.

   1. **Technique for RUG**
      a. An irrigating syringe filled with 10 mL of sterile 30% contrast material is inserted into the urethral meatus.
      b. The penis is stretched slightly to the side.
      c. The urethra is filled with the 10 mL bolus of contrast material.
      d. Two films are acquired – AP and at a 30-degree oblique angle – immediately after injection to demonstrate the prostatic and membranous urethra.

   2. **Alternate technique**
      a. Pass an 8 F Foley catheter into the urethral meatus (approximately 3 to 4 cm).
      b. Position the balloon of the Foley catheter in the distal urethra with sufficient fluid to maintain a tight fit (usually 2 to 4 mL).
      c. Inject the sterile undiluted contrast material (10 mL) in a retrograde fashion, allowing for easy and complete filling of the urethra.

   3. **Findings**
      a. **The most common site of urethral disruption** is the prostate-membranous urethral junction.
      b. **Extravasation of contrast** will be seen at the apex of the prostatic urethra, from the membranous urethra at the triangular ligament.
      c. **Partial visualization** indicates incomplete disruption.
      d. Complete disruption is indicated by an absence of contrast material in the bladder or prostatic urethra.

E. **If the urethrogram is negative, a cystogram is performed.**
   1. **Technique for a cystogram**
      a. Pass a 16 F Foley catheter into the bladder.
      b. Gravity fill the bladder with 300 to 400 mL of sterile undiluted contrast material (i.e., Cystografin).
      c. Frontal and oblique radiographs of the bladder are obtained when the bladder is full.
      d. An AP post-void film is obtained to determine if an extraperitoneal bladder rupture is present.

   2. **Findings**
      a. **Severe pelvic and lower abdominal pain,** caused by extravasation of the contrast material, is a clinical indication of bladder rupture.
      b. **In the unconscious patient,** free flow of the diluted contrast fluid can indicate bladder rupture and intraperitoneal extravasation.
      c. **These films detect bladder rupture with 98% accuracy.**

VIII. IMAGING IN THE INTENSIVE CARE UNIT (ICU). The imaging techniques discussed in this chapter are applicable to the trauma patient in the ICU. Patients requiring ICU care may have many of their imaging studies performed in the ICU.

A. Chest x-rays
   1. A daily chest x-ray may be indicated in any patient who has one or more of the following (can vary with hospital protocol):
   a. Acute respiratory failure
   b. Endotracheal intubation
   c. Positive end-expiratory pressure (PEEP) ≥ 5 cm H_2O
   d. $FiO_2 \geq 0.5$
   e. Chest tube in place
   f. Under treatment for active disease (e.g., pneumonia, atelectasis, etc.)
   2. Selective daily chest x-rays in the ICU for the following patients:
   a. Weaning mode without change in cardiopulmonary status
   3. Chest x-ray is indicated after the following:
   a. Any acute cardiac or pulmonary deterioration
   b. Any invasive chest procedure (e.g., placement of a chest tube, central venous catheter, feeding tube, or endoscopy)
   4. Chest x-rays are not necessary when
   a. A central line was changed over a guidewire without difficulty.
   b. No respiratory care changes in patients with drain tubes or mechanical ventilation.

B. Computed tomography
   1. CT scan of the head is used when an unexplained change occurs in neurologic status or as a follow-up for a previous CT scan of head injury. CT scan for encephalopathy or multiple-system organ failure has a low yield.
   2. CT scan of the chest can be helpful in delineating the pathology involved in acute pulmonary failure (e.g., consolidated lung, loculated collections, empyema, pulmonary embolism).
   3. CT scan of the abdomen without history or physical examination suggesting intraperitoneal pathology is of little benefit. CT scan of the abdomen can be helpful if:
   a. The patient has had previous surgery
   b. It is performed to confirm a presumptive clinical diagnosis
   c. It is necessary to direct a percutaneous study or procedure (i.e., abscess drainage)
   d. Missed intraperitoneal injury is suspected
   e. There is a suspicion of pancreatitis

C. Ultrasound
   1. Bedside US in the ICU is helpful to localize fluid collections and to diagnose acalculous cholecystitis.
   2. Duplex ultrasound can be useful in detecting venous thrombosis or arterial injury.
   3. US is indicated if **pericardial tamponade is suspected.**

D. Fluoroscopy
   1. Fluoroscopy is being used in the ICU to guide the placement of invasive devices such as pulmonary artery catheters, central lines, inferior vena cava (IVC) filters, or enteral feeding tubes.

IX. ADDITIONAL CONSIDERATIONS. (MRI SAFETY, OBESE, MOBILE, RADIATION) Beyond the MOI and patient stability, there are several additional considerations for the optimal planning and interpretation of imaging in trauma patients, including radiation and MRI safety, access to images, and imaging strategies optimized for the obese patient.

A. Radiation safety
   1. The risk–benefit ratio for any study must be considered, especially when it involves ionizing radiation. Radiation reduction practices can be implemented with minimal impact on diagnostic accuracy. The general principle for radiation

exposure is to perform a diagnostic evaluation using a dose as low as reasonably achievable **(ALARA).** Decreasing radiation dose is especially important in the pediatric and pregnant population, as long as it can be done without impairing diagnostic accuracy.

Ways to reduce radiation dose include:

a. Reduction in radiation dose parameters for CT. The two main parameters are the milliamperes (mAs) and peak voltage (kVp). Modern CT scanners can automatically calculate the radiation dose per scan, and this information can be tabulated and compared to recommended dose tables.

b. Eliminating redundant evaluations (e.g., not performing spine radiographs if a CT has been performed)

c. Performing follow-up studies with a technique that uses less or no radiation (e.g., following a pleural effusion with radiographs or ultrasound instead of CT)

d. Not performing multiphase CT scans when not needed (e.g., post-contrast CT of the head serves little role in the evaluation of acute trauma)

e. Not repeating scans that have been performed at an outside institution prior to patient transfer, if the previous scans are of diagnostic quality

B. MRI safety

1. There are many absolute and relative contraindications to MR scanning. 3.0 Tesla MRI involves a magnetic field greater than 30,000 times stronger than that of the earth's magnetic field, which can interfere with implanted medical devices and metallic foreign bodies. As a detailed medical history is not always available in trauma patients, careful screening procedures must take place to prevent injuries to the patient and caregivers. Some metallic foreign bodies can become projectiles, heat adjacent tissue, and if it forms a loop (such as a metal necklace or looped ECG lead) can act as a generator of electrical current in the alternating magnetic field.

2. MRI scans can take more than 30 minutes per study, and significantly longer if multiple body parts are being evaluated (e.g., MRI of the total spine). It must be determined that the patient can safely be away from the ICU or floor for the study, with knowledge that the MRI scanner may have fewer monitoring and resuscitation capabilities than the ICU.

C. Electronic and mobile review of images

1. Modern trauma evaluation is best performed with access to electronic viewing of medical images in a picture archiving and communication system (PACS). This allows ready access to comparison images, image manipulation such as zooming and measuring, allows multiple physicians to simultaneously review images, and essentially negates the chances of a lost film.

2. PACS access can allow subspecialty review of images by physicians not in the hospital or at a different hospital, allowing rapid triage of patients and planning for possible surgical intervention and/or patient transfer.

3. Review of images is currently possible on mobile devices, further increasing the ability to rapidly triage patients and obtain subspecialty input.

D. The obese patient

1. Imaging the obese patient provides challenges for both diagnostic accuracy and patient safety; challenges which are encountered more frequently than in the past.

a. CT scanners previously had a weight limit of approximately 350 lb, varying by model and manufacturer. The bore size of the CT scanner may also prevent patients with large abdominal girth from entering the scanner. If the local scanner does not allow safe performance of the study, an alternate evaluation approach must be taken. If diagnostic information cannot be adequately obtained by other modalities (e.g., radiography, fluoroscopy, ultrasound, DPL, etc.), it may be necessary to transfer a patient to a center than has the capabilities of caring for these patients.

b. MRI scanners typically have smaller bores than CT scanners, and many patients may not fit within the scanner even if they do not exceed the stated weight limit. Patients that barely fit within the scanner may also complain of claustrophobia. As soft tissue acts as an "antenna" in the high field strength of an MRI scanner, obese patients can experience measurable increases in body temperature during a study due to high amounts of energy deposition.

AXIOMS

- The more severely compromised the patient, the more directed the initial radiographic evaluation.
- Specific images should be obtained to answer the most vital and highest priority questions.
- Do not spend time attempting to clear the C-spine in an unstable patient.
- Axial skeletal and pelvic films are not needed in an alert patient without signs or symptoms of these injuries or intoxication/altered sensorium.
- MDCT has revolutionized the radiographic evaluation of the trauma patient, with increased use in the ED but still an evolving thought on best use.

Suggested Readings

Boone DC, Federle MP, Billiar TR, et al. Evolution of management of major hepatic trauma: Identification of patterns of injury. *J Trauma* 1995;39:344–350.

Butela ST, Federle MP, Chang PJ, et al. Performance of CT in detection of bowel injury. *AJR Am J Roentgenol* 2001;176:129–135.

Choudhri AF, Radvany MR. Initial experience with a handheld device dicom viewer: osirix mobile on the iPhone. *J Digital Imaging* 2011;24(2):184–189.

Dyer DS, Moore EE, Ilke DN, et al. Thoracic aortic injury: How predictive is mechanism and is chest computed tomography a reliable screening tool? *J Trauma* 2000;48:673–683.

Fabian TC, Davis KA, Gavant ML, et al. Prospective study of blunt aortic injury: Helical CT is diagnostic and antihypertensive therapy reduces rupture. *Ann Surg* 1998;227:666–677.

Federle MP, Courcoulas AP, Powell M, et al. Blunt splenic injury in adults: Clinical and CT criteria for management, with emphasis on active extravasation. *Radiology* 1998;206:137–142.

Frankel H, Rozycki G, Ochsner M, et al. Indications for obtaining surveillance thoracic and lumbar spine radiographs in injured patients. *J Trauma* 1994;37(4):626–633.

Grogan EL, Morris JA, Dittus RS, et al. Cervical spine evaluation in urban trauma centers: Lowering institutional costs and complications through helical CT scan. *J Am Coll Surg* 2005;200:160–165.

Harris JP, Nelson RC. Abdominal imaging with multidetector computed tomography: State of the art. *J Comput Assist Tomogr* 2004;28:S17–S19.

Holmes JF, Mirvis SE, Panacek EA, et al. Variability in computed tomography and magnetic resonance imaging in patients with cervical spine injury. *J Trauma* 2002;53:524–530.

Image Gently – Alliance for Radiation Safety in Pediatric Imaging. http://www.imagegently.org

Mirvis SE, Shanmuganathan K, Miller BH, et al. Traumatic aortic injury: Diagnosis with contrast-enhanced thoracic CT—five-year experience at a major trauma center. *Radiology* 1996;200:413–422.

Novelline RA, Rhea JT, Rao PM, et al. Helical CT in emergency radiology. *Radiology* 1999;213:321–339.

Phillipp MO, Kubin TM, Hormann M, et al. Three-dimensional volume rendering of multidetector-row CT data: Applicable for emergency radiology. *Eur J Rad* 2003;48:33–38.

Ptak T, Rhea JT, Novelline RA. Radiation dose is reduced in a single-pass whole-body multi-detector row CT trauma protocol compared with a conventional segmented method: Initial experience. *Radiology* 2003;229:902–905.

Shackford SR, Wald SL, Ross SE, et al. The clinical utility of computed tomographic scanning and neurologic examination in the management of patients with minor head injuries. *J Trauma* 1992;33(3):385.

Shanmuganathan K, Mirvis SE, Sherbourne CD, et al. Hemoperitoneum as the sole indicator of abdominal visceral injuries: A potential limitation of screening abdominal US for trauma. *Radiology* 1999;212:423–430.

Shuman WP. CT of blunt abdominal trauma in adults. *Radiology* 1997;205:297–306.

Wechsler RJ, Spettell CM, Kurtz AB, et al. Effects of training and experience in interpretation of emergency body CT. *Radiology* 1996;29:1299–1310.

Yao DC, Jeffrey RB, Mirvis SE, et al. Using contrast-enhanced helical CT to visualize arterial extravasation after blunt abdominal trauma: Incidence and organ distribution. *AJR Am J Roentgenol* 2002;178:17–20.

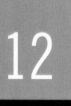

12 Interventional Radiology

J. Scott Williams

I. INTRODUCTION
Interventional radiology is an important part of trauma management across many types of injury. While CT has become the dominant modality in the imaging evaluation of the trauma patient, conventional angiography remains the standard method for definitive vascular diagnosis and guidance during interventional procedures. The most common interventional procedure in the acute setting of trauma is embolization of vascular injuries.

II. THE SPECIAL PROCEDURES ENVIRONMENT
A. The angiography/interventional suite is best constructed, equipped, and staffed as a modified intensive care unit. All nursing staff should have ICU skills and radiologic technologists should be able to meet the demands of the emergency environment. Respiratory technologists and trauma ICU nursing staff should be accessible to assure continuity of emergency trauma care during transfer and intervention.

B. The modern angiography suite uses digital acquisition and is integrated with the hospital radiologic archiving system and the hospital information systems to facilitate the rapid availability of angiographic images and radiologic documentation. While single plane systems are adequate for most trauma applications, intervention in the head and neck and brain is facilitated with biplane technology. Comprehensive bedside imaging system controls, including control of post-processing is required.

III. GENERAL VASCULAR/INTERVENTIONAL TECHNIQUES
A. Access
   1. Prompt uncomplicated access, usually transfemoral, is a key initial step to angiographic intervention. A variety of techniques are available to the operator for reliable safe access, including the Seldinger technique, single wall puncture, and micro-access technique. Use ultrasound guidance, particularly when pulses are difficult to palpate or in those with indistinct landmarks.
   2. For suspected unilateral pelvic injury or lower extremity injury, use the contralateral femoral site.

B. Diagnostic angiography
   1. Principles and planning
      a. Indications for angiography include extravasation or pseudoaneurysm on CT, resuscitation without expected response, and difficulty identifying or controlling hemorrhage.
      b. The approach to angiography begins with the review of prior imaging, particularly CT. Identification of likely sources of bleeding, which may be multiple, permits injured anatomy to be targeted first in the angiographic sequence.
      c. Marking entrance and exit wounds with radio-opaque markers aids care.
      d. A general operational principle of trauma angiography is to start with the least selective angiogram, usually an aortogram. If an embolization target can be localized on the aortogram, proceed with maximal selectivity without wasting time. The offending vessel should be embolized to occlusion, and then complete regional angiography completed.

    e. Optimal aortography requires the use of a flush catheter and a power injector, injecting at about 20 mL/s for 2 seconds. Thoracic aortography requires at least three imaging projections.

    f. Pelvic arteriography

        i. Abdominal aortogram—power injected through flush catheter at 15 mL/s for 2 seconds.

        ii. Selective internal iliac arteries, even if aortogram is normal.

        iii. Care not to miss external iliac branches that may contribute to pelvic hemorrhage.

2. Angiographic equipment

    a. Catheters—Three general categories:

        i. Flush catheters have multiple side holes in addition to the end hole, have a circular shape at the end, and support high injection rates. These are used for thoracic and abdominal aortography as well as pulmonary arteriography. They should be used through an access sheath and advanced and removed over a guidewire.

        ii. Simple curve catheters are angulated near the tip with less than 90-degree angulation. They generally have only one hole, an end hole. They may be used without a sheath and be used to navigate simple branching patterns of anatomy without a guidewire.

        iii. Reverse curve catheters. Reverse curve catheters have a shape angle that exceeds 90 degrees; many have 180-degree shapes and multiple additional curves. Once placed through a sheath over a diagnostic guidewire, a reverse curve catheter must be shaped, a process that converts the catheter, initially extended, to its native unconstrained reverse curve shape. This may be carried out either in the aorta primarily or by advancing the catheter into a side branch of acceptable geometry, withdrawing the supporting guidewire and pushing the catheter forward in the parent vessel as to form the curve.

    b. Guidewires: There are a variety of diagnostic guidewires, commonly 0.035 in. in diameter, appropriate for arteriography. The wires may be generally categorized as those that may be torqued with precision and those that may not be. Shaped tip nitinol wires are examples of the former while outer wire wrap over stainless steel core wires are examples of the latter. Operator preference is the key factor in choosing a guidewire.

    c. Tools for super-selective catheterization

        i. Microcatheters are small diameter catheters passed through diagnostic or guide catheters to selectively catheterize small (1 to 4 mm) vessels. Microcatheters are extremely flexible and generally may not be advanced without guidewire support. They vary in inner diameter from 0.010 to about 0.027 in. and have one or two radio-opaque markers to facilitate fluoroscopic visualization and assist coil positioning and detachment.

        ii. Micro-guidewires are small diameter guidewires varying in diameter from 0.008 to 0.018 in. The most commonly used size is 0.014 in. matched to a 0.021 in. inner diameter microcatheter. Micro-guidewires are made of stainless steel or nitinol and may have a shapeable platinum coil over the distal several cm, outer polymer, and/or hydrophilic coatings.

3. Angiographic findings pertinent to vascular injury

    a. Direct observations include extravasation of contrast material, stenosis, intraluminal filling defect, extension of contrast material outside the expected vascular boundary, and abrupt cut-off of contrast material ("stump").

    b. Seek functional consequences of injuries during angiography. These include identification of important collateral pathways (i.e., vertebral artery occlusion and ipsilateral PICA supply), dynamics over time that may distinguish vasospasm or dysplasia from structural injury, and arteriographically out-of-phase structures that confirm the presence of abnormal arteriovenous shunt. Washout distinguishes intra- from extraluminal contrast material.

    c. Indirect findings such as displacement of otherwise normal vascular structures or organs or segments of organs.

4. The spectrum of arterial dissection

The value of grading dissection is questionable, since the grading system does not reliably predict a continuous spectrum of structural or clinical outcomes. The range of findings includes the following but do not suggest a stepwise progression *per se:*

  a. Stenosis

   i. Vasospasm—no structural injury, but structural injury may be masked. Consider repeat examination.

   ii. Mural thrombus/thrombosis of the false lumen—"subintimal dissection."

  b. Filling defect

   i. Linear filling defect: Intimal flap

   ii. Bulky intraluminal filling defect: Thrombus

  c. Abnormal extension of contrast beyond expected vascular boundaries with washout: Pseudoaneurysm (if there is no washout, then this is extravasation).

  d. Occlusion—"stump" appearance.

  e. Opacification of a vein early in the angiographic sequence: The *sine qua non* of arteriovenous fistula is an arteriovenous shunt.

5. Complications of angiography

  a. Access site complications include bleeding, dissection, pseudoaneurysm, and vascular occlusion secondary to closure device usage. If bleeding is internal, the result is hematoma; if external, hemorrhage. Retroperitoneal hematomata can be nearly eliminated using meticulous access technique.

  b. Contrast nephropathy is a heightened risk in the volume depleted trauma patient. In most instances of hemorrhagic shock warranting angiography, the risks of contrast material usage are outweighed by their benefits. Intravenous N-acetylcysteine may prevent contrast-induced nephropathy and improve outcomes.

  c. True anaphylactic reaction to contrast is rare and in the trauma, the benefits exceed the risk. History of seafood or shellfish allergy is **not** predictive of anaphylactic reaction to contrast material.

  d. Cerebral arteriography has a risk of major neurologic complications as high as 1%, described in populations with atherosclerotic disease and elevated stroke risk. Recent data failed to report a single neurologic complication in almost 800 complete cerebral arteriograms.

6. Many angiographic limitations apply to tomographic vascular imaging as well. Detectable extravasation must occur at about 0.5 mL/min, although CT may detect pooling contrast material that is being leaked at a much slower rate. Vasospasm affects all modalities and may mask underlying vascular injury. Using modern super-selective catheterization techniques, it is rare that selective angiography cannot detect clinically meaningful bleeding.

C. Embolization

 1. General embolization principles

  a. Goal of some embolization (epistaxis) is to diminish tissue perfusion pressure to stop bleeding and facilitate healing.

  b. Most soft tissue vascular territories may be instantly reconstituted by adjacent territories.

  c. Coils and Gelfoam pledgets occlude at the point of deployment. Liquids, when optimally used, occlude the microvasculature, including the capillary bed. Particulates work at some point in between. Gelfoam powder acts like a liquid.

  d. The more selective, the more likely coils are to be effective. Consider particulates when treating bleeding from an array of small branches.

 2. Specific embolics

  a. Coils

   i. Made of stainless steel and platinum

   ii. Available in a wide array of sizes and geometries, including straight, helical, conical, "3D."

   iii. May be coated or fibered (Dacron) to increase thrombogenicity or permanence.

      iv. May be delivered using guidewires, "pusher" wires designed specifically for coil delivery, or by saline flush.

   b. Particulates are suspensions of insoluble particles, either rigid or deformable. Deformable particles are easier to deliver and penetrate more deeply than comparably sized rigid particles.

   c. Gelfoam

      i. Comes as a sheet or powder. Powder is one of the most deeply penetrating embolics.

      ii. Create a slurry from small pieces cut from the supplied sheet. Mix with contrast material and force between two syringes connected by a three-way stopcock. May use whole piece of Gelfoam "pledget" which must be delivered through a diagnostic catheter.

      iii. Absorbable, but powder may cause tissue necrosis.

   d. Avitene, microfibrillar collagen is a deep penetrating particulate embolic.

   e. Liquids such as n-butyl cyanoacrylate, ethanol, Sotradecol, and ethylene vinyl alcohol copolymer have limited use in trauma aside from closing arteriovenous fistulae.

   f. Certain elastomer balloon catheters may be considered temporary embolics, as an endovascular option for rapidly achieving proximal large vessel temporary occlusion or rapidly sealing a large vascular hole to then facilitate surgery.

  3. Complications

   a. Embolization of unwanted territory and resultant tissue ischemia

   b. Tissue necrosis is more common in midline tissues if bilateral embolizations are done or when liquids or Gelfoam powder used.

D. Stents

  1. Stents are endovascular prostheses that secure the injured intima thereby reconstituting the true lumen. They contribute to sealing the intimal rent by apposing the separated layers. Coverings create a barrier across the stent boundaries and exclude aneurysms from flow in the true lumen. If bare metal stent is used in the presence of pseudoaneurysms, coils are frequently required to separately occlude the pseudoaneurysm. There is concern for elevated rates of intimal hyperplasia when covered stents are used.

  2. Types of stents potentially useful in trauma

   a. Bare metal self-expanding

   b. Balloon expandable covered

   c. Self-expanding covered

   d. Stent-grafts

IV. ANATOMICALLY SPECIFIC CONCEPTS

A. Aorta and great arteries

  1. Traumatic injury of the thoracic aorta typically occurs at fixation points that occur near the aortic root, near the isthmus, and the ligamentum arteriosum (most common) or at the diaphragmatic penetration.

  2. Chest radiography is less sensitive in detection of mediastinal hematoma than CT. CT angiography (CTA) is sensitive for the detection of traumatic aortic injury, but may not provide spatial resolution needed to distinguish some developmental abnormalities and variants from injury.

  3. Thoracic aortography remains the gold standard for thoracic aortic imaging and requires images in multiple planes. The field of view should include several centimeters of the great arteries superiorly and the diaphragm inferiorly.

  4. Recent advances make endovascular repair of traumatic aortic injury less risky than surgical repair. Long-term safety and effectiveness of endovascular stents are not defined.

  5. Smaller self-expanding stents can repair innominate artery, subclavian, and common carotid injuries. Elastomer balloon occlusion catheters can aid surgical repair of great artery injuries by providing a reliable endovascular means of temporary vascular occlusion.

B. Craniocervicocerebral arteries
   1. Penetrating carotid and vertebral artery injuries
   a. Clinical examination, CT and CTA detect and characterize zone 1 injuries without the need for conventional angiography in most cases.
   b. Conventional angiography detects injuries, guides treatment planning, and permits intervention in zone 3 and in the intracranial compartment.
   2. Blunt carotid and vertebral artery injuries (BCVI)
   a. Injuries associated with craniocervical vascular injuries include cervical spine fractures; complex facial fractures (Le Fort 2 and 3); skull base fractures, especially those through the carotid canal; Horner's syndrome or anisocoria following blunt trauma; and neck and chest hematoma.
   b. Stroke risk from blunt cerebrovascular injury (BCVI) ranges from 15% to more than 40%.
   c. The screening tool for BCVI at most centers is CTA, but CTA sensitivity is between 49% and 75%. If it can be done with an acceptably low neurologic complication rate, conventional angiography is preferred to detect BCVI. Subtle lesions may devolve into high risk lesions and injuries that do not heal and impart long-term high stroke risk.
   d. Initial management of BCVI is some form of antiplatelet or anticoagulation regimens, although one clear choice does not exist.
   e. After identifying BCVI and initial anticoagulation for a period of days, follow-up imaging can demonstrate healing, stability, or devolution of a lesion. Those lesions that devolve may be treated using endovascular techniques or operatively.
   f. Endovascular treatment of BCVI involves stent placement for the varied manifestations of dissection, with or without coil or covered stent use for those lesions that include pseudoaneurysm.
   g. Carotid "blow-out" is a special case of carotid injury, creating massive carotid extravasation. In most instances the only therapy is carotid sacrifice, either surgical or endovascular, although there may be a role for covered stent placement in this setting.
   3. External carotid injuries
   a. Many vascular injuries of the external carotid system are accessible for manual compression.
   b. Facial, lingual, and internal maxillary extravasation and pseudoaneurysms are treated with endovascular parent vessel sacrifice, including embolization distal to the lesion, if possible, to prevent reconstitution from the contralateral side.
   c. Try to preserve any external to internal carotid arterial connections to limit stroke when donor external carotid branches are embolized.
C. Spleen
   1. Indications for arteriography include high grade splenic injury, splenic injury and hemoperitoneum, active extravasation, or pseudoaneurysm.
   2. There is wide variation among centers in the use of endovascular techniques in splenic injuries. In most patients with splenic injury, surgical treatment is definitive.
   3. An advantage of endovascular techniques in the stable patient with splenic hemorrhage is selective embolization, which permits preservation of portions of the spleen and preservation of immune function. Complications include infection, abscess, and infarction.
   4. Recurrent hemorrhage rate is about 15%; these spleens should be resected.
   5. Long-term vaccination against encapsulated organisms is ideal following nonselective splenic embolization.
D. Liver
   1. Indications include liver injury and hemoperitoneum, extravasation, fistula or pseudoaneurysm on CT.
   2. Hepatic arteriography detects hepatic arterial injury, demonstrates portal venous patency and may identify portal venous injuries.

3. Embolization controls intrahepatic arterial injuries, many of which may be difficult to control surgically without segmental or lobar resection.

4. When embolizing the right hepatic artery, try to embolize distal to the cystic artery to avoid gallbladder necrosis.

5. Complications include infection progressing to abscess, rarely necrosis (liver is resistant secondary to portal supply), biloma, and hemobilia.

E. Pelvis

1. For unstable patients with pelvic fractures, a Trauma Pelvic Orthotic Device (T-POD) or bedsheet helps tamponade hemorrhage. Angiography may be performed through a rent cut into the device or the device may be released during angiography to help target embolization.

2. Consider pelvic arteriography and embolization in the unstable patient with pelvic fracture; when CT demonstrates pelvic hematoma, active extravasation, fistula, or pseudoaneurysm; or in the presence of ongoing or difficult to control pelvic hemorrhage in the OR.

3. In extreme situations (multiple or large bilateral sites of hemorrhage, vasospasm or difficult anatomy preventing selective catheterization, etc.), internal iliac occlusion, even bilaterally, is needed, although the risk of midline and rectal ischemic injury or impotence increases.

4. Recurrent hemorrhage after embolization or negative arteriography occurs in up to 10% of patients; monitor for this and repeat arteriography if needed.

F. Vessels of the extremities

1. In clinically apparent penetrating vascular injury of the extremities, arteriography only delays definitive treatment—emergent surgery is indicated.

2. In penetrating trauma, projectile or path proximity does not alone necessitate arteriography. If many projectiles are present and the path is ambiguous, arteriography provides definitive diagnostic information. CTA may exclude injury in this setting.

3. Large joint dislocations warrant arteriography if any clinical signs of vascular compromise exist.

G. Kidneys

1. Selective embolization of renal hemorrhage is straightforward. Infarction of relatively large portions of a kidney is well tolerated.

2. An entire kidney may be embolized in the presence of a normal contralateral kidney if needed.

H. Chest and abdominal wall

1. Rib fractures and penetrating injuries may affect intercostal and lumbar segmental branches. These are addressed using standard embolization techniques, avoiding proximal spinal branches.

I. Intracranial interventions

1. Blunt or penetrating injury may result in full-thickness tear of the cavernous internal carotid artery segment and create an arteriovenous fistula draining through the cavernous sinus, and causing venous hypertension in the superior ophthalmic vein, the petrosal venous sinuses, or veins draining the brainstem.

2. Chemosis, proptosis, orbital congestion, extra-ocular muscle and visual dysfunction may result.

3. Traumatic carotid cavernous fistulae are managed by endovascular means. The goal is to close the arteriovenous shunt while trying to preserve the injured internal carotid artery.

4. Currently, embolization is carried out using transarterial or transvenous coil embolization. Liquid embolics, specifically Onyx® material or n-butyl cyanoacrylate are options.

5. In some cases, internal carotid artery sacrifice must be performed. Carotid sacrifice should be preceded with internal carotid artery balloon test occlusion, with revascularization carried out before sacrifice if test occlusion fails.

V. "SUBACUTE" INTERVENTIONS

A. Inferior vena cava (IVC) filters

1. The indications for IVC filter placement are discussed elsewhere in this volume, and trauma patients commonly satisfy many criteria for therapeutic or prophylactic IVC filter placement.

2. Filters reduce the rate of symptomatic recurrent PE from about 30% to 50% to 4% to 10%. Filter-related IVC thrombosis rate is 10% to 20%.

3. Retrievable filters permit temporary filtration and reduce the long-term complications of filters. All filters approved in the United States may be used as permanent filters, and increasing experience suggests their safe removal at practically any time point. Only about 5% of filters are removed, with the risks of retention versus removal routinely not well defined.

B. Drainage of fluid collections

1. Abscesses, empyemas, seromas and urinomas are effectively managed with image-guided interventional techniques.

2. A large variety of access and drainage devices are available for the image-guided management of pathologic fluid collections.

AXIOMS

■ Vascular injuries resulting in hemorrhage should take priority in the initial management of the trauma patient.

■ The minimum rate of extravasation required for angiographic detection is about 0.5 mL/min with optimal detection at about 1.0 mL/min.

■ The angiographic goal is the prompt identification of the source of bleeding and selective embolization.

■ Conventional angiography, in high risk patients, is the most sensitive method for detecting BCVI.

Suggested Readings

American College of Radiology Manual on Contrast Reactions, version 7, 2010, ACR Committee on drugs and contrast Media.

Beaty AD, Lieberman PL, Slavin RG. Seafood allergy and radiocontrast media: are physicians propagating a myth? *Am J Med* 2008;121(2):158. e1–4.

Biffl WF, Moore EE, Offner PJ, et al. Blunt Carotid Injuries: implications of a new rating scale. *J Trauma* 1999;47(5):845–853.

Bouras AF, Truant S, Pruvot FR. Management of blunt hepatic trauma. *J Visc Surg* 2010;147(6):e351–e358.

Bynoe RP, Kerwin AJ, Parker HH III, et al. Maxillofacial injuries and life-threatening hemorrhage: Treatment with transcatheter arterial embolization. *J Trauma* 2003;55:74–79.

DiCocco JM, Emmett KP, Fabian TC, et al. Blunt cerebrovascular injury screening with 32-channel multidetector computed tomography: more slices still don't cut it. *Ann Surg* 2011;253(3):444–450.

Katsanos K, Sabharwal T, Carrell T, et al. Peripheral endografts for the treatment of traumatic arterial injuries. *Emerg Radiol* 2009;16(3):175–184.

Keeling AN, McGrath FP, Lee MJ. Interventional radiology in the diagnosis, management, and follow-up of pseudoaneurysms. *Cardiovasc Intervent Radiol* 2009;32(1):2–18.

Marenzi G, Assanelli E, Marana I, et al. N-acetylcysteine and contrast-induced nephropathy in primary angioplasty. *N Engl J Med* 2006;354(26):2773–2782.

Pryor JP, Braslow B, Reilly PM, et al. The evolving role of interventional radiology in trauma care. *J Trauma* 2005;59(1):102–104.

Salazar GM, Walker TG. Evaluation and management of acute vascular trauma. *Tech Vasc Interv Radiol* 2009;12(2):102–116.

Sofocleous CT, Hinrichs C, Hubbi B, et al. Angiographic findings and embolotherapy in renal arterial trauma. *Cardiovasc Intervent Radiol* 2005;28(1):39–47.

Tan EC, van Stigt SF, van Vugt AB. Effect of a new pelvic stabilizer (T-POD®) on reduction of pelvic volume and haemodynamic stability in unstable pelvic fractures. *Injury* 2010;41(12):1239–1243.

13 Sepsis in Trauma

Ayan Sen and Derek C. Angus

I. INTRODUCTION

A. Sepsis is a common, expensive, and frequently fatal condition, likely to increase in frequency as the US population ages.

B. It is a frequent complication in patients who survive initial trauma resuscitation and is largely responsible for the third peak of death based on Trunkey's trimodal death distribution in civilian trauma.

II. DEFINITION OF SEPSIS

Sepsis is a broad term including severe sepsis (infection complicated by acute organ dysfunction) and septic shock (infection leading to shock). When a patient develops an infection, the process that leads to sepsis is widely regarded as a broad innate immune response, consisting of rapid release of multiple cytokines and other inflammatory molecules and activation of immune cells. The clinical manifestation of this response is described as the Systemic Inflammatory Response Syndrome (SIRS). Under the consensus definitions, the different components of sepsis are as follows:

A. Infection is a pathologic process caused by the invasion of normally sterile tissue or fluid or body cavity by pathogenic or potentially pathogenic microorganisms. Caveats include infection by cytopathic toxin producing organisms which do not necessarily invade the host tissue. **SIRS** results from a systemic activation of the innate immune response, regardless of cause. SIRS occurs when patients present one or more of the following findings: Body temperature $>38°C$ or $<36°C$; heart rate >90/min; respiratory rate $>$**20/min, or PaCO$_2$** $<$**32 mm Hg; and white** blood cell count of $>12,000$ cells/mcL or $<4,000$ cells/mcL.

B. Bone et al. defined **sepsis** as SIRS plus infection, **"severe sepsis"** as sepsis associated with organ dysfunction, hypoperfusion, or hypotension, and **"septic shock"** as sepsis with arterial hypotension, despite adequate fluid resuscitation. The 2003 definition was widened to suggest that SIRS was only one of a long list of potential signs of infection and that severe sepsis is simply infection complicated by acute organ dysfunction.

C. Typical acute organ dysfunction includes acute respiratory distress syndrome (ARDS), hypotension or hyperlactemia, acute kidney injury, gastrointestinal ileus and raised transaminases, altered mental status, and thrombocytopenia.

D. None of the findings of the SIRS response is specific for diagnosis. In trauma, the systemic inflammatory response may be due to the injury and not a secondary infection.

III. RISK FACTORS

Patient factors can predispose toward severe sepsis and septic shock.
Risk factors for sepsis in trauma patients—see Table 13-1.

IV. DIAGNOSIS OF SEPSIS IN TRAUMA

The diagnosis and prognosis of sepsis is complicated by the variable and non-specific nature of the signs and symptoms of sepsis in trauma. Early recognition and directed treatment can lower mortality and morbidity.

TABLE 13-1 **Risk Factors for Sepsis in Trauma Patients**

Trauma Severity	Trauma Mechanism	Patient Characteristics	Therapeutic Strategies
High ISS (injury severity score), Low RTS (revised trauma score), TRISS (trauma-related injury severity score) predicting low probability of survival	Burns Penetrating injury Chest injuries— pneumonia Bites—dog, cat, human	Age Male gender Genetic polymorphisms Diabetes mellitus	Laparotomy, splenectomy Invasive procedures, e.g., bladder catheterization, central lines, etc. Blood transfusion Multiple operations

A. Early post-injury inflammatory signs and markers likely reflect tissue damage rather than sepsis.

B. The physical examination is the underpinning to detect the source of infection.

C. Many signs exist to help identify that an infected patient "is septic."

D. Frequently, sources of infection in trauma patients involve the lungs (pneumonia), invasive lines, abdominal sepsis (due to injury or surgery), urinary tract, sinuses, gallbladder and decubitus ulcers (Table 13-2).

E. Biomarkers such as white cell count and C-reactive protein (CRP) have low specificity.

F. Procalcitonin (PCT) may aid as a diagnostic (bacterial infection) or prognostic marker. Current evidence suggests that serum PCT can be used as "an adjunctive diagnostic tool for discriminating infection as the cause for fever or sepsis presentations" in their guidelines for the evaluation of new fever in critically ill adults.

G. Positive blood cultures (BC), if not from a contaminant, are diagnostic of Bacteremia but do not define SIRS. Culture results are not typically available until after treatment with antibiotics, and source control must be initiated prior to these data. Obtain appropriate cultures before starting antibiotics provided this does not delay antimicrobial administration; obtain two or more BCs; one or more BCs should be percutaneous; one BC from each vascular access device in place >48 hours.

H. Other sites should be cultured as clinically indicated.

I. Imaging studies can confirm a source and aid sampling.

J. A specific anatomic site of infection should be established as rapidly as possible and within first 6 hours of diagnosis of sepsis.

K. Formal evaluation for a focus of infection amenable to source control measures (e.g., abscess drainage, tissue debridement) should be done.

L. Implementation of source control measures should be done as soon as possible following successful initial resuscitation. (Exception: Infected pancreatic necrosis, where surgical intervention is best delayed.)

M. Remove intravascular access devices if infected.

N. Microbiology of sepsis in trauma:

    1. In trauma patients, sepsis is caused by gram-positive and gram-negative bacteria in roughly equal proportions. Empiric coverage for both groups may be necessary.

    2. The most prevalent organisms are *Escherichia coli* and *Staphylococcus* (*aureus* or coagulase negative). Meningococcemia and Streptococcemia are comparatively fewer in numbers.

    3. *E.coli* and *Klebsiella* are common but *Pseudomonas* is also a common ICU pathogen. Sixty percent of hospital-acquired isolates of *S. aureus* are methicillin-resistant. *Staph* resistance to vancomycin is rare. *S. epidermidis* has 85% methicillin resistance. Initial antibiotic therapy should take resistance patterns and local antibiograms into account.

TABLE 13-2 **Diagnostic Criteria for Sepsis**

Infection,[a] documented or suspected, and some of the following:[b]
General variables
Fever (core temperature >38.3°C)
Hypothermia (core temperature <36°C)
Heart rate >90 min^{-1} or >2 SD above the normal value for age
Tachypnea
Altered mental status
Significant edema or positive fluid balance (>20 mL/kg over 24 h)
Hyperglycemia (plasma glucose >120 mg/dL or 7.7 mmol/L) in the absence of diabetes
Inflammatory variables
Leukocytosis (WBC count >12,000 uL^{-1})
Leukopenia (WBC count <4,000 uL^{-1})
Normal WBC count with >10% immature forms
Plasma C-reactive protein >2 SD above the normal value
Plasma procalcitonin >2 SD above the normal value
Hemodynamic variables
Arterial hypotension[b] (SBP <90 mm Hg, MAP <70, or an SBP decrease >40 mm Hg in adults or <2 SD below normal for age)
SvO$_2$70%[b]
Cardiac index >3.5 L-min^{-1} M^{-23}
Organ dysfunction variables
Arterial hypoxemia (PaO$_2$/FiO$_2$, <300)
Acute oliguria (urine output <0.5 mL kg^{-1} h^{-1} or 45 mmol/L for at least 2 h)
Creatinine increase >0.5 mg/dL
Coagulation abnormalities (INR > 1.5 or aPTT >60 s)
Ileus (absent bowel sounds)
Thrombocytopenia (platelet count <100,000/μL^{-1})
Hyperbilirubinemia (plasma total bilirubin >4 mg/dL or 70 mmol/L)
Tissue perfusion variables
Hyperlactatemia (>1 mmol/L)
Decreased capillary refill or mottling

WBC, white blood cell; SBP, systolic blood pressure; MAP, mean arterial blood pressure; SvO$_2$, mixed venous oxygen saturation; INR, international normalized ratio; aPTT, activated partial thromboplastin time.
[a]Infection defined as a pathologic process induced by a microorganism.
[b]SvO$_2$ sat >70% is normal in children (normally, 75–80%), and CI 3.5–5.5 is normal in children; therefore, NEITHER should be used as signs of sepsis in newborns or children.
[c]diagnostic criteria for sepsis in the pediatric population are signs and symptoms of inflammation plus infection with hyper- or hypothermia (rectal temperature >38.5 or <35°C), tachycardia (may be absent in hypothermic patients), and at least one of the following indications of altered organ function: Altered mental status, hypoxemia, increased serum lactate level, or bounding pulses.
Updates on Sepsis Definition based on the 2001 ACCP/SCCM criteria
From Levy MM, Fink MP, Marshall JC, et al. 2001 SCCM/ESICM/ACCP/ATS/SIS International Sepsis Definitions Conference. *Crit Care Med* 2003;31:1250–1256.

4. *Enterococcus* causes SSTI, CR-BSI, and UTI. Thirty percent of them are resistant to vancomycin.
5. Seventy percent of *Enterococcus faecium* are VRE; only 3% of *E. faecalis* are. Colonization of VRE precedes invasive infection.
6. Most fungi are opportunistic pathogens in trauma patients. Fungal infections are usually the result of antibiotic overuse. The most common healthcare associated fungal infection is due to Candida species. High risk patients (immune suppressed) or those who need prolonged antibiotics may be susceptible.
7. See Figure 13-1 for common gram-positive and gram-negative bacteria causing sepsis in trauma and Table 13-3 for common organisms and infection syndromes.

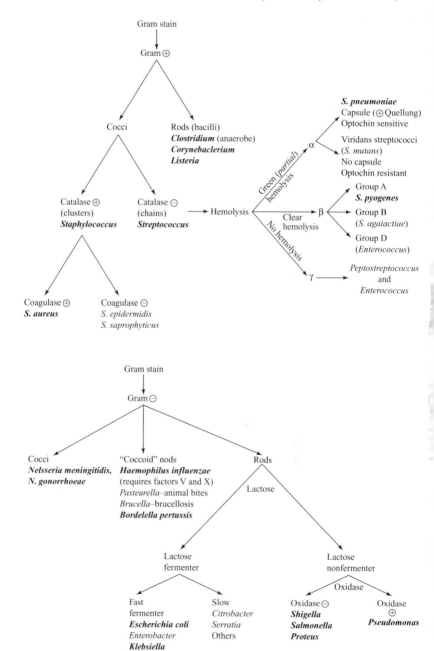

Figure 13-1. Gram stain and types of bacteria commonly implicated in sepsis.

TABLE 13-3	Common Organisms, Infection Syndromes and Antibiotic Therapy	
Source	**Diagnostic criteria**	**Antibiotics**
Lungs (early-aspiration during scene or resuscitation, ARDS from TRALI, contusion; late-nosocomial, ventilator associated)	Pulmonary infiltrate, secretions type with Gram stain and culture	Gram-positive—penicillins, cephalosporins, macrolides, fluoroquinolones with vancomycin for MRSA risk; linezolid for vancomycin resistance or allergies. Gram-negative—cephalosporins, antipseudomonals-3, fourth gen cephalosporins, beta-lactam with beta-lactamase inhibitors
Line (catheter-related)	Differential blood culture (line and peripheral site)purulence, erythema around catheter site	Coagulase negative *Staph* *Staph aureus* responsive to vancomycin *Enterococcus*, VRE—linezolid *Candida*—fluconazole Gram-negative rods—rare (immunosuppressed)
Abdominal (if abdominal trauma, surgery, cirrhosis)	Clinical distension, signs of peritonitis, intolerance of feeds, CT evidence	Gram-positives—cephalosporins, vancomycin, linezolid, tigecycline, daptomycin. Enteric gram-negative organisms—ampicillin/sulbactam; piperacillin/tazobactam; cephalosporins, serious—carbapenems (meropenem); combination (anaerobes)—clindamycin or metronidazole
Urinary tract	Dysuria, bacteriuria, positive urinalysis	Urogenital organisms—gram-negatives usually; gram-positive with *Enterococcus;* coverage with vancomycin, linezolid (VRE) cephalosporins, penicillins, fluoroquinolones,
Skin and soft tissue (skin disruption, diabetics, immunosuppressed)	Tenderness, erythema, fluctuance, subcutaneous emphysema, disruption of fascial planes with gas in tissue	Coverage for gram-positive organisms *Streptococcus, Staphylococcus*
Sinuses (presence of endotracheal tubes, craniotomy, maxillofacial injuries)	Purulent discharge, headache, pain, redness, swelling over sinuses, nasotracheal aspirate, sinus washout	*Streptococcus, Haemophilus, Moraxella, Staphylococcus,* gram-negative *bacilli*, fungus, viruses Empiric community- acquired augmentin, fluroquinoles nosocomial-zosyn, meropenem, amphotericin for mucormycosis
Acalculous cholecystitis (prolonged GI tract non-use, NPO, TPN, ischemia)	Clinical evidence of Murphy's sign; ultrasound findings	cephalosporins
Clostridium difficile associated infection	Diarrhea, positive toxin test, cultures	Metronidazole, vancomycin (enteral, enemas)

V. MANAGEMENT OF SEPSIS IN TRAUMA

Primary approaches to managing patients with sepsis and septic shock post-trauma consist of early resuscitation, identification of the source of infection, and maintenance of organ support and function. The following sections will use recommendations of the Surviving Sepsis Campaign Guidelines, which are based on sepsis in general with additional inputs for a trauma sub-group where evidence exists.

A. Respiratory support:

1. Trauma patients with chest injury, such as rib fracture or pulmonary contusion, have a high incidence of developing pneumonia and sepsis. These patients need monitoring in the ICU and mechanical ventilation for optimum respiratory support at signs of deterioration.

2. Patients with, or at risk of, ARDS should be managed with low tidal volumes. On the basis of the seminal study by the NHLBI ARDS Network, patients should be placed on tidal volumes of 6 mL/kg with plateau pressures kept below 30 mL H_2O to avoid barotrauma. If needed, allow arterial partial pressure of carbon dioxide ($PaCO_2$) to increase above normal to minimize plateau pressures and tidal volumes.

3. Positive end-expiratory pressure (PEEP) is beneficial for alveolar recruitment at end-expiration; this prevents alveolar barotrauma leading to increased release of inflammatory cytokines and worsening of the lung injury.

4. In patients with severe hypoxia and ARDS, consider using prone position if possible.

5. Maintain mechanically ventilated patients in a semi-recumbent position (head of the bed raised to 45°) unless contraindicated, between 30° and 45°.

6. Noninvasive ventilation aids some ARDS patients with mild to moderate hypoxemic respiratory failure. The patients are usually hemodynamically stable, comfortable, easily arousable, able to protect/clear their airways, and expected to recover rapidly.

7. Use a weaning protocol and daily Spontaneous Breathing Trials (SBT) to evaluate the potential for discontinuation of mechanical ventilation. SBT options include a low level of pressure support with continuous positive airway pressure 5 cm H_2O or a T piece.

8. Use a conservative fluid strategy for patients with established ARDS who do not have evidence of tissue hypoperfusion.

9. Use of alternate modes of ventilation such as airway pressure release ventilation (APRV), high-frequency oscillation ventilation with reduced sedation requirements and increased recruitment of the atelectatic lung should only be considered as rescue therapies.

B. Circulatory support:

1. Volume resuscitation:

    Structured and goal-oriented therapy based on central venous pressure, mean arterial pressure, mixed venous oxygen levels and hematocrit levels can reduce mortality in unselected sepsis patients in the emergency department. Adequate volume resuscitation and targeting hemodynamic parameters makes physiologic sense but this should be considered in view of the overall patient trajectory, injuries, and subsequent therapeutic strategies in a trauma patient. Surviving Sepsis Guideline recommendations include:

    a. Target a CVP of >8 mm Hg and >12 mm Hg, if mechanically ventilated.

    b. Use a fluid challenge technique associated with a hemodynamic improvement.

    c. Give fluid challenges of 1,000 mL of crystalloids or 300 to 500 mL of colloids over 30 min.

    d. More rapid and larger volumes may be required in sepsis-induced tissue hypoperfusion.

    e. Rate of fluid administration should be reduced, if cardiac filling pressures increase without concurrent hemodynamic improvement.

2. Fluid selection:

    a. Normal saline or lactated Ringer's is the common choice for fluid resuscitation.

b. Avoid hyperchloremic metabolic acidosis in trauma patients with the use of large volume of normal saline resuscitation.

c. Colloids (with albumin or hetastarch) do not have any benefit over isotonic crystalloid resuscitation (isotonic sodium chloride solution or lactated Ringer's solution).

d. Hypertonic saline has failed to show benefit and should be avoided.

3. Vasopressor/inotrope use:

a. Vasopressor use should be considered after volume resuscitation to keep MAP >65 mm Hg.

b. We recommended norepinephrine. Norepinephrine has predominant alpha-receptor agonist effects and results in potent peripheral arterial vaso-constriction without significantly increasing heart rate or cardiac output. Norepinephrine has been shown to be significantly safer and somewhat more effective in treating septic shock than dopamine, the alternative.

c. Second-line vasopressors for patients with persistent hypotension despite max-imal doses of norepinephrine or dopamine are epinephrine, phenylephrine, and vasopressin.

d. Use epinephrine as the first alternative agent in septic shock when blood pres-sure is poorly responsive to norepinephrine or dopamine.

e. Low-dose vasopressin at 0.04 units/min is not recommended.

f. Dobutamine is an inotropic agent that stimulates beta-receptors and results in increased cardiac output and can be used, if myocardial depression from septic shock is suspected by low cardiac output and elevated cardiac filling pressure after volume resuscitation.

g. Do not use low-dose dopamine for renal protection.

h. In patients requiring vasopressors, insert an arterial catheter as soon as prac-tical.

i. Do not increase cardiac index to supra-normal levels.

4. Hemodynamic goals and devices:

a. Begin resuscitation immediately in patients with hypotension or a serum lactate >4 mmol/L.

b. Maintaining hemodynamic parameters and adequate oxygen delivery: Resusci-tation goals of CVP 8 to 12 mm Hg; mean arterial pressure >65 mm Hg; urine output >0.5 mL/kg/hr; central venous (superior vena cava) oxygen saturation >70% or mixed venous >65%.

c. If venous oxygen saturation target is not achieved, consider further fluid and/or transfuse packed red blood cells if required to hematocrit of >30% (to increase oxygen carrying capacity) and/or start dobutamine infusion, maximum 20 μg/kg/min.

d. Using adjunctive measurement techniques such as ultrasound assessment of inferior vena cava respirographic changes, stroke volume variation, passive leg raising test, and urine output rate may help understand preload responsiveness and guide fluid resuscitation.

e. Lactate clearance (>10% drop over 2 hours) may be an alternative approach to measuring venous saturations to guide therapy.

f. Retrospective analyses of large databases and of several randomized controlled trials have demonstrated either no benefit or an increased risk of death in patients who are managed with a pulmonary artery catheter (PAC). Therefore, use of the PAC should be highly selective.

C. Antibiotics:

1. The choice of empiric antibiotic therapy depends on presumed or known source of sepsis, sensitivity profile of bacteria expected, patient allergies, and the hospital formulary.

2. Cover both gram-positive and gram-negative organisms early in severe illness.

3. Cover anaerobic organisms, if abdominal source is suspected.

4. Incidence or suspicion of MRSA may direct choice of antibiotics.

5. Consider combination therapy in *Pseudomonas* infections and combination empiric therapy in neutropenic patients.

6. Fungal sepsis may be covered with fluconazole.
7. Modification of empiric antibiotics based on culture and sensitivity and de-escalation to narrow spectrum antibiotics is important.
8. Duration of therapy typically limited to 7 to 10 days; longer if response is slow or there are undrainable foci of infection or immunologic deficiencies.
9. Evidence supporting antibiotic prophylaxis is controversial. Antibiotics with shorter half-lives should be used. Only surgical site infection is prevented by prophylaxis. The prophylactic administration of multiple antibiotics for more than 24 hours following severe trauma does not offer additional protection against sepsis.
10. Common infections encountered in the trauma patients and their management is in Table 13-3.

D. Sedation, analgesia, and neuromuscular blockade in sepsis:
1. Use sedation protocols with a sedation goal for critically ill mechanically ventilated patients.
2. Use either intermittent bolus sedation or continuous infusion sedation to predetermined end points (sedation scales), with daily interruption/lightening to produce awakening. Re-titrate if necessary.
3. Avoid neuromuscular blockers where possible. Monitor depth of block with train-of-four when using continuous infusions.

E. Glucose management:
1. Use intravenous insulin to control hyperglycemia in patients with severe sepsis following stabilization in the ICU.
2. Aim to keep blood glucose <150 mg/dL (8.3 mmol/L) using a validated protocol for insulin dose adjustment.
3. Provide a glucose calorie source and monitor blood glucose values every 1 to 2 hours (4 hours when stable) in patients receiving intravenous insulin.

F. Corticosteroids:
1. Patients with vasopressor-refractory hypotension may have temporary adrenal insufficiency of critical illness. Although studies have had mixed results, current guidelines recommend intravenous hydrocortisone for adult septic shock when hypotension responds poorly to adequate fluid resuscitation and vasopressors.
2. ACTH stimulation test is not recommended to identify the subset of adults with septic shock who should receive hydrocortisone.
3. Steroid therapy may be weaned once vasopressors are no longer required.
4. Hydrocortisone is preferred at a dose of 200 to 300 mg/day in divided doses.
5. Do not use corticosteroids to treat sepsis in the absence of shock unless adrenal insufficiency is suspected based on past history of endocrine dysfunction or corticosteroid use.

G. Nutrition:
1. Trauma is also associated with loss, through apoptosis, of both enteric lymphocytes and enteric epithelial cells, compromising the gut barrier function.
2. Early post-operative enteral nutrition is safe and can reduce the incidence of pneumonia, septic complications, and duration of hospital stay in trauma patients.
3. Early parenteral nutrition may increase morbidity due to line-related infection and should be avoided if possible.
4. Gastroparesis is common and should be treated with motility agents (e.g., metoclopramide or erythromycin) or with placement of a post-pyloric feeding tube.
5. There is no established role for immunonutrition in sepsis, such as glutamine, arginine, or omega-3 fatty acids, and their routine use is not recommended.

H. Correction of anemia and coagulopathy:
1. Give red blood cells when hemoglobin decreases to <7.0 g/dL to target a hemoglobin of 7.0 to 9.0 g/dL in adults. A higher hemoglobin level may be required in myocardial ischemia, severe hypoxemia, or acute hemorrhage.
2. Erythropoietin has no role in sepsis-related anemia.
3. Do not use fresh frozen plasma routinely to correct laboratory clotting abnormalities unless there is bleeding or planned invasive procedures.
4. Do not use antithrombin therapy routinely.

5. Administer platelets when counts are $<5,000/mm^3$ regardless of bleeding; counts are 5,000 to $30,000/mm^3$ and with significant bleeding risk; higher platelet counts $>50,000/mm^3$ are required for surgery or invasive procedures.

I. Renal support:
   1. Intermittent hemodialysis and CVVH are considered equivalent.
   2. CVVH offers easier management in hemodynamically unstable patients.
   3. Do not use bicarbonate therapy for the purpose of improving hemodynamics or reducing vasopressor requirements when treating hypoperfusion-induced lactic acidemia with pH >7.15.

J. Deep vein thrombosis prophylaxis:
   1. Use either low-dose unfractionated heparin (5,000 units q12 or q8 subcutaneous) or low-molecular weight heparin (e.g., enoxaparin 30 mg q12 subcutaneous), unless contraindicated.
   2. Use a mechanical prophylactic device, such as compression stockings or an intermittent compression device, when heparin is contraindicated.
   3. Use a combination of pharmacologic and mechanical therapy for patients at high risk for deep vein thrombosis.
   4. In patients at high risk, use LMWH rather than UFH.

K. Stress ulcer prophylaxis:
   1. Provide stress ulcer prophylaxis using an H_2 blocker or a proton pump inhibitor.

L. Adjuvant therapies:
   1. Activated Protein C (Xigris) therapy has no benefit in septic shock with multiorgan failure and was recently withdrawn from the market.
   2. Female sex hormones may be immunoprotective but have not yet been proven effective in humans.
   3. Direct immune enhancement (intravenous immunoglobulin) has no role in routine care of trauma patients with sepsis currently.

M. Consideration for limitation of support:
   1. Discuss advance care planning with patients and families. Describe likely outcomes and set realistic expectations.

AXIOMS

- Sepsis is difficult to identify in the trauma population but must be sought.
- Biomarkers are non-specific in diagnosis.
- Volume resuscitation is paramount in hypotensive patients or those with elevated lactate and should be given with clear targets.
- Use vasopressors such as norepinephrine with caution for profound hypotension during volume resuscitation. Thereafter, use vasopressors to treat hypotension once preload responsiveness to fluids is adequately reduced.
- Hemodynamic monitoring should be used early if vasopressors and inotropes are administered for titration.
- Give antibiotics as early as possible.
- Aim to keep blood glucose <150 mg/dL (8.3 mmol/L) using a validated protocol for insulin dose adjustment.

Suggested Readings

The Acute Respiratory Distress Syndrome Network: Ventilation with lower tidal volumes as compared with traditional tidal volumes for acute lung injury and the acute respiratory distress syndrome. *N Engl J Med* 2000;342:1301–1308.

Angus DC, Linde-Zwirble WT, Lidicker J, et al. Epidemiology of severe sepsis in the United States: Analysis of incidence, outcome, and associated costs of care. *Crit Care Med* 2001;29:1303–1310.

Dellinger RP, Levy MM, Carlet JM, et al. Surviving Sepsis Campaign: international guidelines for management of severe sepsis and septic shock: 2008. *Crit Care Med* 2008;36:296–327.

Hebert PC, Wells G, Blajchman MA, et al. A multicenter, randomized, controlled clinical trial of transfusion requirements in critical care. Transfusion Requirements in Critical Care Investigators, Canadian Critical Care Trials Group. *N Engl J Med* 1999;340:409–417.

Levy MM, Fink MP, Marshall JC, et al. 2001 SCCM/ESICM/ACCP/ATS/SIS International Sepsis Definitions Conference. *Crit Care Med* 2003;31:1250–1256.

Martin GS, Mannino DM, Eaton S, et al. The epidemiology of sepsis in the United States from 1979 through 2000. *N Engl J Med* 2003;348:1546–1554.

Members of the American College of Chest Physicians/Society of Crit Care Med Consensus Conference Committee: American College of Chest Physicians/Society of Crit Care Med Consensus Conference: Definitions for sepsis and organ failure and guidelines for the use of innovative therapies in sepsis. *Crit Care Med* 1992;20:864–874.

Rivers E, Nguyen B, Havstad S, et al. Early goal-directed therapy in the treatment of severe sepsis and septic shock. *N Engl J Med* 2001;345:1368–1377.

Thornhill R, Strong D, Vasanth S, et al. Trauma sepsis. *Trauma* 2010;12:31–49.

Trunkey DD. Trauma. Accidental and intentional injuries account for more years of life lost in the U.S. than cancer and heart disease. Among the prescribed remedies are improved preventive efforts, speedier surgery and further research. *Sci Am* 1983;249:28–35.

14
Infections, Antibiotic Prevention, and Antibiotic Management

Philip S. Barie and Soumitra R. Eachempati

I. EPIDEMIOLOGY

A. Incidence. The incidence of infection following injury approaches 25%. Although most trauma-related deaths within the first 24 hours after injury are from exsanguination or injury to the central nervous system, the leading cause of post-traumatic death after 24 hours is infection, often through the multiple organ dysfunction syndrome (MODS). The high risk of infection is due to the host immune response to injury and stress; challenges of infection control under emergency conditions; direct inoculation of wounds by clothing, dirt, or debris; blood transfusions; catabolism and resultant protein–calorie malnutrition; and poor glycemic control. Appropriate antibiotic prophylaxis reduces the risk, but inappropriate prophylaxis may increase the risk of infection. Early definitive surgical source control (of drainable or resectable foci) and timely, appropriate empiric antibiotic therapy are key to successful management.

B. Patterns of injury. Infections following injury occur in the injured tissue, the surgical site (incision), or as a health care–associated infection (HAI) such as pneumonia or central line–associated blood stream infection (CLABSI) (Table 14-1). Considered together, HAIs are as common as infections of injured tissues. The likelihood of infection is higher with increasing injury severity score (ISS), increasing number of abdominal organs injured, traumatic brain injury, colon injury, shock, increasing number of blood transfusions, prolonged mechanical ventilation, or creation of an ostomy. Traumatic wounds have devitalized, ischemic tissue, with increased risk of infection if contaminated by enteric contents (e.g., penetrating abdominal trauma), fragments of clothing fabric (e.g., gunshot wounds), dirt or gravel (e.g., motor vehicle or farm injuries), or vegetation (e.g., fall from height into a tree). More wound contamination increases the risk of infection of injured tissue.

C. Comparison with critically ill surgical patients (non-trauma). The epidemiology of HAI is changing among critically ill patients, with high (but decreasing) incidences of pneumonia and CLABSI, and fewer urinary tract infections (UTIs) and surgical site infections (SSIs). The epidemiology of infection following trauma differs from other critically ill surgical patients. Trauma patients are both more likely to become infected (Table 14-1) and develop infection earlier post-injury. Pneumonia is the most common HAI following injury. The timing of onset of infection may influence the choice of antimicrobial therapy.

II. RISK FACTORS.
The host is put at risk of invasion by microbial pathogens whenever a natural epithelial barrier (e.g., skin, respiratory tract mucosa, gastrointestinal mucosa) is breached. Colonization of natural epithelial barriers occurs even in healthy hosts. However, invasion does not occur unless injury or some other mechanism of inoculation occurs. Injury, catheterization, or incision creates a portal for tissue invasion by pathogens. Potential pathogens are ubiquitous in the environment. Innate immunity provides continuous surveillance against invasion by foreign antigens, and stimulates a repair response (inflammation), which may result in counterproductive augmentation of the inflammatory response that is destructive to the host. Prolonged or severe inflammation (e.g., the systemic inflammatory response syndrome, SIRS) (Table 14-2) is associated with the MODS.

TABLE 14-1	Rates of Health Care–associated Pneumonia and Catheter-related Bacteremia Among Various ICU Types			
ICU type	CVC use[a] infection rate	TT use[b] infection rate	Mean/median	Mean/median
Medical	0.52	5.0/3.9	0.46	4.9/3.7
Pediatric	0.46	6.6/5.2	0.39	2.9/2.3
Surgical	0.61	4.6/3.4	0.44	9.3/8.3
Cardiovascular	0.79	2.7/1.8	0.43	7.2/6.3
Neurosurgical	0.48	4.6/3.1	0.39	11.2/6.2
Trauma	0.61	7.4/5.2	0.56	15.2/11.4

[a]Number of days of catheter placement/1,000 patient-days in ICU.
[b]Number of days of indwelling endotracheal tube or tracheostomy/1,000 patient-days in ICU.
Infection rates are indexed per 1,000 patient-days.
Based on the National Nosocomial Infection Surveillance System, US.
Centers for Disease Control and Prevention. (From Bercker S, Weber-Carstens S, Deja M, et al. Critical illness polyneuropathy and myopathy in patients with acute respiratory distress syndrome. *Crit Care Med* 2005;33:711–715.)

A. **Injury severity.** Shock and higher ISS increase the risk of infection globally. Thoracoabdominal penetrating injury is associated with a higher risk of infection than either abdominal or thoracic injury alone. The risk of intra-abdominal infection is higher with increasing numbers of abdominal organs injured. Several "local" injuries induce systemic immune, inflammatory, and coagulation responses, including pulmonary contusion and traumatic brain injury (TBI), the latter being the injury most associated with infection, especially pneumonia.

B. **Immune dysfunction**
   1. The immune response to injury is immediate and complex (Table 14-3). The consequences are immediate activation of:

TABLE 14-2	Immune Dysfunction after Trauma

Specific immunity
- Lymphopenia
- Helper: Suppressor T-cell ratio,1
- Downregulated:
  - −T-, B-cell proliferation
  - −NK cell activity
  - −IL-2 receptor expression
  - −IL-4, -10 production
  - −HLA-DR expression
  - −DTH skin test response

Nonspecific immunity
- Monocytosis
- Upregulated:
  - −Acute-phase proteins
  - −TNF, IL-6 production
  - −Eicosanoid production
- Downregulated:
  - −Neutrophil function

NK, natural killer cell; IL, interleukin; HLA-DR, human leukocyte antigen; DTH, delayed topical hypersensitivity; TNF, tumor necrosis factor.

TABLE 14-3   **Systemic Inflammatory Response Syndrome (SIRS)**

Temperature $>38°C$ or $<36°C$
Heart rate >90 bpm
Respiratory rate >20 breaths/min or $PaCO_2$ <32 mm Hg
White blood cell count $>12,000/mm^3$ or $<4,000/mm^3$

[a]In the absence of another explanation (e.g., antineoplastic therapy). SIRS is present if two or more criteria are met. Sepsis is diagnosed when SIRS is caused by infection.

    a. Coagulation as a result of endothelial dysfunction and activation of platelets
    b. Mononuclear and polymorphonuclear leukocytes causing release of both pro- and anti-inflammatory cytokines and activation of host defenses against microbial invasion
    c. Eventual depression of innate and adaptive immunity with host immunosuppression and predisposition to later HAI
  2. Inflammation and the stress response. The stress hormone response that characterizes the "fight or flight" response:
    a. Augments cardiovascular function through the sympathetic nervous system
    b. Enhances glycogenolysis
    c. Mobilizes peripheral lean muscle and fat as fuel (catabolism)
    d. Enhances coagulation to stanch hemorrhage
    e. Stimulates a pro-inflammatory cytokine response to begin the process of tissue repair (Table 14-4). Innate and adaptive immunity are depressed in large part by the actions of cortisol (Table 14-5).
 C. Medical comorbidity. Both very young and elderly patients are at increased risk of infection (Table 14-6). Obesity, malnutrition, diabetes mellitus, hypocholesterolemia, hypothermia, and chronic kidney disease also increase risk of infection.
 D. Transfusion
  1. Blood transfusion cannot be avoided in many, but trauma patients are more than five-fold more likely to develop infection if a blood transfusion is administered. Several theories exist as to why transfusion predisposes to infection:
    a. Transfusion may be immunosuppressive through leukocyte antigen–mediated decreases in innate immunity, specifically a shift to the Th2 (immunosuppressive) response phenotype.
    b. Augmentation of the SIRS response.
    c. Mechanically, the "storage lesion" that develops after 2 weeks of storage in the blood bank depletes erythrocyte 2,3-diphosphoglycerate and cell membrane stores of adenosine triphosphate, decreasing oxygen delivery (DO_2) and RBC deformability, respectively. The latter lesion impairs the ability of the RBC to transit the microcirculation, resulting in rouleaux formation and mechanical obstruction of the microcirculation.

TABLE 14-4   **Overview of the Stress Response to Injury**

Activation of the sympathetic nervous system
Activation of hypophyseal–pituitary–adrenal axis
Peripheral insulin resistance
Production of pro- and anti-inflammatory cytokines
Acute-phase changes of hepatic protein synthesis
Recruitment and activation of neutrophils, monocyte/macrophages, and lymphocytes
Upregulation of procoagulant activity

TABLE 14-5   Principal Hormonal Responses to Surgical Stress

Endocrine gland	Hormones	Change in secretion
Anterior pituitary		
	ACTH	Increased
	Growth hormone	Increased
	TSH	Variable
	FSH/LH	Variable
Posterior pituitary		
	AVP	Increased
Adrenal cortex		
	Cortisol	Increased
	Aldosterone	Increased
Pancreas		
	Insulin	Decreased
	Glucagon	Increased
Thyroid		
	Thyroxine	Decreased
	Triiodothyronine	Decreased

ACTH, adrenocorticotropic hormone; TSH, thyroid-stimulating hormone; FSH, follicle-stimulating hormone; LH, luteinizing hormone; AVP, arginine vasopressin.

    d. Each unit of RBC infusion results in the administration of about 200 mg free iron, which is vital for microbial growth. However, it is unclear whether iron administration *per se* increases the risk of infection.
  2. Transfusion principles are detailed elsewhere in this text.
E. Hyperglycemia
  1. Hyperglycemia was viewed as inevitable following critical illness and injury as a consequence of the counter-regulatory stress hormone response, the mobilization of glucose through glycogenolysis, and the subsequent mobilization of amino acids for glucose synthesis through catabolism of lean tissue. We recognize that hyperglycemia (>200 mg/dL) is associated with an increased incidence of SSI following cardiac or major general surgery.
  2. Despite these observations, little priority was assigned to prevention of hyperglycemia until the publication in 2001 by van den Berghe et al. of a prospective trial of tight glucose control (80 to 110 mg/dL) in critically ill surgical patients

TABLE 14-6   Conditions Known to Increase the Risk of Infection

- Extremes of age
- Malnutrition
- Obesity
- Diabetes
- Prior site irradiation
- Hypothermia
- Hypoxemia
- Remote infection
- Corticosteroid therapy
- Recent operation, especially of the chest or abdomen
- Chronic inflammation
- Hypocholesterolemia

TABLE 14-7	Glucose Dyshomeostasis During Stress and Effects on Cellular Immunity

Effects of stress response on carbohydrate metabolism
- Enhanced peripheral glucose uptake/utilization
- Hyperlactatemia
- Increased gluconeogenesis
- Depressed glycogenolysis
- Peripheral insulin resistance

Effects of hyperglycemia on immune cell function
- Decreased respiratory burst of alveolar macrophages
- Decreased insulin-stimulated chemokinesis
  - Glucose-induced protein kinase C activation
- Increased adherence
  - Increased adhesion molecule generation
- Spontaneous activation of neutrophils

(mostly cardiac surgery) by continuous infusion of insulin. However, the NICE-SUGAR trial noted that tight glucose control as above *increased* mortality in critically ill patients when compared to a target glucose of <180 mg/dL (different from "no glucose control"), primarily through excess cardiac events.

3. Glucose dyshomeostasis has several manifestations during stress (Table 14-7).
   a. Peripheral glucose uptake and utilization are increased.
   b. Glycogenolysis is depressed after initial, short-term mobilization of hepatic glycogen stores.
   c. Gluconeogenesis is increased.
   d. Peripheral insulin resistance.
   e. Importantly, hyperglycemia impairs immune cell function.
      i. Neutrophils may activate spontaneously, with increased generation of adhesion molecules, impairing microcirculatory flow.
      ii. Insulin-stimulated chemokinesis is decreased.
      iii. Phagocytes manifest decreased respiratory burst and thus impaired microbial killing.
4. Given that the stress response is stereotypical and pervasive among critically ill and injured surgical patients, there is indirect evidence that glucose control with insulin therapy seeking <180 mg/dL is as important for trauma patients as it is for surgical patients.

III. PREVENTION OF INFECTION

A. **Principles.** Infection prevention tactics must be utilized as an ensemble; the list of options is not a buffet from which the clinician may select. Infection control is paramount, but often under-emphasized. Traumatic wounds must be cleansed thoroughly and debrided to remove devitalized tissue. Surgical incisions must be handled gently, inspected daily, and dressed if necessary using aseptic technique. Avoid drains and catheters when possible and remove as soon as practical. Use antibiotics in a focused manner to minimize emergence of antibiotic multi–drug-resistant (MDR) pathogens.

B. **Infection control**
   1. Infection control is an individual responsibility as well as a responsibility of the trauma team and trauma unit. **Hand hygiene is the single most effective means to reduce the spread of infection.** Yet, if adherence to hand washing is studied, it is invariably lacking. To be effective, hand cleansing with soap and water requires a minimum of 30 to 45 seconds. Alcohol gel hand cleansers are as effective as soap and water (the notable exception being spores of *Clostridium difficile*, against which alcohol is ineffective), and compliance is

higher. Use universal precautions (i.e., cap, mask, gown, gloves, and protective eyewear) whenever there is a risk of splashing of body fluids (at all times in the trauma bay, and commonly in the ICU).

2. The sources of the bacteria causing infection are the patients' endogenous flora, and skin surfaces, airways, gut lumen, wounds, catheters, and inanimate surfaces within the patient's room (e.g., bed rails, bedside commodes, and computer terminals do become colonized).

3. Whether infection develops is determined primarily by the response of host defenses, as many organisms that cause infection following injury are inherently avirulent (e.g., *Candida, Enterococcus, Pseudomonas*). The fecal–oral route is the most common manner by which auto-infection develops, but health care workers hasten the transmission of pathogens around a unit, with colonizing pathogens recovered from the surfaces of personal communication devices, stethoscopes, and neckties, although defective hand hygiene is the key offender.

4. Contact isolation is an important part of infection control and should be used in targeted patients with methicillin-resistant *Staphylococcus aureus* (MRSA) and vancomycin-resistant enterococci (VRE), or MDR gram-negative bacilli (GNB).

C. Appropriate catheter care includes:

1. Avoidance of insertion when non-essential.
2. Appropriate hand cleansing and barrier protection of the caregiver at all times.
3. Appropriate skin cleansing and barrier protection of the patient during insertion.
4. Selection of the proper catheter.
5. Proper dressings while catheters are indwelling.
6. Removal as soon as possible when no longer needed, or if inserted under less than ideal circumstances. **The benefit of the information gained by catheterization or the relief afforded the patient must always be weighed against the risk of infection.**
7. Any indwelling catheter carries a risk of infection, but non-tunnelled central venous catheters pose the highest risk, including local site infections and blood stream infections (Table 14-1). Other catheters that have a substantial risk of infection include:
   a. Thoracostomy tubes or catheters (particularly if inserted as an emergency procedure).
   b. Ventriculostomy catheters for monitoring of intracranial pressure.
   c. Urinary bladder catheters.
   d. Each day of endotracheal intubation and mechanical ventilation increases the risk of pneumonia (by about 3%/day for the first week, and 1%/day thereafter. It is controversial whether tracheostomy to facilitate pulmonary toilet and decreased work of breathing decreases the risk of infection.
   e. In terms of preventing infection, abdominal drains are the most superfluous.
8. Whenever possible, skin preparation should be with chlorhexidine solution with or without alcohol, which is viricidal and fungicidal as well as bactericidal. Extensive evidence-based guidelines exist for prevention of catheter-related infection.
   a. Chlorhexidine is superior to povidone–iodine solution for skin preparation prior to central venous catheter insertion. When povidone–iodine solution is used, it must be allowed to dry; it is not bactericidal when wet.
   b. Full barrier precautions (i.e., cap, mask, sterile gown, sterile gloves, eye protection, and a large field drape) are mandatory for all bedside catheterization procedures except arterial and urinary bladder catheterization, for which sterile gloves and a sterile field suffice.
   c. The site of central venous catheter insertion influences the risk of infection; the femoral vein site carries a higher risk of infection that either the subclavian or internal jugular vein sites, and should be avoided whenever possible.
   d. Anytime a deep catheter is inserted under less than ideal conditions as described (e.g., a central venous catheter placed during a trauma or cardiac

resuscitation) it should be removed and replaced elsewhere (if needed) within 24 hours.

  e. A single dose of a first-generation cephalosporin (e.g., cefazolin) may prevent some infections following emergency tube thoracostomy or all ventriculostomy placements, but is not indicated for vascular or bladder catheterizations. Topical antiseptics placed post-procedure at the insertion site are of no benefit.

9. The choice of catheter may play a role in decreasing the risk of infection with endotracheal tubes, central venous catheters, and urinary catheters.

  a. An endotracheal tube with an extra lumen that opens to the airway just above the balloon, to facilitate the aspiration of secretions that accumulate in an area that cannot be reached by routine suctioning, below the vocal cords but above the balloon on the endotracheal tube (subglottic secretions), can decrease the incidence of ventilator-associated pneumonia (VAP) by one-half. An endotracheal tube coated with ionic silver reduces the incidence of VAP.

  b. Antibiotic- (e.g., minocycline/rifampin) or antiseptic-coated central venous catheters (e.g., chlorhexidine/silver sulfadiazine) are effective in reducing the incidence of CLABSI; the catheter coated with minocycline/rifampin appears to be most effective.

  c. Urinary bladder catheters coated with ionic silver reduce the incidence of catheter-related bacterial cystitis.

10. Dressings must be maintained clean, dry, and intact. Maintaining an intact dressing is difficult when the patient is agitated or the body surface is irregular (e.g., the neck [internal jugular vein catheterization] as opposed to the chest wall [subclavian vein catheterization].

  a. A simple gauze dressing is best. Occlusive transparent dressings can accumulate moisture beneath that is a usable growth medium for residual skin flora, which re-colonize the skin anyway within a few hours.

  b. Mark the dressing clearly with the date and time of each change.

  c. Dressing carts or trays should not be brought from patient to patient; rather, sufficient supplies should be kept in each patient's room. Inanimate objects (e.g., stethoscopes, scissors) are potential transmission vectors if not cleansed thoroughly after contact with each patient.

11. Evaluate indwelling catheters daily for its continued utility and remove as soon as possible.

  a. Most abdominal drains do not decrease the risk of infection. On the contrary, the risk is probably increased because the catheters hold open a portal for invasion by bacteria and soon become a "two-way street." Other than for hepatic or pancreatic injuries or discrete collections of purulent fluid, abdominal drains are seldom useful. Closed suction drains should not be left in proximity to intestinal suture lines; the negative pressures generated, particularly when such drains are "stripped," may cause disruption.

D. Antibiotic prophylaxis

1. Shock, hypoperfusion, and hemorrhage complicate the pharmacokinetics of prophylactic antibiotic administration immediately following trauma. Shock, hypovolemia, and hypoperfusion also increase the risk of organ dysfunction caused by antibiotics (e.g., aminoglycosides and renal injury).

2. With modern β-lactam antibiotics, the drug needed in the tissues is easily attained with conventional prophylactic doses (e.g., cefazolin 1 g, cefoxitin 1 to 2 g) unless the patient is morbidly obese or bleeding briskly.

IV. DURATION

  A. Antibiotics with short elimination half-lives (e.g., cefazolin and cefoxitin) should be re-dosed intraoperatively (e.g., every 3 hours for cefoxitin and every 4 hours for cefazolin) to ensure that tissue concentrations remain adequate during the vulnerable period when the incision is open. **SSI and only SSI is prevented by antibiotic prophylaxis.** Antibiotic prophylaxis more than 24 hours beyond injury increases the risk of nosocomial infection. Thus, antibiotic prophylaxis in trauma must not extend beyond 24 hours except *perhaps* for grade III open fractures.

B. Numerous randomized prospective trials have shown that 12 to 24 hours of antibiotic prophylaxis for penetrating abdominal trauma is equivalent to 5 days of prophylaxis, even when a colon injury is present, provided surgery is performed within 12 hours of injury. Penetrating abdominal trauma with no intestinal injury requires only a single preoperative dose of antibiotic prophylaxis.

C. Vascular catheter insertion procedures do not require antibiotic prophylaxis. Other catheter insertion procedures require only a single dose of prophylactic antibiotics, except *perhaps* for emergency tube thoracostomy (up to 24 hours). Indwelling catheters otherwise should *never* receive prolonged antibiotic prophylaxis.

V. SPECIFIC INJURIES
A. Abdominal injury

1. The data are unequivocal that prophylaxis of no more than 24 hours of a second-generation cephalosporin (e.g., cefoxitin) is equivalent to a longer course (e.g., 5 days) for penetrating abdominal trauma with injury to a hollow viscus, provided the surgery is performed within 12 hours of injury. Penetrating trauma that does not injure a hollow viscus needs only a single dose of antibiotics given prior to operation.

2. Although not as well studied, the principle is similar for blunt abdominal trauma; if managed non-operatively, no antibiotics are required. If surgery is performed, the duration of prophylaxis (a single dose or 24 hours of prophylaxis) is determined by the pattern of injury.

3. The abdomen may be left open temporarily as part of **damage control** or to prevent or manage the abdominal compartment syndrome. There is no evidence that the open abdomen requires antibiotic prophylaxis even if a prosthesis is employed as part of the temporary closure. Another dose of prophylactic antibiotic aimed against skin flora (e.g., gram-positive cocci [GPC]) is appropriate at the time of abdominal wall closure or reconstruction.

4. There is no evidence that prophylactic antibiotics are required if the liver and spleen are embolized as part of the non-operative management of blunt trauma to those organs.

5. The infection risk associated with the late post-splenectomy period (including bacteremia from encapsulated GPC) is genuine for children but low for adults. Experts often recommend prophylaxis with oral penicillin until age 18 years for splenectomized children, but adults do not require long-term antibiotic prophylaxis.

6. All individuals who undergo splenectomy should receive the polyvalent pneumococcal vaccine, with booster doses at 5-year intervals. Some experts advocate co-administration of vaccines against *Haemophilus influenzae* and *Neisseria meningitidis*; optimal timing of booster doses is unknown. Also unknown is whether patients who have undergone splenic embolization or the increasingly rare splenorrhaphy procedure should be vaccinated against post-splenectomy sepsis. Vaccination of the embolized patient following splenic injury is our practice, especially for children.

B. Chest injuries.
Little data exist to guide antibiotic prophylaxis of chest trauma. For blunt chest trauma, no antibiotic prophylaxis is indicated, even in the presence of pulmonary contusion.

1. Two-thirds of patients who aspirate do not develop pneumonia, so withholding of antibiotics (technically empiric therapy, not prophylaxis in this case) is reasonable until objective evidence of pneumonia is obtained. If antibiotics are started they should be discontinued within 48 to 72 hours if the development of pneumonia is unproven (Section VII.A).

2. Prophylaxis of chest tubes is controversial. The guidelines of the Eastern Association for the Surgery of Trauma recommend 24 hours of prophylaxis only of emergency trauma chest tube insertions as a Level III recommendation (based on expert opinion).

C. Fractures. The guidelines of the Eastern Association for the Surgery of Trauma and the Surgical Infection Society recommend 24 hours of prophylaxis of grade I–II open long bone fractures with an agent active against GPC. For grade III open fractures, the addition of an agent active against GNB is recommended, but for a maximum of 72 hours (*not* 72 hours after each fracture operation, which leads to indefinite antibiotic administration).

D. Skin and soft-tissue injuries. The likelihood of infection is influenced foremost by the degree of contamination of the wound, ranging from approximately 3% for clean wounds to about 25% for wounds with gross contamination. Inspect wounds carefully for foreign material (e.g., clothing, gravel, vegetable matter, wadding from shotgun shells), irrigate with physiologic saline, and debride devitalized tissue.

  1. Risk factors for infection include diabetes mellitus, age (increased risk per year), foreign body, and the width of the incision. Lacerations of the head/neck region and the hand are less likely to become infected. Despite an increased risk of infection posed by some wounds, there is scant evidence that traumatic injuries should receive antibiotic prophylaxis; administration is generally not recommended. The most common pathogens of infected traumatic wounds are aerobic GPC (e.g., *S. aureus*), with aerobic GNB (e.g., *Escherichia coli, Pseudomonas aeruginosa*) being less common.

  2. Animal and human bites are presumed to be infected because of the large bacterial inoculum that is deposited in deep tissues and the resulting challenges inherent in local wound care.

   a. The pathogens differ in bite wounds, with dog and cat bites showing a predilection for *Eikenella corrodens* and *Pasteurella multocida*, respectively. Prophylaxis with amoxicillin/clavulanate is the best strategy, though duration is less well defined (often 5 days.)

   b. Human bites are likely to cause infection with oral anaerobes (e.g., anaerobic streptococci, rarely *Bacteroides fragilis*).

VI. MICROBIOLOGY

  A. Principles of resistance. Bacteria use several different mechanisms to develop resistance to antibiotics.

   1. Cell wall permeability to antibiotics is decreased by changes in porin channels (especially important for gram-negative bacteria with complex cell walls, affecting aminoglycosides, β-lactam drugs, chloramphenicol, sulfonamides, tetracyclines, and possibly fluoroquinolones).

   2. Production of specific antibiotic inactivating-enzymes by either plasmid-mediated or chromosomally mediated mechanisms affects aminoglycosides, β-lactam drugs (β-lactamases), chloramphenicol, and macrolides.

    a. β-lactamases. Members of the family *Enterobacteriaceae* express plasmid-encoded β-lactamase enzymes commonly, which modify or destroy the β-lactam nucleus central to penicillins, cephalosporins, and carbapenems.

   3. Alteration of the target for antibiotic binding in the cell wall (e.g., penicillin-binding proteins, which are important enzymes for formation of the peptidoglycan matrix of the cell wall of gram-positive bacteria) affects β-lactam drugs and vancomycin, whereas alteration of target enzymes can affect β-lactam drugs, sulfonamides, fluoroquinolones, and rifampin.

   4. Drugs that bind to the bacterial ribosome (i.e., aminoglycosides, chloramphenicol, macrolides, lincosamides, streptogramins, and tetracyclines) are also susceptible to alteration of the receptor on the ribosome.

   5. Antibiotics may be extruded actively by efflux pumps once entry to the cell is achieved, in the case of macrolides, lincosamides, streptogramins, fluoroquinolones, and tetracyclines.

  B. The bacterial species of greatest clinical concern for development of resistance may be recalled as the "ESKAPE" pathogens (*Enterococcus faecium, S. aureus, Klebsiella pneumoniae, Acinetobacter calcoaceticus-baumannii complex, P. aeruginosa,* and *Enterobacter* spp.).

1. Certain antibiotic classes are highly associated with emergence of resistance as compared with other antibiotic classes. In the case of MRSA, colonization and infection have been associated with prior exposure to glycopeptides, cephalosporins, and fluoroquinolones. Colonization with C. *difficile* has been associated with cephalosporins, fluoroquinolones, and clindamycin in particular (although any antibiotic, even a single dose of a first- or second-generation cephalosporin used appropriately for surgical prophylaxis and those used for treatment of C. *difficile* infection [CDI], may lead to CDI).

   a. **GPC.** GPC cause most infection following injury. These include infections following neurosurgery (e.g., ventriculitis following invasive monitoring of intracranial pressure), sinusitis, CLABSI, device/implant-associated infections, and complicated skin and skin structure infections (cSSSI). Respiratory tract and UTIs may also be caused by GPC.

      i. *S. aureus* is the most important pathogen among the GPC. Sixty percent of hospital-acquired isolates of *S. aureus* are resistant to methicillin (MRSA), whereas up to 50% of community-acquired strains are now resistant (CA-MRSA) in some regions of the US. Staphylococcal resistance to vancomycin remains rare and is induced only after prolonged exposure to vancomycin among debilitated patients (e.g., dialysis patients). *S. aureus* is a major pathogen in sinusitis, catheter-related bloodstream infections (CR-BSI), cSSSI, and pneumonia.

      ii. *S. epidermidis* is usually resistant to methicillin (MRSE, 85%) and is the major pathogen in CLABSI and device/implant-associated infections.

      iii. *Enterococcus* spp. can cause cSSSI, CR-BSI, and infections of the urinary tract. About 30% of *enterococci* are resistant to vancomycin (VRE), but the pattern is species-specific. Whereas 70% of *E. faecium* isolated are VRE, the same is true for only 3% of *Enterococcus faecalis* isolates. VRE poses a threat primarily to debilitated patients after prolonged hospitalization. Colonization of the feces with VRE usually precedes invasive infection, and cannot be eradicated. Risk factors for the acquisition of VRE include prolonged hospitalization, readmission to the ICU, and therapy with vancomycin or third-generation cephalosporins.

      iv. Because of the high prevalence of MRSA, vancomycin remains the most prescribed antibiotic for resistant GPC despite poor tissue penetration and the risk of toxicity.

      v. Alternatives for therapy of MRSA include linezolid, tigecycline, daptomycin (but **not** for pneumonia), ceftaroline (indicated only for acute bacterial skin and skin structure infections) and quinupristin/dalfopristin (used seldom because of multiple toxicities).

   b. **GNB.** GNB are less common as pathogens than GPC but are important in the pathogenesis of cSSSI (particularly after inoculation of a wound), lower respiratory tract infection, and intra-abdominal infection. Although *E. coli* or *Klebsiella* spp. predominate in intra-abdominal infection, *P. aeruginosa* is the second most common ICU pathogen overall and the bacterium most closely associated with death from HAI. *P. aeruginosa* can infect virtually any tissue, including synovium and vitreous humor. *P. aeruginosa* bacteremia can cause or complicate pneumonia, and other metastatic infections can follow. Antimicrobial resistance is a major problem with *P. aeruginosa*, *Acinetobacter* spp., and *Klebsiella* spp., and increasing among *Enterobacteriaceae* other than *Klebsiella*.

      i. Although resistance to cephalosporins can occur by several mechanisms, the appearance of chromosomally mediated β-lactamases has been identified as a consequence of the use of third-generation cephalosporins. Resistance rates decline when use is restricted. The mutant bacteria develop resistance rapidly to both cephalosporins and entire other classes of β-lactam antibiotics. It is justifiable therefore to restrict the use of ceftazidime, especially when grappling with an ESBL-producing bacterium.

ii. Carbapenems and aminoglycosides generally retain useful microbicidal activity against ESBL-producing strains, but ESBL-producing strains can cause fatal infections because of delayed recognition and consequent delayed empiric antimicrobial therapy. Unfortunately, routine antimicrobial susceptibility testing does not detect ESBL-producing strains. When in doubt, the laboratory now has a bias to label an organism non-susceptible, so as to direct therapy to another agent of a different class.

iii. The resistance problem in GNB is not limited to cephalosporin resistance. Metalloproteinases and carbapenemases threaten the utility of carbapenems to treat *Pseudomonas* and *Acinetobacter*.

iv. The fastest-growing resistance problem for GNB in the US. is quinolone resistance, particularly against *Pseudomonas* and *Enterobacteriaceae*. Quinolone resistance is chromosomally mediated for the most part, primarily by changes in the target sites (DNA gyrase or topoisomerase IV) for the antibiotic.

v. Resistance to one quinolone may also increase the MIC for other quinolones against the organism, so a highly active agent given in adequate dosage is essential for empiric therapy with quinolones.

c. Fungi and yeast

i. Most fungi and yeast are avirulent opportunistic pathogens that do not threaten healthy patients. However, such infections should also be unusual in the "typical" critically ill or injured patient. Unless occurring in a profoundly immunosuppressed patient (i.e., cancer chemotherapy with neutropenia, bone marrow transplant or non-renal solid organ transplant) fungal infections are usually the result of antibiotic overuse. Prolonged broad-spectrum antibiotic therapy suppresses host flora, and creates the opportunity for overgrowth of commensal flora. The most common health care–acquired fungal infections are caused by *Candida* spp., which are part of gut flora in approximately one-quarter of patients.

ii. Although colonization with *Candida* does precede invasive infection, the utility of antifungal prophylaxis remains controversial and unsupported by evidence. However, most surgical patients do not manifest fungemia, the prototypical invasive infection.

iii. Widespread prescribing of fluconazole has led to emergence of resistance among *Candida* spp.

iv. Empiric therapy of suspected invasive fungal infections is probably not necessary in most units that have a low incidence of such infections, but must address the possibility of resistant *Candida* if administered. Therefore, fluconazole should not be used until an organism that is likely to be susceptible to fluconazole is identified (most centers do not perform fungal susceptibility testing). Empiric therapy choices include conventional amphotericin B, lipid formulations of amphotericin B, or the echinocandins, caspofungin or micafungin. Conventional amphotericin B is seldom used currently because of toxicity (e.g., febrile reactions, hypokalemia, renal insufficiency). The lipid formulations mitigate the toxicity, but at high cost. Echinocandins are broadly active against yeast and fungi including *Candida* spp. and *Aspergillus* spp., and a logical, choice for empiric therapy, but data are scant, particularly in surgical patients. Comparative studies suggest that the triazole agent voriconazole may be more effective than amphotericin B for invasive aspergillosis.

VII. NOSOCOMIAL INFECTIONS. Among nosocomial infections, pleuropulmonary infections (e.g., pneumonia, empyema) are more common than bacteremia, which in turn is more common than UTI.

A. Pneumonia. The most common HAI following critical illness or injury is pneumonia (HAP). Trauma patients may be at specific risk for development of pneumonia (or empyema, which complicates 5% of cases of post-traumatic pneumonia) for several reasons.

1. Chest wall injury (e.g., rib fractures) decreases thoracic compliance and impairs pulmonary toilet.
2. Direct (e.g., penetrating injury, pulmonary contusion) or indirect (e.g., acute respiratory distress syndrome, ARDS) pulmonary injury depresses local pulmonary host defenses directly.
3. TBI may impair airway reflexes, leading to an increased risk of aspiration of gastric contents.
4. Iatrogenic risk factors include prolonged bed rest, supine positioning, tracheal or nasogastric intubation, narcotic analgesics and sedatives, and prolonged mechanical ventilation. Even a single day of mechanical ventilation increases the risk of VAP.
5. Pneumonia can be prevented by careful adherence to the principles of infection control included in the "ventilator bundle."
   a. Positioning the head of the bed up 30 degrees at all times
   b. Daily sedation holidays and assessment for liberation from mechanical ventilation
   c. Prophylaxis of stress-related gastric mucosal hemorrhage
   d. Prophylaxis of venous thromboembolic disease
   e. Daily oral hygiene with 0.12% chlorhexidine gluconate mouthwash
6. Some authors describe HAP or VAP as **early-onset** or **late-onset,** with onset more than 5 days after admission or intubation, respectively, being the defining time.
   a. The microbiology of **early-onset HAP/VAP** differs, in that it is more likely to be caused by relatively antibiotic-susceptible bacteria such as *S. pneumoniae, H. influenzae,* or methicillin-sensitive *S. aureus* (MSSA).
   b. **Late-onset HAP** and especially VAP tend to be caused by MRSA, *P. aeruginosa, Acinetobacter* spp., and the *Enterobacteriaceae* (although *E. coli* pneumonia is relatively uncommon).
7. The diagnosis of VAP in particular is controversial.
   a. Routine sputum collection for culture and susceptibility testing by standard endotracheal suctioning can contaminate the specimen with these upper airway "colonists," thereby leading to the over-diagnosis and consequent overtreatment of VAP.
   b. To reduce this risk, **quantitative microbiology testing of sputum** obtained by a technique that minimizes the possibility of contamination has been advocated. Fiberoptic bronchoscopy with bronchoalveolar lavage (BAL) or the use of a protected-specimen brush (PSB) catheter can reduce the risk of contamination of the specimen and increase the accuracy by increasing the specificity of the diagnosis, making antibiotic administration more accurate and affording the opportunity to withhold antibiotic therapy or truncate it.
8. The most common causative organisms for VAP are MRSA and *P. aeruginosa;* effective initial empiric antibiotic therapy must account for both. **Misdirected (against resistant pathogens) and delayed antibiotic therapy of VAP are major causes of therapeutic failure and death.** Data suggest that the duration of therapy for VAP should be as brief as 8 days for most cases of VAP, with the possible exception of cases caused by non-fermenting GNB (e.g., *P. aeruginosa, Acinetobacter* spp., *Stenotrophomonas maltophilia*), which may require up to 2 weeks of therapy.
9. The mortality rate of pneumonia complicating trauma is approximately 20%, whereas it is approximately 35% for VAP in critically ill surgical patients.

B. Central line–associated blood stream infection

1. Trauma and non-trauma ICU patients who are unstable often require reliable large-bore intravenous access. Placed typically into central veins (e.g., femoral, internal jugular, or subclavian vein), these catheters are prone to local infection and blood stream infection, although the incidence are decreasing owing to rigorous infection control practices.
2. When placed under elective (controlled) circumstances, proper insertion technique mandates that the operator prepare the operative field with chlorhexidine

(not povidone–iodine solution), drape the entire bed into a sterile field, and don a cap, mask, and sterile gown and gloves (Table 14-1).

3. When sterile procedure or technique is breached, the risk of infection increases and the catheter should be removed and replaced (if still needed) at a different site using strict sterile technique within 24 hours.

   a. Infection risk for femoral vein catheters is highest, and lowest for catheters placed via the subclavian route.

   b. Peripheral vein catheters, peripherally placed central catheters (PICC), and tunneled central venous catheters (e.g., Hickman, Broviac), pose less risk of infection than percutaneous central venous catheters.

   c. Antibiotic- and antiseptic-coated catheters are controversial, but may decrease the risk of infection.

4. Catheter infection is diagnosed by isolation of >15 cfu from a segment of catheter by the semi-quantitative roll-plate technique. The diagnosis of CLABSI is confirmed when the isolates from blood and the cultured catheter are identical. The pathogens of CLABSI are predominantly GPC, most commonly MRSE, MRSA, and *enterococci. Candida* spp. is the fourth most common pathogen of nosocomial blood stream infections, overall.

   a. Proper technique for the collection and processing of blood cultures should result in a false-positive (contamination) rate of 3% at most. Isolation of MRSE from a single blood culture is likely a contaminant (do not treat), especially if the patient has no indwelling hardware that might become infected secondarily (e.g., prosthetic joint or heart valve).

   b. Gram-negative bacillary pathogens are less common, and fungal CR-BSI are unusual in trauma patients.

   c. Treatment is by removal of the catheter (for peripheral or percutaneous central venous catheters) and parenteral antibiotics initially. Central line–associated blood stream infections caused by MRSA require at least 2 weeks of therapy; some authorities argue for a longer (e.g., 4 to 6 weeks) course because of the risk of metastatic infection. Vancomycin or linezolid may be chosen for MRSA CLABSI (or MRSE when treatment is indicated), with daptomycin as an alternative. Therapy for enterococcal or gram-negative CLABSI is dictated by bacterial susceptibility, without clear consensus as to duration of therapy except that a course of therapy of 2 weeks' duration is probably not necessary. Beyond removal of the catheter, treatment of fungal CLABSI is controversial. Some authorities recommend removal of the catheter as sole therapy; others recommend at least 2 weeks of systemic antifungal therapy after the last positive blood culture. Patients with persistent fungemia receive longer courses of therapy.

C. Peritonitis/intra-abdominal infection

1. The peritonitis associated commonly with perforated viscus is referred to as **secondary peritonitis.** In the trauma setting, secondary peritonitis may occur after penetrating injury to the intestine that is not treated promptly (>12 hours delay). Other causes include dehiscence of a bowel anastomosis with leakage of succus entericus, or development of an intra-abdominal abscess. **Secondary peritonitis is polymicrobial,** with anaerobic GNB (e.g., *B. fragilis*) predominating, and *E. coli* and *Klebsiella* spp. isolated commonly. Any of a number of antibiotic regimens of appropriate spectrum may be appropriate. *Enterococci, Pseudomonas,* and other bacteria may be isolated, but do not require specific therapy if the patient is otherwise healthy (e.g., not immunocompromised) and responding to therapy as prescribed.

   a. Surgical source control is a crucial part of the management of complicated intra-abdominal infection, and must be achieved, whether by percutaneous drainage of a discrete collection, or laparoscopic or open surgery. Antibiotic therapy is necessary, but adjunctive.

2. When secondary peritonitis develops in a hospitalized patient as a complication of disease or therapy, the flora is likely to reflect those encountered in the hospital. For example, *enterococci, Enterobacter,* and *Pseudomonas* are more prevalent, whereas *E. coli* and *Klebsiella* are less common. Antibiotic therapy must be adjusted accordingly for nosocomial peritonitis, with greater emphasis placed on empiric coverage of *enterococci,* MRSA, and yeast. **Surgical source control must be achieved.** Failure of two source control procedures with persistent intra-abdominal collections is referred to as **tertiary peritonitis.**

    a. Tertiary peritonitis represents complete failure of intra-abdominal host defenses. Some authorities recommend that these patients be managed with an open-abdomen technique, so that manual peritoneal toilet can be provided under sedation or anesthesia, possibly at the bedside. At times, there is no alternative to open-abdomen management if the infection extends to involve the abdominal wall, and extensive debridement is required.

D. *Clostridium difficile* **infection (CDI)**

    1. CDI (formerly pseudomembranous colitis) develops because antibiotic therapy disrupts the balance of colonic flora, allowing the selection and overgrowth of *C. difficile*, present in the fecal flora of 3% of normal hosts. Any antibiotic can induce this selection pressure, even as single-dose, although clindamycin, third-generation cephalosporins, and fluoroquinolones have a high predilection. Even antibiotics used to treat CDI (e.g., metronidazole) have been associated with CDI.

    2. CDI is a nosocomial infection. Spores can persist on inanimate surfaces for prolonged periods, and pathogens can be transmitted from patient-to-patient by contaminated equipment (e.g., bedpans, rectal thermometers) or on the hands of health care workers. **The alcohol gel that is used increasingly for hand disinfection is not active against spores of *C. difficile.* Therefore, handwashing with soap and water is necessary when caring for an infected patient or during outbreaks.**

    3. The clinical spectrum of CDI is wide, ranging from asymptomatic (8% of affected patients do not have diarrhea) to life-threatening transmural pancolitis with perforation and severe sepsis or septic shock. The typical patient will have fever, abdominal distension, copious diarrhea, and leukocytosis. Bleeding from the colon is rare, and if observed should prompt strongly the consideration of an alternative diagnosis.

    4. Diagnosis by assay for the enterotoxins in a fresh stool specimen has supplanted colonoscopy. Up to 50% of patients do not have the "characteristic" colonic mucosal pseudomembranes (hence, the change in nomenclature).

    5. Treatment of mild cases consists of withdrawal of the offending antibiotic; oral antibiotic therapy is often prescribed. More severe cases may require parenteral metronidazole or oral or enteral vancomycin (by lavage or enema, if ileus precludes oral therapy); parenteral vancomycin is ineffective. Fidaxomicin is a new non-absorbable macrolide antibiotic that is non-inferior to oral vancomycin for the treatment of mild-to-moderate CDI, and may be associated with a lower risk of recurrence. However, the role of fidaxomicin in treatment of more severe CDI is unknown, if any.

    6. On occasion, patients with severe disease may require total abdominal colectomy. The prevalence of severe disease has increased markedly with the emergence of a new strain of *C. difficile*. The new strain (NAP1–027) has undergone a mutation of a gene that suppresses toxin production, such that far more toxin is elaborated, resulting in clinically severe, systemic disease. Total abdominal colectomy for CDI carries high morbidity and mortality, and worth avoiding if possible, but the indication for colectomy for CDI is not well defined. Higher risk is defined by older age, leukocytosis >20,000/mm^3, and lactic acidosis. If the patient develops septic shock, salvage is unlikely even with a colectomy, so the onset of shock may be too late for effective surgical intervention.

E. Sinusitis

    1. Nosocomial sinusitis is a rare but dangerous closed-space infection that is difficult to diagnose.

    2. Patients with transnasal tubes (particularly nasotracheal intubation, after 7 days of which the incidence is one-third) and maxillofacial trauma are at particular risk. Purulent or foul-smelling nasal discharge is an obvious clue to the diagnosis but not always present. Sinusitis must be sought radiographically by CT of the facial bones to identify sinus mucosal thickening or opacification. Since the process is often occult, the more the diagnosis is sought, the more often it will be found.

3. Sinusitis should be suspected in any patient with sepsis, particularly if initial cultures (e.g., blood, sputum, urine, indwelling vascular catheters) are unrevealing. If sinusitis is suspected, the diagnosis is confirmed by maxillary antral tap, lavage, and culture using aseptic technique. GPC, GNB (including *P. aeruginosa*), and fungi (incidence, 8%) are possible pathogens; initial therapy should be based on local susceptibility patterns. Most antibiotics that might be chosen achieve adequate tissue penetration. The duration of therapy should be based on the clinical response. Refractory cases may require repetitive lavage of the sinus or a formal drainage procedure.

4. Sinusitis is a predisposing factor for VAP and may be a source of pathogens that gain access to the lower respiratory tract.

F. Decubitus ulcer. Infection from decubitus ulcer may be obvious or covert. Patients are at increased risk with prolonged bed rest (>7 days), which may be mitigated by specialized bedding. Morbid obesity is a risk factor, given that routine turning and positioning of such patients is a formidable undertaking. Most decubitus ulcers form in the pre-sacral area, but ulcers can form anywhere unremitting pressure is placed upon tissue. When evaluating a patient for occult infection, the skin must be inspected systematically for decubitus ulcers. **Deep ulcers** (Stage III, involving subcutaneous fat; stage IV, involving fascia, muscle, or bone) may require debridement or systemic antibiotic therapy. In rare cases, a decubitus ulcer may transform into a life-threatening necrotizing soft-tissue infection.

G. Urinary tract infection (UTI)

1. UTI is the leading nosocomial infection among all hospitalized patients, but is not as common as SSI and pneumonia in surgical/trauma patients. By far, the leading risk factor for UTI is an indwelling urinary bladder catheter. Measurement of intra-abdominal pressure via a Foley catheter is also an independent risk factor, owing to interruption of the sterile fluid path.

2. The incidence of bacteriuria/candiduria associated with urinary catheterization is approximately 5%/day. Catheter-associated bacteriuria or candiduria usually represents colonization, is rarely symptomatic, and is an unlikely cause of fever or secondary blood stream infection, even in immunocompromised patients, unless there is urinary tract obstruction, a history of recent urologic manipulation, injury, or surgery; or neutropenia.

3. Effective prevention tactics include avoidance of or brief duration of catheterization (e.g., <24 hours for elective surgery patients), and the use of silver alloy–coated catheters when instrumentation is required.

4. Traditional signs and symptoms (e.g., dysuria, urgency, pelvic or flank pain, fever or chills) that correlate with UTI in non-catheterized patients are rarely reported in ICU patients with documented catheter-associated bacteriuria or candiduria ($>10^5$ cfu/mL). In the ICU, the majority of UTI are related to urinary catheters and are caused by multi-resistant nosocomial GNB, *Enterococcus* spp., and yeasts.

5. When clinical evaluation suggests the urinary tract as a source of infection, a urine specimen should be evaluated by direct microscopy, Gram stain, and quantitative culture. The specimen should be aspirated from the catheter sampling port after disinfecting the port with alcohol, not collected from the drainage bag. Urine collected for culture should reach the laboratory promptly to prevent multiplication of bacteria within the receptacle, which might lead to the misdiagnosis of infection; any delay should prompt refrigeration of the specimen.

6. In contrast to community-acquired UTIs, where pyuria is highly predictive of important bacteriuria, pyuria may be absent with catheter-associated UTI. Even if present, pyuria is not a reliable predictor of UTI in the presence of a catheter.

The concentration of urinary bacteria or yeast needed to cause symptomatic UTI or fever is unclear. Whereas it is clear that counts $>10^3$ cfu/mL represent true bacteriuria or candiduria in catheterized patients, no data to show that higher counts are more likely to represent symptomatic infection.

7. It is appropriate to collect urine specimens in the investigation of fever, but routine monitoring or "surveillance" cultures of urine contribute little to patient management. Rapid dipstick tests, which detect leukocyte esterase and nitrite, are unreliable in the setting of catheter-related UTI.

VIII. PRINCIPLES OF ANTIBIOTIC THERAPY
A. Pharmacokinetics and pharmacodynamics

1. Pharmacokinetics (PK) describes the principles of drug absorption, distribution, and metabolism. Dose–response relationships are influenced by dose, dosing interval, and route of administration. Plasma and tissue drug concentrations are influenced by absorption, distribution, and elimination, which in turn depend on drug metabolism and excretion. Serum drug concentrations may or may not correlate, depending on tissue penetration, but to the extent that they do correlate, relationships between local drug concentration and effect are defined by pharmacodynamic (PD) principles.

2. Basic concepts of PK must be utilized for effective antibiotic prescribing:
   a. *Bioavailability* is the percentage of drug dose that reaches the systemic circulation. Bioavailability is 100% after intravenous administration, but is affected by absorption, intestinal transit time, and the degree of hepatic metabolism after oral administration.
   b. *Half-life* ($T_{1/2}$), the time required for the serum drug concentration to reduce by one-half, reflects both clearance and *volume of distribution* (V_D).
   c. *Clearance* represents the volume of liquid from which drug is eliminated completely per unit of time, whether by tissue distribution, metabolism, or elimination; knowledge of drug clearance is important for determining the dose of drug necessary to maintain a steady-state concentration. In general, if $\geq 40\%$ of administered drug or its active metabolites is eliminated unchanged in the urine, decreased renal function requires a dosage adjustment.

3. PD are unique for antibiotic therapy, because drug–patient, drug–microbe, and microbe–patient interactions all are important. The key drug interaction is with the microbe. Microbial physiology, inoculum size, microbial growth phase, mechanisms of resistance, the micro-environment (e.g., local pH), and the host's response are important factors to consider. Because of microbial resistance, administration of drug may not be microcidal if an adequate concentration is not achieved.

4. Antibiotic PD parameters determined by laboratory analysis include the *minimal inhibitory concentration* (MIC), the lowest serum drug concentration that inhibits bacterial growth (MIC_{90} refers to 90% inhibition). However, some antibiotics may suppress bacterial growth at sub-inhibitory concentrations (*post-antibiotic effect*, PAE). Appreciable PAE can be observed with aminoglycosides and fluoroquinolones for gram-negative bacteria, and with some β-lactam drugs (notably carbapenems) against *S. aureus*. However, MIC testing may not detect resistant bacterial subpopulations within the inoculum (e.g., "heteroresistance" of *S. aureus*). Moreover, *in vitro* results may be irrelevant if bacteria are inhibited only by drug concentrations that cannot be achieved clinically.

B. Empiric antibiotic therapy

Empiric antibiotic therapy must be administered judiciously, meaning at right time, dose, and aimed at specific pathogens. Injudicious therapy could result in undertreatment of established infection, or unnecessary therapy when the patient has only inflammation or bacterial colonization; either may be deleterious. Inappropriate therapy (e.g., delay, therapy misdirected against usual pathogens, failure to treat MDR pathogens) leads unequivocally to increased mortality.

1. *Antibiotic stewardship* includes physician education regarding prescribing patterns, computerized decision support, administration by protocol, and

TABLE 14-8	Factors Influencing Antibiotic Choice

Activity against known/suspected pathogens
Disease believed responsible
Distinguish infection from colonization
Narrow-spectrum coverage most desirable
Antimicrobial resistance patterns
Patient-specific factors
   Severity of illness
   Age
   Immunosuppression
   Organ dysfunction
   Allergy
Institutional guidelines/restrictions

formulary restriction programs. It is crucial for initial empiric antibiotic therapy to be targeted appropriately, administered in sufficient dosage to assure bacterial killing, narrowed in spectrum (*de-escalation*) as soon as possible based on microbiology data and clinical response, and continued only as long as necessary. Appropriate antibiotic prescribing not only optimizes patient care, but supports infection control practice and preserves microbial ecology.

2. Antibiotic choice is based on several interrelated factors (Table 14-8):

  a. Activity against identified or likely (for empiric therapy) pathogens is paramount, presuming infecting and colonizing organisms can be distinguished, and that the narrowest effective spectrum coverage is always desired.

  b. Patient-specific factors of importance include age, debility, immunosuppression, intrinsic organ function, prior allergy or other adverse reaction, and recent antibiotic therapy.

  c. Institutional factors of importance include guidelines that may specify a particular therapy, formulary availability of specific agents, outbreaks of infections caused by drug-resistant pathogens, and antibiotic control programs.

  d. It is important for empiric therapy of any nosocomial infection that may be caused by either a gram-positive or gram-negative infection to include activity against all likely pathogens.

3. Agents available for therapy (Table 14-9): Agents may be chosen based on spectrum, whether broad or targeted (e.g., anti-pseudomonal, anti-anaerobic), in addition to the above factors. If a nosocomial gram-positive pathogen is suspected (e.g., wound or SSI, CLABSI, HAP/VAP) or MRSA is endemic, empiric vancomycin (or linezolid) is appropriate. Some authorities recommend dual-agent therapy for serious *Pseudomonas* infections (i.e., an anti-pseudomonal β-lactam drug plus an aminoglycoside), but evidence of efficacy is mixed.

4. Combination therapy of a specific pathogen (e.g., "double-coverage" of *Pseudomonas*) may worsen outcomes. A meta-analysis of β-lactam monotherapy versus β-lactam-aminoglycoside combination therapy for immunocompetent patients with sepsis found no difference in either mortality or the development of resistance with clinical failure more common with combination therapy.

5. ***Cell wall active agents: β-lactam antibiotics.*** The β-lactam antibiotic group consists of penicillins, cephalosporins, monobactams, and carbapenems. Within this group, several agents have been combined with β-lactamase inhibitors to broaden the spectrum of activity. Several subgroups of antibiotics are recognized within the group, notably several "generations" of cephalosporins and penicillinase-resistant penicillins.

  a. *Penicillins.* Penicillinase-resistant semisynthetic penicillins include methicillin, nafcillin, oxacillin, cloxacillin, and dicloxacillin. These agents are used primarily as therapy for sensitive strains of staphylococci. Hospitalized

TABLE 14-9	Antibacterial Agents for Empiric Use

Anti-pseudomonal
Piperacillin–tazobactam
Cefepime, ceftazidime
Imipenem–cilastatin, meropenem, doripenem
? Ciprofloxacin, levofloxacin (depending on local susceptibility patterns)
Aminoglycoside
Polymyxins (polymyxin B, colistin [polymyxin E])

Targeted-spectrum
Gram-positive
Glycopeptide (e.g., vancomycin, telavancin)
Lipopeptide (e.g., daptomycin; not for known/suspected pneumonia)
Oxazolidinone (e.g., linezolid)
Gram-negative
Third-generation cephalosporin (not ceftriaxone)
Monobactam
Polymyxins (polymyxin B, colistin [polymyxin E])
Anti-anaerobic
Metronidazole

Broad-spectrum
Piperacillin–tazobactam
Carbapenems
Fluoroquinolones (depending on local susceptibility patterns)
Tigecycline (plus an anti-pseudomonal agent)

Anti-anaerobic
Metronidazole
Carbapenems
β-lactam/β-lactamase combination agents
Tigecycline

Anti-MRSA
Ceftaroline
Daptomycin (not for use against pneumonia)
Minocycline (oral only)
Linezolid
Telavancin
Tigecycline (not in pregnancy or for children under the age of 8 y)
Vancomycin

patients should not be treated empirically with these agents, because of high rates of MRSA; virtually all *enterococci* are resistant. However, if the *S. aureus* isolate is susceptible, these drugs are the treatment of choice (TOC). With the exception of carboxy- and ureidopenicillins, penicillins retain little or no activity against most GNB. Carboxypenicillins (ticarcillin and carbenicillin) and ureidopenicillins (azlocillin, mezlocillin, and piperacillin; sometimes referred to as acylampicillins) have some activity against gram-negative bacteria and *P. aeruginosa*. Ureidopenicillins have greater intrinsic activity against *Pseudomonas*, but none are used widely any more without a β-lactamase inhibitor in combination (BLIC) (e.g., sulbactam, tazobactam, clavulanic acid), which enhances the effectiveness of the parent β-lactam agent (piperacillin > ticarcillin > ampicillin), and to a lesser extent the inhibitor (tazobactam > sulbactam ~ clavulanic acid). Spectrum of activity varies, so the clinician must be familiar with each of the drugs. All BLIC drugs are effective against streptococci, MSSA, and anaerobes (except for *C. difficile*). Piperacillin–tazobactam has the widest spectrum of activity, and the most potency among β-lactam drugs against *P. aeruginosa*. Ampicillin–sulbactam is unreliable against *E. coli* and *Klebsiella* (resistance rate ~50%), but is a useful activity against some strains of *Acinetobacter* spp. owing to activity of the sulbactam moiety.

b. *Cephalosporins.* More than twenty cephalosporins are in this class; the characteristics of the drugs vary widely, but are similar within four broad "generations." First- and second-generation agents are useful only for prophylaxis, uncomplicated infections, or for de-escalation after results of susceptibility testing are known. "Third-generation" agents have enhanced activity against GNB (some have specific anti-pseudomonal activity), but most are ineffective against GPC and none against anaerobes. Cefepime, the "fourth-generation" cephalosporin available in the US, has enhanced anti-pseudomonal activity and has regained activity against most GPC, but not MRSA. Ceftaroline (usual dose, 600 mg IV q12h) is unclassified, but has anti-MRSA activity unique among cephalosporins while retaining modest activity (comparable to first-generation agents) against GNB. None of the cephalosporins are active against *enterococci*. The heterogeneity of spectrum, especially among third-generation agents, requires broad familiarity with all of these drugs.

i. *Third-generation cephalosporins* include cefoperazone, cefotaxime, cefpodoxime, cefprozil, ceftazidime, ceftibuten, ceftizoxime, ceftriaxone, and lorcarbicef. They possess a modestly extended spectrum of activity against GNB, but not against gram-positive bacteria (except for ceftriaxone) or anaerobes. Third-generation cephalosporins, particularly ceftazidime, have been associated with the induction of ESBL production among many of the *Enterobacteriaceae*. Activity is reliable only against non–ESBL-producing species of *Enterobacteriaceae* including *Enterobacter, Citrobacter, Providencia,* and *Morganella*. Activity is no longer reliable for empiric use as monotherapy against non-fermenting GNB (e.g., *Acinetobacter* spp., *P. aeruginosa, S. maltophilia*).

ii. *Fourth-generation cephalosporin.* Cefepime has activity more broad than that of the third-generation cephalosporins, (the anti-pseudomonal activity exceeds that of ceftazidime), whereas the anti–gram-positive activity is comparable to that of a first-generation cephalosporin. The safety profile is excellent, and the potential for induction of ESBL production is less. There is no activity against either *enterococci* or enteric anaerobes. Similar to the carbapenems, cefepime appears to be intrinsically more resistant to hydrolysis by β-lactamases, but not enough to be reliable empirically against ESBL-producing bacteria.

c. Monobactams. Aztreonam has a spectrum of activity against GNB that is similar to that of the third-generation cephalosporins, with no activity against either gram-positive organisms or anaerobes. Aztreonam is not a potent inducer of β-lactamases. Resistance to aztreonam is widespread, but the drug may be useful for directed therapy against known susceptible strains, and to treat penicillin-allergic patients because the incidence of cross-reactivity is low.

d. Carbapenems

i. Carbapenems have a configuration of the β-lactam ring that makes these drugs resistant to hydrolysis by β-lactamases. Four drugs, imipenem–cilastatin, meropenem, doripenem, and ertapenem, are available in the US. Ertapenem excepted, carbapenems have the widest (and generally comparable) antibacterial spectrum of any antibiotics, with excellent activity against aerobic and anaerobic streptococci, methicillin-sensitive staphylococci, and virtually all GNB except *Acinetobacter, Legionella, P. cepacia,* and *S. maltophilia*. Activity against the *Enterobacteriaceae* exceeds that of all antibiotics with the possible exceptions of piperacillin–tazobactam and cefepime, and activities of meropenem and doripenem against *P. aeruginosa* are approached only by that of amikacin.

ii. All carbapenems are superlative anti-anaerobic agents, thus there is no reason to treat concurrently with metronidazole. Meropenem and doripenem have less potential for neurotoxicity than imipenem–cilastatin, which is contraindicated in patients with active central nervous system disease or injury (except the spinal cord). With all carbapenems, widespread disruption of host microbial flora may lead to superinfections (e.g., fungi, *C. difficile*, *Stenotrophomonas*, resistant *enterococci*). Ertapenem is not useful against *Pseudomonas* spp., *Acinetobacter* spp., *Enterobacter* spp., or MRSA, but its long half-life permits once-daily dosing. Ertapenem is highly active against ESBL-producing *Enterobacteriaceae*, and also has less potential for neurotoxicity.

6. *Cell wall active agents: Lipoglycopeptides*

  a. Vancomycin, a soluble lipoglycopeptide, is bactericidal to dividing organisms. Tissue penetration of vancomycin is universally poor, limiting its effectiveness. Both *S. aureus* and *S. epidermidis* are usually susceptible to vancomycin, although MICs for *S. aureus* are increasing, requiring higher doses for effect, and leading to rates of clinical failure that exceed 50% in some reports. *Streptococcus pyogenes*, group B streptococci, *S. pneumoniae* (including penicillin-resistant *S. pneumoniae* [PRSP]), and *C. difficile* are also susceptible. Most strains of *E. faecalis* are inhibited (but not killed) by attainable concentrations, but *E. faecium* is increasingly VRE.

  i. Bona fide indications for vancomycin include serious infections caused by MRSA/MRSE, gram-positive infections in patients with serious penicillin allergy, and oral therapy (or by enema in patients with ileus) for serious cases of CDI. Parenteral vancomycin (a starting dose of 15 mg/kg is now recommended for patients with normal renal function, to achieve a minimum trough concentration of 15 to 20 mcg/mL) must be infused over at least 1 hour to avoid toxicity (e.g., "red man syndrome").

  b. Telavancin, a synthetic derivative of vancomycin, is approved for treatment of complicated skin and soft tissue infections. The drug is active against MRSA, pneumococci including PRSP, and vancomycin-susceptible *enterococci* with MICs generally <1 mcg/mL. There appears to be a dual mechanism of action, including cell membrane disruption and inhibition of cell wall synthesis. The most common side effects are taste disturbance, nausea, vomiting, and headache. There may be a small increased risk of acute kidney injury. The usual dose is 10 mg/kg, infused intravenously over 60 minutes, every 24 hours for 7 to 14 days; dosage reductions are necessary in renal insufficiency.

7. *Cell wall active agents: Cyclic lipopeptide.* Daptomycin has potent, rapid bactericidal activity against most gram-positive organisms via rapid membrane depolarization, potassium efflux, arrest of DNA, RNA, and protein synthesis; and cell death. Daptomycin exhibits concentration-dependent killing, and has a long half-life (8 hours). A dose of 4 mg/kg once daily is recommended for complicated soft tissue infections, whereas the dose for bacteremia is 6 mg/kg/day. The dosing interval should be increased to 48 hours when creatinine clearance <30 mL/min. Daptomycin is active against many aerobic and anaerobic gram-positive bacteria, including MDR strains such as MRSA, MRSE, and VRE. Daptomycin is also effective against many anaerobes, including *Peptostreptococcus* spp., *C. perfringens*, and *C. difficile*. Resistance to daptomycin is rare for both MRSA and VRE. Importantly, daptomycin must not be used for the treatment of pneumonia, or empiric therapy when pneumonia is in the differential diagnosis, even if the organism is susceptible, because daptomycin penetrates lung tissue poorly and is also inactivated by pulmonary surfactant.

8. *Cell wall active agents: Polymyxins.* Polymyxins are cyclic, cationic peptide antibiotics that have fatty acid residues. Polymyxin B and polymyxin E (colistin) differ by a single amino acid. Polymyxins bind to the anionic bacterial outer membrane, leading to a detergent effect that disrupts membrane integrity. High-affinity binding to the lipid A moiety of lipopolysaccharide may have an endotoxin-neutralizing effect. Commercial preparations of polymyxin B are standardized, but those of colistimethate (a less-toxic prodrug of colistin that is administered clinically) are not, so dosing depends on which preparation is being supplied. Most recent reports describe colistimethate use, but the drugs are therapeutically equivalent.

    a. Dosing of polymyxin B is 1.5 to 2.5 mg/kg (15,000 to 25,000 U/kg) daily in divided doses, whereas dosing of colistimethate ranges from 2.5 to 6 mg/kg/day, also in divided doses. The diluent is voluminous, adding substantially to daily fluid intake. The drugs exhibit rapid concentration-dependent bacterial killing against most GNB, including *E. coli*, *Klebsiella* spp., *Enterobacter* spp., *P. aeruginosa*, *S. maltophilia*, and *Acinetobacter* spp., including MDR isolates. Combinations of polymyxin B or colistimethate and rifampin exhibit synergistic activity *in vitro*.

    b. Uptake into tissue is poor, but both intrathecal and inhalational administration have been described. Clinical response rates for respiratory tract infections appear to be lower than for other sites of infection. Polymyxins fell out of favor due to nephro- and neurotoxicity, but the emergence of MDR pathogens has returned them to clinical use. Up to 40% of colistimethate-treated patients (5% to 15% for polymyxin B) will have an increase of serum creatinine concentration, but seldom is renal replacement therapy required. Neurotoxicity (5% to 7% for both) usually becomes manifest as muscle weakness or polyneuropathy.

9. Protein synthesis inhibitors. Several classes of antibiotics, although dissimilar structurally and having divergent spectra of activity, exert their antibacterial effects via binding to bacterial ribosomes and inhibiting protein synthesis.

    a. *Aminoglycosides.* Aminoglycoside use is resurgent because resistance to newer antibiotics (especially third-generation cephalosporins and fluoroquinolones) has developed. Gentamicin, tobramycin, and amikacin are still used frequently. Aminoglycosides bind to the bacterial 30S ribosomal subunit, inhibiting protein synthesis. Gentamicin has modest activity against GPC (not MRSA), otherwise the spectrum of activity for the various agents is nearly identical.

    b. Because of the potential for nephro- and ototoxicity, aminoglycosides are seldom first-line therapy, except in a synergistic combination to treat a serious *Pseudomonas* infection, enterococcal endocarditis, or an infection caused by an MDR gram-negative bacillus. As second-line therapy, these drugs are effective against the *Enterobacteriaceae*, modestly so against *Acinetobacter*, but limited against *P. cepacia*, *Aeromonas* spp., and *S. maltophilia*. Aminoglycosides kill bacteria most effectively with a concentration peak: MIC >12, therefore a loading dose is necessary and serum drug concentration monitoring is performed. Synergistic therapy with a β-lactam agent is theoretically effective because bacterial cell wall damage caused by the β-lactam drug enhances intracellular penetration of the aminoglycoside, but evidence of improved outcomes is controversial, especially with conventional dosing.

    c. Conventional dosing for serious infections requires 5 mg/kg/day of gentamicin or tobramycin after a 2 mg/kg loading dose, or 15 mg/kg/day of amikacin after a loading dose of 7.5 mg/kg. Pharmacokinetics are variable and unpredictable in critically ill patients, and higher doses are sometimes necessary (e.g., burn patients). High doses (e.g., gentamicin 7 mg/kg/day, amikacin 20 mg/kg/day) given once daily can obviate these problems in many patients. Marked dosage reductions are necessary in renal insufficiency, but the drugs are dialyzed so a maintenance dose should be given after each hemodialysis treatment.

    d. *Tetracyclines* bind irreversibly to the 30S ribosomal subunit, but unlike aminoglycosides, they are bacteriostatic. Widespread resistance limits their utility in the hospital setting (with two exceptions, doxycycline and tigecycline). Tetracyclines are active against anaerobes; *Actinomyces* can be treated successfully. Doxycycline is active against *B. fragilis*, but used seldom for the purpose. All tetracyclines are contraindicated in pregnancy and for children under the age of 8 years, owing to dental toxicity.

i. Tigecycline is a novel glycylcycline derived from minocycline. With the major exceptions of *Pseudomonas* spp. and *P. mirabilis*, the spectrum of activity is broad, including many MDR gram-positive and gram-negative bacteria, including MRSA, VRE, and *Acinetobacter* spp. Tigecycline overcomes typical bacterial resistance to tetracyclines because its structure facilitates binding to the ribosome with higher affinity. Tigecycline is active against aerobic and anaerobic streptococci, staphylococci, MRSA, MRSE, and *enterococci*, including VRE. Activity against GNB is directed against *Enterobacteriaceae* including ESBL-producing strains, *P. multocida*, *S. maltophilia*, *E. aerogenes*, and *Acinetobacter* spp. Anti-anaerobic activity is excellent.

e. *Oxazolidinones* bind to the ribosomal 50S subunit, preventing complexing with the 30S subunit. Assembly of a functional initiation complex for protein synthesis is blocked, preventing translation of mRNA, therefore linezolid is bacteriostatic against most susceptible organisms. Linezolid is equally active against MSSA and MRSA, vancomycin-susceptible *enterococci* and VRE, and against susceptible and PRSP pneumococci. Most GNB are resistant, but *Bacteroides* spp. are susceptible. Linezolid requires no dosage reduction in renal insufficiency, and exhibits excellent tissue penetration, but it is uncertain whether that provides clinical benefit in treatment. Meta-analysis suggests that linezolid is equivalent to vancomycin for HAP/VAP, but some clinicians are of the opinion that linezolid should supplant vancomycin as first-line therapy for serious infections caused by GPC.

10. Drugs that disrupt nucleic acids

a. *Fluoroquinolones* inhibit bacterial DNA synthesis by inhibiting DNA gyrase, which folds DNA into a superhelix in preparation for replication. The fluoroquinolones exhibit a broad spectrum of activity, excellent oral absorption and bioavailability, and are generally well tolerated (photosensitivity, cartilage and tendon damage). These are potent agents with an unfortunate propensity to develop resistance rapidly. Agents with both parenteral and oral formulations include ciprofloxacin, levofloxacin, and moxifloxacin (which has some anti-anaerobic activity). Fluoroquinolones are most active against enteric gram-negative bacteria, particularly the *Enterobacteriaceae* and *Haemophilus* spp. There is some activity against *P. aeruginosa*, *S. maltophilia*, and GPC. Activity against GPC is variable, being least for ciprofloxacin and best for moxifloxacin. Ciprofloxacin has been most active against *P. aeruginosa*, but rampant overuse of fluoroquinolones is rapidly causing resistance that may limit the future usefulness of these agents. Fluoroquinolone use has been associated with the emergence of resistant *E. coli*, *Klebsiella* spp., *P. aeruginosa*, and MRSA. Fluoroquinolones prolong the QTc interval and may precipitate the ventricular dysrhythmia *torsades de pointes*, so electrocardiographic measurement of the QTc interval before and during fluoroquinolone therapy is important. Also, fluoroquinolones interact with warfarin to cause a rapid, marked prolongation of the International Normalized Ratio (INR), so anticoagulation must be monitored closely during therapy.

11. *Cytotoxic antibiotics*

a. *Metronidazole* is active against nearly all anaerobes, and against many protozoa that parasitize human beings. Metronidazole has potent bactericidal activity against *B. fragilis*, *Prevotella* spp., *Clostridium* spp. (including *C. difficile*), and anaerobic cocci, although it is ineffective in actinomycosis. Resistance remains rare. The drug penetrates well nearly all tissues, including neural tissue, making it effective for deep-seated infections and bacteria that are not multiplying rapidly. Absorption after oral or rectal administration is rapid and nearly complete. The $T_{1/2}$ of metronidazole is 8 hours, owing to an active hydroxy metabolite. Increasingly, intravenous metronidazole is administered every 8 to 12 hours in recognition of the active metabolite, but once-daily dosing is possible. No dosage reduction is required for renal insufficiency, but the drug is dialyzed effectively and administration should be timed to follow dialysis if twice-daily dosing is used. Pharmacokinetics in patients with hepatic insufficiency suggests a dosage reduction of 50% with marked impairment.

b. *Trimethoprim-Sulfamethoxazole (TMP-SMX).* Sulfonamides exert bacteriostatic activity by interfering with bacterial folic acid synthesis, a necessary step in DNA synthesis. Resistance is widespread, limiting use. The addition of sulfamethoxazole to trimethoprim, which prevents the conversion of dihydrofolic acid to tetrahydrofolic acid by the action of dihydrofolate reductase (downstream from the action of sulfonamides), accentuates the bactericidal activity of trimethoprim. The combination of TMP-SMX is active against *S. aureus, S. pyogenes, S. pneumoniae, E. coli, P. mirabilis, Salmonella* and *Shigella* spp., *Yersinia enterocolitica, S. maltophilia, L. monocytogenes,* and *Pneumocystis jerovici.* TMP-SMX is a TOC for infections caused by *S. maltophilia* and outpatient and sometimes inpatient treatment of infections caused by CA-MRSA. A fixed-dose combination of TMP-SMX of 1:5 is available for parenteral administration. The standard oral formulation is 80:400 mg, but lesser and greater strength tablets are available. Oral absorption is rapid and bioavailability is nearly 100%. Tissue penetration is excellent. Ten milliliters of the parenteral formulation contains 160:800 mg drug. Full doses (150 to 300 mg TMP in 3 to 4 divided doses) may be given if creatinine clearance is >30 mL/min, but the drug is not recommended when the creatinine clearance is <15 mL/min.

12. Duration of therapy. The endpoint of antibiotic therapy is largely undefined, because quality data are few. If cultures are negative, empiric antibiotic therapy should be stopped in most cases within 48 to 72 hours. The morbidity of antibiotic therapy also includes allergic reactions; development of nosocomial superinfections, (e.g., fungal, enterococcal, and CDI) organ toxicity; reduced yield from subsequent cultures; and vitamin K deficiency with coagulopathy or accentuation of warfarin effect. If infection is evident, treatment is continued as indicated clinically. Some infections can be treated with therapy lasting 5 days or less. Every decision to start antibiotics must be accompanied by an *a priori* decision regarding duration of therapy. A reason to continue therapy beyond the predetermined endpoint must be compelling. Bacterial killing is rapid in response to effective agents, but the host response may not subside immediately. Therefore, the clinical response of the patient should not be the sole determinant. If a patient still has SIRS at the predetermined endpoint, it is more useful to stop therapy and re-evaluate for persistent or new infection, MDR pathogens, and non-infectious causes of SIRS than to continue therapy uninformed.

AXIOMS

- Choose the most narrow range (per pathogen suspected/known) and adequate antibiotic agent and dose possible; if broad therapy is needed in early severe infection, narrow therapy as soon as possible based on microbiologic data.
- Antibiotic prophylaxis short be done for short intervals—often, just prior to surgery alone.
- Duration of antibiotic therapy is driven by infection location, organism, and response; there is no set interval.
- Hospital infections are best avoided with hand washing and bundled actions regarding catheters and care—treating them is much harder and fraught with morbidity.
- Remove catheters and other indwelling devices as soon as possible, and do not treat all cultures as evidence of infection—correlate the pathogen and the clinical condition to any treatment plan.

Suggested Readings

Barie PS. Multidrug-resistant organisms and antibiotic management. *Surg Clin North Am* 2012;92:345–391.

Burton DC, Edwards JR, Horan TC, et al. Methicillin-resistant *Staphylococcus aureus* central line-associated bloodstream infections in US intensive care units, 1997–2007. *JAMA* 2009;301:727–736.

Centers for Disease Control and Prevention (CDC). Vital signs: Central line-associated blood stream infections–United States, 2001, 2008, and 2009. *MMWR Morb Mortal Wkly Rep* 2011;60:243–248.

Chlebicki MP, Safdar N. Topical chlorhexidine for prevention of ventilator-associated pneumonia: a meta-analysis. *Crit Care Med* 2007;35:595–602.

Darouiche RO, Wall MJ Jr, Itani KM, et al. Chlorhexidine-alcohol versus povidone-iodine for surgical-site antisepsis. *N Engl J Med* 2010;362:18–26.

Gosselin RA, Roberts I, Gillespie WJ. Antibiotics for preventing infection in open limb fractures. *Cochrane Database Syst Rev* 2004;1:CD003764.

Kumar A, Zarychanski R, Light B, et al. Early combination antibiotic therapy yields improved survival compared with monotherapy in septic shock: A propensity-matched analysis. *Crit Care Med* 2010;38:1773–1785.

NICE-SUGAR Study Investigators, Finfer S, Chittock DR, et al. Intensive versus conventional glucose control in critically ill patients. *N Engl J Med* 2009;360(13):1283–1297.

O'Grady NP, Chertow DS. Managing bloodstream infections in patients who have short-term central venous catheters. *Cleve Clin J Med* 2011;78:10–17.

Pronovost P. Interventions to decrease catheter-related bloodstream infections in the ICU: the Keystone Intensive Care Unit Project. *Am J Infect Control* 2008;36:S171.e1–e5.

Prospero E, Barbadoro P, Esposto E, et al.

van den Berghe G, Wouters P, Weekers F, et al. Intensive insulin therapy in the critically ill patients. *N Engl J Med* 2001;345:1359–1367.

15 Trauma Pain Management

Donald M. Yealy

I. BASIC PRINCIPLES OF ANALGESIA. Six basic principles of analgesia apply in all types of pain management.

A. Individualize the route and dose of analgesic.

1. Patients respond differently to painful stimuli based on the type and severity of injury, psychological make-up, and ethnicity. In addition, individual analgesic requirements vary based on the time of day and previous use of analgesics or recreational substances. Although we offer starting doses (Table 15-1), amount and timing should be altered based on the response.

2. Patients may have expectations of being completely pain-free; these expectations are often unrealistic. Provide adequate analgesia, defined as enhancing comfort to a tolerable level without side effect. The expected level of relief should be discussed with each patient to ensure understanding by both the provider and the receiver.

3. Intramuscular injection offers no analgesic advantage over oral or intravenous administration due to erratic absorption and pain on injection. The variable absorption with IM injection (due to hydration, sympathetic tone, muscle site and time of day factors) limits the ability to titrate analgesia to need in a timely fashion, forcing the physician to estimate the correct dose (which is inaccurate in up to two-thirds of cases). This route should rarely be used and can be replaced with subcutaneous injections (which are less painful) in those who cannot tolerate oral medicines and without intravenous access.

B. Offer analgesics on a time-contingent basis during acute pain phases.

1. Time-contingent dosing affords steady blood levels of analgesia, avoiding the wide fluctuations with "prn" dosing. It also avoids making the patient request medication, still allowing for refusal if not needed; this increases the sense of empowerment and satisfaction, augmenting the perceived analgesia.

2. Time-contingent dosing is best for all analgesic preparations, including NSAIDs, acetaminophen and opioid analgesics. When providing oral analgesics, offer the medication based on the pharmacologic profile (e.g., hydrocodone or oxycodone every 4 to 6 hours around the clock) in the acute phase of injury. Parenteral opioids should be administered on a time-contingent basis as well, by hourly infusion (e.g., morphine, 1 to 2 mg/hr in opioid naive patients) or via a patient-controlled analgesia (PCA) device.

C. Opioids are the cornerstone of acute severe pain management.

1. Intravenous opioids offer the best opportunity to deliver rapid, titrated, adequate analgesia. Opioids, given in small increments every 5 to 10 minutes (e.g., morphine 2 to 5 mg, hydromorphone 0.5 to 1 mg, or fentanyl 50 to 100 mcg for most opioid naive adults), based on the pain and physiologic responses, remain the best agents for severe injury or initial postoperative pain. Oral opioids are inexpensive, effective, and tolerated well by patients with ongoing moderate to severe pain in the postoperative period or after the initial injury.

2. PCA—using small patient-triggered boluses of an opioid (usually morphine) every 6 to 10 minutes maximum, with "lock-out intervals" to prevent excess, allows safe and effective relief. PCA requires some initial "loading" – relief gained from bedside titration – before instituting patient maintenance. It can be combined with low dose infusions to decrease needs safely and augment relief. PCA care

TABLE 15-1 Opioid Analgesics

Name	Equianalgesic dose (mg) Oral (mg and hour interval in adults)	IV[a]	Starting oral dose Adults (mg and hour interval)	Children (mg/kg)
Pure agonists				
Morphine	30 q3–4	5 q1–2	15–30 q3–4	0.3
Hydromorphone (Dilaudid)				
Codeine[b]	4–6 q3–4	1 q3–4	2–4 q4–6	0.06
Oxycodone (Roxicodone, Percocet, others)	120–130 q3–4	—	30–60 q3–4	0.5–1
Hydrocodone (Lortab, Lorcet, Vicodin, others)	30 q3–4	—	10–20 q3–4	0.3
Methadone	30 q3–4	—	10–20 q3–4	—
Levorphanol (Levo-Dromoran)	20 q6–8	5 q6–8	5–10 q6–8	0.2
Mixed agonist–antagonists	—	0.05 q0.5–1 (50 μg)	—	—
Nalbuphine (Nubain)	—	5 q3–4	—	—
Butorphanol (Stadol)	—	1 q2–4	—	—

[a]After initial titration, which is done using this dose at 10 min intervals based on response; these are not recommended final doses but equipotent initial doses.
[b]Sedating and constipating in doses >60–90 mg; oxycodone and hydrocodone preferred.
q, every.

paths/plans are best developed together with acute pain practitioners based on local resources.

D. Combination therapy affords the best analgesia, especially in mild to moderate pain syndromes and after acute severe pain is initially controlled.

1. Include an **NSAID** with an opioid whenever possible to provide analgesia by two different and synergistic methods. Avoid if neurologic surgery, existing bleeding disorder or large volume blood loss, or if other anticoagulant/antiplatelet agents are used. All NSAIDs have similar effects when given in equipotent doses—we recommend using the least expensive drug/route for the shortest interval (Table 15-2).

   a. **Ketorolac** (30 to 60 mg i.m. or 15 to 30 mg i.v.) is the only NSAID available for parenteral use. *It is no more effective than oral ibuprofen* (600 mg) or indomethacin (50 mg), although much more expensive than these NSAIDs and generic morphine or hydromorphone. Ketorolac should be reserved for short-term use (<3 days) in those patients who are unable to take an inexpensive NSAID orally.

   b. Newer selective oral NSAIDs (termed **COX-2 inhibitors**) offer analgesic and anti-inflammatory effects similar to traditional NSAIDs with a lower frequency of GI side effects and less anti-platelet effects. However, they are more expensive than traditional NSAIDs, and do not avoid GI or renal side effects; they should be reserved for those patients intolerant of traditional NSAIDs or at high risk for complications who need prolonged therapy. Finally, they increase the risk of cardiovascular events; given the complex issues and limited need in acute pain (compared to other agents), these are not recommended currently for acute pain management.

TABLE 15-2 Non-opioid Analgesics/NSAID

Drug	Usual adult dose	Usual pediatric dose	Comments
Oral			
Acetaminophen	650–1,000 mg q4h	10–15 mg/kg q4h	Acetaminophen lacks anti-inflammatory activity
Aspirin	650–1,000 mg q4h	10–15 mg/kg q4h[a]	The standard against which other NSAIDs are compared. Inhibits platelet aggregation irreversibly (lasts 2 wks); may cause postoperative bleeding
Ibuprofen (Motrin, others)	400–600 mg q4–6h	10 mg/kg q6–8h	Available as several brand names and as generic
Naproxen (Anaprox, Naprosyn others)	500–550 mg initial dose followed by 250–275 mg q6–8h	NA	Available as several brand names and as generic
Parenteral			
Ketorolac tromethamine (Toradol)	30–60 mg i.m. or 15 mg i.v. initial dose followed by 15 or 30 mg q6h		Parenteral use should not exceed 5 d

[a]Contraindicated in presence of fever or other evidence of viral illness.

With the possible exception of trisalicylate and salsalate, all NSAID exhibit reversible antiplatelet effects. Also, these doses are associated with peak analgesic effects, although increased doses cause increased anti-inflammatory affects along with more side effects. NSAID, nonsteroidal anti-inflammatory drug.

2. Similarly, **acetaminophen** augments opioid and NSAID analgesia, allowing greater pain relief with less toxicity. When using acetaminophen/opioid combination preparations, attention to the daily acetaminophen dose is required to avoid toxicity, especially in patients with liver disease. The recent availability of intravenous acetaminophen may aid with management of mild to moderate pain, often in conjunction with an opioid.

3. **Antiemetics and phenothiazine/butyrophenones *do not*** augment analgesia and may increase side effects (especially sedation and hypotension). These agents should be used to treat specific conditions but not routinely added to analgesic regimens.

4. **Benzodiazepines** (midazolam, diazepam, lorazepam) are pure sedatives. These drugs lessen anxiety, produce amnesia and cause skeletal muscular relaxation, augmenting the *perceived* analgesia. However, pure sedatives should not be used alone to treat pain because of lack of analgesia; if used in combination with an opioid (e.g., during orthopedic manipulation), the dose of each should be lowered to avoid clinical respiratory depression or hypotension.

E. **Recognize and treat side effects of analgesic therapy.**

1. NSAID drugs are associated with platelet aggregation inhibition, gastrointestinal dysfunction ranging from dyspepsia to gastrointestinal bleeding, renal insufficiency, and (rarely) mental status changes. These complications occur irrespective

of the route (i.e., parenteral ketorolac causes similar side effects to any equipotent dose of an oral NSAID), and are treated by discontinuation of the drug.

  2. Opioid analgesia is associated with nausea (up to 40% of patients), sedation, itching, constipation, urinary retention and hypotension. Treatment of opioid-induced side effects includes decreasing the dose or changing the route of administration of the drug, as well as treating the side effect.

  a. Opioid-induced hypotension is the result of diminished peripheral sympathetic tone, histamine release, and vasodilation. This usually is mild and transient, but can be dramatic in the sympathetically depleted or hypovolemic patient. Hypotension is best avoided by optimizing volume status and delivering the drug in titrated, small doses. If hypotension occurs, further doses should be withheld and crystalloid bolus infusions given. Opioid antagonists do not reverse opioid-induced hypotension.

  b. Itching after an opioid is poorly understood but may be the result of histamine release or opioid receptor activity. Itching occurs with all agents to varying degrees, especially when given intravenously or in the epidural space. Antihistamines may be effective in relieving itching, with opioid antagonists (naloxone 0.1 to 0.2 mg) used for refractory or severe cases.

  c. Respiratory depression and sedation occur together, with sedation usually preceding clinical respiratory depression. Both can be reversed with incremental doses of an opioid antagonist. We recommend naloxone 0.04 mg every minute if lowered respiratory rate – prepared with 0.4 mg ampule diluted up to 10 cc with saline and given 1 cc at a time – to reverse the excessive effect but maintain analgesia. **For patients with coma or apnea/near apnea, naloxone 0.4 mg IV should be given immediately and repeated every 5 minutes as needed.**

F. Pain is better treated early rather than later.

  1. There is evidence that "pain begets pain" secondary to peripheral and central neuromodulation that occurs after a prolonged painful stimulus such as injury.

  2. Early treatment of pain can decrease the overall need for analgesics and improve patient satisfaction. Similarly, avoiding periods of inadequate analgesia will also help avert up-regulation of pain receptors and thus, improve pain relief.

  3. Early *titrated* pain therapy can alter the sympathetic responses to injury and improve regional blood flow, further aiding resuscitation. Overzealous analgesic administration can produce the opposite response.

II. OVERVIEW: TRAUMA PAIN MANAGEMENT

  A. The principles of pain management in the trauma patient include the basic analgesic principles outlined and principles of acute postoperative pain management.

  B. Certain trauma patients present with special needs: Patients with severe pain during resuscitation, those with substance abuse issues, and those with psychological issues either at the time of the injury or during the rehabilitation phase.

  C. A small number of trauma patients will require analgesia for a prolonged period of time, or may develop a chronic pain syndrome as a result of injury. These patients are best managed with a multidisciplinary approach that includes the trauma and primary care physicians, a physician pain specialist, physical therapists and psychosocial clinicians.

III. ANALGESIA DURING RESUSCITATION

  A. Analgesia should not be withheld during the resuscitation unless one of three conditions exists:

  1. Hemodynamic instability

  2. Respiratory depression

  3. Profound sedation or coma

  In patients without these contraindications, titrated intravenous opioids should be given to attenuate pain with close attention to the physiologic response (especially blood pressure and level of consciousness). **Any opioid or systemic**

sedative/induction agent can cause hypotension, with frequency and degree being the important difference between regimens.

B. Fentanyl causes the least hemodynamic effects and is the agent of choice for pain relief during resuscitation. In doses of 0.25 to 0.50 mcg/kg (50 to 100 mcg for the average adult) every 5 to 10 minutes, it produces safe clinical analgesia up to 60 minutes in most patients. Side effects are treated as noted above. Chest wall rigidity is a rare occurrence, seen mostly with larger doses (>6 mcg/kg boluses). This can compromise ventilation but is extremely rare in the doses recommended for analgesia. It is treated with positive pressure ventilation, opioid reversal agents and (in severe cases) neuromuscular blockade with endotracheal intubation.

C. Other inexpensive opioids (**morphine** 2 to 5 mg, **hydromorphone** 0.5 to 1 mg i.v. increments) produce longer analgesia but are associated with more hemodynamic effects. These drugs are best used in well-resuscitated patients. Other synthetic opioids (alfentanil, sufentanil, remifentanil) offer little advantage at a higher cost.

IV. PROCEDURAL SEDATION AND ANALGESIA

A. Patients usually require pharmacologic assistance when painful or anxiety-provoking procedures are planned. A continuum exists between mild sedation and systemic analgesia to general anesthesia. **In general, the deeper the intended or potential reflex and responsiveness change, the more closely the patient must be monitored by trained experts.**

B. Environmental and other adjuncts will ease the painful perceptions and anxiety. These include:

  1. Comfortable surroundings (dimmed lights, quiet area, distraction, or music if possible).

  2. A calm, clear manner of communication, educating the patient of expected responses and asking for feedback to help improve care (e.g., "If you feel more pain, let me know and I will give more medicine").

  3. Splinting and minimal or gentle handling of injured parts.

  4. Presence of family or friend (if possible, safe and desired).

  5. Attempts to distract patient or help him/her think of other soothing or pleasing settings.

  6. Local or topical anesthetics to ease nociceptive stimuli.

C. Most procedures can be safely and comfortably performed with mild sedation (no pain involved but anxiety provoking, e.g., radiologic studies) or conscious sedation/systemic analgesia (pain and anxiety anticipated, e.g., wound debridement, joint or fracture care). Monitoring of responses, vital signs, pulse oximetry can be performed by either a physician or a nurse with physician supervision.

D. Fasting is often a concern; if the procedure is emergent, life or limb salvaging/maintaining, do not delay. Even with less emergent procedures, the standard preoperative 6- to 12-hour fast is not usually needed, though deep sedation is best avoided in those actively vomiting or known to have a full stomach.

E. Regimens

  1. Opioids are the cornerstone of pain relief during procedures. Titrated fentanyl (0.25 to 0.5 mcg/kg—often 50 to 100 mcg in adults) every 2 to 3 minutes based on the response is a common method. Other opioids – morphine or hydromorphone – are alternates, although the duration and hemodynamic effects differ from the limited amount seen with fentanyl.

  2. Benzodiazepines, especially midazolam (1 to 2 mg increments in adults) or diazepam (2.5 to 5 mg increments), are best for procedures requiring sedation or muscular relaxation. These drugs do not relieve pain, although patients may lack recall of the pain.

  3. Combination of opioids and benzodiazepines are often used for procedures that require pain and anxiety relief or pain relief and muscular relaxation. It is best to deliver the benzodiazepine first, and then add titrated doses of the opioid. Care to the effect is critical, since an additive or synergistic effect can occur, risking airway or hemodynamic complications.

4. Other agents can be used, including ketamine (0.25 mg/kg i.v. increments, creating a "dissociative state" with rare emergence reactions or laryngospasm) and etomidate (0.05 to 0.1 mg/kg increments, creating good sedation but a small risk of deep sedation and some myoclonus on occasion).

5. Titrated **propofol** – a powerful and very short acting agent – can provide sedation plus amnesia and anti-emetic effects, but it is *not* an analgesic. Thus, an opioid – usually fentanyl – is required. The window between desired sedation and complete loss of airway protection or apnea with propofol use can be erratic, although it is short. It should be used only with pulse oximetry, ECG, and capnographic monitoring and an airway expert at the bedside and uninvolved with the procedure. Most often, 50 to 100 mcg IV boluses are used incrementally in an adult until the desired depth is obtained, recognizing the short (minutes) duration.

6. Another new popular approach is called "ketofol", where the local pharmacy mixes 1:1 ketamine 10 mg/cc and propofol 10 mcg/cc, then giving slow doses of 1 to 3 cc each until the desired effect. The combination retains the side effects of each agent but is much less frequent than either alone in equi-effective regimens, and produces good results and short recovery intervals.

F. **General anesthesia is not sought in the trauma bay, emergency department or floor outside of rapid intubation.** Procedures requiring this are best performed in the operating room.

G. In the rare instance **when deep sedation is planned** (e.g., for hip relocation or cardioversion), **it should be done where continuous monitoring equipment** (ECG, automated blood pressure and pulse oximeter mandatory, capnography helpful) **is available, with a physician and nurse dedicated solely to delivering drugs and monitoring the patient.** Those two individuals must be expert in recognizing complications and treatment; this requires knowledge of reversal agents and cardiac drugs plus skill in airway support and endotracheal intubation. The physician performing the procedure **cannot** be responsible for this monitoring. **Deep sedation is usually done with etomidate or propofol and fentanyl as described earlier, usually with larger total doses.**

1. Because of the needs for close monitoring, deep sedation is often carried out in the operating room, although the emergency department and ICU are acceptable if the proper personnel and resources are available.

H. During procedural sedation/systemic analgesia of any level, create a record to document the following.

1. Immediate pre-procedural examination (including noting review of previous examination, allergies, medications and last meal if after initial evaluation).

2. Serial measurement of vital signs, responses to stimuli, oximetry reading and any interventions. This is best done every 5 minutes.

3. Complications, including (but not limited to) vomiting, loss of consciousness or respirations, rhythm changes, rashes, dyspnea, agitation, or any involuntary activity.

4. Clear timing of drugs and doses, including route.

5. Recovery period, including return to pre-procedural state or age appropriate functioning and ability to sit up, walk (if permitted), and take oral liquids.

V. SPECIAL ANALGESIC NEEDS
A. Rib fractures/chest wall pain

1. Rib fractures are in the category of severe pain syndromes; inadequate analgesia may lead to pulmonary compromise and pneumonia. Systemic opioids, especially via scheduled parenteral administration or PCA/continuous drip, are effective in most patients.

2. These patients may benefit from **continuous epidural analgesia.**

   a. Indications: Moderate to severe pain uncontrolled by systemic opioids, in those with preexisting or impending pulmonary compromise.

   b. Contraindications: Coagulopathy, hypovolemia, spinal fracture, or skin infection at site of intended placement, and dural tear. Low molecular weight heparin should not be used in patients with an epidural catheter because of increased risk of epidural hematoma.

   c. Methods: Injection followed by continuous infusion of opioids (preservative free, usually morphine or fentanyl) and local anesthetics (lidocaine or bupivacaine), alone or together. These allow good pain relief at lower doses due to placement of the drug near the active site.

   d. Success is measured by adequate pain relief and improved pulmonary mechanics (or preservation of near normal in those without impairment). When a local anesthetic is infused, the dermatomal level of block can be estimated from a light tough/pin prick examination.

   e. Duration of therapy depends on the clinical response; generally, catheters are removed after 3 to 5 days (although longer intervals are acceptable in the absence of complications or infection). Most patients can be converted to other systemic regimens within 48 hours.

   f. Epidural catheters should be removed immediately if signs of infection develop (erythema, drainage) or if they no longer function properly.

   g. Respiratory depression is rare compared to equipotent systemic doses but can occur early (minutes from injection due to systemic absorption) or late (hours after injection from rostral spread).

   h. Itching is common with epidural opioids. Antihistamines or opioid antagonists (at low doses) can be used to reverse pruritus from epidural opioid administration, with the latter often added in low doses to the infusion.

   i. Continuous thoracic paravertebral blocks also effectively assist in pain control for rib fractures or postoperatively from thoracotomy or laparotomy.

   3. Individual intercostal nerve blocks (using 0.25% to 0.5% bupivacaine with epinephrine) can also be effective in patients with three or fewer rib fractures.

   4. Pleural administration of a local anesthetic (e.g., bupivacaine 10 to 15 mL of a 0.25% to 0.5% solution) can afford good pain relief for 6 to 12 hours. Although it can be instilled through a thoracostomy tube, this is not recommended in the initial phases of management since the tube must be clamped for 20 to 30 minutes to allow contact with the pleura. More commonly, a small bore catheter can be placed in the extrapleural space during an open chest procedure and used postoperatively as a route for pleural anesthesia.

B. Nerve injury

   1. Any trauma may result in direct injury to nerves.

   2. Those patients complaining of pain described as burning, electrical in nature, or those patients with pain complaints that seem out of proportion to the magnitude of traumatic injury, may have neuropathic injury (pain from nerve injury).

   3. Opioid analgesia alone is often not beneficial for long-term treatment. The use of adjuvants is common, including antidepressants and membrane stabilizers (antiseizure medications).

   a. Cyclic antidepressants are best for those with this pain and sleep disturbance, taking advantage of their sedative effects. Amitriptyline (10 to 25 mg), nortriptyline (25 to 50 mg) and trazodone (25 to 50 mg) are the commonly used agents. These are usually started at bedtime and increased in dose and frequency based on the responses, with the lower doses used in the elderly.

   b. Selective serotonin reuptake inhibitor antidepressants can be used for others without sleep disturbance (e.g., fluoxetine 20 mg or sertraline 50 mg once daily initially).

   c. Carbamazepine (100 to 200 mg three times daily), dilantin (1 g initially followed by 100 to 200 mg twice daily) or gabapentin (300 mg daily initially) are also useful, with doses adjusted upward as needed.

   4. Often, the advice of physicians who deal with advanced pain management is necessary to help with the analgesic plan and titration. Blood levels of these various agents generally do not predict success. Monitoring for side effects is necessary (e.g., serial blood counts and liver function studies in those on carbamazepine and ECG for elderly patients or those with conduction abnormalities in those on a cyclic antidepressant).

C. Long-term opioid therapy
1. Those patients requiring multiple surgical procedures, or those with extensive orthopedic injuries (external fixators, pelvic fractures) may require opioid therapy for extended intervals, with the development of opioid tolerance.

2. Patients receiving opioid therapy on a regular basis for more than 2 weeks are at risk for withdrawal if the opioid is abruptly discontinued. Mixed or partial opioid agonists/antagonists (e.g., butorphanol, pentazocine, nalbuphine) may produce withdrawal and should be avoided.

3. Signs of opioid withdrawal include hypertension, tachycardia, tearing, salivation, piloerection, and anxiety.

4. Opioid withdrawal may be avoided by ensuring that opioid therapy is discontinued according to a taper schedule that decreases the amount of opioid by 20% each 24 to 48 hours.

5. You will rarely create an opioid addict from therapeutic use; more likely, long-term opioid prescribing can allow a switch from one unrecognized dependence syndrome to an opioid dependence syndrome. Do not provide ongoing, long-term opioid treatment without seeking the help of a chronic pain specialist.

AXIOMS

■ Pain is best treated early and continuously; do not require awake patients to ask for relief.

■ Intravenous opioids are the cornerstone of acute severe pain management. NSAIDs and acetaminophen are useful adjuncts in moderate to severe pain, and often adequate in mild to moderate pain syndromes.

■ Avoid intramuscular analgesics.

■ Tailor analgesic regimens to each person, with a variation of 5- to 10-fold seen in opioid naive patients and even higher in those using these drugs or other sedatives chronically.

■ The ideal dose of opioid is the one that creates analgesia without excessive sedation or hemodynamic effect, with ceiling doses based on side effects rather than absolute amounts. Switching between opioids before adequate titration offers little benefit.

■ When providing procedural sedation and systemic analgesia, watch for excessive effects (especially respiratory drive and protective reflexes); mishaps are usually related to failure to seek, recognize, or quickly treat excessive/deep sedation.

Suggested Readings
Acute pain management: operative or medical procedures and trauma. Rockville, MD: US Department of Health and Human Services, Agency for Health Care Policy and Research, February 1992.

Arora S. Combining ketamine and propofol ("Ketofol") for emergency department procedural sedation and analgesia: A review. *West J Emerg Med* 2008;9(1):20–23.

Green SM. Fasting is a consideration-not a necessity-for emergency department procedural sedation and analgesia. *Ann Emerg Med* 2003;42:647–650.

Green SM, Yealy DM. Procedural sedation goes Utstein: the Quebec guidelines. *Ann Emerg Med* 2009;53(4):436–438.

Ruth WJ, Burton JH, Bock AJ. Intravenous etomidate for procedural sedation in emergency department patients. *Acad Emerg Med* 2001;8:13–18.

Ward KR, Yealy DM. Systemic analgesia and sedation in managing orthopedic emergencies. *Emerg Med Clin North Am* 2000;18:141–166.

Willman EV, Andolfatto G. A prospective evaluation of "ketofol" (ketamine/propofol combination) for procedural sedation and analgesia in the emergency department. *Ann Emerg Med* 2007;49(1):23–30.

Venous Thromboembolism

Gerard Fulda and Mark Cipolle

I. DEEP VENOUS THROMBOSIS (DVT)

A. Definition. DVT refers to any clot (obstructing or nonobstructing) in any deep venous system, including the upper extremity and the calf.

B. Pathophysiology. The mechanism behind clot development relates to **Virchow's Triad:** Stasis, injury to the vessel wall, and hypercoagulability. Stasis causes interruption of normal laminar flow allowing platelets to come in contact with endothelium; interruption of endothelial integrity exposes the extracellular matrix to platelets; hypercoagulability relates to excess circulating procoagulant factors +/− diminished anticoagulant factors. In trauma, most evidence points to intimal injury as the initial inciting event, followed by platelet adhesion, activation of the procoagulant system and release of thrombin. Hence, direct thrombin inhibitors **(DTIs)** play a strong role in prevention.

C. Epidemiology

1. Incidence. DVT affects >2.5 million people each year in the United States. This is likely an underestimate as many cases go unrecognized by patient and physician. Series have shown the incidence of DVT to be as high as 65% in the untreated major trauma patient.

2. Risk factors. In general, these include age >75, immobilization, acute infectious disease, cancer, general anesthesia, major surgery, estrogen therapy, pregnancy, prior DVT, congestive heart failure, malignancy, hypercoagulable state, and tissue trauma. **Specific to trauma,** risk factors include advanced age, lower extremity fracture, spinal cord injury, head injury (AIS >3), ventilator days >3, shock, multiple blood transfusions, surgery, fracture of the femur or tibia, complex pelvic fracture, venous injury, immobility, and spinal cord injury. Scoring systems have been developed to assess risk factors and better estimate the risk of DVT or pulmonary embolism (PE) (Table 16-1).

3. Location. DVT can occur in any deep venous system.

a. Calf vein thrombosis. Calf vein thrombosis is a clot localized to one or more of the three major named vessels below the knee. Untreated, these can propagate proximally in up to 23% of cases; however, they can also resolve without complications. Treatment is therefore controversial; however, follow-up duplex examination to rule out propagation should be performed.

b. Iliofemoral vein thrombosis. Most common site in the trauma patient. Findings may be subtle. A classical presentation is phlegmasia cerulea dolens (PCD)—painful, swollen, bluish leg. More common on the left. Higher incidence in patients who have had femoral venous lines.

c. Upper extremity thrombosis. The most common cause of upper extremity DVT is subclavian vein catheterization, rates, reported up to 46%. The incidence of PE may be as high as 12%. Treatment is extrapolated from treatment regimens for lower extremity DVT as no good trials exist for this entity specifically. The risk is increased with the length of time the catheter is in place as well as larger or malpositioned catheters.

d. Pelvic vein thrombosis. Missed by commonly used screening modalities.

D. Complications. DVT is a major cause of morbidity and mortality.

1. Local complications. Although rare, local ramifications of DVT include phlegmasia cerulea dolens (edematous, bluish extremity) or phlegmasia alba dolens (blanching "milk leg") with potential ulceration, loss of arterial flow, and/or resultant venous gangrene.

2. **Pulmonary embolism.** Incidence of pulmonary embolism after trauma varies with population, injury pattern, use of prophylaxis, and method of detection. Overall, 1% to 2% of patients with DVT after trauma will have a pulmonary embolism which carries a 30% to 50% mortality risk.

3. **Postphlebitic syndrome.** Venous valves in the lower extremities are destroyed by clot formation when DVT occurs. After the clot dissolves, valvular competence is permanently lost in the affected segment of vein. As a result, nonpitting edema, swelling, discoloration, and pain frequently occur, which can progress to venous hypertension and venous stasis ulceration. The incidence of postphlebitic changes at 12 years post-DVT approximates 28%. Severe sequelae occur in less than 6%.

E. Diagnosis.

1. **Clinical manifestation.** Subjective complaints of pain or swelling of the affected extremity are rare. In fact, only 40% of patients have any clinical signs or symptoms. The classic syndrome of calf discomfort, edema, venous distension, and pain on dorsiflexion of the foot (Homans' sign) is seen in less than 30% of patients.

2. **D-dimer.** D-dimers are a breakdown product of fibrin and should be elevated when venous thrombosis is present. Fibrin degradation products are elevated in

---

TABLE 16-1	**DVT Risk Factor Categories**

A. Risk factors:
- Age 40 years
- Injury severity score (ISS) >9
- Blood transfusion
- Surgical procedure lasting ≥2 h
- Lower extremity fracture
- Pelvic fracture
- Spinal cord injury (SCI)
- Immobilization
- Pregnancy
- Estrogen therapy
- History of DVT/PE
- Malignancy
- Hypercoagulable state (e.g., AT III deficiency)
- Extensive soft tissue trauma
- Congestive heart failure (CHF)

B. High risk factors:
- Age >50 years
- ISS ≥15
- Femoral central venous catheter in trauma resuscitation
- AIS ≥3 (any body region)
- Glasgow coma score (GCS) ≤8
- SCI
- Pelvic fracture
- Femur or tibia fracture
- Venous injury

C. Very high risk factors:
- SCI
- AIS-Head/neck ≥3 + long bone fracture (upper or lower)
- Severe pelvic fracture (posterior element) + long bone fracture (upper or lower)
- Multiple (≥3) long bone fracture

(continued)

TABLE 16-1 **DVT Risk Factor Categories (Continued)**

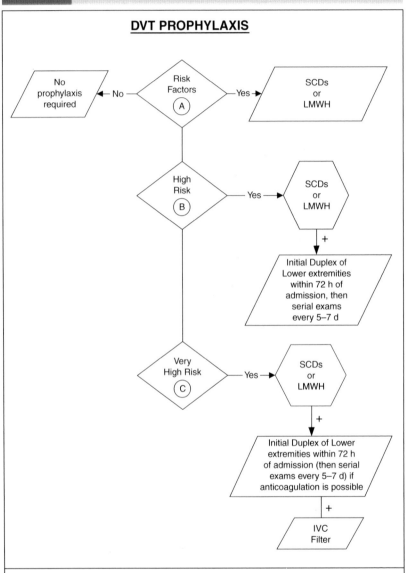

DVT PROPHYLAXIS

SCD, sequential compression device; LMWH, low molecular weight heparin.
Modified from Clinical Management Guidelines, Deep Venous Thrombosis Prophylaxis. Division of Trauma and Surgical Critical Care. Hospital of the University of Pennsylvania. Philadelphia, PA, 2000.

the first 48 hours after traumatic injury. Therefore, there is little utility in using admission d-dimer to diagnose DVT in the trauma patient.

3. **Compression ultrasound.** Duplex ultrasound (DUS) combines real-time B-mode ultrasound with pulsed Doppler capability. In symptomatic patients, the sensitivity and specificity are greater than 95%; thus, DUS is the most commonly performed test for the detection of infrainguinal DVT. The addition of color flow imaging reveals physiologic flow characteristics and may be useful in technically challenging examinations. Whether ultrasound is performed with flow assessment or not, **compression** of the vein along its length is the key aspect in evaluation for DVT. Noncompressibility of the vein is the primary diagnostic criterion for acute DVT. Other DUS findings include an echogenic thrombus within the vein lumen, venous distension, complete absence of spectral or color Doppler signal from the vein lumen, or loss of flow phasicity, response to Valsalva, or augmentation. Limitations of DUS include patient characteristics (obesity, edema, or tenderness), inability to ultrasound through various devices (casts, etc.) or compression of a vein by perivenous pathology (tumor, hematoma). In addition, DUS is unreliable in evaluating iliac veins.

   a. **Surveillance ultrasound.** Routine weekly surveillance of patients at high risk for DVT will increase the yield of discovering asymptomatic DVT. However, there is no strong evidence that the practice decreases PE rates and the cost-effectiveness of this approach has not been demonstrated. Routine use of surveillance is not recommended (CHEST guidelines). Ultrasound is indicated in the evaluation of symptomatic patients.

4. **Contrast venography.** While contrast venography (CV) remains the gold standard for diagnosis of DVT, it is rarely used due to the accuracy of noninvasive testing. CV is invasive and requires intravenous injection of contrast dye with the risks associated; however, it is considered to be 100% sensitive and specific. Diagnosis requires a constant intraluminal filling defect in two views or an abrupt cutoff of a deep vein.

5. **CT venography (CTV).** CTV uses venous phase contrast to directly visualize the inferior vena cava, pelvic veins, and lower extremity veins. It can be timed immediately after a CT pulmonary angiogram (CTPA) or used alone; however, when combined with CTPA, many series report a higher IV contrast dose is necessary for accurate visualization of the vessels. CTV can be plagued by artifact, such as from orthopedic hardware, or poor venous enhancement. The sensitivity and specificity are 89% to 100% and 94% to 100%, respectively. Some advantages of CTV are the readily available of CT scan in most hospitals at off-hours and the ability of a single study to diagnose both PE and DVT.

F. **Prophylaxis.**

   Upper extremity DVT: Early removal of any indwelling central venous catheter is the best way to prevent upper extremity DVT. Chemoprophylaxis is not recommended to prevent upper extremity DVT.

   Lower extremity DVT: As trauma patients are at high risk for the development of VTE, many centers have developed standardized algorithms for prophylaxis. These forms include early ambulation, mechanical devices, such as sequential pneumatic compression devices (PCDs), and pharmacologic therapy, such as low molecular weight heparin (LMWH). All major trauma patients should have some form of DVT prophylaxis. Prophylaxis should begin at the time of admission. If chemoprophylaxis cannot be initiated due to the risk of bleeding, mechanical prophylaxis should be used until chemoprophylaxis can be initiated. Prophylaxis should be continued at a minimum until the patient is fully ambulatory. In some cases of extensive orthopedic injuries, patients should be discharged on chemoprophylaxis. Traumatic brain injury is not an absolute contraindication to chemoprophylaxis; however, the risk of bleeding needs to be assessed prior to initiating therapy. Patients with small stable intracerebral hemorrhages generally can be started on chemoprophylaxis after 3 days.

   1. **Pneumatic compression devices (PCDs).** PCDs prevent VTE primarily by a mechanical mechanism. These devices expand intermittently to increase blood flow and expel blood from the lower extremities. They substitute for the calf

muscle pumps which are inactive in the nonambulatory trauma patient. A second mechanism of action of PCDs is their ability, albeit short-lived, to activate the fibrinolytic system. The intermittent venous compression results in release of plasminogen activators found in all venous walls. This is the means by which they are effective when placed on the upper extremities in cases where the lower extremities are unable to be used. There are no proven benefits of sequential versus nonsequential devices. Unfortunately, PCDs are unable to be used in up to 65% of trauma patients due to fractures or hardware. In addition, although the mechanism of action seems logical, randomized prospective trials in trauma patients have shown no benefit of PCDs over no prophylaxis in the prevention of DVT. However, when the patient cannot receive chemoprophylaxis, PCDs are recommended.

2. **AV foot pumps.** The discovery of a venous pump on the plantar aspect of the foot in 1983 led to the development of a device to reproduce this action. This device is attractive because it can often be used when SCDs cannot be placed or when they are ill-fitting. Also, similar to SCDs, foot pumps can be used when anticoagulant methods are contraindicated. Recent evidence suggests they may be even less effective than other traditional forms of DVT prophylaxis.

3. **Subcutaneous heparin (SCH).** Low dose, unfractionated heparin (5,000u by subcutaneous injection q8–12h) primarily works by enhancement of antithrombin III's ability to block factor Xa, but does not induce a hypocoagulable state. Complications of heparin use primarily include bleeding and heparin-induced thrombocytopenia (HIT) development. Although SCH is used regularly as prophylaxis in trauma patients, Velmahos et al., in a meta-analysis of studies done on trauma patients, reported no benefit of SCH over no prophylaxis. This among other studies has led to the recommendation of chemoprophylaxis other than SCH (unfractionated) as DVT prophylaxis in trauma patients. There are several exceptions patients with: Cr clearance less than 30 mL/min, extremely high BMI, or high risk for bleeding should not receive LMWH due to the difficulty in reversal of LMWH.

4. **LMWHs.** LMWHs are distillates of unfractionated heparin that have better bioavailability and longer plasma half-life. There is a low risk of hemorrhagic complications but not statistically different from SCH. LMWHs have now been widely studied in the trauma population and have been shown to reduce the incidence of DVT more effectively than SCH, SCDs, or AV foot pumps. It is therefore recommended that LMWHs be used for DVT prophylaxis when there is no contraindication to this form of prophylaxis. Of note, the FDA has warned of potential bleeding complications in patients where placement of neuraxial anesthesia is to be initiated.

5. **Vitamin K antagonists (VKAs).** VKAs (e.g., warfarin) have been primarily studied in the pelvic and lower extremity fracture population as well as the total hip replacement population. The dosage must be monitored and an international normalized ratio (INR) of 2.5 is preferred. The risk of hemorrhagic complications is much higher than with LMWH or SCH and so it is not generally recommended in the general trauma population.

6. **Selective factor Xa inhibitors.** This is a class of anticoagulant drugs that specifically provides antithrombin III inhibition of factor Xa. Fondaparinux is the drug most studied to date and has been shown to reduce the relative risk of VTE by 50% compared to LMWH in large orthopedic trials. There is also preliminary evidence that it may have reduced immunomodulator properties when compared to heparin. Unfortunately, although Fondaparinux has many attractive properties, it has not been adequately studied in the major trauma population and so no recommendation for its use can be made at this time.

7. **Oral factor Xa inhibitors.** There are several oral formulations under clinical evaluation. Rivaroxaban has been approved by the FDA for the prevention of DVT in patients for knee undergoing hip replacement surgery. Dose: 10 mg orally, once daily.

Caution: Epidural or spinal hematomas may occur in patients who are anticoagulated especially when receiving neuraxial anesthesia or spinal puncture. Factors which increase the risk of hematomas include:

TABLE 16-2	Heparin Dosing Guidelines

1. Initial order
    Bolus   70 units/kg
    Infusion   18 units/kg/hr
2. Monitor efficacy—6–8 h after initial bolus or change in dosing.
    Check PTT   Therapeutic range 51–68 sec
3. Heparin adjustment

PTT	Adjustment
<41 s	REBOLUS 35 units/kg
	INCREASE infusion 3 units/kg/hr
41–50 s	INCREASE infusion 2 units/kg/hr
51–68 s	No change
69–96 s	DECREASE infusion 1 unit/kg/hr
96–120 s	HOLD infusion 30 min
	DECREASE infusion 2 units/kg/hr
>120 s	HOLD infusion 90 min
	DECREASE infusion 3 units/kg/hr

4. Concomitant orders
    CBC with platelet count qod while on heparin
    No intramuscular injections
    Check all stool for occult blood

Modified from: *Heparin Dosing Protocol.* Hospital of the University of Pennsylvania, Philadelphia, PA, 2000.

    a. Use of indwelling epidural catheters.
    b. Concomitant use of other drugs that affect hemostasis: NSAIDs, platelet inhibitors, other anticoagulants.
    c. A history of traumatic or repeated epidural or spinal punctures.
    These patients should be monitored frequently for adverse neurologic symptoms.
8. Aspirin
    Aspirin is NOT recommended for DVT chemoprophylaxis.
G. Definitive treatment.
    Upper extremity DVT:
    The goals of definitive DVT treatment include preventing clot propagation, reducing the risk of PE, facilitating clot lysis, preserving venous valve function, reducing extremity swelling, alleviating pain, and preventing recurrence.
    1. Anticoagulation. Anticoagulation is the mainstay of DVT treatment, when no contraindication exists. Compared to a few years ago, currently several forms of anticoagulant therapy exist.
      a. Heparin. Full dose heparin by constant intravenous infusion is the standard initial therapy for DVT treatment (Table 16-2). The partial thromboplastin time (PTT) is monitored and heparin is dose adjusted to keep the PTT 60 to 80 seconds. The use of IV heparin is labor intensive and both over- and under-anticoagulation can have devastating consequences. Once therapeutic range is reached and no contraindication to warfarin therapy exists, the initiation of warfarin is begun.
      b. Direct Thrombin Inhibitors (DTIs). These are a class of compounds that directly bind with thrombin to prevent its interaction with enzyme substrates. They include lepirudin, argatroban, desirudin, and others. These compounds tend to be expensive and are reserved to treat DVT or PE in settings where heparin is contraindicated. At this time, no oral form is available; therefore, the patient needs to be converted to warfarin as in initial heparin therapy. While oral DTI have not been approved for this indication, they hold promise in converting

patients to outpatient therapy without the need for frequent blood work and adjustments. Dabigatran is the only FDA approved oral **DTI.** Currently, it is only approved for the reduction of the risk of stroke and systemic embolism in patients with nonvalvular atrial fibrillation.

    c. LMWH. LMWH at higher doses than for DVT prophylaxis has been proven to be an effective treatment of DVT. Due to their cost, however, many centers use this in place of IV heparin until the patient is in therapeutic INR range for warfarin. LMWH is less labor intensive, as PTT does not need to be closely monitored and the patient may be trained and discharged home on subcutaneous injections. Anti-Xa levels may be monitored to document therapeutic levels of LMWH compounds; however, this is not routinely done.

    d. VKA (warfarin). Warfarin is started after therapeutic range for heparin or DTI is achieved or after 24 hours of LMWH, provided no need for anticoagulation reversal is foreseen. Patients are not started on warfarin as first line anticoagulation because of the risk of warfarin-induced skin necrosis. The prothrombin time (PT) and INR are monitored and warfarin is dose adjusted to keep the INR 2.0 to 3.0. The duration of therapy is generally 3 to 6 months.

  2. Other measures. Ambulation is generally acceptable even after initial diagnosis. Elevation of the extremity when at rest helps reduce the swelling. Graded compression stockings may help minimize swelling.

II. PULMONARY EMBOLISM (PE)

  A. Definition. A clot in the main pulmonary artery or its branches that has embolized, traditionally from a venous, noncardiac source.

  B. Incidence. More than 500,000 cases of PE occur annually in the United States. The overall incidence of PE in the injured population is 0.3%; however, it increases to 1% to 2% in patients at risk. The mortality from PE in the severely injured patient may be as high as 20% to 50%.

  C. Diagnosis. The diagnosis of PE in the trauma patient is often clouded by other medical and surgical problems. Patients who have had a PE may have an "impending sense of doom." Dyspnea and pleuritic chest pain are the two most common symptoms. These symptoms are unfortunately frequently present in those who have sustained thoracic trauma. In addition, signs and symptoms of PE often suggest a differential diagnosis that includes many common conditions such as more sophisticated methods of diagnosis are necessary.

    1. Physical examination. Tachypnea and tachycardia are the most frequently encountered physical signs associated with PE. With massive PE, cyanosis and hypotension may occur. These are nonspecific symptoms.

    2. Laboratory tests. An **arterial blood gas** (ABG) is the most useful test to solidify a suspicion of PE. Ninety percent of patients with PE will have a room air PaO_2 <80 mm Hg. Hypocarbia (from tachypnea) and hypoxemia are the initial ABG abnormalities when PE is present. However, in the trauma patient, these abnormalities may be present for a variety of reasons. **D-dimer** can be helpful in distinguishing a DVT, although a positive result is largely nonspecific in the first few days after injury or surgical intervention.

    3. CXR. Classic findings on CXR include atelectasis or pulmonary infiltrate and pleural effusion. These findings can be difficult to differentiate as cause for symptoms or as result of PE or other pathology.

    4. EKG. EKG changes are common, up to 70% of patients will have an abnormality. ST segment or T-wave changes are most common (up to 50%) and R-wave electrical abnormalities are uncommon (6%). An EKG is important in evaluation, as PE and myocardial infarction share similar symptomatology.

    5. Ventilation–perfusion scintigraphy (V/Q Scan). V/Q Scans can be helpful in the diagnosis of PE; however, other pulmonary abnormalities limit its usefulness. V/Q scan is most accurate in the presence of a normal CXR. The trauma patient with pulmonary contusion, aspiration pneumonia, or other pulmonary pathology decreases the effectiveness of the V/Q scan. Even with a normal CXR, a normal V/Q scan carries a 4% PE rate and a high probability scan only carries an 88% PE rate. The patient who can be transported to the nuclear medicine department can receive only the perfusion component of the study due to limitations of venting the radioactive ventilation tracer. These limitations combined with the ease of CT angiography have made the V/Q scan less useful.

6. **CT pulmonary angiography.** The recent generations of multislice spiral CT scanners have allowed CT pulmonary angiography to be performed as a diagnostic test. Advantages include the ready availability of CT imaging in most institutions as well as the ability to diagnose other parenchymal or pleural processes that may cause the physiologic abnormalities that have prompted the workup for a possible PE. Sensitivity and specificity data for the test are reported at greater than 90%, although some recent data suggests that the finding of small, peripheral emboli may be of unclear significance.

7. **Pulmonary angiography.** Formal pulmonary angiography remains the gold standard for diagnosis of pulmonary emboli. The test is invasive, and involves a contrast load. Advantages include the ability for immediate invasive intervention and/or placement of an inferior vena cava filter (IVCF) if indicated.

D. Prophylaxis

1. **DVT Prophylaxis.** Prevention of the initial source clot allows the best prevention of PE.

2. **IVCF.** These are devices placed in the infrarenal IVC that prevent the embolic migration of pelvic or lower extremity clots. Today, these are available as either retrievable or permanent devices. Certain injury complexes that have historically been shown to be associated with high rates of PE **may** lend themselves to the placement of prophylactic IVCF. The ability to place retrievable filters makes IVCF a more attractive option as a prophylactic therapy. Many patients at risk should be able to receive an anticoagulant or will have an acceptable mobility status 2 to 6 weeks from the initial injury, greatly reducing the risk of PE. Unfortunately, little data exists on the effectiveness of this approach to PE prevention and the most recent Chest guidelines recommend against using an IVCF for prophylaxis in the patient with spinal cord injury. There are a number of documented complications from IVCF placement, including DVT, filter migration, and inferior vena caval thrombosis.

E. Treatment

1. **Anticoagulation.** Anticoagulation with heparin, LMWH or warfarin is the mainstay of therapy. If heparin is chosen, a PTT of 2x normal is the goal. If LMWH is chosen, therapeutic (not prophylactic) doses should be used. In cases where heparin or LMWH cannot be used (e.g., patients with heparin-induced thrombocytopenia), DTIs may be used as the initial therapy. When coumadin is started, an INR of 2 to 3 is the goal. Duration of therapy is usually at least 6 months. The newer oral anticoagulants have not been evaluated for this indication.

2. **Thrombolysis.** This is a controversial method of PE treatment and is contraindicated with many injury profiles. Thrombolytics include streptokinase, urokinase, and rTPA (alteplase, reteplase and tenecteplase). In ICU patients, no outcome difference in systemic or catheter-directed therapy has been documented. This therapy should only be considered in severely hemodynamically compromised patients, those with right ventricular hypokinesis and where thrombolysis would not be contraindicated.

3. **Suction embolectomy.** Suction or catheter embolectomy may be warranted in severely compromised individuals with a central PE who has an unquestionable contraindication to thrombolytics. The procedure requires pulmonary angiography and by virtue of the procedure may lead to multiple peripheral emboli, among other complications. There is scant data on this procedure in the trauma population.

4. **Surgical embolectomy.** The surgical extraction of central pulmonary artery thrombosis was largely abandoned and considered heroic but has recently been undertaken with better success rates than in the past. It may be the only option in patients with impending cardiac arrest or severe right ventricular dysfunction/infarction. The procedure requires cardiopulmonary bypass.

AXIOMS

- The incidence of DVT after major trauma remains significant.
- Patients should be evaluated for risk of venous thromboembolism after injury, and treated accordingly.
- DUS is a rapid, portable, and noninvasive technique to diagnose DVT.
- Pulmonary embolism should always be considered with unexplained hypoxia, hypocarbia, or an impending sense of doom.

Suggested Readings

Geerts WH, Code KI, Jay RM, et al. A prospective study of venous thromboembolism after major trauma. N Engl J Med 1994;331:1601–1606.

Geerts WH, Jay RM, Code KI, et al. A comparison of low-dose heparin with low molecular weight heparin as prophylaxis against venous thromboembolism after major trauma. N Engl J Med 1996;335:701–707.

Geerts WH, Pineo GF, Heit JH, et al. Prevention of venous thromboembolism: The Seventh ACCP Conference on Antithrombolytic Therapy. Chest 2004;126:338S–400S.

Knudson MM, Morabito D, Paiemont GD, et al. Use of low molecular weight heparin in preventing thromboembolism in trauma patients. J Trauma 1996;41:446–459.

Knudson MM, Ikossi DG. Venous thromboembolism after trauma. Curr Opin Crit Care 2004;10:539–548.

Patel S, Kazeerooni EA. Helical CT for the evaluation of acute pulmonary embolism. AJR 2005;1185:135–149.

Rosenthal D, Wellons ED, Levitt AB. Role of prophylactic temporary inferior vena cava filters placed at the ICU bedside under intravascular ultrasound guidance in patients with multiple trauma. J Vasc Surg 2004;40:958–964.

Winchell RJ, Hoyt DB, Walsh JC, et al. Risk factors associated with pulmonary embolism despite routine prophylaxis: implications for improved protection. J Trauma 1994;37:600–606.

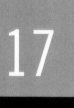

Operating Room Practice

Steven A. Johnson and Michael Rhodes

I. CONDUCTING TRAUMA OPERATION

A. The ideal location for a trauma operating room (OR) is adjacent or in close proximity to the trauma resuscitation unit. **Ideally, it is always better to take the patient to the operating room as opposed to bringing the operating room to the patient.** However, these principles are contingent upon hospital-specific geography, resources, and the scenario faced by the resuscitation team. Optimal situations dictate that the trauma operating room should be located in the main operating room suite to allow more flexibility of equipment and personnel. The so-called *hybrid rooms* with a diverse collection of equipment allow a multidisciplinary approach including full vascular/imaging and interventional technology. Elevator standby and priority transport protocols must be in place. All OR rooms should be stocked with the necessary tools to allow direct OR transport from the scene (in extremis) for continued resuscitation or procedural intervention. These scenarios may dictate bypass of the emergency department.

B. A trauma OR should have adequate space, 400 to 600 sq ft. Safety of the staff with properly configured ORs free of wires, equipment cords, and bulky items in walkways is a priority to avoid personnel injury. The following equipment and drugs should be available:

1. An OR table that is capable of radiography and fluoroscopy (i.e., Jackson table)
2. Warm intravenous fluids and blood products as appropriate (FFP, PRBCS, cryoprecipitate, platelets)
3. A rapid-infusion device
4. High quality OR lights that are adjustable and movable to allow adequate lighting during single or multiple, simultaneous OR procedures
5. Dedicated imaging equipment (built-in if possible) to move in and out of operative field
6. A minimum of four suction canisters
7. A minimum of eight electrical outlets
8. A blood salvage device (Cell Saver, thoracostomy auto-transfusion devices, etc.)
9. A multi-purpose anesthesia machine capable of high minute ventilation (up to 30 L/min.), increased levels of positive end-expiratory pressure (up to 20 cm H_2O), and pressure support inverse-ratio ventilation. A dedicated respiratory therapist may be helpful in those patients with unconventional modes of ventilation such as APRV, high-frequency oscillator ventilation, and single lung ventilation. These modes are frequently utilized in the critically ill patient with severe ventilator-dependent respiratory failure/ARDS
10. Multichannel pressure monitoring
11. High resolution, high definition monitors for viewing radiologic images in the perioperative period
12. Patient external warmers/heating devices
13. Electrocautery with argon beam capability
14. Harmonic scalpel, handheld mesenteric ligation devices
15. Linear stapling devices
16. A general trauma tray with a Finochietto retractor, rib spreader, aortic compressor, sternal saw, Lebsche knife, Fogarty catheters, and a variety of vascular clamps

17. Head light (self-contained battery pack to allow ease of movement around table), face shields and/or goggles, boots, and impervious gowns for the operating team **(UNIVERSAL PRECAUTIONS ARE ALWAYS MANDATORY)**

II. ED TO OR AND OPERATING ROOM ("HAND-OFF") COMMUNICATION

A. The critically injured patient must be accompanied by the resuscitation team to the OR. Notification of the OR charge nurse should be done immediately upon patient arrival to clear the way for potential OR utilization. A point of care analyzer (INR, hemoglobin, and lactate parameters) is essential to continued resuscitation. **Immediate and concise discussion between the operating surgeon, OR circulating/scrub teams, and most importantly, anesthesia personnel should ensue. This "hand-off" communication helps to ensure the availability of blood products and equipment.** It also serves to outline key factors that relate to the patient's medical history, mechanism of injury, and treatment(s) rendered in the ED. Patient safety initiatives using aviation crew resource management and Team-STEPPS principles are recommended. Adequate lifting help must be on hand to move the patient from the stretcher and provide transfer of the patient to the OR table. All equipment such as pelvic binders or backboard equipment should be removed prior to the start of the case.

B. In urgent laparotomy, both arms should be exposed for adequate access and IV access in the central veins should be obtained for the most critically injured (Figure 17-1).

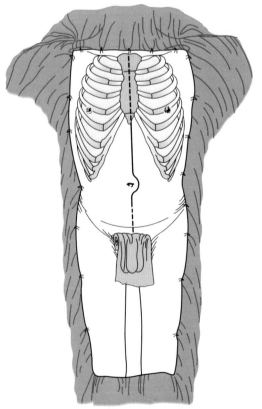

Figure 17-1. OR patient preparation.

A cervical collar or two sandbags with tape across the forehead should be a priority so that cervical spine immobilization is maintained at all times.

C. ECG monitoring, capnometry, pulse oximetry, and arterial pressure monitoring. All monitoring equipment should be placed outside of the operative field as to avoid interference with the operative intervention. The patient should be prepped from chin to knees (chin to mid-thighs and laterally to the table). Draping may be secured in place with staples or sutures. A 15 second prep is superior to no prep in the moribund patient.

III. OPERATING ROOM PRIORITIES

A. Multiple techniques will be employed and decisions should be based on the body region and the stability of the patient. Useful guidelines are as follows:

1. Adequate assistance including a second attending surgeon, lighting, and suction must be ensured; **techniques to ensure correct site surgery are imperative even in emergent situations.** After airway and ventilatory control, major hemorrhage (either external or body cavity) takes priority. External hemorrhage from the face, scalp, and extremities can be controlled by pressure, packing, balloon tamponade, or temporary suture closure until major body cavity hemorrhage is controlled.

2. **The operation should never be compromised by inadequate exposure.** Therefore, an adequate, rapid incision should be made to conduct a thorough exploration.

3. Before opening a body cavity, anesthesia should be prepared to deal with cardiovascular collapse. The abdomen of a hypotensive patient with an obtainable blood pressure should not be opened until blood products are available in the room.

4. Blood salvage capability should be ready before opening a body cavity suspected of massive hemorrhage.

5. Hemorrhage can be controlled by precise packing before attempting definitive repair.

6. In a patient with intraoperative hemodynamic instability, measurements of arterial blood gasses, ionized calcium, and potassium are necessary.

7. Measures should be in place to ensure adequate communication and updates between family and the surgical team.

8. Direct communication between OR and blood bank/laboratory should be available.

9. Generally speaking, uncontrolled thoracic hemorrhage takes priority over uncontrolled abdominal hemorrhage and body cavity hemorrhage (chest, abdomen, pelvis) takes priority over head injury.

10. **In the deadly triad of metabolic acidosis, hypothermia, coagulopathy, and damage control techniques should be used with hemorrhage control via packing and contamination control via stapling of intestine.**

11. Craniotomy without a preceding imaging study in the OR is rarely indicated in the absence of lateralizing signs.

12. A patient with a widened mediastinum and active intra-abdominal hemorrhage should undergo exploratory laparotomy and simultaneous evaluation of the mediastinum by transesophageal echocardiography.

IV. SURGICAL SIMULATION TRAINING AND PERFORMANCE IMPROVEMENT

A. In a high stakes environment such as the trauma resuscitation area and the OR, surgical simulation appears to be crucial to the success of prehospital personnel, trainees and attendings who want the opportunity to be instructed in, or "practice," key aspects of medical care and procedural techniques without fear of costly medical errors.

1. Surgical simulation can be effective with both low and high fidelity models. High fidelity models employ haptic trainers and OR simulation equipment.

2. **Crew resource management and TeamSTEPPS principles** as outlined in the aviation industry and Department of Defense, respectively, are useful adjuncts to organizing surgical care all while teaching teamwork, specific roles, and crucial leadership skills.
3. Collection of OR data and performance improvement models are useful in improving patient care paradigms and providing educational opportunities. The overall positive (or negative) financial impact for the institution may be seen as an improvement of the percentage of total operating expense and revenues generated. From this information, strategic decisions can be made.

Suggested Readings

Arora S, Hull L, Sevdalis N, et al. Factors compromising safety in surgery: stressful events in the operating room. *Am J Surg* 2010;199(1):60–65.

Brogmus G, Leone W, Butler L, et al. Best practices in OR suite layout and equipment choices to reduce slips, trips, and falls. *AORN J* 2007;86(3):384–394.

Caplan RA, Barker SJ, Connis RT, et al. Practice advisory for the prevention and management of operating room fires. *Anesthesiology* 2008;108(5):786–801.

Dagi TF, Schecter W, Napolitano LM. Preparation of the Operating Room. In: ACS Surgery. *Principles and Practice*. Section 1.8 at http://www.acssurgery.com (2012).

Hansen K, Uggen PE, Brattebø G, et al. Training operating room teams in damage control surgery for trauma: a followup study of the Norwegian model. *J Am Coll Surg* 2007;205(5):712–716.

Kneebone R. Practice, rehearsal, and performance. *JAMA* 2009;302(12):1336–1337.

Leach L, Myrtle RC, Weaver FA, et al. Assessing the performance of surgical teams. *Health Care Manage Rev* 2009;34(1):29–41.

Lee BT, Tobias AM, Yueh JH, et al. Design and impact of an intraoperative pathway: a new operating room model for team-based practice. *J Am Coll Surg* 2008;207(6):865–873.

Stepaniak P, Mannaerts GH, de Quelerij M, et al. The effect of operating room coordinator's risk appreciation on operating room efficiency. *Anesth Analg* 2009;108(4):1249–1256.

Turrentine FE, Wang H, Young JS, et al. What is the safety of nonemergent operative procedures performed at night? A study of 10, 426 operations at an acadenic tertiary care hospital using the American College of Surgeons national surgical quality program improvement database. *J Trauma* 2010;69(2):313–319.

Wachtel RE, Dexter F. Review of behavioral operations experimental studies of newsvendor problems for operating room management. *Anesth Analg* 2010;110(6):1698–1710.

18 Disasters, Mass Casualty Incidents

Ronald N. Roth, Amir Blumenfeld and Susan M. Briggs

I. INTRODUCTION

The time, location, or complexity of the next disaster cannot be predicted. Disasters, natural, or human-made, encompass a wide spectrum of threats. Incidents involving weapons of mass destruction (WMD) create a "contaminated" environment and additional challenges to the medical response system. Disasters differ in the degree to which the medical and public health infrastructure of the affected community is disrupted and to which outside assistance is needed. The location of the incident, the availability of local resources, and the number, severity and diversity of injuries are major factors in determining whether a mass casualty incident (MCI) requires resources from outside the affected community. While the spectrum of disasters is endless, all disasters have similar medical and public health concerns.

A. Definitions

1. A **disaster** occurs when the local resources are unable to meet the needs of the event. The required resources may include additional manpower, heavy rescue equipment, or expertise in dealing with an infectious disease outbreak or WMD release.

2. MCIs are events that cause casualties large enough to overwhelm the medical and public health services of the affected community.

B. Scope.
MCIs have traditionally implied a limited geographic location. Many disasters are complex and involve large geographical regions. The earthquake, subsequent tsunami, and nuclear disaster in Japan (2011) is an example of a complex natural disaster involving a large geographic region.

1. Location influences the impact and the ability of medical personnel to respond to an incident.

   a. In an austere environment, resources, transport, access, security, and other aspects of the physical, social, or economic environments impose severe constraints on the adequacy of immediate care for the population.

   b. Incidents in an urban location have a high potential for a large number of injuries, loss of local resources, and destruction of infrastructure.

2. MCIs as a result of the accidental escape of toxic materials (e.g., methyl-isocyanate in Bhopal, India, 1984) or the purposeful release of harmful materials in a WMD incident (Sarin attack on the Tokyo subway, 1995) have the greatest potential to produce chaos and mass casualties.

II. KEY PRINCIPLES

Disaster medical care is not the same as conventional medical care. While the objective of conventional medical care is to do the greatest good for the individual patient, *a key principle of disaster medical care is to do the greatest good for the greatest number of patients.* Disaster medical care requires a fundamental change in the approach to the care of patients (crisis management care/altered standards of care) to achieve this objective.

A. A consistent approach to disasters is the accepted practice throughout the world. This strategy is called MCI response. MCI response has the primary objective of reducing the morbidity (injury/disease) and the mortality (death) associated with the disaster.

B. The basic medical and public health concerns are similar in all disasters, differing by the responses required and need for outside assistance, regional, national, or international.

  1. Basic medical concerns related to MCI responses include:
  - **a.** Search and rescue
  - **b.** Triage and initial stabilization
  - **c.** Evacuation
  - **d.** Definitive care

  2. Basic public health concerns related to MCIs include:
  - **a.** Water
  - **b.** Food
  - **c.** Shelter
  - **d.** Sanitation
  - **e.** Safety/security
  - **f.** Transportation
  - **g.** Communication
  - **h.** Disease surveillance
  - **i.** Endemic/epidemic diseases

III. INCIDENT COMMAND SYSTEM (ICS)

The overall success and safety of a disaster response will largely depend on the quality of the ICS. A well-developed ICS is the most effective method to manage disasters both in the prehospital and hospital environment. Almost all incidents will involve responders from multiple organizations with differing command structures. The ICS is a standardized all-hazards management approach designed to enhance the ability of multiagency organizations (fire, police, emergency medical services, hospitals) and/or multiple jurisdictions to work together effectively in response to a disaster. The ICS uses a common organizational structure and language to achieve this goal and is the accepted standard for all disaster responses. The ICS creates a hierarchy of roles and responsibilities to direct the management of personnel and resources.

  A. ICS comprises five major functional areas. The general responsibilities of each member of the ICS team are predetermined and independent of the nature of the incident. Not all activities are used for every disaster. Functional requirements, not titles, determine ICS hierarchy.

  1. ICS hierarchy
  - **a.** Incident command. Maintains overall responsibility for disaster response and sets objectives and priorities for the disaster response. Several key personnel report to the incident commander (IC). The Liaison Officer assists the IC in communicating with and coordinating the various organizations responding to the disasters. The Public Information Officer provides appropriate information to the public and press. The safety officer is responsible for worker safety.
  - **b.** Operations. Conducts operations, directs disaster resources.
  - **c.** Planning. Develops action plans, maintains status of resources.
  - **d.** Logistics. Provides resources, personnel, and supplies.
  - **e.** Financial/administrative. Monitors costs.

  2. ICS key concepts
  - **a.** Unity of command. Individual responder reports to only one supervisor.
  - **b.** Span and control. An individual should ONLY supervise between three and seven other responders.
  - **c.** Objective related tasks. Specific objectives are ranked and assigned as specific tasks.

  3. Several principles are important for effective use of the ICS in disasters:
  - **a.** The IC and other key positions are identified and trained before a disaster occurs, not chosen at the time of a disaster.
  - **b.** ICS must be started early, before an incident gets out of control.
  - **c.** Medical and public health responders who usually work independently must adhere to the structure of the ICS to avoid negative consequences.

B. The structure of the ICS is the same regardless of the nature of the disaster. The only difference is in the particular expertise of key personnel and the extent of the ICS utilized in a particular disaster. For example, the safety officer will vary by the type of disaster (i.e., an infection control expert might serve as the safety officer during a biologic incident).

IV. MEDICAL RESPONSE TO DISASTERS

A. The National Disaster System (NDMS) is a federally coordinated system that augments the Nation's medical response capability. The overall purpose of the NDMS is to assist State and local authorities in providing disaster relief. Four categories of response teams are part of the NDMS.

  1. Disaster Medical Assistance Teams (DMAT)
  2. International Medical Surgical Response Teams (IMSURT)
  3. Disaster Mortuary Operational Response Teams (DMORT)
  4. National Veterinary Response Teams (NVRT)

B. Disaster Medical Assistance Teams (DMATs) are groups of professional medical personnel (supported by a cadre of logistical and administrative staff) designed to be a rapid-response element to supplement local medical care. There are over 50 DMATs in the United States. IMSURT are teams of medical specialists who provide surgical and critical care during a disaster. Each of the three IMSURT teams is equipped with a rapidly deployable, fully equipped field hospital, including operating rooms (ORs).

C. Search and rescue. Many local response organizations have developed search and rescue teams as integral part of their disaster plans. In large scale incidents, specialized teams from outside agencies may be called upon for assistance. In the United States, a National Urban Search and Rescue System coordinates federal and civilian search and rescue responses.

D. Triage and initial stabilization. Triage is the most important and often the most psychologically challenging mission of disaster medical response. The objective of disaster triage (field triage) is to do the greatest good for the greatest number of people. The goal of disaster triage is to identify the critical patients with the greatest chance of survival and the least expenditure of time and resources (equipment, supplies, and personnel). Both under-triage and over-triage of victims limits the effectiveness of the disaster response. Under-triage is the assignment of critically injured casualties requiring immediate care to a "delayed" category. Over-triage is the assignment of non-critical survivors with no life-threatening injuries to the "urgent" category. Over-triage is more common in MCIs.

  1. Field triage. Victims are categorized on site into two categories, acute and nonacute. Simplified color coding may be done if resources permit. Personnel are typically first responders from the local population or local emergency medical personnel.

  2. Medical triage. Rapid categorization of victims at a casualty collection site or fixed or mobile hospital is performed by experienced medical personnel with knowledge of the medical nature and consequences of various injuries (e.g., burns; blast or crush injuries; or exposure to chemical, biologic, or radioactive agents). Color coding may be used.

  a. Red. Casualties which require immediate lifesaving interventions.

  b. Yellow. Casualties for whom treatment can be delayed. Note that victims of bomb blasts can suffer occult internal injuries. These can be easily missed on initial assessments and patient may be under-triaged. Some facilities in Israel have abandoned the yellow category for victims of a bombing incident.

  c. Green. Individuals who require minimal or no medical care.

  d. Black. Deceased or expected to die. This triage category includes victims not expected to survive due to the severity of injuries and/or lack of resources. Some triage schemes place expectant victims under yellow or in a separate category.

  3. Evacuation triage. Priorities for transfer to medical facilities are assigned to disaster victims. The casualty collection site should have easy visibility for disaster victims and convenient exit routes for air and land evacuation. Victims are matched with available receiving facilities. Often victims with minor injuries can be sent to more distant facilities, keeping closer facilities available for higher priority victims.

E. Definitive medical care. Definitive medical care improves, rather than simply stabilize, a casualty's condition. In some disasters, local hospitals may be destroyed, transportation to medical facilities may not be feasible, or the environment may be contaminated. In these situations, definitive care must be provided outside traditional medical facilities.

1. Hospital teams with mobile equipment that can provide a graded, flexible response to the need for definitive medical care in disasters are keys to a successful disaster response and have been developed by many countries and hospitals.

2. Disaster medical assistance teams must be able to provide care for routine emergencies/diseases as well as disaster-related injuries.

F. Evacuation. Evacuation is useful in a disaster to decompress the disaster area and provide specialized care for specific casualties, such as those with burns and crush injuries.

1. Modes of evacuation from the disaster site to the local hospital and from local facilities to tertiary care centers may include ground transport, helicopter transport, and transport by fixed-wing aircraft.

2. Medical providers must take into account patient stresses of flight that may be encountered during evacuation and affect medical care. These include changes related to the hypobaric environment, decreased partial pressure of oxygen, turbulence, vibration, varying temperatures, and low humidity.

V. PUBLIC HEALTH RESPONSE TO DISASTERS

Medical providers must understand the impact of disasters on the public health infrastructure to have an efficient medical response.

A. The Rapid Needs Assessment (RNA) provides timely evaluation of the impact of the disaster on the affected population. The RNA includes:

1. Assessment of the magnitude of the disaster;

2. Assessment of basic services (water, food, sanitation, and emergency temporary shelter);

3. Assessment of the capacity of the affected community to respond to the disaster needs.

B. Media reports can provide valuable information regarding the magnitude of the disaster, particularly in the area of greatest impact. Media has the ability to direct specific resources (helicopters, reporters, cameramen) to investigate a disaster site. Monitoring media reports and working with the media is important.

VI. HOSPITAL PREPAREDNESS FOR DISASTERS AND MULTI-CASUALTY INCIDENTS

A. Preparation. Mass casualty situations pose challenges for any medical system or hospital. No system will function efficiently without proper preparedness programs. The disaster plan should be applicable to all-hazards and should cover all aspects relevant to such events and provide detailed modes of operation for MCI management including:

1. Pre-designed protocols and standing orders. Each hospital should have written protocols and standing orders pertaining to the various scenarios anticipated during an MCI. Protocols contain series of actions that need to be taken once MCI is declared. Standing orders are translation of these activities into practical orders detailing the sequential actions that need to be executed by different staff members. (e.g., Protocol—All designated relevant personnel should be notified; Standing order—Emergency Department (ED) administrator: Notify hospital director, blood bank, radiology, etc.) Area or person-specific protocols should be clear, concise, and easily accessible.

2. Pre-arranged equipment stocks, and stockpiles. All necessary equipment items including stretchers, medications, medical devices, protection gear, etc. should be prepared in advance. These items should be stored in an accessible location and prepared to be mobilized in time of need.

3. Educational and training programs. Special training programs for various MCI scenarios should be prepared and executed on a periodic basis. Training should involve all staff members that may become involved in these incidents to include physicians, nurses, paramedical personnel, administrators, logistical staff, hospital security personnel, and hospital managerial staff.

B. Following the primary field triage and treatment, casualties are transferred to local hospitals or mobile field facilities. The number and type of hospitals participating in the care of the injured in such events varies, depending on the hospitals available in the vicinity of the MCI and their level of care (trauma center versus nontrauma center).

C. Hospitals must rapidly organize and prepare to operate in an MCI mode. This mode of operation involves multiple elements including:

1. Dedicated admitting areas
2. Presence of trained manpower
3. Immediate availability of logistical means and communication routes

D. Upon receiving an MCI alert, the appropriate hospital plan should be activated. The person with the authority to activate the MCI plan should be specifically stated in the hospital protocol and should be physically present at the hospital on a 24/7 basis (e.g., the on-call senior surgeon, the on-call chief nurse or the emergency medicine attending or chief).

1. Once the MCI alert is activated, the hospital ICS specified in the protocol should be established, and go into action immediately. As communication routes may be congested at emergency time, several alternatives (cell phones, text messages, beepers, runners, etc.) for contacting the staff should be specified.

2. The ED staff should anticipate a 15 to 30 minute period during which they will have to function without additional help or equipment. During this time, existing patients should be evacuated from the ED. Patients can be either transferred rapidly to the hospital wards or discharged according to their condition.

   a. Four sites relating to the triage categories, i.e., critical, immediate, delayed, and deceased should be established. The location of each site depends on the characteristics of each hospital; however, they should be close enough to allow central control, yet keep minimal separation to avoid interference in the management of the severely injured. It is advisable to locate the critical and the immediate zones in proximity to enable quick patient transfer in case of errors in triage.

   b. The necessary equipment should be transferred from the stockpiles and brought to the appropriate sites.

3. All casualties should enter through a single site for initial triage. If there is potential for contaminated victims arriving at the hospital, the triage site should be separated from the hospital to allow decontamination and avoid contaminating the hospital facility. The triage team should include a triage officer, a nurse, and a clerk. The triage officer should be experienced in trauma care, but not necessarily the most experienced surgeon as his/her greatest influence on patient outcome will probably occur at the treatment sites or the OR. The clerk should assign each patient a unique identification number, together with a color tag or bracelet corresponding to the site determined by the triage officer.

4. The treatment sites should be staffed with care giver teams according to severity of injuries. Patient:team ratio should reflect the severity of patients' condition such as one physician and two nurses per critical and immediate patients and one physician and four nurses per twenty delayed patients. This allocation might not be achieved at the beginning of the MCI, but the general concept should be reflected in the activation plan.

5. The intensive care unit (ICU) and OR, should be notified and start preparing for patients arrival. All elective surgical activities should be halted and on-going procedures should be completed as rapidly as possible. The ICU staff is expected to clear as many ICU beds as possible.

6. An emergency communication system should be launched, connecting the key personnel and sites across the hospital. The communication technology should be as reliable as possible, and designed to be minimally influenced by anticipated disturbances such as overload or power failure. Regardless of the chosen technology, a simple back-up system should be ready in case of system failure.

7. Security personnel should be posted in areas designated in the disaster plan to prevent unauthorized people from entering the triage and treatment sites.

8. An information center, operated by administrative staff and social workers should be opened as soon as possible. This center is responsible for providing information and support to family members.

E. Medical management. The medical management at each site should be directed by the site director. This person should be familiar with all aspects of trauma and mass casualty victim care.

1. The basic principles of MCI medical treatment are:

  a. Decontamination as needed

  b. Minimal acceptable care (crisis management care/altered standards of care). In contrast to the routine single patient care, during an MCI a different approach, termed minimal acceptable care, is advised. This approach is intended to keep patients alive by providing lifesaving procedures at the initial phase and providing more comprehensive care at a later date when adequate resources and personnel are available. Minimal acceptable care applies primarily to critical patients, but is extended to less severe ones as well. For example, imaging tests are not performed at the initial phases and treatment is directed by clinical judgment only; until the situation clears and imaging can be performed.

  c. Continuous triage. Triage errors must be expected and planned for in the chaotic state of initial casualty influx. The system should therefore be "error-tolerant" and mitigate these errors by continuous triage.

  d. One directional patient flow

    i. During an MCI it is crucial to strive for a unidirectional flow of patients from the ED to the other hospital services (imaging department, OR, ward). Once a patient leaves the ED, he/she has to have a final destination (OR, ICU, ward), unless the imaging results may influence this decision. Consider performing suturing and splinting at alternative sites.

  e. Meticulous tertiary survey

    i. Due to the chaotic situation, some injuries may be missed during the initial phase. To avoid longer-term harm, plan a mandatory tertiary survey after the initial care. A team of trauma experts should review all the victims within 24 hours of admission and perform the necessary tests for optimal diagnosis and care.

    ii. Prior to discharge from the ED or hospital, every patient should be reviewed to ensure that the patient needs have been met including medications, vaccinations, follow-up instructions, and psychological care.

2. Imaging tests. Only tests that may affect the initial treatment should be performed. CT should be performed only when their results may direct the operative intervention. Following the CT, there should be a controller in the CT area who will decide the need for urgent surgery or ICU/ward admission. Ultrasound may be used liberally during an MCI since it is easily mobilized and performed bedside.

3. Operating room issues. The most experienced available physician should prioritize the surgical intervention during an MCI. No patient should be transported to the OR without clearance from this person. Priorities include patients in hemorrhagic shock followed by those who need neurosurgical procedures. All other surgical procedures should be delayed. The surgical procedures should be as short as possible and damage control surgery is the best operative strategy under these circumstances.

4. Minor procedures including suturing and casting should be delayed unless they are necessary to stabilize the patient's condition.

5. Transfer of patients during MCI is challenging due to the shortage medical personnel and equipment. The level of medical care and monitoring during transport should be determined by the site director, based on the patients' condition and the availability of medical personnel. Inter-hospital transfer due to inadequate services or overwhelmed resources should be planned in advance.

6. Emotional stress is common during MCI. Many patients will exhibit signs of emotional stress with or without mild injuries. Those patients should get support by the hospital psychiatric team.

VII. THE THREAT OF TERRORISM AND WEAPONS OF MASS DESTRUCTION

The spectrum of agents used by terrorist is limitless, but includes conventional weapons, explosives, biologic, chemical, and nuclear agents. Mass casualty events as the result of terrorism are the most challenging for first responders. In addition to the possibility of a large number of victims, responders must be aware of the potential for secondary strikes directed at harming emergency personnel. Contamination from exposure to biologic, chemical, and radiation agents is an additional risk for responders and hospital personnel.

A. Overview. The US Code of Federal Regulations defines terrorism as "…the unlawful use of force and violence against persons or property to intimidate or coerce a government, the civilian population, or any segment thereof, in furtherance of political or social objectives." Three key factors associated with terrorism are violence, fear, and intimidation toward the intended target and the surrounding population.

1. Conventional weapons and explosives are and will probably continue to be the most frequently used instruments of destruction in terrorist attacks.

2. Civilians are less physically and psychologically prepared for injury compared to military personnel. Extremity injuries including fractures and traumatic amputations are common in military and civilian attacks. However, civilians are twice as likely to present with internal wounds, have more severe wounds resulting in higher in hospital mortality rates. Similar findings are seen when comparing victims of motor vehicle accidents versus terrorist attacks.

3. A unique feature of a terrorist incident especially those involving WMDs, is that psychogenic casualties can predominate. Terrorists do not have to kill people to achieve their goals; creating a climate of fear and panic to overwhelm the medical infrastructure achieves their goals. During a 1995 Sarin gas attack in Tokyo 5,000 casualties were referred to hospitals, but less than 1,000 actually had effects of the gas.

   a. WMD incidents have the greatest potential to generate psychogenic casualties large enough to overwhelm most emergency medical systems. Prehospital and hospital systems must have a plan to deal with large numbers of patients with psychological needs. This may include transport of these patients directly to existing or preplanned psychiatric care centers. Hospitals must have the capability to quickly screen these patients and move them out of the ED to a separate area.

B. Scene safety

1. Initial responders should establish a "hot zone" to identify the area of contamination. Access to the hot zone should be limited to rescue personnel in proper protective gear. Medical treatment is very limited in the hot zone. Victims are moved out the hot zone into the warm zone where decontamination and limited medical treatment (antidotes, hemorrhage control, etc.) may be performed by rescuers in proper protective gear. Decontaminated victims are moved to a clean treatment area ("cold zone") away and upwind of the contaminated area.

2. **Personal protection.** WMD events involving chemical, biologic, or nuclear agents may require emergency responders to wear personal protective equipment (PPE). This equipment must be available in sufficient quantity and personnel must know how to properly use the equipment.

   a. Early in a WMD event, the type and extent of contamination may be unknown. It is prudent for initial responders to use the highest level of protection and then scale down as the situation allows.

    b. Receiving facilities should not assume that victims transported to the hospital by emergency personnel have been decontaminated. In addition, potentially contaminated victims may present to these facilities on their own.

C. Blast injuries are the result of the rapid chemical conversion of a liquid or solid material into a gas which results in a release of energy. The highly compressed gasses expand generating a pressure pulse that is propagated by a blast wave. Traditionally associated with military operations, blast injuries are now frequently seen in the civilian population due to terrorism. Bombings and attacks with conventional weapons account for the majority of injuries and fatalities from terrorist incidents. Most terrorist bombings consist of relatively small explosives that produce low casualty rates. Fortunately less common, the bombing of the Murrah Federal building in downtown Oklahoma City is an example of a large amount of explosives placed in a heavily populated areas to create a large number of casualties (168 deaths and over 600 injured).

    1. The effects of the blast wave are increased in a closed space such as a building or bus and underwater. The high morbidity and mortality is related not only to the intensity of the blast, but also to the subsequent structural damage that leads to collapse of buildings, a common phenomenon in large explosions.

    2. Injuries caused by explosives and bombings can be divided into five categories:

        a. *Primary blast injury.* As the blast wave passes through the body.

        b. *Secondary blast injury.* From projectiles either packed in the explosive device or created as the result of the explosion. These injuries are a frequent cause of death.

        c. *Tertiary blast injury.* When the victim becomes a projectile.

        d. *Quaternary blast injury.* As the result of burn or crush injuries.

        e. *Quandary blast injury.* From the addition of chemical, biologic, or radiologic material to the explosive device (dirty bomb).

D. Biologic agents. Biologic terrorism is the use of infectious agents or toxins derived from living organisms to produce death or disease.

    1. The following disease agents are believed to have the greatest potential for bioterrorism:

        a. Anthrax (bacteria)

        b. Tularemia (bacteria)

        c. Plague (bacteria)

        d. Smallpox (virus)

        e. Viral hemorrhagic fevers (virus)

        f. Botulinum (toxin)

    2. The route of exposure of greatest concern with biologic terrorist attacks is inhalation of the agent. Oral routes of exposure for biologic agents are less important but still significant. Ensuring that food and water supply is free of contamination is an important function of public health after a biologic attack. Dermal exposure is unusual but possible, especially if the skin is damaged.

    3. The most effective and important prophylaxis against biologic agents is physical protection. A full-face respirator prevents exposure of the respiratory and mucous membranes to infectious agents. Dermal exposures should be treated immediately by washing with soap and water.

    4. Identification of an attack with biologic agents is often challenging. Symptoms may be delayed during an incubation period, victims may present to a variety of practitioners for care, (i.e., EDs, urgent care centers, or family physicians) and often symptoms may mimic more common disease entities such as influenza. Early recognition of a bioterrorism event is the key to success. The following are indications of a possible biologic attack:

        a. Disease entity that is unusual or does not occur naturally in a given geographic area

        b. Suspected aerosol route of exposure

        c. Massive point-source outbreak

        d. High morbidity and mortality

E. Chemical agents. Chemical agents have been used in warfare and are now part of the terrorist armamentarium. Chemicals used for terrorism may be military chemical weapons, industrial chemicals, or chemicals created *de novo*.

1. The potential results of a chemical attack include:
   a. Inflicting mass casualties
   b. Harm to first responders and hospital personnel
   c. Hysteria, anxiety, and panic in the general population
2. Most chemical warfare agents are liquids. Chemical agents in liquid form must be dispersed in order to be maximally effective. This can be done in three general ways:
   a. Aerosolizing with an aerial sprayer (such as done with pesticides)
   b. Aerosolizing in an explosion
   c. Allowing the liquid to evaporate and dispersing the vapor
3. Often the offending chemical agent is unknown. This can delay the appropriate treatment including the administration of antidotes. Knowing the toxidromes associated with each class of chemical agents may help speed the identification of the agent and provide insight into treatment options.
4. The five principle classes of chemical agents and their toxidromes are:
   a. Nerve agents. Including sarin, tabun, soman, VX
      i. Presentation includes cholinergic crisis: Salivation, lacrimation, urination, gastrointestinal symptoms, miosis, weakness, and seizures.
      ii. Exposure is typically via aerosolized liquid. Toxicity can occur from direct contact with the skin.
      iii. Treatment includes decontamination, symptomatic treatment (benzodiazepines for seizures) and the administration of antidotes including atropine, and 2-PAM.
   b. Vesicants (blistering agents). Mustard agents and Lewisite are examples of vesicants.
      i. Exposure to gas or liquid causes skin erythema, ocular burns, systemic symptoms including shock.
      ii. Treatment includes decontamination and treatment of symptoms.
   c. Blood agents. Cyanide and carbon monoxide are blood agents.
      i. Symptoms include dyspnea, tachycardia, confusion, arrhythmias and coma.
      ii. Exposure varies by the agent but in general can occur by inhalation or ingestion.
      iii. Treatment includes removal from the exposure, oxygen, and the use of antidotes for cyanide (sodium nitrate or hydroxocobalamin).
   d. Pulmonary agents. Chlorine and phosgene are pulmonary agents.
      i. These agents cause cutaneous irritation, ocular burning, and respiratory symptoms that can progress to pulmonary edema. Exposure is typically inhalation.
      ii. Treatment is symptomatic.
   e. Riot control agents
      i. There are a variety of riot control agents (often called "tear gas") that temporarily incapacitate individuals by causing lacrimation, sneezing, and respiratory distress.
      ii. Symptoms are self-limiting and treatment is supportive.

F. Radioactive agents. Radioactive material from medical, industrial, military, or clandestine sources could be used in a terrorist attack. Like all of the other forms of WMDs, radiation has a high potential to cause mass destruction and hysteria. While the detonation of a nuclear weapon is highly unlikely, the possibility of exposure to radioactive material via explosion of a conventional weapon contaminated with nuclear material is real.

1. Nuclear material use by terrorists would likely involve one of four scenarios:
   a. detonation of a nuclear device
   b. meltdown of a nuclear reactor

c. Dispersal of material through use of conventional explosives: A radiation dispersal device (RDD) or "dirty bomb." Some first responder agencies routinely monitor all explosion scenes for radiation.

d. Exposure to nuclear material (i.e., placing radioactive materials in public places).

2. Irradiation versus contamination. A key factor is to understand the difference between irradiation versus contamination.

a. Casualties who have been irradiated but have not had radioactive material deposited on or in their bodies ("fallout") are not themselves radioactive. These patients have been exposed to radiation but do not pose a contamination risk to responders or hospital personnel. Since the clinical effects of all but the most severe radiation exposures are delayed, the clinical presentation of exposed casualties will be primarily related to conventional injuries, and normal trauma triage procedures should be employed.

b. External contamination occurs when radioactive material is deposited on the outside of the body. Internal contamination is the result of radioactive material entering the body via ingestion, inhalation, or wounds. Contaminated victims can expose and contaminate responders and hospital personnel. However, use of standard universal precautions will allow medical personnel to provide life-saving treatments (i.e., establishing an airway, treating a tension pneumothorax, etc.).

  i. The majority of external contamination can be removed by undressing victims. Skin can be cleaned with copious amounts of soap and water. Special attention should be paid to the hair and intertriginous areas where radioactive material can collect.

  ii. Open wounds must be decontaminated to remove radioactive material and protected during total body decontamination.

c. Internal contamination must be prevented. Pharmacologic agents can be used to remove or chelate specific radiologic agents. Consultation of local radiologic experts or the Radiation Emergency Assistance Center/Training Site (REAC/TS 865-576-1005) can guide therapy.

3. Involve local radiation safety experts. Because of military, industrial, and health care experience with radiation, local expertise is often available.

a. Many jurisdictions and most hospitals have radiation safety personnel. They can assist with patient screening, emergency personnel monitoring, and decontamination issues.

b. Radiation oncologists deal with therapeutic exposures to radiation on a daily basis. They can assist with patient monitoring and therapy.

4. Key points with respect to the care of victims from a WMD event with potential radiation exposure/contamination:

a. Consider screening casualties from any event involving an explosion for radiation contamination. Some hospitals have placed screening devices in their EDs. Note that patients and staff that have received diagnostic or therapeutic doses of radiation may also trigger these devices.

b. If possible, remove the victim's clothing prior to or immediately upon arrival at the hospital. This removes a considerable amount of the radioactive contamination. Note that the clothing, once removed, still has the potential to contaminate and irradiate hospital personnel. Potentially contaminated items should be placed in a safe and secure area away from people.

c. Treat life-threatening injuries.

d. Decontaminate wounds and skin.

  i. Protect wounds from re-contamination. Use monitoring devices (i.e., Geiger counters) to measure the need for additional decontamination.

  ii. Address internal contamination if required.

e. Limit the exposure of emergency and hospital personnel.

  i. Exposure can be reduced by the following principles:

    a) Time. Rotate personnel to limit the exposure of any one individual.

    b) Distance. Radiation exposure decreases as the square of the distance from the source. Care givers should stay at a distance from contaminated patients until required to perform an evaluation or intervention.

    c) Shielding. Most low-level radiation will not penetrate standard hospital protective gowns. Protection from higher energy radiation requires significant shielding. (Much more than a standard lead apron.)

  ii. Use monitoring devices to estimate exposure.

f. Avoid contamination of hospital.

  i. Preplan areas of the ED and hospital that will be used to care for potentially contaminated patients.

  ii. Determine paths of entrance and exit from care areas to minimize contamination of the hospital.

g. Involve local radiation safety experts.

AXIOMS

- Disasters are complex events that can include a broad spectrum of threats and challenges. The location and nature of the next disaster cannot be predicted. An all-hazards approach is a key principle of disaster preparedness.
- Disaster medical care is fundamentally different from conventional medical care. Disaster medical care attempts to provide the greatest good for the greatest number of patients.
- While the nature and locations of disasters may vary, there are common themes in every event including the need to address basic medical care and public health concerns.
- Hospitals must be prepared to receive multiple casualties over a short time period. Triage and unidirectional patient flow guidelines must be in place prior to an event.
- Mass casualty events with the accidental or intentional release of toxic or infectious materials are the most challenging for responders. Nuclear, biologic, and chemical weapons can contaminate victims and the environment putting responders and hospital personnel at risk.
- Responders and hospitals must be prepared to deal with psychogenic casualties that may prevail during WMD events.

WEB LINKS

Center for Biosecurity of UPMC http://www.upmc-biosecurity.org/

    Center for Disease Control and Prevention—The National Institute for Occupational Safety and The Emergency Response Safety and Health Database http://www.cdc.gov/NIOSH/ershdb/default.html

    FEMA—Incident Command System http://www.fema.gov/emergency/nims/IncidentCommandSystem.shtm

    International Trauma and Disaster Institute http://www.gs-interactive.net/ITDI/index.html

    National Disaster Medical System http://www.phe.gov/preparedness/responders/ndms/Pages/default.aspx

    Radiation Emergency Assistance Center/Training Site (REAC/TS) http://orise.orau.gov/reacts/

    Wireless Information System for Emergency Responders http://wiser.nlm.nih.gov/

Suggested Readings

Bogucki S, DeAtley C. Incident command system and national incident management system. In: Hauda WE, DeAtley C, Bogucki S, eds. *Special Operations Medical Support.* Dubuque, IA: Kendall/Hunt; 2009:3–10.

Born C, Briggs S, Ciraulo DL, et al. Disasters and mass casualties: II. Explosive, biologic, chemical, and nuclear agents. *J Am Acad Orthop Surg* 2007;15(8):461–473.

Briggs S. Disaster management teams. *Curr Opin Crit Care* 2005;11:585–589.

Briggs SM. Regional interoperability: Making systems connect in complex disasters. *J Trauma* 2009;67:S88–S90.

Briggs SM. *Advanced Disaster Medical Response, Manual for Providers.* Boston, MA: Harvard Medical International; 2003.

Coleman CN, Weinstock D, Casagrande R, et al. Triage and treatment tools for use in a scarce resources-crisis standards of care setting after a nuclear detonation. *Disaster Med Public Health Prep* 2011;5:111–121.

Federal Emergency Management Agency, US Department of Homeland Security. Appendix B: Incident command system. http://www.fema.gov/pdf/emergency/nims/NIMS`AppendixB.pdf. Accessed April 21, 2011.

Halpern P, Tsai MC, Arnold JL, et al. Mass-casualty, terrorist bombings: Implications for emergency department and hospital emergency response (Part II). *Prehosp Disaster Med* 2003;18:235–241.

Lerner EB, Schwartz, RB, McGovern JE. Prehospital triage for mass casualties. In: Hauda WE, DeAtley C, Bogucki S, eds. *Special Operations Medical Support*. Dubuque, IA: Kendall/Hunt; 2009:11–13.

Merin O, Ash N, Levy G, et al. The Israeli field hospital in Haiti – ethical dilemmas in early disaster response. *N Engl J Med* 2010;362:e38.

Nemeth I, Weinstein E, Long C, et al. The federal medical response to disasters. In: Hauda WE, DeAtley C, Bogucki S, eds. *Special Operations Medical Support*. Dubuque, IA: Kendall/Hunt; 2009:67–76.

Page L, Keshishian C, Leonardi G, et al. Frequency and predictors of mass psychogenic illness. *Epidemiology* 2010;21:744–747.

Peleg K, Jaffe D; The Israel Trauma Group. Are injuries from terror and war similar? *Ann Surg* 2010;252(2):363–369.

Singer AJ, Singer AH, Halperin P, et al. Medical lessons from terror attacks in Israel. *J Emerg Med* 2007;32:87–92.

19 Injury Prevention

Charles C. Branas

I. INTRODUCTION. Worldwide, injury is the leading cause of death for the first half of the human life span and a regular source of disability and disfigurement. Every day in the United States, hundreds of thousands of men, women, and children are injured severely enough to seek medical care. Hundreds of these people will sustain a long-term disability due to their injuries and additional hundreds will die.

Injury is among the top three causes of death in the United States. The combined burden of unintentional injury deaths, suicides, and homicides was the leading cause of death in those from 1 to 44 years of age. Unintentional injury alone is the fifth leading cause of death for all US age groups. In 2007, over 180,000 injury-related deaths were documented in the United States. The top five mechanisms of injury deaths in the United States were road traffic, poisonings, firearms, falls, and suffocation.

Around the world, injuries, mainly from motor vehicles and weapons, are rapidly becoming the number one global health threat to children, young adults, and developing nations. In any given year about one out of every three people will be injured severely enough to seek medical care. Injuries thus affect people from all walks of life but are very disproportionately experienced by the poor, creating one of the greatest sources of global health inequity between developed and developing countries. Injuries are the largest contributor to disability in low and lower-middle income countries. People who die from injuries are, on average, more than 30 years younger than people who die from other leading causes. They are children, workers, and young parents, society's most valued and economically productive members.

Over 90% of the world's injury deaths occur in low and middle income countries and injury deaths per capita are three times higher in low as opposed to high income countries. Road traffic deaths are predicted to increase by 83% in low and middle income countries but to drop in high income countries by 27% as soon as 2020. Road traffic crashes are the leading cause of death globally for 10 to 24 year olds. Moreover, for every death due to war, there are three deaths due to homicide and five due to suicide. Yet these same injuries are highly underappreciated as a global health threat and receive inadequate attention and funding. Because injuries so heavily affect individuals in their most productive years, their continued growth is sure to hamper or wipe away economic gains in many developing nations and further health inequities between developed and developing nations.

Mortality alone does not characterize adequately the profound physical, psychosocial, and economic effects of injury. Over one-third of all US emergency department visits, almost 40 million in total, are related to injury. The most common injuries were from falls, nonvehicular strikes (such as assaults), and road traffic. It is estimated that nearly 1 in 6 Americans will require treatment for injuries and over 2 million Americans will be hospitalized for injuries each year. In 2005, total injury-attributable medical costs were estimated to be over $77 billion, or about 5% of all medical costs in the United States. The estimated total cost of injury in the United States in 2005, based on direct medical care and work losses, was estimated at just over $355 billion.

Physicians typically focus on the resuscitation and definitive treatment of injuries. However, recognizing the immense societal burden of injury, and the fact that as much as one-half of all injury deaths take place at the scene of the injury or within minutes of the event itself, necessitates expansion of the medical mission to include prevention of injury before it occurs.

II. UNDERSTANDING INJURY PREVENTION

A. Injury deserves attention as a leading cause of death and disability around the world. Injury also deserves attention because it occurs as part of a unique disease process: Violence, suicide attempts, falls, and traffic crashes are all disease-generating events that can suddenly kill or disable otherwise healthy people. This is in contrast to other leading diseases, which generally become noticeable after months or years of risk exposure and have relatively slow pathophysiologic processes. Thus, injury develops in a fraction of a second, often after a similarly sudden exposure to one or more risk factors, making its study and prevention especially challenging.

B. Injury occurs across a timeline or continuum: From early precursors to the defining disease event to immediate and long-term consequences. Opportunities to prevent or ameliorate injury correspondingly differ across this continuum: **Primary prevention** seeks to completely avert injuries by altering susceptibility or reducing exposure; **secondary prevention** employs early detection and prompt treatment of injuries once they occur; and **tertiary prevention** focuses on limiting disability and restoring function for injured individuals.

Although the medical system is rooted in secondary and tertiary prevention, primary prevention is a potentially more efficient way to relieve the burden of injury. Thus, prevention of all types of injuries is a priority and an expectation of personnel in hospitals, both trauma centers and those that are not. The Committee on Trauma (COT) of the American College of Surgeons mandates that trauma center personnel educate the public about injury as a major public health problem. Physicians are natural leaders in expanding trauma care to include the primary prevention of injury. The COT also suggests that physicians move beyond just public education to activities that include surveillance, epidemiology, intervention research, and evaluation of prevention program effectiveness.

III. THE SCIENCE OF INJURY PREVENTION

A. The science of injury prevention has its roots in many fields including medicine, public health, criminology, engineering, and others. Among the earliest attempts to systematize the approach to injury prevention was put forth by Dr. William Haddon several decades ago in the form of 10 injury countermeasures:

  1. Prevent the creation of the hazard in the first place.
  2. Reduce the amount of the hazard brought into being.
  3. Prevent the release of the hazard that already exists.
  4. Modify the release of the hazard that already exists.
  5. Separate, in time and space, the hazard and that which is to be protected.
  6. Separate, by material barrier, the hazard and that which is to be protected.
  7. Modify the relevant basic qualities of the hazard.
  8. Make that to be protected more resistant to damage from the hazard.
  9. Counter damage already done by the hazard.
  10. Stabilize, repair, and rehabilitate the object of the hazard.

  To the prevention strategist, these countermeasures give basic guidance on when to intervene, what to intervene on, and how to intervene. More important, they offer a system whereby the prevention strategist would leave no stone unturned. That is, by considering all 10 countermeasures, he or she can ensure that no potentially promising or effective intervention is overlooked.

B. Knowledge of successful strategies to reduce the burden of specific injuries has increased. The decline in incidence of motor vehicle injuries is a case in point. Although motor vehicle injuries continue to be the leading cause of injury death in the United States, their rates have declined considerably over the past 25 years (Fig. 19-1). This decrease is the result of systematic and multifaceted prevention efforts that include the implementation of adequate surveillance systems (for instance, the Fatality Analysis Reporting System at the National Highway Traffic Safety Administration), the enforcement of government regulations (such as through updated Federal Motor Vehicle Safety Standards), the introduction of active (such as seat belts) and passive (such as airbags) safety devices, improved roadway design (such as left-turn

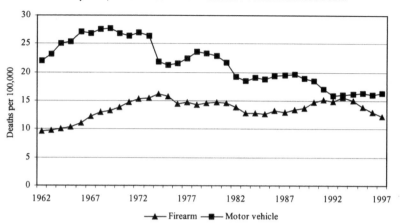

Figure 19-1. Firearm and motor vehicle–related death rates. (From National Center for Injury Prevention and Control, Centers for Disease Control and Prevention, with permission.)

jughandles), advocacy for shifts in social norms (such intolerance of drunk driving), and improved trauma care systems.

C. This success has, however, not extended to all mechanisms of injury, as can be seen in the concurrent increase in firearm injury fatality during the same time period that motor vehicle injury fatalities decreased (Fig. 19-1). Nevertheless, the successful injury prevention strategies used in reducing motor vehicle injuries can also be used to address other major injuries such as those related to firearms and falls. To ensure a high probability of success, these prevention strategies should always be multifaceted, essentially diversifying the prevention strategist's portfolio to defend against failure in any one particular intervention. Moreover, injury prevention strategists should always proceed scientifically, under the mantle of sound evidence, and with the understanding that injuries are not random events. The science of injury deterrence is best founded on epidemiologic surveillance followed by the implementation of prevention strategies that have been thoughtfully designed and systematically evaluated. The following four steps can be taken to more fully understand the epidemiology of specific injuries and mount prevention strategies:

1. Determine the magnitude and characteristics of the problem. Surveillance data provide an indication of the scope of injury. National- and state-level data can assist in identifying trends and allocating resources to address priority injury problems. Many of these databases are available on the internet. It is also important to gain an understanding of injury in the local community. Electronic emergency medical services logs, hospital discharge databases, trauma registries, and electronic death certificate data can be used to study injury specific to a local community.

2. Identify risk factors and determine which of those factors are potentially modifiable. A traditional public health model is a helpful framework to identify and tackle modifiable risk factors for injury (Fig. 19-2). The components of this model are hosts (people and their risky behaviors), agents (automobiles, firearms, knives), and environments (physical [e.g., road design, throw rugs, poor lighting, blighted urban space]; economic [e.g., high unemployment]; social [e.g., access to and use of drugs and alcohol]; and temporal [e.g., season or time of day]). By categorizing injury risks into host, agent, and environment, a comprehensive portfolio of interventions can be created that highlights the complexity

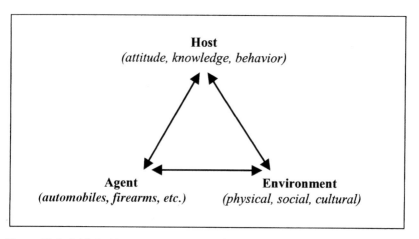

Figure 19-2. Public health model.

of the etiologic chain of events leading to injury. Analysis of these events is an important step in identification of modifiable risk factors. Because the occurrence of injury is often the result of a series of complex, often nonmedical, processes, it is helpful to work with an interdisciplinary team that includes individuals such as other health care providers, epidemiologists, engineers, criminologists, political scientists, economists, and behavioral scientists.

3. **Consider a range of strategies to reduce injury.** All trauma centers are required to participate in trauma prevention. It is important for trauma centers to take the lead in examining the effectiveness of implementing interventions at the local level. In the absence of a program of prevention research, trauma centers can take interventions shown to be effective in other communities and examine if these same interventions can be transferred to their local community. A priori public support, commitment from community and political leaders, and media coverage are indicators that an intervention strategy might be successfully transplanted and implemented. In addition, strategies can best be judged if they are linked to specific, measurable outcomes (e.g., public feelings of safety, injury incidence, mortality) which should be discussed and decided on before actual implementation.

4. **Implement and evaluate the most promising strategies.**
   Strategies that are known to be effective can form the foundation of a new injury prevention program. Strategies such as seat-belt use, child restraints, and designated driver programs are tested interventions that can be implemented in all communities.

IV. RESPONSIBILITIES OF PHYSICIANS

Primary prevention, just like secondary and tertiary prevention, of injury is an important obligation and physicians have two main roles: To spearhead trauma prevention at the community level and to incorporate patient-specific prevention in daily practice. These roles can manifest themselves as part of several day-to-day and long-term activities that physicians and other health care providers can participate in to begin reducing injury in their communities.

A. **Educate the public that injuries are preventable, nonrandom events.**
   Physicians are respected members of the community and can powerfully advocate for injury prevention. A vital first step is to overcome the fatalistic view of injuries as "accidents." Injuries are not random events and should be addressed accordingly. Asking trauma care providers to consider avoiding the word "accident" from their

vocabulary is a key action that can help debunk public fatalism and more appropriately place injuries on solid public health footing with other diseases. Presenting unique profiles of individuals at risk for injury aids in identifying high-risk groups and the factors that contribute to the injury.

B. **Recruit colleagues and collaborate with key players.** Effective prevention efforts require a multitude of skills that extend beyond those typically held by physicians. As leaders of trauma centers and leaders in prevention, physicians can magnify their effectiveness by joining together with other interested parties. For example, involving the hospital media relations department can be key in helping establish contacts with local media and in framing any injury prevention messages that need to be communicated. Making connections with community leaders and elected officials will additionally bring new ideas, new contacts, and new people with nonmedical skills and resources to help solve the problem.

C. **Identify priority injuries to address in the community.** Defining the injury problem specific to the local community helps frame efforts and target resources to those injuries having the greatest impact on the local community. It is important to focus on a targeted at-risk population. A good first step is to use data that are retrievable from trauma center registries. This will provide information on the nature of injuries that reach the trauma center or centers in question. This can be supplemented by other sources of nonfatal and fatal injury data (e.g., hospital discharge data, morgue records, law enforcement, and emergency medical services run data) to create a community-specific profile. Local data analyses can then be placed in context by comparing them with state and national statistics. These data will highlight the injuries of importance to the community served by the trauma center. Injuries that should be prioritized for prevention activities are those that occur most frequently, have the highest mortality, or are most likely to result in prolonged disability. Data that are specific to the local community are the most persuasive in generating sustained interest and commitment from the public and community leaders.

D. **Disseminate injury information of importance to the community.** The general public has a general understanding of injury in their local community. In some cases this understanding of injury can be skewed and is often driven by the most recent high-profile event that received local or national media attention. These high profile cases, however, can be unusual and often do not adequately reflect the nature of the injury problem in a particular community. Furthermore, the general public is constantly exposed to messages that highlight their risks from a variety of threats, but have limited understanding or knowledge of how to weigh the importance of these various risks to their communities or their own lives. Trauma physicians are in a prime position to communicate the actual profile of injury risk in their specific communities and to inform the public of the relative risk of various activities or behaviors. In this way it is important to decide on the main injury prevention messages that will go to the community and to educate fellow professionals to be data-driven, objective spokespeople for these messages.

E. **Secure funding and implement local projects.** In today's health care environment, hospitals often cannot independently fund or implement prevention activities aimed at the community. Therefore, would-be injury prevention strategists would do well to promptly establish an advisory board, composed of community leaders, who can assist in obtaining funds to support community-based interventions. Moreover, although many trauma centers cannot undertake major research agendas in creating and testing injury prevention strategies, they can utilize established prevention programs. Using established programs that have already been shown to be effective is efficient and can secure interest and funding from local leaders. Efficient use of limited funds can also be accomplished by focusing on a specific mechanism of injury, a specific risk factor, or a specific target population. Choosing a specific prevention program is driven both by the data and by the interest and willingness of the community to support and participate. Together with colleagues, advisory board and community partners, develop an implementation plan that will serve as a roadmap for what needs to be accomplished and who is responsible at what timeline milestones. Evaluate frequently to ensure that the planned activities are being carried out and that the program will produce results (including both proclamations of success as well as recognition of unsuccessful strategies that can be discontinued).

F. Help shape reasonable policy decisions

1. The most effective interventions are those that passively safeguard public health rather than those that require active behavioral change. In contrast to active interventions (most typically education campaigns), passive interventions, by definition, do not require individuals to do anything to protect themselves (e.g., better road design, air bags, padded floor in nursing homes). However, passive interventions do meet with public disapproval because they can sometimes limit personal liberties and burden the day-to-day lives of those they are intended to protect. Moreover, as with all interventions, they can have unintended consequences.

2. Policymakers frequently look to experts in the field to secure information and help shape decisions. Physicians can be approached to present testimony before legislative bodies, giving them the opportunity to present relevant data combined with the human aspects of injury. Developing appropriate and reasonable injury prevention policies is an important function that trauma centers can perform in support of this. Physicians can also take a more proactive stance and spearhead efforts to enact legislation that is driven by their data. In this case, it is important to secure the support of one or more key legislators, and their staff, to sponsor the legislation. Injury data are more convincing when they are packaged in a way that presents an understandable, fair, and balanced portrayal of the problem at hand.

G. Work with industry to improve product design and safety. One strategy to reduce the burden of injury is to work directly with industry in creating safer products. Obviously, not all physicians will assume this role. However, this can be an effective intervention to reduce injury. Working with the Consumer Product Safety Commission, automobile manufacturers, child safety seat manufacturers, or firearm manufacturers to establish safety standards for their products are some examples of past industry involvements by health care providers.

H. Incorporate injury prevention into daily practice. Physicians can incorporate injury prevention as a core part of daily clinical practice. Trauma patients can be especially receptive to one-on-one prevention counseling from health care providers during the "teachable moment" that follows an injury. A helpful first step is to document risk factors that potentially contributed to the injury episode. Again, one consideration is to separate risk factors into host, agents, and environments. Documenting specific risk factors will guide potential interventions and might lead to appropriate strategies to reduce future injuries. These strategies can include counseling, teaching, and referrals to abuse counselors.

I. Systematize routine screens to identify patients at risk. Physicians should put systematic routine screens in place to identify patients at risk for recidivism. Screens to capture the presence of interpersonal violence (domestic and child abuse); use of illegal drugs (biologic screens); elderly falls (physical surroundings, comorbid conditions, medications); and abuse of alcohol (CAGE, biologic screens) can help identify patients at high risk. For example, the CAGE screen is one that has proved effective in identifying patients with an alcohol problem. CAGE is a mnemonic of the following four items: Have you ever felt you should **c**ut down on your drinking? Have people **a**nnoyed you by criticizing your drinking? Have you ever felt bad or **g**uilty about your drinking? Have you ever had a drink first thing in the morning to steady your nerves or get rid of a hangover (**e**ye-opener)? A positive reply to any of these questions suggests the need for intervention and a positive response to two or more of these questions should prompt a referral for alcohol treatment.

J. Reduce recidivism by referring patients at high risk to appropriate services. Linking patients identified as high risk with established community services, either through positive routine screens or as indicated by the circumstances surrounding the injury event, allows the routine initiation of appropriate interventions to lessen the potential for recidivism. Such interventions include but are not limited to individual counseling of at-risk patients (e.g., seatbelt and helmet use, safe firearm storage); group counseling by capable professionals; referral to suitable inhospital services (e.g., substance abuse, psychiatric follow-up); and linkages to community-based resources (e.g., domestic abuse hotlines and shelters). Although it will not be possible for all physicians, forays into the community, to visit front-line services and see the living conditions and actual risk factors that generate injuries for patients, are highly educational and will enhance any hospital-based injury prevention program.

V. SUMMARY

Physicians perform a key role in the prevention of injury. Individual physicians can focus on one aspect of prevention that is either clinically or research oriented. The prevention strategist who uses tested interventions in clinical practice is as pivotal as the research-based prevention strategist whose focus is largely in building generalizable knowledge about injury prevention. Prevention activities are a rewarding extension of the acute care trauma mission and hold the promise of greatly reducing the magnitude of injury morbidity and mortality.

Suggested Readings

Anderson GF, Chu E. Expanding priorities – confronting chronic diseases in countries with low income. *New Engl J Med* 2007;356(3):209–211.

Baker SP, O'Neill B, Ginsburg MJ, et al. *The Injury Fact Book*. New York, NY: Oxford University Press; 1992:14–15.

Bonnie RJ, Fulco CE, Liverman CT, eds. *Reducing the Burden of Injury: Advancing Prevention and Treatment*. Washington, DC: Institute of Medicine, National Academy Press; 1999.

Branas CC, Nance ML, Elliott MR, et al. Urban-rural shifts in intentional firearm death: Different causes, same results. *Am J Public Health* 2004;94(10):1750–1755.

Branas CC, Richmond TS, Schwab CW. Firearm homicide and firearm suicide: Opposite but equal. *Public Health Rep* 2004;119(2):114–124.

Branas CC. Injury prevention in the developing world. *Italian J Public Health* 2010;7(2):172–175.

Centers for Disease Control and Prevention. Ten great public health achievements—United States, 1900–1999. *Morb Mortal Wkly Rep* 1999;48(12):241–243.

Cherpitel CJ. Screening for alcohol problems in the emergency department. *Ann Emerg Med* 1995;26(2):158–166.

Haddon W. The basic strategies for reducing hazards of all kinds. *Hazard Prev* 1980:8–12.

Haukeland JV. Welfare consequences of injuries due to traffic accidents. *Accid Anal Prev* 1996;28:63–72.

Kaufmann CR, Branas CC, Brawley ML. A population-based study of trauma recidivism. *J Trauma* 1998;45(2):325–331; discussion 331–332.

Krug EG, Sharma GK, Lozano R. The global burden of injuries. *Am J Public Health* 2000;90(4):523–526.

Meyer M. Death and disability from injury: A global challenge. *J Trauma* 1998;44(1):1–12.

National Center for Injury Prevention and Control. WISQARS (Web-based Injury Statistics Query and Reporting System). http://www.cdc.gov/injury/wisqars/index.html. Accessed June 2011.

Peterson CL, Burton R. U.S. Health Care Spending: Comparison with Other OECD Countries. *CRS Report for Congress*, September 17, 2007.

Richmond TS, Schwab CW, Riely J, et al. Effective trauma center partnerships to address firearm injury: A new paradigm. *J Trauma* 2004;56(6):1197–1205.

Richmond TS, Thompson H, Deatrick J, Kauder DK. The journey towards recovery following physical trauma. *J Adv Nurs* 2000;32:1341–1347.

Rivera FP, Britt J. *You Can Do It: A Community Guide to Injury Prevention*. Available at: http://www.aast.org/YouCan.html. Accessed August 2000.

World Health Organization. *Injury: A Leading Cause of the Global Burden of Disease*. Geneva: World Health Report; 1999.

20 Rehabilitation

John A. Horton III and Gary N. Galang

I. INTRODUCTION

A. Trauma results in injury that can impact the functioning of those involved. Spinal cord injury (SCI), traumatic brain injury (TBI), and severe multiple trauma are among the most life-altering events. These create a need for rehabilitation services during and after acute care to minimize or avoid impairments that affect the ability to care for themselves, to fulfill customary social roles, and to return to daily activities. Some injuries (e.g., SCI, TBI) affect numerous physiologic, psychological, social, and vocational functions to the degree that the individual loses functional independence. The rehabilitation team is responsible to teach the patient the skills and to provide the necessary equipment to optimize function, maximize the return to independence, and enable a reestablishment of a meaningful existence. Beginning this process in the acute care setting and carrying forward into the post-acute continuum is essential to optimize outcomes and ease the adjustment for the patient.

B. Prevention of disabling complications during the acute care phase of treatment minimizes required interventions during the rehabilitation phase of treatment. Secondary injury results in decrement in function and complicates care. Commonly, secondary debility is the result of the prolonged immobilization of the patient. Although rarely life threatening, these secondary concerns can limit eventual functional recovery, can delay patient progression and can contribute to total health care cost.

II. GENERAL EFFECTS OF NEUROTRAUMA AND IMMOBILIZATION AFTER INJURY

A. Cardiovascular deconditioning occurs rapidly with any period of inactivity, with the heart and peripheral vascular mechanisms losing the capacity to respond to stressors. With certain types of injury (e.g., SCI with its associated loss of sympathetic nervous system control), the inability to maintain perfusion pressure with changes in posture can inhibit attempts to mobilize the patient. **The most important approach to this problem is to minimize immobility** and get the patient upright as soon as possible. Additional benefits from this early mobilization include improved respiratory functioning, with decreased atelectasis and complications.

1. A recumbency-induced rise in the resting heart rate of 0.5 beats/min/day adds to any stress rate changes. The combined effect of these changes is resting tachycardia and a reduced ability to meet oxygen demands with activity; this effect is persistent for up to 2 months after return to activity.

2. Many peripheral factors, including decreases in vascular volume, loss of adaptive baroreceptor reflex responses to the upright posture, and increased pooling of blood in lower limb veins, contribute to the intolerance of the patient to an upright posture after immobility.

    a. In healthy individuals, the adaptive response to upright positioning can be totally lost after 3 weeks of complete bed rest. Older patients lose this capacity to respond even more quickly, and return to baseline is slower. Concomitant premorbid disease (e.g., cerebrovascular or cardiovascular lesions) makes older individuals less tolerant of this postural drop in blood pressure.

        Increasing periods of sitting with the feet in a dependent position helps reconditioning efforts for those unable to stand. The use of tilt or recline systems on wheelchairs can facilitate the tolerance to this activity. In severe cases, a tilt table can be used to progressively place the person in an upright position while blood pressure is monitored.

    b. Compressive garments, full-length elastic stockings, (e.g., TED hose, JOBST stockings, Tubigrip stockings, etc.) and abdominal binders may limit venous pooling and provide blood pressure support while adaptation occurs.

    c. Pay attention to nutrition to maintain plasma protein levels, immune system function, and proper hydration to aid combatting hypotension.

    d. In severe cases unresponsive to compression garments, increasing salt intake (up to 1 g PO QID), using sympathomimetic agents (pseudoephedrine, ephedrine, midodrine, or phenylephrine), or giving mineralocorticoids (fludrocortisone) may assist.

    e. In persons with TBI and elevations or fluctuations in intracranial pressure, be careful with aggressive mobilization.

B. Joint contractures result when a joint is not subjected to frequent passive or active range of motion. **Contracture** formation is most often a consequence of untreated muscular spasm because of upper motor neuron impairment. **Spasticity** is defined as a response to velocity-dependent stretch. This involuntary movement causes sustained, uncontrolled muscle tension creating unopposed shortening of the muscles crossing the joint. Muscular tension becomes unbalanced, thereby reducing the mobility of the affected joint. When this limitation of joint range persists, the soft tissues of the joint itself can also become contracted. Remodeling of the connective tissue around the joint contributes to decreased elasticity. The subsequent contracture that is produced is the result of this prolonged shortening and increased stiffness of the soft tissues of the joint.

    1. Contractures contribute to increased morbidity.

        a. Difficulties in positioning the patient can lead to the formation of decubitus ulcers.

        b. Hygiene, particularly in the perineum, palms of the hands, and axillae, is difficult.

        c. Contractures also inhibit functional recovery as motor function or control is regained. This leads to prolonged rehabilitation, potential need for surgical intervention, and higher costs. Contractures may also limit patient long-term functionality, preventing achievement of the full potential for recovery.

    2. Contractures should be prevented.

        a. Fully ranging all joints twice a day is often enough to prevent the formation of these deformities. Active ranging by the patient is preferred when possible as it helps maintain strength and motor control. If weak but voluntary muscle power is present, use active assisted range of motion as the next in preference. In cases of paralysis or coma, use passive range of motion. This may be difficult if severe spasticity or rigidity exist already.

        b. Positioning the patient can help reinforce the gains of therapy after range of motion has been performed. A prone position provides a prolonged stretch to hip flexors. Splinting of the wrists, hands, and ankles is also useful in reinforcement of range of motion gains and prevention of further deformation. Use splints intermittently (not continuously) to avoid skin breakdown in areas of splint contact.

        c. Other physical modalities, in conjunction with range of motion, allow a greater stretch.

            i. Deep heat via use of ultrasound can increase the elasticity of collagen, but may be contraindicated in areas with metallic implants.

            ii. Cooling of the muscle helps to decrease the activity of the muscle spindle mechanism, and thus decrease muscle tone.

        d. Serial casting of an extremity is useful to provide a prolonged stretch. A plaster or fiberglass cast is applied, but must be prepared to pad prominences to prevent skin lesion. Stretch is maintained as the cast material cures. The cast is typically left in place for 3 to 5 days before removal. Once desired positioning is achieved through a series of progressive cast applications, the cast can then be cut into halves longitudinally (bivalve) and used as a resting splint.

e. Focal neurolysis is another tool in the arsenal against contracture formation. Temporary reduction of muscle tone by employment of motor point or peripheral nerve blocks using neurolytic agents (e.g., phenol—approximately 6- to 12-month duration of effect) or neuromuscular blocking agents (e.g., botulinum toxins—approximately 1- to 3-month duration of effect) is useful in cases where tone prevents full range of a joint. These should be performed under EMG, ultrasound, or stimulator guidance and may be required before splinting or serial casting can be successful. Phenol produces a direct neurolysis. Several serotypes of botulinum toxin have been described (A, B, C, D, and E), with only A and B commercially available in the United States.

f. Anti-spasticity medications are used to reduce hyper-reactivity of the skeletal muscle. This phenomenon is common, although usually delayed in onset, in the head-injured patient and those patients with cerebral vascular accident or SCI. Common medications include baclofen, tizanidine, diazepam, and dantrolene sodium.

  i. Baclofen and diazepam are GABA analogue agents and act to provide improved descending inhibition to otherwise disinhibited pathways in the spinal cord. Both of these agents can produce sedation, and baclofen can lower the seizure threshold. Rapid baclofen withdrawal may result in seizures, hyperthermia, and systemic collapse. In general practice, baclofen is most often employed in patients with SCI and perhaps less valuable in patients with spasticity of cerebral origin.

  ii. Tizanidine is an α2-adrenergic agonist, which although sedating, also provides inhibition of descending pathways promoting decreases in muscle tone. Some advocate this for use in more prominent upper extremity tone situations or in decreasing dysesthetic pain. Like baclofen, tizanidine is more often used in SCI patients.

  iii. Dantrolene sodium is a peripheral acting agent that acts at the level of the sarcoplasmic reticulum and appears to produce less cognitive disturbance among those with CNS injury. Use cautiously in those with liver disturbance and monitor for hepatic necrosis (serial transaminases).

C. Decubitus ulcers are a common but preventable complication. Pressure is the primary factor in the development of a skin breakdown. Ulcers occur over bony prominences when the pressure of body weight is unrelieved for prolonged periods. Pressure causes occlusion of perforating blood vessels which results in ischemic damage to the skin and underlying soft tissues. This occurs most commonly at the bone/soft tissue interface. Higher pressures cause breakdown in a shorter time than lower pressures. Evidence of a lesion on the skin surface may only hint at the full extent of the underlying damage which has already taken place.

1. Multiple factors contribute to the development of these dangerous lesions:

  a. Shear either between the skin and supporting surfaces or within the soft tissues causes ischemia at lower pressures than when shear is not present.

  b. Anemia causes increased risk of ischemic damage due to lack of oxygen availability in the deep tissues.

  c. Excessive skin moisture from perspiration or urine reduces the resistance to skin damage.

  d. Poor nutrition predisposes to poor wound healing and also impaired resistance to skin breakdown due to decreased quality of collagen formation.

  e. Infection can lead to skin breakdown with sepsis increasing capillary leak and impaired blood flow to pressure prone areas.

  f. Lack of sensation and altered mental status also contribute to development of pressure ulcers. The normal protective pain sensation or pain awareness, which would otherwise prompt a position change, is missing and thus the pressure is not alleviated, facilitating the development of a lesion.

2. Prevention of ulceration must be the goal.

  a. Careful positioning of the patient. Frequent turning, initially on a schedule of a minimum of every 2 hours, is essential. Increased attention to the occiput, scapulae, sacrum, ischial tuberosities, greater trochanters, malleoli, and heels is key given the frequency of breakdown at these sites. Pillows and foam blocks can relieve pressure over these bony prominences or distribute it to other areas.

  b. Inspection of the skin regularly – at least every shift – is ideal. If signs of breakdown are seen, alleviation of pressure to the area is essential. The earliest sign of damage is an area of non-blanching erythema. Palpation may reveal induration of the underlying soft tissue. If induration is present, more extensive damage may already have occurred, making the situation more critical to treat with increased urgency.

  c. Managing urinary and bowel incontinence to prevent prolonged contact between the skin and urine or feces is important to prevent skin irritation and infection.

  d. For patients at high risk, use of specialized mattresses and seating surfaces are a cost-effective component of a decubitus prevention program.

D. Heterotopic ossification (HO) is a pathologic process during which new bone is formed within periarticular soft tissue. It is hypothesized that trauma promotes the disinhibition of factors allowing multipotential mesenchymal cells to be converted to osteoclast-like cells. Histologically normal bone develops in the soft tissues surrounding a joint.

  1. This process should be distinguished from **traumatic myositis ossificans,** in which bone is formed within traumatized muscles, often because of ossification of intramuscular hematoma.

  2. Populations at risk for HO include those with burns, TBI, SCI, and those with prolonged immobilization. Following SCI or TBI, incidence is from 11% to 79%.

  3. Different distributions of ossification and time course occur in spinal cord versus brain injury. In both cases, the lesions develop below the level of the neurologic injury around major joints. The process appears to be more aggressive in limbs with greater spasticity-related muscular tone.

  4. Upper extremity involvement is more common in brain injury. HO tends to be more extensive and persistent following SCI.

  5. The earliest manifestation of HO is painful loss of range of motion. Otherwise, a striking similarity is seen to the clinical presentation of deep venous thrombosis, with a warm, swollen, erythematous limb. HO may also manifest as "fever of unknown origin."

  6. Diagnostic tools.

  a. Triple-phase bone scan is the earliest, most specific test to confirm the diagnosis. The first and second phases are abnormal in HO.

  b. Alkaline phosphatase can be used to track the relative activity of new bone formation, although elevation of this enzyme tends to be nonspecific.

  c. Additional testing—C-reactive protein and creatine phosphokinase (CPK) have been suggested as useful in the diagnostic spectrum.

  7. Consequences of this process include painful loss of range of motion and compression of vascular or neurologic structures, which can lead to secondary venous thrombosis or significant neuropathic pain due to compression. The bony mass also can lead to development of pressure ulceration of the overlying skin. Perhaps most importantly, HO can simply result in a fixed and immobile joint, leading to an inability to sit or ambulate.

  8. Treatment

  a. The primary modality employed is vigorous range of motion (active or passive). When sensation is preserved (TBI, incomplete SCI), ranging can be painful, leading to increased agitation. Appropriate analgesia can facilitate appropriate physical therapy.

  b. Treatment with disodium etidronate (Didronel) 20 mg/kg enteral dose for 1 to 3 months, followed by 10 mg/kg for 3 months is the most common additional pharmacologic treatment. While not widely practiced, one group has advocated the use of parenteral treatment early in the course of those with SCI and features of HO. HO prophylaxis with Didronel and its utility in long-term treatment is not clear.

    c. Indomethacin and other NSAIDs have also been used. Evidence suggests utility in SCI; its effectiveness is more convincing following total hip replacement than in trauma. In addition, increased risk for gastric erosion, especially given the increased risk in this population, limits the use of this class of agents.

    d. Focal radiation (approximately 500 GY), both as prophylaxis and as treatment, seems to be effective for focused areas of involvement. When early surgical resection is required to reduce compressive phenomenon, radiation early after surgery may prevent recurrence. Employment of this modality is more common following surgical resection and not used commonly for primary treatment.

    e. Surgical resection to improve range of motion may be necessary, particularly when the joint has ankylosed or is preventing functional gains. Operation is usually delayed 12 to 18 months after injury, or until repeat three-phase bone scanning shows no active ossification. With good neurologic recovery, surgery usually provides a good result. Ossification tends to recur in cases of poor neurologic recovery or with resection while ossification is active.

E. Musculoskeletal response to immobilization.

Just as exercise leads to strengthening, immobility leads to weakness of both muscle and bone.

1. Muscle effect

Complete bed rest results in loss of 10% to 15% of muscle strength per week.

Type I (slow twitch) muscle fibers, which predominate in antigravity muscles, are the predominant tissue lost in this process. This reduction of type I capacity, combined with cardiovascular deconditioning, leads to poor endurance when the patient is eventually remobilized.

Type II (fast twitch) fibers and the anaerobic nature of strength-type tasks are relatively preserved in this degenerative process. The result is that with retraining, strength returns rapidly (weeks), whereas endurance requires much longer time to be restored (months).

When immobilization is required for any length of time, maintaining strength through therapeutic exercise is essential. Even when range of motion is not possible, isometric exercises can help prevent weakness. When a patient is awake and cooperative, opportunities for regular upper and lower body exercise can be facilitated by an overhead trapeze and special color-coded bands made from elastic latex sheets with specific thickness (Thera-Band), which can provide controlled resistance exercises for the patient while in bed or sitting in a wheelchair.

Daily contractions of 20% to 30% of maximal voluntary contraction for several seconds are sufficient to maintain strength. Use exercise that includes motion (isotonic or isokinetic), when possible, to aid in the maintenance of joint motion and motor control as well as strengthening.

2. Bone effect

Skeletal strength is dependent on the forces of gravity and muscle pull acting on the bones. With inactivity, osteoclastic activity predominates with resulting breakdown of both cortical and trabecular bone. This breakdown can be profound in acute tetraplegia of young males, resulting in markedly elevated calcium excretion with stone formation and/or hypercalcemia.

Voluntary muscle activity and weight-bearing exercise are important to reverse this disuse osteoporosis. Once activity is resumed, return to baseline bone density may take years. Disuse osteoporosis is particularly problematic in individuals with preexisting osteoporosis from other reasons (post-menopausal women).

Adequate hydration and vigilance for the clinical manifestations of immobilization hypercalcemia are important to prevent the adverse effects of this condition.

Prophylactic use of agents that inhibit either osteoblastic or osteoclastic activity in at-risk patients is not conclusive but does show promise in limiting the degree of disuse osteoporosis.

III. FREQUENT POST-INJURY PROBLEMS

A. Agitation is defined as a set of excessive behaviors that range from motoric restlessness and impulsivity. Behaviors such as emotional lability to verbal and physical aggression are seen, often with post-traumatic amnesia (PTA). It correlates more to a history of premorbid psychiatric illness and substance abuse than to the severity of the injury and/or the presence of hypoxemia. Agitation occurs in 11% to 42% of brain injury patients, depending on the diagnostic criteria used for evaluation. The agitated behavior scale (ABS) is a 14-item test that describes and monitors the patient's agitation which also serves as a measure of the patient's responsiveness to treatment plans. A score of 22 or greater suggests significant agitation.

AGITATED BEHAVIOR SCALE

At the end of the observation period indicate whether the behavior described in each item was present and, if so, to what degree: Slight, moderate, or extreme.

Use the following numerical values and criteria for your ratings.

1 = absent: The behavior is not present.

2 = present to a slight degree: The behavior is present but does not prevent the conduct of other, contextually appropriate behavior. (The individual may redirect spontaneously, or the continuation of the agitated behavior does not disrupt appropriate behavior.)

3 = present to a moderate degree: The individual needs to be redirected from an agitated to an appropriate behavior, but benefits from such cueing.

4 = present to an extreme degree: The individual is not able to engage in appropriate behavior due to the interference of the agitated behavior, even when external cueing or redirection is provided.

1. Short attention span, easy distractibility, inability to concentrate.
2. Impulsive, impatient, low tolerance for pain or frustration.
3. Uncooperative, resistant to care, demanding.
4. Violent or threatening violence toward people or property.
5. Explosive or unpredictable anger.
6. Rocking, rubbing, moaning, or other self-stimulating behavior.
7. Pulling at tubes, restraints, etc.
8. Wandering from treatment areas.
9. Restlessness, pacing, excessive movement.
10. Repetitive behaviors, motor or verbal.
11. Rapid, loud, or excessive talking.
12. Sudden changes of mood.
13. Easily initiated or excessive crying and/or laughter.
14. Self-abusiveness, physical and/or verbal.

Total Score

The treatment of agitation in TBI follows a stepwise progression that uses psychotropic medications as a last resort due to their effects on cognitive and motor performance and recovery. It begins with the exclusion of any organic or metabolic factors (infection, hypoxemia, medications, "sundowning") that could cause or contribute to the behaviors. When possible, establish a normal sleep wake pattern either by promoting proper sleep hygiene (sleep logs, low light environment) or the judicious use of non-sedating/short acting sleep agents (trazodone, ramelteon, melatonin). Non-pharmacologic methods such as environmental modifications and behavioral plans are employed next. The long-term use of antipsychotics and benzodiazepines are not recommended in favor of atypical antipsychotics, mood stabilizers, lipophilic beta blockers, and stimulants.

Many spinal-cord–injured patients, especially those with tetraplegia, will have concomitant brain injury that is often overlooked in favor of resuscitative measures and acute medical management. The diagnosis is based on the observation of cognitive and behavioral deficits that could impact participation and rehabilitation. It is best detected by seeking evidence from the history (loss of consciousness, PTA, hypoxemia, prolonged extraction times) coupled with the neurodeficits. Neuroimaging may show local brain contusions, petechial hemorrhages, or diffuse axonal hemorrhage.

Avoid some common medications (H_2 blockers and dopaminergic blockers) which may adversely affect the recovering brain injury.

B. Autonomic dysreflexia.

Autonomic dysreflexia occurs in patients who have sustained an SCI with a neurologic level of T6 (8) or above. With SCI at lower levels, the intact descending sympathetic control minimizes or prevents the syndrome. It is more common in complete SCI than in incomplete classification injuries. The onset is usually delayed from the initial injury and appears between 2 weeks and up to 2 months post-injury once "spinal shock" has passed allowing for reflex activity propagation. The sequence of events to elicit this life-threatening phenomenon is as follows.

Noxious stimulus occurs below the neurologic level of injury.

Reflexive unopposed sympathetic outflow is elicited. Vasoconstriction and piloerection occurs below the neurologic level of injury. Blood pressure is elevated (>20 mm Hg) above baseline systolic pressures.

In response to elevated blood pressure, the baroreceptors of the great vessels and vagal outflow are still intact and are stimulated; associated bradycardia results. Vasodilation and flushing above the neurologic level is also seen.

1. Causes

Most common causes include over-distended bladder, over-distended bowel, decubitus ulcer, and ingrown toenail.

Other causes include fractures, constricting clothing, wrinkles in underlying sheets, intra-abdominal emergencies, aggressive bowel program stimulation, dysmenorrhea, orgasm with sexual activity, and onset of labor in pregnancy.

2. Treatment

Sit those with autonomic dysreflexia upright. This takes advantage of the tendency to lower blood pressure with upright posture in the SCI patient.

Since this syndrome occurs in response to a noxious stimulus, the first and most important premise is to identify and remove the stimulus; this requires a search for an inciting stimulus. Relief of the distension of bowel or bladder is often the only treatment required, with rapid return of the blood pressure to normal.

When the cause is not readily identified and corrected, control the blood pressure pharmacologically. Nitroglycerine paste is commonly used and applied to the skin. Once the inciting stimulus has been removed, the risk of resulting hypotension is reduced. Sublingual or "bite and swallow" nifedipine (10 mg) is an alternative and can be repeated in 15 to 20 minutes if necessary. Be careful since this can also cause a precipitous drop in blood pressure or cardiac arrhythmia.

In refractory cases, intravenous apresoline, nitroprusside, or spinal anesthesia can be used.

3. Prevention

In cases where the daily bowel or bladder management activities produce autonomic dysreflexia, use of topical anesthetic agents (lidocaine gel or alternatives) limits the cutaneous stimuli and the risk of developing these symptoms.

In recurrent cases (such as with bowel routines), prazosin 1 to 2 mg at night or oral guanethidine, starting with 5 mg daily, can be used prophylactically. Mecamylamine, starting with 2.5 mg twice daily and titrating up to a total dose of 25 mg daily, is an alternative agent. Clonidine patches have also been employed.

Use of anti-cholinergic bladder relaxing medications may also decrease noxious stimulus from bladder distension and aid in decreasing the risk of recurrent dysreflexia.

C. Neurogenic bladder

Neurogenic bladder is one of the most serious alterations of physiologic function following neurologic trauma. In SCI, renal failure from frequent infections combined with reflux and subsequent pyelonephritis was the leading cause of death until the last two decades. Renal failure is less common now because of aggressive management and surveillance of neurogenic bladder function.

In the uninjured, the coordinated function of sensory, reflex, and voluntary motor pathways allows normal elimination. The pathways involved include both autonomic (sympathetic and parasympathetic) and somatic motor tracts.

Classification of the bladder dysfunction requires detailed knowledge of these pathways and is beyond the scope of this chapter. Instead, a protocol of care for acute management of neurogenic bladder in SCI is presented. This protocol allows safe management of the patient while other acute problems are addressed. For definitive management of neurogenic bladder, further workup is necessary and must be balanced with social factors to create the optimal care for the individual.

1. Seeking potential neurogenic bladder is the single most important factor in diagnosis and management. Any process that can affect balanced control of the bladder (TBI, SCI, lumbosacral plexus injury, stroke) may cause neurogenic bladder. The patient with neurologic injury may maintain good urine output with a bladder that is operating at a very high residual volume, which induces a high risk of infection. Check post-void residual volumes to ensure that the bladder is emptying properly. Recurrent post-void volumes of over 100 mL indicate bladder dysfunction. The protocol that follows will suffice in the acute phase of management with all types of trauma.

a. Discontinue Foley or suprapubic catheter unless mandated by coexisting urethral or bladder injury, diabetes insipidus, pharmacologic diuresis, large fluid loads, or other conditions where a high urine volume is expected. Elimination of an indwelling catheter decreases the risk of infection.

b. Institute a timed void/monitoring of urinary volumes. Toileting the patient on a timed basis (q4h or q6h initially) allows a check for appropriate urinary volumes and may achieve continence in this manner alone. If the volumes at these checks are mildly elevated (>300 to 400 cc) then the intake is appropriate; if the patient is unable to volitionally void, intermittent catheterization will be used to empty the bladder and eliminate stasis.

c. For SCI patients, start an intermittent catheterization program as soon as possible after injury unless contraindicated. Do sterile catheterization unless the patient is being taught, where a "clean technique" is used.

d. Catheter urinary volumes should not exceed 300 to 500 mL. Adjust frequency of catheterization/toileting according to the patient's output pattern. Record all output volumes and incontinent episodes on a frequency and volume chart.

e. Restrict patient fluid intake when on intermittent catheterization so that the total urine output is 1,500 to 2,000 mL/24-hour period.

In general, a combination of imaging and sequential testing of bladder pressures is indicated for lifetime surveillance of the patient with neurogenic bladder. This workup is generally deferred to the outpatient setting and initiated approximately 6 months after the acute injury.

Obtain urine cultures with a suspicion of symptomatic infection. Do not administer prophylactic antibiotics or urinary antiseptics unless a complicated urinary tract infection is documented. Complicated urinary tract infection is indicated by symptoms that can include:

i. Fever not attributable to other pathology

ii. Increasing spasticity

iii. Autonomic dysreflexia

iv. Urinary retention or incontinence as a deviation from established patterns

v. Hematuria

vi. More than 50 white blood cells per high-power field on microscopic evaluation

vii. Evidence of stone disease

viii. Bacteriuria—100 colonies in specimen obtained by intermittent catheterization, or any growth in samples obtained from indwelling catheters.

Existence of a "positive" bacterial culture alone is insufficient to prompt treatment in absence of any of the attendant **symptoms** described.

D. Neurogenic bowel

Neurogenic bowel dysfunction usually coexists in patients with a neurogenic bladder since control pathways are similar. The goal of a bowel program is controlled fecal elimination with intervening periods of continence so that the individual can participate in daily activities without concern for social inappropriateness.

All trauma patients can have bowel dysfunction, notably constipation. Since those with SCI usually have impaired or absent rectal and perineal sensation, symptoms of bowel dysfunction may be absent or vague. Lack of appetite or nonspecific malaise may be the only indication that the problem of retained feces exists. Establishment of elimination in all cases will improve patient comfort, and ultimately decrease length of stay.

An ileus typically exists in the initial period after SCI. Once the ileus subsides, often 2 to 3 days, the bowel program (see later) should be initiated. Once the bowel program is producing predictable results, the schedule can be modified as appropriate. The patient's preinjury bowel pattern is the best guide to modification of timing. Individuals who had routine, daily bowel movements usually will continue with this pattern after injury. Individuals who had less frequent bowel movements may require a less frequent bowel program in the long term.

Frequent liquid stools can indicate that bowel motility is too great or inspissated feces is blocking the rectum or colon. Liquid stool from above passes around this blockage and leaks from the anus. It may be possible to detect a full colon on examination, but the most reliable method of detection is to obtain a plain abdominal radiograph. If fecal obstruction is seen, evacuate the colon and institute a routine and reliable bowel program. Use of rectal bags or other external collection devices or use of diapers is strongly discouraged.

1. Classification of neurogenic bowel as either an upper motor neuron or a lower motor neuron injury is essential in appropriate management.

    a. In cases of upper motor neuron injury (tetraplegia), the sacral reflex arcs are intact. Presence of these reflexes helps to initiate bowel evacuation. In some cases, the individual can initiate evacuation with digital stimulation (stretch) of the anal sphincter or use of a suppository. Use of digital stimulation in concert with suppository use is central in initiation of a consistent "on demand" bowel regimen.

    b. In lower motor neuron lesions (conus medullaris or cauda equina injuries), the local reflexes are lost. This situation is more difficult to control, often requiring routine digital disimpaction. Use of stool bulking agents can prevent free leakage of stool, together in combination with consistent lower rectal vault clearance on a periodic basis, is the preferred management.

2. The following bowel program for individuals with SCI also can be applied for other clinical entities in which bowel control is a problem.

    A typical bowel management protocol consists of a stool softener titrated needs and a mild, orally administered stimulant laxative coordinated with a laxative enema (or suppository in selected patients). Use of bulking agents can also facilitate appropriate stool consistency to improve movements. Initially, this is on a daily schedule so that evacuation occurs at a time convenient for the patient and nursing staff.

    Protocol for evening evacuation is Colace (100 mg) twice daily, two tablets of Senokot (Purdue Frederick, Norwalk, Connecticut) at noon, with a Fleet (Lynchburg, Virginia) bisacodyl enema or Dulcolax (Ciba, Woodbridge, New Jersey) suppository, in combination with digital stimulation of the rectum, in the evening.

    If morning evacuation is desired, the Senokot is given at bedtime.

IV. THE SCOPE OF REHABILITATION FOLLOWING TRAUMA

A. Rehabilitation of patients after trauma occurs in several stages, each with a corresponding venue.

    1. Subacute rehabilitation facilities—a phenomenon greatly created with the Medicare policy revisions of 2009 and 2010 and in the implementation of the prospective payment system for inpatient rehabilitation facilities (IRFs). This is a setting for rehabilitative efforts that will provide for a lower overall intensity of therapeutic services over a longer period of time. The capacity of the facility to deal with ongoing medical concerns is variable. If the patient does not meet the criterion for acute inpatient rehabilitative services at an IRF, but cannot care for themselves in the community and would benefit from some degree of therapy to

continue to recover from their injuries, then subacute rehabilitation services are appropriate.

2. Acute inpatient rehabilitation is required when patients are unable to manage their own basic self-care or mobility needs because of physical or cognitive limitations. The goal of inpatient rehabilitation is to reestablish capability for basic routines of daily living so the patient can function safely in the community with a minimal amount of physical assistance or supervision. Ideally, patients are restored to the point where they are both physically and cognitively independent, although this is not always possible. Rehabilitation interventions are directed toward minimizing the amount of physical or cognitive assistance that a patient will require on return to the community. Most facilities follow the Medicare guidelines for admission to the IRF as outlined below.

   a. The patient must require the active and ongoing therapeutic intervention of multiple therapy disciplines (physical therapy, occupational therapy, speech–language pathology, or prosthetics/orthotics therapy), one of which must be physical or occupational therapy.

   b. The patient must require an intensive rehabilitation therapy program; generally consists of at least 3 hours of therapy per day at least 5 days per week.

   c. The patient must reasonably be expected to actively participate in and benefit from the intensive rehabilitation therapy program. The patient is expected to make measurable improvement (that will be of practical value to improve the patient's functional capacity or adaptation to impairments) as a result of the rehabilitation treatment and such improvement is expected to be made within a prescribed period of time.

   d. The patient must require physician supervision.

   e. The patient must require an intensive and coordinated interdisciplinary approach to rehabilitation.

3. Initial phases of outpatient rehabilitation are directed toward enhancing the ability of the patient to return to active participation in the community outside the home and improving the patient's ability to manage more complex instrumental activities of daily living (e.g., cooking, laundry, managing finances, home maintenance). These tasks involve more complex organizational and executive skills that are frequently affected in brain injury. Patients may require assistance with behavioral problems that affect their interpersonal relationships. Residual deficits that limit mobility in the community can also be addressed along with continuing cognitive limitations. This phase of rehabilitation is sometimes referred to as "community reentry."

4. The final phase of rehabilitation involves helping the affected individual (now often referred to as a "client" rather than a "patient") return to some form of competitive employment. Referred to as "vocational rehabilitation," this involves teaching training skills that enable an individual to return to the workplace. It can also involve providing some assistive services (e.g., job placement and job coaching) as well as trial placements in voluntary positions in the community.

AXIOMS

- The rehabilitation team must teach the patient the skills to return to independence.
- Secondary disability is the result of prolonged immobilization of the patient.
- Contractures and decubiti can and should be prevented.
- Complete bed rest result in loss of 10% to 15% of muscle strength per week. Maintaining strength through therapeutic exercise is essential.

Suggested Readings

Acute Management of Autonomic Dysreflexia: Individuals with Spinal Cord Injury Presenting to Health-Care Facilities. Consortium for Spinal Cord Medicine. July 2001.

Banovac K, Sherman AL, Estores IM, et al. Prevention and treatment of heterotopic ossification after spinal cord injury. *J Spinal Cord Med* 2004;27(4):376–382.

Bar-Shai M, Carmeli E, Coleman R, et al. Mechanisms in muscle atrophy in immobilization and aging. *Ann N Y Acad Sci* 2004;1019:475–478.

Bladder Management for Adults with Spinal Cord Injury: A Clinical Practice Guideline for Health-Care Providers. Consortium for Spinal Cord Medicine. August 2006.

Bogner J. The Agitated Behavior Scale. *The Center for Outcome Measurement in Brain Injury.* 2000. http://www.tbims.org/combi/abs (accessed January 25, 2012).

Kirschblum S, Campagnolo DI, Delisa JA, eds. *Spinal Cord Medicine.* Philadelphia, PA: Lippincott Williams & Wilkins; 2002:261–274.

Lombard L, Zafonte R. Agitation after traumatic brain injury: Considerations and treatment options. *Am J Phys Med Rehabil* 2005;84(10):797–812.

Medicare Benefit Policy Manual, Chapter 1 - Inpatient Hospital Services Covered Under Part A (Rev. 119, 01-15-10) Section 110.2 - Inpatient Rehabilitation Facility Medical Necessity Criteria.

Neurogenic Bowel Management in Adults with Spinal Cord Injury. Consortium for Spinal Cord Medicine. March 1998.

Pressure Ulcer Prevention and Treatment Following Spinal Cord Injury: A Clinical Practice Guideline for Health-Care Professionals. Consortium for Spinal Cord Medicine. August 2000.

Silver J, Yudofsky S, Anderson K. Aggressive disorders. In: Silver JM, McAllister TW, Yudofsky SC, eds. *Textbook of Traumatic Brain Injury.* Washington, DC: American Psychiatric Press; 2005.

Wagner AK, Fabio T, Zafonte RD, et al. Physical medicine and rehabilitation consultation: Relationships with acute functional outcome, length of stay and discharge planning after traumatic brain injury. *Am J Phys Med Rehabil* 2003;82(7):526–536.

Zafonte R, Lombard L, Elovic E. Antispasticity medications: Uses and limitations of enteral therapy. *Am J Phys Med Rehabil* 2004;83(10 suppl):S50–S58.

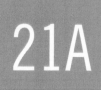

21A Trauma in Children

Daniel J. Grabo, Thane A. Blinman, Michael L. Nance and
C. William Schwab

I. INTRODUCTION

Nearly 8 million children under the age of 15 visit the emergency department yearly for injury in the United States. Advances in injury prevention and healthcare have led to a decrease in the number of deaths from unintentional injury in children from 1997 to 2007 by 30%. Unintentional injury remains the cause of more childhood (ages 1 to 14) deaths than all other childhood diseases combined and is responsible for nearly 30% of all years of potential life lost.

Most pediatric trauma care occurs outside the setting of a designated pediatric trauma center. It is imperative that any treating hospital, knowing the limitations of their institution, transfer severely injured children to a higher level of care when conditions exceed capabilities. Pre-existing transfer agreements between institutions facilitate transfer and care.

II. MECHANISM OF INJURY (Fig. 21A-1)

A. Blunt trauma accounts for more than 90% of pediatric injuries.
   1. Falls are the most frequent type of injury.
   2. Motor-vehicle collisions are the most frequent cause of injury-related mortality.
B. Penetrating trauma accounts for less than 10% of pediatric trauma admissions.
   1. Penetrating trauma is three times as lethal as blunt trauma.
   2. Seventy percent of deaths occur at the scene.
   3. Firearm injuries are the most lethal (case fatality rate of 9% to 17%).

III. ANATOMY AND PHYSIOLOGY

A. Anatomic and physiologic differences between children and adults can have potential clinical consequences (Table 21A-1). In addition, normal measurements of respiratory rate (RR), heart rate, and systolic blood pressure (SBP) differ from adults and vary with increasing age in infants and children (Table 21A-2).

IV. PRIMARY SURVEY.

The goals of initial management of pediatric trauma are the same as adult trauma: Restore and maintain oxygen delivery; discover and manage injuries in order of greatest threat to life; move efficiently to definitive treatment. Specific differences in pediatric anatomy and physiology determine key modifications to the standard age-independent protocols of ATLS®. Rapid access to internet-based resources can help in the management of the injured child and include considerations in Pediatric Trauma (http://emedicine.medscape.com) as well as Pediatric Trauma and Pediatric Resuscitation (www.uptodate.com).

A. Airway
   1. A speaking, crying, or spontaneously breathing child likely has a patent airway. Nasal flaring and sternal retractions are hallmark signs of respiratory compromise. Stridor, hoarseness, and change in the quality of voice can indicate laryngeal spasm or airway edema.
   2. Oropharyngeal obstruction is most commonly caused by the tongue and can be managed in most cases by oral suctioning and head positioning or by placing the chin in the "sniffing position" while taking care to maintain cervical spine (c-spine) immobilization if indicated.
   3. Bag-valve-mask (BVM) ventilation provides adequate oxygenation and ventilation for most pediatric trauma patients.

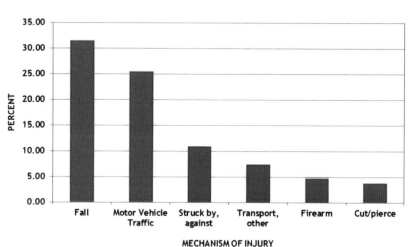

Figure 21A-1. Mechanism of injury for pediatric (age 0 to 19 years) trauma patients. Distribution of the most common causes of pediatric trauma—fall; motor vehicle traffic (occupants, motorcyclists, pedal cyclist, pedestrians struck by motor vehicle); struck by/against (assault); transport/other; firearm; cut/pierce. (Modified and reproduced with permission from the American College of Surgeons Committee on Trauma, National Trauma Databank (NTDB) Pediatric Report 2011.)

4. All trauma centers should have a protocol (Fig. 21A-2) for pediatric rapid sequence intubation (RSI). Indications for intubation include inability to protect the airway (e.g., Glasgow Coma Scale (GCS) score ≤8; significant facial trauma), inability to ventilate (e.g., flail chest), or inability to oxygenate (e.g., smoke inhalation).

5. The pediatric airway differs from the adult as follows: Shorter trachea causing frequent mainstem intubation and easy extubation; prominent occiput, large tongue, and smaller mouth make oral tracheal intubation difficult. An uncuffed

TABLE 21A-1	General Body Differences between Children and Adults and Potential Clinical Consequences
General body difference	**Potential clinical consequence**
Decreased mineralization	Less protection to structures in central nervous system, thorax
Decreased strength	Diminished protection of c-spine, abdomen
Decreased contractility in response to Starling effect	Dependence on increase in heart rate to maintain cardiac output
	Poor tolerance of fluid overload
Distribution of masses	Different injury patterns
	Abdominal contents ride higher in chest Bladder sits above pelvic brim
	Larger heart
	Airway differences
	Altered approach to diagnosis and management
Large surface area to weight ratio	Vulnerable to hypothermia
Shorter neck, larger head, laxity of ligaments, decreased muscle support	Increased risk head injury and flexion injury to the c-spine

TABLE 21A-2   **Age-specific Normal Vital Signs**

Age group weight range	Respiratory rate (breaths/min)	Heart rate (beats/min)	Systolic blood pressure (mm Hg)	Urinary output (mL/kg/h)
Infant: 0–12 mos (3–5 kg)	<60	<160	>60	2.0
Toddler: 1–2 y (10–14 kg)	<40	<150	>70	1.5
Preschool: 3–5 y (14–18 kg)	<35	<140	>75	1.0
School age: 6–12 y (18–36 kg)	<30	<120	>80	1.0
Adolescent: 13 y (36–70 kg)	<30	<100	>90	0.5

Adapted with permission from the American College of Surgeons, Committee on Trauma. Advanced Trauma Life Support for Doctors, ATLS® Student Course Manual, 8th ed. Chicago, IL; 2008. Chapter 10.

tube is recommended in young children to minimize airway trauma (Table 21A-3).

  6. Nasotracheal intubation is not recommended due to the sharp angle between the nasopharynx and oropharynx. Surgical airway is rarely indicated, especially in children less than 8 years. Surgical cricothyroidotomy and translaryngeal jet ventilation (needle) are options in older children (>12 years).
  7. Drug doses for airway and cardiopulmonary support plus device size and care protocols can be gleaned from the age and body mass–based color-coded scheme on the Broselow® Pediatric Emergency Tape.
B. Breathing
  1. Airway or ventilatory compromise is the most common cause of cardiac arrest in children.
  2. Auscultate in the axillae to minimize noise from contralateral chest. Decompress the stomach to avoid its compromising breathing efforts.
  3. If tension pneumothorax is suspected, perform needle decompression followed by chest tube insertion. The preferred placement of the catheter for chest decompression is in the fourth or fifth interspace at the anterior axillary line. Hemothorax or pneumothorax on chest radiograph or suspected clinically is treated with chest tube insertion. Consider insertion of the smallest caliber chest tube or pigtail catheter for isolated pneumothorax (Table 21A-4).

TABLE 21A-3   **Airway Equipment**

Age range weight (kg)	Distance (cm) midtrachea to lip	Endotracheal tube (uncuffed)	Laryngoscope blade
Premie (3)	8.0	2.5–3.0	0 straight
0–6 mos (3.5)	8.0–11.0	3.0–4.0	1 straight
6–12 mos (7)	11–12.5	4.0–4.5	2 straight
1–3 y (10–12)	12.5–14.0	4.5–5.0	2 straight
4–7 y (16–18)	14.0–17.0	5.0–6.5	2 straight
8–10 y (24–30)	17.0–20.0	6.5–10.0	2–3 straight/curved

In adolescents age 12+ and young adults, use adult sized, cuffed endotracheal tubes. Adapted with permission from the American College of Surgeons, Committee on Trauma. Advanced Trauma Life Support for Doctors, ATLS® Student Course Manual, 8th ed. Chicago, IL; 2008. Chapter 10.

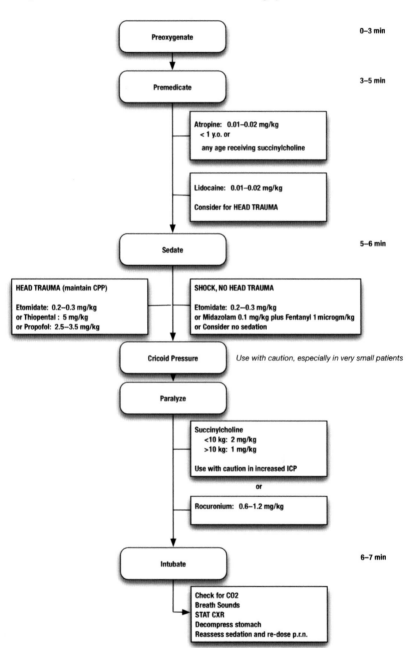

Figure 21A-2. Protocol for pediatric trauma rapid sequence intubation. (Modified and reproduced with permission from Zelicof-Paul A, Smith-Lockridge A, Schnadower D. Controversies in rapid sequence in intubation in children. *Curr Opin Ped* 2005;17:355–362.)

TABLE 21A-4	Supplemental Equipment			

Age range	OG/NG tube	Urinary catheter	Chest tube
Premie	8 Fr	5 feeding	10–14 Fr
0–6 mos	10 Fr	5–8 feeding	12–18 Fr
6–12 mos	10 Fr	8 Fr	14–20 Fr
1–3 y	12 Fr	10 Fr	14–24 Fr
4–7 y	12 Fr	10–12 Fr	20–28 Fr
8–10 y	14 Fr	12 Fr	28–38 Fr

Fr is size in French.
OG, orogastric; NG, nasogastric.
Adapted with permission from the American College of Surgeons, Committee on Trauma. Advanced Trauma Life Support for Doctors, ATLS® Student Course Manual, 8th ed. Chicago, IL; 2008. Chapter 10.

4. Ventilate at a rate and volume according to age and size. Normal spontaneous tidal volumes (TV) range from 6 to 8 mL/kg for infants and children, although larger TV (7 to 10 mL/kg) are frequently required during assisted ventilation. See Table 21A-2 for age-appropriate RR.
5. Inability to hear adequate breath sounds in both lung fields after endotracheal intubation raises the concern for mainstem intubation (most commonly the right) or pneumothorax. Assess the endotracheal tube location and obtain a chest radiograph after intubation, movement or manipulation, or if clinical conditions abruptly change.

C. Circulation
1. Elevated heart rate is the most important early indicator of shock. SBP may not drop until late in volume loss, rendering it an unreliable measure of status or resuscitation endpoints. Cardiac output is maintained by increasing heart rate, as stroke volume is relatively fixed in young children. Hypotension reflects >45% blood loss and is a late and ominous sign of shock. Hypotension is defined as SBP <70 + 2 × age in years. Bradycardia suggests impending cardiovascular collapse (Table 21A-5).

TABLE 21A-5	Systemic Response to Hypovolemic Shock in Children (Table 46-5)		

System	<25% blood loss	25%–45% blood loss	>45% blood loss
Cardiac	Weak, thready pulse; increased heart rate	Increased heart rate	Hypotension; tachycardia to bradycardia
Central nervous system	Lethargic, irritable, confused	Change in level of consciousness; dulled response to pain	Comatose
Skin	Cool, clammy	Cyanotic, decreased capillary refill, cold extremities	Pale, cold
Kidneys	Minimal decrease in urinary output, increased specific gravity	Minimal urine output	No urinary output

Reproduced with permission from Gaines BA, et al. Pediatric trauma. In: Peitzman AB, Rhodes M, Schwab CW, et al., eds. *The Trauma Manual: Trauma and Acute Care Surgery.* 3rd ed. Philadelphia, PA: Wolters Kluwer/Lippincott Williams & Wilkins; 2008.

2. Obtain access to the circulation: Largest size IV possible, one on each side of the patient, in upper or lower extremities.
   a. In the hypotensive child without IV access, start an intraosseous (IO) line for all resuscitative fluids (including blood products) and medications. The preferred site is the proximal tibia below the level of the tibial tuberosity. IO cannulation should not be performed distal to a known fracture site; alternative sites include the distal femur or contralateral proximal tibia. In an awake child, infiltrate with local anesthesia before insertion. Remove the IO line within 4 hours to decrease the risk of osteomyelitis.
   b. Central venous catheter placement provides emergency access to the central venous circulation, monitoring of central venous pressure, and the delivery of medications or resuscitation fluids. Use sterile technique and ultrasound guidance if available, placing the catheter via the Seldinger technique in the internal jugular, subclavian, or femoral vein.
   c. Rarely, venous cutdown may be needed. The preferred cutdown site is the greater saphenous vein anterior to the medial malleolus at the ankle or proximal thigh below the junction with femoral vein.
3. Total circulating volume is approximately 80 mL/kg body weight. Fluid resuscitation begins with 20 mL/kg of Ringer's lactate which may be repeated twice. If no improvement in hemodynamics is noted, transfusion with type O negative packed red blood cells (PRBCs) at 10 mL/kg should be initiated. Look for ongoing sources of bleeding, while planning definitive surgical control (Fig. 21A-3).

D. Disability
1. Quickly assess neurologic function.
2. The best tool is the GCS for children over the age of 5. Modify for the best verbal response in pre-verbal pediatric patients (age <2 to 4 years) (Table 21A-6).
3. Assess and document the GCS, pupillary examination, and a targeted motor examination before any neuromuscular blockade or deep sedation.
4. Maneuvers such as "sternal rub" to provoke a pain response in small children may cause damage and be misinterpreted. Instead, gently pinch the pectoralis muscle or tap the bottom of the foot.

TABLE 21A-6 Pediatric Glasgow Coma Scale

Response	Non-verbal patient age <2–4 y
Eye opening	4 Spontaneous
	3 To voice
	2 To pain
	1 No response
Best verbal response	5 Age appropriate
	4 Consolable
	3 Irritable
	2 Restless
	1 No response
Best motor response	6 Spontaneous
	5 Localizes
	4 Withdraws
	3 Flexion
	2 Extension
	1 No response

Modified from James HE. Neurologic evaluation and support in the child with an acute brain insult. *Ped Annals* 1986;15:16–22.

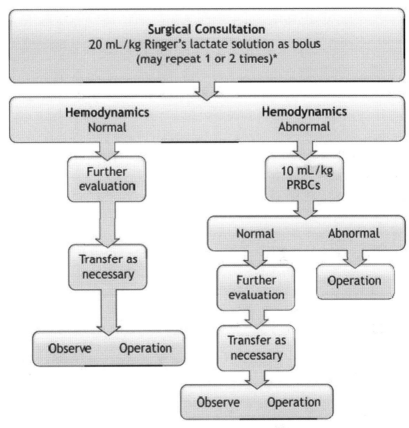

Figure 21A-3. Resuscitation flow diagram for pediatric patients with normal and abnormal hemodynamics. Additional fluid resuscitation is guided by response to initial bolus. (Reproduced with permission from the American College of Surgeons, Committee on Trauma. Advanced Trauma Life Support for Doctors, ATLS®. Chicago, IL; 2008. Chapter 10.)

  5. "Time is brain." Secondary injuries can be prevented by maximizing oxygenation and glucose delivery through optimization of cerebral perfusion pressure. Avoid the following:
      a. Hypoxemia. Keep oxygen saturation ≥98%.
      b. Hypercapnia or hypocapnia. Maintain $PaCO_2$ between 32 and 35 mm Hg.
      c. Hypotension. Maintain blood pressure around 50th percentile for age (80 + 2 × age in years).
      d. Hypoglycemia. Treat blood glucose levels <60 mg/dL with 5 mL/kg of 10% dextrose solution IV push, and start dextrose-containing maintenance fluids.
  6. Manifestation of head injuries in children:
      a. Seizures. Post-traumatic seizures are usually brief and rarely require anticonvulsants.
      b. Vomiting. Treat symptomatically and look for any intra-abdominal or head injury that could have triggered it.
  E. Exposure
      1. Remove all clothing for unobstructed exposure of all injuries and include 360-degree log roll with c-spine immobilization.

2. Infants and children are at risk for hypothermia due to their high body surface area. Protect from exposure to cold (blankets, BairHugger®, warm room, and fluids) taking care to cover the head and extremities.

3. Protect from skin pressure (remove from spine board within 30 minutes).

V. SECONDARY SURVEY

A. Head

1. Head injury causes >75% of pediatric trauma deaths.

2. *CT is the best method to evaluate traumatic brain injury* and is critical for early diagnosis of surgically correctable lesions.

3. There is limited role for plain films of the skull with blunt injury.

4. Scalp lacerations can produce significant hemorrhage. Control bleeding early with temporary sutures or scalp clips and inspect all lacerations for underlying fractures.

5. A bulging or tense fontanelle in an infant suggests increased intracranial pressure (ICP), blood, or hydrocephalus.

6. Coagulation studies are useful only in selected pediatric patients with head injury (e.g., severe injury or known underlying coagulopathy).

B. Neck

1. C-spine) injury is uncommon in children and is usually seen in those sustaining high energy blunt force trauma. Immobilize the c-spine early and quickly assess for injury. Fractures may be found anywhere in the c-spine, but injuries in the upper (C1–C3) vertebrae are most common in children <8 years.

   a. Pseudosubluxation of C3 on C2 is a normal variant occurring in 40% of children <7 years.

   b. True subluxations occur in ~10% to 20% of c-spine injuries and can be found in conjunction with associated fractures.

   c. Atlantooccipital dislocation occurs when the cranium separates from the cervical spinal column (due to the laxity of the transverse ligament in children), produces proximal spinal cord injury, and is nearly 100% fatal.

2. Examination

   a. Apnea or hypoventilation indicates injury at the spinal level for diaphragmatic control (C3, C4, and C5). Hypotension and bradycardia may result from neurogenic shock.

   b. Neck examination includes palpation of the spinous processes for tenderness and deformity while inline stabilization of the c-spine is maintained.

   c. Neurologic examination focuses on overall tone, head position, sensation, muscle strength, and reflexes attempting to identify the spinal level or dermatome of injury.

3. *Most awake, alert children can be cleared of spinal injury by clinical examination.* When clinical clearance is not possible, radiologic evaluation is employed. Initial radiologic assessment includes anteroposterior (AP), lateral, and odontoid views. C-spine CT is sensitive for detection of bony vertebral injury but is inadequate to clear the c-spine in the pediatric patient; it is best used selectively rather than routinely. Often, a plan to maintain immobilization for delayed (i.e., next morning) re-examination and clearance is best. Patients in whom clearance is not possible (e.g., persistent pain, neurologic findings, persistent altered mental status) should undergo MRI to evaluate the spinal cord and adjacent soft tissue structures prior to removal of the cervical collar.

C. Chest

1. Early recognition of life-threatening chest injuries is imperative.

2. An AP chest x-ray should be taken on arrival for any patient who arrives intubated, with chest trauma, or has dyspnea. Repeat films after interventions (intubation, chest tube) and for any deterioration.

3. Tension pneumothorax. Elevation and non-movement of the affected side of the chest is more apparent on physical examination than the classic findings of hyperresonance, distended neck veins, and hypotension.

4. Cardiac tamponade is rarely a source of hypotension in children but does occur. Pericardial ultrasound allows rapid diagnosis.

5. Hemothorax. Initial drainage of around 20% of total blood volume (20% × 80 mL/kg × wt [kg]) or ongoing losses of 1 to 2 mL/kg/h for 4 hours are indications for operative intervention.

6. Tracheobronchial injuries present with crepitus/subcutaneous air in the neck or chest and pneumomediastinum on plain x-ray. Injury occurs most commonly at or above the fourth tracheal ring. Careful endotracheal intubation (with balloon inflated distal to the injury) followed by bronchoscopy and surgical repair (at a center equipped for cardiopulmonary bypass) are indicated. In selected cases, careful observation and time may allow healing. Evaluation for associated injuries such as esophageal tear, c-spine injury, or great vessel injury is necessary.

7. Potentially life-threatening injuries include:

   a. Pneumothorax. Requires chest tube decompression with age appropriate tube size placed in the anterior to mid-axillary line at the fourth interspace.

   b. Rib fractures indicate severity of torso injury (underlying lungs or high abdominal organs) and are associated with 10% risk of mortality from associated injury.

   c. Pulmonary contusion is the most common injury to the chest due to the elasticity of the ribcage and transfer of energy to underlying tissues. Conservative management with supplemental oxygenation and chest physiotherapy is the mainstay of treatment. Fewer than 5% of children with this injury require mechanical ventilation.

   d. Cardiac contusion is a rare injury. Dysrhythmia or hypotension in the context of high energy (e.g., sternal, rib, and scapular fracture) is suggestive. Cardiac monitoring for 24 hours is appropriate if suspected.

D. Abdomen

1. Sixty percent of children with intra-abdominal injuries have a concomitant head injury.

2. Inspection of the abdomen and gentle palpation may help detect intra-abdominal injury. Routine digital rectal examinations provide little information and in most cases should be omitted. Exceptions may include diagnosis of pelvic fracture, perineal ecchymosis, or trans-pelvic penetrating injury with suspicion of rectal injury.

3. Gastric distension from swallowed air is common in crying infants, and in children who have had aggressive bag-valve-mask ventilation. Therefore, tube gastric decompression is indicated (see Table 21A-4 above).

4. CT with oral (when practical) and IV contrast is the most sensitive study to evaluate for the presence of intra-abdominal injury. In addition, CT can provide information regarding location and severity of injuries (e.g., liver laceration) which will guide acute and chronic management decisions.

5. Focused abdominal sonography for trauma (FAST) examination is not sensitive enough to replace CT in the hemodynamically normal child. FAST may be useful when CT is unavailable or the child is hypotensive and an intra-abdominal injury is suspected.

6. In general, order laboratory tests selectively to address specific clinical concerns. A complete blood count (CBC), blood typing and cross-match, and urinalysis (UA) are reasonable initial tests with additional tests ordered if needed but not routinely.

E. Pelvis

1. The "pelvic rock" does not reveal information about stable pelvic fractures, causes pain, and may exacerbate damage in unstable fractures.

2. Obtain pelvic x-rays based on clinical concern from history and physical examination findings; if CT of the abdomen and pelvis are planned, plain films can be omitted.

3. Use bladder catheterization selectively. (See Table 21A-4 above.) Resistance to passage of the tube or blood at the urethra requires a retrograde urethrogram, especially in the setting of pelvic fracture.

F. Extremities
   1. Evaluate the extremities for deformity and compromised perfusion.
   2. Use of extremity imaging is guided by clinical examination (e.g., complaints of pain; examination abnormalities) and should include the joint above and below the area of clinical concern.
   3. Early splinting reduces pain and may restore pulses; heavy splints can exacerbate pain and injury.

VI. Imaging is a vital component of most trauma evaluations. Selection of the appropriate imaging modality (e.g., plain films vs. CT) has attracted interest in recent years due to the increasing recognition of the detrimental effects of ionizing radiation in patients, particularly children. In most studies, CT was the major source of radiation in the pediatric trauma patients. We recommend selective use of CT based on appropriate risk reduction protocols employed. The risk of radiation should not discourage the clinician from obtaining necessary imaging studies but rather discourage obtaining images for convenience. The routine "pan-scanning" (whole body CT) of children may not create more good than harm. Information regarding risk reduction protocols for pediatric imaging exists at www.pedrad.org.

VII. Tertiary Survey is a thorough re-examination of the entire child within the first 24 hours after admission with the objective of identifying overlooked injuries or progression of known injuries. Up to 4% to 10% of children admitted for trauma will have an occult injury discovered later, most of which require intervention.

VIII. SPECIFIC INJURIES
   A. Traumatic brain injury (TBI)
   1. Epidural hematomas (EDHs) are more common than subdural hematomas; these often present with a lucid interval 30 to 60 minutes after injury, followed by abrupt decline in mental status.
   2. Subdural hematoma (SDH) may "blossom" over the first 48 hours.
   3. Rapid decline in mental status is an indication for urgent CT (or repeat CT) and neurosurgical consultation.
   4. Diffuse injuries (concussion, diffuse axonal injury) are more common in children.
   5. In most cases, GCS of 8 or less is an indication for intubation, immediate head CT, and ICP monitoring.
   6. Ventriculostomy offers some control of ICP in addition to monitoring and is preferred in severe TBI. Cerebral perfusion pressure should be maintained above 40 mm Hg in young children.
   7. Increases in ICP can be managed by drainage, neuromuscular blockade, sedation, or 3% saline at 0.1 to 1.0 mL/kg/h. Serum osmolarity should be maintained <320 mOsm/L. In the setting of herniation, use aggressive hyperventilation (PaCO$_2$ <30 mm Hg) and/or mannitol 0.25 to 1 g/kg. Decompressive craniectomy also permits ICP reduction. Outside of herniation, do not routinely use mannitol or hyperventilation for ICP prophylaxis.
   8. Use anticonvulsants such as phenytoin and valproate selectively.
   9. Minor head injury can lead to measurable cognitive deficits that persist for months after the injury. Routine follow-up is encouraged.
   B. Concussions and sports-related c-spine injuries (See Chapter 23 Head Injury and Chapter 25 Injury to the Spinal Cord and Spinal Column).
   1. Concussions are mild traumatic brain injuries, with many sports-related. Neuroimaging results (head CT) are, by definition, normal. Neuropsychological testing can provide objective data to patients, families, and the health care team. Cognitive and physical rest is the mainstay of treatment until symptoms (headache, nausea, poor sleep, distraction, behavioral problems) resolve, usually 7 to 10 days. Return-to-play decisions are based on symptom resolution. Premature return to play can have disastrous consequences since re-injury can happen at a lower force threshold.

    2. Ligamentous injury and muscle strain are the most common types of sports-related minor neck injuries in children. Severe injury that involves vertebral body fracture and dislocation and spinal cord injury can also result. The most common symptoms associated with minor neck injury include burning pain, numbness, and motor weakness. Keep the c-spine immobilized from the time of injury until cleared, using care when removing protective helmets and pads.

C. Penetrating trauma
    1. Fifty percent of gunshot wounded (GSW) young patients will have injuries to multiple body regions.
    2. GSW to the abdomen generally require exploratory celiotomy.
    3. Laparoscopy may be both diagnostic and therapeutic in the hemodynamically stable pediatric patient with penetrating abdominal trauma. The identification of injury most often warrants open celiotomy for definitive repair and evaluation of all abdominal viscera and peritoneal surfaces.

D. Spleen and Liver
    1. The spleen is the most commonly injured solid abdominal organ (40% of solid organ injuries); liver injury represents 15% to 30% of solid abdominal organ injuries in children.
    2. Most are lower grade injuries (American Association for the Surgery of Trauma Grades I, II, and III), and more than 95% do not require operative intervention. Few (<5%) require transfusion.
    3. IV contrast enhanced CT scan is >98% sensitive, and provides injury grading useful for management decisions.
    4. Operation is indicated for those patients with hemodynamic instability, ongoing need for transfusion, diaphragmatic injury, or hollow viscus injury.
    5. In the case operative intervention is indicated, splenectomy is usually required but splenorrhaphy may be attempted in low grade polar injuries and if few other injuries are present. For operative liver injuries, packing and temporary abdominal closure is often indicated.
    6. Exact indications for angiography and splenic artery embolization (SAE) are not clear in the pediatric population. SAE, however, may be valuable with isolated and higher grade injury (Grade 3 or higher).
    7. Non-operative management of injury to the liver includes angiographic embolization of actively bleeding hepatic vessels in the hemodynamically stable child in centers with the appropriate expertise.
    8. Overwhelming post-splenectomy infection (OPSI) occurs in up to 5% (lifetime risk) with 50% of patients acquiring infection in the first 6 months after splenectomy. Mortality estimates are 38% to 69%. Immunization against *Streptococcus pneumoniae, Haemophilus influenzae* type B, and *Neisseria meningitidis* are required.
    9. Long-term management does not mandate repeat radiologic studies. Indications for "return to play" are similar for splenic and liver injuries in children. For example, normal activity may resume after CT grade plus 2 weeks (e.g., Grade II splenic injury = 4 weeks restriction). Contact sports may require longer periods of restriction.

E. Duodenum and Pancreas
    1. Duodenal and pancreatic injuries result from similar mechanisms and although uncommon, are associated with serious complications. Suspect duodenal and pancreatic trauma in a patient with pain and nausea in the context of focal epigastric trauma (e.g., bicycle handle-bar; punch or foot stomp to the anterior torso).
    2. CT with IV contrast aids delineation of the severity of laceration and at times, the status of the main pancreatic duct. In cases with suspected ductal injury, endoscopic retrograde cholangiopancreatography (ERCP) provides information on ductal anatomy and allows possible intervention (e.g., stenting). Magnetic resonance pancreatography (MRP) details the duct but does not provide a therapeutic option. Both ERCP and MRP typically require sedation or anesthesia.

3. Duodenal hematomas or pancreatic contusions and minor lacerations are treated with bowel rest (nasogastric decompression). For prolonged obstruction or enzyme abnormalities, total parenteral nutrition (TPN) or nasojejunal feeds may be necessary.
4. Morbidity and mortality from duodenal injury (60% and 25%, respectively) result from perforation and are related to delay in diagnosis and definitive treatment.
5. Management and outcome are largely a function of the status of the pancreatic duct. An intact duct will typically heal with conservative management. A disrupted duct can be managed either operatively or non-operatively, both with challenging courses.

F. Intestinal injury
1. The most common sites of intestinal injury are at points of fixation with the jejunum, terminal ileum, and descending and sigmoid colon.
2. The appropriate mechanism, a tender abdomen or external bruising, and the presence of free fluid in the absence of solid organ injury suggest an intestinal injury.
3. Using CT to diagnose intestinal injury from blunt abdominal trauma is challenging even when both oral and IV contrast are given.
4. The "seat belt" complex includes abdominal wall ecchymosis above the anterior iliac spine and intestinal injury. It is often associated with a lumbar Chance fracture (transverse fracture of the vertebral body).

G. Pelvic fractures
1. Twenty percent of children with pelvic fracture also sustain abdominal injury.
2. Associated urethral injury or hemodynamic instability is rare.

H. Kidney
1. Grade by CT with IV contrast (assure obtaining delayed images). For Grade 4 and above with extravasation, re-assess by CT or ultrasound (US) at 48 to 72 hours. Evidence of expanding urinoma necessitates stenting or percutaneous nephrostomy.
2. Ninety-five percent can be managed without operative nephrectomy or nephrorrhaphy.
3. Hypertension can develop 6 months to 15 years after injury to the renovascular pedicle.

I. Bladder
1. There is a higher risk of bladder rupture from blunt trauma in young children, with 50% of bladder injuries associated with other abdominal injuries and most seen with pelvic fractures.
2. CT cystogram with delayed images is the most accurate diagnostic modality.
3. Most isolated extraperitoneal bladder perforation can be managed with Foley catheter drainage for 7 days, antibiotics, and pain control.
4. Intraperitoneal injury requires primary repair (layered; absorbable monofilament suture).

J. Genital injuries
1. Straddle injury is the compression of the soft tissue of the perineum against the bony pelvis and is sustained from falls, bicycle-related crashes, abuse, or playground activities.
2. Bleeding from the perineum occurs in 50%.
3. Examination under anesthesia is frequently indicated to allow full assessment of perineal injuries.
4. Urethral and vaginal strictures can result from missed injuries.

IX. BURNS (See Chapter 33 Burns)

A. Burns resulting from house fires are the leading cause of accidental death in the home for children <14 years. Twenty percent of burned children are victims of abuse, a result of neglect. Scald burns are the most common form of burn injury.

B. Resuscitation. Ringer's lactate is the resuscitation fluid of choice in the first 24 hours, guided by the Parkland/Baxter formula. Additional fluids should be given

| TABLE 21A-7 | Pediatric Burn Rule of Nines (Table 46-7) |

	Age (years)				
Body area	0	1	5	10	Adult
Head	19	17	13	11	7
Neck	2	2	2	2	2
Anterior trunk	13	13	13	13	13
Posterior trunk	13	13	13	13	13
Buttocks	2.5	2.5	2.5	2.5	2.5
Genitalia	1	1	1	1	1
Upper arm	2.5	2.5	2.5	2.5	2.5
Lower arm	3	3	3	3	3
Hand	2.5	2.5	2.5	2.5	2.5
Thigh	5.5	6.5	8	8.5	9.5
Leg	5	5	5.5	6	7
Foot	3.5	3.5	3.5	3.5	3.5

All values are percent body surface area (BSA).
Reproduced with permission from Gaines BA, et al. Pediatric trauma. In: Peitzman AB, Rhodes M, Schwab CW, et al., eds. *The Trauma Manual: Trauma and Acute Care Surgery.* 3rd ed. Philadelphia, PA: Wolters Kluwer/Lippincott Williams & Wilkins; 2008.

to achieve set endpoints of resuscitation such as age-appropriate HR, BP, and urine output (Table 21A-2). Because of differences in body surface area, appropriate tables should be used when estimating severity of burn injury (Table 21A-7).

C. Hypothermia is a risk; do not cover burns with wet, saline soaked dressings—use dry gauze or clean sheets.

D. Refer all children with burns to a burn center if any of these exist.
   1. Greater than 15% total body surface area burn (second or third degree)
   2. Burns to genitals or perineum
   3. Complex burns to face, hands, feet, or circumferential burns
   4. Thermal injury plus inhalation injury

X. NON-ACCIDENTAL TRAUMA (CHILD ABUSE)
   A. 1 to 1.5 million children are abused annually. As many as 1 in 10 of ED visits are thought to be from non-accidental injury, with 60,000 serious injuries. Head and abdominal trauma carry high mortality risk.
   B. All medical professionals have a duty to report suspected child abuse. This obligation supersedes doctor–patient relationships, carries penalties for failure to report, and provides immunity if reported in good faith.
   C. Suspicious history
   1. Unwitnessed injury, delay in seeking care, changing or evasive history, other evidence of neglect
   2. Implausible history (e.g., "rolled-off couch" in a child who cannot turn over; severity of injury discordant with reported mechanism)
   3. Multiple visits to ED; multiple injuries in different stages of healing
   D. Suspicious patterns of injury
   1. Head. Missing hair; torn lip frenulum (or other perioral injuries); retinal hemorrhages; bruising behind ears.
   2. Intracranial injury (most common cause of death). Chronic subdural or bilateral subdural bleeding; multiple hemorrhages in different stages of healing.
   3. "Shaken Baby Syndrome" is better understood as "Shaken Impact Syndrome" and is a pattern of injury seen after repeated blunt force to the head, not simply shaking. It includes cerebral edema, intracranial hemorrhage, and retinal hemorrhage and is commonly accompanied by multiple rib fractures.

TABLE 21A-8	Pediatric Trauma Score (PTS)		
Component	**+2**	**+1**	**−1**
Weight	>20 kg	10–20 kg	<10 kg
Airway	Normal	Maintained with oral or nasal airway	Intubated; cricothyroidotomy
Systolic blood pressure	>90 mm Hg; good peripheral pulses	50–90 mm Hg; carotid/ femoral pulses palpable	<50 mm Hg; weak or no pulses
Level of consciousness	Awake	Obtunded; any loss of consciousness	Comatose
Cutaneous	No injury	Minor: Contusion; laceration <7 cm not through fascia	Major: Penetrating wound through fascia
Fractures	None	Single; closed	Open; multiple

Modified and reproduced with permission from Tepas JJ 3rd, Mollitt DL, Talbert JL, et al. The pediatric trauma score as a predictor of injury severity in the injured child. *J Ped Surg* 1987;22:14–18.

   4. Musculoskeletal. Spiral fractures attributed to a fall; multiple fractures in various stages of healing; bucket-handle fractures (epiphyseal–metaphyseal separation produced by shaking or jerking); multiple bruises in various stages of resolution.
   E. Thoracoabdominal injuries associated with abuse
   1. Rib fractures (especially if multiple, or in varying stages of healing)
   2. Duodenal and pancreatic injuries and small bowel perforation are seen with punching or stomping.
   F. Injuries in the pattern of household objects (e.g., lighters, belt buckles, etc.)
   G. Suspicious perineal injuries. Multiple bruises to perineum, multiple lacerations to vulva, linear lacerations to vaginal walls, and rectal injuries

XI. SCORING SYSTEMS IN PEDIATRIC TRAUMA
   A. Scoring systems are intended to yield predictive power for outcome and to create relatively objective measures of injury severity. Commonly used scoring systems, such as Injury Severity Score (ISS), tend to overestimate risk of morality in children.
   B. Pediatric-specific scores
   1. Pediatric Trauma Score (PTS) is the most common scoring system applied to pediatric trauma patients. The PTS considers both anatomic and physiologic parameters as well as injuries and is used to predict outcomes. An injured child with a PTS score of less than 8 should be triaged to a pediatric trauma center as they are most at risk for preventable mortality, morbidity, and disability (Table 21A-8).
   2. Age-specific Pediatric Trauma Score (ASPTS) uses the same methodology but incorporates age-specific values for SBP, pulse, and RR. The ASPTS is the sum total of coded values for all variables. A threshold score of less than 10 is a predictor of increased mortality and suggests the need to transfer to a pediatric-capable center (Table 21A-9).

AXIOMS
- Trauma is the leading cause of death in children.
- Know the anatomic and physiologic differences in children to optimally give care.
- Bag-valve-mask ventilation is best for most and is a better urgent solution than intubation for the provider with limited pediatric experience.
- Hypoventilation is the most common cause of cardiac arrest in the pediatric trauma patient.

TABLE 21A-9	Age-Specific Pediatric Trauma Score (ASPTS)

GCS	SBP	Pulse	RR	Coded score
14–15	Normal	Normal	Normal	3
10–13	Mild-moderate hypotension (SBP < mean − 2SD)	Tachycardia (HR > mean + SD)	Tachypnea (RR > mean + SD)	2
4–9	Severe hypotension (SBP < mean − 3SD)	Bradycardia (HR < mean − SD)	Hypoventilation (RR > mean − SD)	1
3	0	0	0 or intubated	0

GCS, Glasgow Coma Scale; SBP, systolic blood pressure; RR, respiratory rate .
Modified and reproduced with permission from Potoka DA, Schall LC, Ford HR. Development of a novel age-specific pediatric trauma score. *J Pediatr Surg* 2001;36(1):106–112.

- Tachycardia is the most common initial manifestation of hypovolemia; hypotension is a late finding.
- Traumatic brain injuries are the most common cause of pediatric trauma death (75%).
- Solid organ injuries can be managed non-operatively in the majority of children (95%) irrespective of grade.
- Child abuse is common—consider it when the history does not fit the injuries or when unusual injuries exist.

Suggested Readings

Alexiou GA, Sfakianos G, Prodromou N. Pediatric head trauma. *J Emerg Trauma Shock* 2011;4:403–408.

Alterman DM. Considerations in pediatric trauma. Medscape Reference. Editor: Geibel J. Updated June 2011.http://emedicine.medscape.com/article/435031-overview. Accessed February 2, 2012.

Halstead ME, Walter KD. The Council on Sports, Medicine, and Fitness. Sport-related concussion in children and adolescents. *Pediatrics* 2010;126:597–611.

James HE. Neurologic evaluation and support in the child with an acute brain insult. *Pediatr Ann* 1986;15:16–22.

Mayglothling JA, Haan JM, Scalea TM. Blunt splenic injuries in the adolescent trauma population: the role of angiography and embolization. *J Emerg Med* 2011;41:21–28.

UpToDate®. Pediatric Resuscitation. Accessed online February 2, 2012. www.uptodate.com/home/clinicians/toc.do?tocKey=table_of_contents%2F3%2F1115

UpToDate®. Pediatric Trauma. Accessed online February 2, 2012. www.uptodate.com/home/clinicians/toc.do?tocKey=table_of_contents%2F3%2F1119

Zelicof-Paul A, Smith-Lockridge A, Schnadower D, et al. Controversies in rapid sequence in intubation in children. *Curr Opin Pediatr* 2005;17:355–362.

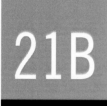

21B Trauma in Pregnant Women

Daniel J. Grabo and C. William Schwab

I. INTRODUCTION

Trauma complicates 6% to 7% of all pregnancies and accounts for 46% of maternal deaths. It is the leading non-obstetrical cause of maternal morbidity and mortality. Maternal injury severity is directly related to trauma-related fetal demise. The optimal early management of the pregnant trauma patient affords the best outcome for the fetus, that is, save the mother; save the fetus. While initial treatment priorities remain the same, anatomic and physiologic changes that accompany pregnancy alter the mother's response to injury and modify trauma care.

II. ANATOMIC AND PHYSIOLOGIC CHANGES OF PREGNANCY

A. Anatomic and physiologic changes involve essentially every organ system occur throughout all trimesters of pregnancy (Table 21B-1).
B. Abdomen and pelvis
   1. Enlarging uterus displaces viscera cephalad and alters injury patterns.
   2. Engorgement of pelvic veins increases the risk of bleeding with pelvic fracture.
   3. Pelvic ligaments relax and can alter radiographic appearance of pelvis.
   4. Location of gastro-esophageal junction is altered and gastric emptying is delayed, increasing risk of reflux and aspiration.
C. Uteroplacental unit
   1. The uterus increases in size, assuming a full pelvic and intra-abdominal location, and the muscular wall becomes progressively thinner increasing the susceptibility to direct uterofetal injury. The mother's inferior vena cava (IVC) is compressed in the supine position.
   2. There is increased uterine blood flow as pregnancy advances, increasing the potential for hemorrhage.
   3. The placenta lacks elasticity and is prone to separation (abruption).
   4. The uteroplacental unit lacks autoregulation and is sensitive to catecholamines and vasopressors. This means maternal hypovolemia or use of vasoconstrictor can compromise placental blood flow and fetal perfusion and should be avoided.

III. MECHANISMS OF INJURY

A. Blunt trauma
   1. Blunt abdominal trauma is associated with up to 38% incidence of fetal mortality and can be associated with obstetrical complications such as preterm labor, placental abruption, and fetomaternal hemorrhage.
   2. Falls are more common later in pregnancy as the center of gravity shifts and increases spinal lordosis.
   3. Domestic violence is prevalent and associated with 5% risk of fetal death.
   4. Motor vehicle collisions (MVCs) account for 50% to 80% of all traumas in pregnant women.
B. Penetrating trauma
   1. GSW are more common than stab wounds (SWs), again often from domestic violence.
   2. As pregnancy progresses, the risk of uterine and fetal injury increases due to enlargement and intra-abdominal location. Upper abdominal penetrating wounds can be associated with gastrointestinal injury (visceral displacement and abdominal crowding).

TABLE 21B-1	Anatomic and Physiologic Changes of Pregnancy and Potential Clinical Consequences	
System or anatomic location	**Anatomic/physiologic change**	**Potential clinical consequence**
Neurologic	Eclampsia	Increase in ICP; seizures; can mimic head injury
Cardiovascular system	Increase cardiac output, heart rate, blood pressure (second trimester) Decrease CVP, peripheral vasodilation	Altered vital signs Hyperdynamic state Peripheral edema
Pulmonary/thoracic	Increase tidal volume, minute ventilation (30–50%) Decreased function residual capacity Airway edema Diaphragm elevated (4 cm) with increased excursion	Decreased $PaCO_2$ (32 mm Hg) Decreased tolerance for hypoxemia Airway obstruction Difficult intubation Altered anatomic landmark (e.g., misplaced chest tube)
Renal	Increase renal blood flow, glomerular filtration rate Dilation of collecting system	Altered sodium reabsorption and water retention Decreased serum creatinine Radiographic abnormalities
Hematologic	Intravascular volume expansion Larger increase in plasma volume than RBC volume Increase procoagulant factors	Anemia of pregnancy Blood loss volume of up to 1,500 mL before manifesting signs of hypovolemia Hypercoagulable state Incidence of DVT/PE higher.
Endocrine	Pituitary enlarges with increased blood flow	Sheehan's syndrome: Shock-related pituitary insufficiency

3. GSW to the abdomen that cause uterine injury result in fetal injury in up to 70% of cases as well as preterm labor; 40% to 70% result in fetal death.

IV. PRINCIPLES OF MANAGEMENT
  A. General considerations
    1. Consider pregnancy in all female trauma patients between 10 and 50 years and perform beta-human chorionic gonadotropin (HCG) testing unless known inability to conceive.
    2. Initial treatment priorities remain the same as American College of Surgeons Committee on Trauma Advanced Trauma Life Support (ATLS®) protocols and focus on assuring maternal oxygenation and cardiopulmonary stability.
    3. In cases of maternal blood loss, the mother will shunt blood from the fetus, so volume resuscitation and early fetal monitoring are key.
    4. Early obstetrical consultation and fetal assessment are necessary.
    5. Transport to a trauma center if any concerns of moderate to severe trauma.
  B. Primary survey modifications
    1. Place women in the second and third trimesters on the left side with a torso bump (15% leftward roll with pillow or bump under the right buttock and back) to displace the gravid uterus off the IVC and maximize venous return to the heart.
    2. Give supplemental oxygen, and intubate if this fails or severe compromise exists to minimize fetal hypoxia. Laryngoscopy and intubation may be difficult due to airway edema and body habitus.

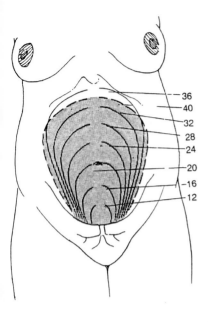

Figure 21B-1. Uterine Size. 1 cm = 1 week gestational age. Reproduced with permission from Knudson MM. Trauma in pregnancy. (From Blaisdell FW, Trunkey DD, eds. *Trauma Management—Abdominal Trauma.* 2nd ed. New York, NY: Thieme Medical Publishers; 1993.)

    a. Pregnant women are at increased risk of aspiration. For rapid sequence intubation, use smaller doses of succinylcholine (1 mg/kg max) because of placental production of pseudocholinesterases.
  3. Invasive diagnostic and therapeutic procedures must consider altered anatomy. Higher diaphragmatic position and enlarged breast tissue change chest tube placement and enlarged uterus require a supraumbilical open diagnostic peritoneal lavage.
  4. Due to physiologic hypervolemia the pregnant woman can lose up to 1,500 mL of blood without clinical manifestations.
  5. If needed, upper extremity venous access in the upper extremities is best.
  6. If needed early, use Type O, Rh-negative blood to avoid Rh isoimmunization.
  7. Think of eclampsia when seeing a third trimester woman with altered mental status if head CT is normal and blood pressure is above 120 mm Hg systolic.
C. Secondary survey modifications
  1. Obstetric history should include:
    a. Date of last menstrual period (LMP) and expected date of delivery
    b. Perception of fetal movement
    c. State of current pregnancy including related complications; previous obstetric history
  2. Fundal height as measured in centimeters from the pubis (Fig. 21B-1) provides a rapid approximation of gestational age.
  3. Abdominal examination includes assessment of uterine tenderness, presence of contractions, and determination of fetal lie and movement. The presence of vaginal blood or amniotic fluid on pelvic examination is important. Nitrazine paper color change (from blue-green to deep blue) suggests the presence of amniotic fluid. Obstetric consultation to identify cervical dilation, effacement, or fetal station is recommended.
D. Fetal assessment
  1. Fetal viability is usual after 22 to 24 weeks' gestation.
  2. Fetal heart tones (FHT) can be auscultated with a stethoscope beyond 20 weeks' gestation; use a Doppler before this time. Normal fetal heart rate is from 120 to 160 beats/min. Bradycardia indicates fetal distress.

TABLE 21B-2 | **Absorbed Radiation Dose from Radiographic Study**

Radiographic study	Absorbed dose (rad)
Cervical spine series	0.0005
Anteroposterior chest	0.0025
Anteroposterior pelvis	0.2
Lumbosacral spine series	0.75–1.0
Head CT scan	0.05
Chest CT scan	1.0
Abdomen CT scan (including pelvis)	3.0–9.0
Limited upper abdomen CT scan	3.0

Modified and reproduced with permission from Tinkhoff, G. Care of the pregnant trauma patient. In: Peitzman AB, Rhodes M, Schwab CW, et al., eds. *The Trauma Manual: Trauma and Acute Care Surgery*. 3rd ed. Philadelphia, PA: Wolters Kluwer/Lippincott Williams & Wilkins; 2008.

3. Start continuous fetal monitoring at or beyond 20 to 24 weeks gestation with trauma, having trained personnel interpret the tracings for signs of fetal distress (abnormal baseline, repetitive decelerations, absence of accelerations, or variability).

4. Fetal ultrasound is excellent in assessment of the fetus for gestational age, cardiac activity, movement, and placental evaluation.

E. Diagnostic modalities

1. Standard laboratory evaluation includes hematocrit and coagulation studies. Kleihauer–Betke (KB) testing is performed to determine the amount of mixing of maternal and fetal blood. The KB blood test allows quantification of the amount of fetal red blood cells introduced into the maternal circulation.

2. Despite displacement of abdominal viscera and enlarged uterus, the sensitivity and specificity of FAST examination for free fluid or blood in the abdomen in pregnant trauma patients is similar to non-pregnant patients.

3. Diagnostic peritoneal lavage (DPL) is more challenging in the pregnant patient with displaced abdominal viscera and gravid uterus. For DPL, a supra-umbilical approach is used if the uterus is palpated above the pubic symphysis; use an open technique to minimize uterine or fetal injury.

4. Indications for radiographic imaging including CT are the same as the non-pregnant patient.

   a. The uterus should be shielded with lead aprons when possible.

   b. Radiation doses above 20 rad increase the risk of teratogenesis. The early weeks of fetal growth and organogenesis (weeks 2 to 7) are the most sensitive for teratogenic, growth retarding, and postnatal neoplastic effects of radiation (Table 21B-2).

   c. Patients within the first trimester, especially those who are close by dates to 8 weeks' gestational age (GA), should have limited radiographs if clinically well. Obstetric and radiology consultation can help to determine risks and alternatives to radiographic investigation.

F. Medications in pregnancy

1. Tetanus toxoid administration is not contraindicated in pregnant patients.

2. Use standard antibiotic prophylaxis and treatment.

   a. Penicillins, cephalosporins, and clindamycin are safe.

   b. Avoid aminoglycosides (fetal ototoxicity), sulfonamides (neonatal kernicterus), quinolones, and metronidazole.

G. Exploratory laparotomy

1. Indications are the same as for the non-pregnant injured patient.

2. Handle the uterus gently; excessive twisting and traction compromises blood flow to and within the uterus.

3. Exploratory laparotomy is not an indication for cesarean delivery; do this with a consulting obstetrician when available.
H. Emergency cesarean delivery
1. Indications
   a. The risk of fetal distress exceeds the risk of prematurity
   b. Placental abruption with fetal distress; uterine rupture
   c. Fetal malposition with premature labor
   d. Severe pelvic or lumbosacral spine fractures
   e. The gravid uterus interfering with exposure for other injuries during laparotomy.
   f. Disseminated intravascular coagulation
2. Perimortem cesarean delivery can be considered in situations of gestational age ≥26 weeks and <15-minute interval between maternal death and delivery. Continue maternal cardiopulmonary resuscitation during delivery. Neonatal ICU support must be immediately available.
3. Technique
   a. Vertical midline abdominal incision.
   b. Incise the uterus vertically.
   c. Expose the infant's head; suction oropharynx with bulb syringe.
   d. Deliver the infant.
   e. Clamp and divide the umbilical cord. (3 to 5 cm from the infant's body.)
   f. Manually remove the placenta.
   g. Inspect the endometrial surface and ensure removal of all membranes.
   h. Close the uterus in layers with absorbable suture.
   i. Oxytocin (20 U IV) to treat postpartum uterine bleeding.

V. PROBLEMS UNIQUE TO THE PREGNANT TRAUMA PATIENT

A. Preterm labor can complicate up to 25% of trauma patients with a viable fetus.
   1. Approximately 40% of pregnant trauma patients have contractions.
   2. Only 11% are associated with preterm labor which is treated with standard obstetric protocols.
B. Placental abruption can occur with minor injuries and is common after multi-system trauma or severe direct abdominal injury.
   1. Next to maternal death, abruption is the most common cause of fetal death.
   2. Shearing injuries can separate the myometrium from the placenta and cause DIC.
   3. Evaluation includes electronic fetal monitoring (cardiotocography; 100% negative predictive value with reassuring monitoring and the absence of significant clinical findings) for 4 hours in the patient of 20 weeks' gestational age who has experienced abdominal or multi-system trauma. Non-reassuring fetal heart tones in conjunction with clinical evidence of placental abruption are indications for emergent cesarean delivery.
   4. Minor degrees of placental separation are compatible with fetal survival.
C. Fetomaternal hemorrhage occurs more commonly in women with abdominal trauma.
   1. A small amount (1 mL) of Rh-positive fetal blood can sensitize an Rh-negative woman.
   2. All Rh-negative pregnant trauma victims should receive 300 micrograms (mcg) of Rh-immune globulin within 72 hours of injury and another 300 mcg for each 30 mL of estimated fetal blood identified in the maternal circulation via the Kleihauer–Betke test.
D. Disseminated intravascular coagulation is often the result of amniotic fluid embolism and thromboplastin release during placental abruption.
   1. Maternal shock and death can quickly ensue.
   2. Treatment includes emergent cesarean delivery and uterine evacuation in addition to blood component therapy to reverse coagulopathy.
E. Uterine rupture is a rare but devastating complication of blunt abdominal trauma that can result in maternal mortality rate (10%).
   1. Risk factors include rapid deceleration injuries, direct uterine injury, prior cesarean delivery, and advanced gestational age.

2. Uterine wall rupture results in extrusion of the fetus into the abdominal cavity and extensive hemorrhage.

3. Uterine and abdominal tenderness and abnormal uterine shape.

4. Diagnosis can be confirmed with abdominal x-ray or more often ultrasound.

5. Emergent surgical and obstetrical management is often required.

AXIOMS

- "Save the mother; save the fetus."
- The best early treatment of the fetus is optimal resuscitation of the mother.
- Large blood loss can occur in the pregnant patient without changes in vital signs.
- Routinely perform HCG on all women of child-bearing age.
- Displace the uterus to the left side with torso bump in late pregnancy.
- The fetus can be in jeopardy, even with apparent minor maternal injury.
- Early consultation with an obstetrician is optimal.

Suggested Readings

Chames MC, Pearlman MD. Trauma during pregnancy: outcomes and clinical management. *Clin Obstet Gynecol* 2008;51:398–408.

Hill CC, Pickinpaugh J. Physiologic Changes in Pregnancy. *Surg Clin N Am* 2008;88:391–401.

Katz VL, Balderston K, Defreest M. Perimortem cesarean delivery: were our assumptions correct? *Am J Obstet Gynecol* 2005;192(6):1916–1920.

Mattox KL, Goetzl L. Trauma in pregnancy. *Crit Care Med* 2005;33(10):S385–S389.

Shah AJ, Kilcline BA. Trauma in pregnancy. *Emerg Med Clin North Am* 2003;21:615–629.

UpToDate®. Trauma in pregnancy. Accessed online. February 2, 2012. www.uptodate.com/contents/trauma-in-pregnancy.

21C | Trauma in Older Adults

Daniel J. Grabo and C. William Schwab

I. INTRODUCTION. Unique anatomic and physiologic characteristics can affect the older individual's response to injury. Modifications in standard ATLS management are based on age-related anatomy and physiology as well as the presence of chronic medical conditions and medications.

In the United States, the number of adults over the age of 65 is expected to increase by 70 million by the year 2030. When compared with younger cohorts, trauma in the elderly results in sicker patients with lower ISS, increased hospital length of stay, and mortality. Those providing emergency care must have an understanding of the age-related physiologic changes, the common mechanisms of injury, and the management of specific injuries.

II. AGE-RELATED APPROACH TO PATIENT CARE. The response to injury and illness changes with increasing age. A number of treatment guidelines have been developed for the care of the older trauma patient.

  A. Age 55 to 64 years
  1. Assume mild decrease in physiologic reserve to hemodynamic or respiratory stressors.
  2. Expect more frequent presence of chronic diseases (diabetes mellitus, cardiovascular disease, hypertension, previous surgery, blood transfusion).
  3. Suspect the use of prescription or over-the-counter (OTC) medications.
  4. Assume the patient is competent to provide an accurate medical history.
  5. Look for subtle signs of organ dysfunction, especially cardiovascular and respiratory systems.
  6. Proceed with standard diagnostic and management schemes.

  B. Age 65 to 74 years
  1. Accept the presence of age-related and acquired disease-induced physiologic alteration of organ systems.
  2. Expect frequent presence of chronic disease and medications to treat them. Assume a higher incidence of previous surgery and blood transfusion.
  3. Evaluate the patient for competency to provide a reliable medical history. Early review of the history with the patient's relatives or personal physician is often helpful.
  4. Provide early, appropriate resuscitation to optimize cardiac performance and oxygen delivery.
  5. Any history of loss of consciousness, alteration in mental status, cognitive or sensory function indicates the presence of brain injury and requires brain imaging with CT.
  6. Standard diagnostic and management schemes should be pursued, including early aggressive operative management.
  7. Poor outcomes, especially with severe injury to the central nervous system (CNS) or marked physiologic deterioration secondary to injury, are more frequent.
  8. Check for advance directives guiding care.

  C. Age 75 years and older
  1. Proceed as in 2.
  2. Poor outcome should be assumed with moderate to severe injury, especially with the CNS injury or any injury causing physiologic dysfunction.

3. After aggressive initial resuscitation and diagnostic maneuvers, reassess the magnitude of the patient's injuries and discuss appropriateness of care with the patient (if competent) and family members.
4. Check for advanced directives.
5. Consider early consultation with experts in ethics and social services to help the family and medical team with difficult decisions.

III. PHYSIOLOGIC CHANGES IN THE ELDERLY

A. Nervous system
1. Decrease in brain tissue mass can result in loss of intracranial volume which results in more "space" needed to fill before intracranial pressure elevation and increased vascular shearing injury which can result in frequent intracranial hemorrhage.
2. Decreased cerebral blood flow can manifest as blunted sensation (visual, auditory, tactile). Cognitive function is often altered, and the perception of pain can be blunted. Alterations in cerebellar function, gait, and balance increase susceptibility to injury, such as falls.
3. Cognition and sensorium may be altered by CNS active medications or preexisting neurologic disease (e.g., dementia) which can significantly impact neurologic evaluation after injury.

B. Cardiovascular system
1. Cardiovascular disease is common. Myocardial dysfunction impairs the ability to improve cardiac contractility in response to stress and catecholamine surge. Conduction abnormalities develop and results in different forms of dysrhythmias; atrial fibrillation is the most common.
2. Arteriosclerotic vascular disease can impair blood flow to organs and tissues in the CNS and peripheral arterial system. Baseline peripheral pulse examination can be diminished or absent.
3. Cardiovascular medications are common, including beta-blockers. Undesirable side-effects include blunting of reflexive or catecholamine-induced tachycardia and increases in cardiac output. Elders are preload dependent, and hypovolemia (from dehydration, diuretic use, blood loss, etc.) is poorly tolerated. Blood pressure measurement may be misleading due to underlying chronic hypertension, anti-hypertensive medication use, diuretics, or dehydration.

C. Respiratory system
1. Declining chest wall compliance, respiratory muscle strength, and lung elasticity results in alveolar collapse and decreased arterial oxygenation.
2. Injury-related torso pain can hasten the development of poor inspiratory effort, atelectasis, and pneumonia; this makes adequate treatment of pain important. Epidural anesthesia/analgesia and non-steroidal anti-inflammatory drugs (NSAIDs) are good options. Opioids in titrated doses and carefully monitored for respiratory effects are helpful; these can be given in continuous fashion or short interval boluses via patient-controlled analgesia (PCA) pumps.

D. Renal
1. Decrease in renal cortex mass results in as much as 25% functional cortical loss. Glomerular filtration rate (GFR) decreases, and renal tubule reabsorption is impaired resulting in problems with solute clearance and water balance.
2. Lean body mass decreases with age and creatinine production declines. Serum creatinine levels can remain within normal range even though renal function may be impaired. Therefore, calculate creatinine clearance (C_{Cr}) to assess function: C_{Cr} (mL/min) $= (140 - \text{age}) \times \text{mass (kg)}/\text{serum creatinine} \times 72$.
3. Use nephrotoxic agents such as intravenous contrast, aminoglycosides, diuretics, and vasopressor with care and after optimizing volume status.

E. Musculoskeletal system
1. Osteoarthritis is the second most common chronic medical condition in adults over 65 years in the United States. Pain often compromises mobility and impairs the ability to avoid injury. As a result of diminished muscle mass, strength, and

TABLE 21C-1 **Premorbid Illness Criteria**

Chronic disease	Historical questions
Hypertension	Any hypertensive medication
	Documented prior history
Cardiac disease	History of cardiac surgery
	Any cardiac medication
	MI within 12 months of admission
	MI more than 12 months before admission
Diabetes mellitus	Insulin dependent
	Non-insulin dependent
Liver disease	Bilirubin >2 mg/dL (on admission)
	Cirrhosis
Malignancy	Documented history
Pulmonary disease (Asthma, COPD)	Bronchodilator therapy
Obesity	Female >200 lb
	Male >250 lb
Renal disease	Serum creatinine >2 mg/dL (on admission)
Neurologic (CVA)	Documented prior history

MI, Myocardial infarction; COPD, chronic obstructive pulmonary disease.
Modified and reproduced with permission from Kauder DR. Geriatric trauma. In: Peitzman AB, Rhodes M, Schwab CW, et al., eds. *The Trauma Manual: Trauma and Acute Care Surgery.* 3rd ed. Philadelphia, PA: Wolters Kluwer/Lippincott Williams & Wilkins; 2008, Table 48-1.

agility, they have an inability to avoid obstacles and serious injury, especially when falling (altered righting reflex).

2. Analgesics, often in the form of over the counter medications (aspirin, nonsteroidals, etc.) are commonly used and often not be perceived as "medications" when history is taken despite the impact on bleeding or renal function.

IV. INFLUENCE OF COMORBID CONDITIONS

A. Roughly 80% of Americans over the age of 65 are found to have at least one chronic medical condition and 50% have two. Hypertension, osteoarthritis, coronary artery disease, and diabetes mellitus are the most common. Resuscitation and management strategies should be influenced by knowledge of current disease states. Table 21C-1 provides a helpful listing of the more common conditions encountered.

V. MECHANISMS OF INJURY

A. Falls

1. Falls are the most frequent cause of injury in the elderly. Ground level falls (GLF) are low energy mechanisms, but often result in severe injury.

2. Falls may be the result of age-related changes such as impaired vision, postural instability, gait disturbances, poor balance, and decreased muscle strength. The sequelae of chronic medical conditions such as immobility from osteoarthritis and syncope from cardiovascular disease can contribute to falls. The effects of chronic medications can be a risk factor for falls, such as orthostatic hypotension from antihypertensive agents, and can lead to devastating consequences from falls, such as life-threatening bleeding from anticoagulation use. The reason for the fall must be sought and treated.

3. Fall intervention programs include environmental modifications, monitoring for polypharmacy, and physical strength and conditioning programs and have been found to be beneficial in attenuating risk factors for falls and injury prevention (reduction of fall incidence by 19%).

B. Motor vehicle crashes
   1. Those patients over 75 years have the highest fatal crash rate.
   2. Declines in reaction time, vision, and mobility in addition to comorbid conditions, and medications have effects on driving skills, and recurrent crashes may indicate the need to restrict driving.
   3. In contrast to younger drivers, older drivers are more likely to have vehicular crashes during daylight hours and in good weather. Currently, there are no federal or state mandated driving restrictions for advanced age.
C. Pedestrian–automobile collisions
   1. More than 20% of all pedestrian–automobile fatalities in the United States occur in the elderly.
   2. Declines in vision, hearing, and walking speed are predisposing factors. Impaired cognition and judgment play a critical role.
   3. Measures to identify dangerous intersections and to provide crossing guards may bring about a reduction in older pedestrian fatalities.
D. Injuries related to violence
   1. Injuries resulting from assault account for 4% to 14% of elderly trauma admissions. Suicide is the most common reason for gun-related deaths in older individuals.
   2. In excess of 240,000 cases are reported annually, likely an under-representation of the actual occurrence. Look for elderly abuse, especially in those with frequent ED visits for "minor" injuries, multiple bruises in various healing stages, poor nutrition, an unkempt appearance, and poor personal hygiene are warning signs. Social services agency consultation is required.
E. Burns (See Chapter 33 Burns)
   1. The elderly are particularly vulnerable to burn injury.
   2. Thinning of the skin leads to deeper burn injury.
   3. Scalding appears to be the most common form of burn injury.
   4. Burns exceeding 50% of total body surface are uniformly fatal, and inhalation injuries are poorly tolerated.
   5. Large resuscitation volumes are poorly tolerated due to limited cardiopulmonary reserve; monitor the cardiopulmonary status closely.

VI. PRINCIPLES OF MANAGEMENT

A. General considerations
   1. The management of elderly trauma patients follows the principles of ATLS®.
   2. Early awareness of a blunted physiologic response to injury and blood loss (chronic medical conditions and medications) is important.
   3. During the initial resuscitation phase, try to contact family members, caregivers, and the patient's pharmacy for medical information and advanced directives. Hospital-based pharmacists can be helpful in acquiring medication records from commercial pharmacies and undertake a prompt medication reconciliation. The pharmacy records may have other valuable information, for example, allergies, home address, etc.
B. Primary survey modifications
   1. Airway. Due to lack of pulmonary reserve and high probability of underlying cardiovascular disease, mild hypoxia is poorly tolerated.
   2. Breathing. Seek chest wall injuries and obtain early chest radiograph and adequate pain control.
   3. Circulation. Deviations in blood pressure and heart rate are inadequate predictors of shock in the elderly blunt trauma patient. Almost 60% of elderly patients with severe injuries (ISS >15) and 25% with critical injuries (ISS >25) do not manifest significant hypotension (SBP <90 mm Hg). Blood transfusion is needed early and large volume crystalloid resuscitation should be limited. Invasive monitoring devices, bedside ultrasound, and echocardiography are adjuncts to determine volume status and response to therapy.

4. Disability. Neurologic assessment can be difficult because of dementia, cerebrovascular disease, or other conditions. Head CT scan is the best to diagnose CNS injury early.

5. Exposure

    a. Information can be learned about medical history from inspection of the location of surgical incisions.

    b. Large quantities of blood can be sequestered in the elastic tissues of the elderly (back and buttocks).

    c. Due to thinning of the skin and poor temperature regulation, the elderly are susceptible to hypothermia and care must be taken to provide a warm environment (increased room temperature, BairHugger®, and blankets).

    d. Extra padding and frequent repositioning of the patient helps avoid skin breakdown.

C. Survey modifications

    1. The effect of medical history, medical conditions, and medications must be considered with the history and mechanism of injury. For example, a series of falls and MVCs in the elderly are often the sequelae of undiagnosed and treated medical conditions (cardiac dysrhythmias, transient ischemic attacks, non-insulin–dependent diabetes mellitus, etc.).

    2. Look for coagulopathic conditions.

    3. Implantable devices, notably cardiac, should be identified.

    4. In addition to the routine laboratory measurements and monitoring, obtain arterial blood gasses, electrocardiogram, cardiac enzymes, blood cultures, and urinalysis if ambiguity exists or deterioration occurs.

VII. MANAGEMENT OF SPECIFIC PROBLEMS

A. Antiplatelet and warfarin (or newer non-warfarin anticoagulants) increase bleeding; some can be reversed, especially if CNS bleed, massive soft tissue injury, or significant visceral bleeding exists.

    1. Platelet-associated coagulopathy from aspirin and clopidogrel is often treated with platelet transfusion (5 to 10 units of platelet concentrate), although outcome data are lacking. Desmopressin 0.03 mcg/kg IV is an alternative.

    2. Reversing warfarin-induced coagulopathy requires large volumes of plasma (10 to 15 mL/kg; 4 to 6 units; 800 to 1,200 mL) which can result in pulmonary edema in the setting of limited cardiopulmonary reserve.

    3. Prothrombin complex concentrates contain plasma-derived Vitamin K–dependent coagulation factors, use less volume, and are effective in decreasing time to reversal of warfarin-related coagulopathy. These are still not widely available in the United States.

    4. Intravenous Vitamin K (5 mg to 10 mg) can be used an adjunct to other warfarin reversal options but is slower.

    5. Recombinant factor VIIa (rFVIIa) enhances thrombin generation and has been shown to be both safe and effective in the elderly with moderate coagulopathy and traumatic brain injury.

B. Dabigatran and rivaroxaban are shorter acting oral anticoagulants; neither has reversal agents although dialysis can decrease dabigatran effects and PCC may temper rivaroxaban bleeding. Traumatic brain injury (TBI) in the elderly is associated with a high mortality (12% to 19%).

    1. Underlying dementia, previous cerebrovascular accident (CVA), or the presence of sedatives or antipsychotics alter mental status examination and mandate early CT brain and spine imaging.

    2. At times, head CT precedes full evaluation of the stable patient after a quick survey reveals altered mental status. For example, in the patient with dementia taking warfarin and a history of a ground level fall, CT is likely the only way to accurately detect intracranial bleeding in need of immediate surgical care.

C. Pre-existing degenerative joint disease in the cervical spine can predispose to cervical injuries, with odontoid fractures being the most common.

1. Falls from standing can result in cervical hyperextension, acute compression of the spinal cord, and injury to the central portion of the spinal cord.
2. "Central cord syndrome" carries poor prognosis with approximately 50% mortality rate, which is likely related to respiratory failure that arises from complications of cervical immobilization.
3. CT is the best initial imaging modality, with magnetic resonance imaging (MRI) obtained in those patients with cord injuries present or still possible.

D. Minor mechanisms of injury can cause significant torso injury, and physical examination is often unreliable.
1. CT of the chest and abdomen is the best way to detect injury.
2. IV contrast enhanced CT scanning in elderly trauma patients has not been shown to increase the risk of acute kidney injury (AKI); however, avoidance of iodinated contrast solutions is recommended for patients at risk of AKI (e.g., chronic kidney disease, dehydration).

E. Early celiotomy is recommended in the elderly patient with solid abdominal organ injury, hemoperitoneum, and hemodynamic instability.

F. Improved survival of elderly patients with severe injury occurs with damage control resuscitation and surgical strategies, although outcomes from these extreme injuries are less than in younger cohorts.

VIII. OUTCOMES

A. Immediate post-injury and long-term trauma morbidity and mortality rates are higher in elderly trauma patients than their age-matched cohorts. Re-injury and death are more frequent for 5 years from the time of initial injury.

B. Trauma-related mortality risk increases with the presence and number of chronic medical conditions. As ISS rises above 15, these cease to be significant. ISS above 25 is an independent risk factor for increased mortality.

IX. ETHICS AND END-OF-LIFE ISSUES

A. The medical ethics issues surrounding the care of the injured elderly are difficult.
1. It is appropriate to begin aggressive resuscitative efforts and to sustain them until some insight can be gained into the patient's functional status, state of health, and wishes.
2. Living wills or advanced directives are uncommon and are even less likely to be on their person at the time of a serious injury.
3. Early contact with a family member or a personal physician can yield crucial information that can influence medical decision making.
4. The patient's and family's interpretation of end-of-life documents may be different from what is written or understood by the medical providers, and open repetitive communication with all parties is necessary.

B. Social service personnel and chaplains help identify and communicate with family members and other loved ones.

C. A realistic presentation of injuries, care, and prognosis for the patient and family is imperative for decision making.

D. Gerontology and ethics consultation may help.

AXIOMS

- Accurate information about comorbid conditions, medications, functional capacity, and advanced directives is key.
- Hypoxia and hypercapnia are poorly tolerated; treat these early.
- Normal heart rate and blood pressure do not imply normovolemia; consider early invasive monitoring.
- Loss of consciousness or altered mental status is a TBI and requires urgent evaluation with CT of the head.
- Hypovolemia is poorly tolerated, and early operative or angiographic control of bleeding is recommended over repeated transfusion.

Suggested Readings

Bhullar IS, Roberts EE, Brown L, et al. The effect of age on blunt traumatic brain-injured patients. *Am Surg* 2010;76:966–968.

Dossett LA, Riesel JN, Griffin MR, et al. Prevalence and implications of preinjury warfarin use. *Arch Surg* 2011;146:565–570.

Harrington DS, Thakkar RK, Monaghan SF, et al. Factors associated with survival following blunt chest trauma in older patients: results from a large regional trauma cooperative. *Arch Surg* 2010;145:432–437.

McQuay N, Cipolla J, Franges EZ, et al. The use of recombinant factor VIIa in coagulopathic traumatic brain injury requiring emergent craniotomy. Is it benefical? *J Neurosurg* 2009;111:666–671.

Newell MA, Schlitzkus LL, Waibel BH, et al. "Damage control" in the elderly: futile endeavor or fruitful enterprise? *J Trauma* 2010;69:1049–1043.

Zarzaur BL, Croce MA, Magnotti LJ, et al. Identifying life-threatening shock in the older injured patient: an analysis of the National Trauma Databank. *J Trauma* 2010;68:1134–1138.

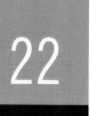

22

Introduction to Trauma: Mechanism of Injury

Gregory J. Jurkovich and L.D. Britt

MECHANISM OF INJURY

Trauma, or physical force injury, occurs from blunt, penetrating, or thermal mechanisms. The distinction of the cause of the injury is more than just nomenclature: The mechanism of injury often dictates specific management approaches. These mechanisms of physical force injury are divided into more specific categories (Table 22-1). While each trauma registry has their own shorthand nomenclature for injury mechanism, this table outlines the most commonly used shorthand descriptors.

BLUNT TRAUMA

I. MOTOR VEHICLE CRASHES (MVCs) (Fig. 22-1)
   A. Injuries are produced by the rapid decrease in velocity over a short distance (deceleration). Severity of injury depends on energy transferred during deceleration as a result of a crash.
   1. MVCs account for 30% to 40% deaths from unintentional causes.
   2. MVCs cause at least half of closed head and spinal cord injuries.
   3. The risk of a major injury increases 3- to 5-fold if the patient is ejected (including a 1 in 13 risk of spinal column injury).
   4. Highest risk of injury in MVCs occurs if there is a death of another occupant, partial or complete ejection of the patient, or >12 in. of intrusion on the occupant side and >18 in. of intrusion anywhere, including the roof.
   5. MVCs involve three types of collisions:
      a. Primary collision—motor vehicle impacts another object
      b. Secondary collision—patient strikes internal components of the car
      c. Deceleration-induced deformation—results in differential movement of fixed and nonfixed anatomic parts (e.g., shearing injury to the brain or transection of the thoracic aorta)
   B. Determinants of injury
   1. Magnitude of force (force = mass × acceleration)
   2. Location of patient (front seat vs. back seat; driver vs. passenger)
   3. Restraint devices (Table 22-2)
      a. Injury risk is greatest in the unrestrained patients.
      b. Lap belts alone decrease mortality by 50% (but with an increased rate of abdominal injury).
      c. The lap belt is designed to fit across the pelvis (the anterior superior iliac spines). If inappropriately worn high over the abdomen, anterior compression fractures of the upper lumbar spine (chance fractures) can occur. Lap belt contusions ("seat-belt sign") are associated with pancreatic, bowel, mesentery, and aortic injury. Lap belt contusion and chance fracture in children are associated with a 65% incidence of bowel injury.
      d. Three-point constraints plus airbags provide the optimal protection, especially in front-end collisions.
      e. Secondary collisions of occupant with the vehicle are reduced with the utilization of three-point restraints. Ejection is prevented and mortality is substantially decreased.

TABLE 22-1	Major Mechanisms of Injury and Their Subheadings as Identified in Most Trauma Registries			
Blunt trauma	**Penetrating trauma**	**Thermal trauma**	**Other/MSC**
Motor vehicle crash (MVC)	Gunshot (GSW) or firearm	Burn (BU), flame	Hanging, strangulation or suffocation (ST)
Motorcycle crash (MCC)	Shotgun (SGW)	Burn, chemical	Drowning (DR)
Pedestrian versus automobile (PV)	Stab (SW) or knife (KN) or cut, pierce	Burn, inhalation injury	Electrocution (ES)
Fall (FL)			Poisoning
Assault (AS)			
Blunt instrument (B)			
Bicycle (BI) or pedal cycle			
Nonaccidental trauma (NAT) or child abuse (CH)			
Machinery or equipment (ME)			
Sports or play (SP)			

    f. Three-point constraints are not designed to prevent extremity injuries. Also, there is no effect on major injury patterns with side impact collisions.

    g. Shoulder belt should not be worn without the lap component; the driver and passengers can slip under this restraint.

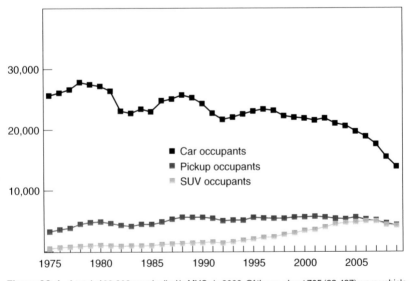

Figure 22-1. A total of 33,808 people died in MVCs in 2009. Of these, about 705 (23,437) were vehicle passengers. Car occupant deaths have declined 45% since 1975, while pickup occupant deaths have risen 29% and SUV occupant deaths are more than 9 times as high. Passenger vehicle occupant deaths by vehicle type, 1975–2009. (Source: Fatality Facts, 2009. Insurance Institute for Highway Safety.) http://www.iihs.org/research/fatality_facts_2009/occupants.html Accessed Oct 21, 2011

TABLE 22-2	**Restraint Devices**

A. Lap belt
B. Shoulder belt
C. Shoulder and lap belts
D. Airbags (frontal and side impact)

    h. Shoulder belt injuries are associated with multiple vascular injuries, including intimal damage or thrombosis of innominate, subclavian, carotid, or vertebral arteries.

    i. Airbags allow a less traumatic deceleration when compared to three-point restraints. The proportion and severity of lower extremity injuries are increased relative to torso and head injuries. However, airbags can cause injuries to occupants who are facing backward or leaning against the steering wheel or into another passenger's compartment.

4. Unrestrained

    a. The majority of injuries in frontal crashes are a result of impact with the steering wheel, windshield, dashboard, or floorboards. These injuries include the head and neck (10% to 37%), thorax (46%), abdomen (5% to 10%), upper extremities (46%), and lower extremities (33% to 66%).

    b. Frontal impacts account for slightly greater than 50% of motor vehicle occupant fatalities, side impacts for 27%, and rollover impact for about 20%.

    c. Lateral crashes ("T-bone")

        i. A lateral crash can result in direct impact between the vehicle and the occupant because of the limited space between the driver and the colliding vehicle.

        ii. Because there is little substantive material to blunt such an impact, lateral impact collisions are associated with twice the mortality of frontal impacts.

        iii. Greater than 12 in. of intrusion on the occupant side signify a greater than 20% chance of significant injury.

        iv. The occupant is projected into the next compartment.

    d. Rear-end impact collisions

        i. Rear-end impact collisions do not usually cause severe injuries, with only 8% of crashes resulting in serious injury.

        ii. An extension–flexion injury ("whiplash") is common.

    e. Rollover collisions

        i. Because of the random nature of these collisions, force vectors vary.

        ii. Kinetic energy of the car is usually dissipated over a long distance.

        iii. Roof collapse can produce severe head injury, and >18 in. of roof or any sidewall intrusion is associated with 20% likelihood of severe injury.

        iv. Axial load forces can result in compression fractures of the spine.

    f. Ejection

        i. Partial or complete ejection of an occupant is highly associated with severe injury. Along with death of an occupant, this is the leading indicator of likelihood of severe injury.

II. MOTORCYCLE CRASHES

    A. Unlike MVCs, the driver or passenger usually absorbs all the impact and the associated kinetic energy.

    B. The majority (75%) of motorcycle deaths are from head injury.

    C. Spine, pelvis, and extremity injuries are also common, with pelvic fractures particularly severe and life-threatening.

    D. There is a high risk of limb loss with open or severe injury to the tibia and fibula.

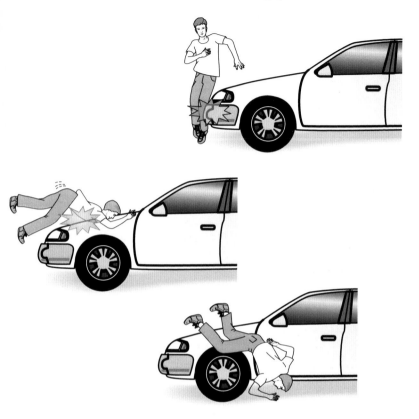

Figure 22-2. Pedestrian–automobile impact.

III. PEDESTRIAN–AUTOMOBILE IMPACTS

A. Although pedestrian–automobile impacts account for only 2% of traffic injuries, they account for 13% of traffic-related deaths. Children, the elderly, and the intoxicated are more at risk for this mechanism of injury. The pattern of injury is depicted in Figure 22-2. Torso trauma (chest, abdomen, and pelvis) represents 6% of the injuries; however, musculoskeletal and intra-abdominal are more common (35% and 27%, respectively).

B. This type of impact often results in **Waddle's triad** of injury: (1) Tibiofibular or femur fracture, (2) truncal injury, and (3) craniofacial injury. Therefore, a patient with two components of Waddle's triad of injury should be assumed to have the third component as well.

C. In general, small children tend to be "run over" and adults "run under" or thrown over the car with impact onto the street.

D. A lateral compression pelvic fracture can occur as a result of contact between the hip and the fender of the motor vehicle.

IV. FALLS

A. Falls in the elderly, including ground level falls, are the leading cause of unintentional injury fatality in the United States, having recently surpassed MVC for this distinction. Anticoagulation medications and other comorbidities contribute.

B. Injuries sustained in falls depend on distance of fall, surface struck, and the position on impact.

C. Energy at impact is the product of the patient's weight times distance of fall times gravitational forces.

    1. Kinetic energy is dissipated on impact throughout the skeleton and soft tissues.

    2. Duration of impact (i.e., how quickly the patient stops) is critical in determining injury severity.

        a. Impact force over a shorter time increases the magnitude of injury.

        b. Harder surfaces increase severity of injury because of immediate deceleration and transfer of all energy to the body (e.g., concrete vs. grass, sand, or snow).

D. Falls of 2 to 3 times the height of the patient are associated with more injury: >20 ft in adults and >10 ft in children. Three story falls have a mortality of 50%. Survival is rare in free falls from above five stories.

E. Injury patterns differ depending on how the patient lands. If the patient lands on his or her feet from a height above 10 to 15 ft, the injuries may include calcaneal, lower extremity, pelvis, and spine fractures. Thoracic aorta and renal injuries can also occur.

F. Falls with a horizontal orientation result in greater energy dissipation and fewer injuries. This is a less predictable injury pattern and includes craniofacial trauma, hand and wrist fractures, along with abdominal and thoracic visceral injuries.

V. ASSAULTS (fisticuffs, kicking, stomping, striking with an object)

A. Young males are the most commonly injured by this mechanism, with injury patterns being variable (depending on the weapon, position of the person being assaulted, and the magnitude and intensity of the attack).

B. Head and facial injuries are more common (72%).

C. Defensive posturing of the patient usually results in lower extremity injuries (10%).

D. Severe torso injuries (including pancreatic and hollow viscus injuries) can occur from a stomping or kicking injury.

E. An intoxicated assault patient with a depressed level of consciousness has an intracranial injury until proven otherwise.

PENETRATING TRAUMA

I. GUNSHOT WOUNDS (GSWS)

A. Introduction

To understand the mechanisms of gunshot injuries, it is important to understand the nature of firearms and their projectiles. **Ballistics** is defined as the scientific study of projectile motion and is divided into three categories: Internal, external, and terminal ballistics. Internal ballistics has to do with the projectile within the firearm. External ballistics describes the projectile in the air. Terminal ballistics relates to actions of the projectile in its target. Wound ballistics is a subset of terminal ballistics; it is the most important aspect of ballistics for physicians to understand. However, to completely understand the wounding process some knowledge of all aspects of ballistics is necessary.

B. Types of firearms

    1. Handguns, rifles, airguns, and shotguns are the major firearms encountered in civilian injuries in the United States. The wounding potential of each is different; it is important to be aware of these differences. Fully automatic weapons are illegal in the United States, and injuries from these weapons are infrequent. Fully automatic weapons differ only from rifles and handguns in their ability to autoload and the resultant rapidity of fire. The injuries caused by the individual projectiles are essentially the same as those of handgun and rifle injuries. Handguns and rifles have many characteristics in common and will be discussed together. Airguns and shotguns differ in their wounding characteristics from other weapons and will be discussed separately.

    2. Handguns and rifles. Handguns and rifles fire bullets. Before firing, the lead bullet is held firmly in the end of a brass cartridge case. This cartridge case contains

TABLE 22-3   Ballistic Data for Four Handguns

Caliber (in.)	Weapon type	Bullet weight (grains)	Muzzle velocity (ft/s)	Kinetic energy (ft-lb)
0.25	25 automatic	50	810	73
0.354	9-mm Luger	115	1,155	341
0.357	357 magnum	158	1,410	696
0.44	44 magnum	240	1,470	1,150

in., inches; ft/s, feet per second; ft-lb, foot-pounds.

a flammable propellant (the charge) and has a primer at its base. When the firing pin of the gun strikes the primer, the primer is detonated, igniting the charge within the cartridge case. The burning gasses expand and propel the bullet from the cartridge case and along the barrel of the gun. Spiral grooves within the barrel of the gun (rifling) grip the bullet causing it to spin around its long axis. This spinning creates a gyroscopic effect, which prevents yaw, or the deviation of the longitudinal axis of the bullet from its line of flight. This gives the bullet directional stability in the air, enabling it to travel more accurately than a nonspinning projectile, analogous to the stable flight of a football when a long pass is thrown with a "perfect" spiral, as compared with the wobble when thrown imperfectly. The longer the barrel, the more time the bullet has to accelerate and the faster it will be going when it leaves the gun. Because rifles have longer barrels than handguns, rifle bullets leave the gun with much higher velocities than handgun bullets (Tables 22-3 and 22-4).

a. Since the kinetic energy of the bullet is equal to half its mass multiplied by the square of its velocity, high-velocity bullets have much higher kinetic energy than low-velocity bullets.

$$KE = 1/2\,mv^2$$

(KE = kinetic energy in Joules; m = mass in grams; v = velocity in feet/second.)
This higher kinetic energy gives rifle bullets greater wounding potential than the handgun bullets.

b. Wounding potential is only part of the equation. The type of projectile, type of tissue injured, and the distance (range) between the weapon and the patient all have major effect on these injuries. In direct contact injuries, both the energy of the bullet and much of the combustion gasses enter the patient, causing considerable tissue expansion and more severe injuries than noncontact injuries. The same handgun or rifle can often fire several different types of projectiles. The construction of these projectiles has a major effect on wounding.

TABLE 22-4   Ballistic Data for Four Rifles

Caliber (in.)	Weapon type	Bullet weight (grains)	Muzzle velocity (ft/s)	Kinetic energy (ft-lb)
0.22	Remington 22	40	1,180	124
0.223	M-16	55	3,200	1,248
0.270	270 Winchester	150	2,900	2,810
0.308	30-0	150	2,910	2,820

in., inches; ft/s, feet per second; ft-lb, foot-pounds.

c. It is important to be aware not only of the behavior of projectiles before and after impact, but also of the manner in which various tissues respond to gunshot injuries. More elastic tissues, such as lung or fat, dissipate energy well. Less elastic tissues, such as brain, liver, or spleen (solid organs) do not dissipate energy well, with more tissue damage resulting from similar kinetic energy of the missile.

d. Although rifle bullets have greater energy available for wounding than handgun bullets, the wounding mechanisms of both are similar in many respects. When the bullet strikes human tissue, it ceases spinning. Having lost its directional stability, it is now able to "tumble" (rotate around its short axis). A nondeformed bullet will usually be tapered at its tip and hence have more mass concentrated at its base. Momentum will cause the bullet to tumble through 180 degrees and continue through the tissue with its heavier base leading. If the bullet is deformed by impact with the tissue, this tendency to tumble will be modified and may even be eliminated completely. If there is sufficient width of tissue for the bullet to complete its 180-degree tumble, it will carve an elliptical-shaped tunnel of tissue damage, known as the *permanent cavity*. A shockwave is generated by this damage, compressing the adjacent tissue. This is known as the *temporary cavity* and is also elliptical in shape. Damage in the temporary cavity varies from one tissue to another and generally increases with increasing tissue-specific gravity.

e. Bullets are classified by caliber, which is a measurement of the diameter of the bullet, most commonly in decimals of an inch (e.g., 0.357) or in millimeters (e.g., 9 mm). The measurement of caliber does not address the weight of the bullet, construction of the bullet, or the size of the charge, all of which are important factors in determining the wounding potential (Tables 22-3, 22-4, 22-5, and 22-6). Most bullets are made of lead. In some low-velocity weapons, the bullet is made entirely of lead. In medium- and high-velocity weapons, bullets usually have a metal jacket surrounding the lead to protect it from deformity, while the bullet is in the gun barrel. A copper jacket is most common, but occasionally other metals are used. If the bullet is entirely encased, it is said to have a *full metal jacket;* if the bullet is partially encased, it is said to be *semi-jacketed.* Semi-jacketed bullets typically have exposed lead at the tip, are also referred to as *soft-point bullets,* and are designed to deform on impact. Some bullets have an open cavity in their tips and are referred to as *hollow-point bullets.* Hollow-point bullets are also designed to deform on impact and typically transform into a mushroom shape. When bullets deform

TABLE 22-5	Blunt Trauma: Documented and Possible Associated Injuries
Documented injury	**Possible associated injuries**
Neck hyperextension	Carotid artery injury
Sternal, scapular, or upper thoracic trauma	Thoracic aortic injury, pulmonary and myocardial contusion, atrial rupture
Lower chest wall injury (rib 6–12)	Left side—splenic injury Right side—hepatic injury
Lap belt sign and lumbar fracture	Pancreatic contusion/transection, intestinal rupture
Lap belt sign	Intestinal rupture, mesenteric rent/contusion
Severe pelvic fracture	Bladder rupture, urethral transection, rectal/vaginal injury
Shoulder dislocation (anterior)	Axillary nerve injury
Knee dislocation (posterior)	Popliteal artery injury (intimal tear/thrombosis) supracondylar femur fracture
Bilateral calcaneal fractures	Spinal column fractures, renal injury, aortic injuries, lower extremity fractures

TABLE 22-6	Penetrating Trauma: Documented and Possible Associated Injuries

Documented injury	Possible associated injuries
Cervical (platysma penetration)	Jugular vein/carotid artery injury, tracheal/ injuries, esophageal injury
Transmediastinal injury	Cardiac/tracheobronchial and pulmonary/vascular/ diaphragmatic/gastrointestinal injury
Thoracoabdominal injury	Pulmonary/diaphragmatic/cardiac/gastrointestinal injury
Transabdominal injury	Gastrointestinal/hepatic/vascular injury
Transpelvic injury	Bladder/intestinal/uterine/vascular injury
Flank injury	Genitourinary/intestinal injury

on impact, they decelerate more quickly, delivering more of their energy to a smaller volume of tissue. This is intended to increase tissue damage, making deforming bullets more effective at wounding than nondeforming bullets. A deformed bullet, particularly one with a mushroomed tip, tends not to tumble. High-velocity rifle bullets, particularly the soft- and hollow-point varieties, tend to fragment on impact with tissue. This fragmentation leads to an expanding conical pattern of permanent injury, as the fragments separate from one another.

f. Bullet injuries are most severe in friable solid organs (e.g., the liver and brain), where damage may be caused by temporary cavitation remote from the actual bullet track. Dense tissues (e.g., bone) and loose tissues (e.g., subcutaneous fat) are more resistant to bullet injury. Bones modify the behavior of bullets markedly, altering their course, slowing them down, and increasing their deformity and fragmentation.

g. In general, bullets and bullet fragments follow a straight trajectory, even after entering tissue. Bullets that strike rigid changes in tissue density, such as bone cortices and dense fascia, will often be deflected from their initial course. After this deflection the fragments will continue in a relatively straight trajectory unless they encounter another solid interface. Bullets that pass through intermediate targets (e.g., a door or wall) may already be deformed before they strike the patient and will always have reduced energy.

3. **Airguns.** Airguns do not use a flammable charge to propel their projectiles down the barrel but rely simply on air pressure from pumps, springs, or gas canisters. These weapons usually fire pellets in the form of round BBs or waisted lead slugs. In general these weapons have low muzzle velocity and therefore low wounding potential. The construction of airguns may resemble either rifles or handguns and once again, longer barreled weapons will impart more kinetic energy to their projectiles.

a. Low-velocity weapons, including both airguns and small-caliber handguns, have much lower wounding potential than high-velocity weapons. Whereas close-range injuries with low-velocity projectiles can be fatal, medium- and long-range injuries are often superficial. The subcutaneous tissue offers the path of least resistance for low-velocity projectiles, which may travel long distances through the subcutaneous tissue but fail to penetrate the fascia. This phenomenon is most common at medium to long range and when the entry wound is at a shallow angle to the skin surface.

4. **Shotguns**

a. Shotgun injuries differ substantially from rifle and handgun wounds. Unlike the single bullet of a rifle or handgun cartridge, shotgun shells usually contain multiple metal pellets, also known as shot. Typically, the shotgun shell is made of plastic with a brass cap at the base containing the primer. The charge is separated from the pellets by a wadding material that may be either paper or plastic. In contact or very close range injuries the wadding will be projected into the patient along with the pellets and expanding gasses. Shotguns do not have rifled barrels, hence their pellets do not spin.

b. The size of shotgun cartridges is measured *gauge*, not caliber. The higher the gauge, the smaller is the diameter. Shotgun shells are much larger than rifle or handgun cartridges and generally containing a much bigger charge and a greater total mass of projectiles. However, shotgun pellets separate after leaving the barrel of the gun and their velocity rapidly decreases. As the pellets spread their area of distribution increases and the energy in each pellet decreases. Thus, range differences affect the wounding potential of shotgun pellets far more than they affect the wounding potential of bullets. At close range (less than 15 ft) shotgun injuries are usually far more severe than bullet injuries because the total energy available is much greater, but further away the damage decreases substantially.

c. The combined mass of multiple pellets spread over a small area can produce massive destruction of soft tissue and bone. At long range, the wider spread and lower velocity of the pellets produce multiple, widely separated, superficial injuries that are often painful but rarely life threatening. At intermediate range, shotgun injuries are less predictable, with severity being mainly a function of anatomic location and pellet density. Pellets come in many sizes, but each individual cartridge usually contains only one size. Larger pellets are known as *buckshot,* and smaller pellets are called *birdshot.* Most injuries encountered in clinical practice involve birdshot.

d. As with bullet injuries, the severity of shotgun injuries varies with tissue type and local anatomy. Vascular injuries are of particular concern because the smaller size of the pellets makes embolization more likely than with bullets. Such emboli can result in tissue infarction.

e. In the past, all shotgun pellets were made of lead. However, recent wildlife regulations require shotgun pellets to be made of steel, when they are used on waterfowl. Steel pellets are ferromagnetic and can move if the patient is exposed to a strong magnetic field, thus causing additional damage. Therefore, magnetic resonance (MR) imaging may be contraindicated in such patients. Fortunately, steel and lead pellets can usually be distinguished from one another at radiography. Lead pellets tend to be deformed and fragmented by impact with soft tissues and bone, whereas steel shot usually remains round. Simple analysis of a radiograph is all that is needed to determine if a patient with a shotgun injury can be safely placed in the MR imaging magnet.

II. GUNSHOT INJURY ASSESSMENT

A. Prompt and accurate clinical and radiographic assessment of the injuries is essential. While entrance and exit wounds have differing characteristics, distinguishing one from the other is unreliable. It is best to refer to both simply as surface wounds and characterize their appearance and location carefully. Both the surgical approach and planning of imaging are aided by the prompt acquisition of initial plain radiographs. Metallic markers should be put beside each surface wound, before obtaining the radiographs. Two perpendicular projections of the injured area are essential. If the projectiles are a long distance from the entry site, they may not be included in the field of view of the initial radiographs. If a low-velocity projectile is not found on the initial radiographs and there is no exit wound, additional radiographs over a wider field of view should be obtained.

B. With good imaging data, the organs at risk can be determined and the best possible action plan formulated. In unstable patients, there is often time only for conventional radiography before the patient must be taken to the operating room; these essential initial films can provide important information as to bullet quality, fragmentation, pathway, or other unsuspected foreign bodies. In stable patients computed tomography (CT) offers a more accurate road map of the injury. A rapid and accurate assessment of the path of the projectile and its direction of travel often aids the planning of surgical approach, particularly if the fragment has crossed body cavities, such as trans-mediastinal, transdiaphragmatic, or transpelvic. Any time the bullet or pellets are close to major vessels, conventional or CT angiography should be considered. Significant vascular injuries may be present, even when peripheral pulses are normal. To emphasize, **hemodynamic instability from presumed hemorrhagic shock precludes detailed imaging.**

C. In general, bullets that are not causing mechanical problems can safely be left in the tissues, with one exception. Bullets left within synovial joints result in slow leeching of lead by the synovial fluid. This leads to chronic inflammatory changes within the synovium and to a gradual increase in serum lead levels. After many years, the patient will develop not only a chronic, debilitating lead arthropathy but also systemic lead poisoning. Therefore, remove bullets and pellets within synovial joints.

D. Imaging details. Evaluation of bone injuries and the distribution of bone and bullet fragments on radiographs can be helpful in determining the direction of travel, which is important not only for clinical assessment but also for forensic evaluation of the incident. Bone and bullet fragments are usually distributed along the bullet track within the soft tissues, beyond the defect in the bone. Careful examination of the images should reveal beveling of the bone toward the direction of travel.

    1. The degree of bullet fragmentation is also visible on radiographs. Bullets with full metal jackets often remain in one piece and usually do not deform. These projectiles typically do not leave a trail of lead fragments along their path. On the other hand, hollow-point, nonjacketed, and soft-point bullets tend to deform on impact or break apart, leaving a trail of metal fragments through the soft tissues. Hollow-point handgun bullets usually deform by simply mushrooming with minimal fragmentation, whereas high-velocity soft-point rifle bullets often undergo marked fragmentation. This fragmentation of high-velocity bullets creates a "lead snowstorm" appearance on radiographs. The area over which the lead snowstorm fragments are deposited in the soft tissues widens as the distance from the entry site increases. A conical distribution of lead fragments in radiographs will have the apex of the cone pointing toward the entry site.

    2. While the makeup of shotgun pellets (lead vs. steel) can usually be determined based on their radiographic image as stated previously, the same is not true for jacketed bullets. The type of metal used for the jacket cannot be determined from radiographs. Because bullet jackets are occasionally made of steel, it may not be safe to place a bullet wound patient into an MR imager when the nature of the bullet construction is unknown.

III. STAB WOUNDS

A. Stab wounds result from "hand-driven" weapons, such as knives, but also include more unusual weapons or offending agents such as ice picks, glass shards, sharp edges of metal, or even wooden posts. A description of the stab wound includes the length, width, and the depth of penetration of the offending agent, although this last dimension is seldom known at the time of initial evaluation. It is helpful to have direct examination of the weapon, as the patient's or witnesses' perceptions may not be accurate given the heightened emotional states at the time of injury. Wound size and history of type of weapon do not necessarily correlate to depth of wound or wound trajectory.

B. Slash wounds are usually long lacerations of relatively shallow depth. These wounds tend to gape, allowing easy visual inspection of their depth. **Impalement wounds** are those in which the offending agent is plunged into the patient along the long axis of the blade, resulting in a small puncture wound of the skin and unknown depth. In common use, "stab" implies the use of a knife, whereas "impalement" connotes a larger object driven into the torso. If the wounding agent is still in the patient on arrival at the treatment facility, it is best removed in the operating room. An impaling object can be providing tamponade of major vessels and therefore should be removed under direct vision. Of stab wounds, 4% mortality rate is primarily from direct injury to the great vessels or the heart.

C. **Impalement** usually occurs secondary to a fall onto a piercing object or sustained from machinery or pneumatic tools (nail guns), but also includes low-velocity missiles such as arrows. The wound can be complicated by blunt deceleration from the fall, by secondary injuries resulting from extraction by untrained personnel, or by unintentional shifts of the impaling object during transport.

D. Arrows are fired for hunting and recreational pursuit. **Crossbows** generate bolt velocity of 61.0 to 84.4 m/s (200 to 275 ft/s). Bolts are usually unable to pass through weight-bearing bone, but easily penetrate ribs, sternum, posterior vertebral elements, and calvarium. **Archery and hunting bows** can generate arrow velocities up to 74 m/s (240 ft/s). Arrow penetration is a function of arrow momentum (weight and velocity) and type of tip (target vs. hunting). These wounds should be treated as an impalement.

AXIOMS

- Patterns of injury are associated with specific mechanisms.
- Severity of injury depends on the energy transferred to the injured person.
- Falls of 25 to 30 ft (three stories) have a mortality of 50%.
- Trajectory defines anatomic injury.
- Follow the entire trajectory/pathway of the penetrating agent to find all the injuries.
- Do not describe bullet wounds as exit or entrance wounds; describe location and appearance of wounds only.
- Objects that are impaled in the patient should be removed in the operating room.

Suggested Readings

Adams DB. Wound ballistics: A review. *Mil Med* 1982;147:831–835.

Benoit R, Watts DD, Dwyer K, et al. Windows 99: A source of suburban pediatric trauma. *J Trauma* 2000;49(3):477–482.

Centers for Disease Control and Prevention. Deaths resulting from firearm- and motor-vehicle-related injuries—United States, 1968–1991. *JAMA* 1994;271:495–496.

Centers for Disease Control and Prevention. Firearm-related deaths—Louisiana and Texas, 1970–1990. *JAMA* 1992;267:3008–3009.

Centers for Disease Control and Prevention. Wonder Web site. Available at: http://wonder.cdc.gov. Accessed October 3, 2006.

Choi CH, Pritchard J, Richard J. Path of bullet and injuries determined by radiography. *Am J Forensic Med Pathol* 1990;11:244–245.

Collins KA, Lantz PE. Interpretation of fatal, multiple, and exiting gunshot wounds by trauma specialists. *J Forensic Sci* 1994;39:94–99.

Dimaio VJM. *Gunshot Wounds: Practical Aspects of Firearms, Ballistics, and Forensic Techniques.* Boca Raton, FL: CRC Press; 1985:163–226, 257–265.

Dischinger PC, Cushing BM, Kerns TJ. Injury patterns associated with direction of impact: Drivers admitted to trauma centers. *J Trauma* 1993;35:454.

Fackler ML. How to describe bullet holes. *Ann Emerg Med* 1994;23:386–387.

Feliciano DV, Wall MJ Jr. Patterns of injury. In: Moore EE, Mattox KL, Feliciano DV, eds. *Trauma.* Norwalk, CT: Appleton & Lange; 1988:81–96.

Glezer JA, Minard G, Croce MA, et al. Shotgun wounds to the abdomen. *Am Surg* 1993;59:129–132.

Hollerman JJ, Fackler ML, Coldwell DM, et al. Gunshot wounds. I. Bullets, ballistics, and mechanisms of injury. *AJR Am J Roentgenol* 1990;155:685–690.

Hollerman JJ, Fackler ML, Coldwell DM, et al. Gunshot wounds. II. Radiology. *AJR Am J Roentgenol* 1990;155:691–702.

Lowenstein SR, Yaron M, Carrero R, et al. Vertical trauma: Injuries to patients who fall and land on their feet. *Ann Emerg Med* 1989;18:161–165.

Macpherson AK, Rothman L, McKeag AM, et al. Mechanism of injury affects 6-month functional outcome in children hospitalized because of severe injuries. *J Trauma* 2003;55(3):454–458.

McGwin G Jr, Metzger J, Porterfield JR, et al. Association between side air bags and risk of injury in motor vehicle collisions with near-side impact. *J Trauma* 2003;55(3):430–436.

Padra JC, Barone JE, Reed DM, et al. Expanding handgun bullets. *J Trauma* 1997;43:516–520.

Peng RY, Bongard F. Pedestrian versus motor vehicle accidents: An analysis of 5,000 patients. *J Am Coll Surg* 1999;189:343.

Phillips CD. Emergent radiologic evaluation of the gunshot wound victim. *Radiol Clin North Am* 1992;30:307–324.

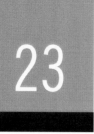

23 Traumatic Brain Injury

Meredith S. Tinti, Vicente H. Gracias and Peter D. Le Roux

TRAUMATIC BRAIN INJURY

Central nervous system (CNS) injury is the most common cause of death from injury. Two million people per year in the United States suffer traumatic brain injuries (TBIs), many as the result of motor vehicle crashes and falls. Approximately 50,000 deaths per year and 500,000 hospital admissions are attributable to head injury. Most of these victims are between the ages of 16 and 30 years and motor vehicle crashes are responsible for the majority of these injuries. The increasing use of seat belts and airbags has resulted in an estimated 20% to 25% reduction in traffic fatalities. However, the incidence of penetrating injury to the brain and spinal cord is increasing. As awareness of literature based methods for brain injury management grows, guidelines for TBI have been developed and have been shown to improve the outcome.

I. ANATOMY AND PHYSIOLOGY

A. The **skull** is particularly thin in the temporal region and thick in the occiput. The floor of the cranial cavity or the skull base is divided into three regions: Anterior (houses the frontal lobes), middle (contains the temporal lobes), and posterior cranial fossa (houses the lower brainstem and cerebellum).

B. The **meninges** cover the brain in three layers: Dura mater (fibrous membrane that adheres to the internal surface of the skull), arachnoid membrane, and pia mater (attached to the surface of the brain). Cerebrospinal fluid (CSF) circulates between the arachnoid membrane and pia mater in the subarachnoid space.

C. The **brain** is comprised of the cerebrum, cerebellum, and the brainstem.

  1. The **cerebrum** is the largest and most well developed portion of the brain. It is responsible for language/communication, learning/memory, movement and sensory processing.

  2. The **cerebellum** is located at the bottom of the brain. It is responsible for motor coordination and motor learning.

  3. The **brainstem** consists of the posterior portion of the brain that adjoins the spinal cord. It consists of the midbrain, pons, and medulla. The reticular activating system (responsible for state of alertness) is within the midbrain and upper pons. The cardiorespiratory centers reside in the medulla.

D. The **Monro–Kellie doctrine** states that the total volume of intracranial contents must remain constant because of the rigid bony cranium. With an expanding mass lesion or cerebral edema, **CSF** and blood volume within the skull decrease to compensate and maintain intracranial pressure (ICP) within normal limits. This occurs until the point of decompensation on the pressure–volume curve is reached and then ICP dramatically increases.

E. **Cerebral perfusion pressure (CPP) = Mean arterial pressure – ICP.** Maintenance of cerebral perfusion is essential in the management of patients with severe closed head injury.

  1. Normal **cerebral blood flow (CBF)** is approximately 50 mL/100 g brain/minute or 15% of cardiac output and this flow rate is tightly regulated to maintain the metabolic activity of the brain. CBF <20 mL/100 g brain/minute causes cerebral ischemia, and cell death occurs at approximately 5 mL/100 g brain/minute. CBF >65 mL/100 g brain/minute causes hyperemia of the brain and raises ICP. CBF is determined by many factors, the most important of which is CPP.

2. Under normal circumstances, CPP is relatively constant due to the brain's intact autoregulatory system. With TBI, this autoregulation can be lost and the practitioner must regulate the CPP, goal 60 to 70 mm Hg.

II. TBIs are categorized as mild (80%), moderate (10%), or severe (10%), depending on the level of neurologic dysfunction at the time of initial evaluation. Loss of consciousness (LOC) is an important indicator of TBI. Determination of the **Glasgow Coma Scale (GCS)** score as early as possible and then serially is essential. Classification of TBI is based on the GCS.

A. Mild head injury = GCS 13 to 15

1. Brief period of LOC or other signs of concussion (10% to 35% will have a lesion detected on CT)
2. Most prevalent type of brain injury
3. Diagnosis often missed at time of injury
4. Prognosis is excellent (although may have long lasting consequences)
5. Mortality rate 1%

B. Moderate head injury = GCS 9 to 12

1. Confused and may have focal neurologic deficits
2. Prognosis is good but 12% will progress to severe TBI
3. Mortality rate 5%

C. Severe head injury = GCS ≤8

1. Generally, the accepted definition of coma
2. Until recently, mortality was 40%. Mortality is still approximately 20%
3. Most survivors have significant disabilities
4. Early airway control is essential
5. Elevated ICP is a common cause of death and neurologic disability
6. Requires multi-modality treatment

III. INITIAL EVALUATION AND TREATMENT OF BRAIN INJURY

A. General

1. Patients suspected of having a head injury, particularly if confused or unresponsive, require emergency evaluation and treatment at a center with capabilities for immediate neurosurgical intervention. General objectives are rapid diagnosis and evacuation of intracranial mass lesions, expedient treatment of extracranial injuries, and avoidance of secondary brain injury.
   a. **Secondary brain injury** is due to hypoxia or hypotension. Other secondary insults such as hyperglycemia, hypothermia, and anemia may also exacerbate outcome during the hospital course.
   b. All patients with clinical signs of brain injury should be evaluated with CT. Those with findings on CT scan require admission to the hospital and serial neurologic examinations.
2. Severe brain injury is associated with cerebral ischemia. Therefore, a principal therapeutic goal is to enhance cerebral perfusion and oxygenation and avoid further ischemic injury to the brain.
3. ICU admission should be considered in all patients with moderate to severe TBI.
   a. Changes in motor score portion of GCS are most prognostic.

B. Initial management of the unresponsive patient with brain injury—ABCs

1. **A**irway/**B**reathing—intubation with controlled ventilation
   a. If possible, perform a focused neurologic examination, including assessment of GCS, pupillary response, and all four extremity movements, before intubation and pharmacologic paralysis.
   b. Avoid routine hyperventilation. Hyperventilation causes cerebral vasoconstriction and can worsen cerebral ischemia. Hyperventilation is indicated only in the setting of abrupt neurologic deterioration with suspected herniation and is used as a short-term rescue therapy.
2. **C**irculation—venous access

    a. Restore intravascular volume, blood pressure, and perfusion.

    b. Avoid hypotonic and dextrose-containing solutions.

  3. Disability—immobilization and serial neurologic examinations

    a. Immobilize the patient with full spine precautions and cervical spine (C-spine) collar. Assume that all patients with TBI have a spine injury until proven otherwise.

    b. Repeat neurologic examination and assessment of GCS. Documentation of the GCS in patients who are intubated or "tubed" should be noted by a T (i.e., GCS 11T) and in patients who are intubated and pharmacologically paralyzed, with TP (i.e., GCS 3TP). This allows meaningful interpretation of the GCS score.

  4. Add pharmacologic agents if agitated or combative

    a. Short-acting agents are recommended.

      i. Analgesia: Fentanyl or morphine

      ii. Sedation: Propofol, avoid long-acting benzodiazepines

      iii. Paralytics: Vecuronium bromide, cisatracurium, or succinylcholine

  5. Monitoring—monitor and record blood pressure and O_2 saturation continuously.

  6. Laboratory evaluation—check arterial blood gasses (ABGs), blood glucose, electrolytes, prothrombin time (PT), partial thromboplastin time (PTT), hematocrit, and platelet count. With active therapy for elevated ICP, serum sodium levels and osmolality should be tracked frequently.

  7. Radiologic diagnosis of brain injury. Rapid acquisition of a computed tomographic (CT) of the head and complete C-spine (if time permits) should be obtained for all classifications of brain injury. On the basis of time, distance, and local capabilities, transfer may be necessary. Rapid referral to a center capable of immediate neurosurgical intervention may be required. Do not delay transport to definitive care to obtain a CT of the head. Early diagnosis and evacuation of cranial mass lesions are critical.

C. Secondary management of brain injury

  1. The avoidance of secondary brain injury is essential. Secondary brain injury is produced by hypoxia and hypotension. A single episode of hypotension (systolic blood pressure <90 mm Hg) in the adult will worsen prognosis and can increase mortality up to 50%.

  2. The GCS obtained in the emergency department may be a more reliable assessment of the severity of brain injury than the GCS obtained in the field.

  3. The GCS cannot be assessed by simple observation and requires stimulation of the patient. In cases of asymmetry in either eye opening or motor scores, the best score is used.

  4. Should emergent operative intervention be required and CT capabilities not available, a lateral C-spine x-ray study should be obtained to evaluate for gross injury or malalignment of the C-spine (Fig. 23-1). If available, and time permits, rapid C-spine CT should be used to detect fractures as well.

IV. TREATMENT OF SEVERE TBI

A. Intensive care management of patients with severe TBI (GCS ≤8). The goal is to prevent secondary brain injury by limiting focal cerebral ischemia, preventing cerebral hypoxia, and maintaining adequate cerebral perfusion. This can be accomplished only by the continuous monitoring of several physiologic parameters and the judicious use of therapies to lower elevated ICP.

  1. Physiologic monitoring

    a. Arterial blood pressure. Noninvasive monitoring can be used, but an arterial catheter is preferred.

    b. Heart rate, electrocardiogram (ECG), temperature, and pulse oximetry.

    c. Central venous pressure or pulmonary artery catheter monitoring

    d. Fluid balance (intake and output).

    e. Laboratory evaluation. ABGs every 4 to 6 hours initially; electrolytes, glucose, and serum osmolality (if receiving mannitol) every 6 hours; hemoglobin/hematocrit, PT, PTT, platelets every 12 hours.

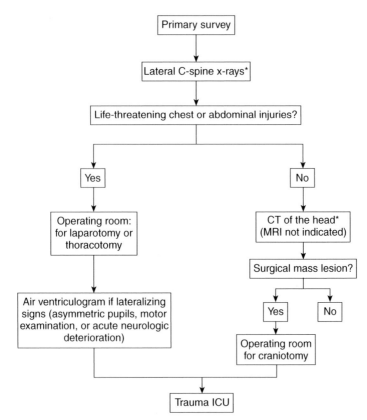

Figure 23-1. Emergency department triage of severe brain injury. *can be deleted if CT of the C-spine can be accomplished rapidly with CT of the brain

    f. ICP monitoring.

    g. Brain tissue O_2 and/or cerebral microdialysis (if available)

    h. Jugular venous O_2 saturation or O_2 content (if available)

2. Initial treatment

    a. Blood pressure. Mean arterial blood pressure >80 mm Hg. **No** role for antihypertensive medications in TBI before brain CT and ICP monitoring performed. If mass effect, treat elevated ICP rather than elevated BP.

    b. Oxygenation/Ventilation. Keep pO_2 >60 torr. Aim for arterial oxygen saturation 100%. Hyperventilation ONLY with impending herniation. Target normocapnia (pCO_2 34 to 40 torr).

    c. Volume status. Keep central venous pressure 8 to 15 cm H_2O and hematocrit ≤32%.

    d. Glycemic control/Tonicity. Avoid dextrose-containing intravenous solutions for first 24 hours; avoid free water for extent of active therapy unless diabetes insipidus is present. Tight glucose control; avoid hyperglycemia.

    e. Coagulation profile. Correct coagulopathy rapidly. Ensure normal PT, PTT, and platelet count.

    f. Normothermia. Maintain a normal temperature (<99°F)

    g. Anticonvulsant prophylaxis. Current recommendations are for the prophylactic use (dosing without levels) of phenytoin during the first 7 days following injury in patients at high risk for early posttraumatic seizures. These risk factors include cortical contusion, subdural hematoma, penetrating head wound, epidural hematoma, depressed skull fracture, intracerebral hematoma, or seizure within 24 hours of injury but not at the time of injury. Seizure activity not related to acute injury event requires prolonged anticonvulsant therapy. Phenytoin should always be administered by giving a test dose and subsequently, monitoring for myocardial depression.

h. Steroids. There is **no** indication for the use of steroids in TBI.

i. Nutrition. Begin nutritional supplementation within 48 hours of the injury. TBI may increase caloric requirements by 25%. Aim for approximately 25 to 30 kcal/kg/day with either enteral (preferred) or parenteral supplementation. Most of these patients will tolerate gastric or postpyloric feeding.

j. Repeat CT of the head should be obtained within 24 hours after the initial scan to detect delayed posttraumatic hematomas and should be obtained with any abrupt increase in ICP, worsening of the neurologic examination (GCS declines by 2 or motor score decreases) or the patient develops hypoxia.

3. ICP monitoring

a. Indications for ICP monitoring. As a general approach, liberal use of ICP monitoring in patients with severe TBI (GCS ≤8) is recommended. An ICP monitor should be used with a brain oxygen monitor (if available). ICP monitoring is not routinely indicated for patients with moderate or mild closed head injury. An ICP monitor should also be considered in a patient with moderate head injury who is going to the OR for other injuries.

　i. Severe closed head injury (GCS ≤8) and abnormal CT of head

　　a) Abnormal CT: Hemorrhage, intracerebral hematoma, parenchymal contusion

　ii. Severe closed head injury (GCS ≤8) and normal CT of head, if two or more of the following exist: Age >40 years, unilateral or bilateral flexor or extensor posturing, systolic blood pressure <90 mm Hg

b. Types of ICP monitors

　i. Fiberoptic parenchymal catheters are transducers (not truly catheters) that are inserted through a bolt. They monitor ICP and allow the use of direct brain oxygen monitoring. They are easier to insert than ventricular catheters and are associated with a lower risk than ventriculostomies. However, they are more expensive and do not allow for CSF drainage (Fig. 23-2).

　ii. Ventriculostomy catheters coupled with a strain gauge can be used to monitor ICP, particularly when there is hydrocephalus. This system is relatively inexpensive, accurate, and allows CSF drainage when needed to control ICP.

　　a) Continuous CSF drainage is not recommended; the ventricular walls can collapse around the catheter tip and occlude its ports.

B. Treatment of elevated ICP

1. Positioning—elevate head of bed and loosen C-collar to decrease ICP.

2. Control of the environment—monitor room temperature to maintain normothermia, decrease ambient lighting, and limit external stimuli.

3. Analgesia/Sedation—these medications decrease external stimuli to the brain and decrease the metabolic demand, therefore decreasing ICP.

a. Use short-acting agents that allow frequent neurologic examinations.

b. Remember that sedatives do not have analgesic effects, so both agents should be used.

4. Optimize CPP—volume resuscitate to CVP 10 to 12 mm Hg and initiate vasopressors as needed to keep CPP 50 to 70 mm Hg.

5. Mannitol—causes an osmotic diuresis that decreases intracerebral edema. Bolus therapy (0.25 to 1.0 g/kg) should be used with observed effect in 20 to 60 minutes. A repeat dose may be given if no effect within 20 minutes of the initial dose and every 6 hours after that for ICP >20. Osmolality should be maintained at <320 milliosmol (mOsm).

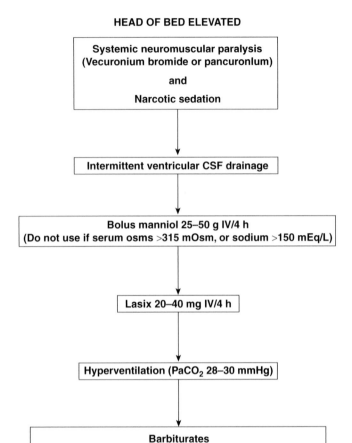

Figure 23-2. Steps for the management of elevated ICP.

    a. Mannitol has no effect above 320 mOsm.
    b. Should not be given as continuous infusion or dosed more frequently than every 6 hours as this will allow equalization of the mannitol molecules across the membranes.
    c. Contraindicated in patients with poor renal perfusion.
    d. Must monitor for hypovolemia and hyperosmolality during use.
  6. Hypertonic saline—given as either a bolus dose or continuous infusion after mannitol failure and persistently elevated ICPs. Must be administered via a central line and requires close monitoring of central volumes as this is a vasoactive solution (concentration varies between institutions). Titrate to sodium 155 to 160 mEq/L.
  7. Acute hyperventilation—may be used to treat some patients with high ICP when there is hyperemia (elevated brain oxygen or narrow arteriovenous oxygen content difference) as detected on adjunctive monitoring systems. It should be

used **only** when a measure of its effects (e.g., brain oxygen or CBF) is in place; hyperventilation should be stopped if it adversely affects these parameters.

8. **Barbiturate coma**—second line therapy for ICP control in pediatric population when all other treatments have failed. No current indication for use in adults.

   a. When using barbiturates, patients should receive a pulmonary artery catheter and undergo continuous EEG monitoring. The depression of myocardial contractility can be minimized by maintenance of a high-normal intravascular volume. All patients receiving barbiturate therapy (for elevated ICP) should have frequent measurements of cardiac output and preload. EEG monitoring to observe burst suppression should be used.

9. **Hypothermia**—in theory, decreasing temperatures to $33°C$ for 48 hours is neuroprotective and prevents ischemia/reperfusion injury. Not proven to be effective in TBI.

10. **Decompressive craniectomy**—craniectomy for refractory elevation in ICP without a surgical lesion (therapeutic surgical intervention such as craniotomy, craniectomy, or burr holes should be the first step in management of patients with extra-axial blood). Minimal literature to support this practice and unclear outcomes.

C. Adjunctive monitoring

1. **Brain tissue oxygen monitoring ($PbtO_2$)**—a fiberoptic catheter is placed into the white matter of the brain in the penumbra of the injury to measure brain tissue oxygenation. Adjustments in FiO_2, PEEP, and ICP management can be made based on the $PbtO_2$ readings. Cerebral Cortical Oxygen monitoring has been shown to decrease mortality in severe TBI patients.

2. **Jugular venous bulb oximetry (SjO_2)**—a catheter is placed in the IJ and is directed upward toward the jugular venous bulb. Intermittent blood samples are drawn from the catheter to measure venous saturation of blood leaving the brain. Goal is to balance oxygen consumption and oxygen delivery. Normal is 50% to 75%.

3. **Transcranial Doppler**—noninvasive method of assessing intracranial circulation. It is a good prognosticator but has limited use in clinical management at this time.

D. Prognosis after severe TBI

1. The outcome following severe TBI is strongly correlated with initial GCS score, pupil reactivity and size, age, ICP (pressures >20 mm Hg or inability to reduce elevated ICP), surgical intracranial mass lesions (extent of midline shift), hypotension (systolic blood pressure <90 mm Hg), and jugular venous O_2 saturation <50%.

2. The establishment and availability of dedicated head injury rehabilitation facilities have greatly improved long-term outcome for these patients. Every effort should be made to transfer these patients to such a rehabilitation facility for aggressive inpatient therapy once they are medically and neurologically stable.

V. TREATMENT OF MILD TO MODERATE TBI

A. All patients with signs of concussion of more severe TBI should receive a CT for evaluation and diagnosis.

B. Most patients with **mild head injury** can be observed safely in the emergency department and discharged, although a few are at risk for delayed posttraumatic intracerebral hematomas or brain swelling. Identification of these patients requires careful neurologic assessment and liberal use of the CT.

1. Clinical characteristics associated with an increased risk for subsequent brain swelling or hemorrhage are LOC associated with posttraumatic or retrograde amnesia.

2. Patients with an abnormal CT or those who have a focal neurologic deficit on evaluation in the emergency department should be admitted for serial examinations.

3. Patients in a coagulopathic state or taking anticoagulants are at increased risk for progression and should be admitted to the hospital.

TABLE 23-1 Grading of Sports-related Head Injury

Author	Grade I	Grade II	Grade III
AAN, 1997	No LOC	No LOC symptoms <15 min	LOC symptoms >15 min
Cantu, 1998	No LOC PTA <1 h	LOC <5 min PTA 1–24 h	LOC >5 min PTA >24 h
Colorado Medical Society, 1991	No LOC Confusion No amnesia	No LOC Confusion and amnesia	LOC
Torg, 1985	No LOC PTA only	LOC <few min PTA or retrograde amnesia	LOC Confusion and amnesia

C. Postconcussion Syndrome
   1. Postconcussion syndrome can result from relatively minor head injuries.
   2. Most commonly involves headaches, tinnitus, vertigo, gait unsteadiness, emotional lability, sleep disturbances, intermittent blurring of vision, and irritability.
   3. Symptoms can continue for weeks, months, or several years, but are rarely permanent.
   4. Of patients who suffer postconcussion syndrome, 90% have spontaneous resolution of their symptoms within 2 weeks of injury.
   5. Beta-blocking agents, tricyclic antidepressants, or nonsteroidal anti-inflammatory agents may be beneficial, as well as psychotherapy and physical therapy for those that have prolonged symptomatology.
   6. For those with persistent symptoms, referral to a brain rehabilitation specialist is necessary.
D. Return to play after **sports-related head injuries** is determined by LOC or amnesia (Tables 23-1 and 23-2). The following guidelines are recommended (asymptomatic refers to no symptoms after provocative testing (e.g., a neurologic examination after ten pushups or ten sit-ups) and based on their grade:
   1. No LOC and no amnesia following a minor head injury: The patient can return 5 to 15 minutes after becoming completely lucid and asymptomatic.
   2. Posttraumatic amnesia but no LOC or retrograde amnesia: No return to play that day.
   3. Posttraumatic and retrograde amnesia with LOC: No return to play for 1 week after becoming completely lucid and asymptomatic and only after a detailed neurologic examination and CT scan.
   4. Posttraumatic and retrograde amnesia and prolonged LOC: No return to play for 1 month and only after detailed neurologic evaluation and CT scan.

TABLE 23-2 Return to Competition

Concussion grade	First concussion	Second concussion	Third concussion	
Grade I	Return if asymptomatic >30 min	Return after 2 wk and asymptomatic for 1 wk	End season	
Grade II	Return after 2 wks and asymptomatic for 1 wk	Return after 4 wks and asymptomatic for 1 wk	End season?	
Grade III	Return in 1 mo and End career? 1 wk	End season	End season	asymptomatic for

E. The likelihood of sustaining one or more head injuries after an initial minor head injury is increased, and subsequent head injuries have an additive, deleterious effect on complex processing abilities and reaction times.

VI. PENETRATING BRAIN INJURIES

A. Penetrating injuries can be subcategorized into gunshot wounds and lower velocity injuries; the prognosis between the two is very different.

1. Gunshot wounds to the brain carry a high mortality rate. As the bullet traverses the brain tissue, it causes a cylinder of tissue destruction extending perpendicular from the bullet tract to a distance of as much as 10 times the diameter of the bullet.

a. General management of gunshot wounds to the brain follows the same principles of cerebral resuscitation as other brain injuries. The incidence of elevated ICP is high.

b. Superficial debridement of the entrance and exit wounds is generally recommended, although it is usually not necessary to retrieve all deep-seated bullet and bone fragments.

c. Broad-spectrum intravenous antibiotics and prophylactic anticonvulsant therapy are recommended.

d. Prognosis depends largely on the trajectory of the bullet through the brain. If the bullet traverses deep brain structures (e.g., the basal ganglia or brainstem), traverses the posterior fossa, or has a transcranial trajectory, the mortality rate is high. If the bullet avoids these structures, the outcome can be more optimistic.

e. Patients with an initial GCS score of 3 to 4 will have a high mortality rate (>80%). Conversely, 80% of patients who are able to follow commands on admission to the hospital (GCS >8) will have mild or no disability.

2. Lower velocity missile wounds. The most important factor determining outcome from lower velocity missile wounds (e.g., stab or arrow wounds) to the head is the location of brain injury. If the missile damages the motor cortex, for example, contralateral motor weakness should be confined to the area of cortex that was damaged.

a. The missile may be tamponading a major intracranial arterial injury, so it is best to remove protruding knives or other objects only in the operating room and only when the surgeon is prepared to deal with the consequences of major arterial bleeding.

b. A 7- to 14-day course of broad-spectrum antibiotics and prophylactic anticonvulsants (7 days) is indicated.

B. Following a penetrating head injury – including high- or low-velocity missile or nonmissile injury (e.g., stab wound) – it is important to perform an angiogram to exclude a traumatic aneurysm.

VII. SKULL FRACTURES

A. Linear skull fractures are most common and typically occur over the lateral convexities of the skull.

1. The squamous portion of the temporal bone in this region is thin and closely associated with the middle meningeal artery. Fractures in this area can tear the artery, which is the most common cause for epidural hematoma.

2. For most skull fractures, it is not the fracture but rather the underlying blood clot or brain contusion that raises concern.

3. Since these associated lesions are best detected with CT and are not recognized with plain skull x-rays, a CT of the head is the diagnostic study of choice for patients suspected of having a skull fracture.

B. Depressed skull fractures. These fractures are usually the result of blunt force trauma. They are comminuted fractures with the fragments displaced inward. These fractures may be open (associated with an overlying scalp laceration) or closed.

1. Indications for surgical repair of depressed skull fractures are evidence of CSF leak, cosmetic deformity, or contaminated bone or scalp fragments pushed into the brain. In addition, when a dural tear is suspected – usually indicated by the bone being depressed beyond the inner table – then repair should be considered.

 a. The surgical elevation and repair of these fractures will not lead to a change in associated neurologic deficit or a decrease in the risk for subsequent seizures.

 2. Broad-spectrum antibiotics for 7 to 14 days if the wounds are contaminated or the fracture involves a facial sinus.

 3. Prophylactic anticonvulsant therapy for 7 days.

C. Basilar skull fractures, which occur most commonly through the floor of the anterior cranial fossa, can disrupt the ethmoid bones and lead to CSF leak through the nose (rhinorrhea). Fractures also can occur through the petrous bones posteriorly, leading to CSF drainage through the ear (otorrhea). Cranial nerve injuries are commonly associated with posterior basilar skull fractures, and findings should be sought on clinical examination.

 1. The primary concern with basilar skull fractures is associated CSF leak and risk of meningitis.

 2. Prophylactic antibiotic treatment is not recommended.

 3. Control of CSF leak. Begin with elevation of the head of the bed to 60 degrees. If the leak does not stop within 8 hours, a lumbar CSF catheter should be placed (provided there are no contraindications on CT such as edema or mass lesion), and 50 to 100 mL of CSF should be drained every 8 hours. If this fails to stop the leak within 72 hours, the patient should be taken for surgical repair of the dural laceration.

  a. Overdrainage of CSF and meningitis are complications of CSF drainage catheters. The drain should be clamped if the patient is decompensating or showing clinical signs of overdrainage.

AXIOMS

- LOC is an important indicator of brain injury.
- Determine the GCS score as early as possible.
- A principle therapeutic goal is to enhance cerebral perfusion and avoid further ischemic injury.
- Early diagnosis and evacuation of mass lesions are critical.
- CT is the diagnostic test of choice for patients with all brain injuries.

Suggested Readings

American College of Surgeons Committee on Trauma. *Advanced Trauma Life Support.* 8th ed. Chicago, IL: American College of Surgeons; 2008.

Bouma GJ, Muizelaar JP, Choi SC, et al. Cerebral circulation and metabolism after severe traumatic brain injury: The elusive role of ischemia. *J Neurosurg* 1991:685–693.

Chesnut RM, Marshall LF, Klauber MR, et al. The role of secondary brain injury in determining outcome from severe head injury. *J Trauma* 1993;34:216–222.

Chesnut RM, Marshall SB, Piek J, et al. Early and late systemic hypotension as a frequent and fundamental source of cerebral ischemia following severe brain injury in the traumatic coma data bank. *Acta Neurochir Suppl (Wien)* 1993;59:121–125.

Clifton GL, Kreutzer JS, Choi SC, et al. Relationship between Glasgow outcome scale and neuropsychological measures after brain injury. *Neurosurg* 1994;33:34–39.

Clifton GL, Valadka A, Zygun D, et al. Very early hypothermia induction in patients with severe brain injury (the Nation Acute Brain Injury Study: Hypothermia II): a randomized trial. *Lancet Neurol* 2011;10:131–139.

Cooper DJ, Rosenfeld JV, Murray L, et al. Decompressive craniectomy in diffuse traumatic brain injury. *NEJM* 2011;364:1493–1502.

Fletcher JM, Ewing-Cobbs L, Miner ME, et al. Behavioral changes after closed head injury in children. *J Consult Clin Psychol* 1990;58:93–98.

Gracias VH, Gullomondegui OD, Steifel MF, et al. Cerebral cortical oxygenation: A pilot study. *J Trauma* 2004;56(3):469–474.

Joint Section on Neurotrauma and Critical Care. *Guidelines for the Management of Severe Head Injury.* 3rd ed. New York, NY: Brain Trauma Foundation; 2007.

Levin HS, Grossman RG, Rose JE, et al. Long-term neuropsychological outcome of closed head injury. *J Neurosurg* 1979;50:412–422.

Levin HS, Williams DH, Eisenberg HM, et al. Serial MRI and neurobehavioral findings after mild to moderate closed head injury. *J Neurol Neurosurg Psychiatry* 1992;55:255–262.

Marion DW, Carlier PM. Problems with initial Glasgow Coma score assessment caused by the prehospital treatment of head-injured patients: Results of a national survey. *J Trauma* 1994;36:89–95.

Marion DW, Darby J, Yonas H. Acute regional cerebral blood flow changes caused by severe head injuries. *J Neurosurg* 1991;74:407–414.

Marion DW, ed. *Traumatic Brain Injury.* New York, NY: Thieme Medical Publishers; 1999.

Muizelaar JP, Marmarou A, Ward JD, et al. Adverse effects of prolonged hyperventilation in patients with severe head injury: A randomized clinical trial. *J Neurosurg* 1991;75:731–739.

Palmer S. Cerebral oxygen desaturation with normal ICP and CPP in severe traumatic brain injury. *Open Critical Care Med J* 2008;I:28–32.

Smith MJ, Stiefel MF, Gracias VH, et al. Packed red blood cell transfusion increases local cerebral oxygenation. *Crit Care Med* 2005;33(5):1104–1108.

Stiefel MF, Spiotta A, Gracias V, et al. Reduced mortality rate in patients with severe traumatic brain injury treated with brain tissue oxygen monitoring. *J Neurosurg* 2005;103:805–811.

Sydenham E. Hypothermia for traumatic brain injury. *Cochrane Database of Syst Rev* 2009;2.

Vollmer DG, Torner JC, Jane JA, et al. Age and outcome following traumatic coma: Why do older patients fare worse? *J Neurosurg* 1991;75:S37–S49.

24 Maxillofacial Injury

William L. Chung, James M. Russavage and Mark W. Ochs

I. EVALUATION OF THE PATIENT WITH SUSPECTED MAXILLOFACIAL TRAUMA

A. Treatment principles of hard- and soft-tissue injuries

1. Contusions or lacerations often accompany underlying bony injuries; consider imaging, especially if tenderness or deformity exists.
2. Treat fractures of the maxillofacial complex before definitive soft-tissue management to avoid repetitive damage to the latter. It may be possible to repair open fractures exposed through any lacerations rather than the standard incision for fracture repair.
3. Tissue that is contaminated or damaged by crush or contusion is at risk for infection if primary repair is performed. The likelihood of contamination increases proportional to the length of time elapsed since the injury.
4. The history and mechanism of injury provide evidence of the possibility of retained foreign bodies.

B. Initial survey

1. Relieve airway obstruction/ensure adequate oxygenation and ventilation.
2. Control hemorrhage.
3. Search for immediately life-threatening injuries (thoracic, abdominal, intracranial, extremity).
4. Assume cervical spine (C-spine) injury exists and stabilize until it is cleared.
5. Perform a neurologic assessment.

C. Secondary survey

1. Complete head, eye, ear, nose, throat (HEENT) examination.
   a. Scalp and skull evaluation (palpate).
   b. Cranial nerve evaluation (especially optic, CN II). Evaluate structural function(s) in the vicinity of the injury.
   c. Ophthalmologic evaluation (pupil symmetry, reactivity, visual acuity, and ocular movement).
   d. Otologic evaluation (external ear structures and otoscopic examination).
   e. Evaluate nasal structures, sinuses, salivary glands, and associated ducts.

D. Photography. Useful for:

1. Accurate record keeping and documentation.
2. Insurance and legal purposes.
3. Assess efficacy of therapy.

II. DENTOALVEOLAR TRAUMA

A. Anatomy

1. Adult dentition is composed of 32 teeth, including bilateral maxillary and mandibular central and lateral incisors, canines, first and second bicuspids, and three molars. Typically, the third molars (wisdom teeth) are impacted or absent. The teeth are numbered from the right maxillary third molar (no. 1) moving forward and across the arch to the left maxillary third molar (no. 16), then the mandibular left third molar (no. 17) and across to the right wisdom tooth (no. 32) (Fig. 24-1A).
2. The pediatric dentition consists of 20 total deciduous teeth, including bilateral maxillary and mandibular central and lateral incisors, canines, and two molars

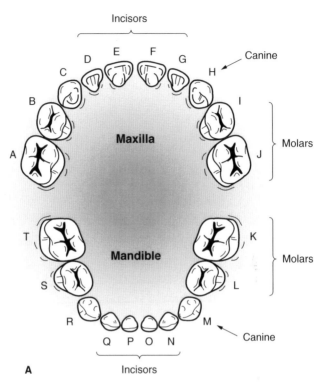

Figure 24-1. A: Pediatric dental arches. **(*continued*)**

(Fig. 24-1B). The primary dentition is named by capital letters. Exfoliation of the deciduous teeth begins at approximately 6 years of age and the mixed dentition stage continues until 12 to 14 years of age. The teeth are attached to the alveolar processes of the maxilla and mandible by periodontal ligaments. Alveolar bone in younger age groups undergoes plastic deformation when subjected to trauma.

B. Evaluation

  1. Clinical

  a. Count all of the teeth; attempt to locate any missing teeth at the location of the injury. With unaccounted or missing teeth, look for traumatic impaction into the local bone or surrounding soft tissues. Also, dislodged teeth can be aspirated or swallowed. Chest or neck imaging can help locate swallowed teeth.

  b. Evaluate the occlusion and ask the patient if the bite feels normal; this is a sensitive screening tool to detect a dentoalveolar or facial fracture. Assess next for stability and symmetry. Occlusal discrepancies, new gaps in the dental arch, or lacerations of the usually pink, firm, attached gingival raise the suspicion of a fracture.

  c. Evaluate damaged or displaced teeth. Fractured teeth can be classified by the depth and location of the fracture (Fig. 24-2A, B). Dislocated teeth can be totally avulsed or subluxated or an associated alveolar fracture may be present.

  2. Radiographs

  a. A panorex is a good screening radiograph for most dentoalveolar trauma. If not available, obtain a CT scan. Isolated tooth fractures are best evaluated

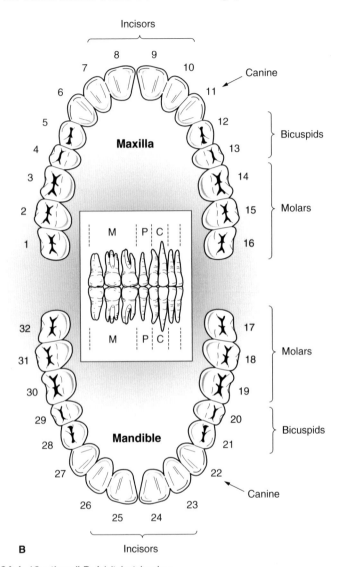

B

Figure 24-1. (*Continued*) **B:** Adult dental arches.

with intraoral dental radiographs. If these are not available, early dental referral should be sought.

C. Management

1. Age of the patient, type of tooth (deciduous or permanent), status of tooth development, condition of tooth before trauma, patient motivation, time elapsed since injury, and associated injuries all influence the management of dentoalveolar trauma.

2. Intraoral soft-tissue lacerations are usually best treated by conservative debridement, irrigation, and primary repair with resorbable sutures after stabilization or definitive treatment of the dentoalveolar fracture.

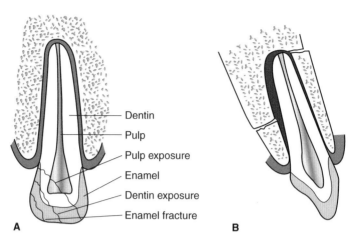

Figure 24-2. A and B: Level of tooth fractures.

3. In general, isolated tooth crown fractures need emergent referral if the dental pulp (dark pink or red appearance) is exposed or if teeth are sensitive.

   a. Dislocated or subluxed teeth and dentoalveolar fractures need to be emergently reduced and stabilized with wire and composite resin bonding. Composite resins are opaque white filling material (similar to what orthodontists use to bond brackets to teeth) that is either chemically or UV light activated.

   b. Avulsed deciduous (pediatric) teeth should not be reimplanted because of low success rate and the possibility of damage to the underlying developing permanent dentition.

   c. Avulsed permanent teeth should be replaced into the tooth socket as soon as possible after the trauma. Immediate reimplantation is ideal. If this is not possible, the tooth should be stored in an appropriate storage medium (avulsed tooth storage system, buccal vestibule, milk, saline, or moist towel) and replaced as soon as possible, with less than 30 minutes ideal. A delay of 2 hours or desiccation of the tooth root markedly drops the overall success of reimplantation. Once reimplanted, the tooth requires composite resin splinting to the adjacent stable teeth, and tell patients to avoid heavy chewing/solid ingestion until seen in follow-up within a week.

III. MANDIBULAR FRACTURES

Mandibular fractures are the second most common of bony maxillofacial fractures. The mechanism of injury is usually blunt trauma from an assault or a motor vehicle crash.

A. Anatomy and location of injury. Fractures tend to occur at the local site of impact, areas of weakness, and are often multiple. The anatomic regions and associated incidence of fracture are shown in Figure 24-3. In edentulous patients, the incidence of subcondylar fractures accounts for 37% of all mandible fractures and is often paired with a contralateral body fracture. The inferior alveolar neurovascular bundle enters the mandible on the medial aspect of the mid-ramus through the mandibular foramen and traverses an intrabony canal, exiting through the mental foramen located just inferior to the mandibular bicuspid root tips. It is strictly a sensory nerve (V_3) supplying the ipsilateral lower lip, teeth, and gingiva.

B. Evaluation

1. Clinical

   a. Emergent situations

      i. Airway obstruction. Foreign bodies (e.g., dentures, avulsed teeth) can cause airway obstruction; remove them at the time of initial evaluation.

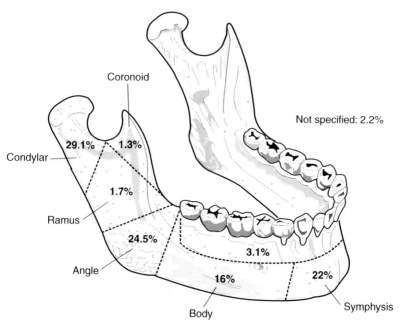

Figure 24-3. Mandibular anatomy and fracture zones.

In addition, airway obstruction can occur with bilateral mandibular parasymphyseal or body fractures. Manual anterior distraction of the flail anterior mandibular segment, allowing the patient to be semi-supine or to sit up, and oral suctioning can provide temporary relief, but a definitive airway should be secured urgently.

ii. Hemorrhage is rarely a significant problem with mandibular fractures.

  a) The inferior alveolar artery traveling in the mandibular canal can be lacerated during the initial injury, but simple fracture reduction, direct pressure, or infiltration with an epinephrine containing local anesthetic is usually adequate for hemostasis.

  b) Persistent or profuse bleeding is often associated with penetrating injury and a secure airway is the primary concern. Then, control bleeding with direct surgical exploration, or rarely, by interventional radiology. Fracture reduction and temporary stabilization are preferred for hemorrhage control. Local packing can cause fracture distraction, allowing continued bleeding.

b. Occlusion. Malocclusion is one of the first clinical signs detected in patients with a mandibular fracture. If the fracture is in the tooth-bearing segment of the mandible, a noticeable step deformity or interdental gap may be detected.

c. Floor of mouth ecchymosis is pathognomonic for a mandibular parasymphyseal or body fracture. If the fracture is located in the subcondylar region, a shift of the chin toward the affected side or an anterior or lateral open bite may be present (Fig. 24-4).

d. Soft-tissue signs, such as ecchymosis, edema, pain, and gingival or mucosal lacerations, may be present at the fracture site.

e. Sensation. Lower lip and chin paresthesia or anesthesia is common in patients with mandible fractures located between the mid-ramus and canine region. Greater bony displacement increases the risk for inferior alveolar nerve injury or even transection.

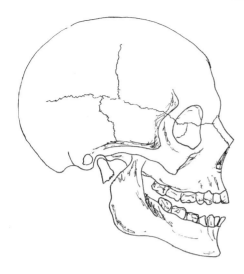

Figure 24-4. Anterior open bite caused by a condyle fracture with posterior vertical collapse.

2. Radiographs. Plain radiographs usually suffice for evaluation of mandibular fractures. At least two views at 90 degrees should be used to evaluate most injuries. This is especially important in the subcondylar region, where superimposition of other structures can mimic or obscure a fracture.
   a. The best initial radiograph is the panorex, accompanied by an open mouth Towne's view. Other radiographs that can be used to evaluate mandibular fractures are the posteroanterior (PA) and lateral oblique views.
   b. Computed tomography (CT) aids the evaluation of patients with condylar or subcondylar fractures. This is particularly true in children because their condyles are developing and incompletely ossified, making plain radiology detection difficult. Patients (especially children) with a chin laceration and preauricular pain or swelling should be evaluated for a condylar or subcondylar fracture. Coronoid fracture accounts are uncommon and are generally associated with an overlying zygomatic complex fracture that was displaced medially, creating the injury.

C. Management

1. Cervical immobilization
   a. Cervical immobilization should be maintained until C-spine injury is excluded unless a trivial mechanism exists.

2. Management of emergent problems
   a. Initial management should be control of the airway and bleeding. Control of the airway is performed with distraction of flail bony segments, if possible. In the event of a compromised airway, perform endotracheal intubation or surgical airway before stabilization and repair of the mandibular fracture.

3. Temporary immobilization
   a. Temporary partial reduction and stabilization of the fracture segments can provide symptomatic relief, help control bleeding, and minimize damage to the inferior alveolar neurovascular bundle. This can be performed with a modified Barton's bandage (circumferential wrap from chin to skull vertex) or by placing a stainless steel bridal wire (24 to 26 gauge) around the necks of two teeth on either side of the line of fracture (Fig. 24-5).

4. Definitive treatment
Fractures should be reduced adequately, fixated, and immobilized for adequate healing to occur. This is typically accomplished by open reduction and internal screw fixation. Without immobilization, fracture segments usually become

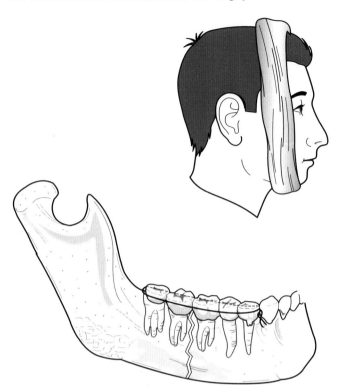

Figure 24-5. Bridal wiring to stabilize an anterior mandibular fracture site.

displaced by the pull of muscles of mastication, leading to a malunion or nonunion. Isolated minimally displaced fractures, particularly those of the condylar region, can be treated by wiring the teeth, or maxillomandibular fixation (MMF). The period of MMF for subcondylar fractures is 2 to 3 weeks to avoid the risk of ankylosis; 6 weeks for all other mandibular fractures.

5. **Prophylactic antibiotics.** Mandibular fractures that include tooth-bearing segments are considered compound fractures because of the egress of saliva, bacteria, and other contaminants through the periodontal ligament or fracture site. Prophylactic antibiotics that cover most oral microorganisms (e.g., penicillin, amoxicillin with clavulanate) or a first-generation cephalosporin are recommended, along with oral saline or antimicrobial (Peridex) rinses. In the penicillin-allergic patient, clindamycin is an alternative.

IV. **MIDFACE FRACTURES** are any fracture of the orbital–zygomatic–maxillary complex. The mechanism of injury is usually blunt trauma from either an assault or motor vehicle crash.

A. **General midfacial fracture management**

1. **Anatomy and location of injury.** The midface is divided into the maxilla, the zygomatic complexes, and the nasal–orbital–ethmoid (NOE) complex (Fig. 24-6). Fractures tend to occur at the site of impact and inherently weak regions of the midfacial complex, including bony sutures, foramina, and apertures.

a. The infraorbital neurovascular bundle enters the midfacial complex via the orbital region through the inferior orbital fissure and then traversing

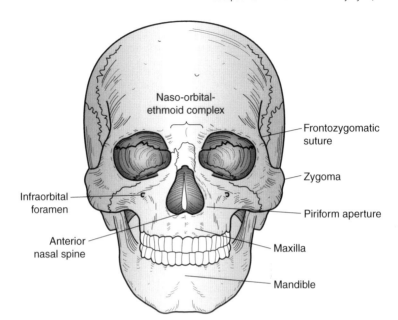

Figure 24-6. Midfacial anatomy.

partially through a bony canal along the floor of the orbit to exit through the infraorbital foramen on the anterior surface of the maxilla. The infraorbital nerve (V_2) supplies general sensation to the ipsilateral lower eyelid, lateral nose, upper lip, and anterior maxilla.

2. Evaluation

  a. Clinical

    i. Emergent situations

      a) Airway obstruction. In most clinical situations, airway obstruction occurs in patients with panfacial trauma, including significant mandibular fractures.

      b) Hemorrhage. Significant hemorrhage is more common with midfacial fractures than mandibular fractures. The descending palatine arteries, which travel in a bony canal along the posterior surface of the nasal cavity within the palatine bone, can cause profuse posterior nasal bleeding. Other vessels that may be injured include the nasal septal, sphenopalatine, and pterygoid plexus.

    ii. Occlusion. Occlusal discrepancies are one of the first clinical signs detected in patients with certain midfacial fractures. Mobility of the maxillary teeth relative to other midfacial structures is pathognomonic of a maxillary fracture. A posteriorly directed force of significant magnitude can cause a posteriorly impacted maxilla. Either an anterior or posterior open bite is indicative of a maxillary or midfacial fracture.

    iii. Soft-tissue signs include ecchymosis, edema, pain, and mucosal lacerations.

    iv. Palpation. Palpate all bones of the midface, including maxilla, orbital rims, zygomas, and nose; often, the patient is too sensitive to allow a complete examination. However, grasping the anterior maxillary teeth with the thumb and forefinger and attempting upward or side-to-side movement while stabilizing the entire forehead with the opposite hand is crucial in detection of a midfacial fracture.

v. Sensation. Upper lateral lip, nose, and cheek paresthesia or anesthesia is common in patients with a fracture extending through the infraorbital foramen. Complete transection of the infraorbital nerve is uncommon in blunt trauma.

vi. Ophthalmologic examination. Any fracture involving the bony orbit or zygomatic complex can cause injury to the globe or other orbital contents. Complete examination includes pupils, visual acuity, range of motion of the globe, globe position, and the globe itself, including a funduscopic examination. Extraocular movements in multiple fields of gaze are often diminished in patients with significant orbital edema, but tend to be mild without a firm fixed sudden stop. Blowout fracture of one of the orbital walls (most commonly the medial orbital floor) can cause entrapment of the extraocular muscles (inferior rectus muscles or inferior oblique). A firm, fixed and reproducible point of limitation in upward gaze or, more likely, downward gaze should alert the practitioner to this possibility. An urgent specialist consultation is appropriate because prolonged muscle ischemia and resultant fibrosis can lead to long-term impairment of movement.

vii. Nasal examination. Nasal trauma can be associated with nasal airway obstruction and epistaxis.

  a) Epistaxis from anterior vessels is controlled with upright positioning, cold compresses, topical nasal vasoconstrictor sprays, local direct pressure, or, infrequently, anterior nasal packing.

  b) Posterior epistaxis may require compression tamponade (often done with balloon devices or manual packing).

  c) Evaluate the nasal septum for a septal hematoma, which (if untreated) can lead to a "saddle nose" deformity.

viii. Examination for cerebrospinal fluid (CSF) leak. CSF leaks most commonly occur with midfacial, frontal sinus, or basilar skull fractures.

  a) Fractures involving the NOE complex occasionally involve the cribriform plate in the superior aspect of the nasal cavity and floor of the anterior cranial fossa.

  b) Basilar skull fractures can involve the petrous temporal bone, resulting in leakage of CSF.

  c) Various tests, including the "ring test" and fluid chloride or glucose sampling, have been offered to detect CSF, but these are not accurate. Measuring fluid for *beta$_2$-transferrin* (positive with CSF leak) is the best test but often not rapidly available.

ix. Radiographs

  a) CT is the diagnostic modality of choice for the complete evaluation of midfacial trauma with thin sections (1.5 mm) in axial planes through the midface and the orbits. Direct coronal views are particularly helpful with orbital fractures but the patient's C-spine status may preclude obtaining them.

  b) The panoramic radiograph is of little use in the evaluation of midfacial trauma, except in determining if a concomitant mandibular fracture exists.

3. Management

  a. With severely displaced or multiple midfacial fractures, cervical immobilization is maintained until C-spine injury is excluded.

  b. Management of emergent problems

  i. As above, first priorities are control of the airway and bleeding.

  ii. Ongoing posterior nasal hemorrhage is controlled with posterior nasopharynx occlusion with a balloon catheter inserted transnasally into the nasopharynx, inflated with water or saline. Some devices have two balloons to compress posterior and anterior; if using a urinary catheter, gently apply anterior traction and insert anterior nasal packing.

    iii. Persistent deep hemorrhage may require surgical ligation of branches of the external carotid artery in the neck if bleeding is massive or, in the setting of less active bleeding, with interventional radiology.

    iv. Because of risk of inadvertent intracranial placement, **do not attempt blind** (non-fiberoptic) **nasal intubation** with endotracheal tubes or nasogastric tubes in patients with suspected midfacial trauma involving the NOE complex.

  c. Treatment of ophthalmologic problems. Obtain ophthalmologic consultation for individuals with potential globe injuries. Fat herniation through an upper eyelid laceration or an irregular (not round) pointing pupil suggests a penetrating globe injury.

  d. Decongestants. Topical decongestants (e.g., phenylephrine or oxymetazoline) can provide symptomatic relief for nasal airway obstruction and to minimize epistaxis.

  e. Edema prevention. Open surgical treatment of midfacial trauma is difficult when significant edema exists. It may be best to delay operative repair until edema has resolved. Prevention of facial edema can provide symptomatic relief for the patient and expedite definitive treatment.

    i. Steroids. Pharmacologic administration of glucocorticoids may hasten the resolution of facial edema in patients with maxillofacial trauma. Dexamethasone (4 to 8 mg) administered intravenously (IV) every 6 hours or methylprednisolone (125 mg) IV every 6 hours for 24 to 48 hours may be used. Once edema is established, steroids are not helpful. Caution should be used when administering high dose steroids in diabetic patients or multiply injured patients.

    ii. Elevate the head of the bed to 30 to 45 degrees for the first several days after sustaining facial trauma.

    iii. Intermittent application of cold compresses for the first 24 hours only may minimize facial edema (20 minutes on and 20 minutes off).

  f. Osseous healing can start as early as 7 days after the injury. Reduction and repair can be difficult if surgery is delayed for more than 2 weeks. Contemporary treatment of midfacial fractures involves open reduction and internal fixation using titanium miniplates and screws. Minimally or nondisplaced nasal, orbital, zygomatic complex (tripod), and zygomatic arch fractures may not require surgical treatment. Nonunion of these isolated fractures is rare.

B. Le Fort fractures are those of the midface that involve the maxillary dentoalveolar segment. The mechanism and location of impact usually determine the type of fracture sustained. Fractures tend to occur in certain patterns of the midface and are traditionally classified by the highest level of fracture (Fig. 24-7). Most Le Fort fractures are not "pure" and can have comminution, additional levels or lines of fracture, and other associated facial fractures.

C. Zygomaticomaxillary complex fractures. Zygomaticomaxillary complex (ZMC, tripod or malar) fractures usually are sustained with direct blunt trauma to the zygomatic buttress of the face. The zygoma has four major stability points, with connections as follows: (a) The frontal bone at the frontozygomatic suture; (b) the maxilla at the medial inferior orbital rim; (c) at the zygomaticomaxillary buttress; and (d) the temporal bone at the zygomatic arch. A complete fracture of the complex usually involves all four of these major stability points (Fig. 24-8). Anteriorly, the fracture usually occurs in the maxilla obliquely through the infraorbital foramen because of the relatively weak nature of this bone resulting in a high incidence of V_2 sensory division paresthesia. Other significant physical findings associated with ZMC fractures are depression of the zygomatic eminence, lateral subconjunctival hemorrhage, ocular dystopia (uneven pupillary levels), lateral canthal ptosis, enophthalmos, and palpable fractures at the inferior and lateral orbital rims. With extreme medial and posterior displacement, the patient can exhibit limited mouth opening because of impingement of the fractured complex against the coronoid process of the mandible. For oral access or intubation, initial deviation

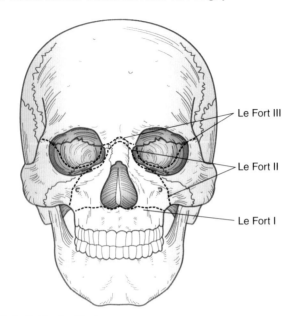

Figure 24-7. Le Fort levels of fracture.

of the mandible toward the uninjured side can sufficiently clear this mechanical obstruction.

D. Zygomatic arch fractures. Isolated zygomatic arch fractures usually are sustained by focal direct blunt trauma to the zygomatic arch, creating three breakpoints with a classic W-pattern (Fig. 24-9). Common physical findings are a depression at the location of trauma and pain on mandibular opening caused by masseteric muscle pull. Limited mandibular opening can also exist because of mechanical obstruction of the coronoid process. A submental vertex or "jug-handle" view is

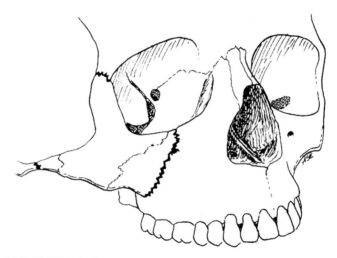

Figure 24-8. Right ZMC fracture.

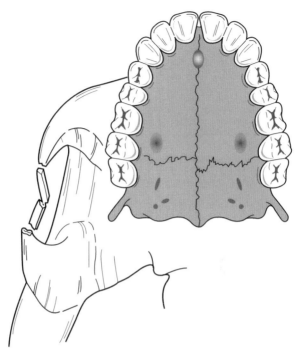

Figure 24-9. Right zygomatic arch fracture viewed from below.

usually sufficient to identify this fracture. Early (24 hours) surgical reduction without internal fixation via a lateral brow, temporal hairline (Gille's), or maxillary vestibular incision is optimal. Later stabilization often is complicated by fracture sagging, thus requiring a more extensive exposure (e.g., a hemicoronal incision) for direct access and plating.

E. Orbital blowout fractures occur from direct impact to the orbit or globe (Fig. 24-10). The floor of the orbit and the medial orbital wall are the thinnest walls and most commonly involved with this type of fracture. The surrounding maxillary sinus and

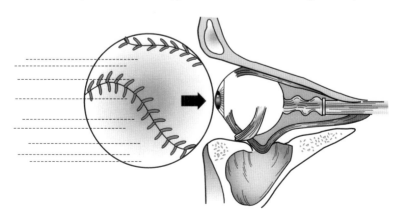

Figure 24-10. Orbital floor blowout fracture.

ethmoid air cells act as "airbags of the orbit," cushioning the blow and absorbing the force, protecting to some degree against globe rupture. The prolapse of some of the orbital contents into these spaces can produce enophthalmos or orbital dystopia because of a relative increase in the orbital volume. In addition, suspensory fascia (Tenon's capsule) or extraocular muscles can be entrapped in the fracture line, leading to restricted eye movement and diplopia in certain fields of gaze.

1. Coronal CT is invaluable in evaluation of this injury and should be correlated with clinical findings.
2. Indications for surgical correction include a significant cosmetic or functional deformity. A relative indication is 25% to 50% of the surface area of an orbital wall being involved in the fracture. If edema allows, optimal time for repair is within 24 hours.
3. If significant edema exists, reevaluation and repair within 5 to 7 days is desirable. Patients should be cautioned not to blow the nose, which can cause significant orbital emphysema. Repair usually entails open reduction or removal of the fractured segments, then reduction of the orbital contents with possible autogenous or alloplastic implant reconstruction.

F. **Nasal fracture** is the most common facial fracture. Complete examination should include evaluation for a septal hematoma. Epistaxis should be controlled with direct pressure, upright positioning, and topic vasoconstrictors.

1. The diagnosis of a nasal fracture is primarily a clinical one. Nasal deformity, deviation, and bony crepitus with movement are the usual findings.
2. Occasionally, radiographs can aid in the diagnosis.
3. If edema allows, early reduction (within 24 to 48 hours) of isolated nasal and septal fractures affords the greatest stability. If not, repair should be performed within 5 to 7 days after sufficient resolution of the edema. Reduce septal fractures and dislocations at that time.

G. **Fractures of the entire NOE complex** occur after direct high impact to the region. Diagnosis usually can be made by clinical observation and direct palpation in the region of nasal dorsum and medial canthal tendons.

1. Findings can include lateral displacement of the medial canthal tendons (telecanthus) causing an increased distance (normal medial intercanthal distance is 30 to 34 mm). Significant disruption in this region can lead to epiphora secondary to swelling or damage of the lacrimal drainage system.
2. Primary surgical repair of fractures includes open reduction and plating of the bony segments, with direct repair of the canthal tendons. Repair should be done within the first 7 to 10 days, because secondary repair is difficult and often leads to compromised results. Globe injuries and CSF leaks should be sought when evaluating an NOE injury.

V. FRONTAL SINUS FRACTURES

A. **Anatomy and location of injury.** The frontal sinus is usually divided into left and right halves by a midline septum; both sides drain into the middle meatus of the nose through their respective nasofrontal ducts or foramina. Of adults, 5% have no frontal sinus and 5% have only a unilateral sinus. Trauma to the forehead region can fracture the anterior or posterior walls of the frontal sinus or damage the nasofrontal ducts. With fracture of the posterior wall of the frontal sinus, consider the potential for a dural laceration or cerebral injury.

B. **Evaluation**
   1. **Clinical**
      a. Emergent situations
         i. Open fracture of the anterior and posterior table of the frontal sinus are emergencies because of the high risk of meningitis from direct cerebral exposure. Emergent surgical intervention is indicated.
         ii. Cerebral contusions are common with injuries to the frontal sinus.
      b. Local signs include ecchymosis, edema, pain, and cutaneous lacerations at the location of fracture, and fractures and deformity of the forehead and superior orbital rims.

   c. Sensation. Forehead and scalp paresthesia or anesthesia. The supraorbital and supratrochlear nerves (V_1) supply this region.

   d. Nasal examination and CSF leaks. NOE complex trauma can be associated with frontal sinus fractures. CSF leaks can occur in patients with frontal sinus fractures. Any ongoing nasal discharge should be submitted for a b_2-transferrin level to detect CSF.

2. Radiographs. CT is the diagnostic modality of choice for frontal sinus trauma. Thin sections (1.5 to 0 mm) in the axial plane through the paranasal sinuses are usually adequate for most purposes. Both the anterior and posterior tables of the frontal sinus should be categorized as **fractured or noninvolved** and **displaced versus nondisplaced.** Displacement is defined as overlap by the amount of thickness of the adjacent cortical bone. Intermediate distinctions such as mild or moderate displacement are confusing and have no clinical relevance.

   a. A displaced posterior table (overlapped fracture margins) is often associated with dural tears or cerebral injury requiring neurosurgical intervention.

   b. Plain radiographs can be used as initial screening for bony injury but will not evaluate the underlying brain. The best plain radiographic series includes the Caldwell view and the lateral cephalogram.

C. Management

1. Airway and cervical spine care as noted with other injuries.

2. Management of **emergent problems.** Open fractures of the anterior and posterior tables of the frontal sinus require emergent exploration and treatment. They can be treated with primary cutaneous repair and delayed treatment of the frontal sinus injury.

3. Prophylactic antibiotics. Most frontal sinus fractures fill with blood and mucus early after trauma. The use of prophylactic antibiotics is controversial; sinus infection or meningitis can occur between 5% and 50% of cases, but evidence does not support a benefit from routine prophylaxis. If chosen, use agents that cover most sinus microorganisms (e.g., ampicillin with clavulanate) or a first-generation cephalosporin. Posterior table involvement is covered with antibiotics that can cross the blood–brain barrier.

4. Decongestants. Because of mucosal edema and the potential for compromised frontal sinus drainage, decongestants should be used in patients with significant frontal sinus trauma.

5. Definitive treatment of frontal sinus fractures depends on the extent of the fracture. If the drainage system of the sinuses is significantly compromised, obliteration or cranialization is usually recommended. If only the anterior table is involved and nondisplaced, no surgical treatment is generally necessary. A displaced frontal sinus that is either extensive or creates a cosmetic deformity can be accessed directly through the fracture or via a liberal sinusotomy. The mucosal lining is then completely removed with curettage and drilling to deter formation of a mucocele at a usually much later date—such as years later. The nasofrontal ducts can then be obliterated with fascia or bone grafts and the frontal sinus can be obliterated with autologous fat, bone, pericranium, or alloplastic materials. If only the anterior table is displaced without involvement of the nasofrontal ducts, primary repair without obliteration can be performed. Significant involvement or displacement of the posterior table usually requires direct exploration, with repair or cranialization depending on the degree of damage. Smaller frontal sinuses in young patients can be cranialized by simply removing the posterior sinus wall, smoothing the edges, removing the mucosal lining, and obliterating the frontonasal ducts. This treatment in older patients and those with large frontal sinuses may predispose them to developing chronic subdural fluid accumulations. With displaced posterior table fractures, associated dural tears requiring neurosurgical repair is the rule rather than the exception.

VI. ANATOMIC CONSIDERATIONS IN REPAIRING SOFT TISSUE

A. Facial nerve. It is often impractical and unnecessary to identify and suture the terminal branches of the facial nerve. The plexus of nerve fibers makes regeneration

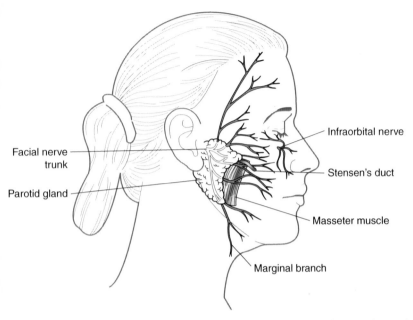

Figure 24-11. Deep anatomy of the cheek showing facial nerve, parotid gland, Stensen's duct, and masseter muscle.

of activity common even without direct facial nerve suturing. Approximation of the tissues usually allows some element of nerve regeneration by neurotization of muscle.

1. Nerve repair need not be performed anterior to a line drawn at the lateral canthus of the eyelids.
2. Larger branches (all the named ones) of the facial nerve should be identified and sutured (Fig. 24-11). Primary repair at the time of the initial treatment is recommended.

B. Trigeminal nerve. The sensory branches of the trigeminal nerve (Fig. 24-12) in the region of the skin are small, and approximation is impractical and unnecessary. Partial or complete recovery of sensation usually occurs within a few months to a year, with slight hypesthesia often present. Contusion of trigeminal nerve branches also occurs as a result of fractures.

C. Parotid duct lacerations. Seek and repair lacerations of the parotid duct at the time of wound closure to prevent fistula to the skin or to the mucous membrane of the mouth.

1. To identify the course of the parotid duct, draw a line drawn from the tragus of the ear to the midportion of the upper lip. The duct traverses the middle third of the line.
2. The parotid duct travels adjacent to the buccal branch of the facial nerve. Buccal branch paralysis with an overlying laceration suggests the possibility of a parotid duct injury.
3. The parotid duct empties into the mouth opposite the maxillary second molar.
   a. Insert a silastic tube or silver probe into the opening of the duct and the course of the duct followed. Irrigate the duct with saline using a no. 22 angiocath sleeve. The appearance of saline in the wound indicates that the duct is injured. Identify the proximal end of the duct by expressing secretion of saliva.

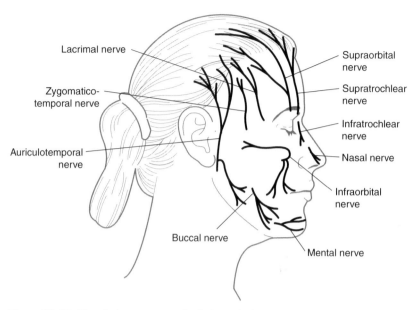

Figure 24-12. Trigeminal sensory nerve distribution to the face.

    b. Place a silastic catheter in the duct and the wound repaired with fine sutures. The tube is left in for a 2-week period, as tolerated (Fig. 24-13).

D. Forehead and brow considerations
    1. Preserve the eyebrow. **Do not shave the eyebrow.**
    2. Be sure to repair the muscle layer.

E. Ears. Assess adjacent wounds and the middle and inner ear. The presence of hearing loss, hemorrhagic otorrhea, CSF leak, or facial nerve injury suggests middle- or inner-ear injury.
    1. Ecchymosis over the mastoid area is known as **Battle's sign,** a finding associated with basilar skull fracture.
    2. The ear may be involved in abrasions, contusions, lacerations, and hematomas.
        a. Abrasions heal with the continued application of light dressing and ointment. A well-designed dressing, suitably padded (with mineral oil–soaked cotton), minimizes edema and hemorrhage. Avoid inordinate pressure that prevents circulation to the auricle.
        b. Lacerations of the auricle are usually associated with lacerations of the cartilage. The ear can be totally or incompletely avulsed, but is often viable when even a small pedicle remains. Appropriate debridement and cleansing of the wound minimizes the likelihood of subsequent chondritis or deformity.
            i. The ear should be sutured into place and supported with dressings.
            ii. Stent the ear canal with Xeroform (Sherwood-Davis & Geck; St. Louis, Missouri) gauze.
            iii. Trim cartilage to the skin margin.
            iv. The auricle has numerous landmarks that allow accurate placement of skin sutures, providing excellent realignment and minimal deformity.

    3. Repair
        a. Conservative debridement.
        b. Return tissues to point of origin.
        c. Repair cartilage with 5-0 **clear** monofilament nonabsorbable suture.
        d. Repair skin with 6-0 monofilament nonabsorbable suture.

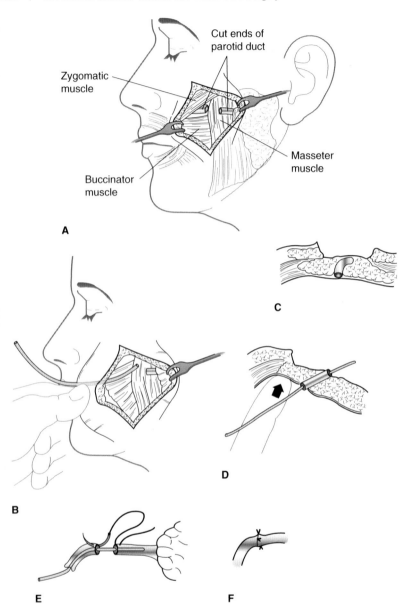

Figure 24-13. Repair of a severed parotid duct **(A)**, severed duct **(B)**, silastic tube in duct **(C)**, angulation of Stensen's duct in cheek **(D)**, stretching of mucosa facilitating stent placement **(E)**, suturing of duct under magnification **(F)**, stent remaining in 10 to 14 days.

F. Nose. Lacerations of the nose can involve the skin, the lining in the vestibule of the nose, or the mucous membrane of the nasal cavity, most commonly at the junction of the bone and the cartilages.

1. **Approximate all wounds with anatomic accuracy,** aligning the nostril borders precisely.
2. Septal hematomas are diagnosed easily with a nasal speculum examination. Immediately evacuate the hematoma through a small mucosal incision or by needle aspiration. An untreated septal hematoma will typically resorb and destroy septal cartilage, especially if becoming infected.
3. When treating injury that penetrates all soft-tissue layers of the nose, it is easiest to repair the mucous membrane lining first, with 4-0 plain catgut or other resorbable suture.
4. Torn septal, upper lateral, alar, and columellar cartilages usually can be reapproximated under direct vision through the wound and held in position by accurate repair of the underlying mucoperichondrium and the overlying skin. Interrupted sutures with 6-0 monofilament polypropylene are ideal for such skin closure.
   a. The nose is sometimes packed with a petroleum-impregnated gauze to maintain position of cartilaginous or bony fragments.

G. Lips
1. Lacerations of the lips can involve only the superficial skin and subcutaneous tissues or extend into the orbicularis oris muscle. Full thickness lacerations are possible.
2. Bleeding is profuse if the labial artery is severed. Local pressure or ligation of the vessel controls the bleeding.
3. The vermilion–cutaneous margin and the vermilion–mucosal margin provide accurate landmarks **that must be accurately approximated.**
   a. Close the lip musculature first, using 4-0 or 5-0 absorbable sutures.
   b. Clear all blood and debris from the vermilion border to ensure accurate approximation.
   c. Close the mucous membrane with 4-0 or 5-0 absorbable suture.
   d. Skin closure is with 6-0 nonabsorbable suture (Fig. 24-14).

VII. ANESTHESIA. Reassurance and empathy along with sedation permits extensive procedures to be performed under local anesthesia.
   A. Nerve blocks can establish regional anesthesia in a wide field with reduced dosage of medication and less discomfort. Less complicated wounds (e.g., small lacerations) and some uncomplicated fractures of the facial bones (e.g., nasal fractures) are treated under local anesthesia in an emergency department or in an outpatient office.
   B. More extensive injuries usually require general anesthesia.

VIII. DEBRIDEMENT AND CARE. Thorough cleansing of soft-tissue wounds is imperative before any definitive treatment is attempted. Wash all blood and debris with copious amounts of water or saline, using mild detergents if needed. Remove any foreign materials such as glass, hair, clothing, tooth structures, pieces of artificial dentures, paint, grease, gravel, or dirt.
   A. **Except for the removal of obviously devitalized portions of tissue, extensive debridement of soft tissue has little place in management of maxillofacial injuries.** Otherwise, retain as much tissue in the repair.
   1. Err on the side of retaining tissues that may not survive rather than debriding or destroying any tissues that might be important in a final result. The excellent blood supply of the face usually makes extensive debridement unnecessary.

IX. CLEANING OF THE WOUND. All wounds should be carefully inspected for foreign material. Its removal is imperative to prevent separation, infection, delayed healing, and subsequent pigmentation of the skin. The presence of foreign material and hematoma reduces the bacterial inoculum necessary for infection to develop.

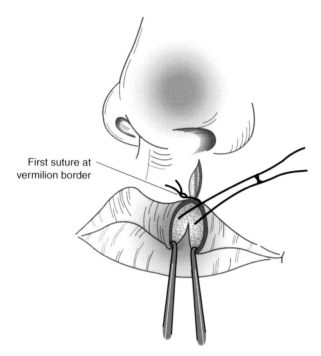

First suture at
vermilion border

Figure 24-14. Repair of vertical laceration of lip.

A. The tissue edges can be cleansed with dilute antiseptics, detergent soaps, and water.
B. In rare cases, solvents (e.g., ether, benzene, or alcohol) are necessary to remove materials not soluble in water or removable by scrubbing or debridement. Scrubbing with a brush under anesthesia may be required to remove foreign material and prevent the development of infection or "traumatic tattoo." The material can be removed initially with scrubbing, the point of a no. 11 blade, or a small dermatologic curette.

X. WOUND TYPE
A. Abrasions
1. Clean with a mild, nonirritating soap or Betadine (Purdue Frederick; Norwalk, Connecticut). When available, dilute Hibiclens (Zeneca; Wilmington, Delaware) can be used in patients sensitive or allergic to Betadine.
2. Carefully scrub dirt, grease, carbon, and other materials out of the wound.
3. Apply a light lubricating dressing.
4. Apply moist compresses (wet to wet) or an antibacterial ointment to prevent drying and desiccation of the exposed wound surfaces.

B. Contused wounds
1. Most hematomas absorb gradually and subside without the need for active treatment.
2. Eyelid, cheek, or forehead hematoma may require drainage.
3. A nasal septal hematoma needs to be evacuated through a small incision in the septal mucosa or with a large-bore needle.

C. Simple lacerations
1. Repair after assessing underlying structures and removing foreign bodies.
2. Time lapse between injury and repair is important relative to risk of infection and choice of repair technique.

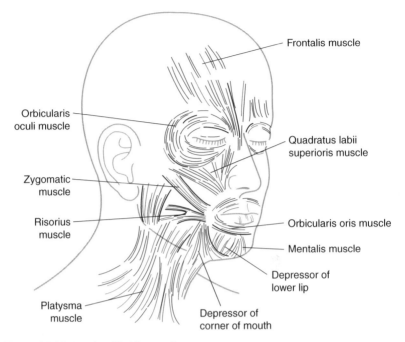

Figure 24-15. Muscles of facial expression.

3. With the exception of animal bites and traumatic tattoo, most soft-tissue wounds of the face, properly cleansed and dressed, can await primary repair up to 24 hours without serious risk of infection.

4. Devitalized tissue must be excised, regardless of its location or importance.
   a. Although debridement should be conservative, it must be adequate. Cautiously excise ragged, severely contused wound edges to provide perpendicular skin edges that will heal primarily with minimal scarring.

5. Convert closely parallel lacerations to a single wound by excising the intervening skin bridge, facilitating repair and reducing scar formation.

6. Displaced tissue should be returned to its original position.

7. Occasionally, immediately changing the direction of a wound by Z-plasty or making tissue allowance for scar contracture at the time of primary wound repair is appropriate.

8. If the contused marginal tissues are of anatomic importance, avoid debridement and consider secondary reconstructive surgery.

D. **Deep lacerations.** The muscles of facial expression (Fig. 24-15) are so closely associated with the skin that careful closure of the wound in layers gives adequate approximation of the muscle.

1. If possible, identify facial muscle layers and close separately with fine absorbable sutures.

2. Closure of the muscle and fascia in layers, including the subcutaneous tissue, restores adequate function and prevents adherence of cheek skin to the muscle.

E. **Delayed primary wound closure**

1. **Indications**
   a. Patient seen late after injury.
   b. Extensive tissue edema.
   c. Subcutaneous hematoma.
   d. Crush injury.

e. Wound edges are badly contused.
f. Tissue is devitalized.
2. Treatment
  a. Limited debridement to remove devitalized tissue.
  b. Wet dressings.
  c. Antibiotic therapy.
3. Treatment continues until resolution of edema and acute inflammation and a clean appearance of the wound. Delayed primary closure is then more likely to be successful.
F. Primary closure under unsatisfactory conditions can contribute to increased tension, soft-tissue loss, infection, and soft-tissue necrosis. Healing by secondary intention should be avoided if possible.

XI. NONSUTURE TECHNIQUE OF WOUND CLOSURE. Some superficial wounds, especially in children, respond well to approximation with commercially available sterile adhesive strips or skin adhesive (cyanoacrylate). Benzoin or Mastisol can be placed along the wound edges to assist tape adherence. The tape is reinforced and provides strong resistance to traction in the lateral direction. When using tissue adhesive, apply a barrier of gel just adjacent and dependent to the wound to avoid the material pooling in an unwanted area (notably the eyelids).
A. Adhesive strapping can provide uniform approximation of tissue margins and eliminates trauma from sutures.
B. The disadvantage is the potential for uneven alignment of the wound edges. Adhesive strips may be left in place for 2 to 3 weeks if indicated, and the wound, thus reinforced, prevents lateral pull on the incision.

XII. SUTURE TECHNIQUE. The most satisfactory scars after repair of facial lacerations are seen when the laceration parallels the relaxed skin tension lines (Fig. 24-16). The basic techniques are best described in Figure 24-17. Choice of suture materials and surgical needles is wide.

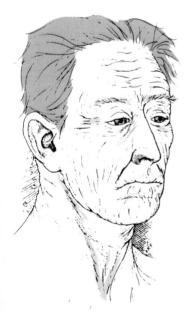

Figure 24-16. Relaxed skin tension lines.

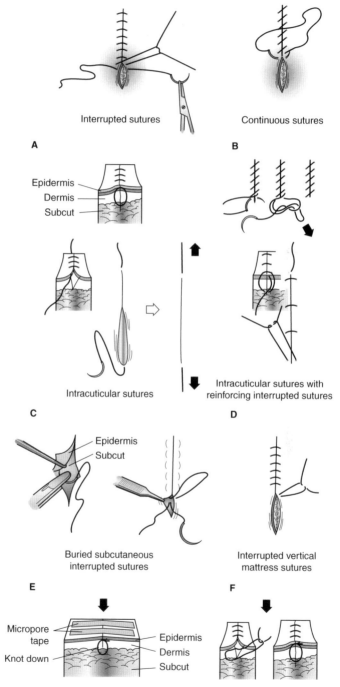

Interrupted sutures

Continuous sutures

A

Epidermis
Dermis
Subcut

B

Intracuticular sutures

Intracuticular sutures with
reinforcing interrupted sutures

C

Epidermis
Subcut

D

Buried subcutaneous
interrupted sutures

Interrupted vertical
mattress sutures

E

Micropore
tape
Knot down

Epidermis
Dermis
Subcut

F

Figure 24-17. Basic suture techniques.

A. With proper closure of the subcutaneous and dermal tissues, minimal tension in the skin should result. Skin sutures should be removed as soon as possible to prevent suture hole scarring.

XIII. REMOVAL OF SUTURES. Facial wounds have the advantage of a rich vascular supply, which contributes to early healing. Where the skin is thin, as in the eyelids, sutures can be removed in 3 days. Elsewhere on the face, sutures can be left in 4 to 6 days. Sutures in ears can remain 10 to 14 days when associated with injury to underlying cartilage.

XIV. ANIMAL AND HUMAN BITES

A. The surgical creation of a clean wound is an essential prerequisite prior to primary wound closure. Irrigate the wound with large amounts of water or saline under pressure (19 g or smaller catheter to create 5 psi).

B. Alternatively, surgical debridement and excision of the wound can convert the wound to a clean injury.

C. Broad-spectrum antibiotic coverage is mandatory, often with ampicillin/clavulanate.

D. Since the risk of infection from human bites is high, routine secondary closure of such injuries is an accepted approach.

AXIOMS

- Control of both the airway and hemorrhage is the immediate goal in the management of maxillofacial injuries.
- Assume that all patients with facial fractures have concomitant cervical spine injury.
- Malocclusion is an important clinical sign of mandibular or maxillary fractures.
- A nasal septal hematoma must be identified and evacuated to avoid a saddle nose deformity.
- Extensive debridement of soft tissues is rarely required for facial injuries; preserve as much tissues as possible.
- Scars from facial wounds are determined less by suture materials and needles than by the character of the wound, appropriate debridement, and skill of the surgeon.

Suggested Readings

Larsen PE. Maxillofacial trauma. In: Miloro M, ed. *Peterson's Principles of Oral and Maxillofacial Surgery.* 2nd ed. Hamilton, Ontario, ON: BC Decker; 2004:327–562.
Marciani RD, Hendler BH. Trauma. In: Fonseca RJ, ed. *Oral and Maxillofacial Surgery.* Philadelphia, PA: WB Saunders; 2000.
Ochs MW. Mandible fractures. In: Myers EN, Eibling DE, eds. *Operative Otolaryngology-Head and Neck Surgery.* 2nd ed. Philadelphia, PA: Elsevier Science; 2005.

25 Spinal Cord and Spinal Column

Matthew Sanborn, Lachlan J. Smith and Neil R. Malhotra

INTRODUCTION

Each year, nearly 250,000 individuals will suffer an injury involving the spine. In the United States, approximately 10,000 new patients with spinal cord injury (SCI) are seen yearly. The impact of SCI is disproportionately large relative to its incidence given the frequency of disability and occurrence in a relatively young population in the prime of productivity. Since 2005, the mean age of a patient with a SCI is 40 years with 80% of injuries occurring in men. The estimated cost of SCI in the United State is $9.7 billion.

Of patients with spinal cord injuries, 44% also suffer from other significant injury, with 14% having head and facial injury. Half of all spinal cord injuries involve the cervical spine, most occurring between C4 and C7, with a 3-month mortality of 20%. One-half of spinal cord injuries involve complete quadriplegia.

The median age of patients with SCI has increased in recent years, reflecting an increase in the median age of the US population. This increase in median age is reflected in falls (27.9%) superseding violence (15.0%) as the second most common cause of SCI. The most common cause remains motor vehicle crashes (40.4%).

Anatomy

The human spinal cord has 31 segments including 8 cervical, 12 thoracic, 5 lumbar, and 6 sacro-coccygeal segments. The spinal canal is surrounded by bony structures: The vertebral body anteriorly, the pedicles laterally, and the lamina posteriorly. With the exception of the sacral vertebra, the vertebral bodies articulate with each other across the intervertebral disc anteriorly and facet joints posteriorly, forming a functional spinal unit. The facet joints, associated ligamentous structures, and other bone articulations (e.g., the rib cage) determine the motion across two vertebral bodies (Fig. 25-1). Motions can be in the sagittal plane (flexion and extension), coronal plane (lateral flexion), and in the transverse plane (rotation).

The adult spinal cord begins at the level of the cervicomedullary junction as the spinal cord passes through the foramen magnum of the skull to join the medulla of the brainstem. The spinal cord is surrounded by the three layers of the meninges which are contiguous with the cranial compartment. The dura mater is the outermost, tough layer, followed by the arachnoid that loosely invests the spinal cord and contains space for the cerebrospinal fluid (CSF). The pia mater is tightly adherent to the spinal cord itself. The spinal cord tapers to an end at the conus medullaris posterior to the L1–L2 vertebral body.

The spinal cord contains white matter tracts consisting of axons originating from upper motor neurons (UMNs) within the brain. These axons synapse with lower motor neurons (LMNs) within the gray matter of the spinal cord that send axons out in the form of nerve roots and the cauda equina. Lesions of the UMNs or their axons result in spasticity, while lesions of the LMNs or their axons result in flaccid paralysis. Generally speaking, UMN lesions carry a worse prognosis than LMN lesions, as nerve roots have better capacity for repair than the spinal cord. Further, because LMN have overlapping motor and sensory distributions, minor injuries may have limited sequela. After exiting the spinal canal, the nerve roots in the cervical and lumbar regions fuse as the cervical and lumbar plexuses before separating again as specific nerves.

In the cervical spine nerve roots exit above the like-numbered pedicle, with C1 exiting between the cranium and the pedicle of C1, and C8 exiting beneath the pedicle of C7. The spinal canal in the cervical region is generally more capacious than in the thoracic or lumbar

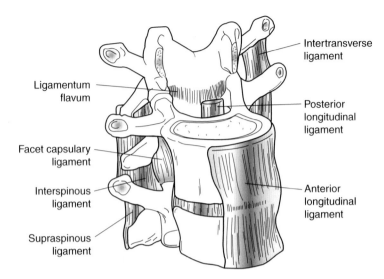

Figure 25-1. Basic osseous and ligamentous anatomy of spine.

regions. Facets are oriented in a coronal plane and overlap one another like roof-tiles, thus coupling ipsilateral bending with contralateral axial rotation. In the cervical spine, about 50% of flexion and extension occurs between the occiput and C1, whereas 50% of rotation occurs between C1 and C2. The remainder of cervical movement takes place in the subaxial (below C2) region.

In the thoracic spine, nerve roots exit beneath like-numbered pedicles with the T1 nerve root exiting beneath the pedicle associated with the T1 vertebral body. The thoracic spine has little motion because of the facet joint orientation and added stabilization of the rib cage.

Lumbar nerve roots exit beneath like-numbered pedicles, as in the thoracic spine. The facet joints of the lumbar spine have a more sagittal orientation and allow moderate motion in the sagittal plane while resisting rotation. The transition from the stiff thoracic spine to a mobile lumbar area accounts for the high number of injuries at the thoracolumbar junction.

Mechanics of Vertebral Column Injury

Injuries to the spinal column occur as a result of excessive forces applied to the spine. These forces can cause axial loading, hyperflexion, hyperextension, distraction, rotation, or a combination of forces. Injury to the spinal column can cause spinal instability, which can be defined on either radiographic or clinical grounds. In the acute setting, radiographic features are most commonly used to determine spinal stability (see later).

The conceptualization of the spine as a series of support columns provides a framework for our understanding of biomechanical stability. Denis first described the three column model of the spine for thoracolumbar fractures. The anterior column (anterior longitudinal ligament and the anterior two-thirds of the vertebral body and disc), the middle column (posterior third of the vertebral body and disc and the posterior longitudinal ligament), and the posterior column (the facet joints, capsule, ligamentum flavum, and posterior ligaments) describe the main columns of overall biomechanical support (Fig. 25-2). Injuries to two of three columns suggest biomechanical instability.

Spinal cord injuries can be distinct from spinal column injuries. Spinal column injuries are bone or ligamentous disruptions that result in bone fractures or ligamentous instability. The loss of these stabilizing and supporting elements can result in compression and injury of neural elements. The diagnosis of spinal column injury is based on both clinical (pain,

Posterior Element   Middle Element   Anterior Element

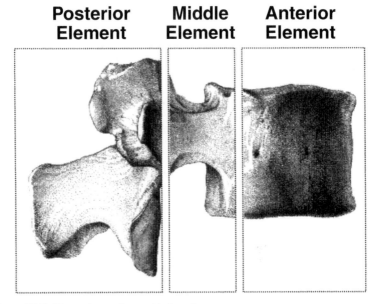

Figure 25-2. Three columns of support in the spine.

tenderness, or ecchymosis) and radiographic criteria on plain films or tomography. Spinal column injuries can occur without SCI, just as SCI can occur without spinal column fracture.

The diagnosis of a SCI is made on clinical grounds and supplemented with imaging studies. The level of SCI frequently correlates with the level of spinal column injury. However, SCI can occur without spinal column injury. Spinal cord injury without radiographic abnormality (SCIWORA) tends to happen in the very young or the elderly in whom ligamentous laxity or canal stenosis, respectively, are predisposing factors. This term developed before the era of magnetic resonance imaging (MRI) and retrospectively these cases may have shown imaging abnormality today.

Certain comorbidities can alter the usual biomechanics of the spine and predispose the trauma patient to unusual fracture patterns. Ankylosing spondylitis can lead to fusion across multiple spinal levels, known as "bamboo spine." This increased rigidity causes the spine to act like a tubular long-bone, with fractures resulting from relatively minor trauma and frequently leading to significant instability. Osteoporosis is found in 38% of women over 75 and is characterized by a decrease in density of normal bone. This decreased density increases risk for fractures from even minor trauma, particularly of the vertebral body. These vertebral compression fractures are rarely associated with neurologic deficit but can lead to progressive kyphosis, ongoing pain, and loss of height.

Prehospital Measures

Initial treatment of patients directed to establish an adequate airway, ventilate the lungs and maintain circulatory support to prevent secondary hypoxic neurologic injury. All patients with a suspected SCI should be immobilized. An estimated 3% to 25% of spinal cord injuries occur after the initial trauma, either in transport or during early resuscitation. A rigid cervical collar alone does not adequately prevent translation in the upper cervical spine, where instability has dire consequences. Use of bilateral sandbags and tape immobilization is more effective in achieving cervical immobilization than any device, especially in conjunction with a rigid collar. When turning is necessary (e.g., active emesis), three members of the treatment team should logroll the patient.

Flat, firm backboards are typically used to facilitate immobilization of the spine but are not optimal in all situations. These boards can lead to skin breakdown over bony prominences. In the rare case of a patient with ankylosing spondylitis, the patient should be transported in the most comfortable position rather than exacerbating spine injury by forcing the spine into a "normal" position.

A scoop stretcher or similar backboard with supportive blocks and straps should be used rather than logrolling to prevent uncontrolled motion. Transport to a definitive treatment center should be the goal, as delays can incur worse outcomes, longer hospitalization, and higher costs. The patient should remain on a backboard until evaluated in the emergency department.

Trauma patients with a mechanism of injury severe enough to cause spinal injury frequently require airway protection. This is discussed in Chapter 3.

Hypovolemic and neurogenic shock can occur in the setting of SCI. Hypotension should be considered first to be from abdominal bleeding, aortic or cardiac injury, or external blood loss before considering neurogenic shock. Neurogenic shock is a diagnosis of exclusion; it is caused by interruption of sympathetic outflow tracts with resultant unopposed vagal tone. Bradycardia is a classic but not always present, as is true for warm, dry skin.

Regardless of cause, shock should be appropriately treated to prevent further ischemic injury to the spinal cord. Treatment consists of crystalloid fluid administration first with vasopressors to maintain adequate blood pressure only once certain that euvolemia is achieved. This is covered in Chapter 5.

Neurologic Evaluation and Physical Examination

At the conclusion of the primary survey, a focused neurologic examination should be performed examining level of consciousness with Glasgow Coma Score (GCS), pupillary size and reaction, lateralizing signs and SCI level.

During the secondary examination, a more detailed neurologic examination, external assessment for spinal tenderness or deformity (e.g., spinous process step-off) and radiologic evaluation guided by the results of the neurologic and physical examinations is performed. Evaluate the mental status, cranial nerves, motor testing, sensory testing, and reflexes to assess global functioning, and repeat this to detect any changes over time.

Motor evaluation is performed by asking the patient to move all extremities individually and assessing strength using the American Spinal Injury Association/International Medical Society of Paraplegia (ASIA/IMSOP) protocol. Normal strength is graded 5/5, with mild weakness graded as 4/5. Grades 4 and 5 are determined based on amount resistance overcome and grade 4 is the only grade that is sometimes subdivided into three divisions to further clarify amount of power (−4, 4, 4+). The ability to fully overcome gravity through a full range of motion, but not overcome any applied resistance by the examiner, is graded 3/5. Movement throughout a range of motion but unable to overcome gravity is graded 2/5. Flicker motion of muscles is 1/5 and no movement is 0/5. Patients with C5 levels of spinal cord function will be able to flex only their arms and should not be confused with pathologic flexor posturing.

Sensory testing of light touch and pain perception can aid determining radiographic target for imaging (Fig. 25-3). Useful examination tools include a cotton swab broken in half or safety pins. Pay close attention to the level of sensation and asymmetry.

Reflex testing is performed at the biceps (C5), triceps (C7), brachioradialis, knee (L4), and ankle areas (S1). Special reflex testing includes jaw jerk, deltoid (C5), pectoral, superficial abdominal (T9–T12), bulbo- or cliterocavernositis (S3–S4), anal wink (S5), and Babinski. The extremity reflexes are graded on a scale of 0 to 4, where 0 represents absent reflex activity, 1 is decreased reflex activity, 2 is normal reflex activity, 3 represents increased reflex activity, and 4 is grossly exaggerated reflex activity with sustained clonus. An exaggerated jaw jerk indicates injury at or above the pons. Deltoid and pectoral reflexes are usually associated with significant hyperreflexia. Bulbo- or cliterocavernosis reflexes may be retained in complete injury, but lost during spinal shock. Their reappearance may indicate that a period of spinal shock has ended. Babinski responses are recorded as present or absent. The presence of UMN findings (hyperreflexia, loss of superficial abdominal reflexes, Babinski responses) indicates spinal cord or conus medullaris injury. Decreased reflexes imply LMN (cauda equina and

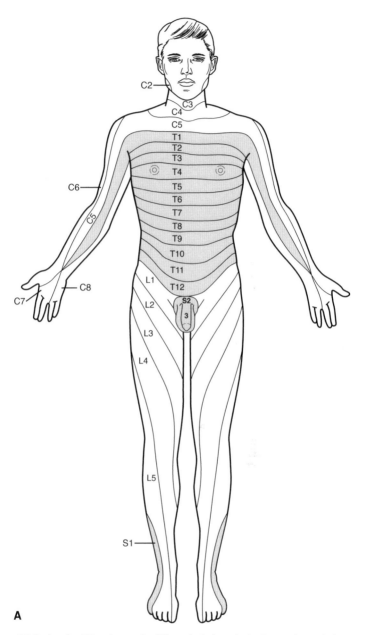

Figure 25-3. Anterior **(A)** and posterior **(B)** cervical, thoracic, lumbar, and sacral dermatomes. (*continued*)

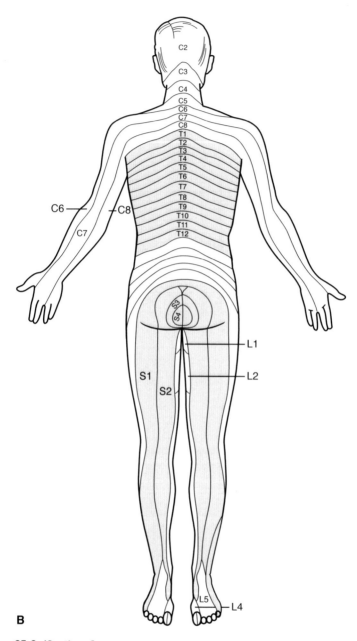

B

Figure 25-3. (*Continued*)

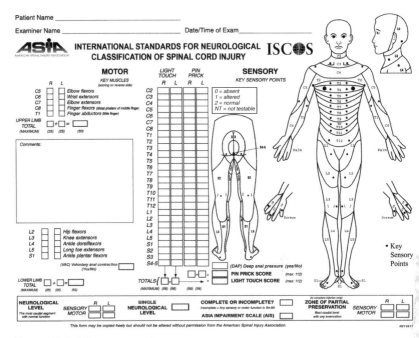

Figure 25-4. ASIA assessment form.

nerve root) injury. Weakness, sensory loss, and bladder, bowel, and sexual dysfunction can be seen with either UMN or LMN injuries. Of note, acute UMN injuries often present with reflex stunning or areflexia, mimicking a LMN injury, and may last for 24 to 48 hours.

The most sensitive predictor of prognosis is the severity of neurologic injury as characterized by level and completeness of deficit. The neurologic sensory levels are determined and recorded based on the lowest segment with normal sensory and full motor function bilaterally. Complete injury is seen in the patient without sensory or motor function below the level of neurologic injury, including loss of perianal sensation and sphincter function. The patient with incomplete injury has partial preservation of sensory or motor function below the level of neurologic injury, with preservation of perianal sensation and motor function called "sacral sparing"; the latter does not include an intact bulbo/clitorocavernosus reflex which can be present in complete injuries.

In the acute setting, the use of specific terms denoting neurologic level is preferable to more general terms (e.g., paraparesis, quadriplegia). The ASIA impairment scale, consisting of a five-point grading scale demarcated A–E (Fig. 25-4), is as follows:

A. Complete loss of sensory and motor function (including the sacral area) below the neurologic level. Even patients with ASIA A scores can improve neurologically, although few of these patients will achieve functional motor recovery.

B. Incomplete injury, whereby sensory function is preserved below the level of neurologic injury including the sacral area.

C. Incomplete injury with motor function preserved below the neurologic level and most preserved groups exhibiting strength of <3 (gravity).

D. Incomplete injury with motor function preserved below the neurologic level and most preserved groups exhibiting >3 strength.

E. Normal sensory and motor examination.

Spinal cord injuries can often present with characteristic constellations of findings indicating the region of the spinal cord affected and reflecting the mechanism of injury.

1. **Posterior cord injury** with loss of position sense resulting from injury to the posterior columns is rarely traumatic. This injury is usually related to vitamin deficiencies and infections (e.g., syphilis). The patients develop a loss of position and vibratory sense.
2. **Central cord injury** is common in the cervical spine of patients who experience excessive motion in the sagittal plane, particularly in those with pre-existing stenosis of the spinal canal. These injuries are thought to result from vascular compromise to the central areas of the spinal cord. The hallmark features are hand weakness that is more pronounced than lower extremity weakness, bladder dysfunction, and variable degrees of sensory loss below the lesion.
3. **Anterior cord injury** often occurs in the setting of vascular compromise and suggests anterior spinal artery occlusion. Infarction of the spinal cord results in loss of all motor and sensory function other than proprioception.
4. **Brown-Sequard syndrome** is rarely seen in its pure form and is a result of injury to one-half of the spinal cord. It is characterized by loss of ipsilateral motor function, ipsilateral position sense, and contralateral loss of pain and temperature sensation two to three segments below the level of injury.
5. **Conus medullaris and cauda equina syndromes** occur at the thoracolumbar levels and result in varying degrees of weakness, sensory loss, bladder, bowel, and sexual dysfunction. Conus injuries affect UMNs, which may precipitate hyperreflexia. Conus injuries may also cause reflex stunning with the loss of the bulbocavernosus reflex. The cauda equina syndrome typically results from a compressive lesion below the level of the spinal cord with resultant bowel/bladder dysfunction, saddle paresthesias, and lower extremity weakness. This represents one of the few operative emergencies in spinal trauma; compression should be alleviated as soon as safely possible to attain maximal recovery and prevent further deterioration.

Radiographic Examination

The cervical spine can be clinically cleared without radiography in patients who present with a GCS of 15, with no evidence of drug or alcohol use, normal neurologic examination, without midline cervical pain/tenderness, and without distracting or significant injuries. The Canadian C-spine rule (Fig. 25-5) is a well-validated algorithm to avoid unnecessary imaging. For the majority of trauma patients who do not meet these guidelines, evaluation in the past started with plain films.

The sensitivity of plain cervical x-rays to detect fracture is low, with pooled data from meta-analysis showing a sensitivity of 52% versus 98% for CT. With a 14.5% probability of paralysis for missed injuries, CT has emerged as the diagnostic modality of choice. In select circumstances, plain films can aid evaluation of the spine.

While cost remains a point of contention, in moderate- to high-risk patients in urban trauma centers, CT can be cost-effective. Of note, the most commonly missed cervical fractures are at the C1 to C2 and C7 to T1 levels, usually the result of inadequate imaging.

The basic lateral radiographic studies must include the skull base and T1 vertebral body for adequate interpretation. A "swimmer's view" may be required to fully assess C7 to T1. Oblique views may also help assess C7 to T1, although CT should be obtained after two attempted failures to obtain adequate plain films.

Lateral plain films are reviewed with careful attention to three lines:

a. Posterior vertebral body line
b. Anterior vertebral body line
c. Spinolaminar line (Fig. 25-6)

These lines should be uninterrupted and smooth. The appearance of a straight spine (loss of the normal cervical lordosis) indicates extensor muscular spasm and is suggestive of spinal injury. A rigid cervical collar can also cause loss of lordosis. The vertebral canal is defined as the distance from the spinolaminar line to the posterior vertebral body line. This represents the space available for the cord and should be at least 13 mm at every level. A narrower canal may represent injury or congenital cervical stenosis.

Soft tissues are then examined. The trachea contains air and provides a line of contrast against the vertebral bodies. Prevertebral swelling indicates a hematoma suggestive of spinal

For Alert (Glasgow Coma Scale Score = 15)
and Stable Trauma Patients Where
Cervical Spine (C-Spine) Injury is a Concern

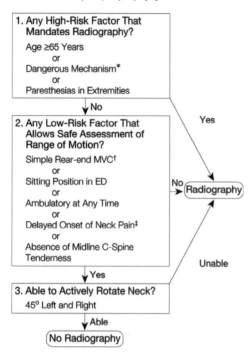

Figure 25-5. Canadian C-spine rule. (From Stiell IG, Clement CM, McKnight RD, et al. The Canadian C-spine rule versus the NEXUS low-risk criteria in patients with trauma. *N Engl J Med* 2003;349:2512).

column injury. The soft-tissue space should be no greater than 6 mm in front of the C2 vertebral body and no greater than 22 mm anterior to C6.

Atlanto-occipital dislocation (AOD) is suggested by a distance of >8.5 mm between the basion of the skull and the tip of the dens on CT. Similarly the distance between the occipital condyle and the superior articular surface of C1 should be less than 1.4 mm

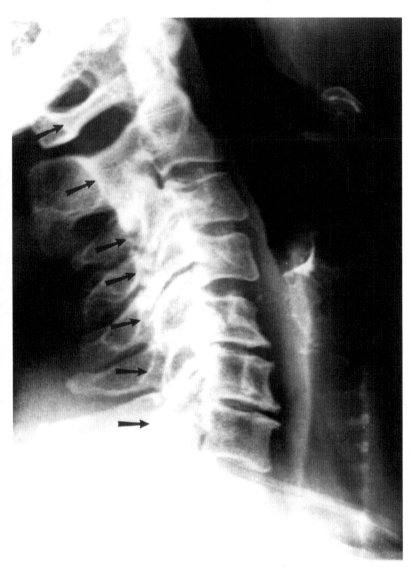

Figure 25-6. Normal cervical spine lateral radiograph demonstrating spinolaminar line (*arrows*).

on sagittal reconstructed CT scans. Missed or delayed diagnosis of this injury can have catastrophic consequences.

Another important distance is the atlantodental interval. This is the space between the anterior aspect of the odontoid (dens) and the ring of C1. This space should not exceed 3.5 mm in the adult and 5 mm in the child. Distances greater than those indicate disruption of the transverse ligament, with resultant instability.

The lateral masses of C1 are examined with regard to their relationship to C2. Little or no overhang of the lateral masses should be seen. A combined, bilateral overhang >6.9 mm on anteroposterior (AP) x-ray indicates a fracture of the ring of C1, with probable disruption of the transverse ligament. However, transverse ligament disruption may occur without overhang greater than 6.9 mm. The odontoid bone should be symmetrically located between the lateral masses of C2.

The dens may be evaluated with either CT or through an open mouth odontoid radiograph and should be inspected for the present of type I, II, or III odontoid fractures (see later).

Vertebral height is examined next, including vertebral body morphology. The vertebral bodies should be similar in appearance, without evidence of compression or fracture. The distance between the posterior spinous processes, or interspinous distance, should be similar at each level.

The AP view of the spine is examined for the distance between spinous process, alignment, and rotation. Facet anatomy is more closely observed with oblique views of the cervical spine. Areas suspected of fracture should be further evaluated with fine-cut CT if one has not been performed.

MRI is indicated in patients with neurologic deficits and to assess ligamentous integrity or other soft tissues including the spinal cord and canal contents. The MRI also detects subtle compression fractures, traumatic disc rupture, and SCI. Signal change on long TR images helps differentiate acute from chronic injury.

All patients with neurologic deficits should be evaluated in consultation with a spine expert.

Patients with neck pain in the setting of normal preliminary x-rays require further studies. In the past, flexion and extension films were utilized; must less so currently. In patients with pain, dynamic studies are often delayed until resolution of neck pain in cervical immobilization. These must visualize C7 to T1. Further radiographs, including MRI and even bone scan, can be appropriate to rule out possible bone or ligamentous injury. The rigid collar should remain in place until the neck is cleared clinically and radiographically.

Patients with suspected vertebral artery injury should have computed tomography angiography (CTA), or MR angiogram. The slightly lower sensitivity of CTA is balanced by the ease with which it is obtained. Indications for angiogram may include complete cervical spine injury, fracture of the foramen transversarium, facet dislocation, subluxation, C1–C2 injury, or suspicious neurologic examination suggesting dissection.

The thoracolumbar spine is commonly injured at the T12 to L1 levels. This occurs because of the large lever arm created by the inflexible thoracic spine as it joins the lumbar spine. AP and lateral films are indicated in those patients with symptoms referable to the thoracic area who are not undergoing thoracoabdominal CT already. Three lines are observed along the anterior and posterior aspects of the vertebral bodies, and along the posterior aspect of the spinous processes. The distance between these processes should also remain equal. On the AP view, the distance between pedicles is determined as is the distance between the posterior spinous processes. The transverse processes and ribs are evaluated for fractures and the soft tissues are examined for swelling. Plain x-rays are being used much less often.

More specialized imaging studies are obtained as necessary. Thoracic spine CT is indicated for those patients with fractures noted on x-ray film or when the anatomy is not well seen on plain films. MRI is indicated for all patients with neurologic findings when primary injury does not mandate emergent surgical intervention.

The spinal cord ends at L1–L2 level and so true SCI from lumbar fractures is rare. Injuries to the conus medullaris and cauda equina can occur if the spinal canal is compromised. Commonly, no neurologic injury is noted with lumbar spine fractures. CT can be useful to determine the amount of canal compromise in cases of burst fracture. MRI and myelography are also helpful in cases of traumatic nerve root injury, canal compression, and conus medullaris or cauda equina syndromes.

Medical Management of Spinal Cord Injury

The goal is to prevent secondary cord injury, which can be exacerbated by hypotension, shock, hypoxia, hypercoagulability, or hyperthermia. Management protocols include definitive treatment of other injuries, maintenance of adequate blood pressure, high-dose steroids if appropriate, determination of the need for surgical intervention, and postoperative rehabilitation.

Injury to the cervical or thoracic spinal cord above T6 has the potential to cause neurogenic shock by interrupting sympathetic outflow tracts with resultant autonomic instability. This typically manifests as hypotension and bradycardia. Nearly all patients with severe high cervical cord injuries will exhibit persistent bradycardia and 68% will have hypotension. If untreated, this hypotension can result in an increased risk for morbidity, mortality, and the potential for secondary ischemic cord injury.

Evidence-based guidelines for the cardiovascular management of the SCI patient include monitoring of cardiac and hemodynamic parameters following acute SCI, maintaining a mean-arterial pressure (MAP) of greater than 85 mm Hg for 7 days following SCI, timely detection and treatment of neurogenic shock and associated cardiac dysrhythmias and immediate treatment of episodes of autonomic instability.

Although the NASCIS II and III studies demonstrated a modest clinical benefit of corticosteroids (methylprednisolone 30 mg/kg intravenously over 45 minutes within 8 hours after injury followed by 5.4 mg/kg/h IV continuous 23-hour infusion), other studies using a similar protocol failed to show this benefit. High-dose corticosteroids are associated with an increase in pulmonary and gastrointestinal complications and increased risk of infection. The modest and inconclusive clinical benefit and the complications associated with high-dose corticosteroids have resulted in a growing ambiguity regarding their role in SCI. Currently, the administration of steroids "is recommended as an option in treatment of patients with acute spinal cord injuries that should be undertaken only with the knowledge that the evidence suggesting harmful side effects is more consistent than any suggestion of clinical benefit." The American College of Surgeons has altered the Advanced Trauma Life Support Guidelines from stating that methylprednisolone is "the recommended treatment" to "a recommended treatment."

Hypoxia from respiratory dysfunction must also be assiduously avoided following SCI. Acute SCI can result in impairment of respiratory muscles, ineffective cough and clearing of secretions, reduced lung and chest wall compliance. The phrenic nerve, with contributions from nerve roots at C3, C4, and C5, innervates the diaphragm and SCI at this level is associated with ventilator dependence. SCI below this level can impact respiration by disrupting function in intercostal muscles and other accessory muscles of inspiration or expiration. Early tracheostomy can reduce length of stay and facilitate care. In 178 patients with ASIA A SCI, 70% required a tracheostomy; 100% for injuries at or above C3 and none at or below C8.

Patients with complete SCI require diligent monitoring in the subacute and chronic setting to prevent development of additional comorbidities. Urinary tract infections are common in paralyzed patients because of repeated catheterization. Decubitus ulcers can occur rapidly in insensate patients. Aggressive nursing care is the mainstay of treatment. Stress gastric and duodenal ulcers are common and prophylaxis is recommended. Joint contractures and heterotopic ossification are common in paralyzed patients. These complications can be reduced by physical therapy.

SCI patients are more sensitive to succinylcholine, which can precipitate a hyperkalemic crisis. Autonomic dysreflexia occurs in up to 90% of patients with lesions above T6. Distension of hollow viscera or cutaneous stimulation can produce rapid fluctuations in blood pressure, vasoconstriction, bladder spasm, flushing, sweating, encephalopathy, seizures, congestive heart failure, or arrhythmias. Treatment involves removal of the stimulus and aggressive blood pressure control.

In the absence of prophylaxis, patients with acute SCI have a 12% to 64% incidence of clinical DVT and PE; the rate increases to 81% within the first 3 weeks when screened using arterial impedance plethysmography. Duplex ultrasonography is used to diagnose DVT. Current evidence-based guidelines call for the use of compression stocking or pneumatic compression devices bilaterally for at least 2 weeks following SCI. In cases without active bleeding or coagulopathy, low-molecular weight-heparin or low-dose unfractionated heparin prophylaxis should be instituted within 72 hours. Consensus guidelines recommend continuation of pharmacologic therapy in patients with complete motor SCI for a minimum of 8 weeks and possibly longer (12 weeks or until discharge from rehabilitation) in patients

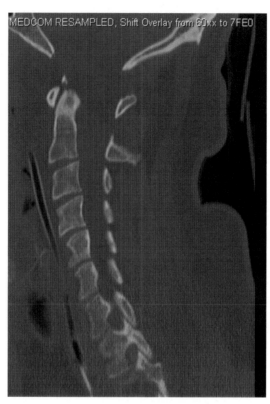

Figure 25-7. AOD.

with risk factors for DVT such as lower limb fractures, obesity, age >70 years, heart failure, cancer or history of thrombosis.

Cervical Spine Fractures

At the top of the cervical spine rests the atlas, providing articulation between the spine and occiput at the occipital condyle. Condylar fractures are commonly a result of axial load and are frequently missed on cervical radiograph. Patients are usually neurologically intact, but may present with delayed lower cranial nerve palsy. These injuries require CT scan for proper evaluation and rarely require anything more than cervical orthosis, except in the setting of avulsion of the alar ligament where halo vest or surgery may be indicated.

AOD (Fig. 25-7), results from disruption of the ligamentous connections between occipital condyles and C1. Patients who survive typically exhibit lower cranial neuropathies, mono/para/quadriplegia, and respiratory dysfunction, although 20% may have normal examinations. Craniocervical subarachnoid blood or cervical prevertebral edema can provide an early clue to the diagnosis. Treatment involves craniocervical fusion with internal fixation.

Atlas fractures account for 10% of cervical spine fractures and are rarely associated with neurologic deficit; in 50% of cases, these are associated with other cervical spine fractures. Jefferson fractures occur when an axial load is placed on the head and the C1 bony ring is forced apart. Stability depends on the integrity of the transverse ligament. A fracture with evidence of ligamentous disruption can be treated with a halo orthosis for 3 months or a C1–C2 fusion depending on the injury pattern. Stable fractures can be treated with a rigid cervical collar for 2 to 3 months.

Stability of the atlantoaxial complex is dependent on the integrity of the ligamentous structures, the most important being the transverse ligament. Injury to the transverse ligament, suggested by an atlantodental interval of >3.5 mm (Fig. 25-8), or total overhang of the lateral masses of C1 on C2 is greater than 6.9 mm (Fig. 25-9) implies instability and may require immobilization with a halo vest or C1–C2 fusion.

The bony odontoid fractures can be divided into types I, II, and III (Fig. 25-10).

a. **Type I fractures** are oblique fractures through the upper portion, or tip, of the odontoid process. This usually cause pain alone and are rarely a neurologic threat.
b. **Type II fractures** occur at the base of the dens. These fractures are unstable, although most can be managed with external stabilization (rigid cervical collar or halo-vest device). Nonunion with external mobilization is more common in older patients (>50). Fractures with posterior displacement provide increased morbidity from impingement on the spinal cord. Surgical options include an odontoid screw, posterior fixation transarticular screws, or a C1–C2 construct. Close airway attention is critical in these patients as upper airway swelling and respiratory compromise can occur (Fig. 25-11).
c. **Type III fractures** extend from the odontoid into the vertebral body and joints of C2. They generally have a better healing rate than type II fractures with external fixation due to the increased surface area of fracture. Type III fractures rarely need surgery.

Hangman's fractures are bilateral through the pars interarticularis of C2. This type of fracture is generally stable and treated in a hard cervical collar. Surgical stabilization including anterior C2–C3 fusion or posterior fusion should be considered in cases of severe angulation, C2–C3 disc disruption, fracture/dislocation, or failure to achieve anatomic alignment with external fixation.

In the subaxial cervical spine flexion injuries can result in **disruption of the facet joints.** The presence of 25% subluxation of one vertebra on another can represent a unilateral facet fracture or dislocation. Subluxation of 50% generally means that a bilateral facet injury has occurred. There is debate with regard to the utilization of an MRI scan before closed reduction. Certainly MRI should be considered if closed reduction is unsuccessful and the patient is being considered for open reduction. Patients with traumatic disc herniation may need anterior discectomy and subsequent intraoperative reduction and stabilization.

Unilateral facet fractures (Fig. 25-12) can be stable, with pure bony injuries handled by external mobilization. An irreducible dislocation, progressive deformity, or neurologic compromise may require surgical stabilization. **Bilateral facet injuries** are unstable and intraoperative reduction and surgical stabilization is the treatment method of choice if awake closed reduction fails.

Burst fractures generally occur as a result of flexion or axial loading. The columns may appear well aligned at first glance on the lateral radiograph. Generally noted is an expansion of the prevertebral space and loss of vertebral height. The CT scan will show the vertebral comminution, which can cause canal compromise and subsequent neurologic deficit. Fracture compression of 40% or more and subluxation of 20% or more have been associated with instability as is neurologic compromise. These often require surgical stabilization; traction may be helpful for preoperative decompression and stabilization.

MRI can detect posterior ligamentous disruption and the **"tear drop" fracture.** Teardrop fractures are typically the result of hyperflexion or axial loading of the neck in a flexed position, with ligamentous disruption and injury to both the facet joints and disc space below. The "teardrop" is a small chip of bone displaced from the anterior inferior edge of the involved vertebral body. These injuries are unstable, typically present with severe neurologic impairment, and must be differentiated from the less ominous extension injury with a small fragment off the anterior cortex of the vertebral body. CT will usually demonstrate a sagittally oriented fracture through the vertebral body. MRI will often demonstrate an early spinal cord contusion. Surgical stabilization is required in most cases.

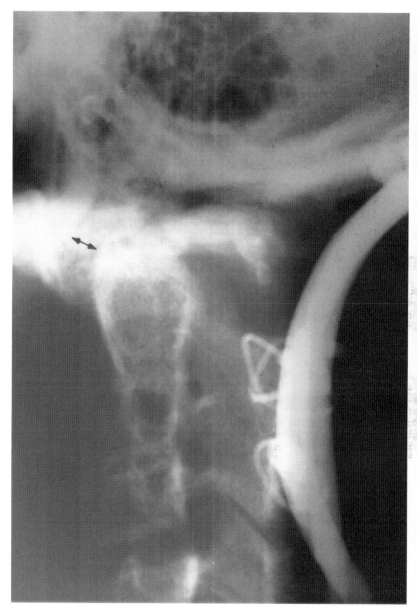

Figure 25-8. Lateral radiograph demonstrating excessive atlantodens interval.

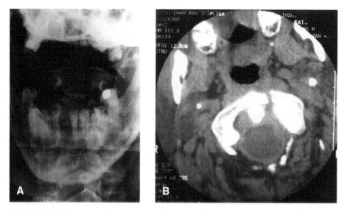

Figure 25-9. C1 fracture with overhanging of the C1 lateral masses as seen on anteroposterior plain film **(A)** and axial computed tomography scan **(B)**.

Thoracolumbar Spine Fractures

Wedge compression fractures (Fig. 25-13) are the most common fracture seen in this region of the spine. Usually considered stable, a wedge fracture involves the anterior column alone most frequently. Posterior column involvement in wedge fractures via distraction can result in instability.

    Thoracolumbar burst fractures are similar to wedge fractures but result from both anterior and middle column failure from the addition of axial compression to the flexion

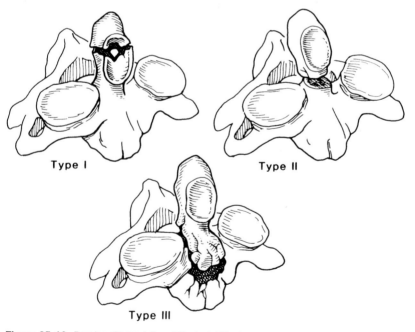

Figure 25-10. Drawing of types I, II, and III odontoid fractures.

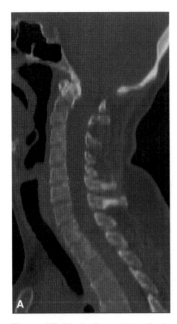
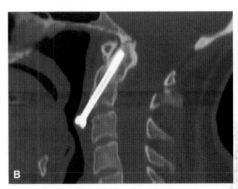

Figure 25-11. Radiograph type II odontoid fracture.

of the wedge fracture. Neurologically intact patients without evidence of damage to the posterior osteoligamentous complex may be managed in an extension brace for 3 months. Patients receive close radiographic follow-up with concern for progressive kyphosis. Patients with a progressive deficit require operative intervention.

Another common fracture observed is the **seatbelt or "Chance" fracture,** an axially oriented injury caused by a flexion injury around an anterior fulcrum (lap belt without shoulder harness). The excessive flexion motion places the spine in kyphosis. This injury is associated with a 33% incidence of abdominal injury and 13% risk of paralysis. Some of the pure bony injuries can be managed non-operatively by placing the patients in an extension brace to bring the fractured bony elements into apposition, but ligamentous injuries require surgery.

Fracture dislocation injuries account for nearly 20% of thoracolumbar injuries and must be addressed based on specifics of the injury. Most occur at the thoracolumbar junction and are highly unstable. The more cephalad the injury, the more likely paraplegia will result (90% above T10 and 60% below T10). These injuries require surgical stabilization.

Surgical Management of Spine Injury

Intervention is indicated to decompress the neural elements and to provide stabilization to an unstable spinal column thus eliminating secondary injury, facilitating rehabilitation and reducing pulmonary complications. Intervention may take the form of closed reduction and cervical traction or surgery for open decompression and internal fixation.

Traction is applied in a variety of settings, but early placement is most important when clear abnormality on plain films exists with a declining neurologic examination. Traction can play a major role in correction of cervical spine abnormalities but is ineffective in lower spine regions.

Gardner-Wells tongs can be applied at the bedside with local anesthetic and permit serial addition of weights to achieve reduction. A torque sensitive pin allows determination of degree of pressure displaced to the skull at insertion site, which is generally 2 cm above

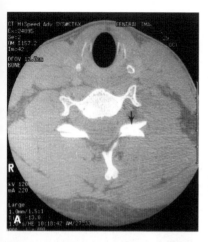
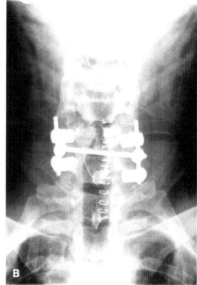
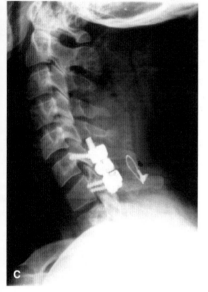

Figure 25-12. Preoperative axial computed tomography scan demonstrating a unilateral jumped and locked facet fracture and dislocation **(A).** The left jumped facet has the appearance of two opposing hamburger buns (*arrow*). Anteroposterior **(B)** and lateral **(C)** radiographs demonstrating the instrumented fusion using lateral mass screws and rods with interspinous wiring and bone grafting.

the pinna of the ear. Thirty pounds of compressive force is applied to the skull at maximal setting and is confirmed again at 24 hours to ensure this is unchanged; thereafter no pressure adjustments are performed. Accepted indications for cervical traction include facet joint subluxation (e.g., unilateral perched, or bilateral jumped facet), as well as burst type fractures.

Slow addition of weight is the most effective and safe approach to closed reduction when a distracting injury is not present. Prior to weight addition, both traumatic disc herniation and ligamentous injury with distraction must be ruled out. Failure to recognize

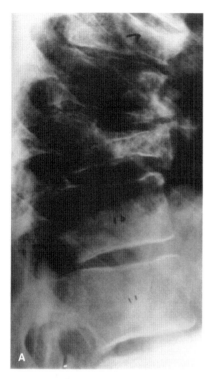
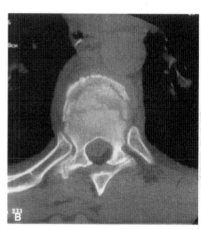

Figure 25-13. T9 compression fracture as seen on lateral radiograph **(A)** and axial computed tomography scan **(B).**

AOD could result in patient demise upon application of weight. Initially, a small amount of weight (10 lb or 3 × cervical vertebral level) is used. Every 10 to 15 minutes serial imaging is acquired and another 5 to 10 lb may be added until either reduction or a pre-determined maximum weight is achieved. Most guidelines recommend not exceeding either 5 or 10 lb per vertebral body level below the occiput. Titrated IV diazepam can be an effective adjunct but should not inhibit breathing or serial neurologic examinations. Lateral radiographs should be completed for each incremental addition of weight to demonstrate correction or over distraction. Extensive distraction is a contraindication to further addition of weight, especially at sites away from goal distraction site, and suggests open correction of deformity will be required. Progression of neurologic deficit is a clear contraindication to continuance of cervical traction.

Surgical decision-making in cervical spine trauma is complex and dependent on multiple variables. There are many classifications of cervical fractures to codify the surgical decision-making process—the most recent being the subaxial cervical spine injury classification system proposed by Vaccaro et al. In this scoring system, points are assigned for fracture morphology, integrity of the disco-ligamentous complex and neurologic injury (Table 25-1). If the total points assigned are less than 3 the patient may be managed non-operatively; if the total is greater than or equal to 5 then operative treatment is recommended.

The thoracolumbar injury classification and severity score (TLICS) helps classify thoracolumbar fractures and guide surgical decision-making in a manner analogous to the SLIC system. Similar to the SLIC, points are assigned based on injury morphology, neurologic injury, and integrity of the posterior ligamentous complex. A score of 3 or less suggests a non-operative injury, while 5 or more suggests the need for surgery (Table 25-2).

TABLE 25-1	The Subaxial Cervical Injury Classification and Severity Score (SLICS)	
Injury Morphometry		
Compression		1
Compression (burst)		2
Distraction (e.g., facet perch, hyperextension)		3
Rotation/translation (e.g., facet dislocation, unstable teardrop or advanced flexion/compression injury)		4
Disco-ligamentous Complex		
Intact		0
Suspected/indeterminate		2
Injured		3
Neurologic Status		
Intact		0
Nerve root		2
Cord (complete)		2
Cord (incomplete)		3
Continuous cord compression in setting of neuro deficit (neuro modifier)		+1

The timing of surgical intervention in spinal trauma remains controversial with the preponderance of data coming from studies limited to the cervical spine. Currently, most spine surgeons advocate surgical decompression within 24 hours for SCI. Early fixation of unstable spinal injuries in the polytrauma patient, even in the absence of neurologic injury, is associated with shorter hospital stays and improved patient outcomes. Surgical decision-making must be balanced against hemodynamic stability and each patient's ability to tolerate surgery. Patients with central cord syndrome and spondylosis but no unstable fracture are a particularly controversial population. Current guidelines recommend early surgical decompression for the most seriously injured (ASIA C) and delayed decompression for those with more minor neurologic deficits (ASIA D).

Penetrating Spinal Column Injury

Penetrating injuries to the spine should be treated as elsewhere in the body. The standard surgical principles of debridement and closure can be applied. The caveat is that patients

TABLE 25-2	The Thoracolumbar Injury Classification and Severity Score (TLICS)	
Injury Morphometry		
Compression		1
Compression (burst)		2
Translational/rotational		3
Distraction		4
Integrity of the Posterior Ligamentous Complex		
Intact		0
Suspected/indeterminate		2
Injured		3
Neurologic Status		
Intact		0
Nerve root		2
Cord/conus (complete)		2
Cord/conus (incomplete)		3
Cauda equina		3

with CSF leaks are at risk of meningitis and paravertebral abscess formation, unless CSF egress is controlled. Steroid therapy is contraindicated in this population due to the risk of infection.

Passage through the esophagus, pharynx, or colon before traversing the spine has the potential to cause spinal sepsis. Radical debridement of the spine is no longer advocated in this situation. Minimal debridement of bullet tract and 1 to 2 weeks of broad-spectrum antibiotics is sufficient to decrease the chance of spinal infection to about 10% of cases when the bullet traverses the colon, esophagus, or pharynx.

Surgery is indicated in situations of nerve root or spinal compression with neurologic deficit, CSF leak, spinal instability, debridement to reduce risk of infection in cases of extensive damage or coincident injury to the GI or respiratory tract. Lead toxicity from bullets occurs only when the bullet is lodged within a joint, bursae or disc space and may also necessitate removal. These procedures can be facilitated if performed in a delayed fashion to allow easier dural repair. CSF diversion may be required for persistent leakage. Neurologic deterioration obviously mandates a more urgent approach.

AXIOMS

- The diagnosis of a SCI is made on clinical grounds and supplemented with imaging studies.
- Neurogenic shock is a diagnosis of exclusion; assume the patient has cavitary bleeding until proven otherwise.
- Hypoxemia and hypotension must be avoided in the patient with SCI; extension of the injury may result.

Suggested Readings

Blood pressure management after acute spinal cord injury. *Neurosurgery* 2002;50:S58–S62.

Boswell HB, Dietrich A, Shiels WE, et al. Accuracy of visual determination of neutral position of the immobilized pediatric cervical spine. *Pediatr Emerg Care* 2001;17:10–14.

Bracken MB, Shepard MJ, Collins WF, et al. A randomized, controlled trial of methylprednisolone or naloxone in the treatment of acute spinalcord injury. Results of the Second National Acute Spinal Cord Injury Study. *N Engl J Med* 1990;322:1405–1411.

Denis F. The three column spine and its significance in the classification of acute thoracolumbar spinal injuries. *Spine* 1983;8:817–831.

Dimar JR, Carreon LY, Riina J, et al. Early versus late stabilization of the spine in the polytrauma patient. *Spine* 2010;35:S187–S192.

Fehlings MG, Rabin D, Sears W, et al. Current practice in the timing of surgical intervention in spinal cord injury. *Spine* 2010;35:S166–S173.

Grogan EL, Morris JA Jr, Dittus RS, et al. Cervical spine evaluation in urban trauma centers: lowering institutional costs and complications through helical CT scan. *J Am Coll Surg* 2005;200:160–165.

Holmes JF, Akkinepalli R. Computed tomography versus plain radiography to screen for cervical spine injury: a metaanalysis. *J Trauma* 2005;58:902–905.

Lenehan B, Fisher CG, Vaccaro A, et al. The urgency of surgical decompression in acute central cord injuries with spondylosis and without instability. *Spine* 2010;35:S180–S186.

Pharmacological therapy after acute cervical spinal cord injury. *Neurosurgery* 2002;50:S63–S72.

Ploumis A, Yadlapalli N, Fehlings MG, et al. A systematic review of the evidence supporting a role for vasopressor support in acute SCI. *Spinal Cord* 2010;48:356–362.

Rojas CA, Bertozzi JC, Martinez CR, et al. Reassessment of the craniocervical junction: normal values on CT. *AJNR Am J Neuroradiol* 2007;28:1819–1823.

Stiell IG, Clement CM, McKnight RD, et al. The Canadian C-spine rule versus the NEXUS low-risk criteria in patients with trauma. *N Engl J Med* 2003;349:2510–2518.

Stiell IG, Wells GA, Vandemheen KL, et al. The Canadian C-spine rule for radiography in alert and stable trauma patients. *JAMA* 2001;286:1841–1848.

Vaccaro AR, Hulbert RJ, Patel AA, et al. The subaxial cervical spine injury classification system: a novel approach to recognize the importance of morphology, neurology, and integrity of the discoligamentous complex. *Spine (Phila Pa 1976)* 2007;32:2365–2374.

Ophthalmic Injuries

S. Tonya Stefko and Donald M. Yealy

I. INTRODUCTION

A. Eye injuries require prompt evaluation and treatment to minimize the risk of loss of sight. These injuries may be obvious (as with penetrating trauma) or more subtle, yet still sight threatening. In addition, competing injuries and altered responsiveness can hinder ophthalmic assessment.

B. Prompt consultation with an ophthalmologist is recommended when ocular injury exists or any suspicion of injury exists. Patients with periorbital or ocular trauma may have sight-threatening injuries with little superficial evidence.

II. HISTORY. Key features specific to the eye injury.

A. Obtain a complete history regarding the mechanism of the injury. What type of object (e.g., ball, metal, etc.) hit the eye? Was it thrown or hit by a bat, and from how far away?

B. Obtain a history of preexisting ocular disease. Does the patient normally wear eyeglasses? Is there a history of ocular surgery or previous trauma?

C. Was the patient wearing eye/face protection?

D. What are the patient's complaints? Specifically, ask regarding a change in vision, pain, photophobia, or other new visual symptom or change (such as floaters or sensation of a curtain obscuring the vision).

III. PHYSICAL EXAMINATION

A. Visual acuity is the "vital sign" of the eye. Regardless of how minor an injury may appear, documentation of visual acuity is the first step in evaluation of any patient with possible ocular trauma. In general, the ultimate visual outcome is directly related to the presenting visual acuity.

1. Test each eye separately for vision by covering the opposite eye with either the palm of the patient's hand or an occlusive device.

a. In the emergency setting, patients are often supine. A description of the ability to see letters on a card, a pen, or name tag is sufficient. In the case of a patient with reduced vision, the distance at which the patient can count fingers, see a hand wave, tell the direction of a light (light projection), or detect the presence of a light (light perception) provides an adequate preliminary assessment.

b. If the patient has eyeglasses, check visual acuity with them in use. For older patients with bifocal glasses, test near vision with the patient looking through the bifocal portion at the bottom of the glasses.

i. If the glasses have been lost or are not with the patient, a pinhole device (in a piece of paper or cardboard or a commercial device) may be used to approximate corrected vision.

ii. Documentation in the medical record of "vision intact," "vision okay," "fine," or "the same" is inadequate.

2. Test pupillary reactivity and compare one pupil to the other; note the shape and reactivity. Documentation of the presence or absence of a relative afferent pupillary defect (RAPD) is important in characterization of injury.

a. RAPD refers to a difference in reactivity of the pupils when a bright light is swung briskly from one eye to the other. The affected pupil will react less strongly, not at all, or perhaps even dilate when presented with the same light that produces a normal constriction of the unaffected pupil. **Presence of**

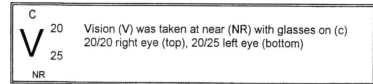

Figure 26-1. Documentation of visual acuity.

an RAPD indicates serious optic nerve or ophthalmic damage, as it is a bulk response of the visual apparatus. Absence of an RAPD indicates no significant optic nerve damage or bilateral optic nerve damage (note, however, that in its absence severe eye injury may still be present).

3. Obtain visual field evaluation by confrontation testing (asking the patient to count fingers in all four quadrants of each eye separately) and document whether the patient is cooperative enough to undergo the test (Fig. 26-1 and Table 26-1).
4. Examine the extraocular movements and report any decrease or pain.
5. Document the gross appearance of the eye: Does it appear to be intact and quiet? If further evaluation is possible, assess the following:
   a. **Eyelids.** Assess for edema, laceration, ptosis, or other evidence of injury.
   b. **Palpate the orbital rim** for deformity or crepitus.
   c. **Examine the globe without applying pressure.** Assess the globe for possible displacement or entrapment, and describe the movement of the eye.
   d. **Conjunctivae.** Evaluate for subconjunctival hemorrhage, chemosis (swelling), or foreign bodies.
   e. **Cornea.** Assess for integrity, opacity, abrasions, foreign bodies, or contact lenses.
      i. **Contacts should be removed from trauma patients.** If unsure whether a patient wears contact lenses, a small amount of fluorescein will make the presence obvious. An unconscious patient can develop a perforating bacterial corneal ulcer from a contact lens left in the eye for several days.
      ii. Abrasions may be visualized with fluorescein instilled into the conjunctival sac. A cobalt blue light will cause bright yellow fluorescence of the injured area.
   f. **Anterior chamber.** Using a light directed at varying angles (direct and from side), assess for blood (hyphema) or abnormal depth. A shallow anterior chamber can result from an anterior penetrating wound, and a deep anterior chamber from injury to the posterior portion of the globe. A slit lamp examination is ideal for anterior chamber and corneal evaluation but can be difficult in immobilized or severely injured patients.
   g. **Iris** should be reactive and the pupil should be round.
   h. **Lens** should be in the normal location and transparent. A dislocated lens will often be apparent only because the edge will be visible in the pupil.
   i. **Vitreous** should be transparent. Blood in the vitreous will obscure the normal red reflection of the slit lamp or ophthalmoscope light from the retina. Assess for foreign bodies.
   j. **Retina.** Assess for hemorrhage or detachment. Use of an ophthalmoscope with papillary dilation allows only part of the retina to be visualized and will

TABLE 26-1	Documentation of Pupillary Responses

PERRL—APD
Normal pupil responses to light, negative afferent pupillary defect

miss noncentral lesions. Again, a dilated examination using magnification performed by an ophthalmologist is ideal, but sometimes impractical in the severely injured patient. Dilating agents should be used only with ophthalmic and neurosurgical input, given the potential impairment of the examination and potential complications in certain settings (e.g., open globe or elevated intraocular pressure).

IV. COMMON INJURIES
A. Chemical injury. Chemical injury is a true ocular emergency, with care in the first minutes altering the outcome. A patient with chemical exposure to the eye must be irrigated copiously with saline (liters of normal saline connected to IV tubing with the needle end removed works well). Usually 15 minutes of constant irrigation is necessary before further examination takes place. The nature of the chemical is important in prognosis and further treatment. However, **the specific nature is irrelevant in the first 15 minutes and all injuries should be irrigated with saline or water.** Do not attempt to neutralize any acid or base by additions to the irrigating fluid. After the first large volume irrigation, test the pH in the conjunctival sac fluid—if abnormal, continue irrigation. Consult an ophthalmologist early.
B. Open globe. An open globe is the most serious sight-threatening ocular injury occurring in blunt maxillofacial trauma. It refers to a laceration or rupture of the eye wall with extrusion of intraocular contents.
1. With a suspected open globe, immediately place a rigid shield over but not touching the eye and consult an ophthalmologist. **Never place pressure or drops on the globe.** Even slight pressure can cause extrusion of intraocular contents and reduce the chance of restoring useful vision or avoiding enucleation. This includes the pressure exerted by the eyelids in a forced squeeze, local anesthesia injection into the periocular region, or inadvertent pressure while closing lacerations on the face.
2. Prehospital care of a suspected open globe involves protecting the eye with a plastic or metal shield taped from the forehead to the cheekbone.
3. Additional maneuvers that may help save sight include administration of pain medication and antiemetics if needed to avoid grimacing and Valsalva.
4. An ophthalmologist should perform ocular explorations under general anesthesia without local anesthetics.
5. The most common rupture site for an open globe is at the limbus, the junction between the cornea and sclera. The second most common site for a scleral laceration is just posterior to the insertion of the four recti muscles.
6. **Signs that suggest a ruptured globe include (not all may be present):**
   a. Any distortion of the front of the eye
   b. Loss of vision
   c. A pupil that is not round
   d. Displaced lens
   e. Traumatic hyphema
   f. Hemorrhagic chemosis (hemorrhagic swelling of the conjunctivae, generalized or localized)
   g. Shallow or deep anterior chamber
7. After the initial evaluation, obtain computed tomography (CT) scan of the orbit.
8. In the emergency department, give a prophylactic intravenous (IV) antibiotic, usually a cephalosporin. Wounds contaminated with soil or dirt require clindamycin to prevent *Bacillus cereus* endophthalmitis.
C. Traumatic hyphema. This refers to blood in the anterior chamber of the eye, which can obscure the detail of the iris or lens. A hyphema may be associated with a more serious injury (e.g., a ruptured globe). The hemorrhage will be visible as a layer or wisps of red blood. A microhyphema is suspended red blood cells without layering, visible only with a slit lamp.
1. A hyphema is treated with the following:
   a. Rigid shield to the affected eye
   b. Bed rest with the head elevated

TABLE 26-2   **Outpatient Management of Hyphema**

Medications
—Atropine 1% three times daily
—Prednisolone acetate 1% one drop four times daily
—Topical antibiotics, if epithelial defects are present
—Acetaminophen—no aspirin or nonsteroidal anti-inflammatory drugs
—Acetazolamide or beta-blocker if intraocular pressure is elevated

Activities
—Bed rest with head elevated
—Limited activity—no bending, lifting (straining)
—Shield over injured eye

Follow-up
—See daily for 4–5 d

     c. Avoidance of aspirin or other NSAIDs
     d. Dilation/cycloplegia (e.g., atropine 1% three times daily)
     e. Topical anti-inflammatory (e.g., prednisolone acetate 1% 4 to 6 times daily)
     f. Serial examinations with intraocular pressure checks by an ophthalmologist for at least the first 5 days postinjury
   2. Consider a sickle screen if the patient is African American.
   3. Imaging studies to disclose associated injuries are based on other factors.
   4. Most patients with microhyphemas and small hyphemas are treated as outpatients (Table 26-2). Patients with larger hyphemas, other periocular trauma, and sickle-cell disease or trait usually are treated as inpatients (Table 26-3).
D. Intraocular foreign bodies (IOFBs) may be present despite excellent visual acuity. Small metallic fragments can enter the eye without the patient experiencing much discomfort. These metallic pieces are often small and multiple. Consider these in any eye injury, especially in a patient with a history of metal-on-metal hammering. The most useful imaging test is high-resolution, thin-cut CT through the globe. Obtain axial and coronal views. Small IOFBs may indicate that other ocular injuries are present and a detailed ophthalmologic examination must be performed. Surgical removal is usually accomplished by vitrectomy (Table 26-4).

TABLE 26-3   **Inpatient Acute Management of Hyphema**

Medications
—Atropine 1% three times daily
—Prednisolone acetate 1% four times daily
—Antiglaucoma medication: Timolol maleate 0.5% twice daily, acetazolamide 500 mg twice daily
—Acetaminophen for pain: As needed
—Aminocaproic acid (50 mg/kg liquid every 4 h; maximum dose 30 g/24 h)

Activities
—Bed rest with bathroom privileges and decreased activity
—Shield full time to injured eye

Indications for surgery
—Blood staining of the cornea
—Elevated intraocular pressure of 50 mm Hg for 5 d, 35 mm Hg for 7 d, or eight ball hyphema. In patients with sickle cell, surgery recommended with intraocular pressure over 24 mm Hg for 24 h on maximal medications.

TABLE 26-4	**Intraocular Foreign Body Evaluation**

Visual acuity
Dilated fundus examination
Shield
Computed tomography
Operating room

E. **Corneal abrasions and foreign bodies.** Abrasions are common and cause pain, tearing, a foreign body sensation, photophobia, and decreased visual acuity. Fluorescein will stain the corneal abrasion bright yellow when viewed with a cobalt blue filter.
   1. Superficial corneal foreign bodies can be removed with irrigation. If the foreign bodies are embedded in the cornea, these can be removed with a needle tip or cotton tip under slit lamp examination by a trained provider or can be referred to an ophthalmologist after instilling ophthalmic ointment in the eye. An abrasion will usually exist after removal.
   2. Patching the eye may be dangerous as it allows bacteria in dirty abrasions to multiply and does not increase comfort.
   3. Any abrasion should be treated with application of ophthalmic antibiotic ointment, erythromycin or polymyxin, (do not use broader agents or aminoglycoside drops) at least once daily until the epithelium is healed. Refer the patient to an ophthalmologist for follow-up and counsel the patient to seek immediate treatment if symptoms persist for more than 24 hours, or if a central abrasion or defect larger than 2 mm is detected.
F. **Eyelid lacerations.** Perform an ophthalmic examination on every patient with an eyelid laceration and consider this for lacerations around the orbits. In general, the closer to the eye, especially if any symptoms, the more detailed the examination needed. Soft-tissue injuries are repaired only after globe injuries are excluded and imaging studies performed. Even the most complex eyelid laceration repairs can be delayed for 24 to 48 hours with excellent surgical results.
   1. Specific eyelid complications include canthal tendon disinsertion, lacrimal drainage system (canalicular) laceration, and levator aponeurosis laceration. These and transmarginal eyelid lacerations require special attention.
   2. Any laceration in the medial aspect of the eyelid, particularly if caused by a tearing injury, is likely to result in a canalicular laceration. Careful inspection, probing, and irrigation of the lacrimal apparatus are required to detect this injury. Irrigate and examine all wounds for the presence of foreign bodies.
   3. Complicated injuries and pediatric patients are best repaired in the operating room under monitored sedation or general anesthesia. Most superficial lacerations can be repaired with local eyelid blocks in the emergency department. With severe eyelid disruption, the medial canthus should be addressed first with repair of the canalicular injury, silicone intubation of the lacrimal system, and repair of the deep head of the medial canthal tendon before closure of any other eyelid lacerations. These are best repaired by an ophthalmologist or plastic surgeon skilled in lid repair, in a procedure room or an operating room.
   4. Lacerations of the eyelid margin require a two-layered closure with 6-0 absorbable sutures in the deep tissue and nonabsorbable sutures in the eyelid margins (6-0 silk or 8-0 silk). Take care when closing deep eyelid tissue—**never place sutures in contact with the surface of the eyeball.**
   5. Superficial skin closure is best accomplished with 7-0 or 8-0 monofilament or chromic gut sutures.
   6. Ptosis secondary to the trauma is best observed for 6 to 12 months and then treated by a levator resection or advancement. Mechanical ptosis from hematoma or tissue edema usually improves slowly.

7. Topical antibiotic ointments offer bacterial prophylaxis and corneal protection in circumstances of poor eyelid closure. Ice packs and nondependent head positioning are important post-treatment maneuvers.

8. Avoid occluding the eye with pressure patching because of the risk of orbital hemorrhage. Check vision and pupils at regular intervals. The skin sutures usually are removed in 4 to 5 days. However, leave lid margin sutures in place 10 to 12 days.

G. Hemorrhage and orbital bone fractures. Orbital fractures can lead to acute, compressive orbital hemorrhage, an ophthalmologic emergency. The increasing intraorbital pressure resulting from an expanding hemorrhage can quickly lead to vascular compromise of the retina and optic nerve, resulting in permanent vision loss. Timely decompression with a lateral canthotomy and cantholysis can save vision in an eye with an expanding orbital hemorrhage. **An emergency physician or trauma surgeon must perform canthotomy** if vision is decreased and no ophthalmologist is available. (Go to http://emedicine.medscape.com/article/82812-overview to see text and video on this procedure.)

1. Of orbital fractures, 40% are associated with serious ocular injuries, including retinal tears and detachments, retinal hemorrhage, vitreous hemorrhage, dislocation of the lens, hyphema, glaucoma, or traumatic cataract. Ocular injuries occur with midface, supraorbital, and frontal fractures. An open globe, retinal detachment, or traumatic optic neuropathy presents contraindication to early bony repair. As a general guideline, fix the globe first. The bone can then be repaired in approximately 2 weeks.

2. Elevated intraocular pressure suggests increased orbital pressure, whereas lower intraocular pressure suggests a penetrating or perforating injury with globe disruption. Recognition of these ocular injuries is essential. Repair of isolated orbital fractures is rarely an operative emergency, and a complete ocular evaluation should be done before any orbital bone surgery.

3. Exception to this rule occurs in young patients who have greenstick fractures (trapdoors) of the orbital floor with inferior rectus entrapment. These patients often have a relatively white, quiet-looking eye, severe deficiency of upgaze, pain, and nausea. These must be repaired in the operating room as soon as safely possible, preferably within 24 hours.

H. Traumatic optic neuropathy. Traumatic vision loss with complete blindness occurs in approximately 3% of patients suffering blunt maxillofacial injury. Of midface, supraorbital, or frontal sinus fractures, 4% are associated with severe optic nerve injuries. Early diagnosis and treatment of optic nerve injury may minimize vision loss.

1. With a greater number of patients with closed head trauma surviving, more surviving patients have permanent loss of vision. Decreased visual acuity or visual fields with an afferent pupillary defect in the involved eye indicates optic nerve injury. It is sometimes difficult for the non-ophthalmologist to make this determination because multiply injured trauma patients are often uncooperative or unconscious. In addition, the optic disc may appear normal on ophthalmoscopy. Look carefully for an afferent pupillary defect to help detect this injury.

2. Obtain thin-section CT through the orbit and optic canal to exclude the possibility of a bone fracture compromising the optic nerve.

3. Treatment of optic neuropathy in this setting is controversial. Although used previously, steroids have no proven benefit. A surgical optic nerve decompression may be performed if bone fragments appear to be compromising the canal, but is realistic only in the hands of an experienced surgeon. Otherwise, observation is the mainstay currently.

I. Cataract. A blunt injury to the eye can result in clouding (cataract) or displacement of the lens. A sharp injury to the lens capsule can also cause a cataract, but lens particles can also leak into the anterior chamber, resulting in severe uveitis, lens-induced glaucoma, and on occasion **lens anaphylaxis** (severe inflammation from exposure to lens proteins). A leaking lens must be removed.

J. Retinal detachment. Blunt trauma can cause retinal detachment, especially in patients who are nearsighted, have had previous ocular injury, or have had cataract surgery.

1. Most retinal detachments caused by trauma do not occur at the time of injury, but occur days to months later. Although the risk never drops to zero, most detachments occur within 6 months of injury.

2. The diagnosis is suspected when a patient presents with complaints of flashing lights and a curtain or shade interfering with some portion of the visual field. Confrontation visual fields may detect the field loss. The diagnosis is made by indirect ophthalmoscopy through a dilated pupil.

K. Commotio Retinae. A finger or other object directly hitting the eye or orbit can cause retinal damage that has the appearance of edema around the optic nerve or macula on ophthalmoscopy. This is caused by a shearing injury of the retina, and recovery is usually quick (weeks) and complete. Blood may also appear under the retina. Recovery can be complete or very limited.

AXIOMS

- Measure visual acuity early to detect serious eye injury.
- Sutures are never placed in direct contact with the globe.
- If an open globe is suspected, put no pressure on the eye and use no drops in the eye.
- Never wait to perform lateral canthotomy when vision is impaired and orbital hematoma exist.

Suggested Readings

Catalano R, Belin M. *Ocular Emergencies.* Philadelphia, PA: WB Saunders; 1992.
Eagling E, Roper-Hall M. *Eye Injuries: An Illustrated Guide.* Philadelphia, PA: JB Lippincott Co; 1986.
Kanitkar KD, Makar M, Kunimoto DY, eds. *The Wills Eye Manual: Office and Emergency Room Diagnosis and Treatment of Eye Disease.* 4th ed. Philadelphia, PA: JB Lippincott Co; 1990.
Linberg J. *Oculoplastic and Orbital Emergencies.* Norwalk, CT: Appleton & Lange; 1990.
McInnes G, Howes DW. Lateral canthotomy and cantholysis: a simple, vision-saving procedure. *CJEM* 2002;4(1):49–52.
Spoor T, Nesi F. *Management of Ocular, Orbital and Adnexal Trauma.* New York, NY: Raven Press; 1988.

27 Neck Trauma

Tiffany K. Bee and Martin A. Croce

Injuries to the neck can cause morbidity and mortality. Initial evaluation and management differ depending on the mechanism of injury. This chapter will discuss the evaluation and management of penetrating and blunt neck injuries.

Anatomy: The neck encompasses the area bounded superiorly by the base of the mandible and a line running from the angle of the mandible to the mastoid process of the skull base, inferiorly by the clavicle, anteriorly by the anterior median line that includes the cricoid cartilage and posteriorly by the anterior margin of the trapezius.

The neck contains a diversity of vital structures in a relatively small space. Vital portions of many organ systems are represented in the neck.

1. Respiratory
   a. Trachea
   b. Larynx
2. Cardiovascular
   a. Carotid arteries
   b. Jugular veins
   c. Vertebral arteries
3. Neurologic
   a. Cervical spinal cord
   b. Vagus nerve
   c. Phrenic nerve
   d. Recurrent Laryngeal nerves
4. Digestive
   a. Pharynx
   b. Esophagus
5. Endocrine
   a. Thyroid
   b. Parathyroids
6. Musculoskeletal
   a. Spine and its ligaments

Historically, the neck is divided into triangles mainly by muscle location. The anterior triangle is bounded by the median line of the neck anteriorly, the anterior margin of the sternocleidomastoid muscle laterally, the inferior portion of the mandible superiorly, and the clavicles and manubrium inferiorly. The posterior triangle is bounded by the sternocleidomastoid muscle anteriorly, the anterior edge of the trapezius posteriorly, the middle third of the clavicle inferiorly and superiorly between the attachment of the sternocleidomastoid and trapezius to the occiput (Fig. 27-1).

The neck is divided into zones in trauma situations (Fig. 27-2).

1. **Zone I:** Clavicle to cricoid injuries. Structures include the lung apices, trachea, brachiocephalic vein, subclavian artery, common carotid artery, thoracic duct, cervical nerve roots, and esophagus.
2. **Zone II:** Cricoid to angle of the mandible. Structures include common carotid and vertebral arteries, jugular veins, esophagus, thyroid, cervical spine, pharynx, trachea, and larynx.

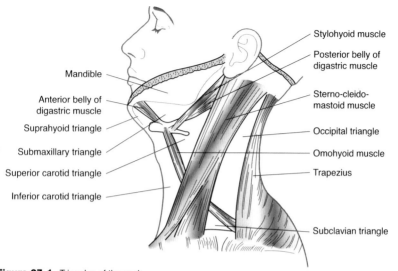

Figure 27-1. Triangles of the neck.

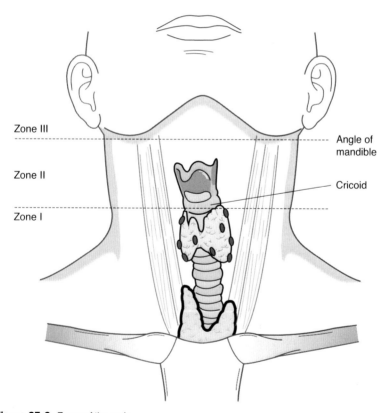

Figure 27-2. Zones of the neck.

316

3. **Zone III:** Angle of mandible to skull base. Structures include external carotid and internal carotid arteries, vertebral arteries, jugular veins, salivary glands, cranial nerves IX–XII, and hypopharynx.

PENETRATING NECK INJURY

I. INTRODUCTION. No longer is platysmal penetration an absolute indication for neck exploration. Instead, diagnostic testing and observation is used in many cases absent of signs of vascular or aerodigestive disruption and with hemodynamic stability. A major vascular injury may be easily identified but injury to the aerodigestive, neurologic, or musculoskeletal system may be more difficult to identify, but is nonetheless life-threatening. A multidisciplinary approach to these injuries is often necessary bringing in the expertise of trauma surgeons, interventional radiologists, ear, nose, and throat surgeons, plastic surgeons, neurosurgeons, and oral maxillofacial surgeons.

II. INITIAL EVALUATION

A. A systematic evaluation should be performed. A rigid cervical collar is not necessary unless blunt trauma occurred or neurologic signs or symptoms are present. The "ABCD" evaluation, well described in the initial trauma evaluation, is the cornerstone in initial care.

B. Immediately operate on those patients with severe active bleeding, hemodynamic instability, expanding or pulsatile neck hematoma, massive subcutaneous air, or air bubbling from wound.

C. Patients without indication for immediate operation should undergo a primary survey then followed by a full secondary survey:
1. Inspection-evaluate for hematoma, platysmal penetration (do **not** probe wound), crepitance, stridor, hoarseness, odynophagia, dysphagia, or tracheal deviation.
2. Auscultation-listen for a bruit, bilateral breath sounds.
3. Palpation-feel for a thrill along vessels or subcutaneous emphysema. Determine pulse examination.
4. Chest radiograph-check for pneumo or hemothorax, pneumopericardium, retropharyngeal air, enlargement of superior mediastinum, or apical cap.

III. DIAGNOSTIC TESTING

A. In the hemodynamically stable patient, further evaluation can determine injury. Patients who have dysphonia, dysphagia, retropharyngeal air, odynophagia, hemoptysis, hematemesis, or slight pulse discrepancy require further diagnostic testing. Some centers advocate observation alone if none of the above signs is present. This can vary by institution. At our institution the algorithm in Figure 27-3 is used for penetrating neck injury patients.

B. Diagnostic testing options available include
1. Four-vessel angiography, esophagography with or without laryngotracheobronchoscopy (if subcutaneous emphysema or retropharyngeal air). This method is accurate but does put the patient at risk for morbidity due to angiography.
2. Color flow Doppler imaging. This can aid diagnosis of vascular injury.
3. Helical CTA. CTA technology is quickly becoming the choice of modalities to detect vascular injury. It may not be reliable for esophageal injury detection, although any retropharyngeal air should trigger further investigation.
4. Esophagography and esophagoscopy. Contrast esophagography under fluoroscopic guidance has a sensitivity of nearly 90%. Use of barium instead of water-soluble contrast to distend the esophagus is beneficial. Many authors are now reporting good results with flexible esophagoscopy as well.
5. Observation and physical examination. This may be adequate for vascular injuries in zone II. However, the zone I and III vascular injuries may be missed by physical examination alone. Also esophageal injuries are difficult to determine by physical examination.

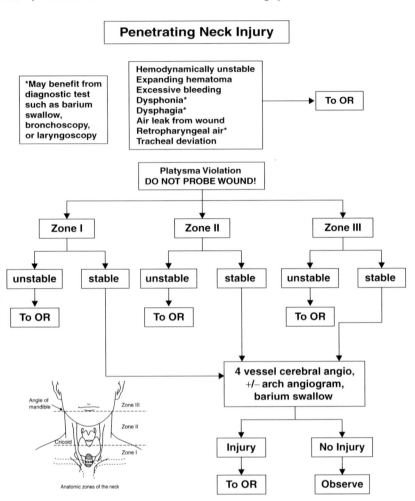

Figure 27-3. Penetrating neck injury algorithm.

IV. SURGICAL MANAGEMENT OF SPECIFIC INJURIES

A. The patient should be positioned supine with the neck extended and rotated opposite the injury side (assuming the cervical spine is cleared). The patient should be prepped earlobe to umbilicus with special attention to the same side lateral chest. A portion of the thigh for a possible saphenous vein graft should also be included.

B. Vascular injury approaches (Fig. 27-4)

　　1. Carotid

　　　　a. Ascertain neurologic status. If patient is comatose but has prograde flow or significant back bleeding, attempt repair. If the patient is neurologically intact, attempt repair. If the patient is unstable, ligation may be necessary.

　　　　b. Obtain exposure by an anterior sternocleidomastoid incision. High carotid injuries may require anterior subluxation of the mandible or division of the omohyoid and digastric muscles. Placement of a Fogarty catheter into the distal artery may also help with bleeding control.

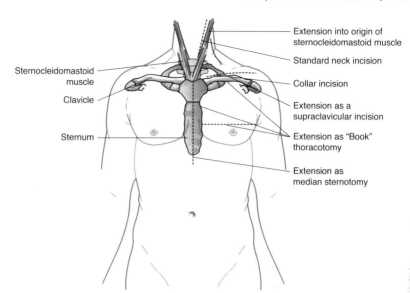

Figure 27-4. Incisions for exposure of penetrating neck injuries.

    c. Repair can often be done primarily with some additional length gained by dividing the superior thyroid artery. If the defect is longer than 2 cm, use a saphenous vein graft. Transposition of the external carotid to the internal carotid artery is another option. Prosthetic grafts do not have good patency and should not be used.

2. Innominate and proximal subclavian arteries

    a. Expose the proximal right subclavian artery and innominate artery through a median sternotomy. A proximal left subclavian artery is approached through a left thoracotomy, although a "trap-door" incision that combines a left antero-lateral thoracotomy with a partial median sternotomy and left supraclavicular incision may be needed to fully expose. Resection of the medial clavicle to visualize the thyrocervical trunk helps. In unstable patients, ligate the subclavian artery distal to the take off of the vertebral artery.

3. Vertebral artery

    a. In a patient with vertebral artery injury, treatment options include surgical ligation or radiologic embolization. Ligate through the C1–C2 interspace for the distal vertebral or a supraclavicular incision with medial clavicle removal for the proximal vertebral.

4. Venous injury

    a. Ligation is the management of most venous injuries unless easily repaired.

    b. Carefully avoid any air embolism; large air emboli require hyperbaric oxygen therapy acutely, especially if symptomatic.

C. Esophageal injury

    1. Ideal exposure is via an anterior sternocleidomastoid incision, with a nasogastric tube placed in advance when possible. Instilling methylene blue or air into the nasogastric tube may help visualize the injury.

    2. Most injuries can be repaired primarily in two layers with interrupted absorbable suture approximating the mucosa and a nonabsorbable suture approximating the muscular layer. If possible, surrounding tissue (e.g., the head of the sternocleido-mastoid or strap muscles) can be used to cover the repair.

3. If the injury is discovered more than 24 hours after it occurred, drainage and/or cervical esophagostomy with feeding tube will be necessary as the friable tissue and contamination make primary repair contraindicated.

D. Tracheal injury

    1. Exposure through a sternocleidomastoid or collar incision.

    2. Repair can often be done primarily with a single interrupted polyglycolic or vicryl suture. If a portion of trachea is completely destroyed length may be obtained by mobilization of the anterior trachea avoiding injury to the lateral vascular supply. A tissue buttress should be placed around the repair. A tracheostomy may be needed for severe injury but should not be placed through the injured area.

BLUNT NECK INJURY

I. INTRODUCTION. Blunt neck trauma is common, but significant injury (excluding that to the cervical spine) is relatively uncommon, but life-threatening if present. The unrestrained driver hitting a steering wheel or a direct blow to the neck are two common mechanisms. Violent torsion, flexion, or extension of the neck also may result in blunt neck injury without external signs of trauma. Patients with non-emergency airway control measure (intubation, etc.) have a higher degree of iatrogenic injury to the pharynx and upper esophagus. Often the signs and symptoms of blunt neck trauma are subtle.

II. INITIAL EVALUATION

A. Use the primary and secondary survey approach noted earlier in this text. Maintenance of cervical stability is important in the discussion and evaluation of patients with possible blunt cervical injury.

    1. Airway

        a. Patients having difficulty with oxygenation, ventilation, or decreased sensorium must be intubated, preferably orally. If unable to be intubated, a cricothyroidotomy should be performed. Be careful—obtaining a secure airway in patients with laryngotracheal injuries is challenging.

    2. Breathing

        a. Pneumothorax may occur with laryngotracheal or esophageal trauma, and on occasion result in tension pneumothorax. If a tension pneumothorax is present, do needle decompression followed by tube thoracostomy. Pneumomediastinum may be present, but usually does not compromise breathing by itself.

        b. Tracheal or laryngeal disruption alone may lead to breathing difficulty.

    3. Circulation

        a. As always, place large bore peripheral IVs and resuscitate.

        b. Monitoring the peripheral pulses to detect signs of deficit.

        c. Apply direct pressure to bleeding areas in the neck *without* probing or blind clamp placement.

    4. Disability

        a. Seek evidence of spinal cord injury

        b. Neurologic abnormalities not always associated with intracranial or spinal cord injury include:

            i. Anisocoria and/or Horner's syndrome

            ii. Weakness of extremity

            iii. Change in mental status

B. Physical Examination

For adequate examination, remove the cervical collar while maintaining in-line traction.

    1. Inspection

        a. Look for lacerations, abrasions, contusions, crepitance, jugular venous distension, asymmetry, "seatbelt sign," or other gross deformities.

    2. Auscultation

        a. Seek any bruit over a carotid vessel; if found in the presence of a hematoma, assume an acute injury.

    b. Stridor, hoarseness, odynophagia, and dysphagia are suggestive of laryngotracheal or aerodigestive injury.

  3. Palpation

    a. Presence of a pulse deficit, expanding pulsatile hematoma or thrill suggests a vascular injury.

    b. Loss of the normal anatomic contours of the anterior neck, thyroid cartilage, and cricoid cartilage suggest laryngeal fracture.

    c. Be sure that the trachea is in the midline (and not pushed by hematoma, tension pneumothorax, or another mass). A defect in the tracheal wall ("step-off") indicates tracheal disruption. Tracheal injury usually presents with subcutaneous emphysema.

    d. Subcutaneous emphysema suggests pneumothorax or airway injury. It is unlikely that an esophageal injury will cause significant subcutaneous emphysema, but retropharyngeal air is often present.

C. Radiographic evaluation

  1. Plain cervical spine radiograph—look for:

    a. Tracheal deviation, increased soft tissue density and swelling are signs of hematoma.

    b. Pretracheal soft tissue thickness greater than 6.0 mm at C2 or greater than 22 mm at C6 suggests cervical spine fracture.

    c. Signs of subcutaneous emphysema or retropharyngeal air suggest laryngotracheal or esophageal injury.

    d. Malalignment and or abnormal spacing of the vertebral bodies and their processes.

    e. Continue cervical immobilization until the spine is cleared radiographically and clinically.

  2. Chest radiograph

    a. Look for pneumothorax, subcutaneous emphysema, pneumomediastinum, and pneumopericardium.

    b. Enlargement of the superior mediastinum and apical cap indicates great vessel injury at the thoracic outlet or base of the neck.

III. DIAGNOSTIC MODALITIES. Take patients with expanding hematomas or active hemorrhage immediately to the operating room. For hemodynamically stable patients, further diagnostic evaluation is necessary.

A. CT and CT angiogram

  1. Strengths

    a. Excellent for identifying injuries to the larynx, vertebral column, and vessels.

    b. May identify small collections of extraluminal air in the unusual case of blunt esophageal injury.

    c. Detection of soft tissue injury.

    d. Excellent study for tracheal injury.

  2. Weaknesses

    a. Sensitivity for ligamentous and vascular injuries is controversial (see MRI).

    b. Requires IV contrast.

B. Laryngoscopy/bronchoscopy

  1. Strength

    a. Direct visualization of larynx and trachea.

  2. Weakness

    a. Injury to larynx or trachea may be obscured by endotracheal tube.

C. Duplex ultrasound

  1. Strength

    a. Noninvasive test for occlusive carotid disease.

  2. Weakness

    a. Operator dependent.

    b. Difficult to visualize anatomy in the presence of a hematoma or subcutaneous emphysema.

    c. Unreliable for identification of acute blunt ICA dissection.

    d. Inadequate examination common when using cervical immobilization devices.

D. Angiography

  1. Strengths

    a. Long history of use in the diagnosis of carotid or vertebral artery injuries.

    b. May perform therapeutic interventions at the same time.

    c. Provides information on intracerebral anatomy.

  2. Weaknesses

    a. Invasive and may cause bleeding or neurologic injury in rare cases.

    b. Requires IV contrast.

E. Esophagram

  1. Strength

    a. Barium adequately distends the esophagus for easier identification of injury; water-soluble contrast is inadequate.

  2. Weakness

    a. Technically difficult in the intubated patient.

    b. Poor visualization of pharynx and high esophagus.

F. Flexible esophagoscopy

  1. Strengths

    a. Good visualization of esophagus, especially mid and distal portions.

    b. May safely be performed in patients with cervical immobilization (unlike rigid esophagoscopy).

  2. Weakness

    a. May be difficult to adequately distend esophagus to identify small injuries.

    b. Poor visualization of pharynx, esophageal introitus, and high esophagus.

G. MRI

  1. Strengths

    a. Good for evaluation of cervical spine ligamentous injury.

    b. Good for evaluation of spinal cord.

  2. Weakness

    a. Time consuming.

    b. Difficult to perform in the unstable patient.

IV. SPECIFIC INJURIES

A. Blunt cerebral vascular injuries

  1. Incidence

    a. Increasing with awareness and screening.

    b. Estimate of incidence of blunt carotid injury is 0.5% of all blunt trauma admissions, the incidence of vertebral injuries is considered higher by a factor of 1.5 to 3.

  2. Mechanism best described by Crissey and Bernstein.

    a. Crissey 1: Direct blow to the neck.

    b. Crissey 2: Blow to head with neck rotation and hyperextension causing the internal carotid to stretch.

    c. Crissey 3: Intraoral trauma.

    d. Crissey 4: Damage to intrapetrous portion of ICA.

B. Carotid artery

  1. Common carotid

    a. Usually due to direct blow to neck, with surrounding soft tissue hematoma or contusion.

    b. May present with hemiparesis that is unexplained by brain CT findings.

    c. Associated facial (LeFort II and III) and cervical fractures are signs of severe trauma and should increase suspicion of vascular injury.

    d. Diagnosis is with angiography. A complete four-vessel angiogram is necessary to evaluate the presence or lack of cross filling, since only one-third of patients will have an intact circle of Willis. CT angiography may have an increased role in the diagnosis as the technology continues to improve.

    e. CT and CT angiogram are emerging as the initial preferred imaging procedure.

f. Injury grades of carotid injuries
- **i.** Grade I: Arteriographic appearance of irregularity of the vessel wall or dissection/intramural hematoma with less than 25% luminal narrowing.
- **ii.** Grade II: Arteriographic appearance of an intimal flap or intramural hematoma with greater than 25% narrowing or dissection.
- **iii.** Grade III: Arteriographic appearance of a pseudoaneurysm.
- **iv.** Grade IV: Arteriographic appearance of occlusion.
- **v.** Grade V: Transection or hemodynamically significant injuries.

2. Internal carotid
- **a.** Usually due to rapid deceleration with neck rotation and hyperextension. This causes the internal carotid to stretch over the second to third cervical transverse process, resulting in an intimal injury. Typically, there is dissection extending up to the skull base. There may be associated pseudoaneurysm.
- **b.** May present with hemiparesis or other neurologic deficit that is unexplained by brain CT findings. The complete Horner's syndrome is not usually present, but miosis is typically present from injury to sympathetic fibers nearby.
- **c.** Angiography is used to detect internal carotid injury.

C. Vertebral Artery
1. Associated with flexion and rotation of the neck, also cervical spine fractures or subfixation. Fractures of the foramen transversarium are likewise associated with vascular injuries.
2. With associated cervical injury, a cerebral angiogram is indicated.

D. Larynx/trachea
1. Usually due to direct blow to neck.
2. Perforation of the upper aerodigestive tract is a result of the laryngeal cartilage being compressed by the vertebral bodies.
3. Usually associated with subcutaneous emphysema and loss of the normal contour of the thyroid cartilage. A palpable defect may be felt in the tracheal wall.
4. Awake patients with laryngotracheal injuries will assume a position in which they have a patent airway.
5. The airway *must* be secured. The best option is a surgical airway using local anesthesia in the operating room.
6. Non-obvious diagnosis is by direct laryngoscopy or bronchoscopy. 3D multislice CT diagnosis is another option.

E. Esophagus
1. Usually due to direct blow to neck; these injuries are rare.
2. Diagnosis is by barium swallow.

V. TREATMENT
A. Carotid artery (Fig. 27-5)
1. Reserve operative management for injuries to the common carotid or the proximal internal carotid. Blunt injuries, which are usually dissections (with or without associated pseudoaneurysm), typically extend distally, making primary repair impractical. Interposition grafting is usually necessary, and a long segment may be required.
2. Nonoperative therapy with anticoagulation to or embolization is the primary treatment for blunt traumatic ICA dissections. Continuous heparin is the preferred treatment, although it must be used with caution in patients with associated injuries, and is relatively contraindicated in patients with cerebral intraparenchymal hemorrhage or contusion. Monitor the partial thromboplastin time (PTT) with a goal of 40 to 45 seconds. Follow-up angiography at 7 to 14 days will assess for progression of injury. If no progression, convert to warfarin or antiplatelet therapy with aspirin and continue for approximately 6 months. Follow-up studies, including magnetic resonance or CT angiography, can detect persistent injury and mandate continued antithrombotic treatment or possible stent placement.

Treatment for pseudoaneurysms involves stent grafts with antiplatelet therapy until the stent has endothelialized about 6 months. Aspirin is generally continued for the life of the stented patient.

Evaluation for Blunt Carotid Artery Injury

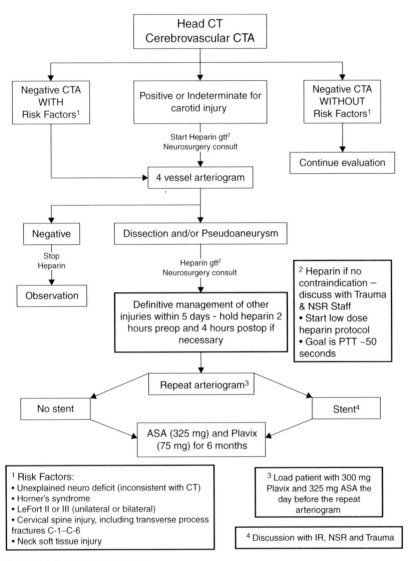

Figure 27-5. Blunt injury algorithm.

B. Vertebral artery (Fig. 27-6)

1. Operative management is usually not necessary.
2. Nonoperative management is similar to the anticoagulation and antiplatelet therapy for internal carotid injuries.
3. Radiologic embolization should be reserved for arteriovenous fistula or active extravasation.

Evaluation for Blunt Vertebral Artery Injury

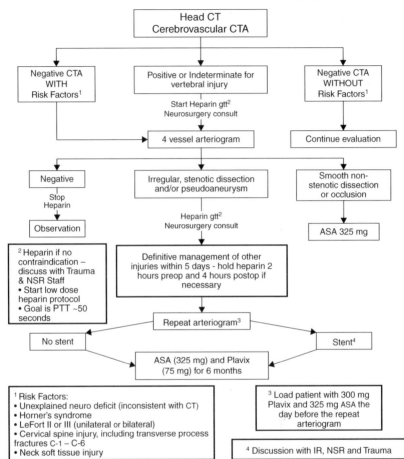

Figure 27-6. Blunt vertebral artery injury algorithm.

C. Larynx/trachea

1. An emergent incision and intubation of the disrupted distal trachea may be needed.
2. For destructive injuries, tracheal reconstruction may be necessary. Mathison and Grillo have established basic management principles.
   a. Avoid searching for recurrent laryngeal nerves.
   b. Separation of tracheal and esophageal suture lines.
   c. Conservation of viable trachea.
   d. Avoidance of tracheostomy through the repair.
   e. Flexion of the neck to avoid tension on the repair.
3. Less destructive injuries (usually to the larynx) may be managed with tracheostomy distal to the injury and primary repair of the injury.
4. Mild injuries with minimal swelling or nondisplaced cartilage may be treated with observation, voice rest, and humidified air.

    5. Hoarseness from bilateral vocal cord paralysis in laryngotracheal disruption may improve with time.

D. Esophagus

    1. Operative repair should be undertaken when the diagnosis is made. The esophagus should be repaired in two layers (inner mucosal, outer muscularis), buttressed by surrounding strap muscles. If a drain is necessary, it should be a closed suction drain.

AXIOMS

■ The first priority is to obtain a secure airway, and may be difficult in a patient with severe neck trauma.
Significant injuries to the larynx, trachea, carotid, or esophagus are not common, but are associated with high morbidity and mortality.

■ Look hard for these injuries using multiple modalities, and operate when instability or clear anatomic disruption exists.

Suggested Readings

Asensio JA, Chahwan S, Forno W, et al. Penetrating esophageal injuries: multicenter study of the American Association for the Surgery of Trauma. *J Trauma* 2001;50(2):289–296.

Bhojani RA, Rosenbaum DH. Contemporary assessment of laryngotracheal trauma. *J Thorac Cardiovasc Surg* 2005;130(2):426–432.

Bynoe RP, Miles WS, Bell RM, et al. Non-invasive diagnosis of vascular trauma by duplex ultrasonography. *J Vasc Surg* 1991;14:346–352.

Demetriades D, Theoforou D, Cornwell E, et al. Evaluation of penetrating injuries of the neck: Prospective study of 223 patients. *World J Surg* 1997;21(1):L41–L47.

Emmett KP, Fabian TC. Improving the screening criteria for blunt cerebrovascular injury: the appropriate role for CT angiography. *J Trauma* 2011;70(5):1058–1063.

Fabian TC, George SM, Croce MA, et al. Carotid artery trauma: Management based on mechanism of injury. *J Trauma* 1990;30(8):953–961.

Ginzburg E, Montalvo B. The use of duplex ultrasonography in penetrating neck trauma. *Arch Surg* 1996;131:691–693.

Hirshberg A, Wall MJ. Transcervical gunshot injuries. *Am J Surg* 1994;167:309–312.

McConnell DB, Trunkey DD. Management of penetrating trauma to the neck. *Adv Surg* 1994;27:97–127.

Munera F, Cohn S, Rival LA. Penetrating injuries of the neck: Use of helical computed tomographic angiography. *J Trauma* 2005;58(2):413–418.

Sclafani SJ, Scalea TM. Internal carotid artery gunshot wounds. *J Trauma* 1996;40:751–757.

Srinivasan R, Haywood T, Horwitz B, et al. Role of flexible endoscopy in the evaluation of possible esophageal trauma after penetrating injuries. *Am J Gastroenterol* 2000;95(7):1725–1729.

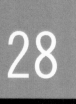

28 Thoracic Injuries

Juan A. Asensio, Federico N. Mazzini and Thai Vu

I. INTRODUCTION. Thoracic injuries are responsible for approximately 25% of all trauma deaths and in addition contribute to 25% of deaths annually in the United States. Immediate deaths usually involve blunt disruption of the heart or great vessels or penetrating injuries to the thoracic vessels. Deaths within a few hours are frequently caused by airway obstruction, tension pneumothorax, hemorrhage, or cardiac tamponade. Pulmonary complications, sepsis, and missed injuries account for late mortality.

Although thoracic injuries are often life threatening, the majority of thoracic injuries are managed nonoperatively. Treatment options include analgesia, aggressive respiratory therapy, endotracheal intubation, and tube thoracostomy. Only 10% to 15% of patients with chest injury will require thoracotomy or sternotomy.

Hemodynamic instability from a chest wound indicates a major vascular or cardiac injury that mandates immediate control of hemorrhage. Ideally, emergency operations on the chest should be performed in the operating room (OR) after a brief resuscitation. However, cardiac tamponade or exsanguination will require definitive procedures in the trauma resuscitation area.

The chest cavity is more compartmentalized than the abdomen. The bony chest wall, clavicles, and shoulders make operative exposure of injured viscera difficult. Large, relatively fixed structures limit exposure of the posterior mediastinum. Thus, the choice of thoracic incision is determined by the expected anatomic injury, the urgency with which surgical access is required, and the patient's hemodynamic stability.

II. IMMEDIATE EVALUATION
   A. Physical examination includes evaluation of upper airway, chest wall symmetry and stability, breath sounds, and heart sounds. Findings of decreased breath sounds, subcutaneous emphysema, jugular venous distension (JVD), and tracheal deviation are specifically sought early in the evaluation.
   B. Begin resuscitation while performing concurrent diagnostic procedures. **Administer oxygen** by high flow, non-rebreathing mask. If the patient does not respond adequately to volume resuscitation as evidenced by persistent hypotension, tachycardia, or decreased mental status, consider ongoing blood loss, and re-assess for the presence of cardiac tamponade, tension pneumothorax, and cardiogenic shock from blunt cardiac injury (BCI).
   When a major thoracic vascular injury is suspected, initiate prompt resuscitation while searching for the cause.
   1. Perform immediate endotracheal intubation.
   2. Place two large-bore intravenous (IV) lines for volume infusion, ideally one above and one below the diaphragm. Avoid central lines on the side of injury.
   3. Infuse pre-warmed crystalloids. Consider transfusing warmed blood immediately, and other blood products as needed (see Chapter 7).
   4. Have rapid-infusion and cell-saver devices immediately available.
   5. Administer tetanus prophylaxis and preoperative antibiotics.
   C. Monitor pulse oximetry and electrocardiogram (ECG) continuously.
   D. Obtain a **chest x-ray (CXR)** early in the evaluation of all patients sustaining thoracic injury. Sites of missile entry or penetration should be identified with radiopaque markers (e.g., metallic markers, paper clips).

E. In patients with significant injury, an arterial blood gas (ABG) is useful to determine adequacy of ventilation and acid–base status.

F. Identify **indications for immediate operation.**

1. Massive hemothorax (1,000 to 1,500 mL blood returned on insertion of chest tube)

2. Ongoing hemorrhage from chest (>200 mL/h for ≥4 hours)

3. Presence of cardiac tamponade

4. Penetrating transmediastinal chest wounds with hemodynamic instability

5. Open thoracic injuries or impalement wounds to the chest

6. Massive air leak from the chest tube or major tracheobronchial injury identified on bronchoscopy

7. Mediastinal hematoma or radiographic evidence of great vessel injury with hemodynamic instability.

8. Suspected or confirmed air embolism

III. IMMEDIATE MANAGEMENT OF PENETRATING THORACIC WOUNDS

A. DO NOT PROBE the wound to determine depth or angle, which can produce pneumothorax or hemothorax.

B. Obtain a **CXR** with metallic markers placed on all penetrating wounds.

1. Attempt to **determine trajectory to delineate anatomic injury.**

2. Perform immediate tube thoracostomy for pneumothorax or hemothorax.

  a. Administration of prophylactic antibiotics such as cefazolin or cefoxitin, as a single dose before the start of the procedure, has been recommended to decrease the risk of empyema and pneumonia.

3. If negative, repeat film in 6 hours; approximately 7% to 10% of this population will develop delayed pneumothorax.

C. Administer tetanus prophylaxis.

D. Routine antibiotics **are not** used for penetrating wounds treated without an operation or procedure.

IV. IMMEDIATE EVALUATION OF TRANSMEDIASTINAL PENETRATING WOUNDS (Fig. 28-1)

A. Diagnosis of transmediastinal penetration is based on clinical suspicion, trajectory of the missile, or CXR findings. Rapidly assess airway, hemodynamic status, and need for hemorrhage control.

B. Classify the patient, based on hemodynamics, as **in extremis, unstable, or stable** (Fig. 28-2).

C. The patient in **extremis** has agonal respirations without measurable blood pressure.

1. Intubate, oxygenate, and start volume resuscitation.

2. Perform immediate left anterolateral resuscitation thoracotomy to control hemorrhage or relieve cardiac tamponade. If needed, extend across sternum to a right thoracotomy ("clamshell thoracotomy").

3. Control bleeding from pleural cavities or heart injuries as necessary.

D. The **unstable patient** has a measurable blood pressure but is hypotensive, with a systolic blood pressure <90 mm Hg. These patients, with associated transmediastinal trajectory, often have injuries to the following organs (in descending frequency): Lung, heart, chest wall vessels, great vessels, esophagus, trachea or bronchi, and pulmonary artery or vein or their branches.

1. Assess the need for intubation, oxygenate, and start volume resuscitation.

2. Obtain a CXR.

3. Perform tube thoracostomy for pneumothorax or hemothorax.

4. Perform a **focused abdominal sonography for trauma (FAST) ultrasound examination** to diagnose pericardial effusion.

  a. A **positive** pericardial view on the FAST in an unstable patient is an indication to proceed with immediate median sternotomy.

  b. An **equivocal** pericardial view on the FAST examination necessitates either sub-xiphoid window or an exploratory median sternotomy.

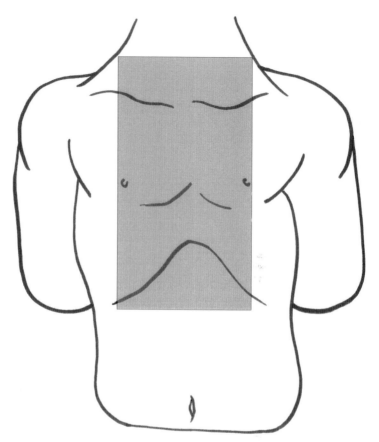

Figure 28-1. The box of death. *Shaded area* represents the danger zone for transmediastinal injury.

  c. A **negative** FAST can be falsely negative secondary to decompression of pericardial blood into the pleural space. Consider sub-xiphoid pericardial window if there is a suspicion of middle mediastinal trajectory.
  d. If FAST is **not available,** proceed to the OR for sub-xiphoid pericardial window.
  5. Thoracotomy is performed, as indicated, based on the output of chest tube and the hemodynamic status of the patient (see II.F.)
  6. After major hemorrhage is controlled, perform flexible esophagoscopy and bronchoscopy to diagnose aerodigestive tract injury. A gastrografin swallow study can be used in lieu of esophagoscopy with about the same sensitivity (see V.B.5). The two tests in combination yield sensitivity >90%.
  7. If great vessel injury is suspected by trajectory and the patient remains hemodynamically stable without any other operative indication, perform **angiography** to evaluate potential vascular injury.
E. In the **stable patient,** evaluate possible cardiac injury or great vessel injuries as well as injuries to the esophagus, trachea, and bronchi.
  1. Assess the need for intubation, oxygenate, and start volume resuscitation.
  2. Obtain a CXR.

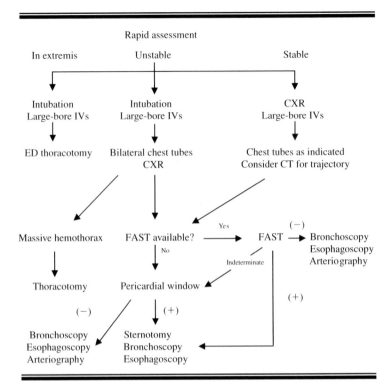

Figure 28-2. Diagnostic algorithm for transmediastinal penetrating trauma. FAST, focused abdominal sonography for trauma; CXR, chest x-ray; ED, emergency department; CT, computed tomography.

3. Perform tube thoracostomy for pneumothorax or hemothorax.
4. If available, perform a **FAST ultrasound examination** to diagnose pericardial effusion (see IV.D.4).
5. A search for mediastinal injury can be guided by presenting signs and symptoms. A combination of the following tests may be needed to exclude injuries.
   a. Computed Tomography of the chest (CCT), ideally CTA (CT angiography), can be used to determine trajectory and thus guide subsequent diagnostic procedures.
   b. Esophagoscopy or esophagography for posterior mediastinal trajectories or in patients with hematemesis.
   c. Bronchoscopy for patients with large air leaks after tube thoracostomy or those which present with hemoptysis.
   d. Angiography for patients with mediastinal, thoracic inlet/zone I of the neck or axillary hematomas if CTA is not diagnostic.

V. MAJOR THORACIC INJURIES can be divided into those that are immediately life threatening and those more difficult to diagnose (Table 28-1).
   A. Immediate life-threatening injuries
      1. **Airway obstruction.** Control of the airway is foremost in trauma resuscitation. The airway must be secured quickly, with attention to the possibility of associated cervical spine injury.

TABLE 28-1	Major Thoracic Injury

Lethal seven	Hidden six
Airway obstruction	Traumatic rupture of the aorta
Tension pneumothorax	Major tracheobronchial disruption
Cardiac tamponade	Blunt cardiac injury
Open pneumothorax	Diaphragmatic tear
Massive hemothorax	Esophageal perforation
Flail chest	Pulmonary contusion
Commotio cordis	

    a. Causes
        i. Relaxation of the tongue into the posterior pharynx in the unconscious patient occludes the airway.
        ii. Loose dentures, avulsed teeth, lacerated tissue, secretions, or blood pooling in the mouth and hypopharynx.
        iii. Bilateral mandibular fractures allowing the tongue to collapse into the hypopharynx.
        iv. Expanding neck hematoma producing deviation of the larynx and mechanical compression of the trachea.
        v. Laryngeal trauma (e.g., thyroid or cricoid cartilage fractures) producing submucosal hemorrhage and edema.
        vi. Tracheal tear or transection.
    b. Physical findings include stridor, hoarseness, subcutaneous emphysema, altered mental status, accessory muscle use, air hunger, apnea, and cyanosis (sign of preterminal hypoxemia).
    c. Any suspicion of airway obstruction or inability to exchange air adequately mandates early intubation.
    d. Management (see Chapter 3).
        i. When in doubt, intubate using a controlled rapid sequence intubation (RSI).
        ii. Provide in-line cervical spine immobilization during intubation.
        iii. Intubate early, especially in the presence of neck hematomas in either zone I or II or possible airway edema. Airway edema can be insidious and progressive and can make delayed intubation more difficult.
        iv. Must always have equipment for emergency cricothyroidotomy readily available if endotracheal intubation fails.
        v. Rescue airway techniques such as the **combitube** or **laryngeal mask airway** (LMA) should be used only by personnel who have had formal training in the use of these devices.
            a) These are **not definitive airways,** as defined as a cuffed tube traversing the vocal cords.
            b) If patients arrive with these airways in place, they should only be exchanged by practitioners familiar with their design and use.
2. Tension pneumothorax occurs when air enters the pleural space from lung injury or through the chest wall without a means of exit. Pressure develops within the pleural space, compressing the superior and the inferior vena cava, impairing venous return and decreasing cardiac output (CO).
    a. Most common causes
        i. Penetrating injury to the thorax
        ii. Blunt trauma with parenchymal lung injury
        iii. Mechanical ventilation with high airway pressures
        iv. Spontaneous pneumothorax with blebs that fail to seal

b. Diagnosis

    i. Clinical diagnosis

        a) Severe respiratory distress

        b) Hypotension

        c) Unilateral absence of breath sounds

        d) Hyperresonance to percussion over affected hemithorax

        e) JVD (can be absent in hypovolemic patients)

        f) Tracheal deviation (late finding—not necessary to confirm clinical diagnosis)

    ii. CXR will usually show a pneumothorax (PTX) large enough to cause tension, however, in a few cases a large anterior or posterior collapse will not be evident on plain film.

    iii. Bedside ultrasound is now being applied to the diagnosis of pneumothorax with good results.

c. Treatment

    i. Immediately decompress the affected hemithoracic cavity by inserting a 12 or 14 gauge IV catheter into the second intercostal space in the midclavicular line or fifth intercostal space in the anterior axillary line. This converts the tension pneumothorax into a simple open pneumothorax.

    ii. Follow immediately with tube thoracostomy.

3. Pericardial tamponade is commonly the result of penetrating trauma, but can also be present with blunt chest trauma. The pericardial sac does not tolerate acute distension, approximately 75 to 100 mL of blood can produce tamponade physiology in the adult.

a. Diagnosis (Fig. 28-3)

    i. If awake, these patients are extremely anxious and even combative; they are reluctant to lie flat, and will often state that they sense "impending doom," and may appear "deathlike."

    ii. Suspect the presence of tamponade in the patient with persistent hypotension, acidosis, or base deficit, despite adequate blood and fluid resuscitation, especially if ongoing blood loss is not evident.

    iii. Classic signs. JVD, hypotension, and muffled heart sounds **(Beck's triad)** are present in only 10% to 30% of patients with confirmed tamponade. JVD may not be present secondary to hypovolemia. **Pulsus**

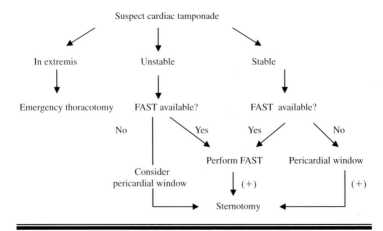

Figure 28-3. Diagnostic algorithm for suspected cardiac tamponade. FAST, focused abdominal sonography for trauma.

paradoxus is a decrease in systolic pressure of >10 mm Hg during inspiration and also suggests tamponade. **Kussmaul's sign** is a hard and true sign of tamponade; inspiration in a spontaneously breathing patient results in an increase of the JVD. The classic signs of cardiac tamponade are uncommon—**shock or ongoing hypotension without evident blood loss is the usual trigger to suggest this injury.**

    iv. If a pulmonary artery catheter is present, right- and left-side heart pressures will equalize. Central venous pressure approaches the pulmonary wedge pressure, and both will be elevated.

    v. If available, a **FAST ultrasound examination** should be performed to identify pericardial fluid.

      a) A **positive** pericardial view on the FAST in an **unstable** patient is an indication to proceed immediately to median sternotomy or left anterolateral thoracotomy.

      b) An **equivocal** pericardial view on the FAST examination or a positive examination in a **stable** patient necessitates a sub-xiphoid operative pericardial window.

      c) A **negative** FAST with a cardiac injury can be falsely negative secondary to decompression of pericardial fluid into the pleural space.

  b. Treatment. Generally, the multiple interventions mentioned below are instituted simultaneously. These can be performed in either the emergency department (ED) or the OR, based on the clinical condition of the patient.

    i. Assess the need for intubation, oxygenate, and start volume resuscitation.

    ii. If a surgeon is not available, pericardiocentesis can be used only as a temporizing maneuver to relieve tamponade. This is often difficult to successfully perform because of the "blind" nature of the procedure and relatively small blood volume in the sac. Similarly, it cannot evaluate pericardial clot (see VII.C).

    iii. If the patient is **in extremis,** an emergent left anterolateral thoracotomy should be performed to open the pericardium, relieve the tamponade, and repair the underlying cardiac injury.

    iv. If the patient is **unstable,** emergency median sternotomy should be performed in the OR.

    v. If the patient is **stable,** a diagnostic sub-xiphoid pericardial window can be performed in the OR to confirm the diagnosis. If this reveals blood in the sac, the incision is converted to a median sternotomy.

4. Open pneumothorax (sucking chest wound)

  a. Usually caused by impalement injury or destructive penetrating wound (shotgun).

  b. Large open defect in chest wall (>3 cm diameter) with equilibration between intrathoracic and atmospheric pressure.

    i. If the opening is greater than two-thirds the diameter of the trachea, air follows the path of least resistance through the chest wall with each inspiration, leading to profound hypoventilation and hypoxia. Signs and symptoms are usually proportional to the size of the defect.

  c. Management

    i. Intubate, if patient is unstable or in any respiratory distress.

    ii. Temporarily close the chest wall defect with a sterile occlusive dressing taped on three sides to act as a flutter-type valve. Avoid securing the dressing on all four sides in the absence of a chest tube, as this can produce a tension pneumothorax.

    iii. Perform tube thoracostomy on the affected side. Avoid placing the tube near or through the traumatic wound.

    iv. Perform urgent thoracotomy to evacuate blood clot and treat associated intrathoracic injuries.

      a) Irrigate, debride, and close the chest wall defect in the OR.

      b) Large defects may require musculocutaneous flap closure, often in a delayed fashion.

5. Massive hemothorax

  a. Common in penetrating trauma with hilar or systemic vessel disruption

    i. Intercostal and internal mammary vessels are most commonly injured.

    ii. Each hemithorax can hold up to 3 L of blood.

    iii. Neck veins can be flat secondary to hypovolemia or distended because of the mechanical effects of intrathoracic blood.

    iv. Hilar or great vessel disruption will present with severe shock.

  b. Diagnosis

    i. Hemorrhagic shock

    ii. Unilateral absence or decreased of breath sounds

    iii. Unilateral dullness to percussion

    iv. Flat neck veins

    v. CXR will show unilateral "white out" (opacification)

  c. Treatment

    i. Intubate patients in shock or with any respiratory difficulty.

    ii. Establish large-bore IV access (ideally a femoral line in this setting) and have blood available for transfusion before decompression.

    iii. If available, have an autotransfusion setup for the chest tube collection system.

    iv. Perform tube thoracostomy with a large chest tube (36F or 40F) in the fifth intercostal space, anterior to mid-axillary line.

      a) A second chest tube may occasionally be necessary to adequately evacuate the hemothorax.

    v. Thoracotomy is indicated for:

      a) Hemodynamic decompensation or ongoing instability because of thoracic bleeding

      b) 1,000 to 1,500 mL blood evacuated initially

      c) Ongoing bleeding of >200 mL/h for ≥4 hours

      d) Failure to completely drain hemothorax, despite at least two functioning and appropriately positioned chest tubes

    vi. Consider early video-assisted thoracoscopy (VATS) for incompletely drained or clotted hemothorax.

6. Flail chest usually results from direct high energy impact. The flail segment classically involves anterior (costochondral cartilage) or lateral rib fractures. Posterior rib fractures usually do not produce a flail segment because the heavy musculature of the posterior chest wall provides stability.

  a. Diagnosis

    i. Diagnosis is made when two or more ribs are fractured in two or more locations, which may lead to paradoxical motion of that chest wall segment. Patients on positive pressure ventilation may not show this paradoxical motion.

    ii. Blunt force of injury typically produces an underlying pulmonary contusion. Morbidity and mortality are generally related to the pulmonary parenchymal injury rather than the chest wall injury.

    iii. The patient is at high risk for pneumothorax or hemothorax, either as an immediate or delayed presentation.

    iv. The flail segment, underlying pulmonary contusion, and splinting caused by pain all exacerbate hypoxemia.

    v. Associated abdominal injuries occur in approximately 15% of patients with flail chest.

  b. Management

    i. Immediately intubate for shock or signs of respiratory distress, such as:

      a) Labored breathing requiring use of accessory muscles of respiration

      b) Respiratory rate >35/min or <8/min

      c) Oxygen saturation <90%, PaO_2 <60 mm Hg

      d) $PaCO_2$ >55 mm Hg

    ii. Consider intubation for patients with hemodynamic instability, need for other surgical interventions, chronic obstructive pulmonary disease (COPD), cardiac disease, or advanced age.

    iii. Admit the patient to the surgical intensive care unit (SICU). The natural progression of the injury is worsening hypoxemia and respiratory insufficiency.

    iv. Control pain (see Chapter 15).

      a) Regional analgesia in the form of an epidural block is the most effective way to deliver pain relief for patients with chest wall trauma. Paravertebral catheters are also effective.

      b) Systemic opioids by continuous infusion or patient-controlled anesthesia (PCA).

      c) Intercostal nerve blocks.

    v. Monitor pulse oximetry and, if available, monitor continuous end tidal CO_2.

    vi. Provide aggressive pulmonary therapy, including incentive spirometry and cough-deep breathing. Adequate pain control and continuous positive airway pressure (CPAP) may preclude intubation. Promote removal of pulmonary secretions.

7. Commotio Cordis is sudden death after a blunt injury to the chest. The injury most often occurs during sporting events where a direct blow to the chest is caused by a fast moving ball, such as a baseball or lacrosse ball.

  a. Patients will not necessarily have a structural injury such as BCI.

  b. The most common dysrhythmia is ventricular fibrillation, possibly caused by massive activation of the Sodium–Potassium–ATP channels.

  c. Treatment consists of following ACLS procedures and aggressive cardiopulmonary resuscitation. Despite prompt and skillful resuscitation, some patients not able to be resuscitated.

B. Potentially life-threatening injuries

1. Traumatic rupture of the aorta is defined as a tear in the wall of the aorta that is contained by the adventitia of this artery and the parietal pleura.

  a. The mechanism of injury is rapid deceleration, such as falls from significant heights, high-speed motor vehicular collisions, or ejection. Thoracic aortic injury may also occur with significant lateral impacts, especially in older patients. Approximately, 80% of these patients die at the scene. The remaining patients are at risk for delayed free rupture into the mediastinum or pleural space.

  b. Patients may be asymptomatic or complain of chest pain. Survivors have contained ruptures. Since free rupture of the transected aorta is rapidly fatal, persistent or recurring hypotension usually results from secondary hemorrhage from other source and not the aortic injury.

  c. Laceration is usually located near the ligamentum arteriosum (85%). Less often, injury is situated in the ascending aorta, at the diaphragm, or in the mid descending thoracic aorta.

  d. Diagnosis (Fig. 28-4)

    i. Clinical signs

      a) Asymmetry in upper extremity blood pressures and upper extremity hypertension

      b) Widened pulse pressure

      c) Chest wall contusion

      d) Posterior scapular pain, interscapular murmur

      e) One-half of patients with great vessel injury from blunt trauma have no external signs of blunt chest injury.

    ii. Signs on **CXR**

      a) Widened mediastinum (>8 cm); this is the most consistent finding

      b) Fracture of first three ribs, scapula and/or sternum

      c) Obliteration of the aortic knob

      d) Tracheal deviation to the right

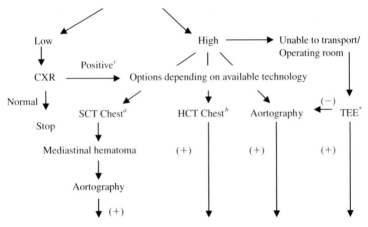

Early medical management to decrease aortic wall tension and operative repair

*a*Standard conventional computed tomography; *b*Helical computed tomography;
*c*Positive = findings listed in (IV.B.1.d.(2)). TEE = *Transesophageal echocardiogram

Figure 28-4. Diagnostic algorithm for suspected traumatic rupture of the aorta (TRA). SCT, standard computed tomography; HCT, helical computed tomography.

> **e)** Presence of pleural cap, usually on the left but occasionally bilaterally
> **f)** Elevation and rightward shift of the right mainstem bronchus
> **g)** Depression of the left mainstem bronchus >40 degrees from horizontal
> **h)** Obliteration of aortopulmonary window
> **i)** Deviation of nasogastric tube (esophagus) to right. This is one of the most infrequent but highly reliable sign.
> **j)** Left pleural effusion
> **k)** No single sign reliably confirms or excludes aortic injury. However, a widened mediastinum is the most consistent finding on CXR and should prompt further evaluation.
> > **1)** Up to 15% of patients with traumatic rupture of the aorta will have a *normal CXR*
>
> **iii.** Historically, **aortography** was the gold standard for diagnosis. Approximately 10% of all angiograms are positive when liberal indications are used, and only 2% to 3% are falsely negative.
> **iv.** **Chest computed tomography** (CT) has recently become a most common diagnostic tool for aortic injury. Standard CT imaging can characterize mediastinal hematomas that are suggestive of aortic injury. Helical and new high-speed, high-resolution scanners can provide definitive diagnosis of the aortic injury, rivaling angiography with respect to overall accuracy.
> > **a)** Nonspecific mediastinal hematomas found on chest CT mandate aortography for definitive diagnosis; an uncommon circumstance with current CTA technology.

b) Definitive diagnostic aortic injuries found on helical scanners may be sufficient characterization for treatment or may require aortography, depending on the practices of the surgeon who will perform the repair.

c) Negative scans rule out aortic injury with a 92% sensitivity.

v. Transesophageal echocardiogram (TEE) is not as reliable as angiography in the diagnosis of aortic injury (sensitivity of 63% and specificity of 84%). A positive TEE will confirm the location of the injury and expedite management. If the TEE is negative, CTA or aortography is required to reliably exclude the injury. TEE is an excellent alternative for unstable patients who:

a) Must be transported directly to the OR for other surgical interventions

b) Have a wide mediastinum and a high suspicion of thoracic aortic injury

c) Patients in the ICU at high risk for transport to radiology.

e. Management

i. Establish airway, as needed.

ii. Control and prevent hypertension. Maneuvers to decrease systolic wall tension in the aorta preoperatively decrease risk of rupture. Beta blockade should be instituted only after significant hemorrhage from other injuries has been ruled out. The goal for systolic blood pressure should be approximately 100 mm/Hg.

a) Esmolol is a short-acting beta-blocker that can be easily titrated to desired blood pressure. The loading dose is **500 μg/kg** followed by a continuous infusion of **50 μg/kg/min** titrated to a systolic blood pressure of 100 mm Hg and a heart rate <100 beats/min.

b) Labetalol is a longer-acting beta- and alpha-blocker that can decrease wall tension. An initial IV dose of **20 mg** is given. Additional doses can be given to obtain parameters as above, up to **300 mg total.**

c) Sodium Nitroprusside can be added as a second agent if blood pressure is not controlled with beta blockade. It is administered as a continuous infusion at **0.1 μg/kg/min** titrated to effect up to a dose of 10 μg/kg/min.

iii. If the patient has a stable mediastinal hematoma and concomitant abdominal injury, perform definitive or damage control laparotomy first. If damage control is required, do not pack the abdomen tightly or clamp the aorta, causing increased proximal aortic pressure. An intraoperative TEE can be used to evaluate the thoracic aorta.

iv. Exposure. The proximal innominate artery and aortic arch are best approached by a median sternotomy. Early ligation of the innominate vein and associated thymic tissue in the anterior mediastinum will aid in exposing the aortic arch. The proximal descending aorta is approached by posterolateral thoracotomy. Traumatic blunt ruptures of the aorta are typically found in this location distal to the ligamentum arteriosum.

v. Technique

a) With an open approach, control of the aorta at the arch is difficult. Small injuries can be controlled initially with finger occlusion and at times with a partially occluding Satinsky clamp. Primary repair can be accomplished using nonabsorbable monofilament sutures with or without pledgets. Treat proximal innominate artery injuries by ligating proximally and performing a bypass from the aorta to the distal innominate.

b) Blunt, traumatic rupture of the aorta is repaired either primarily or with an interposition graft. Best option is to use a femorofemoral bypass with a biomedicus pump. Other options include direct repair without distal shunting, repair with passive shunting of blood distally using a Gott shunt, or repair using full or partial cardiopulmonary bypass.

vi. Definitive repair is performed at the discretion of the cardiothoracic or vascular or trauma surgeon. Several techniques are available.

a) Repair after full cardiac bypass often requires large doses of heparin and cannot be done in cases with many associated solid organ injury, pelvic fractures or traumatic brain injuries. Major chest injury also precludes the single lung ventilation which is necessary for open repair.

b) Repair during passive bypass with heparin-bonded shunts, or no bypass at all is possible although less often used.

c) **Endovascular** aortic stent grafts are now available at some centers and offer the advantage of avoiding a thoracotomy in patients who may have significant associated pulmonary compromise. These have become the most common method of repair of blunt thoracic aortic transection. The benefit is a significantly lower mortality and risk of paraplegia compared to open repair. Five percent of patients treated with an endovascular stent will have technical issues requiring a second procedure. In addition, the long-term durability of these stents is unknown.

2. Tracheobronchial injuries

a. Most patients with major airway injuries die at the scene as a result of asphyxia. Those who survive to reach the hospital are usually *in extremis.* Minor injuries can cause late sequelae such as granuloma formation with subsequent stenosis, persistent atelectasis, and recurring pneumonia.

b. Location

i. Cervical tracheal injuries

a) Usually present with upper airway obstruction and cyanosis unrelieved with O_2 supplementation

b) Symptoms include local pain, dysphagia, cough, and hemoptysis

c) Subcutaneous emphysema

d) Blunt transection is uncommon and tends to occur at the cricotracheal junction

ii. Thoracic tracheal or bronchial injuries

a) Of major bronchial injuries, 80% occur within 2 cm of the carina.

b) Intrapleural laceration. The patient develops persistent dyspnea, massive air leak, and massive pneumothorax that do not re-expand with chest tube drainage. Intraparenchymal injuries usually seal spontaneously if the lung is adequately expanded.

c) Extrapleural rupture into the mediastinum. The patient will present with pneumomediastinum and subcutaneous emphysema. Respiratory distress may be minimal, especially with partial bronchial transection. Of partial bronchial disruptions, 25% go undetected for 2 to 4 weeks, but persistent atelectasis, recurrent pneumonia, and suppuration should prompt further investigation.

d) Radiographic signs on CXR

1) An abnormal admission CXR will be seen in 90% of cases; findings include pneumothorax, hemothorax, pleural effusion, subcutaneous emphysema, fractures of ipsilateral ribs 1 to 5, and mediastinal hematoma.

2) Specific findings
- Peribronchial air
- Deep cervical emphysema; radiolucent line along prevertebral fascia (early and reliable sign)
- "Fallen lung" refers to a pattern of lung collapse sometimes seen with these injuries. The lung collapses laterally with a medial pneumothorax.

e) Management

1) Endotracheal intubation is almost always indicated, although conversion to positive pressure often exacerbates the massive air leak.

2) Perform immediate bronchoscopy to localize the injury.

3) On occasion it may be possible during bronchoscopy to guide the endotracheal tube past a tracheal injury or into the uninjured mainstem bronchus to improve ventilation of the uninjured lung.

4) Double lumen intubation by anesthesiologists will provide optimal operative exposure for these injuries.

5) Definitive treatment includes primary repair with mucosa-to-mucosa closure using nonabsorbable, interrupted polypropylene sutures. Exposure of the injury depends on location:

- Median sternotomy provides access to the anterior or left lateral portion of the mediastinal trachea.
- Right posterolateral thoracotomy provides exposure of the right lateral or posterior aspect of the trachea or right lung bronchi or parenchymal injury.
- Left posterolateral thoracotomy provides access to the left lung bronchi or parenchymal laceration.

3. Cardiac Injuries

a. Blunt cardiac injury (BCI)

i. Definition. BCI is a phrase used to describe a spectrum of injury to the heart. It can range from asymptomatic myocardial muscle contusion to clinically significant dysrhythmia, acute heart failure, valvular injury, or cardiac rupture. Critical BCI, particularly that causes hemodynamic instability, is rare.

a) The most common complication of blunt injury to the myocardium is dysrhythmias such as sinus tachycardia, premature atrial contractions (PACs), atrial fibrillation (AF), and premature ventricular contractions (PVCs). Other ECG changes that may be seen are right bundle branch block or acute current of injury with ST elevation and T-wave flattening.

ii. Diagnosis. Ample debate is present in the literature regarding the criteria for the diagnosis and significance of BCI (Fig. 28-5).

a) An admission 12-lead ECG should be performed as a screening test for all patients suspected of having BCI.

1) An ECG is considered positive if it demonstrates dysrhythmia, atrial or ventricular ectopy, ST changes, bundle branch block, or hemifascicular blocks. Reminder that sinus tachycardia is the most common rhythm abnormality with BCI.

b) Echocardiography (ECHO) can be used to assess wall motion and valvular competency. Transthoracic echocardiogram (TTE) is convenient and noninvasive, although sometimes is technically limited. TEE is more invasive, however, may be necessary when the echocardiography is inadequate.

c) We do not obtain troponin levels in younger patients with suspected BCI. In the middle age or older population (>45 years), where ischemic cardiac disease is the concern, cardiac enzymes may be helpful in the diagnosis of ischemic cardiac disease.

d) The presence of a sternal fracture does not correlate with the presence of BCI.

iii. Treatment

a) Admit patients with suspected BCI to an ECG-monitored bed/telemetry unit. Dysrhythmias are treated as necessary according to Advanced Cardiac Life Support (ACLS) protocols.

1) Patients with ischemic changes on the ECG or elevated cardiac enzyme levels are treated similarly to those with myocardial infarction.

2) If echocardiographic-proved contusion (hypokinesis or abnormal wall movement) is seen, admit the patient to an ICU.

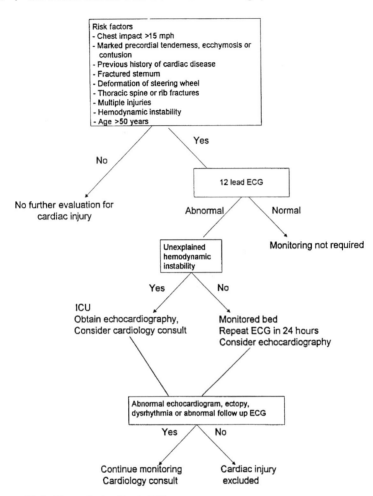

Figure 28-5. Diagnostic algorithm for BCI.

3) If the patient develops signs and symptoms of acute heart failure, begin invasive monitoring with a pulmonary artery catheter.

b) Obtain follow-up ECG only for those with an initial abnormal tracings initially or new signs.

c) BCI is not an absolute contraindication to surgery. If the patient with BCI requires noncardiac surgery, invasive monitoring perioperatively is usually needed (arterial line, pulmonary artery catheter).

b. Penetrating cardiac injury

i. Presentation. Pericardial tamponade, mediastinal hematoma, or massive hemothorax with wounds that communicate through the pericardium.

ii. Exposure. Median sternotomy or left anterolateral thoracotomy. Extension of the left thoracotomy across to the right (clamshell) provides excellent exposure to the entire middle mediastinum.

    iii. Technique. Wounds of the atria and auricles can be controlled with a partial occluding Satinsky clamp and repaired primarily with 2-0 or 3-0 polypropylene sutures with or without pledgets. Wounds on the ventricles are repaired with individual horizontal mattress sutures with 2-0 polypropylene, ethibond, or tevdek. Pledgeted sutures are often required to repair gunshot (GSWs) of the heart.

4. Vascular injuries

Major thoracic or cardiac injuries will frequently present with hemodynamic instability. The goal is to quickly determine that a major injury exists and to prepare for emergent exploration and repair. Patients who arrive unresponsive without a measurable blood pressure are *in extremis* and should undergo immediate emergency department thoracotomy (EDT) (see Section VI).

  a. Clinical signs of thoracic vascular or cardiac injury
    i. Hemodynamic instability (hypotension, altered sensorium, or other signs of shock) in the presence of a penetrating chest wound
    ii. Massive hemothorax (1,000 to 1,500 mL) on insertion of a chest tube, persistent hemothorax on CXR, or >200 mL/h for 4 hours)
    iii. Cardiac tamponade
    iv. Large mediastinal hematoma

  b. Diagnosis
    i. Use **CXR** to diagnose a hemothorax or mediastinal hematoma. Penetrating wound sites should be marked with metallic clips to help determine trajectories. Anteroposterior and lateral views can help to determine trajectory. The cardiac silhouette generally does not change appreciably in acute tamponade.
    ii. Ultrasound. FAST examination, with special attention to the pericardial view, can determine the presence of fluid in the pericardium or abdomen.
    iii. Tube thoracostomy can be both diagnostic and therapeutic. Pneumothorax or hemothorax can be confirmed by tube thoracostomy. For patients in shock, tube thoracostomy should be used as the initial diagnostic and therapeutic intervention, rather than CXR.

  c. Injury complexes. Certain thoracic vascular injuries can be predicted by the injury mechanism, trajectory, and findings on the initial CXR.
    i. Massive hemothorax involves injury to pulmonary hilum, proximal subclavian artery on the left, proximal innominate and/or subclavian artery on the right, heart with a communication through the pericardium, intercostal artery, internal mammary artery, and azygos vein. For unstable patients who do not respond to chest tube drainage, the choice of incision is a **thoracotomy** on the side of hemothorax.
    ii. Superior mediastinal hematoma involves injury to innominate artery and vein, subclavian vessels and carotid arteries bilaterally, superior vena cava, or heart. The best approach is through a median sternotomy with extension into the neck at the anterior border of the sternocleidomastoid muscle or subclavicular, depending on the vessels injured.
    iii. Middle mediastinal hematoma includes cardiac injury with intact pericardium, aortic arch, proximal innominate, or left proximal carotid and subclavian arteries. Best approach is through a median sternotomy.

  d. Specific injuries
    i. Carotid artery
      a) Presentation. Superior mediastinal hematoma or neck hematoma. Hemiplegia on physical examination is suggestive of a carotid injury.
      b) Exposure. Median sternotomy with either a right or left cervical extension along the anterior border of the sternocleidomastoid muscle (with proximal carotid artery injury).
      c) Technique. Primary repair or interposition graft with vein or polytetrafluoroethylene (PTFE). Consider simple ligation without bypass for injuries that show no prograde flow preoperatively.

ii. Subclavian artery

a) Presentation. Superior mediastinal hematoma or neck hematoma. Proximal injuries can present with massive left hemothorax.

b) Exposure. The proximal subclavian artery is accessed by a median sternotomy. An infra- or supraclavicular extension is used to gain distal control with or without removal of the clavicle.

c) Technique. Primary repair or interposition graft with PTFE. If possible based on patient stability, an endovascular stent is an excellent option.

iii. Pulmonary hilum

a) Presentation. Massive hemothorax on the side of injury.

b) Exposure. Anterolateral thoracotomy on the side of injury. Control can also be gained initially through a median sternotomy.

c) Technique. Control of hilar hemorrhage can be accomplished initially by manual compression. Quick dissection of the inferior pulmonary ligament aids in the isolation and identification of the bleeding site. Exsanguinating hemorrhage can then be definitively stopped by placing a clamp across the entire hilum.

1) Intrapericardial control of hilar vessels is used for proximal injury to the pulmonary artery or vein, if necessary. Primary repair is desirable; however, lobectomy should be considered early if bleeding is not easily controlled.

2) With the advent of stapled pulmonary tractotomy and stapled pneumonectomy, approximately 85% of pulmonary injuries will be spared resection.

3) Pneumonectomy is rarely required to stop hilar bleeding and carries high postoperative morbidity and mortality.

iv. Intercostal arteries

a) Presentation. Hemothorax or subcutaneous hematoma.

b) Exposure. Thoracotomy on the side of injury.

c) Technique. Simple ligation proximal and distal to the injury.

v. Internal mammary artery

a) Presentation. Hemothorax, superior or middle mediastinal hematoma.

b) Exposure. Median sternotomy or anterolateral thoracotomy.

c) Technique. Simple ligation proximal and distal to the injury. Bilateral internal mammary artery ligation can be performed safely in most patients.

vi. Azygos and hemiazygos veins

a) Presentation. Hemothorax

b) Exposure. Thoracotomy on the side of hemothorax

c) Technique. Suture ligation proximal and distal to injury. Take care to avoid inadvertent injury to the thoracic duct on the left.

5. Diaphragmatic injury

a. Blunt trauma. Diaphragmatic injury from blunt forces is classically large, radial, and located posterolaterally. The left hemidiaphragm is involved in 65% to 80% of cases. Diaphragmatic ruptures are markers for associated intraabdominal injuries.

b. Penetrating trauma. Wounds are smaller but tend to enlarge over time. Left-sided injuries still predominate. These injuries required operative repair when diagnosed as they do not heal spontaneously and can produce herniation or strangulation of hollow viscera as late sequelae.

c. Diagnosis

i. Diagnosis can be difficult; therefore, a high index of suspicion based on mechanism is required.

a) Rapid deceleration or direct crush to the upper abdomen

b) Severe chest trauma, lower rib fractures

c) Penetrating injuries to the chest and upper abdomen

ii. CXR is diagnostic in only 25% to 50% of cases of blunt trauma. Possible findings include:

  a) Hemidiaphragmatic elevation or lower lobe atelectasis

  b) Nasogastric tube in left hemithorax

  c) Stomach, colon, or small bowel herniated into chest

  d) In penetrating trauma and small defects, the diaphragm appears normal.

  e) Positive pressure can tamponade visceral herniation and make the CXR appear normal. After extubation, herniation may become apparent on CXR.

iii. Right hemidiaphragm tears are less likely to be diagnosed by CXR because of the presence of the liver in the defect.

iv. CT scan may miss diaphragmatic injury in the absence of gross hollow visceral herniation.

v. Diagnostic peritoneal lavage (DPL) yields false-negative results in 25% to 34% of diaphragmatic injuries. If an ipsilateral chest tube is present, DPL fluid may be observed exiting the chest tube, although this finding is rare.

vi. Direct visualization of the injury by laparotomy, laparoscopy, or thoracoscopy remains the standard for diagnosis.

d. Treatment

  i. Diaphragmatic tears require repair.

  ii. Acute repair is accomplished via laparotomy, in most cases, with nonabsorbable, interrupted horizontal mattress sutures.

  iii. Thoracotomy may be needed to reduce large defects in chronic herniation.

  iv. Prosthetic material or flaps are rarely needed to close the defect.

  v. The mortality rate is 25% to 40% because of the severity of associated injuries.

6. Esophageal injury

  a. Most injuries result from penetrating trauma. Blunt injury is rare (<0.1% incidence). Presentation varies according to location of injury:

  i. Cervical esophagus. Subcutaneous emphysema, hematemesis.

  ii. Thoracic esophagus. Mediastinal emphysema, subcutaneous emphysema, pleural effusion, retroesophageal air, unexplained fever within 24 hours of injury.

  iii. Intraabdominal esophagus. Commonly asymptomatic initially; may present with pneumoperitoneum, hemoperitoneum, or acute peritoneal signs.

  b. Diagnosis

  i. Penetrating trajectory involving the mediastinum or neck mandate diagnostic workup to exclude injury to the esophagus.

  ii. Many penetrating injuries are detected at the time of emergency neck exploration, thoracotomy, or laparotomy.

  iii. Esophagoscopy and **esophagogram** are used with equal sensitivity (60%). Combining both studies will detect almost all esophageal injuries.

  iv. CT scan may have a role in determining trajectory in stable patients.

  c. Management

  i. Operative exposure

   a) Cervical. Unilateral neck incision along the anterior border of the left sternocleidomastoid muscle

   b) Proximal thoracic. Right posterolateral thoracotomy in the fifth intercostal space

   c) Distal thoracic. Left posterolateral thoracotomy in the sixth intercostal space

  ii. Definitive repair

   a) Injury <6 hours old. Close primarily in two layers. The inner layer with absorbable sutures and the outer layer with nonabsorbable sutures. Buttress suture lines with pleural or intercostal muscle flap. Distal esophageal repair can also be reinforced with Nissen wrap. Drain.

  b) Complex injury or >12 hours old. Repair wound as above. Diverting cervical esophagostomy and oversewing of the distal esophagus may be considered with signs of mediastinitis. Wide drainage with chest tubes and feeding gastrostomy are both indicated. Avoid resection if possible.

  c) Injury 6 to 12 hours old. Repair primarily. Buttress repairs with muscular or pleural flaps. Drain widely.

7. Pulmonary contusion

  a. The most common potentially lethal thoracic injury

  b. Caused by hemorrhage into lung parenchyma

  c. Commonly, this accompanies a flail segment or multiple fractured ribs. Pulmonary contusion can also accompany a penetrating injury.

  d. Children may have a pulmonary contusion in the absence of rib fractures because of the resilience of their chest wall.

  e. The natural progression is worsening hypoxemia for the first 24 to 48 hours.

    i. Diagnosis. CXR findings are typically delayed in appearance and non-segmental. If abnormalities are seen on the admission CXR, the pulmonary contusion is considered to be severe. Hemoptysis or blood in the endotracheal tube is a sign of pulmonary contusion.

    ii. Treatment

      a) Although excessive extravascular lung water can exacerbate pulmonary contusions, adequate volume resuscitation should not be withheld in patients with other injuries. The goal is euvolemia.

      b) If the fluid status is in question, hemodynamic invasive monitoring either a pulmonary artery catheter or central line (CVP) may guide fluid management.

      c) Prophylactic antibiotics or steroids are **not** indicated.

      d) Mild contusion. Administer supplemental oxygen, monitor oxygen saturation, provide aggressive pulmonary therapy, and administer analgesia.

      e) Moderate to severe contusion. In addition to the above, intubate and mechanically ventilate with positive end-expiratory pressure.

      f) Catastrophic contusion. If the patient is not responsive to conventional ventilation, consider pressure-limiting ventilatory modes, such as pressure control, airway pressure release ventilation (APRV), inverse ratio ventilation, or high frequency jet ventilation. Extracorporeal membrane oxygenation (ECMO) is an option in centers with this expertise. For severe unilateral contusions, consider independent lung ventilation through a double lumen tube.

VI. OTHER THORACIC INJURIES

A. Traumatic asphyxia

1. Definition

  a. Occurs with a severe crushing injury to the chest or upper abdomen. Intrathoracic and superior vena cava pressures increase and, together with reflux closure of the glottis, produce reversal of flow in the valveless veins of the head and neck with subsequent capillary disruption.

  b. Chest wall, intrathoracic, and intraabdominal injuries (heart, lung, liver) are frequently associated injuries.

  c. Increased intracranial pressure, cerebral edema, and hypoxic brain injury are rare sequelae.

2. Diagnosis

  a. Craniocervical cyanosis, followed by craniocervical rubor

  b. Facial edema

c. Petechiae over the face, neck, and torso

d. Subconjunctival hemorrhage

e. Neurologic symptoms (e.g., loss of consciousness, seizures, confusion, and temporary or permanent blindness) occur occasionally.

f. Hematuria, hemotympanum, or epistaxis occurs rarely.

3. Treatment

a. Elevate head of bed at a 30-degree angle.

b. Administer oxygen.

c. Treat any underlying injuries.

d. Perform adequate pulmonary hygiene.

B. Chest wall injury

1. Fractures of the scapula or first or second rib result from significant force. The risk of associated intrathoracic injury is >50%.

2. Sternal fractures. Of these, 40% will have associated rib fractures and 25% will have associated long-bone injury.

3. Fractures of ribs 3 to 8

a. The main clinical issues are pain and restriction of ventilation with impairment of both static and dynamic compliances.

b. Search for pulmonary contusion and BCI.

c. Provide adequate pain relief by epidural anesthesia, PCA, or intercostal nerve blocks.

4. Fractures of ribs 9 to 12. A 10% risk exists of associated hepatic (right-sided fractures), and a 20% risk of splenic (left-sided fractures), or renal injuries.

VII. EMERGENCY THORACIC PROCEDURES

A. Tube thoracostomy (Fig. 28-6)

1. The usual insertion site is the fifth intercostal space at the anterior to mid-axillary line. Identify the space between the pectoralis major anteriorly and the latissimus dorsi posteriorly (Fig. 28-6A). Do not insert tubes through traumatic wounds. Use a large caliber chest tube ($\geq$36 to 40 Fr) to ensure adequate drainage of the pleural space.

2. Administer a single dose of prophylactic antibiotics such as cefazolin or cefoxitin.

3. Prepare and drape the chest.

4. Anesthetize the site locally with 1% lidocaine (10 to 20 mL), including the skin, periosteum, subpleural space, and pleura. Except under the most life-threatening circumstances, proper local anesthesia must be used to minimize patient discomfort.

5. Commence with 3 to 5 cm horizontal skin incision below the selected interspace and continue the incision down to the chest wall (Fig. 28-6B).

6. With a large curved Kelly clamp, carefully puncture the parietal pleura just above the rib, avoiding the neurovascular bundle coursing along the inferior border. Spread the intercostal muscles.

7. Remove the clamp and insert a finger into the pleural space to confirm appropriate position and to clear any adhesions that may be present (Fig. 28-6C).

8. Use the clamp or a finger as a guide to advance and position the tube into the pleural space. Guide the tube posteriorly and toward the apex of the pleural space (Fig. 28-6D–F).

9. If correctly placed, the tube should "fog" with expiration. After placement, run a finger along the tube to confirm proper placement. Confirm that all of the holes are within the pleural space. Rotating the tube 360 degrees ensures that it is not kinked in the chest.

10. Connect the tube to an underwater-seal apparatus and apply at 20 cm of water suction. For known hemothoraces, use an autotransfusion reservoir.

11. Secure tube with 0-silk sutures. Tape all tube connections to prevent separation.

12. Obtain a CXR to confirm proper placement.

B. Pericardiocentesis (Fig. 28-7)

1. Indications

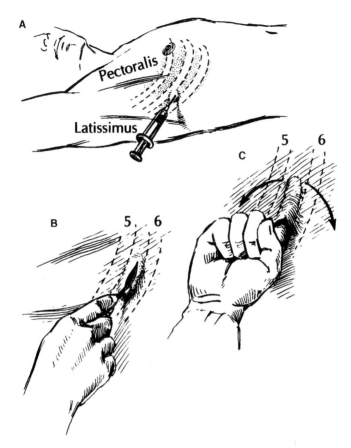

Figure 28-6. Steps for chest tube insertion (Figures A–F). (From Trunkey DD, Guernsey JM. Surgical procedures. In: Blaisdell FW, Trunkey DD, eds. *Trauma Management—Cervicothoracic Trauma.* New York, NY: Thieme Medical Publishers; 1986:310, with permission.) **(continued)**

    a. Acute distension of the pericardial sac with as little as 75 to 100 mL of blood can produce cardiac tamponade. Withdrawal of this fluid is lifesaving. However, it is difficult to aspirate fluid, especially if it accumulates posteriorly. Similarly, clot cannot be aspirated.

    b. When used for diagnosis, pericardiocentesis can produce false-negative results in 50% to 60% of cases because of pericardial blood clotting or needle misplacement.

    c. In acute cardiac tamponade, pericardiocentesis can be used as a temporizing maneuver until definitive pericardiotomy is possible.

    d. Pericardiocentesis is rarely indicated in a level I trauma center.

2. Technique

    a. A 16 or 18 gauge long (6″) needle is connected to a 30 mL syringe. The needle is introduced at the left xiphisternal junction (Larrey's point) and directed toward the left shoulder and at a 45-degree angle to the skin. Back pressure is placed on the plunger of the syringe as the needle is advanced.

    b. Blood (30 mL) is withdrawn and the clinical situation is reassessed. If no improvement is noted, aspiration is repeated.

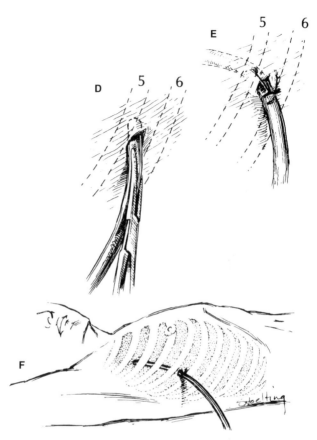

Figure 28-6. (*Continued*)

3. Complications
   a. Iatrogenic coronary artery injury, myocardial laceration, pneumothorax, hemothorax, and mediastinal hematoma can occur.
   b. False-positive return can occur when the ventricle or a hemothorax is inadvertently entered.
C. Pericardial window (Fig. 28-8)
   1. Sub-xiphoid pericardial window should be considered in the patient who is at risk of cardiac injury but who has maintained adequate vital signs. As mentioned, pericardial tamponade is rapidly fatal. If the patient is *in extremis* or hypotensive, prompt left anterolateral thoracotomy is indicated. However, in a more stable patient with a parasternal penetrating wound suggestive of possible cardiac injury, a sub-xiphoid pericardial window is safer and more definitive than pericardiocentesis.
2. Technique
   a. Sub-xiphoid pericardial window is performed in the OR under general anesthesia.
   b. Prepare the patient from chin to midthighs before induction of general anesthesia in anticipation of acute hemodynamic decompensation.
   c. A 10 cm incision is made over the xiphoid process and extend cephalad and caudal the upper midline of the abdomen.

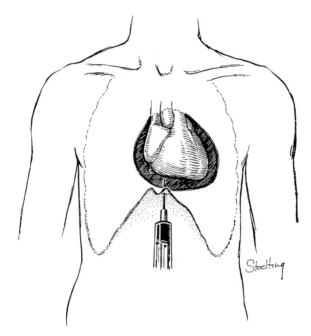

Figure 28-7. Pericardiocentesis. (From Rich NM, Spencer FC. *Vascular Trauma*. Philadelphia, PA: WB Saunders; 1978:409, with permission.)

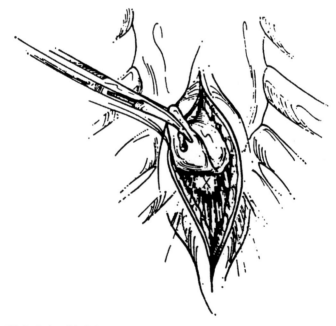

Figure 28-8. Pericardial window.

d. Excision of the xiphoid process may facilitate the procedure. The diaphragmatic attachments immediately deep to the sternum should be freed by blunt dissection. The diaphragm can then be retracted downward with Allis clamps. Reverse Trendelenburg position helps to expose the pericardium. A Kittner dissector can be used to mobilize the pericardial fat off the anterior surface of the pericardium. The tense, fibrous, white pericardium is then identified.

e. A 1 to 2 cm incision is made with scissors or knife on the anterior surface of the pericardium.

   i. If blood is found in the pericardial sac, the procedure should be rapidly converted to median sternotomy to perform cardiorrhaphy.

   ii. If no gross blood is aspirated, a catheter is placed to gently irrigate the pericardium with warm saline to obtain clots from the pericardial recesses.

D. Emergency department thoracotomy (EDT). Enthusiasm for EDT has waned over the past several years since the overall mortality of patients receiving EDT is high. Patients most likely to benefit from EDT are young, have isolated penetrating injury to the chest, preferably a cardiac wound with tamponade that can be easily released. Patients with blunt injury, exsanguination below the diaphragm or associated head injury have very low survival rates.

1. Indications (Table 28.2)

   a. EDT is indicated for patients who are *in extremis* or in cardiopulmonary arrest without **vital signs,** which is defined as a measurable blood pressure or pulse. Patients should be evaluated for when signs of life (SOL) were present and lost. SOL include:

   i. Spontaneous movements

   ii. Pupillary response, eye movement

   iii. Spontaneous respirations

   iv. Electrical complexes >40/min on ECG

   b. In patients with cardiopulmonary arrest from **blunt trauma,** EDT is indicated only if the patient has SOL **on arrival to the hospital.** Patients who have SOL in the field and lose them in route are considered dead on arrival (DOA).

   c. In patients with cardiopulmonary arrest from **penetrating trauma,** EDT is indicated if the patient had SOL in the field. Patients with penetrating injury should receive EDT even if SOL are lost en route. This expanded indication (compared with blunt trauma arrest) is specific because of the higher frequency of reparable lesions being present.

   d. Patients **without SOL in the field,** regardless of mechanism are DOA.

2. Technique

   a. Perform a left anterolateral thoracotomy at the fifth intercostal space. The incision begins at the left sternocostal margin, it is curvilinear and is extended to the latissimus dorsi posteriorly (Fig. 28-9). In females, displace the breast cephalad to perform the skin incision in the inframammary crease. Incise the intercostal muscles with scissors and insert a finochietto retractor. Take care

TABLE 28-2	Indications for Emergency Department Thoracotomy				
No measurable blood pressure or pulse					
Blunt mechanism			**Penetrating mechanism**		
No SOL	**SOL field only**	**SOL arrival**	**No SOL**	**SOL field only**	**SOL arrival**
DOA	DOA	EDT	DOA	EDT	EDT

SOL, signs of life (eye movement, pupillary response, spontaneous respiration, electrical activity >40 complexes/min on electrogram); DOA, dead on arrival; EDT, emergency department thoracotomy.

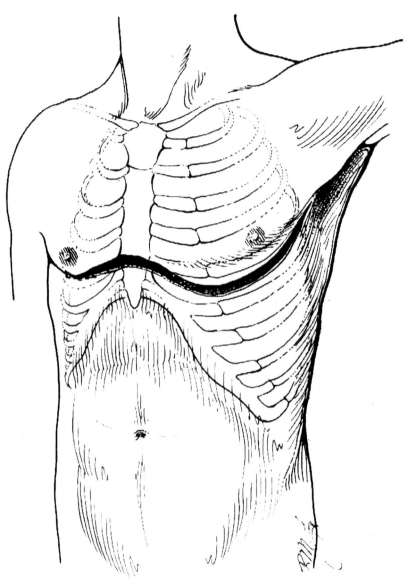

Figure 28-9. EDT. Extend the incision to the right side below the right nipple for easy access to the right chest. (Adapted from Moore EE, Eiseman B, Van Way CW. *Critical Decisions in Trauma.* St. Louis, MO: Mosby; 1984:524, with permission.)

to insert the retractor with the "T" bar posteriorly near the bed; this will allow free access to extend the thoracotomy across the sternum to the right side if necessary (Fig. 28-10).

b. The pericardium is opened anterior to the phrenic nerve. This relieves tamponade and allows more effective internal compressions. This should be done

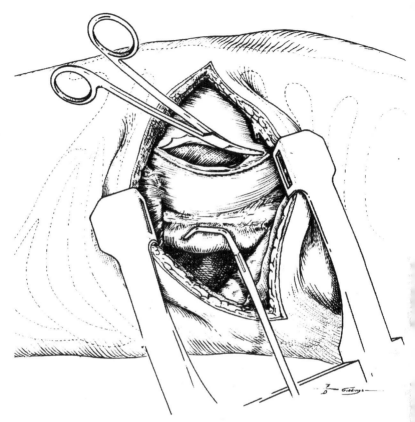

Figure 28-10. A view into the left chest during EDT. A clamp is shown on the descending aorta and a sharp pericardiotomy is shown proceeding cephalad anterior to the phrenic vessels. (Adapted from Moore EE, Eiseman B, Van Way CW. *Critical Decisions in Trauma*. St. Louis, MO: Mosby; 1984:529, with permission.)

in the anterior portion of the pericardium in a caudal to cephalad plane, avoiding injury to the phrenic nerve. The opening should extend from the cardiac apex to the root of the aorta.

c. If the heart is not beating, perform internal massage with open hands spanning the left ventricle—do not squeeze with one hand, as this can lead to ventricular injury. If the heart is fibrillating, attempt internal cardioversion at 20 J followed by 30 J. Cardioversion may be repeated after internal compression to perfuse the coronaries.

d. If the myocardium is ruptured or injured, digitally occlude the injury. Cardiorrhaphy should be performed with 2-0 sutures with horizontal mattress sutures.

    i. Although some surgeons recommend placing a balloon catheter into a cardiac injury, this maneuver should not be performed as the maneuver often exacerbates the injury.

    ii. If the wound is adjacent to a coronary artery, the cardiorrhaphy must not compromise the coronary artery. The horizontal mattress sutures should be placed underneath the coronary artery to avoid coronary narrowing.

      iii. Atrial wounds can be controlled with a Satinsky partial occlusion clamp followed by repair with 2-0 horizontal mattress sutures.

    e. If the thoracic aorta is bleeding, compress and clamp with a partial occlusion vascular clamp. Check for the possibility of a posterior injury.

    f. In cases of massive hemorrhage from the pulmonary parenchyma or the hilum, clamp the hilum. This is best performed by releasing the inferior pulmonary ligament, passing a hand around the vascular structures, and safely guiding a vascular clamp to gently occlude the hilum.

    g. If no reparable thoracic injury is found, the patient is unlikely to survive. With the chest open, clamp the descending thoracic aorta and continue open cardiac massage. If this successfully restores a palpable carotid pulse in a short period of time, rapidly transport to the OR for repair of injuries below the diaphragm.

E. Median sternotomy

    1. Advantage. Provides excellent exposure of the heart and proximal great vessels, but not the posterior mediastinal structures. The incision can be extended into the neck or supraclavicular are for more distal vascular control and repair (Fig. 28-11).

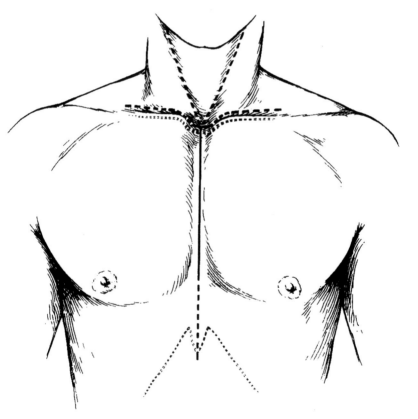

Figure 28-11. Extensions of the median sternotomy. Supraclavicular and neck extensions are shown (*dotted lines*). (Adapted from Rutherford RB. *Atlas of Vascular Surgery: Basic Techniques and Exposures.* Philadelphia, PA: WB Saunders; 1993:235, with permission.)

    2. Disadvantages. Requires a sternal saw or Lebsche knife and usually takes more time to perform than left anterolateral thoracotomy; because of this, it is not recommended for EDT. Also, access is limited to the esophagus and descending aorta.

    3. Technique

       a. The patient is placed supine on the OR table with both arms abducted to 90 degrees.

       b. The skin and subcutaneous tissues are incised from the sternal notch to inferior to the xiphoid.

       c. A plane on the posterior surface of the sternum is developed bluntly from above and below before division of the sternum with a sternal saw or Lebsche knife. Begin this at the upper edge of the sternum, and lift the saw or knife and sternum as you proceed in the caudal direction. (Procedure may also be performed from caudal to cephalad direction.) Stay in the center of the sternum to avoid injury to the costal cartilages and entry into either hemithorax.

       d. Bone wax may be required for cancellous bone bleeding.

       e. To facilitate exposure of the great vessels, this incision can be extended laterally into the neck, dividing sternocleidomastoid, platysma, strap, and anterior scalene muscles (protecting the phrenic nerve).

       f. Further exposure of the second and third portions of the subclavian vessels can be enhanced by resection or division of the clavicle.

       g. Extension into the abdomen with a midline incision is easily accomplished.

F. Left anterolateral thoracotomy

    1. Advantage. Permits rapid access to the chest, especially for decompression of pericardial tamponade and for repair of the heart, left lung and hilum, or aorta. This can be extended across the sternum (bilateral or clamshell thoracotomy) to access the right chest. Left anterolateral thoracotomy is the best initial operative approach for unstable patients requiring resuscitation or when the location of the intrathoracic injury is unclear.

    2. Disadvantage. Poor access to the posterior mediastinum, distal subclavian vessels, and right chest.

    3. Technique

       a. The left arm should be fully extended over the patient's head to provide extension of the incision on the posterior chest wall.

       b. An incision is made in the fifth intercostal space, from the sternal edge to the scapula.

       c. The muscles of the anterior chest wall are divided with electrocautery and the intercostal muscles are also sharply transected while avoiding injury to the neurovascular bundle.

       d. A Finochietto rib retractor is inserted with the "T" bar toward the back and opened widely.

       e. A thoracoabdominal incision can be carried out by performing a midline laparotomy. We do not recommend costal margin transection.

G. Left or right posterolateral thoracotomy

    1. Advantages. Provides excellent access to the hemithorax. The left posterolateral thoracotomy permits access to the aorta and proximal left subclavian artery, the left lung, the left chest wall, and the distal esophagus. The right posterolateral thoracotomy provides access to the trachea, the right lung, the right chest wall, and the proximal esophagus.

    2. Disadvantages. The lateral position for the posterolateral thoracotomy is time consuming and leaves little flexibility in gaining access to opposite hemithorax or abdominal structures, thus injuries elsewhere cannot be accessed.

    3. Technique

       a. Use the standard skin incision for elective thoracic surgery. By varying the interspace entered, all regions of the thoracic cavity can be exposed.

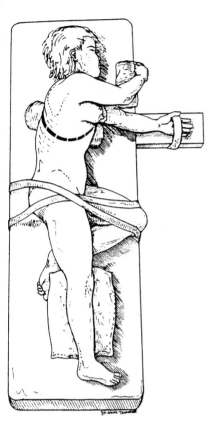

Figure 28-12. Position for an urgent right posterolateral thoracotomy. (From Champion HR, Robbs JV, Trunkey DD. Trauma surgery (parts 1 and 2). In: Dudley H, Carter D, Russell RCG, eds. *Rob and Smith's Operative Surgery.* London: Butterworth; 1989:273, with permission.)

b. The patient is placed in full lateral decubitus position with the upper arm supported over the head, the lower arm extended and padded with an axillary roll, the lower leg is flexed, and the upper leg extended with padding between the knees. The pelvis should be secured with adhesive tape and a sandbag (Fig. 28-12).

c. Using the tip of the scapula as a landmark, the muscles of the lateral chest wall are divided down to and including the intercostal muscles. In more stable patients requiring less exposure, sparing of the latissimus dorsi muscle is possible.

H. Bilateral thoracotomy (clamshell thoracotomy) (Fig. 28-13)

1. Advantage. Permits wide exposure to all structures in the chest. Best incision for patients with multiple gunshot wounds that violate both pleural spaces, bilateral hemothoraces, and superior mediastinal hematomas.

2. Disadvantage. Large incision, extensive heat loss from wound, both internal mammary arteries are ligated.

3. Technique. After the anterolateral thoracotomy, the sternum is divided transversely with heavy scissors, Lebsche knife, or sternal saw. The sternal incision is opened with a Finochietto rib retractor. The incision is extended through the fifth interspace as far into the contralateral chest as possible.

a. Care is taken to ligate the internal mammary arteries on each side of the sternum. Often these arteries will start to hemorrhage heavily with successful resuscitation and return of an adequate blood pressure

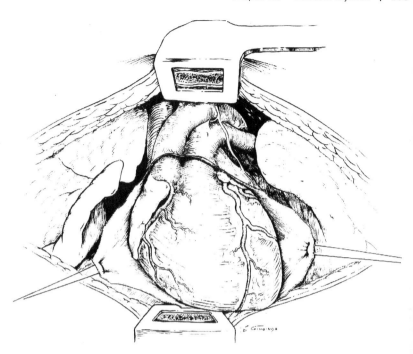

Figure 28-13. A view into the chest during a bilateral "clamshell" thoracotomy. Note the excellent exposure of the heart and great vessels. (Adapted from Moore EE, Eiseman B, Van Way CW. *Critical Decisions in Trauma.* St. Louis, MO: Mosby; 1984:528, with permission.)

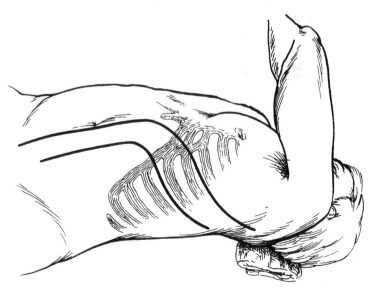

Figure 28-14. The "taxi-hailing" position that allows for access to the abdomen and left chest. (Adapted from Rutherford RB. *Atlas of Vascular Surgery: Basic Techniques and Exposures.* Philadelphia, PA: WB Saunders; 1993:223, with permission.)

   I. Other approaches include:

      1. Right thoracotomy can be useful for isolated right hemothorax. It is also the incision of choice with high esophageal wounds and wounds to the trachea and tracheobronchial tree.

      2. Thoracoabdominal incision is useful to expose the inferior thoracic and supraceliac aorta on the left side. It is also indicated to gain control of the proximal thoracic inferior vena cava on the right side (Fig. 28-14).

AXIOMS

- Hemodynamic instability from a chest wound indicates a major vascular or cardiac injury that mandates immediate control of hemorrhage.
- The choice of thoracic incision is determined by the expected anatomic injury, urgency with which surgical access is required, and the patient's hemodynamic stability.
- Diagnosis of transmediastinal penetration is based on clinical suspicion, trajectory of the missile, or CXR findings.
- Suspect the presence of tamponade in the patient with persistent hypotension, acidosis, or base deficit, despite adequate blood and fluid resuscitation.

Suggested Readings

Asensio JA, Arroyo H, Veloz W, et al. Penetrating thoracoabdominal injuries: ongoing dilemma-which cavity and when? *World J Surg* 2002;26:539–543.

Asensio JA, Berne JD, Demetriades D, et al. One hundred five penetrating cardiac injuries: a 2-year prospective evaluation. *J Trauma* 1998;44:1073–1082.

Asensio JA, Chahwan S, Forno W, et al. Penetrating esophageal injuries: multicenter study of the American Association for the Surgery of Trauma. *J Trauma* 2001;50:289–296.

Asensio JA, Demetriades D, Murray J, et al. Penetrating cardiac injuries: a prospective study of variables predicting outcomes. *J Am Coll Surg* 1997;186:24–34.

Asensio JA, Petrone P, Costa D, et al. An evidenced based critical appraisal of emergency department thoracotomy. *Evidence-Based Surgery* 2003;1:11–21.

Biffl WL, Moore FA, Moore EE, et al. Cardiac enzymes are irrelevant in the patient with suspected myocardial contusion. *Am J Surg* 1994;169:523–528.

Demetriades D, Velmahos GC, Scalea TM, et al. Operative repair or endovascular stent graft in blunt traumatic thoracic aortic injuries: results of an American Association for the Surgery of Trauma Multicenter Study. *J Trauma* 2008;64:561–571.

Fabian TC, Davis KA, Gavant ML, et al. Prospective study of blunt aortic injury: helical CT is diagnostic and antihypertensive therapy reduces rupture. *Ann Surg* 1998;227:666–676.

Link MS. Mechanically induced sudden death in chest wall impact (commotio cordis). *Prog Biophys Mol Biol* 2003;82:175–186.

Maenza RL, Seaberg D, DiAmico F. A meta-analysis of blunt cardiac trauma: ending myocardial confusion. *Am J Emerg Med* 1996;14:237–241.

Moon RM, Luchette FA, Gibson SW, et al. Prospective, randomized comparison between epidural versus parenteral opioid analgesia in thoracic trauma. *Ann Surg* 1999;229:684–692.

Ott MC, Stewart TC, Lawlor DK, et al. Management of blunt thoracic aortic injuries: endovascular stents versus open repair. *J Trauma* 2004;56:565–570.

Richardson JD, Flint LM, Snow NJ, et al. Management of transmediastinal gunshot wounds. *Surgery* 1981;90:671–676.

Richardson JD, Miller FB, Carillo EH, et al. Complex thoracic injuries. *Surg Clin North Am* 1996;76:725–748.

Rozycki GS, Feliciano DV, Oschner MG, et al. The role of ultrasound in patients with possible penetrating cardiac wounds: a prospective multicenter study. *J Trauma* 1999;46:543–552.

Velmahos GC, Baker C, Demetriades D, et al. Lung-sparing surgery after penetrating trauma using tractotomy, partial lobectomy, and pneumonorrhaphy. *Arch Surg* 1999;134:186–189.

29 Abdominal Trauma

Matthew D. Neal, L.D. Britt, Greg Watson, Alan Murdock and
Andrew B. Peitzman

I. Abdominal injuries are divided into two broad categories: *Blunt* and *penetrating* abdominal trauma, based on the mechanism of injury. Expedient diagnosis and treatment of intraabdominal injuries are essential to avoid preventable morbidity and death. Since management guidelines are different for blunt and penetrating abdominal trauma, they will be discussed separately.

II. *Blunt abdominal trauma.* Common mechanisms include falls, motor vehicle crashes, motorcycle or bicycle crashes, sporting mishaps, and assaults.
   A. *Intraabdominal injuries result from:*
   1. Compression causing a crush injury
   2. Abrupt shearing force causing tears of organs or vascular pedicles
   3. Sudden rise in intraabdominal pressure causing rupture of an intraabdominal viscus
   B. *Evaluation*
   1. Clinical. Information regarding the mechanism of injury is essential to determine the likelihood of an intraabdominal injury (see Chapter 22). Abdominal examination after blunt trauma is often unreliable. Altered level of consciousness, spinal cord or other distracting injury, and medication or substance effects can further confound the physical examination. Although adjunctive tests are important in the evaluation of blunt abdominal trauma, *careful, repeated physical examination of the patient remains essential in the early diagnosis of abdominal injury.* The choice of adjunctive diagnostic tests depends, in part, on the hemodynamic stability of the patient, the associated injuries and the patient volume at the treating institution (i.e., extremely busy centers may not have the personnel to perform serial physical examinations reliably) (Fig. 29-1).

   In the hemodynamically unstable patient or the patient with ongoing fluid requirements, rapid evaluation of the abdomen while the patient is in the trauma resuscitation area is mandatory. Ultrasound (focused abdominal sonography for trauma [FAST]), diagnostic peritoneal aspiration (DPA), or diagnostic peritoneal lavage (DPL) are appropriate diagnostic tools to determine the presence of hemoperitoneum; in recent years, the safety and rapidity of surgeon-performed focused ultrasound have substantially diminished the role of DPL. *In the stable patient without immediate need for the operating room* (OR), computed tomography (CT) is the investigation of choice.
   a. Physical examination. Evaluation of the patient will often uncover signs of hypoperfusion (e.g., obtundation, cool skin temperature, mottling, diminished pulse volume, or delayed capillary refill), which should initiate a search for a source of blood loss. Factors associated with abdominal injury requiring laparotomy include chest injury, base deficit, pelvic fracture, or hypotension in the field or trauma resuscitation area.
      i. Evaluation of the abdomen may detect distension or signs of peritoneal irritation (usually associated with injury to a hollow viscus). On the other hand, blood in the peritoneum often does not produce peritoneal signs, and massive hemoperitoneum may be present without abdominal distension.
      ii. Commonly injured abdominal organs are generally solid organs: Liver, spleen, bowel mesentery, or kidney. If the patient is a restrained victim in a

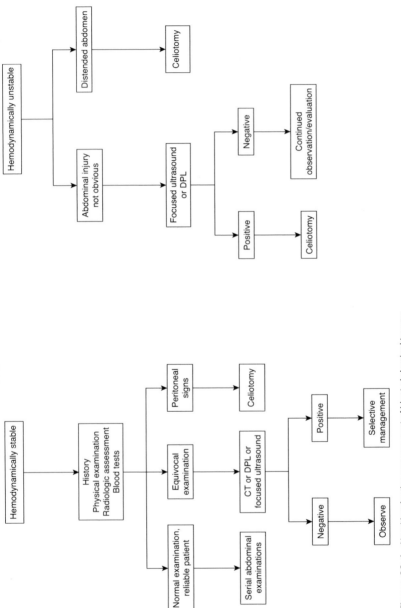

Figure 29-1. Algorithm for the management of blunt abdominal trauma.

motor vehicle crash, particularly with a visible contusion on the abdomen from a lap belt, or a lumbar vertebral body fracture (especially a Chance fracture), suspect hollow viscus injury, an injury commonly missed.

2. *Diagnostic tests.* The goal of the initial evaluation of the abdomen is to identify quickly the patient who requires laparotomy. Victims of blunt trauma with hypotension and abdominal distension or peritoneal signs should proceed immediately to laparotomy without further workup.

For patients without an obvious indication for laparotomy, various modalities are available to evaluate the abdomen further. Ancillary evaluation beyond physical examination should be considered for patients with:

a. Abnormal or equivocal abdominal evaluation

b. Concurrent injury to the chest or pelvic ring

c. Gross hematuria

d. Diminished level of consciousness

e. Spinal cord injury

f. Other injuries requiring a long general anesthetic for management, rendering repeat abdominal examination impossible.

g. Diminished capacity to tolerate a delay in diagnosis of abdominal injury (e.g., extremes of age)

The diagnostic test used depends upon the mechanism of injury, associated injuries, and hemodynamic stability. ***Remember that control of cavitary bleeding takes precedence over further diagnostic testing. Delays to control bleeding increase mortality.***

a. *Plain radiographs.* The chest radiograph may reveal a ruptured hemidiaphragm or pneumoperitoneum. Plain abdominal films are rarely productive, but may show retroperitoneal gas or findings associated with abdominal injury (e.g., fractures of the lumbar spine or lower rib cage).

b. *Laboratory evaluation.* Patients with blunt injury received promptly from the scene may not be anemic or acidotic on presentation. Similarly, amylase levels can be normal with significant pancreatic or intestinal injury, or can be elevated from extra-abdominal injury such as head and neck trauma.

c. *Focused assessment by sonography in trauma* (FAST) is a rapid, noninvasive means to identify hemoperitoneum in the trauma resuscitation area and, as such, has replaced DPL in many centers (Fig. 29-2).

  i. *Indications* include a hemodynamically unstable patient without obvious indication for laparotomy; any patient requiring prompt transfer to the OR for nonabdominal cause; or use as a screening test for all others requiring abdominal evaluation.

  ii. *Contraindications* include obvious need for laparotomy or lack of FAST expertise.

  iii. *Accuracy.* Sensitivity and specificity (60% to 85%) are generally less than those of CT in detection of hemoperitoneum. It is not accurate for the detection and anatomic characterization of solid organ injury. FAST is most valuable when positive in the hemodynamically unstable patient; prompt transfer to the operating room is thus facilitated. On the other hand, with a false-negative rate as high as 40%, a negative FAST should generally be followed by a more definitive diagnostic test (CT or DPL) in the patient incurring high-energy injury.

  iv. *Advantages.* Ultrasound is rapid and noninvasive; no need to transfer the patient to the radiology suite; can be performed by a trained member of the trauma team; can be repeated; is less expensive than CT.

  v. *Disadvantages.* Can miss solid organ injury in the absence of hemoperitoneum or small amounts of hemoperitoneum; cannot distinguish between ascites, succus entericus and blood; requires specialized training and competency; and is difficult to interpret in the obese or patients with extensive subcutaneous emphysema.

  vi. *Technique of FAST.* A 3 to 5.0 MHz transducer is placed in the subxiphoid region in the sagittal plane to set the machine gain. Sagittal views of

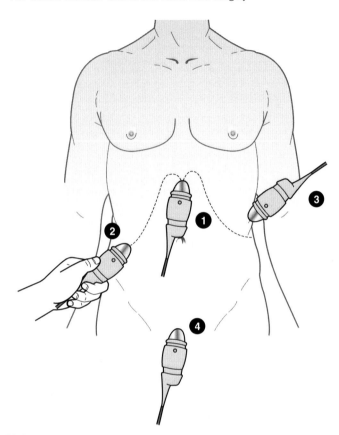

Figure 29-2. Ultrasound.

Morison's pouch and the splenorenal recess are performed, followed by a pelvic transverse view. Free fluid appears anechoic (black) compared with the surrounding structures.

d. *CT* can evaluate solid organ injury; intraabdominal fluid, blood, air; and retroperitoneal organ injury in hemodynamically stable patient suspected of intraabdominal injury. CT of the abdomen and pelvis (upper abdominal cuts will show caudad pulmonary parenchyma and may reveal occult pneumothorax; pelvic cuts may reveal dependent hemoperitoneum) should be obtained, using intravenous (IV) contrast, and currently less so, oral contrast.

   i. *Indications.* Hemodynamically stable patients requiring abdominal evaluation

   ii. *Contraindications.* Hemodynamically unstable patients or those with an obvious need for laparotomy

   iii. *Accuracy.* Recent experience with modern high-resolution CT technology shows accuracy rates of 92% to 98%. Hollow viscus and pancreatic injuries are those most likely to be missed by CT.

   iv. *Advantages*

      a) Noninvasive

      b) Reveals solid organ injury with anatomic characterization

      c) Estimates free fluid volume

      d) Provides assessment of retroperitoneal injuries

  v. *Disadvantages*
   a) Need for specialized personnel
   b) Cost
   c) Time
   d) Radiation
   e) Not an ideal environment for ongoing evaluation and resuscitation
   f) Variable reliability in detection of hollow viscus injury and pancreatic injury
   g) Intravenous contrast
 e. DPL, a rapid and accurate modality for the diagnosis of intraabdominal injury in blunt trauma victims, has been supplanted by ultrasound at most centers for the rapid evaluation of the hemodynamically unstable patient. Briefly, a catheter is placed into the peritoneal cavity for aspiration of blood or fluid. If this is negative, a liter of warmed normal saline solution is infused (or 10 mL/kg in children) into the abdomen and allowed to drain by gravity. The effluent is sent for laboratory analysis.
  i. *Criteria for positive DPL*
   a) 10 mL gross blood on aspiration
   b) >100,000 red blood cells/mm^3
   c) >500 white blood cells/mm^3
   d) Bacteria
   e) Bile
   f) Food particles
  ii. *Indications* in general are as for FAST, but the utility of FAST has limited the benefit of DPL to situations where the rapid determination of the nature of free intraabdominal fluid is necessary, such as the patient with FAST- or CT-documented intraperitoneal fluid in the absence of solid organ injury, particularly if physical examination is unreliable for the diagnosis of peritonitis.
  iii. *Contraindications* are obvious need for laparotomy, previous abdominal operations (relative), pregnancy, or pelvic ring fracture (relative, may be performed supraumbilically).
  iv. *Accuracy.* The sensitivity and specificity of DPL approach 95%. The false-negative rate is 4%.
  v. *Advantages.* DPL is quick, accurate, sensitive, and low cost.
  vi. *Disadvantages.* DPL is invasive and results in nontherapeutic laparotomy in 15% to 27%. DPL can fail to detect diaphragmatic or retroperitoneal injury.
  vii. Technique. DPL can be performed in an open or closed technique. In the open technique, skin, subcutaneous tissue fascia, and peritoneum are incised under direct vision for catheter insertion. Seldinger technique is used for the closed method. Pre-DPL gastric and urinary bladder drainage are mandatory, regardless of the technique utilized.
 f. DPA has been used in lieu of DPL at many centers. This is a rapid technique to simply determine the presence of gross hemoperitoneum. Ironically, DPL evolved in 1965, because of the inaccuracy of DPA. Certainly, a grossly positive aspiration is useful information. The false-negative rate of DPA is not well defined in the literature.

III. *Penetrating abdominal trauma* is usually by gunshot wound (GSW) or stab wound. The likelihood of injury requiring operative repair is higher for abdominal GSW (80% to 95%) than for stab wounds (25% to 33%) and the management algorithms differ. Abdominal organs commonly injured with penetrating wounds include small bowel, liver, stomach, colon, and vascular structures. Any penetrating wound from the nipple line anteriorly or scapular tip posteriorly to the buttocks inferiorly can produce an intraperitoneal injury.
 A. *Gunshot injury.* In most instances, patients sustaining transperitoneal GSWs to the abdomen require laparotomy as their diagnostic and therapeutic modality.

1. *Physical examination.* Carefully inspect the patient to avoid missing wounds. Bullets that do not strike bone or other solid objects generally travel in a straight line. *Trajectory determination is the key to injury identification.* Hemodynamically unstable patients with abdominal GSW should not have extensive evaluation before celiotomy. Carefully examine the patient paying special attention to the body creases, perineum, and rectum. Bullet wounds should be counted and assessed. An odd number of wounds suggest a retained bullet; elongated wounds without penetration typify graze injuries. Palpate the abdomen for signs of tenderness. A neurologic examination should be performed to exclude spinal cord injury.

2. *Plain radiographs* assist in determining trajectory. Mark cutaneous bullet wounds with radiopaque markers. In addition, the presence of pneumoperitoneum, spinal fractures, pneumo-, or hemothorax can be appreciated.

3. *CT* has a limited role in the evaluation of patients with abdominal GSW. However, in the hemodynamically stable patient in whom it is questioned, peritoneal penetration can be excluded by visualizing the path of the bullet on CT. If any doubt exists, laparotomy or laparoscopy is mandatory. In addition, selected patients with right upper-quadrant GSW isolated to the liver may be candidates for nonoperative management (NOM).

4. *FAST,* similarly, has a limited role in evaluation of abdominal GSW. It can be useful to assess the pericardium or assist in operative planning in hypotensive patients with multi-cavity wounds.

5. *Laparoscopy* can be useful in assessing hemodynamically stable patients with tangential GSW, especially in the thoracoabdominal region.

B. *Stab wounds.* Indications for immediate exploration include hypotension, peritoneal signs, and evisceration. If these are not present, a selective management approach is justified. Anterior stab wounds refer to those in front of the anterior axillary line. One-third is extraperitoneal, one-third is intraperitoneal requiring repair, and one-third is intraperitoneal not requiring visceral repair. Flank stab wounds lie between the anterior and posterior axillary lines from the scapular tip to the iliac crest. Back stab wounds are posterior to the posterior axillary line (Fig. 29-3). Abdominal organs are at risk with thoracic wounds inferior to the nipple line anteriorly (ICS 4) and scapular tip posteriorly (ICS 7).

1. *Serial examination (selective management)* can be used to detect the development of peritoneal signs in a hemodynamically stable patient. The same surgeon should repeat abdominal examinations also documenting temperature, pulse rate, and white blood count.

2. *Local wound exploration* can be performed in the trauma resuscitation area on patients without indication for operation after anterior abdominal stab. The skin is prepared and anesthetized and the original wound is enlarged. Exploration is considered positive if anterior fascial penetration is observed. Patients with positive local wound explorations progress to laparoscopy or laparotomy.

3. *CT with triple contrast* (oral, IV, and rectal) can be used to evaluate back and flank SW with a sensitivity of 89%, specificity of 98%, and accuracy of 97%. CT is not very helpful in the evaluation of anterior abdominal stab wounds, especially in thin patients with slight abdominal musculature.

4. *FAST* is minimally useful in the workup of stable patients with abdominal stab wounds. If positive, visceral injury can be inferred.

5. *DPL* can be performed to evaluate abdominal stab wounds. The criteria for red blood cell (RBC) counts are generally lower than that for patients with blunt injury (i.e., 1,000 vs. 100,000/mm^3). Lower threshold values will improve the sensitivity of the modality, but increase the negative or nontherapeutic laparotomy rate.

C. *Shotgun wounds.* Close-range shotgun wounds are high-velocity injuries. As such, they can result in blast and penetrating abdominal wounds. Shotgun wounds with peritoneal penetration mandate laparotomy. Those delivered from a distance can be evaluated with CT to determine peritoneal penetration by pellets.

D. *Impalement injuries.* The impaled object is secured in place and removed in the OR under direct visualization with the abdomen open.

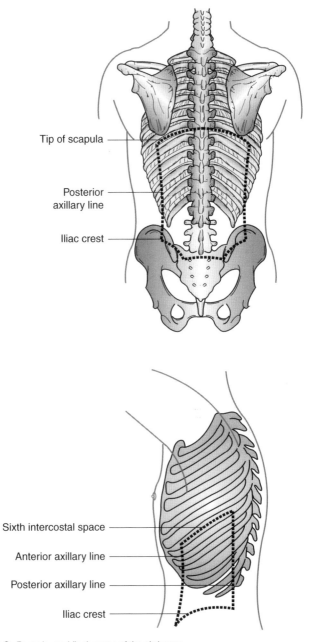

Figure 29-3. Posterior and flank zones of the abdomen.

IV. *Conduct of an exploratory laparotomy.* Refinements in diagnostic capabilities have allowed a more selective application of laparotomy, reducing the number of nontherapeutic laparotomies.

A. *Indications for exploratory laparotomy.* Performed on the basis of physical examination findings or on the results of diagnostic tests.

  1. *Clinical*
    a. Obvious peritoneal signs on physical examination
    b. Hypotension with a distended abdomen on physical examination
    c. Abdominal GSW with peritoneal penetration
    d. Abdominal stab wound with evisceration, hypotension, or peritonitis
  2. *Diagnostic tests*
    a. Positive FAST with hemodynamic instability or DPL
    b. Findings with any other diagnostic intervention (e.g., chest x-ray [ruptured diaphragm, pneumoperitoneum], abdominal ultrasound, abdominal CT, or laparoscopy suggestive of an intraabdominal injury requiring repair)

B. *General setup*

  1. An OR appropriately stocked with appropriate anesthesia, nursing, and support staff should be immediately available 24 hours a day.
  2. Once the decision is made to operate, the patient must be rapidly transported directly to the OR with appropriate airway support personnel, trauma team surgeons, and trauma team nursing staff in attendance. This is direct transfer to the operating room—**not** the preoperative holding area.
  3. If possible, informed consent is obtained from the patient or relative before laparotomy. This is not always possible or practical; the operation should proceed without delays to obtain consent in life-threatening circumstances.
  4. *Intravenous lines, tubes, and spinal precautions*
    a. The patient should already have at least two large-bore IVs placed; other IV and arterial access can be placed as necessary in the OR. Control of cavitary bleeding should not be delayed by attempts at fluid resuscitation.
    b. Administer broad-spectrum, Gram-negative, and anaerobic antibiotic coverage (e.g., an extended spectrum penicillin or a third-generation cephalosporin).
    c. Place chest tubes to underwater seal, *not clamped,* during transport and to suction drainage on arrival in the OR. Place the canisters where they are readily visible and blood loss from the chest tubes can be observed.
    d. Place nasogastric or orogastric tube and a bladder catheter before laparotomy. No procedure should be performed in such a way as to delay control of bleeding and contamination.
    e. Move the patient onto the operating table with appropriate cervical spine and thoracolumbar spine precautions; in many cases, spinal injury will not be excluded before arrival in the OR. If the patient is still immobilized on a backboard, logroll the patient and remove the board before beginning the operation. *Occult penetrating wounds must be sought before beginning laparotomy.*
    f. Sequential compression devices can be used for hemodynamically stable patients, if readily available.
  5. *Rapid-infusion system.* Prime the infusion system to infuse blood products and "cell-saved blood" quickly via large-bore lines before the incision releases the tamponade. Ascertain that packed RBC are in the OR and plasma and platelets are available for the patient with active hemorrhage. In the exsanguinating patient, the massive transfusion protocol should be activated to facilitate availability of blood products.
  6. *Preparation of the patient.* The patient is shaved (if time allows), and the entire anterolateral neck (remove anterior portion of cervical collar and then sandbag to maintain cervical spine immobilization), chest to the table bilaterally, abdomen, groin, and thigh region (to the knees bilaterally) are prepared and draped in sterile fashion (see Fig. 17.1).

C. *Initial goals.* **Stop bleeding and control gastrointestinal contamination**. The exploratory laparotomy for trauma is a sequential, consistently conducted, operative procedure.

1. *Incision.* For urgent laparotomy, a generous midline incision is preferred. Alternative abdominal incisions can be useful for known injuries in stable patients. Adequate exposure is critical. Self-retaining retractor systems and headlights are invaluable.

2. *Bleeding control.* Scoop-free blood and rapidly pack all four quadrants to control bleeding as a first step. *With blunt injuries,* the likely sources of bleeding are the liver, spleen, and mesentery. Pack the liver and spleen, and quickly clamp the mesenteric bleeders. *With penetrating injuries,* the likely sources of significant bleeding are the liver, retroperitoneal vascular structures, and mesentery, based on trajectory of the weapon or bullets. Pack the liver and retroperitoneum, and quickly clamp mesenteric bleeding vessels. *If packing does not control a bleeding site, this source of hemorrhage must be controlled as the first priority.*

3. *Contamination control.* Quickly control bowel content contamination using Babcock clamps, Allis clamps, a stapler, rapid temporary sutures, or ligatures.

4. *Systematic exploration.* Systematically explore the entire abdomen, giving priority to areas of ongoing hemorrhage to definitively control bleeding:
   a. Liver
   b. Spleen
   c. Stomach
   d. Right colon, transverse colon, descending colon, sigmoid colon, rectum, and small bowel, from ligament of Treitz to terminal ileum, looking at the entire bowel wall and the mesentery
   e. Pancreas, by opening lesser sac (visualize and palpate)
   f. Kocher maneuver to visualize the duodenum, with evidence of possible injury
   g. Left and right hemidiaphragms and retroperitoneum
   h. Pelvic structures, including the bladder
   i. *With penetrating injuries,* exploration should focus on following the track of the weapon or missile.

5. Injury repair (section V)

6. *Closure*
   a. Running non-absorbable or absorbable monofilament suture (e.g., No. 1 nylon or No. 1 looped absorbable suture)
   b. Leave skin open with delayed secondary closure if there is contamination or shock
   c. If gross edema of abdominal contents precludes closure, absorbable mesh, sterile IV bags, or intestinal bags can be used with moist gauze and an impermeable dressing (e.g., Op-Site, VAC dressing) to prevent possible abdominal compartment syndrome. Recognize the combination of complex injuries (often liver, pelvis, or major vascular injury) and physiologic signs ("the lethal triad": Hypothermia, acidosis, and coagulopathy) that dictate abbreviated laparotomy (damage control).

V. **SPECIFIC ORGAN INJURIES.** Treatment of an organ injury is similar whether the injury mechanism is penetrating or blunt. An exception to the rule is a retroperitoneal hematoma. Explore all retroperitoneal hematomas caused by penetrating injury.

A. **Diaphragm**

1. The diaphragm, a dome-shaped muscular structure with an aponeurotic sheath ("central tendon"), effectively separates the thoracic and abdominal cavities. It attaches to the first three lumbar vertebrae, the ribs, and the posterior aspect of the lower sternum. Because of the decussation of its crura and hiatal architecture, the diaphragm provides an avenue for many vital structures, including the aorta, esophagus, thoracic duct, vagus nerves, azygos vein, and the inferior vena cava. Physiologically, the wide excursion of the diaphragm during inspiration and expiration contributes to both respiratory function and venous return.

2. Blunt Injury
   Blunt trauma accounts for up to 30% of diaphragmatic ruptures in the United States. Motor vehicle collisions and falls from heights are the most common mechanisms of injury. Diaphragmatic rupture occurs as a result of an acute increase

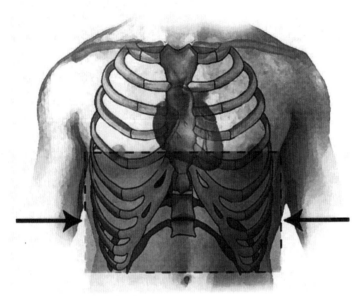

Figure 29-4. Thoracoabdominal region.

in the intraabdominal pressure. Right-sided diaphragmatic ruptures occur less frequently than those on the left.

3. Penetrating Injury

In addition to excluding possible cardiac injury if the penetrating wound is more central, the paramount reason that the thoracoabdominal region (Fig. 29-4) presents such a diagnostic challenge to the acute care surgeon is the possibility of an occult diaphragmatic injury. Patients who are hemodynamically labile or have peritoneal signs require mandatory exploration. Clinically stable patients should undergo a more selective approach. No conventional diagnostic modality consistently makes the definitive diagnosis of diaphragmatic injury. Making the diagnosis of a diaphragmatic injury is important for two reasons. First, the presence of an acute injury to the diaphragm mandates abdominal exploration with high risk for an associated intraabdominal injury. Second, there are risks, both acutely and long-term, of diaphragmatic herniation and possible incarceration/strangulation. Because of this diagnostic challenge, the thoracoabdominal region was correctly underscored as "the ultimate blind spot" in penetrating trauma. Patients who present with indications for exploration (Table 29-1) require no essential

TABLE 29-1	**Absolute Indication for Celiotomy/Thoracotomy**

1. Hemodynamic lability
2. Peritoneal signs
3. Free air
4. Bleeding from an orifice
5. Massive hemothorax (thoracotomy required)
   Chest tube >1,500 cc initial output
   Chest tube >200 cc/h for more than 4 h
6. Impaled object

diagnostic studies. An expectant approach (observation only) does not address potential for the presence of an injury to the diaphragm and its sequela, such as the increased risk for the development of a herniation of abdominal viscera. Although the injury occurs acutely, clinical signs of a hernia are usually lacking and a "high index of suspicion" is imperative to prompt optimum investigation. The time from injury to presentation of a symptomatic diaphragmatic hernia may vary from days to years postinjury. The patient may present with signs and symptoms of bowel obstruction or even peritoneal signs due to necrosis of the incarcerated bowel; mortality rate is high in this setting. This further emphasizes the importance to diagnose and repair these injuries in the acute setting.

4. Several **diagnostic modalities** have been used in the evaluation of thoracoabdominal trauma in both the blunt and penetrating settings.

   a. Chest x-ray is the usual screening diagnostic modality. However, the diagnostic accuracy for diaphragmatic injury ranges from 13% to 94%. The accuracy may increase when the CXR is repeated after the placement of a radiopaque nasogastric tube.

   b. Computed tomography has a sensitivity of 63% and a specificity of 100% for diaphragmatic "rupture" with blunt injury. Computed tomography fails to diagnose diaphragmatic injuries without associated visceral herniation. Patients with penetrating injuries are less likely to have visceral herniation and, therefore, their injuries can easily be missed on CT.

   c. Diaphragm injury as a result of penetrating trauma ranges from 0.8% to 15%. Mandatory exploration of all penetrating thoracoabdominal injuries has been advocated for many years on the premise that it is the only way to assess definitively the diaphragm. Adequate visualization is critical, considering the increased morbidity and mortality as a result of a missed diaphragmatic injury.

   d. However, mandatory celiotomy for an injury with such a low incidence results in a high number of nontherapeutic explorations, prompting the need for an alternative approach. Thus, diagnostic laparoscopy has been applied as the definitive modality for identification of diaphragmatic injury in penetrating thoracoabdominal trauma. In the acute setting of penetrating thoracoabdominal injuries, there are few (if any) indications for diagnostic thoracoscopy to determine the integrity of the diaphragm. Such an intervention would likely require a double-lumen endotracheal tube insertion and lateral decubitus positioning of the patient. Diagnostic laparoscopy is more appropriate and efficient management for these injuries. The ability to evaluate adequately the diaphragm with the laparoscope provides an attractive diagnostic modality that benefits those patients with diaphragmatic injury and avoids an unnecessary celiotomy.

5. **Treatment**
   In the acute setting, diaphragmatic injury is preferentially repaired primarily with a heavy non-absorbable suture. Although the indications are infrequent, a non-absorbable mesh can be incorporated in the diaphragmatic closure where there is significant tissue destruction, which usually occurs in blunt trauma. In the event of a gross contamination, endogenous tissue can be utilized for a definitive repair. Such tissue includes a latissimus dorsi flap, tensor fascia lata, or omentum. There are some who advocate using biologic tissue grafts, such as AlloDerm (human acellular tissue matrix; Life Cell Corporation). The durability of such a repair is questionable. Irrigate the thoracic cavity through the defect in the diaphragm; leave a chest tube. Figure 29-5 is a treatment algorithm for penetrating thoracoabdominal injury, the most common mechanism for diaphragmatic injury.

6. **Outcomes**
   Overall, the expected outcomes for diaphragmatic injuries are good (Table 29-2). Mortality and significant morbidity are related to associated organ injury.

B. Stomach
The stomach is the second most common intraperitoneal hollow viscus injury. Its size and intraperitoneal location makes this organ a vulnerable target, with size being affected by the intraluminal volume. Gastric injury secondary to blunt trauma

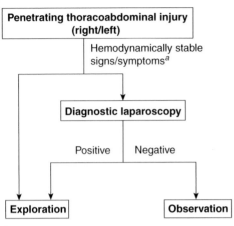

Figure 29-5. Treatment algorithm.

is infrequent. When it does occur, it is often the result of increased intraluminal pressure and distension; seat belt injuries and direct blows to the epigastrium are common causes. Penetrating wounds of the stomach are a more frequent mechanism of injury; the anterior and posterior aspects of the stomach need to be meticulously inspected for through-and-through injuries. Injury of the stomach should be repaired

TABLE 29-2	Diaphragmatic Injury			
Organ	**Incidence**	**Diagnosis**	**Specific management**	**Outcome**
Diaphragm	6% of all intraabdominal injuries resulting from penetrating trauma	■ Physical examination: Chest pain and shortness of breath Scaphoid abdomen Bowel sounds on auscultation of the hemithorax ■ Plain radiography Hollow viscus noted in the left hemithorax Nasogastric tube in the left hemithorax ■ FAST examination Unreliable ■ DPL Inconclusive; high false-negative ■ CT scan Inconclusive ■ Laparoscopy, the diagnostic modality of choice	■ Preoperative antibiotics ■ Primary closure is the preferred definitive management ■ With documentation of a diaphragmatic rent (laceration), exploratory laparotomy is necessary	■ Associated injuries dictate morbidity and mortality

TABLE 29-3	CT Findings of Blunt Bowel Injury

Direct	Indirect
Oral contrast extravasation	Mesenteric hematoma
Free air	Mesenteric blush
	Bowel wall edema
	Unexplained free fluid
	Fat streaking
	Unopacified (vascular contrast media) bowel loops

primarily after debridement of nonviable edges. The primary repair can be performed in either a single layer with non-absorbable suture or as a double-layer closure with an absorbable suture with the first layer and the second layer with non-absorbable sutures (e.g., silk). It is unlikely that primary repair of a through-in-through stomach injury would compromise the gastric lumen. It is uncommon that gastric injuries require a major resection. Since gross contamination is usually associated with stomach wounds, copious irrigation of the abdominal cavity is an essential component of the operative strategy.

C. Small Intestine

Small bowel wounds are the most common intraperitoneal hollow viscus injury. As with other hollow viscus injuries, there is no place for NOM of a small bowel perforation or rupture.

1. The small bowel is commonly injured from penetrating trauma; 5% to 15% of small bowel injury is as the result of blunt trauma. CT evaluation can be helpful in detection of a possible blunt bowel injury. There are two basic types of findings of bowel injury on CT: Direct and indirect (Table 29-3).

2. The management of injury to the small intestine is well established, with control of bleeding and gross spillage as the major goals. If bowel viability is questioned, a segmental resection should be performed. Isolated small bowel enterotomies can be closed primarily with non-absorbable sutures as a one-layer closure. If the edges of the enterotomy appear nonviable, gently debride them prior to primary closure. However, multiple contiguous small bowel holes or an intestinal injury on the mesenteric border with associated mesenteric hematoma will likely necessitate segmental resection and anastomosis of the remaining segments of small bowel. The operative goal is always the reestablishment of intestinal continuity without substantial narrowing of the intestinal lumen, along with closure of any associated mesenteric defeat. Application of non-crushing bowel clamps can minimize ongoing contamination while the repair is performed. Although a hand-sewn or stapled anastomosis is operator dependent, trauma laparotomies are time-sensitive interventions and expeditious management is imperative. In the immediate postoperative period, bowel decompression for 12 to 24 hours is prudent. As in most trauma laparotomies, antibiotics should be routinely given in only the perioperative period, unless there is an ensuing infectious complication in the postoperative period.

D. Colon/rectum

Penetrating trauma accounts for most of the colon and rectal injuries in the civilian setting. Even today, there remains debate regarding the optimal treatment of colon injuries, with the preponderance of evidence supporting primary closure of the colonic wounds and segmental resection (with primary anastomosis) in the majority of the settings. Most colonic injuries are quickly diagnosed during the initial exploration and mobilization of the colon. With two-thirds of the rectum being extraperitoneal and bordered by the bony pelvis, detection and direct management of a localized rectal injury is a challenge. Rectal injuries are usually a result of pelvic fractures or penetrating trauma. Generally, extraperitoneal rectal injuries are managed with proximal diversion. With intraperitoneal injury, the segment of injured bowel should be thoroughly inspected, particularly missile injuries that are most common, through-and-through injury. This requires adequate mobilization of the colon to visualize the entire circumference of the bowel wall. As highlighted above, initially controversial, right- or left-sided injury of the colon can be closed primarily. If the colon injury is so extensive that primary repair is not possible or would compromise the lumen, a segmental resection should be performed. Depending on the setting, the remaining proximal segment can be anastomosed to the distal segment or a proximal ostomy and Hartmann's procedure can be performed. If the distal segment is long enough, a mucous fistula should be established. Documented rectal injuries, below the peritoneal reflection necessitate a diverting colostomy. Presacral drainage (exiting from the perineum) is not universally endorsed; it can be considered for lower one-third rectal injuries only.

A capsule summary of the incidence, diagnosis, management options, and related outcomes for injuries of the stomach, small intestine, colon, and rectum is depicted in Table 29-4.

E. Duodenum and pancreas. Pancreatic and duodenal injuries are listed together because of their shared blood supply and high incidence of concomitant injury (Fig. 29-6). Preoperative diagnosis of these injuries is often difficult and management challenging.

1. *Pancreatic injury*

    a. *Incidence*

        i. Uncommon, 0.2% to 2% of all trauma patients and 3% to 12% of patients with abdominal trauma; in the United States most are caused by penetrating injury but outside the United States blunt trauma is the leading cause of injury. GSWs and stabbings account for the majority of penetrating injuries, while motor vehicle collisions and assaults account for most of blunt injuries in adults. Blunt pancreatic injuries most commonly occur from a crushing force to the upper abdomen resulting in the compression of the pancreas between the spine and another object (e.g., steering wheel, handlebar, or blunt weapon).

        ii. Associated injuries are found in 50% to 100% of pancreatic injuries with an average of 3.4 organ systems involved. The liver, major vascular structures, colon or small bowel, duodenum, stomach, spleen, or kidney are the most commonly associated intraabdominal injuries. Associated major vascular injury (aorta, portal vein, or inferior vena cava) is the leading cause of death and is associated with 50% to 75% of penetrating pancreatic injuries and 12% of blunt pancreatic injuries.

    b. *Anatomy*

        i. The pancreas is almost entirely retroperitoneal. The head of the pancreas lies to the right of the midline originating at the level of L2. The body crosses the midline with the pancreatic tail ending in the hilum of the spleen at the level of L1. The superior mesenteric artery (SMA) and superior mesenteric vein (SMV) lie posterior in a groove in the neck of the pancreas.

        ii. The main pancreatic duct of Wirsung usually runs the length of the pancreas. The accessory duct of Santorini usually branches from the pancreatic duct within the pancreas and empties separately into the duodenum; in 20%, the accessory duct drains into the main pancreatic duct and in 8% it is the sole drainage of the pancreas.

    c. *Diagnosis*

        i. Early diagnosis of pancreatic injury, especially in patients with blunt injury, without an indication for emergent laparotomy remains a challenge. Beyond diagnosis of the injury itself, the integrity of the main pancreatic duct is the most important diagnostic question as injury to the main duct is associated with higher mortality and morbidity. Furthermore, delay in diagnosis is associated with higher risk of complications. Therefore, it is important to maintain a high index of suspicion based on the mechanism of injury and perform repeat examinations and diagnostic studies in patients without obvious signs of pancreatic injury on initial evaluation.

TABLE 29-4 Injury of the Stomach, Small Intestine, Colon, and Rectum: Incidence, Diagnosis, Management, and Outcomes

Organ	Incidence	Diagnosis	Management	Outcome

Stomach	■ More common injury in penetrating trauma than blunt 10% of penetrating injuries of the abdomen	■ Physical examination
		– Epigastric tenderness
		– Peritoneal signs
		– Bloody gastric aspirate
		■ Plain radiography
		–Free air under the diaphragm
		■ FAST examination
		–Unreliable
		■ DPL
		– + lavage
		  RBCs
		  WBCs
		  Gross contamination
		– Pneumoperitoneum
		■ CT scan
		■ Laparoscopy
		– Operator dependent
			■ Preop antibiotics
			■ Debridement when necessary
			■ Primary closure (two layers)
				■ Associated injuries dictate morbidity and mortality

Small bowel	■ Highest incidence of injury of the intraabdominal organ from penetrating injury	■ Physical examination
		■ Cannot rely on tenderness/peritoneal signs in the early stage of injury
		■ Plain radiography
		■ FAST examination: Free fluid with CT demonstrating no solid organ injury
		■ CT
		  High false-negative rate
		  Pneumoperitoneum
		  Free fluid, especially without associated solid organ injury
			■ Preoperative antibiotics
			■ Primary closure of simple lacerations
			■ Segmental resection of complex injuries with functional end-to-end tension-free anastomosis
			■ One (or double) layer closure/anastomosis or stapled anastomosis
				■ Outcome is good
				  Negligible leak rate even in contaminated field

Colon	■ Majority
	  ■ Stab wounds
	  ■ Gunshot
	  ■ Instrumentation
	  ■ Blunt trauma
	  – Infrequent
		■ Physical examination
		■ Tenderness/peritoneal signs
		■ Gross blood on rectal examination
		■ Proctoscopy
			■ Preoperative antibiotics
			■ Primary closure of simple injuries (avoid narrowing the lumen)
			■ Segmental resection and fecal diversion of complex colonic wounds
				■ Overall, favorable outcome
				■ Complications
				  Low leak rate
				  Wound infection
				  Intraperitoneal abscess

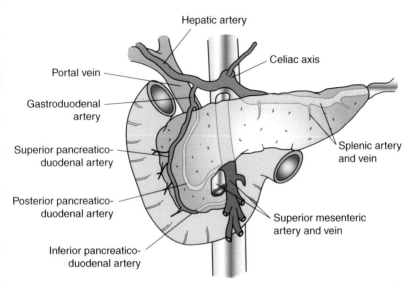

Figure 29-6. Anatomy of the pancreas.

ii. Generally, laparotomy is indicated for patients with pancreatic injury because of concomitant abdominal injuries since isolated pancreatic injuries are uncommon. If laparotomy is not indicated, the diagnosis of pancreatic injury can be challenging since clinical signs may be subtle and only become apparent later in the postinjury course (23% between 6 and 14 hours, 19% >24 hours from time of injury to diagnosis).

iii. Serum hyperamylasemia is neither sensitive nor specific on initial presentation and may be elevated in only 14% to 80% of patient with blunt pancreatic injury, even in the presence of complete pancreatic duct transection.

iv. Due to the retroperitoneal location of the pancreas, physical examination, DPL, and FAST are relatively insensitive in detection of pancreatic injury. Physical signs and symptoms at presentation such as abdominal pain (78%), tenderness (79%), and ecchymosis (34%) may suggest the presence of pancreatic injury but their absence does not exclude injury (34% negative or unreliable abdominal examination). Furthermore, measurement of amylase in DPL fluid has been shown to be of low yield in diagnosing pancreatic injury.

v. CT is the primary imaging modality used in the diagnosis of blunt pancreatic injury. As with early amylase determination, CT is an imperfect test for early diagnosis of injury. Reported sensitivity of CT for detecting pancreatic injury has varied widely (28% to 85%). Even newer imaging techniques with helical scanning have been shown in multicenter retrospective studies to be only moderately sensitive (50%) with either 16-slice or 64-slice multidetector CT on initial presentation. The sensitivity of CT may improve with time after injury; therefore, repeat CT during the course of observation may be warranted for patients with persistent symptoms or hyperamylasemia.

vi. Endoscopic retrograde cholangiopancreatography (ERCP) is the most sensitive technique short of operative exploration for diagnosis of pancreatic ductal injury. However, the logistics of obtaining ERCP in acutely injured patients make it of limited use in the initial assessment phase of injury. In addition, ERCP is associated with a complication rate of 3% to 5%.

However, ERCP may be useful in patients managed initially nonoperatively, in whom demonstration of a ductal injury would alter management by prompting a laparotomy. Recently magnetic resonance cholangiopancreatography (MRCP) has been used increasingly in the diagnosis of pancreaticobiliary disease. However, its role in trauma has not been fully delineated.

vii. Intraoperative diagnosis of pancreatic injury depends on visual inspection and bimanual palpation of the pancreas by opening the gastrocolic ligament and entering the lesser sac, and by performing a full Kocher maneuver. Mobilization of the spleen along with the tail of the pancreas and opening of the retroperitoneum to facilitate palpation of the substance of the gland may be necessary to determine transection versus contusion. *Identification of injury to the major duct is the critical issue in intraoperative management of pancreatic injury.*

  a) Although reported, we do not recommend intraoperative pancreatography (IP). IP may be performed through the ampulla of Vater via a duodenotomy or through the distal main pancreatic duct via amputation of the tail of the pancreas. *However, careful inspection of the pancreas appears to be adequate to determine the presence of ductal injury.*

d. *Treatment.* Suspected pancreatic injury should be surgically explored. The status of the pancreatic duct, the location of injury (proximal vs. distal), and the overall status of the patient are the major determinants of the management required for pancreatic injury. Literature suggest that more conservative management protocols utilizing external drainage and distal pancreatectomy result in lower mortality and morbidity compared to more radical procedures utilizing complex resections and pancreaticoenteric anastomoses. These treatment principles include

  i. Control hemorrhage
  ii. Debride devitalized pancreas, which may require resection
  iii. Preserve maximal amount of viable pancreatic tissue
  iv. Wide drainage of pancreatic secretions with closed-suction drains
  v. Feeding jejunostomy for postoperative care with significant lesions

e. *Treatment options*

  i. *Pancreatic contusion or capsular lacerations without ductal injury (AAST Grade I to II) are best managed by debridement of devitalized tissue and wide external drainage alone. Suturing of injured capsule or parenchyma in these injuries is unnecessary and may result in pseudocyst formation.* An operative goal is to ensure that if a pancreatic fistula develops postoperatively, it will be a controlled fistula. These usually close spontaneously.

  ii. *Pancreatic transection distal to the SMA (AAST Grade III) → distal pancreatectomy.* Recommend attempting splenic conservation in patients who are hemodynamically stable. Control the resection line by stapling the pancreatic stump or closing with non-absorbable sutures in a horizontal mattress fashion. The main pancreatic duct should also be ligated if identified. Place closed-suction drains.

  iii. *Pancreatic transection to the right of the SMA (not involving the ampulla) or massive disruption of pancreatic head (Grade IV to V) → no optimal operation.* The options include wide drainage of the area of injury to develop a controlled pancreatic fistula or complex procedures such as onlay pancreaticojejunostomy or pancreaticoduodenectomy. We favor simple drainage alone since a controlled pancreatic fistula is easier to deal with and less morbid that the complications arising from more aggressive approaches.

  iv. Combined duodenal and pancreatic injuries are especially demanding. Severe injury to both the head of the pancreas and the duodenum may require pancreaticoduodenectomy; however, this is rarely indicated. In a reported series of patients with combined injuries, 24% to 46% were managed with simple duodenal repair and drainage of the pancreatic injury,

41% to 61% required more complex pancreatic repairs or resections most often done with pyloric exclusion and 7% to 10% required pancreatico-duodenectomy. Indications for pancreaticoduodenectomy include massive disruption of the pancreatic head with uncontrolled hemorrhage, massive hemorrhage from adjacent vascular structures, and severe combined duodenal, pancreatic, and biliary injuries. If pancreaticoduodenectomy is indicated, it is suggested that a staged approach with initial resection and delayed reconstruction (24 to 48 hours) may facilitate anastomotic reconstruction.

   v. Although several recent papers suggest NOM of documented pancreatic duct injury, we do not believe this approach is appropriate.

f. *Outcome*

   i. Ten percent to twenty percent incidence of pancreatic fistula as defined as >100 cc/day for 14 to 31 days (minor) or greater than 31 days (major). Most minor and major fistulae will spontaneously resolve with only 0% to 7% requiring further operative intervention.

   ii. Ten percent to twenty-five percent incidence of pancreatic abscess. Pancreatic duct and colon injury are independent predictors of abscess formation.

   iii. Post-traumatic pancreatitis should be expected in the patient with persistent abdominal pain, nausea, vomiting, and hyperamylasemia and complicates 3% to 8% of pancreatic injuries.

   iv. Pancreatic pseudocysts occur in 1.6% to 4%. Most related to missed or inadequately treated ductal injuries.

   v. Postoperative hemorrhage may occur in 3% to 10% and requires reoperation in most.

   vi. Overall mortality ranges from 12% to 32% with pancreatic-related mortality alone ranging from 1.6% to 3%.

2. *Duodenal injury*

a. *Incidence.* Most injuries to the duodenum are from penetrating trauma. Blunt mechanisms account for 20% to 25% of duodenal injuries due to similar mechanism causing pancreatic injuries. The second portion of the duodenum is the most commonly injured. Delays in diagnosis are common and significantly increase morbidity and mortality, which can be as high as 50%. Duodenal injury is rarely an isolated abdominal injury, with up to 98% having associated abdominal injuries. Commonly associated injuries include liver, pancreas, small bowel, colon, IVC, portal vein, and aorta.

b. *Anatomy.* The anatomy of the duodenum is complex due to its close relationship to adjacent structures and shared blood supply with the pancreas. Lying deep in the abdomen, the duodenum is well protected in the retroperitoneum. It extends from the pylorus to the ligament of Treitz (25 cm in length) and consists of four portions: The first portion (superior) of the duodenum is intraperitoneal; the second portion of the duodenum (descending) contains the orifices of the bile and pancreatic ducts; the third portion of the duodenum (transverse) extends from the ampulla of Vater to the mesenteric vessels, with the ureter, IVC, and aorta posterior and SMA interiorly; the fourth portion of the duodenum (ascending) begins at the mesenteric vessels and ends at the jejunum, to the left of the lumbar column. Bile (1,000 mL/day), pancreatic juices (800 to 1,000 mL/day), and gastric juices (1,500 to 2,500 mL/day) combine and flow through the duodenum making injuries and leaks difficult to control.

c. *Diagnosis*

   i. Duodenal injury has no specific clinical signs and symptoms. Therefore, clinical suspicion is based on the mechanism of injury. With blunt injury, the patient usually has mid-epigastric or right upper-quadrant pain or tenderness and may have peritoneal signs. The symptoms and findings can be understated. Retroperitoneal air or obliteration of the right psoas margin may be seen on abdominal x-ray study. The diagnosis is generally made at laparotomy for associated injuries.

    ii. CT findings include paraduodenal hemorrhage and air or contrast leak; oral contrast and fastidious technique are important.

    iii. With equivocal CT findings, an upper gastrointestinal (UGI) study may be essential. The contrast enhanced UGI study is first done with water-soluble contrast; if this is negative, barium is then used.

    iv. DPL has a low sensitivity for duodenal injury but will often detect associated injuries.

    v. Adequate intraoperative exposure is vital; duodenal injuries are among the most commonly missed at laparotomy. They should be exposed in a manner similar to that used for the pancreas, including a wide Kocher maneuver. Bile staining, air in the retroperitoneum, or a central retroperitoneal hematoma mandates a thorough exploration of the duodenum.

d. *Treatment*

    i. *Intramural duodenal hematoma* is more common in children than in adults and up to 50% are related to child abuse. A "coiled spring" or "stacked coins" appearance is seen on UGI series. Follow-up UGI with Gastrografin should be obtained every 7 days, if the obstruction persists clinically.

      a) Treated nonoperatively with nasogastric suction and IV alimentation. Operative decompression may be necessary to evacuate the hematoma if it does not resolve after 2 to 3 weeks.

      b) Treatment of an intramural hematoma found at early laparotomy is controversial.

        1) One option is to open the serosa, evacuate the hematoma without violation of the mucosa, and repair the wall of the bowel. The concern is that this may convert a partial tear to a full-thickness tear of the duodenal wall.

        2) Another option is to explore the duodenum to exclude a perforation, leaving the intramural hematoma intact and planning nasogastric decompression postoperatively.

        3) Recommend placement of a jejunal feeding tube for postoperative enteral feeding.

    ii. *Duodenal perforation* must be treated operatively. Many options are available, depending on injury severity.

      a) Transverse primary closure in one or two layers is applicable in 71% to 85% of duodenal injuries. This requires debridement of the edges of the duodenal wall and closure that avoids narrowing of the duodenal lumen. Longitudinal duodenal injury can usually be closed transversely if the length of the duodenal injury is <50% of the circumference of the duodenum. More severe injuries may require repair using pyloric exclusion, duodenal decompression, or more complex operations.

      b) Several techniques may be applied to help protect a tenuous duodenal repair. Decompression of the duodenal repair is the first option. *Of the various decompression options, retrograde jejunostomy drainage is preferred over lateral tube duodenostomy.* If more protection is required, the stomach contents may be diverted by pyloric exclusion with gastrojejunostomy. Recent data have questioned the need for pyloric exclusion in the management of duodenal injury and repair. Exclusion can be accomplished by oversewing the pyloric outlet through a gastric incision (absorbable or non-absorbable suture) and using the incision as the gastrojejunostomy site (Fig. 29-7). Similarly, the pylorus can be stapled directly and a separate incision made to perform gastrojejunostomy. Truncal vagotomy to prevent marginal ulceration is not indicated since the pyloric exclusion opens within a few weeks.

      c) If primary closure would compromise the lumen of the duodenum, buttress the injury with a jejunal serosal patch or omental patch.

      d) A three-tube technique may also be used. This consists of a gastrostomy tube to decompress the stomach, a retrograde jejunostomy to decompress the duodenum, and an antegrade jejunostomy to feed the patient.

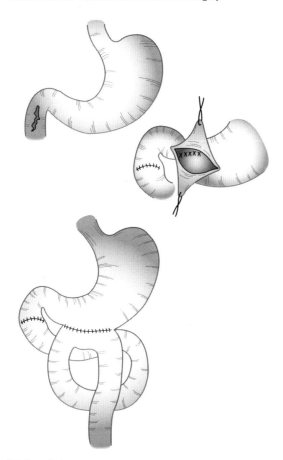

Figure 29-7. Pyloric exclusion.

    e) If complete duodenal transection or long lacerations of the duodenal wall are found, perform debridement and primary closure. Derotation of the small intestine can facilitate this. With duodenal injury where end-to-end anastomosis is made difficult by proximity to the SMA/SMV, a more proximal side-to-side duodenojejunostomy is technically easier. If a primary anastomosis cannot be accomplished without tension, a Roux-en-Y jejunostomy over the defect or closure of the distal duodenum and Roux-en-Y duodenojejunostomy proximally may be required (uncommon).

    f) The uncommon circumstance of destructive combined injuries to the duodenum and the head of the pancreas may necessitate pancreatico-duodenectomy (discussed in pancreatic injury section)

e. *Outcome*

    i. The mortality rate reaches 40% if diagnosis is delayed >24 hours, but it is 2% to 11% if the patient undergoes repair within 24 hours of injury. Duodenal dehiscence with resultant sepsis accounts for nearly one-half of the deaths. Complications occur in 64% of patients with duodenal injuries.

    ii. Retrograde-tube decompression of the duodenum can be associated with a decreased mortality rate (9% with tube decompression vs. 19.4% without).

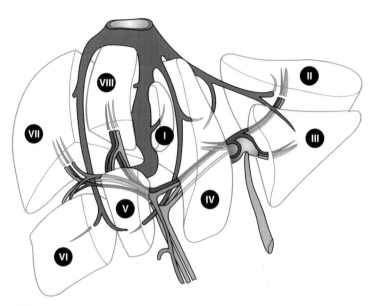

Figure 29-8. Hepatic anatomy.

The duodenal fistula rate was 2.3% with decompression versus 11.8% without decompression in the same review.

F. *Liver*

1. *Incidence.* The liver is the most commonly injured intraabdominal organ; injury occurs more often in penetrating trauma than in blunt trauma. The mortality rate for liver injury is 10%, generally from bleeding.

2. *Anatomy.* An understanding of hepatic anatomy is essential to manage complex liver injuries. A sagittal plane running from the IVC to the gallbladder fossa separates the right and left lobes of the liver (Cantlie's line). The segmental anatomy of the liver is shown in Figure 29-8.

a. The right and left hepatic veins have short extrahepatic courses before they empty directly in the IVC. The middle hepatic vein usually joins the left hepatic vein within the liver parenchyma (85%). The intrahepatic portions of the hepatic veins are 8 to 12 cm in length. The retrohepatic IVC (8 to 10 cm in length) has multiple, small hepatic veins that enter the IVC directly (average 5–7 short hepatic veins; may be 1 cm in diameter); this area is difficult to access and control.

b. The portal triad, which consists of portal vein, hepatic artery, and bile duct, is encased within a tough extension of Glisson's capsule. The portal triads run centrally *within* the segments of the liver. On the other hand, the major hepatic veins run *between* segments of the liver, within the *portal scissurae*, and are not protected by an investing sheath. Thus, hepatic vein injury is a common component of liver injury.

c. The right and left hepatic arteries usually arise from the common hepatic artery. Anomalies are frequent and include the right hepatic artery originating from the SMA and the left hepatic artery originating from the left gastric artery.

d. Adequate mobilization of the liver requires division of the ligamentous attachments.

e. The falciform ligament divides the left lateral segment (segments II, III) of the liver from the medial segment of the left lobe (segment IV).

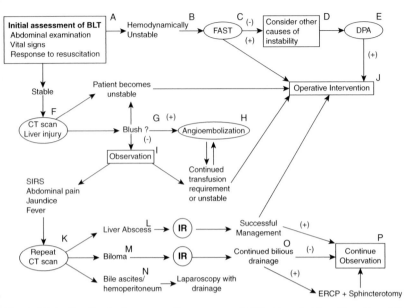

Figure 29-9. Algorithm for the nonoperative management of blunt hepatic injury. (From Kozar RA, Moore FA, Moore EE, et al. Western Trauma Association critical decisions in trauma: nonoperative management of adult blunt hepatic trauma. *J Trauma* 2009;67:1145.)

- **f.** The coronary ligaments are the diaphragmatic attachments to the liver (anterior and posterior leaflets); they do not meet on the posterior surface of the liver (the bare area). The triangular ligaments (left and right) are the more lateral extensions of the coronary ligaments. Injury to the diaphragm, phrenic veins, and hepatic veins must be avoided when mobilizing the liver.

3. *Diagnosis*
- **a.** The appropriate diagnostic modality depends on the hemodynamic status of the patient on arrival in the trauma resuscitation area. If the patient is hemodynamically stable with a blunt mechanism of injury, CT is preferred. The vast majority of hemodynamically stable patients with liver injury can be treated nonoperatively (Fig. 29-9).
- **b.** DPL is sensitive but not specific for liver injury. Of liver injuries, 70% are no longer bleeding at the time of laparotomy for a positive DPL, depending on the patient population.

4. *Treatment*
- **a.** The hemodynamically stable patient with blunt injury of the liver, without other intraabdominal injury requiring laparotomy, can be treated nonoperatively, regardless of the grade of the liver injury. This may represent up to 85% of patients; the vast majority with grade I to III liver injury. The presence of hemoperitoneum on CT does not mandate laparotomy. *Arterial blush or pooling of contrast* on CT or high-grade (grades IV and V) hepatic injuries are most likely to fail NOM. Nonetheless, embolization can circumvent the need for laparotomy; angioembolization has assumed an increasing role in the management of liver injury. The criteria for NOM of blunt liver injury includes:
  - **i.** Hemodynamic stability
  - **ii.** Absence of peritoneal signs
  - **iii.** Lack of continued need for transfusion for the hepatic injury; bleeding can be addressed with angioembolization.

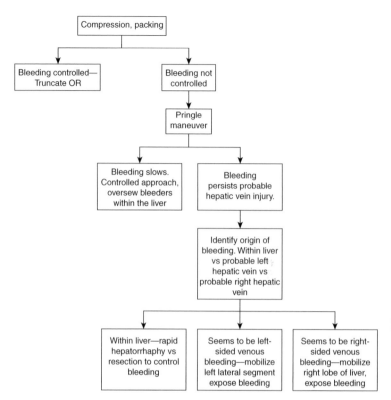

Figure 29-10. Flow chart for the operative management of major liver injury.

b. Posterior right-lobe injuries (even if extensive) and the split-liver type of injuries (extensive injury along the relatively avascular plane between the left and right lobes) can generally be managed successfully nonoperatively. Injuries to the left hemiliver are often not as well contained and more likely to bleed.

c. No support is seen for frequent hemoglobin sampling, bed rest, or prolonged intensive care unit (ICU) monitoring in NOM of blunt liver injury. Similarly, re-imaging the asymptomatic hepatic injury by CT scan is not necessary. Follow-up CT can be deferred, except to document healing (at ~8 weeks) in physically active patients (e.g., athletes) before resumption of normal activities.

d. Immediate laparotomy or angiographic intervention is required for those patients who fail nonoperative therapy by demonstrating enlarging lesions on CT scan, hemodynamic instability, or continual blood product requirement (<10%).

e. If the patient is hemodynamically unstable or has indications for laparotomy, operative management is required. The operative approach to major hepatic injury should be systematic and logical (Fig. 29-10). Management principles include the following:

i. *Adequate exposure of the injury is essential.* Exploration is through a long midline incision or bilateral subcostal incision. Use of a self-retaining retractor (Rochard, Thompson, or Upper Hand) to lift the upper edges of the wound cephalad **and** anteriorly facilitates exposure of the liver. Complete mobilization of the liver is performed, including division of the ligaments if access to bleeding sites is necessary. A right subcostal extension off the midline incision is often necessary to treat extensive right-lobe injury or retrohepatic caval injury. On rare occasion, an extension of the midline incision to sternotomy is needed for complex suprahepatic IVC injury. Thoracotomy is rarely a useful maneuver.

ii. Most blunt and penetrating hepatic injuries are grades I to III (70% to 90%) and can be managed with simple techniques (e.g., electrocautery, simple suture, or hemostatic agents). Complex liver injuries can produce exsanguinating hemorrhage. The approach to major liver injury should be systematic and logical (Fig. 29-9). Rapid, temporary tamponade of the bleeding by manual compression of the liver injury immediately after entering the abdomen allows the anesthesiologist to resuscitate the patient. How the liver is initially packed is important; attempt to restore normal anatomy by compressing the left lobe back into the right lobe. Simultaneously, direct the liver posteriorly to slow any hepatic vein or IVC bleeding. Do **not** stuff packs into the liver laceration, as this will distract the injury and may exacerbate the bleeding. After resuscitation, the liver injury can be repaired. The ultimate operative goals with a major liver injury are control of hemorrhage, control bile leak, debridement of nonviable liver, and drainage. The only essential goal at the first operation is to stop the bleeding. If packing successfully stops the bleeding in a hemodynamically unstable patient, this is all that is necessary at the first operation.

iii. If packing does not control the bleeding liver, next occlude the portal triad with an atraumatic clamp (Pringle maneuver). This is both a diagnostic and therapeutic maneuver. If the Pringle maneuver substantially slows the bleeding, proceed to rapid direct oversew of the injuries within the parenchyma of the liver. If bleeding persists with the porta hepatis clamped, the source of bleeding is from retrohepatic IVC, major hepatic vein, or short hepatic vein injury. Intermittent application of the Pringle maneuver (10 to 15 minutes on, 5 minutes off) produces less hepatic ischemia than continuous clamping.

iv. Hepatorrhaphy with individual vessel ligation is recommended instead of large ischemia-producing mass parenchymal sutures.
   a) Glisson's capsule is incised with the electrocautery.
   b) The injury within the liver is approached by the finger fracture technique (Fig. 29-11), by division of the liver tissue over a right-angled clamp with ligation of the hepatic tissue with 2-0 silk sutures, or even more rapidly with the staplers. A vascular load of the stapling device is preferred.
   c) With gentle traction on the liver edges, expose the injury site. Blood vessels and bile ducts are directly visualized and ligated or repaired.
   d) Debride nonviable liver tissue.
   e) Pack the defect in the liver with viable omentum.

v. As mentioned, if bleeding persists despite a Pringle maneuver, the source of blood loss is the IVC or hepatic veins. If the origin is within the laceration in the liver, a direct approach is preferred. Remember this is a low pressure system and restoration of containment by the liver is generally sufficient to control the bleeding. If the bleeding is extrahepatic, quickly determine whether the origin is over the dome of the liver → middle or left hepatic vein versus behind the liver → retrohepatic IVC or right hepatic vein. On the basis of these findings, mobilize the appropriate lobe of the liver and obtain expedient exposure and control of the bleeding.

vi. Perform closed-suction drainage of grade III to V injuries. Drains are not necessary for grade I and II injuries if bleeding and bile leakage are controlled.

vii. Perform resectional debridement of nonviable tissue rather than formal anatomic resections. A nonanatomic lobectomy can be performed rapidly

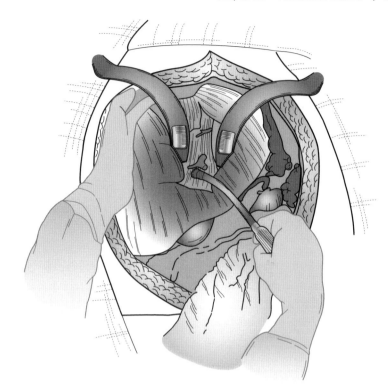

Figure 29-11. Blood vessels and bile ducts are directly visualized and ligated or repaired.

and safely with the staplers. It is critical to avoid injury to vascular structures or bile ducts in the normal liver. Be certain to be 1 to 1.5 cm off Cantlie's line **toward** the lobe being resected; avoid injury to the middle hepatic vein which simply adds another bleeding site. Anatomic hepatic resection (segment or lobe) is not commonly required for liver injury; resectional debridement and direct suture control of the vessels and ducts can generally accomplish the same objectives, with lower mortality. Planned, delayed anatomic resection is also an approach for major hepatic injury, if packing sufficiently controls hemorrhage during the initial laparotomy.

viii. Perform perihepatic packing in cases of hemorrhage, hypothermia, and coagulopathy. Approximately 5% of patients with hepatic injury require perihepatic packing (i.e., damage control laparotomy). Indications include coagulopathy, subcapsular hematomas, bilobar injuries, and hypothermia, or to allow transfer of the patient to a higher level of care.

ix. Selective hepatic artery ligation has been reported in 1% to 2% of hepatic injury cases. The liver will generally tolerate this; but the bile ducts less so. Hepatic abscess or biloma may be the result. Direct suture control of bleeding within the liver is preferable to hepatic artery ligation. Nonetheless, patients with significant central hepatic laceration who have damage control laparotomy may be candidates for arteriography with possible embolization postoperatively. Cholecystectomy is required with interruption of the right hepatic artery.

   x. With major hepatic resection, an intraoperative cholangiogram via the cystic duct (perform a cholecystectomy) will define biliary anatomy. In addition, injection of saline through the cystic duct helps identify bile leaks and avoid them as a postoperative complication. This maneuver is often at the second operation after an initial damage control approach.

  f. Hepatic vascular isolation with occlusion of the suprahepatic and infrahepatic venae cavae, as well as application of the Pringle maneuver, may be required for major retrohepatic venous injury. As mentioned above, do not hesitate to make a subcostal extension off the midline incision to expose these difficult injuries. Thoracotomy or atrial–caval shunt is rarely necessary or helpful. Alternatively, complex retrohepatic vascular injury in which tamponade does not achieve hemostasis can be repaired in an avascular field on venovenous bypass with total hepatic vascular isolation. Survival depends on prompt recognition of this anatomic site of injury.

  g. Bleeding from penetrating wounds of the liver that are not easily accessed, at times, can be controlled with internal tamponade. This is accomplished by using Penrose drains tied at each end (as a balloon) over a red rubber catheter. The end of the Penrose drain is brought through the skin. Finally, in wounds where tamponade does not achieve hemostasis, consider repair under vascular isolation by experienced personnel.

5. *Outcome.* Mortality correlates with the degree of injury. Since most hepatic injuries are grade I or II, the overall mortality for liver injury is 10%. However, the mortality rates for high-grade liver injury and retrohepatic caval injury in most series are still high (>50%).

  a. *Complications*

    i. With recurrent bleeding (occurs in 2% to 7% of patients) → return the patient to the OR or in selected patients, obtain an angiogram and perform embolization. Recurrent bleeding is generally caused by inadequate initial hemostasis. Hypothermia and coagulopathy must be corrected. Preparations to control retrohepatic hemorrhage (i.e., vascular bypass) should be made.

    ii. Hemobilia is a rare complication of liver injury. The classic presentation is right upper-quadrant pain, jaundice, and hemorrhage; one-third of patients have all three components of the triad. The patient may present with hemobilia days or weeks after injury. Treatment is angiogram and embolization.

    iii. Intrahepatic or perihepatic abscess or biloma (7% to 40% of patients) can generally be drained percutaneously. Meticulous control of bleeding and repair of bile ducts, adequate debridement, and closed-suction drainage are essential to avoid abscess formation.

    iv. Biliary fistulas (>50 mL/day for >2 weeks) usually resolve nonoperatively if external drainage of the leak is adequate and distal obstruction is not present.

      a) If >300 mL of bile drains each day, further evaluation with a radionuclide scan, a fistulogram, ERCP, or a transhepatic cholangiogram may be necessary. Major ductal injury can be stented to facilitate healing of the injury or as a guide if operative repair is required. Endoscopic sphincterotomy or transampullary stenting may facilitate resolution of the biliary leak.

G. *Extrahepatic biliary tract injury* is uncommon. The gallbladder is the most common site; cholecystectomy is the usual treatment. Injury to the extrahepatic bile ducts can be missed at laparotomy unless careful operative inspection of the porta hepatis is performed. A cholangiogram through the gallbladder or cystic duct stump helps define the injury. The location and severity of the injury will dictate the appropriate treatment. Simple bile duct injury (<50% of the circumference) can be repaired with primary suture repair. Complex bile duct injury (>50% of the circumference) may require Roux-en-Y choledochojejunostomy or hepaticojejunostomy. Primary end-to-end anastomosis of the bile duct in this setting is not advised; the stricture rate approaches 50%.

H. *Spleen*

1. *Incidence.* Blunt splenic injury is produced by compression or deceleration force (e.g., from motor vehicle crashes, falls, or direct blows to the abdomen). Penetrating injury to the spleen is less common.

2. *Anatomy and function.* The spleen is bounded by the stomach, left hemidiaphragm, left kidney and adrenal gland, colon, and chest wall. These relationships define the attachment of the spleen: Gastrosplenic ligament, splenorenal ligament, splenophrenic ligament, splenocolic ligament, and pancreaticosplenic attachments. The spleen receives 5% of the cardiac output, primarily through the splenic artery. The splenic artery usually courses superior and anterior to the splenic vein in a groove along the superior edge of the pancreas and supplies portions of the stomach and pancreas through the left gastroepiploic, short gastric, the dorsal and greater pancreatic arteries, and ultimately bifurcates into superior and inferior polar arteries. The spleen has an open microcirculation without endothelium. It filters blood-borne bacteria, particulate matter, and aged cells. The spleen produces antibodies, properdin, and tuftsin.

3. *Diagnosis*

a. The patient may have signs of hypovolemia with tachycardia or hypotension and complain of left upper-quadrant tenderness or referred pain to the left shoulder (Kehr's sign).

b. Physical examination is insensitive and nonspecific in the diagnosis of splenic injury and may be unreliable due to concomitant injuries and altered mental status. The patient may have signs of generalized peritoneal irritation or left upper-quadrant tenderness or fullness.

c. Of patients with lower left-rib fractures (ribs 9 to 12), 25% will have a splenic injury.

d. In the unstable trauma patient, ultrasound (or DPL) will provide the most rapid diagnosis of hemoperitoneum, the source of which is commonly the spleen.

e. In the stable patient suffering from blunt injury, CT of the abdomen allows delineation and grading of the splenic injury. The most common finding on CT in association with splenic injury is hemoperitoneum.

4. *Treatment.* Management of splenic injury depends primarily on the hemodynamic status of the patient on presentation. **Hemodynamically unstable patients with splenic injury require intervention.** Other factors to be considered include the age of the patient, associated injuries, and the grade of the splenic injury (Fig. 29-12).

a. Nonoperative management (NOM). The use of abdominal CT and an understanding of the importance of splenic function have resulted in the preservation of many injured spleens.

i. NOM of splenic injury is successful in >90% of children irrespective of the grade of splenic injury (Table 29-5); however, children who present in shock still warrant operative management.

ii. NOM of blunt splenic injury in adults is common, with approximately 60% to 80% of adults ultimately managed nonoperatively.

iii. Neither advanced age nor associated head injury is absolute contraindication to NOM but age >55 years has been suggested as a relative contraindication due to a higher failure rate and an increased mortality and length of stay in those who fail.

iv. NOM failure rates correlate with severity of splenic injury. According to the multi-institutional study by the Eastern Association for the Surgery of Trauma (EAST), 61.5% of adult patients with blunt splenic injury were initially observed. Of these, 11% failed observation with 61% of failures occurring within 24 hours and 90% within 72 hours. Failure of NOM by grade was grade I—5%; grade II—10%; grade III—20%; grade IV—33%; and grade V—75%. In adults, the risk of NOM failure also

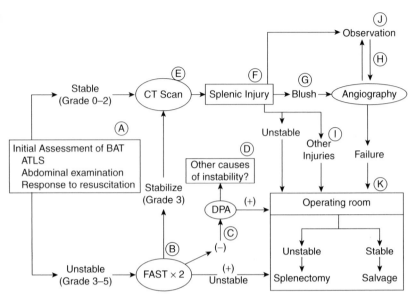

Figure 29-12. Management of adult blunt splenic injury. (From Moore FA, Davis JW, Moore EE Jr, et al. Western Trauma Association critical decisions in trauma: management of adult blunt splenic trauma. *J Trauma* 2008;65:1008.)

correlates with the quantity of hemoperitoneum. Recent data from the National Trauma Data Bank report 40% to 50% failure rate for grade IV or V splenic injury.

v. Patients with significant splenic injuries treated nonoperatively should be observed in a monitored unit and have *immediate access to CT, blood and blood components, a surgeon, and an OR*. Changes in physical examination, hemodynamic stability, or ongoing blood or fluid requirements indicate the need for laparotomy.

vi. No consensus exists for NOM and practice patterns vary widely from institution to institution. At a minimum, serial hemoglobin levels should be monitored until they remain stable and patients initially placed on bedrest during this interval.

vii. Our practice is follow-up CT at 48 hours. One large study identified 7% of patients with either early or delayed pseudoaneurysms using a protocol that obtained a repeat CT 48 hours following injury. The authors

TABLE 29-5	Management of Pediatric Splenic Injury			
CT grade of injury	I	II	III	IV
ICU stay (days)	None	None	None	1
Hospital stay (days)	2	3	4	5
Activity restrictions post-discharge (wk)	3	4	5	6

Adapted from Stylianos S. Evidence-based guidelines for resource utilization in children with isolated spleen or liver injury. The APSA Trauma Committee. *J Pediatr Surg.* 2000;35(2):164–167; discussion 167–169.

reported successful angioembolization of these pseudoaneurysms >90% of the time and an overall splenic salvage rate of >97%. The role of follow-up imaging in children is unclear but is used less frequently than in adults.

viii. Splenic artery embolization (SAE) has been reported to improve the success rate of NOM although this finding is controversial and no randomized study exists to guide decision making.

a) Suggested indications for SAE include active extravasation, traumatic pseudoaneurysm, grade III injury with large hemoperitoneum, and grade IV injuries (all in the hemodynamically *stable* patient). The use of SAE for these indications has been associated with a greater success rate of NOM.

b) Multiple studies suggest that patients who undergo successful SAE have preserved immunologic function of the spleen.

c) The failure rate associated with SAE is highly variable between studies, ranging from 2% to 29% but with multiple authors suggesting that failure rates increase with increasing grade of injury.

b. Operative management

i. If the patient is not hemodynamically stable, operative treatment is required. Operative therapy may also be considered in higher grade injuries based on imaging characteristics and the predicted rate of NOM failure as discussed above. Splenorrhaphy may be considered for lower grade, isolated injuries to preserve splenic function. Unstable patients or those with multiple other injuries, especially other sources of bleeding and bowel injury, should undergo splenectomy.

a) Exploration is through a long midline incision. The abdomen is packed and explored. Exsanguinating hemorrhage and gastrointestinal soilage are controlled first.

b) Mobilize the spleen to visualize the injury. The operator's nondominant hand will provide medial traction on the spleen to facilitate the operation. The splenocolic ligament can be vascular and require ligation. The splenorenal and splenophrenic ligaments are avascular and should be divided with blunt and sharp technique; avoid injury to the splenic capsule as this is performed (Fig. 29-13).

c) Further mobilize the spleen by bluntly freeing it from the retroperitoneum. It is important to stay in the plane posterior to the pancreas as the spleen and pancreas are mobilized. The hilum of the spleen can then be controlled with manual compression.

d) The gastrosplenic ligament with the short gastric vessels is divided and ligated near the spleen to avoid injury or late necrosis of the gastric wall.

e) Next mobilize the spleen medially into the operative field.

f) Splenectomy may now be performed by dividing the splenic vessels. The vessels may be taken individually if hemodynamics permit or en masse in an unstable patient. Methods of division include vascular staple loads, suture ligation, or ligation between clamps.

g) Splenorrhaphy may be contemplated when circumstances permit. Because of the increased reliance on NOM of splenic injury, splenorrhaphy is rarely employed and experience with the technique is dwindling.

1) Nonbleeding grade I splenic injury may require no further treatment. Topical hemostatic agents, an argon beam coagulator, or electrocautery may suffice.

2) Grade II to III splenic injury may require the aforementioned interventions, suture repair, or mesh wrap of capsular defects. Suture repair in adults often requires Teflon pledgets to avoid tearing of the splenic capsule (Fig. 29-14).

3) Grade IV to V splenic injury may require anatomic resection, including ligation of the lobar artery. A small rim of capsule at the resection line

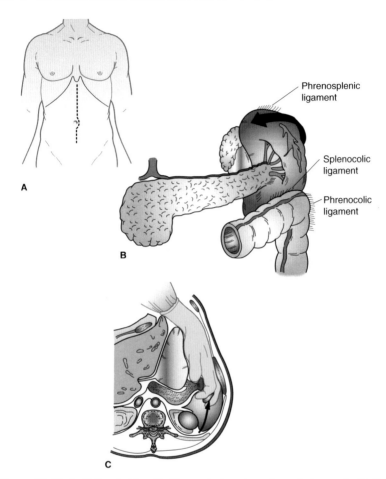

Figure 29-13. A: Midline incision. **B:** Phrenosplenic, splenocolic, and phrenocolic ligaments. **C:** Mobilization of spleen.

may help reinforce the resection line. Pledgeted horizontal mattress sutures may also be necessary. In general, splenorrhaphy in Grade IV injuries should be considered only in rare circumstances and Grade V splenic injury usually requires splenectomy.

4) When considering splenorrhaphy, it is important to note that one-third of the splenic mass must be functional to maintain immuno-competence.

h) Drainage of the splenic fossa is associated with an increased incidence of subphrenic abscess and should be avoided. The exception is when concern exists about injury to the tail of the pancreas.

5. *Outcomes and complications*

a. Choice of therapy determines specific outcomes and rates of failure, as addressed above. Rates of rebleeding following both splenectomy and splenorrhaphy performed for low-grade injuries are generally low.

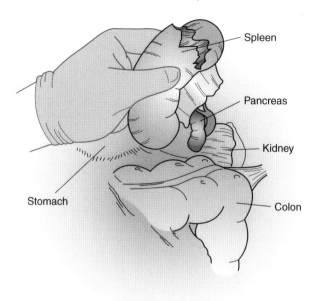

Figure 29-14. Splenic repair. The mobilized spleen in the operative field.

b. Pulmonary complications, which are common in patients treated operatively and nonoperatively, include atelectasis, left pleural effusion, and pneumonia. Left subphrenic abscess occurs in 3% to 13% of postoperative patients and may be more common with the use of drains or with concomitant bowel injury.

c. Thrombocytosis occurs in as many as 50% of patients after splenectomy; the platelet count usually peaks 2 to 10 days postoperatively. The elevated platelet count generally abates in several weeks. Treatment is usually not required.

d. The risk of overwhelming postsplenectomy infection (OPSI) is greater in children than in adults; the overall risk is less than 0.5% but the mortality rate approaches 50%. The common organisms are encapsulated bacteria: Meningococcus, *Haemophilus influenzae*, and *Streptococcus pneumoniae*, as well as *Staphylococcus aureus* and *Escherichia coli*. After splenectomy, pneumococcal (Pneumovax), *H. influenzae*, and meningococcal vaccines should be administered. The timing of injection of the vaccine is controversial. Some authors recommend giving the vaccine 3 to 4 weeks postoperatively because the patient may be too immunosuppressed in the immediate postinjury period, although many centers vaccinate patients within 2 weeks of splenectomy (before the patient may be lost to follow up). Current recommendation is to repeat the pneumococcal vaccination at 5 years. The patient should be discharged from the hospital with a clear understanding of the concerns about OPSI, should wear a tag alerting healthcare providers of his/her asplenic state, and should begin penicillin therapy with the development of even mild infections. Consideration should also be given to vaccinating patients with higher grade injuries (III to V) in whom NOM is attempted, although this remains controversial.

    e. Complications of SAE include re-bleeding requiring repeat SAE or splenectomy, splenic necrosis or delayed rupture, reports of pancreatic necrosis with proximal SAE, iatrogenic vascular injury, hematoma at the catheter insertion site, and contrast reactions/nephropathy.

ABDOMINAL VASCULAR INJURY

I. The patient who is hemodynamically labile with increasing abdominal distension has a vascular injury, either secondary to a mesenteric rent or specific vessel wound. There are several major intraabdominal vessels that, if injured, can result in substantial bleeding (Fig. 29-15). In the central area (Zone I), these include the abdominal aorta, the celiac axis vessels, the superior mesenteric artery/vein, portal vein, and the inferior vena cava. The perinephric region (Zone II) encompasses the renal artery and vein, bilaterally. Zone III represents the pelvic region where the iliac arteries/veins and their tributaries lie (Fig. 29-16).

    A. Although blunt trauma can result in mesenteric avulsion with associated bleeding, the majority of vascular injuries occur secondary to penetrating abdominal and transpelvic trauma.

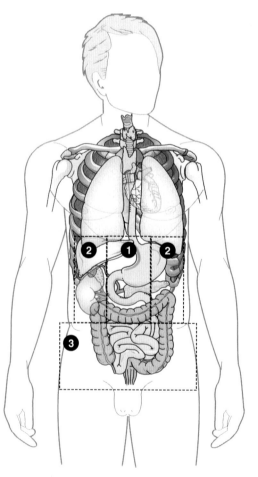

Figure 29-15. Zones of retroperitoneum. *1.* Central-medial retroperitoneal zone. *2.* Lateral retroperitoneal zone. *3.* Pelvic retroperitoneal zone.

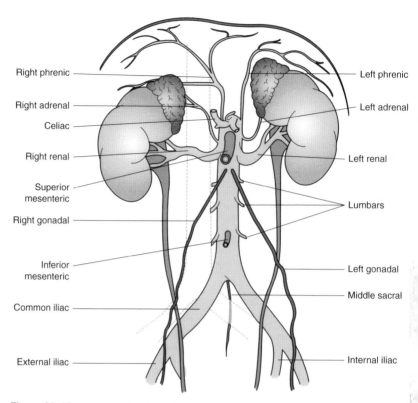

Figure 29-16. Abdominal vascular anatomy.

B. Less aggressive fluid resuscitation, with minimization of crystalloids, is the current practice, particularly in situations in which the time between the prehospital setting and the definitive hospital management is relatively short. In the trauma bay, the quickest method to confirm intraabdominal hemorrhage is by performing FAST examination. Such an assessment can be done while the patient is undergoing expeditious ATLS protocol, with the establishment of an optimal airway and the insertion of large-bore intravenous catheters.

C. Upon entering the abdomen, free blood and clots should be removed followed by gauze (laparotomy pads) packing of each of the four quadrants. Areas of concern should be manually compressed as the pads are carefully removed from the other quadrants (Table 29-6). Also, operative prioritization of intraabdominal hemorrhage should be, expeditiously identify and control aortic and inferior vena caval injuries, followed by management of bleeding solid organs. After which, contained retroperitoneal hematomas should be addressed. The fundamental principle of proximal and distal control of an injured vessel prior to repair remains applicable in this setting. Definitive management of specific arterial and venous injuries is elucidated in Tables 29-7 and 29-8.

  1. Two fundamental maneuvers in gaining access to the central vasculature are medial mobilization of right-sided and left-sided intraabdominal viscera (Figs. 29-17 and 29-18). In addition to having a prepared blood bank, a trauma surgeon encountering a major abdominal vascular injury should have certain adjuncts (e.g., conduits for establishment of temporary shunts and material for silo development in the open abdomen) to assist in the management of the injured patient.

Preparation
- Identify trauma operating room in advance, with anesthesia and operating equipment in place.
- Maintain operating room temperature at 27°C.
- Have cell-saver and rapid-infusion devices in room.

Position
- Patient supine, both arms out
- Multiple, large-bore intravenous lines above the diaphragm
- Urinary catheter with collection bag beneath head of bed
- Chest tubes, if present, to suction and in view of nurses and anesthesiologists and surgeons
- Skin preparation from chin to knees, drape to expose torso and thighs, and laterally on the chest to allow thoracotomy
- Extra operating room help (i.e., scrub assistant or extra physician) to help operating surgeon

Incision
- Midline, xiphoid to symphysis pubis
- If patient is agonal and aortic control is needed, consider left thoracotomy with aortic occlusion first

First maneuvers: Assessment
- Use four-hand retraction, evacuate blood and clot, pack all four quadrants.
- Look for bleeding; if easy, control large bleeding sites.
- Note hematomas and sites of contamination.
- Place large, self-retaining retractor (e.g., Bookwalter, Thompson).

Second maneuvers: Exposure
- With retroperitoneal hematoma, perform right or left medial visceral rotation, or other necessary maneuvers to expose retroperitoneal vascular structures.

Third maneuvers: Control and repair
- Control hemorrhage: Decide on the "best" approach for proximal and distal control, or for control of an active bleeding site directly or through a hematoma.
- Control contamination: After arterial and venous control is obtained, control all hollow visceral injuries.
- Vascular repair: Reestablish vascular continuity with repair or graft. If patient is in extremis; cold, coagulopathic, acidotic—consider damage control (with intravascular shunt), or vessel ligation.

Site of abdominal vascular injury	Principle route of operative exposure	Preferred management options
Infrarenal aorta	Midline inframesocolic retroperitoneum	Lateral suture, patch repair, or interposition graft (rare). Ligation requires extra-anatomic bypass reconstruction.
Suprarenal aorta	Left-to-right medial visceral rotation (spleen, pancreas, and left colon)	Lateral suture or patch repair. Interposition graft requires bypass to celiac, SMA, and/or renal arteries (rare). No ligation.
Celiac axis	Left-to-right medial visceral rotation (spleen, pancreas, and left colon)	Lateral suture if feasible; ligation otherwise preferred; interposition graft if collaterals disrupted (rare).
Hepatic artery	Hepatoduodenal ligament	Lateral suture, interposition graft, or ligation (may require bypass graft).
Splenic artery	Through lesser sac	Ligation preferred.
Superior mesenteric artery	Left-to-right medial visceral rotation (spleen, pancreas, and left colon); base of mesentery	Lateral suture, patch repair, or ligation and distal bypass.

(continued)

Inferior mesenteric artery	Midline inframesocolic retroperitoneum	Ligation preferred.
Proximal renal arteries	Midline inframesocolic retroperitoneum, right-to-left medial visceral rotation (right colon and left duodenum), or left-to-right medial visceral rotation	Lateral suture, patch repair, ligation and bypass, or nephrectomy.
Distal renal arteries	Right-to-left medial visceral rotation (right colon and duodenum) on right; left-to-right medial visceral rotation on left	Lateral suture, patch repair, interposition graft, or nephrectomy.
Common and external iliac arteries	Midline pelvic retroperitoneum; medial reflection of sigmoid colon on left	Lateral suture, patch repair, interposition graft, or ligation with bypass to external iliac artery (may be extra anatomic).
Internal iliac arteries	Midline pelvic retroperitoneum	Ligation preferred.

Adapted from Kokinos PG, Thompson RW. In: Soper NJ, Thompson EC, eds. *Abdominal Vascular Trauma in Problems in General Surgery.* Vol. 15, No. 2. Philadelphia, PA: Lippincott-Raven; 1998:84.

TABLE 29-8 Abdominal Venous Injuries: Exposure and Management Options

Site of abdominal vascular injury	Principal route of operative exposure	Preferred management options
Infrarenal inferior vena cava	Midline inframesocolic retroperitoneum or right-to-left medial visceral rotation (right colon)	Lateral suture, patch repair, or ligation.
Renal veins	Right-to-left medial visceral rotation (right colon and duodenum) on right; midline inframesocolic retroperitoneum on left	Lateral suture or patch repair, ligation if collaterals intact on left; interposition vein graft on right or on left if no collaterals; nephrectomy.
Juxtarenal inferior vena cava	Right-to-left medial visceral rotation (right colon and duodenum)	Lateral suture or patch repair.
Retrohepatic inferior vena cava	Right-to-left medial visceral rotation (right colon, duodenum, and right liver) with vascular exclusion of the liver (Pringle maneuver)	Lateral suture or patch repair.
Portal vein	Hepatoduodenal ligament; right-to-left medial visceral rotation (right colon and duodenum); lesser sac and transpancreatic	Lateral suture, patch repair (vein), splenic vein bypass to superior mesenteric vein, or ligation.
Iliac veins	Midline pelvic retroperitoneum; medial reflection of sigmoid colon on left; divide iliac artery (rare)	Lateral suture, patch repair, or ligation.

Adapted from: Kokinos PG, Thompson RW. In: Soper NJ, Thompson EC, eds. *Abdominal Vascular Trauma in Problems in General Surgery.* Vol. 15, No. 2. Philadelphia, PA: Lippincott-Raven; 1998:85.

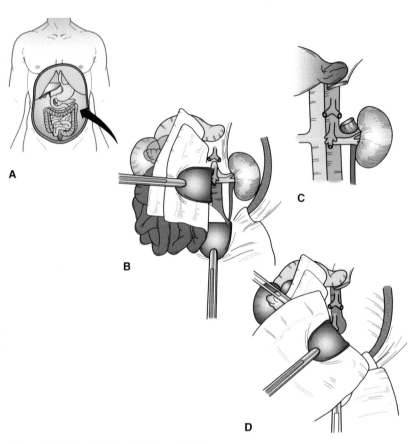

Figure 29-17. Left-sided medial visceral rotation.

Approximately 25% with major abdominal injuries will have significant vascular trauma. There is no other intraabdominal presentation that defines time-sensitive management as this cohort of injuries.

RETROPERITONEAL HEMATOMA

I. The retroperitoneum contains several vital structures, including portions of the duodenum, the pancreas, the kidneys/adrenals, major vessels (aorta, inferior vena cava, and other vasculature), along with other organs. The specific retroperitoneal injury is usually easily detected by advanced diagnostic imaging, such as computed tomography. However, there are occasions when such injuries are found while performing an abdominal exploration for blunt or penetrating trauma. In this setting, the only suggestion of an injury to a structure in this region might be a discovery of a retroperitoneal hematoma.

II. Management of the retroperitoneal hematoma is dictated by mechanism of injury and location of the hematoma (Fig. 29-15). All penetrating injuries resulting in retroperitoneal hematoma should be explored when found in the operating room. The trajectory of the weapon must be traced to avoid missed injury. Management of retroperitoneal hematoma from blunt injury is dictated by location of the hematoma (zone).
   A. In the central region (Zone I) of the retroperitoneum resides the abdominal aorta, celiac axis, and the superior mesenteric artery, vena cava, and proximal renal

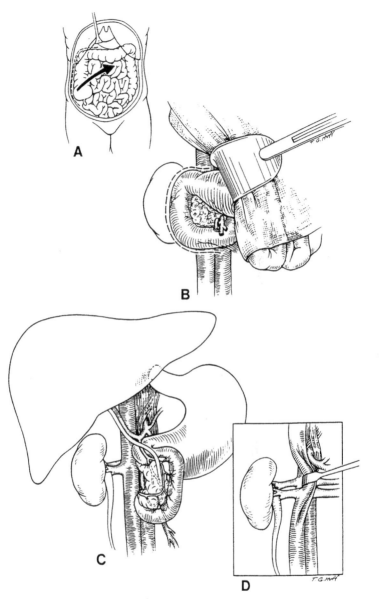

Figure 29-18. Right-sided medial visceral rotation. (From Frey W. Abdominal arterial trauma. In: Blaisdell FW, Trunkey DD, eds. Trauma Management-Abdominal Trauma. 2nd ed. New York, NY: Thieme Medical Publishers; 1993:345, with permission.)

vasculature. The lateral retroperitoneum (Zone II) encompasses the proximal genitourinary system and its vasculature. The pelvic retroperitoneum (Zone III) contains the iliac arteries, veins, and their tributaries. In addition to the vasculature and the kidneys (plus ureters) highlighted above, the retroperitoneum contains the second, third, and fourth portions of the duodenum, along with the pancreas, the adrenals, and the intrapelvic portion of the colon and rectum. Ideally, proximal (and when applicable, distal) control needs to be achieved before exploring a retroperitoneal hematoma.

1. For retroperitoneal hematomas in Zone I, irrespective of a penetrating or blunt mechanism, mandatory exploration is required. Also, a retroperitoneal hematoma in any of the three zones requires exploration for all penetrating injuries. For Zone II retroperitoneal hematomas resulting from blunt trauma, all pulsatile or expanding hematomas should undergo exploration. Gross extravasation of urine also necessitates exploration. Be certain to find any injury to the retroperitoneal colon. Zone III (pelvic retroperitoneum) hematomas should be explored only for penetrating injuries to determine if there is a specific intrapelvic colorectal, bladder, ureteral, or vascular injury. However, such an approach should not be taken for blunt trauma, for the injury would likely be venous and application of an external compression device would be the preferred intervention. An arterial injury could be addressed by arteriography/embolization.

AXIOMS

- Mechanism of injury is essential to determine the likelihood of an intraabdominal injury.
- In the hemodynamically unstable patient or the patient with ongoing fluid requirements, rapid evaluation of the abdomen in the trauma resuscitation area is mandatory.
- Unstable patients need to be in the operating room; NEVER the CT scanner.
- Identification of injury to the major duct is the critical issue in intraoperative management of pancreatic injury.
- Do not hesitate to make a subcostal extension off the midline incision to expose major hepatic injury.
- NOM is never appropriate for the hemodynamically unstable patient.

Suggested Readings

Asensio JA, Chahwan S, Hanpeter D, et al. Operative management and outcome of 302 abdominal vascular injuries. *Am J Surg* 2001;180:528.

Asensio JA, Feliciano DV, Britt LD, et al. Management of duodenal injuries. *Curr Probl Surg* 1993;30:1021–1100.

Blaisdell FW, Trunkey DD, eds. *Abdominal Trauma*. New York, NY: Thieme; 1993.

Bradley EL, Young PR, Chang MC, et al. Diagnosis and initial management of blunt pancreatic trauma: guidelines from a multi-institutional review. *Ann Surg* 1998;227:861–869.

Britt LD, McQuay N Jr. Laparoscopy in the evaluation of penetrating thoracoabdominal trauma. *Am Surg* 2003;69(9):788–791.

Buckman BF Jr, Miraliakbari R, Badellino MM. Juxtahepatic venous injuries: a critical review of reported management strategies. *J Trauma* 2000;48:978–984.

Davis TP, Feliciano DV, Rozycki GS, et al. Results with abdominal vascular trauma in the modern era. *Am Surg* 2001;67:565.

Demetriades D, Murray AJ, Chan L, et al. Penetrating colon injuries requiring resection: diversion or primary anastomosis? An AAST prospective multicenter study. *J Trauma* 2001;50(5):765–775.

Demetriades D, Velmahos G. Indications for Laparotomy. In: Feliciano DV, Moore EE, Mattox KL, eds. *Trauma*. 5th ed. New York, NY: McGraw-Hill; 2004:593–610.

George SM, Fabian TC, Voeller GR, et al. Primary repair of colon wounds. *Ann Surg* 1989;209:728–734.

Ivatury RR, Simon RJ, Weksler B. Laparoscopy in the evaluation of the intrathoracic abdomen after penetrating injury. *J Trauma* 1992;33:101.

Kozar RA, Moore FA, Moore EE, et al. Western Trauma Association critical decisions in trauma: non-operative management of adult blunt hepatic trauma. *J Trauma* 2009;67:1144–1149.

Moore FA, Davis JW, Moore EE Jr, et al. Western Trauma Association critical decisions in trauma: management of adult blunt splenic trauma. *J Trauma* 2008;65:1007–1011.

Phelan HA, Velmahos GC, Jurkovich GJ, et al. An evaluation of multidetector computed tomography in detecting pancreatic injury: results of a multicenter AAST study. *J Trauma* 2009;66:641–647.

Smego DR, Richardson JD, Flint LM. Determinants of outcome in pancreatic trauma. *J Trauma* 1985;25(8):771–776.

Smith J, Armen S, Cook CH, et al. Blunt splenic injuries: have we watched long enough? *J Trauma* 2008;64:656–665.

Watson GA, Rosengart MR, Zenati MS, et al. Nonoperative management of severe blunt splenic injury: are we getting better? *J Trauma* 2006;61:1113–1119.

I. INTRODUCTION

A. Approximately 10% of trauma patients sustain a genitourinary (GU) injury, with the kidney most commonly involved. The mechanism of injury, physical findings, and urinalysis alert the evaluating physician to the probability of such injuries and guide the initial evaluation.

B. Hematuria is the hallmark of GU injury and can originate from injury anywhere along the GU tract. However, substantial urologic injury can exist in the absence of blood in the urine.

II. HEMATURIA (Fig. 30-1)

A. Hematuria is either microscopic (presence of blood noted only with the aid of microscope or urine dipstick) or macroscopic (visible presence of blood).

  1. Any degree of **macroscopic hematuria** warrants GU evaluation of the upper urinary tract. Degree of macroscopic hematuria **does not** correlate with degree of injury.

  2. **Microscopic** hematuria may indicate injury or infection. Testing of the initial aliquot of urine is important as hematuria can clear quickly and be missed.

   a. Guidelines to further evaluate based on microhematuria include:

    i. Proximity of penetrating injuries

    ii. Children less than 15 years of age with $>$**30 RBC/high power field**

    iii. Adults with blunt trauma, microhematuria **and**

     a) any recorded systolic blood pressure <90 mm Hg

     b) rapid deceleration injuries (e.g., falls from great heights)

     c) selected patients with high risk mechanism (e.g., straddle injury, flank blow) or multiple coexistent injuries

III. IMAGING TECHNIQUES

A. Retrograde urethrogram (RUG)

  1. Performed primarily in male patients to evaluate for **urethral injury** after straddle injury, pelvic fracture, or penetrating mechanism.

  2. To perform, place patient in 30-degree oblique position with upper leg straight and lower leg flexed slightly forward. Insert Foley catheter into the meatus and partially inflate balloon – with 2 to 3 cc of water – to occlude urethra. Stretch penis to straighten anterior urethra. Slowly inject undiluted contrast with plain film or fluoroscopic images at 10 cc intervals.

  3. Evidence of contrast extravasation or occlusion of the urethra implies urethral injury. With these findings, do not place a urinary catheter until urologic consultation is done.

B. Cystography

  1. **Plain film cystogram.** With urinary catheter in bladder, obtain a **scout film.** Fill bladder with 350 cc of 30% dilute sterile contrast and obtain a **filled bladder AP film.** After seeing the view with a distended bladder, drain the bladder entirely and obtain a **postdrainage** AP film. Many small bladder injuries are appreciated **only** on postdrainage films. It is important to differentiate **intraperitoneal versus extraperitoneal** bladder rupture since the management differs.

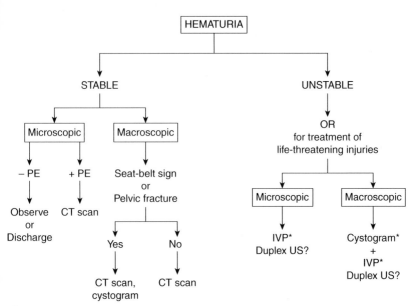

*Rapid portable study in the operating room, or evaluate after initial surgery.

Figure 30-1. Hematuria workup. PE, flank mass, flank pain, lower rib fractures, spine fracture, hypotension (even transient).

2. **CT cystography.** Preferred method of imaging. The study requires a Foley catheter and a **complete fill** scan after gravity instillation of 30% contrast at 30 cm H_2O height to tolerance in awake patients or to 350 cc in unresponsive patients. Postdrainage scans are not required with CT.

3. **CT** scan during the excretion phase following intravenous injection of contrast is **not sufficient** to exclude bladder injury.

C. Renal Trauma **CT Scan**

1. This is the best method to evaluate and stage injury to the kidneys and ureters.

2. Examine the early (venous) phase from the diaphragm to the ischial tuberosities to assess vascular and parenchymal integrity of the kidney.

3. Examine the 10 minute delayed phase to detect urinary contrast extravasation from kidney, renal pelvis, or ureter.

D. **Arteriography**

1. The arteriogram is selectively used in the setting of renal trauma to delineate the vascular integrity of the kidney, particularly in the setting of suspected renal arterial thrombosis or segmental renal arterial injury.

2. Arteriography followed by stenting or embolization may be therapeutic in cases of thrombosis or bleeding.

E. **One-shot intravenous pyelography (IVP)**

1. Much less commonly used now with wide CT availability, this can be rapidly obtained, especially in patients being taken directly to the OR **prior** to radiologic investigations.

2. The purposes of the one-shot IVP are to assess for major renal injury or contrast extravasation and to demonstrate and document contralateral renal function.

3. It has limited utility during the initial resuscitation and should not delay the transport of a patient to the operating room (OR). Its primary use is as an intraoperative study. Hypotension will limit the effectiveness of the study and is best performed when the patient is normotensive.

    4. To perform, give 2 cc/kg (or 150 cc) of 50% contrast given as an IV bolus followed by a single-shot flat plate film 10 minutes later.

F. Ultrasound
    1. Ultrasound can rapidly outline the kidney parenchyma and surrounding tissues and provide evidence that an additional study may be necessary.
    2. The imaging study of choice in the evaluation of testicular injuries.
    3. Useful in the evaluation of the transplanted kidney.

IV. RENAL INJURIES (Fig. 30-2)
A. Mechanism and diagnosis
    1. In the United States, approximately 80% of renal injuries are the result of blunt trauma and 20% penetrating trauma.
    2. Suspect renal injury in patients with hematuria or a mechanism of injury or physical findings suggestive of renal trauma (Section II).
    3. Significant renal injury **can** exist in the absence of hematuria—specifically, major injury to the renal pedicle or transection of the ureteropelvic junction (UPJ).
    4. Staging of renal trauma is by CT or intraoperative findings.

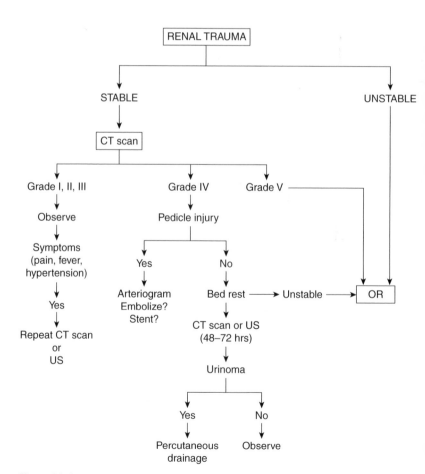

Figure 30-2. Renal trauma workup.

B. Treatment

1. **Nonoperative management** is common for **hemodynamically stable** patients with grade I to IV renal injuries.

2. **Operative exploration** is indicated in unstable patients and those with renal hilar or pedicle injuries (selected vascular grades IV and V).

3. If the patient is explored for other reasons prior to appropriate imaging evaluation, examine the retroperitoneum for evidence of expanding or pulsatile hematomas, the presence of which should prompt renal exploration. A **one-shot IVP** can be performed **prior** to renal exploration to document function of the contralateral side should nephrectomy become necessary.

4. The treatment of nonpulsatile, nonexpanding retroperitoneal hematomas found at the time of exploratory laparotomy is controversial. Generally, watch these if they are the result of blunt trauma. Explore all retroperitoneal hematomas from penetrating trauma, irrespective of the zone.

5. Early vascular control of the injured renal unit maximizes chances of renal unit salvage, best accomplished through a midline transperitoneal approach. Incision of the mesentery just medial and inferior to the inferior mesenteric vein allows exposure of the right- and left-sided renal vessels (Fig. 30-3). Alternatively, reflection of the ipsilateral colon allows exposure of the hilum, but avoids entry into Gerota's fascia before controlling the renal vessels.

6. Nephrectomy is used when renal injuries are considered unreconstructable or when patients are unstable from other injuries or have high grade actively bleeding injuries.

7. In stable patients with nonhilar vascular injuries or parenchymal injuries, renal reconstruction is frequently successful and **should be considered by experienced surgeons.** Principles include debridement of devascularized tissues, careful closure of collecting system injuries, and reinforcement of the site of repair with omentum or perinephric fat. Use of fibrin glue may limit parenchymal bleeding. Postoperative drainage of the retroperitoneum is mandatory (Fig. 30-4).

C. Complications

1. Prolonged urine extravasation may follow renal reconstruction or nonoperative management of grade IV renal lacerations, typically resolving spontaneously. Ureteric stents may facilitate antegrade drainage.

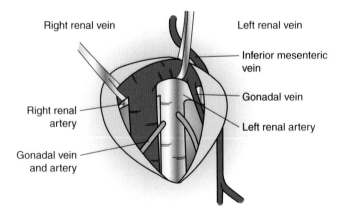

Figure 30-3. Incision of the mesentery just medial and inferior to the inferior mesenteric vein.

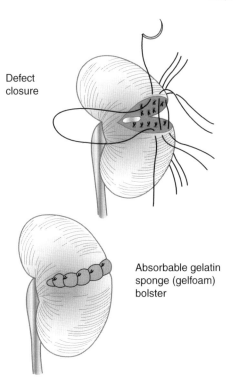

Defect closure

Absorbable gelatin sponge (gelfoam) bolster

Figure 30-4. Repair of the renal paren-chyma.

2. Urinoma formation can occur days to weeks after repair. Treat retroperitoneal urinomas or perinephric abscesses with percutaneous drainage.
3. Postinjury hypertension can occur in up to 5% of patients following renal trauma and may occur up to 6 months after injury. This may resolve spontaneously, but antihypertensive treatment is frequently required. Nephrectomy is the most common treatment if hypertension cannot be controlled.

V. URETERAL INJURIES
A. Mechanism and diagnosis
1. Ureteral injuries are rare. The majority occurs from penetrating trauma; gun-shots outnumber stab wounds. Blunt injuries to the ureter are rare and are usually seen at the level of the UPJ.
2. **Hematuria is not a consistent finding with ureteral injuries; thus, the absence of blood in the urine does not exclude a ureteral injury.**
3. Stable patients are best evaluated with a CT with IV contrast and delayed views. Cystoscopy and retrograde pyelography are sensitive and specific, but can be logistically difficult in the setting of multiple injuries and/or active resuscitation or exploration. It is reserved for defining suspected ureteral or renal pelvic injury when operative exploration is not planned or difficult.
4. Intraoperative exploration of retroperitoneal hematomas or periureteral injury is mandatory if ureteral injury is suspected and retrograde ureteral study or stenting are not possible.
B. Treatment
1. Treatment options are largely guided by location and extent of injury. Frequently, injuries can be treated with stent placement and primary repair.

    a. Distal ureteral injury below the pelvic brim may require ureteral reimplantation possibly along with psoas hitching to create a tension-free anastomosis.

    b. Midureteral injury is often amenable to primary ureteroureterostomy. Injury involving loss of long tissue segments may require formation of a Boari bladder flap or transureteroureterostomy.

    c. Proximal ureteral injury may be amenable to ureteroureterostomy. However, more complex reconstructive efforts may be required including ureteropyelostomy, ureterocalicostomy, transureteroureterostomy, or ileal segment interposition.

    d. In the unstable patient with a high-grade ureteral injury, establish temporary external drainage until the patient is better suited for operative reconstruction. Options include creation of a cutaneous ureterostomy, or simple ureteral ligation with subsequent percutaneous nephrostomy tube (PCN) placement.

    e. In the rare circumstance of long segment ureteral injury to a solitary kidney, successful autotransplantation has been reported in a delayed setting.

  2. Keys to successful repair include the debridement of devitalized tissue, proximal and distal mobilization, spatulation allowing for a tension-free repair, use of an indwelling ureteral stent, creation of a watertight anastomosis using interrupted absorbable sutures, and postoperative retroperitoneal and bladder drainage.

C. Complications following repair of ureteral injuries include urine leak or fistula formation, abscess formation, and stricture formation. Perform follow-up ultrasound or radionuclide scintigraphy to identify late development of hydronephrosis.

VI. BLADDER INJURIES

A. Mechanism

  1. The majority of bladder injuries are ruptures from blunt trauma; 80% are extraperitoneal and 20% are intraperitoneal.

  2. Most **(95%) of the bladder injuries are associated with gross hematuria.**

  3. Bladder injuries are highly associated with fractures of the pelvis, in particular, pubic diastasis and obturator ring fractures (i.e., superior and inferior pubic rami).

B. Diagnosis

  1. CT cystography is the study of choice (Section III. B). Plain film cystography has comparable accuracy but is less easily integrated into the trauma imaging sequence than CT.

  2. Excretion or cystographic phase CT scanning is **NOT** sufficient as there is a high rate of false negative results due to inadequate distension of the urinary bladder.

  3. **It is important to differentiate between intraperitoneal and extraperitoneal** injury as management differs.

    a. An **extraperitoneal** bladder rupture usually has a typical distribution in the retroperitoneal space surrounding the urinary bladder and demonstrates a characteristic molar tooth appearance as contrast extravasates into the perivesical space of Retzius.

    b. An **intraperitoneal** bladder rupture will reveal contrast outlining loops of bowel in the peritoneum. Such injuries are frequently associated with blunt trauma with a full bladder causing rupture at the dome, pelvic fractures, or gunshot wounds.

C. Management

  1. Contusions – injuries to the bladder causing **hematuria without obvious signs of contrast extravasation** – can be managed **conservatively** either with or without a bladder catheter.

  2. Extraperitoneal rupture of the bladder can generally be managed nonoperatively with a catheter and repeated cystography in 7 to 10 days to confirm healing. Large defects with marked contrast extravasation may be best repaired operatively in a similar manner to that performed for intraperitoneal injuries.

3. **Contraindications to the nonoperative management of extraperitoneal bladder ruptures include:**
   a. Associated injuries to the urethra, vagina, or rectum
   b. Active urinary tract infection
   c. Inadequate bladder drainage via urethral catheter
   d. Presence of bone fragments in the bladder
   e. Patients undergoing internal fixation of pelvic injuries (due to potential for infectious risk)
   f. Open pelvic fractures
   g. Laparotomy for nonurologic injuries is a relative indication for repair in the stable patient

4. **Explore penetrating injuries** to the bladder and repair due to the high likelihood of complications.

5. **Intraperitoneal rupture requires exploratory laparotomy and repair because of the large size of the defects and propensity for urinary ascites and its complications.**

6. Operative management includes preliminary exploration to identify additional bladder or urethral injuries. Bladder repair consists of a two-layer closure of the bladder wall using a continuous slowly absorbable suture. Use of a 20 Fr Foley catheter allows adequate bladder decompression; perioperative antibiotics and postoperative perivesical drainage are essential components of management.

7. Bladder drainage is maintained for 7 to 10 days after both operative repair and nonoperative management. Obtain a cystogram prior to catheter removal to document healing. Continued contrast extravasation should prompt continued bladder drainage. Repeat imaging studies can be obtained at 7 to 14 day intervals. Antibiotic prophylaxis need only be maintained if the patient is at risk for seeding other sites (e.g., orthopedic hardware, cardiac valves, etc.).

D. Complications include persistent bladder extravasation leading to urinoma or pelvic abscess formation, fistula formation, and osteomyelitis or infection of orthopedic hardware. Delayed complications of incontinence, urinary retention or bladder dysfunction are most often related to sacral nerve root or local soft tissue injury.

VII. URETHRAL INJURIES

A. **Mechanism**
   1. Urethral injury is more common in males than females. The mechanism of urethral injury is usually blunt; frequently associated with significant concurrent injuries.
   2. The **posterior urethra** is injured in males and females in association **with pelvic fracture.** In contrast, the male anterior urethra may be injured in penetrating trauma or a straddle-type injury causing a crush of the bulbar urethra against the pubic ramus.
   3. A straddle injury can cause urethral trauma in the absence of a pelvic fracture.
   4. Injury to the female urethra and bladder neck occurs in <5% of pelvic fractures.

B. **Diagnosis**
   1. **The best test is the RUG in men.**
   2. Seek this injury in men with blunt pelvic trauma and
      a. an inability to void
      b. blood at the urethral meatus
      c. a high-riding or indiscreet prostate on digital rectal examination
      d. swelling or ecchymosis of the penis, scrotum, or perineum
   3. In females, urethral injuries are less frequent but often missed initially and diagnosed incidentally or at time of examination under anesthesia.

C. **Treatment**
   1. **Posterior urethral injury** management requires immediate bladder decompression. Suprapubic cystostomy remains the standard of care for male pelvic fracture urethral injury with complete disruption. Initial resuscitation, stabilization, and management of life-threatening injuries take initial priority. Immediate primary repair has been condemned because of high rates of incontinence,

impotence, and stricture formation. Thus, such injuries are managed with placement of a large-caliber suprapubic tube followed by definitive repair 3 to 6 months later. Endoscopic urethral realignment may be attempted in the hemodynamically stable patient within 0 to 7 days of injury. When successful, this approach may reduce the incidence of urethral stricture and reduce the distance of the gap of urethra seen in complete disruptions.

2. **Anterior urethral injury** can be also managed in a variety of ways. Partial disruption due to blunt trauma can be managed with endoscopic or fluoroscopic urethral catheter placement followed by a pericatheter urethrogram 10 to 14 days later to assess for healing prior to removal. Injury causing complete disruption or large hematoma is treated with suprapubic tube placement followed by endoscopic or radiologic assessment of the urethra weeks to months later. Immediate repair of a urethral injury can be challenging and should be limited to stable patients with penetrating injuries requiring simple closure.

D. Complications of urethral injuries include urethral stricture formation, incontinence, and erectile dysfunction.

VIII. SCROTAL INJURY

A. Mechanism

1. 85% of injuries to the scrotum are the result of blunt injuries—often sports-related injuries.

2. **Relationship of scrotum and urethra make concurrent injuries possible**—do a RUG unless certain no urethral injury exists.

B. Diagnosis

1. **Physical examination** is difficult due to pain; however, a mechanism of injury and examination consistent with significant testicular injury warrants **prompt** surgical exploration.

2. Scrotal ultrasound is the single best study for evaluation of scrotal injury as it can evaluate testicular size, location, blood flow, and injury patterns.

C. Management

1. Except for superficial scrotal injury, **all penetrating injuries warrant surgical exploration.**

2. Indications for scrotal exploration following **blunt** trauma include testicular rupture, torsion, presence of a large hematocele, and testicular dislocation.

3. Operative goals are evacuation of hematoma with copious irrigation, conservative debridement of nonviable tissue, closure of the tunica albuginea of the testis with absorbable suture, epididymal repair, and scrotal closure. A scrotal drain should be used.

4. Orchiectomy is reserved for shattered testicles with limited remaining viable tissue.

5. Due to its extensibility, even large losses of scrotal skin can often be closed primarily. Exposed testicles following substantial scrotal skin loss are classically buried in the subcutaneous tissue of the thigh or abdomen. More recently, use of saline dressings to wrap the testicles has been used effectively. Following the development of healthy granulation tissue, split-thickness skin grafting can be performed with good cosmetic results.

IX. PENILE INJURIES

A. Mechanism

1. Penile injuries can be penetrating or blunt including trauma during sexual intercourse and avulsion injuries.

B. Penile fracture

1. Penile fracture is a rupture of the tunica albuginea surrounding the corpora cavernosa (erectile bodies) of the penis.

2. **This injury occurs almost exclusively to the erect penis** when a substantial angulation or blunt force is applied. Most frequently this results in the patient experiencing pain and hearing a loud "pop," followed by almost immediate detumescence.

3. Large penile hematomas, referred to as **"eggplant deformities,"** are typical.
4. Concurrent urethral injuries are frequent, therefore a high level of suspicion must be maintained and RUG performed routinely.
5. Management involves operative repair—immediate urologic consultation should be obtained.
C. Penetrating injuries to the penis require exploration, copious irrigation, and repair.

X. VAGINAL INJURIES
A. Mechanism
1. Usually occurs through blunt trauma and is frequently associated with pelvic fracture. In females, straddle injuries can involve the vulva.
B. Diagnosis
1. In females with pelvic fracture, a pelvic examination with speculum inspection of the vault **is mandatory** to avoid missing occult injuries.
2. Examination is best obtained with an anesthetized patient placed in lithotomy position.
C. Treatment
1. Most frequently, treatment is simple closure and, occasionally, drainage.

AXIOMS

- Hematuria is the hallmark of injury to the genitourinary system; however, significant injury may exist without blood in the urine.
- All trauma patients with gross hematuria require further evaluation.
- The evaluation of trauma patients with microscopic hematuria is based on mechanism of injury and physical examination findings.
- CT scan with IV contrast is essential in the evaluation of stable patients with suspected renal injuries.
- Most ureteral injuries are from penetrating trauma.
- Extraperitoneal bladder ruptures can frequently be managed with catheter drainage.
- Do a **RUG** before attempting urethral catheter placement if any suspicion of urethral injury exists.

Suggested Readings
Avey G, Blackmore CC, Wessells H, et al. Radiographic and clinical predictors of bladder rupture in blunt trauma patients with pelvic fracture. *Acad Radiol* 2006;13(5):573–579.
Basta A, Blackmore CG, Wessells H. Predicting urethral injury from pelvic fracture patterns in male blunt trauma patients. *J Urol* 2007;177(2):571–575.
Black P, Miller E, Porter JR, et al. Urethral and bladder neck injury associated with pelvic fracture in 25 female patients. *J Urol* 2006;175(6):2140–2144; discussion 2144.
Brandes S, Coburn M, Armenakas N, et al. Diagnosis and management of ureteric injury: An evidence-based analysis. *BJU Int* 2004;94(3):277–289.
Chapple C, Barbagli G, Jordan B, et al. Consensus statement on urethral trauma. *BJU Int* 2004;93(9):1195–1202.
Gomez RG, Ceballos L, Coburn M, et al. Consensus statement on bladder injuries. *BJU Int* 2004;94(1):27–32
Santucci RA, Wessells H, Bartsch G, et al. Evaluation and management of renal injuries: consensus statement of the renal trauma subcommittee. *BJU Int* 2004;93:937–954
Wessells H, Long L. Penile and genital injuries. *Urol Clin North Am* 2006;33(1):117–126.

31 Orthopedic Trauma, Fractures, and Dislocations

Samir Mehta and L. Scott Levin

I. PRINCIPLES AND DEFINITIONS OF ORTHOPAEDIC TRAUMATIC INJURIES

A. Evaluation of the trauma patient with a potential fracture or dislocation should include a complete musculoskeletal evaluation, led by the mechanism of injury.

1. **Dislocation** is a complete loss of articular contact between two bones in a joint; this occurs with severe injury to ligamentous and capsular tissues. **Define the direction of the dislocation** with the distal piece described in relation to the proximal joint or bone (Fig. 31-1). Dislocations should be identified during the secondary survey and should be promptly reduced.

   a. Findings on examination with joint dislocation include pain, loss of motion, shortening of the extremity, and associated neurovascular injuries (Table 31-1).

   b. **Reduction of major joint dislocation must occur as soon as possible after completion of a secondary survey.** Reduction is performed with intravenous sedation, analgesia, and (in rare, major joints) chemical relaxation; use finesse rather than force. Occasionally, deep sedation or general anesthesia is needed for relocation.

      i. Prereduction x-rays identify associated pathology. For example, a patient with a dislocated shoulder may have a non-displaced proximal humerus fracture, which may displace during reduction, leading to complications.

2. **Subluxation** refers to the *partial* loss of articular congruity; capsular and ligamentous structures remain to prevent complete dislocation. On a continuum, subluxation represents less injury than dislocation, although a complete dislocation that has partially reduced from the elastic recoil of the soft tissue can appear to be a subluxation.

3. **A fracture** is a structural break in bone continuity. Clinical signs include pain, displacement, shortening, swelling, and loss of function. Fractures are classified as either **open** (communicates with the external environment, Fig. 31-2) or **closed. Describe the** clinical deformity, soft tissues, and neurovascular structures, using this **universal scheme.**

   a. The distal piece is described in relation to the proximal piece.

   b. Fractures classifications include (Fig. 31-3):

      i. **Pattern.** Transverse, oblique, spiral, other
      ii. **Morphology.** Simple (two parts) or comminuted (three or more parts)
      iii. **Location.** Proximal, middle, or distal; extraarticular or intraarticular
      iv. Radiographic parameters. **Displacement, angulation, rotation, shortening, apposition**

   c. Assessing the degree of soft-tissue injury is important. Extensive soft-tissue injury increases the risk of the development of infection or compartment syndrome.

4. **Pediatric** fractures are classified according to their **physical (growth plate) involvement** (Salter–Harris classification).

   a. **Type I.** Displaced or nondisplaced through growth plate
   b. **Type II.** Small metaphyseal fragment
   c. **Type III.** Intraarticular through epiphysis
   d. **Type IV.** Through metaphysis and epiphysis
   e. **Type V.** Severe crush to growth plate (cannot be determined acutely, only after growth arrest)

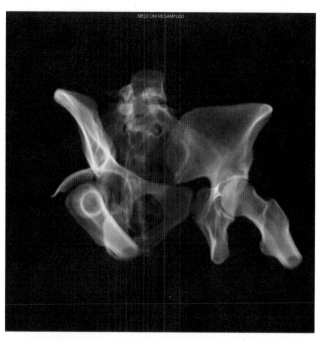

Figure 31-1. Obturator oblique view of the right acetabulum (rendered from axial CT scan) showing a posterior hip dislocation with displacement of the posterior wall.

B. Be familiar with the events surrounding the injury (mechanism of injury) and with the patient's underlying medical conditions and current complaints. In the multiply injured patient, 15% to 20% of minor fractures (e.g., hand, foot, clavicle) are missed initially. The physical examination should:
   1. Visually **inspect** for obvious soft-tissue abnormalities, including breaks in the skin, and deformities or asymmetry of the extremities.
   2. Inspect the extremity throughout and turn the patient to the side (e.g., for spinal injuries, pelvic ring injuries extending to the anus).

TABLE 31-1	Neurovascular Injuries Associated with Fractures or Dislocations
Orthopedic injury	**Neurovascular injury**
Anterior shoulder dislocation	Axillary nerve injury, axillary artery injury
Humeral shaft fracture	Radial nerve injury
Supracondylar humeral fracture	Brachial artery, ulnar nerve injury
Distal radius fracture	Median nerve injury
Perilunate dislocation	Median nerve injury
Posterior hip dislocation	Sciatic nerve injury
Supracondylar femoral fracture/posterior	Popliteal artery injury/thrombosis
Knee dislocation/tibial plateau fracture/proximal fibular fracture	Peroneal nerve
Mangled extremity/tibial fracture	All neurovascular structures of the lower leg/compartment syndrome

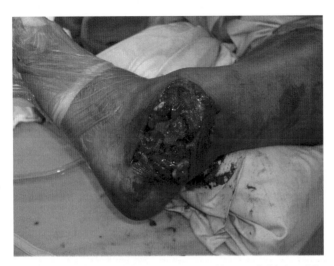

Figure 31-2. Open ankle fracture–dislocation with exposed bone and violation of the soft-tissue envelope.

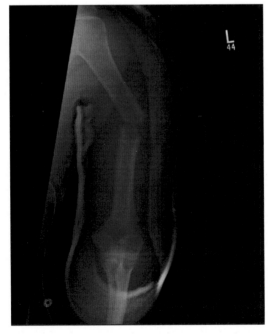

Figure 31-3. Using a descriptive classification system, this humerus would be described as "mid-shaft transverse simple fracture with approximately 45 degrees of varus angulation, and medial bony apposition."

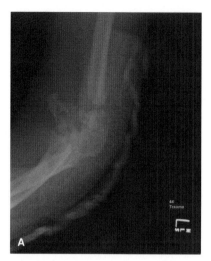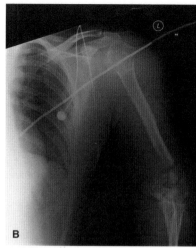

Figure 31-4. A: Oblique non-traction radiograph of an open elbow fracture/dislocation with the splint already applied. It is difficult to visualize the boney architecture of the elbow, assess bone loss, or realize normal anatomy. **B:** The same elbow with the splint removed, adequate sedation provided to the patient, and traction during the radiograph. The condyles of the elbow can be visualized, the fracture of the articular surface is noted, and the significant bone loss can be better anticipated for the operating room.

3. Palpate bone and soft tissues to evaluate tenderness, crepitus, and firmness of compartments.
4. Test active and passive **range of motion** to detect bony injury, ligamentous injury, or weakness.
5. **A neurovascular examination** records quality of peripheral pulses, sensation (pinprick, light touch), and motor function.
6. Perform an additional **tertiary orthopedic survey** after the initial 24 to 48 hours or when the patient is more responsive to detect additional injuries.

C. **Radiographic evaluation**
   1. **Obtain at least two views at right (orthogonal) angles** (generally antero-posterior and lateral views) of the involved extremity.
   2. A **traction x-ray** of involved extremity may provide more information than a radiograph of displaced, subluxed, or dislocated joint. This is particularly helpful with the elbow (Fig. 31-4), distal femur, or the hip. In general, once the joint is reduced and out to length, computed tomography (CT) is essential to define periarticular fractures and to prepare for the operating room.
   3. Imaging **must include** the joint above and the joint below the site of injury. For example, if the patient has a humeral shaft fracture, image the shoulder and elbow on the ipsilateral side.
   4. Other views (e.g., stress views of the ankle or knee) may be necessary to assess joint stability.
   5. Additional imaging, such as an MRI for a multi-ligamentous injury to the knee or arthrography for a shoulder dislocation, can be obtained later.

D. **Emergent treatment of fractures or dislocations**
   1. **Reduce** the fracture or dislocation.
   2. **Splint/stabilize** the extremity.
   3. **Irrigate** open fractures with saline and cover with sterile saline-soaked gauze.
   4. **Administer parenteral antibiotics** for open fractures or perioperatively in patients who require open reduction and internal fixation (ORIF).

5. Administer tetanus prophylaxis if >5 years since last dose for patients with open fractures or who require ORIF.

E. Definitive treatment of fractures or dislocations. The goal in treatment of musculoskeletal injury is to restore normal anatomy and function and relieve pain as quickly as possible. The early reduction and internal fixation in the multiply injured patient has reduced morbidity and mortality. The method of fixation should be adapted to the general condition (i.e., external fixation in unstable patients). Stabilization of the spine, pelvis, and long bone fractures (femur, tibia) allows early mobilization of patients.

  1. Reduction can be accomplished by either closed (external realignment) or open (direct operative approach).

  2. Immobilization of the extremity by splint, cast, traction, orthosis, external fixation, or internal fixation.

F. The most important measures in the care of open fractures are delivery of antibiotics, extensive and appropriate debridement followed by skeletal stabilization. Prevention of infection is of paramount importance. Development of osteomyelitis because of lack of antibiotic administration or inadequate debridement can be a devastating complication and will greatly increase the morbidity and potential for loss of function or limb. **Antibiotics are not a substitute for effective debridement of necrotic and contaminated tissues.**

  1. Classification of open fractures (Gustilo and Anderson)

  a. Type I. Low energy, <1 cm wound caused by protrusion of the bone through the skin or a low-velocity bullet

  b. Type II. Moderate energy, >1 cm with flap or avulsion wound in the skin with minimal devitalized soft tissue and minimal contamination

  c. Type III. High energy, extensive soft-tissue injury (usually >10 cm), "barnyard injury"

  i. IIIa. Adequate soft-tissue coverage, no vascular injury necessitating repair

  ii. IIIb. Significant soft-tissue loss with exposed bone that requires tissue transfer for coverage (Fig. 31-5)

  iii. IIIc. Vascular injury **requiring** repair for limb preservation; amputation rates reported from 25% to 50%

  2. Management after initial evaluation

  a. Open fractures require urgent operative debridement and irrigation, with the orthopedic standard within 6 hours if the patient is physiologically stable.

  b. Wounds require repeated irrigation and debridement in the operating room (OR) every 48 to 72 hours until definitive stabilization and soft-tissue coverage can be achieved (within 7 days of injury). **Minimize multiple inspections of the wound outside the operating room except by the surgeon making critical management decisions.** Continue antibiotics until 48 hours after definitive coverage.

  c. Antibiotic-impregnated bone cement "beads" and "blocks" may benefit delivery of antibiotics to spaces that do not receive the systemic antibiotics (Fig. 31-6). This local delivery has few systemic effects. The general mix dose is two vials of tobramycin (1.2 g each, 3.6 g total) per bag of cement and two vials of vancomycin (1 g each, 2 g total). The beads are strung on a stainless steel wire or heavy suture, allowed to harden, placed into the wound and covered with a liquid-sealed dressing (e.g., OpSite, Ioban). This "bead pouch" retains the fluid bathing the beads and is rich in antibiotic concentration.

  d. Internal fixation of type I open fractures after adequate debridement and irrigation can be accomplished with infection rates of <10%. If soft-tissue loss is minimal and coverage is adequate, select type II and IIIa open fractures can be treated with intramedullary fixation. External fixation may be necessary to stabilize type III open fractures, where infection rates can range from 20% to 50%. **A staged, planned redebridement may be necessary in open fractures with severe soft-tissue damage.**

  e. Wound closure may not be possible in all cases. Temporary closure with negative-pressure wound therapy may be required to provide temporary

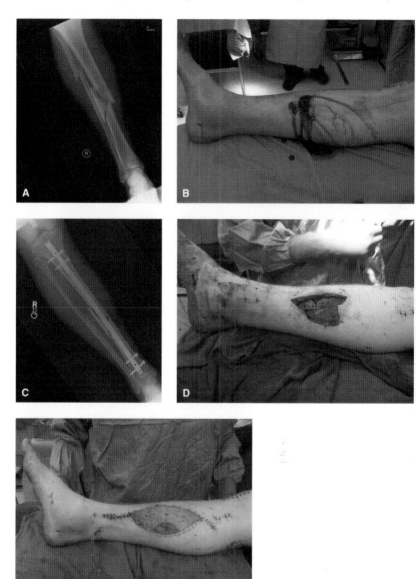

Figure 31-5. (A) AP radiograph of a Type IIIb mid-shaft tibia fracture sustained in a motorcycle crash with **(B)** associated, full thickness soft-tissue defect over the medial tibia. The patient was stabilized with an intramedullary nail **(C)** after a significant debridement of the devitalized soft-tissue **(D)** necessitating a free-tissue transfer for the soft-tissue defect **(E).**

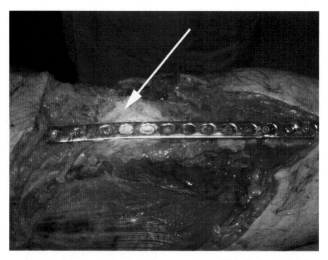

Figure 31-6. Antibiotic-impregnated cement spacer (*white arrow*) in a Type IIIb open tibia with delayed soft-tissue coverage.

coverage. At the end of the debridement, coverage of the bone is essential. However, negative-pressure **should not be applied directly to exposed bone, tendon, nerve, or vessel.** If adequate soft-tissue coverage cannot be achieved, an orthopedic or plastic surgeon skilled in managing extremity reconstruction should be consulted.

3. Gunshot injuries

  a. Low-velocity gunshot injuries cause less soft-tissue destruction than high-velocity wounds. Because of the splintering effect of gunshot injuries, bone is often unstable and requires operative fixation. Debridement of the skin wounds and treatment of the bone as a closed injury is generally accepted. Prolonged antibiotic use is controversial; our practice is to administer 24 to 48 hours of intravenous antibiotics versus oral antibiotics for 5 to 7 days.

  b. High-velocity gunshot wounds and **close-range shotgun blasts** cause significant soft-tissue injury, nerve and vascular injury, and should be treated as severe type III open fractures (Fig. 31-7). These wounds often require extensive reconstruction.

II. IDENTIFICATION AND MANAGEMENT OF SPECIFIC ORTHOPAEDIC INJURIES

A. Pelvis

  1. The pelvis is the supporting structure for the peritoneal contents and retroperitoneal structures. It connects the appendicular skeleton to the axial skeleton.

  2. Because the pelvis lies in close proximity to vessels, the colon, and genitourinary structures, pelvic injuries can be associated with retroperitoneal bleeding and neurologic, bowel, and bladder injuries.

  3. The sacrum and posterior ring are critical to the overall stability of the pelvic ring as the sacrum is the "keystone" to maintaining the biomechanics of ring congruity through force transmission.

  4. Pelvic fractures may be defined as stable, rotationally unstable, or rotationally and vertically unstable.

  5. All unstable injuries involve disruption of the posterior portion of the pelvic ring. Unstable pelvic fractures result from high-energy injury and are associated with 50% mortality in the multiple trauma patient. They require rapid assessment for stabilization and triage.

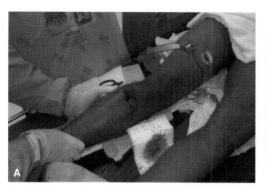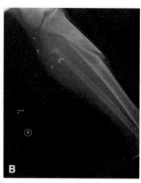

Figure 31-7. (A) Type IIIc proximal third tibia fracture resulting from a gunshot wound from an assault rifle. Despite the "small" wound **(B),** the patient had a vascular injury requiring vascular repair and delayed boney reconstruction.

6. The anterior and the posterior pelvis should be inspected for open wounds. In males, the scrotal contents are palpated for testicular displacement and the penile meatus is examined for blood, which would suggest urethral injury. Assess rectal tone and possible laceration or prostate displacement. Women should undergo both bimanual and speculum examinations to rule out vaginal, urethral, and bladder injury. Vaginal or rectal laceration requires specific treatment.

7. Pelvic ring injury causing hypotension requires prompt diagnosis and treatment. Reducing the volume of the pelvis with a binding device (see later) is often effective in tamponading pelvic bleeding, which most commonly is from a venous source.

8. Posterior pelvic disruption can result in 3 to 4 L of blood loss and hemodynamic instability (Table 31-2). Concomitantly, aggressive intravenous resuscitation is necessary and may require blood product administration to achieve adequate hemodynamic stability. Patients who do not respond to resuscitative efforts should be continually re-evaluated to avoid a missed diagnosis for the underlying hypotension. If the working diagnosis remains hypotension secondary to pelvic ring disruption and hemorrhage, do angiography of the pelvic vasculature next after binding. In this scenario, a "blush" or active arterial bleeding source may be identified via angiogram and embolized at the time of the study. The most common source of arterial bleeding in the pelvis is injury to the superior gluteal artery.

9. Pelvic volume reduction ("binding") can be done with a circumferential binder (either a bed sheet or a commercially available wrap [e.g., T-pod]) placed around

TABLE 31-2	Occult Blood Loss in Acute Fractures
Location of fracture	**Blood loss (units)**
Ankle	0.5–1.5
Elbow	0.5–1.5
Femur	1.0–2.0
Forearm	0.5–1.0
Hip	1.5–2.5
Humerus	1.0–2.0
Knee	1.0–1.5
Pelvis	1.5–4.5
Tibia	0.5–1.5

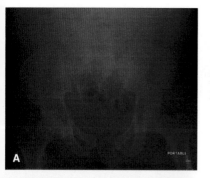

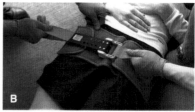

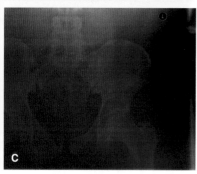

Figure 31-8. (A) AP pelvic radiograph of a 32-year-old patient who jumped from three-stories showing a disruption of the symphysis as well as widening of the sacroiliac joint. After application of a circumferential binder around the pelvis **(B)**, the pelvis (and the pelvic volume) reduce dramatically as seen on the post-application AP pelvis radiograph **(C)**.

the pelvis and greater trochanters to reduce the intrapelvic volume (Fig. 31-8). It is imperative that the commercially available binders be assessed for soft-tissue pressure necrosis after every 24 hours. Percutaneous external fixation is a temporary measure before definitive ORIF. If pelvic stabilization is not possible or bleeding continues despite application of external fixation, angiography and embolization are therapeutic alternatives.

10. Radiographic assessment includes an anteroposterior view of the pelvis, along with inlet and outlet views. Further evaluation of identified fractures is obtained with pelvic computed tomography, and a cystogram and retrograde urethrogram may also be indicated.

11. The use of a circumferential binder, although often adequate to reduce the fracture and control bleeding, does not provide secure mechanical stability. Be careful mobilizing the patient with binding alone given the potential for resumption of bleeding with disruption of any clot.

12. Once the patient is stabilized, return to the operating room for definitive care of unstable pelvic fractures. Stabilization of these fractures leads to earlier patient mobilization, minimizes the risk of pulmonary complications, decreases ventilator time, and improves morbidity and mortality.

B. Acetabular (hip socket) fractures are complex and can be associated with a hip dislocation. Acetabular fractures can create lifelong disability. Most acetabular fractures require temporary skeletal traction to maintain the reduction and prevent soft-tissue contracture, with eventual ORIF of the articular injury. The acetabulum is divided into the anterior and posterior columns, which together provide stability.

1. Types

a. Central (obturator) fracture–dislocations often require temporary skeletal traction.

b. **Posterior wall/column fracture–dislocations** require urgent reduction under anesthesia. Sciatic nerve injuries occur in 10% to 30% of patients. A careful neurologic examination must be performed before and following reduction of the dislocation. Superior gluteal artery injuries can occur, usually presenting when the fracture exits into the greater sciatic notch. **Closed reduction may not be achieved if an associated fracture to the femoral head or neck is present. In these cases, or if the fracture pattern causes re-dislocation, operative treatment is best.**

c. **Anterior fracture–dislocations** are rarer and often associated with more severe acetabular fractures.

2. **Radiographic evaluation** includes anteroposterior (Fig. 31-9A) and obturator oblique (Fig. 31-9B) and iliac oblique (Fig. 31-9C) views (collectively called Judet views) of the pelvis. After reduction of the dislocation, CT of the acetabulum is performed with 1 to 2 mm cuts. The radiologist should provide reconstructions in multiple views.

3. **Treatment**

a. Temporizing skeletal traction

b. Delayed ORIF is the treatment of choice for displaced fractures, instability, or incongruent reductions of the joint. Definitive operative intervention is usually 2 to 7 days postinjury, which reduces the chance for bleeding complications at the operative site (Fig. 31-10).

c. Posttraumatic arthritis, chondrolysis, or heterotopic ossification are the common complications (Fig. 31-10B). **Meticulous intraoperative rinsing and muscular dissection are key to prevent heterotopic ossification.** Postoperatively, indomethacin (75 mg/day for 2 weeks) or radiation (single 700 [gray or Gy] dose) can help prevent heterotopic ossification.

C. **Hip dislocation,** with or without associated acetabular fracture, occurs through the capsular area containing the blood supply to the femoral head.

1. **Types** (based on orientation of the femoral head to the acetabulum)

a. **Posterior dislocation** is most common. Sciatic nerve injuries occur (10% to 30%). The leg is usually flexed and adducted.

b. **Anterior dislocation.** The femoral head sits on top of the pubis or in the obturator foramen. The leg is generally abducted and externally rotated.

2. Radiographic evaluation in the trauma resuscitation area includes anteroposterior and Judet views. CT is required postreduction.

3. **Treatment.** Dislocation of the hip requires urgent reduction because of the risk of avascular necrosis (AVN) of the femoral head which can manifest as early as 12 weeks after injury. Reduction with intravenous sedation and analgesia (with a qualified physician monitoring that alone and the cardiopulmonary status) can be attempted (by an orthopedist) once the patient is in the trauma resuscitation area. If not achieved, an urgent closed reduction under general anesthesia is necessary. If the latter fails, open reduction is necessary.

a. Postreduction CT (1 to 2 mm cuts) is obtained to exclude associated fracture of the posterior wall or loose bodies in the joint.

b. A careful neurologic examination testing femoral, posterior tibial, and peroneal nerve sensory and motor function is mandatory before and after reduction of the dislocation.

D. Stabilization of **long bone fractures,** including the femur and tibia, has allowed patients to mobilize early and avoid complications. Advances in orthopedic hardware, including the development of statically locked intramedullary nails, have improved outcomes. The most common injuries are discussed below.

1. **Femoral neck fractures** in young patients are the result of high-energy impact. They commonly occur in the elderly, often from low-energy injuries (falls from a standing position). Femoral neck fractures are generally displaced and occur concurrently with 10% of femoral diaphyseal fractures. For this reason, radiographic evaluation of the hip is essential before femoral shaft fracture fixation.

a. **Treatment.** Displaced femoral neck fractures require urgent ORIF to reduce the complication rates of AVN and nonunion (Fig. 31-11). Elderly patients

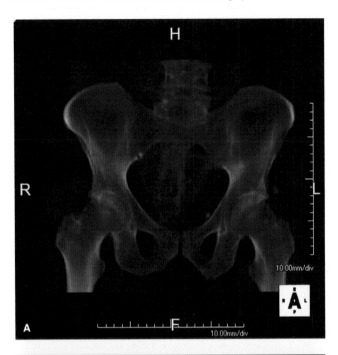

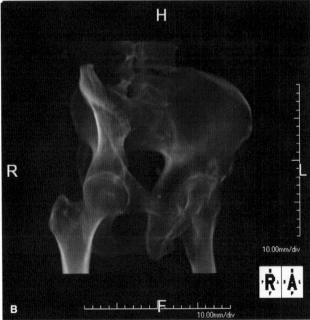

Figure 31-9. A: AP view of the pelvis and bilateral acetabuli. **B:** Obturator oblique view of the right acetabulum showing the anterior column and posterior wall. **(continued)**

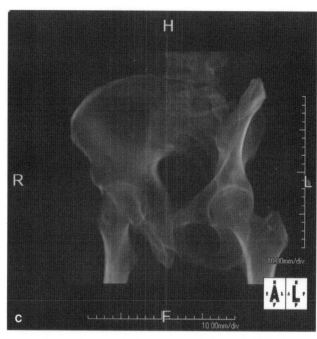

Figure 31-9. (*Continued*) **C:** Iliac oblique view of the right acetabulum showing the posterior column and anterior wall.

with significant medical problems may benefit from delayed hemiarthroplasty. Morbidity and mortality of hip fractures in the elderly are related to pre-injury cognitive function and associated medical illnesses.

2. **Pertrochanteric femur fractures** are more common in elderly patients. If they occur in young patients, high-energy trauma is present. Treatment is generally operative, but because the vascular supply is usually spared, ORIF is not as

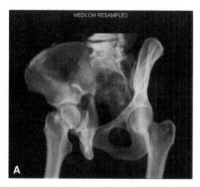
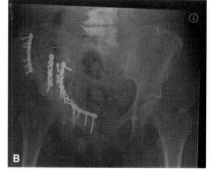

Figure 31-10. (A) Iliac oblique view of the right acetabulum showing a both-column fracture–dislocation of the right hip. After several days and stabilization of the patient, an ORIF was performed. Six months after ORIF, an AP radiograph **(B)** shows a concentrically reduced hip with minimal degenerative changes. However, the patient has developed heterotopic bone medial to his acetabulum.

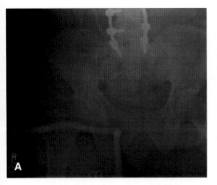 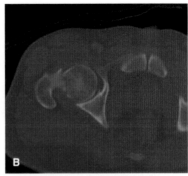

Figure 31-11. (A) Pelvis showing a right-sided femoral neck fracture. It is essential to obtain a CT to assess the amount of displacement. After CT showing the displacement **(B),** the patient was taken for an emergent ORIF of his femoral neck.

urgent as in femoral neck fractures; immediate or delayed ORIF is acceptable. Temporary skin traction is used for comfort before ORIF. Similar to other femur fractures, these in the elderly have high morbidity and mortality.

   a. Treatment is typically with intramedullary implants that permit immediate weight bearing in most cases, allowing more independence and more efficient care postoperatively. If operative intervention is delayed, skeletal traction should be employed.

3. **Femoral shaft fractures** are defined as 5 cm distal to the lesser trochanter and 6 cm proximal to the knee joint. They result from high-energy forces. Image the hip and pelvis to seek an associated femoral neck fracture.

   a. Treatment. Early intramedullary nailing is the treatment of choice. This is generally performed without actual exposure of the fracture site. This operative approach reduces the incidence of malrotation, shortening, and pulmonary complications.

4. **Supracondylar femur fractures** occur within 6 cm of the knee joint. They can either be intraarticular or extraarticular. They may have superficial femoral artery or popliteal artery injury.

   a. Treatment. Complex, intraarticular closed fracture requires careful preoperative planning and may be delayed. If delayed, use external fixation or the skeletal traction through the tibia or calcaneus.

5. **Knee dislocation** requires urgent reduction and immobilization (Fig. 31-12). **Despite immediate reduction, important complications can occur: Compartment syndrome, arterial injury, or neurologic complications (peroneal and tibial nerve injury).** Injury to the popliteal artery is common (20%), and the symptoms from intimal tears may be secondary occlusion or embolus. Arteriography or immediate operation is essential if pulse asymmetry is found in the neurovascular examination. Even in the absence of clear signs of arterial injury, consider arteriography for documented knee dislocation because of the risk of undetected intimal injury with late occlusion.

   a. Types. Anterior, posterior, medial, lateral, or rotatory.

   b. Treatment. Early reconstruction is not necessary but can be performed. Acute treatment can be achieved with a splint, hinged brace, or external fixator.

6. **Patellar fractures**

   a. Usually result from direct blow to the flexed knee. Displacement results in loss of continuity of the quadriceps mechanism. May be associated with a femur fracture or posterior hip dislocation.

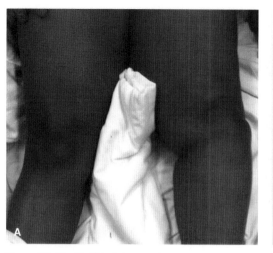
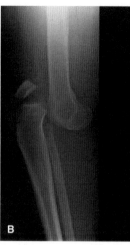

Figure 31-12. (A) Clinical photograph of a patient with a left knee dislocation. The left limb is clearly asymmetric compared the right side. A lateral radiograph **(B)** shows anterior dislocation of the tibia relative to the femur. The patient had an associated popliteal artery requiring immediate external fixation and vascular repair.

b. Nonoperative treatment for nondisplaced fractures or with an intact extensor mechanism (ability to perform a straight leg raise). Operation is necessary to restore quadriceps function and articular surface integrity. Repair requires ORIF or partial patellectomy, with patellar repair.

7. **Tibial plateau fractures** most frequently occur to the lateral tibial plateau. They usually involve depression of articular surface and/or displacement (2 mm) requiring operative fixation (Fig. 31-13). Associated knee ligament injury or vascular injury occurs in many with high-energy tibial plateau fractures. Compartment syndrome occurs in up to 25% of patients with high-energy tibial plateau fractures.

   a. **Treatment.** ORIF is preferred for displaced fractures. Treat nondisplaced fractures nonoperatively or with percutaneous screw fixation. In the elderly, tibial plateau fractures are usually minimally displaced and can be treated nonoperatively. In young adults with high-energy injury, the fracture often extends to the tibial diaphysis and may require staged treatment with external fixation followed by definitive fixation.

8. **Tibial shaft fractures** occur as high-energy injuries (e.g., motorcycle crashes, pedestrian–automobile impacts, crush injuries). Open tibial fractures are best treated by intramedullary nailing. Compartment syndrome occurs in 10% of tibia fractures, more commonly in diaphyseal tibia fractures. Tibial fractures are described based on location (proximal third, middle third, or distal third), displacement, comminution, and open versus closed.

   a. **Treatment**

      i. Closed fractures may be treated with closed reduction and casting if anatomic alignment can be achieved and maintained. ORIF with intramedullary nailing is required for unstable fracture patterns, segmental fractures, or tibial fractures associated with ipsilateral femur fractures unless severe soft-tissue injury is present.

      ii. Open tibial fractures are treated based on the type of the open fracture and degree of soft-tissue injury. Consider external fixation (Fig. 31-14) in fractures with significant soft-tissue injury because it provides adequate

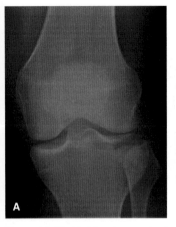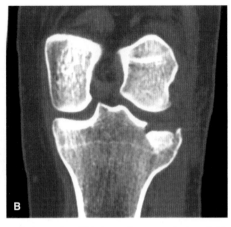

Figure 31-13. (A) AP radiograph showing a split-depression tibial plateau fracture on the lateral side after a motor vehicle collision. The coronal CT scan **(B)** shows the severe depression in the articular surface.

stability, minimizes the foreign body burden (metal implant), and allows access to the limb for soft-tissue reconstruction.

a) Early soft-tissue coverage of open fractures has decreased the incidence of secondary infection. Flaps commonly include (*a*) rotation of the gastrocnemius for proximal one-third fractures (Fig. 31-15), (*b*) rotation of the soleus for middle one-third fractures, and (*c*) free-tissue transfer of the rectus, latissimus, or gracilis for distal one-third fractures.

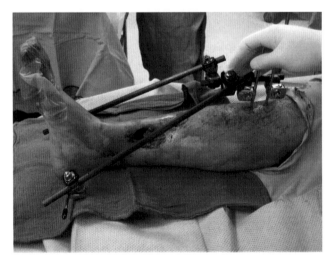

Figure 31-14. Clinical photograph of an open Type IIIb open tibial shaft fracture with bone loss treated in a staged fashion. External fixation was applied until definitive fixation (including free-tissue transfer) could be performed. Note the external fixator pins being away from the zone of injury, planned surgical incisions, and necessary definitive hardware.

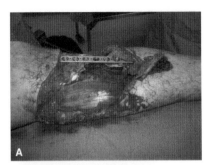

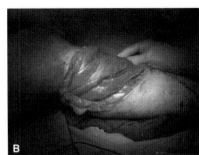

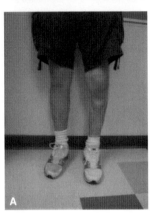

Figure 31-15. (A) Open Type IIIb proximal third tibial shaft fracture after crush injury to the limb. After multiple debridements, irrigation, and definitive stabilization, the patient received a gastrocnemius rotational flap **(B).** After 1 year, the appearance of the leg **(C)** with a well-healed flap is evident.

- **b)** Early amputation may be indicated in severely crushed limbs or type IIIc open fractures without possibility of vascular repair. Lack of plantar sensation is **NOT** an indication for immediate amputation as nearly 50% of patients will regain their sensation.
- **c) Mangled extremity** (Table 31-3). When the injured extremity has such severe injury that its salvageability is in question, decisions regarding immediate amputation require input from the trauma surgeon and orthopedist. The mangled extremity may be an open or closed fracture. Prognostic scoring systems exist for the lower extremity; the most commonly used is the mangled extremity severity scoring (MESS) system. A limb with a MESS >7 is ultimately likely to undergo amputation of the extremity, whereas limbs with MESS <7 can generally be successfully salvaged. **The scoring system should be used as a guide, not as a rule of clinical practice.** Ability to salvage an extremity depends on the status of the skin, bone, muscles, vessels, and nerves. Prolonged attempts at limb salvage are inappropriate in the multiply injured patient with immediately life-threatening injuries of the chest, head, or abdomen.
- **d) Damage control** principles have been applied to the unstable, multiply injured patient with orthopedic injury. This approach involves rapid external fixation of extremity fractures to temporarily stabilize them. Certain clinical parameters predispose the patient to adverse outcome (Table 31-4). Intramedullary nailing is done when the patient is stabilized.

TABLE 31-3	Mangled Extremity Severity Score	
Criteria	**Description**	**Points**
Skeletal/soft-tissue injury	Low energy (stab, simple fracture, pistol gunshot wound)	1
	Medium energy (open or multiple fractures, dislocation)	2
	High energy (high speed MVC or rifle GSW)	3
	Very high energy (high speed trauma + gross contamination)	4
Limb ischemia[a]	Pulse reduced or absent but perfusion normal	1
	Pulseless; paresthesias, diminished capillary refill	2
	Cool, paralyzed, insensate, numb	3
Shock	Systolic BP always >90 mm Hg	0
	Hypotensive transiently	1
	Persistent hypotension	2
Age (years)	<30	0
	30–50	1
	>50	2

MVC, motor vehicle collision.
[a]Score doubled for ischemia >6 h.

9. **Tibial plafond (pilon) fractures** occur in the distal tibia, usually involving the articular surface from an axial load. CT can be useful to define the character of the fracture. The fibula may be involved, indicating a higher energy of injury. Pilon fractures generally involve concomitant soft-tissue injury with high risk of associated soft-tissue loss and infection.

   a. **Treatment** is dictated by the status of the soft-tissue envelope as wound complication rates are high. Temporary skeletal stabilization with an external fixator may be necessary until the soft-tissue edema decreases at which time ORIF can be performed safely. Posttraumatic arthritis usually requires late ankle arthrodesis.

10. **Ankle fractures** are mostly commonly produced by external rotation with a fracture to the fibula or an injury to the interosseous membrane (Maisonneuve injury). Ankle fractures are classified based on fracture location of the lateral malleolus (fibula) and the presence (or absence) of a medial malleolus fracture.

    a. Radiographic evaluation includes anteroposterior, lateral, and mortise views, both initially and after reduction.

    b. **Treatment** requires ORIF if any subluxation (>1 mm) or incongruity of the ankle joint is found. Perform this immediately (before soft-tissue swelling develops) or on a delayed basis (7 to 14 days).

TABLE 31-4	Parameters Associated with Adverse Outcome in Polytrauma Patients
Criteria	

ISS >40 in the absence of additional thoracic injury
ISS >20 and additional thoracic trauma (AIS 2)
Multiple long bones 1 truncal injury AIS 2 or more
Polytrauma with abdomen/pelvic trauma (Moore 3) and hemorrhagic shock (initial RR, 90 mm Hg)
Bilateral lung contusions on first plain film
Presumed operation time >6 h
Initial mean pulmonary arterial pressure 24 mm Hg (if available)

11. **Calcaneus fractures** are usually the result of high falls and are often bilateral. Look for associated tibial plateau or spine injuries. Calcaneal fractures are disabling injuries and patients are often unable to return to labor.

    a. **Radiographic evaluation** includes anteroposterior, lateral, and axial views. Obtain CT (3 mm cuts) in two planes (axial and coronal) for adequate delineation of the fracture and joint.

    b. **Treatment.** Displaced intraarticular fractures require ORIF when the soft-tissue swelling subsides (10 to 21 days). Use elevation and a foot pump to reduce swelling. For fractures that are not reconstructible, primary arthrodesis may be an option. If the soft-tissue injury is extensive, external fixation or simple percutaneous pinning can also be used. The complication rate with ORIF is approximately 10% and often results in the need for tissue transfer flaps with risk of associated infection. This high risk of infection has prompted many to use only limited reductions and in situ pinning. This approach allows restoration of the hindfoot architecture and reconstructive procedures on a delayed basis, when less chance exists for soft-tissue complications.

12. **Talar neck fractures** are usually caused by forced hyperdorsiflexion of the foot on the ankle. Because of the precarious blood supply, talar neck fractures require anatomic reduction. Associated subtalar or talar dislocations **should be reduced immediately** to minimize risk of AVN (up to 85% to 100%), which is related to fracture severity. Displaced fractures require ORIF, and nondisplaced fractures can be treated with percutaneous screw fixation.

13. **Tarsometatarsal (Lisfranc) fractures** are usually associated with midfoot tenderness and swelling; these are commonly missed at initial presentation. Foot compartment syndrome can occur and results in significant disability. ORIF is indicated for displaced fractures. These are devastating injuries and can be associated with significant injury to the plantar ligamentous structures, which can result in late deformity (e.g., planovalgus). Posttraumatic degenerative joint disease (DJD) is common and requires delayed arthrodesis.

14. **Metatarsal fractures** can usually be treated in a short leg walking cast. Open reduction is indicated for intraarticular displacement or severe soft tissue swelling. Closed reduction and pin fixation is indicated for significant plantar displacement.

E. **Upper extremity fractures** also have an impact on the outcome of trauma patients. Upper extremities are necessary for activities of daily living and as weight-bearing structures when the lower extremities are compromised.

    1. **Sternoclavicular dislocation** can be anterior or posterior.

        a. Anterior dislocation is of minimal clinical significance. Perform a single attempt at closed reduction, recognizing this often fails or recurs.

        b. Posterior dislocation of the clavicle can be associated with life-threatening mediastinal injuries; do a CT or arteriography if any concern exists. Perform any closed reduction in the OR under general anesthesia, reserving open reduction if unsuccessful.

    2. **Clavicle shaft fractures** are generally of minimal clinical significance. They are classified according to location of the fracture: Medial one-third, middle one-third (most common), and distal one-third. Associated injuries include brachial plexus injury, pneumothorax, and sternoclavicular or acromioclavicular joint injury.

        a. **Treatment.** These fractures are generally treated symptomatically with a sling; expect healing in 6 to 8 weeks. Figure-of-eight straps are not well tolerated. ORIF is indicated for open fractures, neurovascular compromise, and skin compromise. Also, selected fractures of the distal one-third of the clavicle may require ORIF. Patients who are polytraumatized may require fixation of their clavicle for early weight bearing.

    3. **Acromioclavicular joint sprains (separated shoulder)** are usually treated symptomatically with a sling. ORIF is indicated for severe displacement with trapezoid ligament entrapment. Late distal clavicle excision may be necessary for symptomatic arthritis.

4. **Scapula fractures,** which are produced by high-energy impact, are frequently associated with intrathoracic injuries. Symptomatic treatment in a sling is usually sufficient with early motion. ORIF is indicated for the following:
   a. Large, displaced coracoid or acromial fragments
   b. Ipsilateral, displaced glenoid neck, and displaced clavicle fracture (floating shoulder)
   c. Intraarticular glenoid (subluxation of the glenoid >25% surface)

5. **Glenohumeral dislocation (shoulder)** is usually anterior. Posterior dislocations can occur with seizures, electrocution, or dashboard injury. Careful neurovascular examination is needed to exclude axillary nerve or artery injury.
   a. Obtain **radiographs**—anteroposterior and axillary views (the latter needed to detect luxation).
   b. **Treatment.** Early closed reduction with adequate sedation followed by sling protection with supervised active range-of-motion when pain abates. Associated rotator cuff injuries are common in patients >40 years of age, but do not change the initial management.

6. **Proximal humerus fractures** usually occur in elderly osteoporotic bone. When occurring in young patients, they are usually caused by high-energy trauma and often come with associated injuries.
   a. **Types.** Anatomic classification is based on four parts: Head, greater tuberosity, lesser tuberosity, or metaphysis fractures. Displacement is defined as 1 cm of displacement or 45-degree angulation.
      i. One-part fracture. All undisplaced fractures, regardless of the number of fracture lines
      ii. Two-part fracture. Fractures involving the anatomic neck, surgical neck, isolated lesser or greater tuberosity fractures
      iii. Three-part fracture. Fracture of the neck and a tuberosity fracture
      iv. Four-part fracture. Fracture of the neck, greater tuberosity fracture, and lesser tuberosity fracture
   b. **Treatment.** In young patients, efforts are aimed at anatomic reduction of the fracture, often surgically, to maximize function. In the elderly or less active individuals, nonoperative management or hemiarthroplasty allows adequate pain relief and function.
      i. Stable, two-part impacted neck fractures may be treated in a sling
      ii. Two-part neck or unstable require ORIF rather than closed reduction and percutaneous pinning
      iii. Displaced greater tuberosity fracture requires ORIF
      iv. Three-part in younger patients with good bone stock requires ORIF

7. **Humeral shaft fractures** have a high rate of union with nonoperative management using fracture braces. In the multiply injured patient, ORIF or intramedullary nailing may facilitate nursing care and use for the activities of daily living. Distal third fractures can be associated with radial nerve palsy (usually a neurapraxia).

8. **Distal humerus fractures** are more common in children than in adults. The classification scheme is as complex as the fractures themselves, based on intraarticular versus extraarticular, degree of comminution, and displacement. Intraarticular fractures mandate an anatomic reduction.
   a. **Pediatric distal humerus fractures** may be associated with neurovascular injury and compartment syndrome. Urgent (not emergent) closed reduction should be performed in the OR. Percutaneous pinning is necessary for unstable fractures or those with significant soft-tissue swelling. Open reduction is required if closed reduction is unsuccessful. Cubitus varus is a common complication.
   b. **Adult distal humerus fractures** require ORIF in almost all cases. Heterotopic ossification can occur, especially in head-injured patients. Stiffness and ulnar neuropathy can occur.

9. **Olecranon fractures** usually occur as traction injuries. ORIF with tension band techniques is indicated if displacement is greater than 2 mm. Olecranon fractures

may be associated with more complex fracture–dislocations of the elbow included radial head as well as trans-olecranon.

10. **Coronoid fractures** are treated with early motion if the elbow is stable; however, clinical series are revealing that these injuries are often associated with elbow instability and require fixation.

11. **Radial head fractures** occur from a fall on an outstretched hand.

    a. **Treatment.** Treat nondisplaced fractures with early motion. ORIF is performed if angulation is greater than 30 degrees, 3 mm displacement, or depression greater than one-third of the articular surface. Radial head replacement is reserved for severely comminuted fractures. Manage associated dislocations first; suspect distal radioulnar joint (DRUJ) injury.

12. **Elbow dislocations** are common and most often posterior. Dislocations and fractures of the elbow usually result from a fall on an outstretched arm or direct impact on the elbow. A careful neurovascular examination is needed to assess the ulnar, radial or median nerves, and the brachial artery; most nerve injuries are neuralpraxia. Associated fractures of the coronoid, radial head, and medial epicondyle can occur; obtain radiographs to exclude an associated fracture. Treatment consists of immediate closed reduction and application of a posterior splint. Document median and ulnar nerve function before and after reduction; nerve entrapment can occur with reduction. The splint should be removed at 7 to 10 days and start active range of motion. In unstable cases, maintain suspicion of a coronoid or radial head fracture. Elbow instability after dislocation often requires ligamentous and boney reconstruction.

13. **Combined radius and ulna fractures** in an adult should be treated with ORIF. Fractures of both bones in the forearm risk a compartment syndrome. Posterior interosseous nerve injury is common with proximal third fractures. Severely contaminated open fractures may require external fixation.

14. **Ulnar shaft fractures** occur as a result of a direct blow. These fractures are generally treated with functional bracing, but delayed union is common. ORIF should be performed with angulation greater than 10 degrees or displacement greater than 50%. Associated injuries to the wrist and elbow should be suspected. **Monteggia fracture–dislocations** are a proximal ulnar fracture with an associated radial head dislocation; this mandates ORIF.

15. **Radius fractures** are treated in a long arm cast in supination if they are nondisplaced and in the proximal one-fifth with range of motion starting within 2 weeks of injury. Fractures distal to this in the radial shaft should be treated by ORIF. **Galeazzi fracture** is a radial shaft fracture, at the junction of the middle and distal third of the radius, associated with dislocation of the DRUJ. Treatment is anatomic fixation of the radial shaft fracture and re-assessment of the DRUJ with fixation as needed.

16. **Distal radius fractures** usually occur from a fall on an outstretched arm. Associated median or ulnar nerve injury, DRUJ disruption, and carpal instability can occur. Extensor pollicis longus rupture can also occur and is usually seen 5 to 8 weeks after injury.

    a. **Colles fracture** is a fracture of the distal radius with displacement of the carpus.

    b. **Smith's fracture** is a reversed Colles fracture—a fracture of the distal radius with the distal fragment and accompanying carpal row displaced volarly.

    c. **Barton's fracture** is a distal radius fracture with displacement of a dorsally based triangular segment from the radius. **Reversed Barton's fracture** is a distal radius fracture with displacement of a palmary based triangular segment from the radius.

    d. **Radiographic evaluation** includes anteroposterior, lateral, and oblique views. Also obtain radiographs of the hand and elbow.

    e. **Treatment** starts with closed reduction and casting. Fractures involving an intraarticular step-off, shortening, or severe comminution require anatomic reduction and fixation with pins or plates, with or without external fixation. ORIF is required with large, displaced articular fragments.

17. **Scaphoid fractures** can be associated with other carpal injuries. For nondisplaced (less than 2 mm) fractures, treat with a long arm thumb spica. Treatment duration varies with fracture location, but ranges from 8 to 20 weeks. For displaced fractures, perform closed reduction and pinning or ORIF. An anatomic reduction is necessary to reduce the risk of nonunion and AVN. AVN and nonunion are more common with scaphoid waist and proximal pole fractures.

18. **Perilunate dislocations** are commonly missed at initial presentation---look closely at the radiographs. Associated scaphoid fractures are common. Reduction and pinning are necessary, and dorsal ligament repair may also be required. Associated median nerve injury is also common and early carpal tunnel decompression may be required.

III. **CONSIDERATIONS DURING AMPUTATION** can result in morbidity and potentially dysfunctional limbs. Therefore, amputation injuries should be handled only at institutions under the direction of a team whose care is directed by a microvascular surgeon. **Amputations are true limb- and life-threatening injuries and should be handled as such, with no delays in treatment.** Unsuccessful replantations can result in disability. Realistic expectations should be provided to the patient only after evaluation by the multidisciplinary team.

   A. The physician responsible for replantation should be notified as soon as possible, preferably before arrival.

   B. Necessary historical data includes the patient's name, age, occupation, handedness for upper extremity, **time of injury,** mechanism of injury, level of injury (bone, soft tissue), exact neurovascular status, concomitant injuries and associated medical conditions, and the location and telephone number of the nearest relative, especially if the patient is a minor.

   C. The OR should be prepared as soon as potential need is present (i.e., before arrival).

   D. The patient should be transported quickly.

   E. Preserve amputated parts by wrapping in a sterile gauze moistened with sterile saline solution. Place in a watertight plastic container or re-sealable plastic bag, which should then be placed into an iced saline bath. **DO NOT use dry ice. DO NOT place the amputated part in direct contact with ice.** Clearly label the container with the patient's name and time placed.

      1. Administer tetanus prophylaxis (if needed) and broad-spectrum antibiotics as for open fractures.

   F. The replantation team should be present at time of arrival to the emergency department. Evaluate the limbs and amputated parts clinically and radiographically. Amputated parts are replaced in container (as previously discussed).

   G. Transfer the patient to the OR. A two-team approach is used if associated injuries require intervention.

   H. Factors associated with a poor outcome include crush injury, long ischemia time (>6 hours), proximal amputations, nerve injuries (axonotmesis), systemic hypotension, severe contamination, concomitant injuries or medical conditions, advanced age, poor nutrition, or is psychologically compromised (Fig. 31-16).

IV. **BASIC SPLINTING.** Splinting should never be harmful, and adequate knowledge of relevant anatomy and potential complications is necessary. Follow the principles of splinting described below.

   A. The **purpose for splinting is immobilization.** This provides temporary stabilization of bone and soft tissue, aids in control of hemorrhage, and helps reduce pain and prevent further injury.

   B. **Principles** of splinting include splinting open fractures as they lie. Gross angulation in closed fractures should be reduced by longitudinal traction. Neurovascular status must **always** be re-assessed after the splint is applied. If neurovascular compromise is present, remove or loosen the splint. When splinting, include the joint above and joint below, and make sure the splint is rigid enough to provide immobilization. It should not be circumferentially compressive unless ongoing hemorrhage is present.

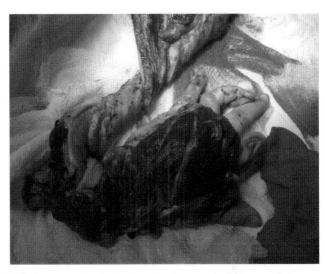

Figure 31-16. Severely crushed left upper extremity traumatically amputated after a motor vehicle collision with prolonged extraction presenting with gross contamination, loss of neurologic structures, limited soft-tissue coverage, and no remaining bony anatomy. Salvage is not possible.

C. Types of commercial splints
1. Extremity splints
   a. Air splints for extremity fractures can induce compartment syndrome but have little structural stability.
   b. Structural aluminum malleable (SAM) splints consist of semirigid cardboard; they are useful for upper extremity, ankle, and foot fractures in the acute setting.
   c. Silicone splints function similar to air splints, but with less chance for compartment syndrome. They are useful for distal extremities.
   d. Hare and Thomas traction splints are useful for femur fractures by providing longitudinal traction from foot to ischial tuberosity. Traction splints should be removed in a timely fashion to prevent neurologic and soft-tissue injury.
2. Other types of splints include plaster. It is readily available, relatively inexpensive, and easy to use. Newer premade fiberglass splints are more rigid than the plaster counterpart. Pillow splints are easy to use, and they can be secured with ace wrap or roll gauze. They are effective, comfortable, and an excellent choice for distal extremities. Splints can also be fashioned with cardboard, blankets or towels, and aluminum.

D. Specific areas
1. C-spine may require a cervical collar and sandbags.
2. The spine may require a backboard.
3. The shoulder may require a sling, sling and swathe, and ace wrap arm to chest.
4. Splints for the humerus are the same as for the shoulder and also may include a SAM splint or plaster U-splint.
5. Elbows should be splinted at a 90-degree angle with a posterior plaster splint.
6. Splinting of the forearm, wrist, and hand should include the elbow at a 90-degree angle. Plaster U-splint or pillow splint can also be used.
7. Circumferential binders may be used initially to splint pelvic fractures.
8. Splinting of the proximal femur and femoral shaft can include Hare traction, posterior plaster splint, pillow splints, or traction pins.

9. Splinting of the distal femur, knee, and proximal tibia may require a knee immo-bilizer, posterior plaster splint, pillow splints, or traction.

10. Splinting of the tibial shaft should include posterior plaster or U-splint, pillow splints, or silicone splints.

11. Ankle and foot splinting can be performed with posterior plaster or U-splint, pillow splints, or silicone splints.

AXIOMS

■ Up to 25% of fractures may be occult in the multiple-injured patient
■ Obvious severe open fractures may be distracting in patients with coexisting life-threatening injuries
■ Fractures are a source of occult blood loss
■ Reduction of a major joint dislocation should be reduced as soon as possible after com-pletion of the secondary survey
■ Key steps in open fracture management include antibiotics, debridement, and stabilization
■ Unstable pelvic fractures can be a source on massive hemorrhage. Management may include compression, stabilization, and angiography
■ Closed tibial fractures must be monitored closely for compartment syndrome
■ All fractures should be carefully assessed for associate neuro-vascular injuries
■ Mangled extremity scoring systems provide guidelines for limb salvage efforts
■ The indication for early amputation should be documented by at least two treating physi-cians when possible (i.e., EM, trauma, ortho, vascular, etc.)
■ Vascular shunting may be a temporary bridge to skeletal fixation

Suggested Readings

Flynn J. *Orthopaedic Knowledge Update 10*. Rosemont, IL: American Academy of Orthopaedic Surgeons; 2011.

Gustilo RB, Anderson JT. Prevention of infection in the treatment of 1025 open fractures of long bones. *J Bone Joint Surg Am* 1976;58A:453–459.

Hunt JP, Weintraub SL, Wang Y, et al. Kinematics of trauma. In: Moore EE, Feliciano DV, Mattox KL, eds. *Trauma*. 5th ed. New York, NY: McGraw-Hill; 2004:141–158.

Johansen K, Daines M, Howey T, et al. Objective criteria accurately predict amputation following lower extremity trauma. *J Trauma* 1990;30:568–573.

Pape HC, Giannoudis P, Rockwood C. *Rockwood and Green's Fractures in Adults*. 6th ed. Philadelphia, PA: Lippincott Williams & Wilkins; 2005.

Schmidt AH, Teague DC. *Orthopaedic Knowledge Update Trauma 4*. Rosemont, IL: American Academy of Orthopaedic Surgeons; 2010.

32 Peripheral Vascular Injuries

Louis J. Magnotti, John P. Sharpe and Timothy C. Fabian

I. **INTRODUCTION.** To optimize outcomes following peripheral vascular injuries, prompt recognition is crucial. This mandates accurate diagnosis of those injuries requiring operation. Delays in either the recognition or subsequent treatment of these injuries can contribute to preventable limb loss.

Mandatory operative exploration is no longer required for all potential vascular injuries. Reliance on the physical examination findings of "hard" signs (Table 32-1) coupled with the selective use of arteriography has become the mainstay to guide operative and other therapy. After recognition, the best outcomes emanate from timely reperfusion and avoiding the factors associated with limb loss (Table 32-2).

II. **ETIOLOGY**
   A. Vascular trauma is classified according to the general mechanism of injury (blunt or penetrating); different mechanisms typically produce different types of injuries and injury patterns. In urban trauma centers, peripheral vascular injuries are most commonly (75% to 80%) caused by penetrating trauma. Approximately 50% of these injuries are caused by handguns, 30% from stab wounds, and 5% from shotgun wounds. In the past, most gunshot wounds were small-caliber low-velocity bullets, although currently those are largely replaced by semiautomatic and automatic large-caliber weapons discharging higher-velocity missiles. The resulting vascular injuries are more devastating and are often associated with substantial associated soft-tissue and skeletal injuries. Peripheral vascular injuries from blunt trauma to the extremities including fractures, dislocations, crush injuries, and traction account for 5% to 25% of vascular injuries.
   B. Penetrating injuries can result in complete transection and may present as thrombosis from vessel spasm or bleeding. In contrast, partially transected vessels may contract and continue to bleed. Even if controlled initially, the injured vessel may re-bleed as the patient is resuscitated and the arterial pressure rises. In the majority of cases, the location of a presumed vascular injury is estimated by following the path of the penetrating object.
   C. The mechanism is critical to determine the risk of vascular injury and potential for amputation. Stab wounds are unlikely to lead to amputation. However, high-velocity injuries with associated blast effect and tissue loss are at an elevated risk of vascular injury and limb loss.
   D. Blunt trauma usually results in an avulsion type injury where the artery is stretched. This stretching disrupts either the tunica intima alone or the tunica intima and tunica media together; the highly thrombogenic tunica externa is left to maintain vessel continuity. Significant intimal damage leads to thrombosis and eventually complete occlusion of the vessel. Those injuries that do not occlude can instead produce intimal flaps, pseudoaneurysms, or arteriovenous (AV) fistulas. While blunt trauma represents the minority of peripheral vascular injuries, delays in diagnosis and revascularization are more common, and generally result in a higher amputation rate than penetrating mechanisms. For blunt trauma, it is important to recognize that specific vascular injuries are commonly associated with distinct orthopedic injures (Table 32-3). Those skeletal injuries should prompt the clinician toward early recognition of vascular injury.

TABLE 32-1	Hard Signs of Arterial Injury

Absent distal pulses
Active hemorrhage
Large, expanding, or pulsatile hematoma
Palpable thrill or audible bruit
Signs of distal ischemia: 5 P's—pain, pallor, paralysis, paresthesias, poikilothermia (coolness)

III. ARTERIAL INJURIES

A. Diagnosis. Delays in diagnosis or therapy can be prevented through careful history and physical examination combined with the appropriate use of diagnostic modalities. The clinical manifestations of major peripheral vascular injuries (hard signs) must be recognized promptly and addressed early. A defined algorithm for management of penetrating vascular trauma should be utilized (Fig. 32-1).

1. **History.** Assessment of the injured extremity begins with a detailed history in conjunction with the physical examination. Pertinent information includes the estimation of blood loss at the scene (including pulsatile blood loss), time of injury, mechanism of injury, type of projectile, and the vital signs during the pre-hospital period. These details can provide important clues in identification of major vascular injury. Primary survey and stabilization of life-threatening injuries takes precedence over evaluation of the extremity; active hemorrhage from an injured extremity is addressed in the primary survey.

2. **Physical examination.** Detailed vascular, neurologic, soft-tissue, and skeletal examinations will determine the potential for vascular injury and the risk for limb loss.

   A careful extremity evaluation provides information on the location and severity of the vascular injury.

   a. Vascular examination. The presence of any hard signs (see Table 32-1) should prompt immediate search for a vascular injury.

   i. All pulses proximal and distal to the area of potential injury should be palpated and documented. The injured extremity should be compared to the contralateral, uninjured extremity and any pulse differences noted.

   ii. For uncomplicated penetrating extremity trauma, the presence of any hard sign should trigger immediate surgical exploration. In general, evaluating such patients with further diagnostic modalities is unnecessary and delays definitive therapy; nearly all of these patients will have injuries requiring operative repair.

   a) When a patient presents with hard signs of vascular injury in the face of multilevel trauma to the extremity, it can be difficult to determine the level of arterial injury. In this situation, arteriography is indicated,

TABLE 32-2	Factors Associated with Higher Rates of Limb Loss in Vascular Trauma

Treatment delay—6 h
Blunt mechanism of injury
Lower extremity injuries, especially of the popliteal artery
Associated injuries: Nerve, vein, bone, soft-tissue loss
High-velocity gunshot wounds and close-range shotgun wounds
Preexisting chronic peripheral vascular disease and other comorbidities
Failure or delay in performing fasciotomy
Clinical presentation in shock or obvious limb ischemia

TABLE 32-3   **Vascular Injuries Associated with Specific Orthopedic Injuries**

Orthopedic injury	Associated vascular injury
Knee dislocation	Popliteal artery
Femur fracture	Superficial femoral artery
Supracondylar humerus fracture	Brachial artery
Clavicle fracture	Subclavian artery
Shoulder dislocation	Axillary artery

preferably intra-operative angiography, to minimize delay in repairing the injury and facilitate intra-operative decision-making.

b) The absence of hard signs in an injured extremity virtually excludes the presence of a major vascular injury as reliably as arteriography or any other imaging modality.

iii. Soft signs of vascular injury include a history of severe hemorrhage at the scene, unexplained hypotension, a stable, small hematoma that is not expanding or pulsatile, diminished or unequal pulses, a neurologic deficit, or a wound in proximity to vascular structures. Such findings may require diagnostic modalities beyond physical examination.

b. Neurologic evaluation. Motor and sensory examination of the affected extremity should be performed, documented, and compared to the uninjured extremity. It is important to remember that vascular injury may initially manifest sensory, "stocking or glove anesthesia," and motor deficits secondary to

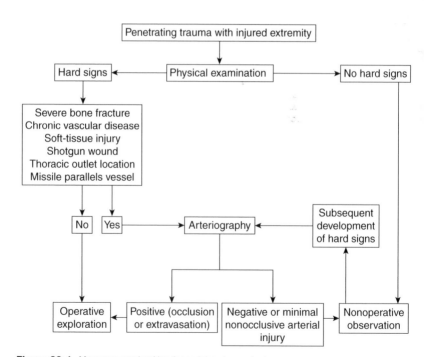

Figure 32-1. Management algorithm for peripheral vascular trauma.

peripheral nerve ischemia. A nerve injury can only be diagnosed once vascular perfusion is restored or a nerve injury is directly visualized.

3. **Non-invasive tests.** These tests are not required for the evaluation of patients with hard signs of arterial injury. Such modalities can be helpful for the intra-operative or post-operative evaluation of vessel patency. They do not have advantages over physical examination in the initial diagnostic evaluation of injured extremities for vascular injury. Moreover, the information non-invasive tests yield in this setting can be misleading and falsely exclude a vascular injury on the basis of flow signals.

   a. **Ankle–brachial index (ABI).** The ABI is obtained by placing a blood pressure cuff on the supine patient proximal to the ankle or wrist of the injured limb. The systolic blood pressure is determined with a Doppler probe at the respective posterior tibial and dorsalis pedis arteries or at the ulnar and radial arteries. The ratio of the highest systolic pressure obtained in the affected extremity to the systolic pressure in the unaffected extremity (most often the brachial artery) comprises the ABI. An ABI lower than 0.90 has a sensitivity and specificity of 87% and 97%, respectively for arterial injury. It is important to remember that there are certain clinical situations in which a vascular injury may not result in an abnormal ABI. For example, a non-axial injury, a lesion that does not disrupt arterial flow (intimal flap or transected artery with pseudoaneurysm), or an AV fistula may not lower the ABI and thus be missed.

   b. Duplex imaging can aid intra-operative and post-operative evaluation of vessel patency. However, this modality is operator dependent and not routinely available.

4. **Conventional contrast arteriography.** Diagnostic angiography has a sensitivity of 95% to 100% and a specificity of 90% and 98%; it remains the diagnostic standard for evaluation or confirmation of arterial injury. With extremity trauma, non-selective angiography is not cost effective. It is often overly sensitive, detecting minimal injuries that do not require further management. Arteriography can be time consuming, delay definitive treatment, and lead to complications, including renal contrast toxicity and pseudoaneurysm formation.

   There is little reason to perform angiography in a patient with hard signs of injury, unless an intra-operative angiogram is necessary to delineate anatomy. Operative intervention should never be delayed for arteriography in patients with hard vascular failure signs.

   Also, unstable patients should not be sent from the trauma bay, operating room, or ICU for diagnostic arteriography. For these patients, arteriography may be performed in the primary setting, although the operating room is best when this constellation exists. The technique for lower extremity angiography is as follows:

   a. Access the contralateral (unaffected) common femoral artery percutaneously with an 18 gauge arterial entry needle.
   b. Insert a 5 french introducer sheath.
   c. Pass a 260 cm 0.035 in guidewire through the introducer sheath.
   d. Using fluoroscopy, pass an angiographic catheter, over the guidewire from the unaffected limb navigating the aortic bifurcation to the affected limb.
   e. Hand inject full strength contrast while imaging (under fluoroscopy) defined segments of the affected limb. Then, observe for evidence and location of occlusion or gross extravasation of contrast.

5. **Computed Tomographic Angiography (CTA).** In recent years, CTA has shown levels of accuracy, resolution, and cost comparable to conventional arteriography. Rapid data acquisition facilitates the diagnostic work-up in critically injured patients who will require imaging for injuries to structures in which the vessel traverses, avoiding the delay for formal angiography. The three-dimensional reconstructions of CTA may be superior to conventional angiography. CTA represents a viable challenge to conventional angiography.

B. **Blunt and complex vascular injury** involves combined injuries to extremity vessels, bone, soft tissue, and nerves, and are associated with high amputation rates.

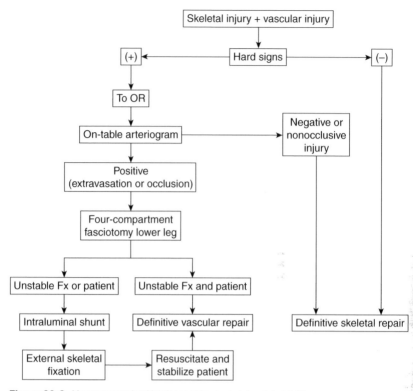

Figure 32-2. Management algorithm for combined arterial and skeletal trauma.

These injuries can result from blunt or destructive penetrating (shotgun and high-velocity firearm wounds) mechanisms. Application of a defined management algorithm for combined arterial and skeletal trauma is advantageous (Fig. 32-2).

1. Obtain as complete a history as possible from the pre-hospital providers (field blood loss, joint dislocation). Examine the extremity, being sure to document any change in the examination over time.

2. Delay in the treatment of complex extremity vascular injury represents the most common cause of limb loss, especially in the setting of the multiply injured trauma patient. Re-establishment of arterial flow should be the first priority after life-threatening injuries have been stabilized to maximize limb salvage. Skeletal, nerve, or soft-tissue trauma should be addressed only after revascularization has been accomplished.

3. Comminuted fractures or joint dislocation can temporarily obstruct arterial flow. A careful vascular examination should be performed before and after fracture reduction/realignment or splinting and relocation of dislocated joints with care to document pulses pre- and post-intervention.

4. The presence of hard signs mandates immediate vascular evaluation by arteriography, as many hard signs are due to findings from associated injuries in the setting of blunt trauma (high false positive rate of physical examination). Adhering to this practice helps avoid a high rate of negative limb exploration which may complicate associated injuries. To avoid potential delays in therapy, perform arteriography in the OR in conjunction with orthopedic management.

5. Dressings, wraps, or splints can restrict venous or arterial flow; carefully apply and monitor these to avoid harm. Swelling and edema can increase over time, leading to constriction. Injured extremities should be periodically checked for signs of compartment syndrome and changes in perfusion.

6. There is an increased risk of compartment syndrome in the setting of blunt and complex vascular injury. This is best confirmed by physical examination findings (pain on passive movement) and direct measurement of compartment pressures. Prophylactic fasciotomy is preferable to delaying fasciotomy until overt signs of extremity compartment syndrome develop.

C. Basic principles of operative management. Arterial injuries should be repaired immediately after resolution of more life-threatening injuries (life over limb). Ideally, flow to an injured extremity should be restored within 6 hours of injury to maximize limb salvage.

1. Do not blindly clamp bleeding vessels prior to obtaining adequate exposure, preferably in the OR. Any active hemorrhage should be controlled with direct pressure en route to the OR. Tourniquets have been discouraged for many years; however, experiences from the recent Middle East wars show they can be beneficial and are associated with few complications when *properly* utilized. They are currently being re-introduced to hospitals and EMS systems. They can control hemorrhage during stabilization and transport to the OR. Incorrectly applied tourniquets can increase bleeding from an extremity wound and increase the risk of exsanguination by occluding low-pressure venous outflow while incompletely occluding high-pressure arterial inflow.

2. Prepare and drape the uninjured extremity, anticipating the need to harvest a saphenous or cephalic vein conduit. Never "prep yourself out of an operation."

3. Repair the vascular injuries before other associated injuries in the involved extremity. Restoration of blood flow *always* takes priority. Temporary intraluminal shunts may be used to re-establish perfusion in those patients with unstable fractures or dislocations, life-threatening injuries, or ongoing hemodynamic instability prior to definitive arterial repair.

4. It is important to gain proximal control of the injured vessel (control at a point one level higher than the injured area) before assessing the site of injury. In situations where proximal control cannot be obtained, an intraluminal balloon may be used to achieve temporary control.

5. Following isolation of the injury, systemic heparin should be given in cases of isolated injury with obvious ischemia. Do not use early heparin with massive blood loss, extensive soft-tissue injury, or multiple injuries; consider once vascular control has been obtained to minimize thrombosis.

6. Debride the injured vessel to remove areas of contused arterial wall or intimal flap. This is best done by transecting the injured vessel through the contusion and continuing to trim the vessel proximally and distally until healthy vessel is reached.

7. Perform proximal and distal balloon catheter thrombectomy before completing repair to ensure adequate inflow and appropriate back-bleeding.

8. Primary repair is usually appropriate for uncomplicated stab wounds and many low-velocity missile injuries. The blood vessel should be mobilized proximal and distal to the site of injury. If the injury is so extensive that primary repair is under tension, repair should be done with a graft. In the case of lower extremity injury, a reversed interposition saphenous vein graft harvested from the **contralateral** extremity provides good results. When veins are not satisfactory, expanded polytetrafluoroethylene is an alternative but should not be smaller in diameter than 6 mm. Many surgeons use the interrupted suture technique for vessels below the elbow or below the knee.

9. Perform arteriography following restoration of flow and prior to leaving the OR. This may be accomplished via cannulation of the native uninjured vessel with a small catheter proximal to the repair or via the diagnostic angiography catheter if intra-operative angiography occurred earlier.

10. Consider fasciotomy in the presence of ischemic time exceeding 4 to 6 hours, uncertain limb viability, shock, combined vascular and skeletal injury, or simultaneous arterial and venous injury. ***Prophylactic rather than therapeutic fasciotomy offers the best opportunity for limb salvage and preservation of limb function.***

11. Post-operatively, these patients must be closely monitored for any change in vascular examination and compartment syndrome. Loss of palpable pulse or Doppler signal or development of compartment syndrome mandates immediate return to the OR for evaluation and repair. No other diagnostic tests are necessary in the immediate post-operative period.

12. **Management of asymptomatic non-occlusive arterial injuries.** Select extremity arterial injuries in the absence of hard signs and without extravasation or occlusion on arteriography are successfully managed non-operatively in 90% of cases. These clinically occult, minimal arterial injuries include small intimal flaps or other intraluminal irregularities. Typically, these injuries have a benign natural history and may be safely observed with serial examination and close follow-up. The rare asymptomatic, non-occlusive arterial injury that worsens during follow-up is readily repaired without increased complications or limb loss.

D. Outcomes and complications

1. Long-term outcome for successful arterial repair is good (>95% salvage rates under optimal conditions). Limb loss increases with delays in diagnosis and restoration of flow, high-velocity or destructive gunshot wounds with substantial tissue loss, injury to smaller (more distal) vessels, pre-existing peripheral vascular disease, and in multiply injured or hemodynamically unstable patients.

2. Combined vascular and skeletal extremity injuries have higher rates of infection and amputation (70%) in some series (e.g., open tibia or fibula fractures with trifurcation injury).

3. Peripheral nerve injuries are present in up to 50% of patients with extremity vascular trauma and are the most significant determinant of long-term disability.

4. Most **preventable** complications are associated with prolonged ischemic times or failure to perform fasciotomy. Complications are both early and late and include:

   a. **Early.** Thrombosis or graft failure (often related to technical problems), bleeding, compartment syndrome, infection, limb loss, rhabdomyolysis with associated renal failure, venous thromboembolism related to immobility or venous injury, and death.

   b. **Late.** Pseudoaneurysm, arteriovenous fistula, infection, and occlusion.

IV. COMPARTMENT SYNDROME

A. **Etiology.** Any injury resulting in severe tissue edema within the fascial compartments or associated with tissue ischemia can produce compartment syndrome. This situation compromises perfusion and can create myoneural necrosis, loss of function, and require amputation. In trauma patients, compartment syndrome is most often associated with vascular or orthopedic injury.

1. **Ischemia-reperfusion injury.** Vascular injury with associated limb **ischemia** leads to tissue edema. Following vascular repair, **reperfusion** generates reactive oxygen species, increases capillary permeability, and produces significant swelling. Concomitant shock increases the degree of damage in the affected extremity.

2. **Crush injuries** with significant musculoskeletal trauma are at high risk for the development of compartment syndrome.

B. **Pathophysiology.** Increasing compartment pressure results in complete venous obstruction. Continued arterial inflow further elevates intra-compartmental pressure. As venous obstruction becomes more extensive, accompanying arterioles undergo reflex spasm, resulting in tissue ischemia. Progressive ischemia worsens tissue edema, contributing to further elevation of compartment pressure. A vicious cycle is created that continues until compartment release or tissue necrosis occurs.

C. **Diagnosis.** Diagnosis of compartment syndrome can be difficult. Diagnosis is usually established by a collection of symptoms, serial physical examination, and measurement of a compartment pressure.

1. **Symptoms.** Pain out of proportion to physical examination is a classic symptom. Paraesthesias and paralysis are late findings and develop with continued hypoperfusion.

2. **Signs.** Compartment syndrome is often characterized by a swollen, tense compartment. In the awake patient, pain on passive stretching occurs early. As the syndrome progresses, conscious patients may manifest sensory deficits and progressive motor weakness of the involved neuromuscular structures. Although loss of function may be the earliest sign, loss of peripheral pulses is a late finding usually accompanied by irreversible damage. A palpable distal pulse does not exclude compartment syndrome.

3. **Compartment pressures.** Elevation of compartment pressure precedes development of symptoms. For this reason, measurement of compartment pressures is paramount to diagnosis, especially in patients with impaired consciousness in whom subjective information is limited and physical examination is unreliable. Most consider compartment pressure >30 mm Hg an indication for fasciotomy. Compartment pressure between 20 and 30 mm Hg in the symptomatic patient or in the face of prolonged hypotension also warrants fasciotomy. *Delay in performing fasciotomy worsens outcome—if doubt exists regarding the diagnosis, do a fasciotomy.*

   a. Measurement devices include the needle catheter or Stryker handheld monitor.

   b. **Technique.** The skin overlying the compartment to be measured is prepared in a sterile fashion and infiltrated with local anesthetic. The needle is advanced through the skin until it pops through the fascia and into the muscular compartment. A small amount of saline is flushed to eliminate interference from catheter plugging, and the pressure is recorded. Correct needle position can be confirmed by noting a brief increase in pressure with compression of the compartment being measured. Measurements should be repeated to confirm elevated pressures.

D. **Treatment of compartment syndrome** requires adequate decompressive fasciotomy of the affected limb. This will both normalize compartmental pressures and restore adequate tissue perfusion. At the time of fasciotomy, debride only frankly necrotic tissue. If tissue viability is questionable, the compartment should be reexamined within 24 hours to assess viability.

1. **Lower leg fasciotomy** should release all four compartments (anterior, lateral, superficial, and deep posterior) and is accomplished with a double incision technique (Fig. 32-3). Make an incision on the lateral leg from just below the head of the fibula to just above the ankle, approximately 1 cm anterior to the fibula. Avoid injury to the peroneal nerve as you extend the incision cephalad. Identify the septum dividing the anterior and lateral compartments and open the fascia on either side of this septum to release these compartments. Make a second incision of similar length on the medial side of the leg, 2 cm posterior to the tibia. Open the fascia here to release the superficial posterior compartment. Partially detach the proximal soleus from the back of the tibia, incise the fascia, and release the deep posterior compartment.

2. **Thigh fasciotomy** should release three compartments (quadriceps, hamstrings, and adductors). Access and release the quadriceps compartment through an anterolateral incision on the thigh. Decompress the hamstring compartment by dividing the intermuscular septum posteriorly. Release the adductor compartment through a separate incision medially along the length of the compartment.

3. **Forearm fasciotomy** involves release of the volar compartment through an incision along the volar aspect of the forearm curving across joint spaces to avoid contracture with healing (Fig. 32-4). Most advocate a carpal tunnel release with this procedure. Once the volar compartment is released, measure the dorsal compartment pressure; if still elevated, perform a dorsal fasciotomy. Release the

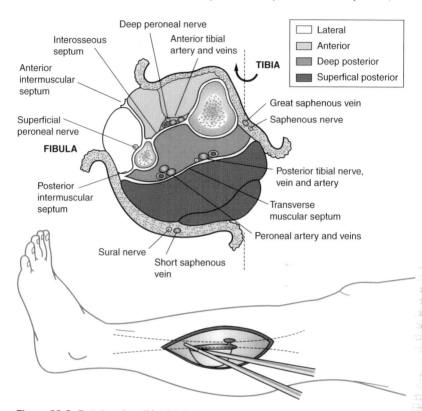

Figure 32-3. Technique for calf fasciotomy.

dorsal compartment through a single straight incision on the back of the forearm from the lateral epicondyle to the wrist.

4. **Closure.** These wounds are closed once the swelling has improved and there is no longer evidence of ongoing necrosis with either primary closure or skin grafting. The goal is to avoid closing the wound under tension and thereby recreating compartment syndrome.

E. **Complications.** The major complications of compartment syndrome include infection and rhabdomyolysis.

1. Infection occurs secondary to the presence of necrotic muscle. Control requires debridement of all non-viable tissue. This is best accomplished through repeated daily debridement in the operating room.

2. Rhabdomyolysis can lead to acute kidney injury and renal dysfunction. This occurs when toxins released from damaged muscle enter the systemic circulation. Early recognition and treatment reduces the incidence of acute kidney injury and renal dysfunction.

   a. **Etiology.** Any injury associated with skeletal muscle damage (either directly or indirectly) can produce rhabdomyolysis. Direct compression of skeletal muscle (with or without concomitant orthopedic or vascular injury) leading to a local crush injury is most commonly associated with the development of rhabdomyolysis. Electrical injury and ischemia-reperfusion following vascular injury can also damage muscle, leading to the release of myoglobin and other toxins into the systemic circulation.

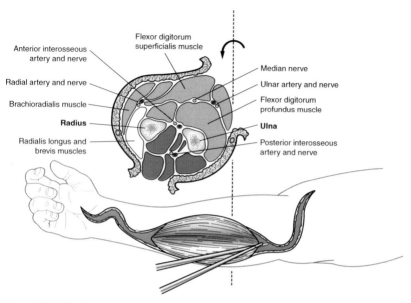

Figure 32-4. Technique for forearm fasciotomy.

- **b. Diagnosis.** A combination of signs, symptoms, and laboratory findings in the appropriate clinical setting is key—and considering it with any crush or reperfusion injury.
- **c. Signs and symptoms.** Physical examination can be normal in up to 50% of patients. Tea-colored urine – or "dip stick positive for blood" urine absent red blood cells on analysis – in the appropriate clinical setting is suggestive of rhabdomyolysis with associated myoglobinuria.
- **d. Laboratory findings.** Elevated serum creatine phosphokinase is the most sensitive marker of muscle damage. Urine myoglobin is usually positive and is easily followed. If urine myoglobin is not available, urinalysis that is dipstick positive for blood with few or no red cells on microscopic examination is highly suggestive of rhabdomyolysis.
- **e. Treatment of rhabdomyolysis** centers on prevention of renal dysfunction with adequate hydration and forced diuresis, correction of electrolyte abnormalities, and correction of the underlying cause.

V. VENOUS INJURIES

Venous injuries are commonly recognized at the time of exploration for arterial injury. The decision regarding repair versus ligation of a venous injury depends on the physiologic status of the patient and the adequacy of venous outflow. There is benefit in repairing select venous injuries, especially the popliteal vein. Repair should also be undertaken if the patient is stable and there is evidence of venous hypertension with excessive venous and soft-tissue bleeding on completion of the arterial repair. Ligation should be performed in patients who are unstable, coagulopathic, acidotic, hypothermic, or have other life-threatening problems. Ligation does not usually produce significant chronic problems or adversely affect limb salvage.

A. Diagnosis

1. Clinical signs of venous injury include hemorrhage, venous engorgement, and swelling of the extremity. Do not image patients to detect asymptomatic venous injury.

B. Treatment
1. Venous injury without active bleeding or hematoma does not require operation.
2. Venous injury found at the time of arterial exploration can often be repaired by lateral venorrhaphy with minimal narrowing of the vessel. Occasionally, interposition grafting is necessary. Although long-term patency results are lower than arterial repair, short-term patency reduces post-operative complications of swelling and edema, allowing time for re-canalization and formation of collaterals.
3. If ligation is necessary, fasciotomy or leg elevation and compression stockings should be used depending on the level of ligation.
4. There is no need to perform follow-up imaging of venous repairs unless clinically significant symptoms of venous insufficiency develop.

VI. SPECIAL CONSIDERATIONS
A. Immediate amputation—the mangled extremity. Indications for immediate amputation without attempting arterial repair include the following:
1. Nerve destruction, resulting in an insensate and paralyzed extremity, confirmed by direct examination of the nerve at exploration to exclude simple nerve contusion.
2. Extensive concomitant bone and soft-tissue loss or destruction.
3. Non-viable muscles in all compartments at fasciotomy.
4. Severe comorbidities.
5. Any setting in which arterial repair is deemed futile or has failed without viable option for revascularization.
6. Prolonged attempts at revascularization result in myonecrosis, rhabdomyolysis, and occasional preventable deaths from those complications.
B. Autogenous saphenous vein remains the conduit of choice for vascular reconstruction (highest long-term patency rates and lowest infection risk). However, associated injuries and inadequate size can preclude its use. In this setting, alternatives include polytetrafluoroethylene (should be utilized with caution in contaminated fields) and extra-anatomic bypass.
C. Use of temporary conduits as a "damage control" bridge (intraluminal shunts) combined with external fixation of skeletal injuries allows rapid restoration of distal blood flow and provides the option to take the multiply injured patient to the intensive care unit for further resuscitation. Definitive vascular repair may then be accomplished later when the patient has been stabilized.
D. Optimal sequence of repair. Restoration of distal perfusion is the first priority with any vascular injury. Use of an intraluminal shunt allows temporary restoration of flow while the fracture is realigned. Once the fracture has been stabilized (either with external fixation or intramedullary rod), definitive vascular repair should be undertaken provided the patient remains hemodynamically stable. For stable fractures, without anticipated need for extensive manipulation, definitive vascular repair is the preferred method of immediate reperfusion. The trauma surgeon should be available during the orthopedic procedure to assist with any problems that may develop in the initially repaired or shunted vessels.

VII. MANAGEMENT OF SPECIFIC ARTERIAL INJURIES
A. Axillary artery
1. The axillary artery originates at the lateral border of the first rib and ends at the inferior border of the teres major muscle. The axillary artery has three segments from which six branches originate (Fig. 32-5). The axillary vein and brachial plexus course along with the axillary artery.
2. Given the proximity of the axillary vein and brachial plexus, concomitant venous and nerve injury occurs in 40% and 50% of cases, respectively.
3. The operative field should include the entire arm, neck, and chest. This allows the surgeon to manipulate the arm during repair to aid in reducing tension on the repair. Expose the axillary artery via an S-shaped incision, beginning at the midclavicle, following the deltopectoral groove and continuing to the groove between

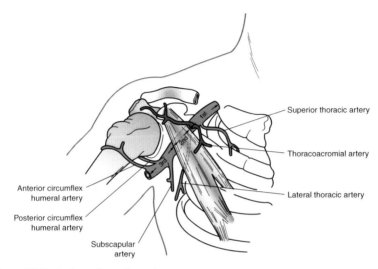

Superior thoracic artery

Thoracoacromial artery

Lateral thoracic artery

Anterior circumflex
humeral artery

Posterior circumflex
humeral artery

Subscapular
artery

Figure 32-5. Anatomy of an axillary artery.

biceps and triceps muscles. Perform primary repair or resection with primary anastomosis, if possible. Often by adducting the arm, a primary anastomosis can be performed without undue tension, making an interposition graft unnecessary.

B. Brachial artery

1. These injuries are usually produced by penetrating injuries. The brachial artery begins at the border of the teres major muscle and ends 1 cm below the antecubital fossa. Major branches include the profunda brachii, ulnar, and radial arteries (Fig. 32-6). The median nerve courses with the brachial artery. In addition, the radial and ulnar nerves are also in proximity. The degree of ischemia depends on whether injury is proximal or distal to the profunda brachii. The more proximal the injury, the more likely distal ischemia will develop.

2. Exposure is undertaken along the groove between the triceps and biceps muscles, via an S-shaped extension if the incision crosses the antecubital fossa. End-to-end repair is often possible; however, tension may require use of a saphenous vein interposition graft.

C. Forearm vascular injury

1. The brachial artery divides into the radial and ulnar arteries 1 in. below the antecubital fossa. Eighty percent of patients will have a dominant ulnar artery supplying their hand. Ten percent of patients have an incomplete palmar arch. Sixty percent of patients with either a radial or ulnar artery injury will have a concomitant nerve injury.

2. Operative repair is through a longitudinal incision overlying the artery. If only the radial or ulnar artery is injured and distal neurologic function is intact and the palmar arch is intact, the injured vessel may be ligated. Even with early successful repair, long-term patency of a repaired single vessel is only 50%.

D. Common, profunda, and superficial femoral arteries (Fig. 32-7)

1. These proximal lower extremity vessels are commonly injured in civilians, comprising 20% of vascular injuries. The majority of injuries are secondary to penetrating trauma.

2. Operative approach involves prepping the abdomen, entire injured leg, and proximal contralateral leg in case saphenous vein harvest is needed. Proximal control may require division of the inguinal ligament or retroperitoneal control of the

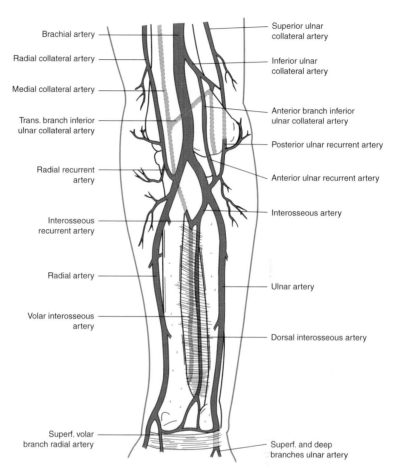

Figure 32-6. Anatomy of a brachial artery.

external iliac artery. Begin with a longitudinal incision over the course of the femoral vessels. Approach to the superficial femoral artery involves a longitudinal incision along the anterior border of the sartorius muscle. Repair all arterial injuries except for distal injuries to the profunda femoris artery.

E. Popliteal artery

1. The popliteal artery begins at the adductor hiatus as a continuation of the superficial femoral artery. The proximal popliteal artery lies posterior to the femur while the distal aspect is situated behind the capsule of the knee joint (Fig. 32-8). Its fixation at the adductor hiatus proximally and soleus arch distally make it vulnerable to blunt injury. The popliteal vein courses from the lateral to the medial side of the artery in its mid-portion.

2. Injuries to the popliteal artery comprise 5% to 10% of civilian vascular trauma overall. Due to its relatively fixed anatomy, nearly 50% of popliteal injuries follow blunt trauma. Amputation can be as high as 25% with blunt injury (compared to only 4% following penetrating injury), primarily as a result of

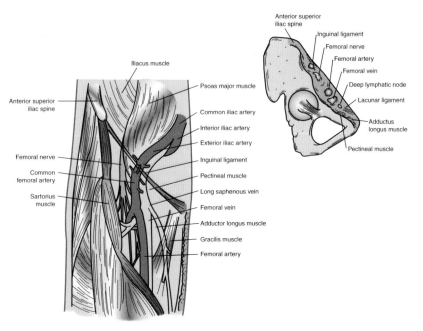

Figure 32-7. Anatomy of a femoral artery.

the degree of associated skeletal and soft-tissue injuries. The collateral blood supply provided by the geniculate arteries is rather sparse, which further contributes to a higher amputation rate than that from other extremity arterial injuries.

3. Operative approach is generally via a medial exposure. The contralateral leg must be prepared so that saphenous vein can be harvested if necessary. Most blunt injuries cannot be repaired primarily. Attempt should be made to preserve the ipsilateral saphenous vein as this may be the only venous drainage from the injured extremity. The medial head of gastrocnemius muscle can be detached to improve distal exposure. Repair venous injuries if possible. Plan to perform fasciotomies (>60% of patients will ultimately require fasciotomy). In cases of extensive associated perigeniculate soft-tissue or skeletal injury, or prolonged ischemia, revascularization can be more expeditiously accomplished by above knee to below knee saphenous vein bypass rather than dissecting out the injured artery which always has substantial destruction. Completion arteriography is recommended after repair.

F. Anterior tibial, posterior tibial, and peroneal arteries

1. The anterior tibial artery is the first branch of the below knee popliteal artery. The tibio-peroneal trunk then bifurcates into the peroneal artery and the posterior tibial artery.

2. Penetrating trauma is responsible for injury to the shank vessels in two-thirds of cases. Injury to the tibio-peroneal trunk or all three shank vessels carries an amputation rate of >50%. A single-vessel injury does not usually require repair. The presence of limb ischemia, injury to the tibio-peroneal trunk, or injury to multiple vessels requires restoration of flow through at least one vessel. Bypass or interpositional grafting is usually necessary.

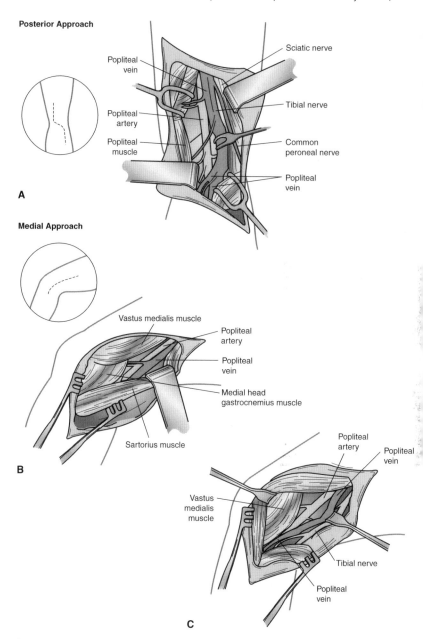

Figure 32-8. Anatomy of a popliteal artery.

AXIOMS

- Physical examination is the mainstay for the diagnosis of vascular injury.
- In uncomplicated penetrating trauma, hard signs of arterial injury mandate immediate operative exploration.
- In blunt or complex extremity trauma, arteriography in the OR is best to minimize delay in revascularization.
- The absence of hard signs in any setting reliably excludes surgically significant arterial injury and eliminates the need for imaging.
- For arterial repairs requiring interposition grafts, harvest saphenous vein from the contralateral, uninjured extremity.
- Most preventable amputations are associated with delayed diagnosis and treatment of arterial injury or delayed or inadequate fasciotomy.
- For combined skeletal and vascular injury, restoration of arterial flow always takes precedence. The use of intraluminal shunts can be invaluable for these cases as well as the unstable patient requiring ongoing resuscitation.
- Compartment syndrome is challenging to diagnose early; however, therapy is most effective when performed early. In any with a crush or ischemia injury, look for compartment syndrome—starting with pain with passive stretch.
- It is much better to perform an ultimately unneeded fasciotomy than fail to provide one when needed.

Suggested Readings

Anderson RJ, Hobson RW 2nd, Padberg FT, et al. Penetrating extremity trauma: identification of patients at high-risk requiring arteriography. *J Vasc Surg* 1990;11:544.

Attebery LR, Dennis JW, Russo-Alesi F, et al. Changing patterns of arterial injuries associated with fractures and dislocations. *J Am Coll Surg* 1996;183:377–383.

Busquets AR, Acosta JA, Colon E, et al. Helical computed tomographic angiography for the diagnosis of traumatic arterial injuries of the extremities. *J Trauma* 2004;56:625.

Dennis JW, Frykberg ER, Veldenz HC, et al. Validation of nonoperative management of occult vascular injuries and accuracy of physical examination alone in penetrating extremity trauma: 5 to 10 year followup. *J Trauma* 1998;44:243–253.

Frykberg ER, Schinco MA. Peripheral vascular injury. In: Feliciano DV, Mattox KL, Moore EE, eds. *Trauma*. 6th ed. New York, NY: McGraw-Hill; 2008:941–971.

Hafez HM, Woolgar J, Robbs JV. Lower extremity arterial injury: Results of 550 cases and review of risk factors associated with limb loss. *J Vasc Surg* 2001;33:1212–1219.

Inaba K, Potzman J, Munera F, et al. Multi-slice CT angiography for arterial evaluation in the injured lower extremity. *J Trauma* 2006;60:502–506.

Kostler W, Strohm PC, Sudkamp NP. Acute compartment syndrome of the limb. *Injury* 2004;35:1221–1227.

Malinoski DJ, Slater MS, Mullins RJ. Crush injury and rhabdomyolysis. *Crit Care Clin* 2004;20:171–192.

Rozycki GS, Tremblay LN, Feliciano DV, et al. Blunt vascular trauma in the extremity: diagnosis, management, and outcome. *J Trauma* 2003;55:814–824.

Wallin D, Yaghoubian A, Rosing D, et al. Computed tomographic angiography as the primary diagnostic modality in penetrating lower extremity vascular injuries: a level I trauma experience. *Ann Vasc Surg* 2011;25:620–623.

33 Burns/Inhalation Injury

James H. Holmes IV

I. INTRODUCTION

A. Epidemiology

1. Approximately 45,000 people in the United States require hospitalization each year for burn injuries, with 10% suffering a concomitant inhalation injury.
2. Overall mortality rate is 4%, with the LD_{50} (50% lethal dose) occurring at 70% total body surface area (TBSA).
3. Most burn deaths occur in residential fires and nearly half are smoking-related or due to substance abuse.
4. Suspect abuse and report when seeing a patient with unusual burns like a child (e.g., immersion burns, odd shape/distribution, recurrent injuries, etc.), or when the history and injury do not match (see Chapter 21).
5. Approximately 5% of burn patients have concomitant non-thermal injuries.

B. Transfer to burn center

1. American Burn Association (ABA) criteria for transfer to a dedicated burn center:
   a. Partial-thickness burns >10% TBSA
   b. Burns involving the face, ears, hands, feet, genitalia, perineum, or major joints
   c. Full-thickness burns of any size
   d. Electrical burns or injuries, including lightning
   e. Chemical burns
   f. Inhalation injury
   g. Burns in patients with preexisting medical conditions
   h. Burns associated with concomitant non-thermal trauma in which the burn injury poses the greatest risk of morbidity or mortality
   i. Burned children in hospitals without qualified personnel
   j. Burns in patients requiring special social, emotional, or long-term rehabilitation interventions

II. PREHOSPITAL

A. History

1. Time of injury (start time for calculating fluid resuscitation)
2. Open or closed space (inhalation injury is more likely in closed space)
3. Source of burn: Flame, liquid, steam, chemical, explosion, electrical
4. Duration of exposure
5. Mechanism of any associated injury: Motor vehicle crash (MVC), fall, etc.
6. Quantity of prehospital fluid

B. Care at scene

1. Safely remove patient from source of injury.
2. Extinguish flames and remove clothing.
3. Burn patients are trauma patients and receive full evaluation until proven otherwise.
4. Assess for immediate life-threatening injuries, as per advanced trauma life support (ATLS) and advanced burn life support (ABLS).
5. Provide supplemental oxygen and airway protection.
6. Apply dry dressings.
7. Maintain normothermia.
8. Initiate transport to hospital.

III. INITIAL ASSESSMENT AND RESUSCITATION

A. General

1. Burn injury can be dramatic and distract the resuscitation team from concomitant non-thermal injuries.
2. Patients with severe burn injury may appear **deceptively stable on arrival.** A patient may be talking on admission with stable blood pressure and mild tachycardia. Within 24 hours, the patient is frequently critically ill.
3. Provide early pain control with frequent small doses of intravenous (IV) opiates.
4. Elevate the ambient room temperature to avoid heat loss from the burn wound.
5. Burns are tetanus-prone and mandate prophylaxis.

B. Airway

1. **Note:** Although urgent endotracheal intubation is sometimes necessary, time usually exists to assess the airway and provide a semi-elective intubation, when necessary.
2. Provide supplemental oxygen to all patients.
3. Criteria for intubation are the same as in all trauma patients. The following clinical conditions may require immediate or early intubation in a burn patient:
   a. Apnea, respiratory failure, or profound hypoxia.
   b. Patients with severe facial burns may appear initially stable. Consider semi-elective intubation because profound orofacial swelling over the next few hours can make intubation very difficult.
   c. Signs and symptoms of inhalation injury:
      i. Injuries sustained in a closed-space fire
      ii. Carbon deposits in the naso/oropharynx
      iii. Expectorated, carbonaceous sputum
      iv. Wheezing
      v. Hoarseness
      vi. Stridor
      vii. $PaO_2:FiO_2$ <300
   d. Upper airway injury and obstruction frequently occur in patients with burns of the face and neck. Soft-tissue swelling of the face, oropharynx, glottis, and trachea can be dramatic, precluding safe intubation and making cricothyroidotomy/tracheostomy difficult. Any patient with phonation changes or stridor should be considered for immediate intubation.

C. Breathing

1. If intubated, deliver 100% oxygen (generally with 5 to 10 cm H_2O of positive end-expiratory pressure [PEEP]) with a goal to avoid high airway pressures while maintaining patient comfort. Perform arterial blood gasses (ABGs) to ensure adequate oxygenation, ventilation, and clearance of acidosis.
2. Perform a chest radiograph to look for associated trauma, early signs of inhalation injury, and position of tubes/lines.
3. Bronchoscopy may be necessary to assess inhalation injury.
4. Circumferential torso burns causing elevated airway pressures may require escharotomy. **Note:** Patients without complete circumferential torso burns may also require escharotomy to provide adequate ventilation at lower airway pressures.

D. Circulation

1. **Intravenous access** is ideally obtained with large-bore (14 to 16 gauge in adults) peripheral catheters placed through unburned tissue. In severe burns (>30% TBSA), it is optimal to obtain central venous access early before massive swelling and edema occur. Placement through burned tissue is acceptable, if it is the only option.
2. **Initial fluid resuscitation**
   a. Typically, only burns ≥20% TBSA in adults require formal IV fluid resuscitation.
   b. Start with and use only **Lactated Ringer's (LR).** Do not use normal saline (NS), as profound hypernatremia and hyperchloremia may result when a large burn resuscitation is completely done with NS.

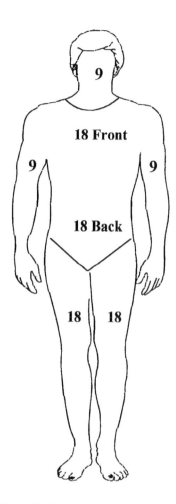

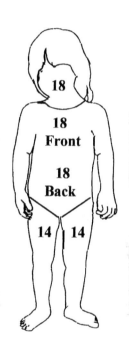

Figure 33-1. Rule of nines.

    c. The **Parkland/Baxter formula (4 mL LR/kg body weight/% TBSA burn)** is used to guide initial resuscitation.

    d. How to use the Parkland/Baxter formula:

        i. The formula is only a guide for fluid requirements in the first 24 hours following injury. Fluid resuscitation should be adjusted based on the patient's physiologic response to treatment, notably urine output and blood pressure.

        ii. Only partial- and full-thickness burns (aka second and third degree) are included in the TBSA estimation.

        iii. TBSA is determined by the rule of nines (Fig. 33-1) or age-appropriate burn diagrams.

        iv. Give one-half of the calculated requirement in the first 8 hours from the time of injury. The second half is given over the subsequent 16 hours.

        v. The first 8 hours begin at the time of burn, not at the time the patient is first seen.

vi. For example, a 35% TBSA burn in a 70 kg person gets 9,800 mL LR over 24 hours, 4,900 mL over the first 8 hours (613 mL/hour), and 4,900 over subsequent 16 hours (306 mL/hour).

vii. Once started, use urine output to guide the fluid rate to obtain 30 to 50 mL/hour in an adult.

viii. In the second 24 hours post-burn, a patient's maintenance fluid requirements are ~1.5 to 2 times normal maintenance fluid volumes. This volume should be given as crystalloid, with the composition of the fluid determined by serum electrolyte levels. Any colloid supplementation (i.e., albumin) should occur >24 hours post-burn.

e. A subset of patients (inhalation injury, high-voltage electrical, delayed resuscitation, massive deep burns) may require additional fluid over that estimated by the Parkland/Baxter formula. Hemoconcentration (i.e., hematocrit >55%) may be an early clue to increased fluid requirements.

f. Any patient who does not respond with adequate urine output during the first few hours of resuscitation, is elderly, or has a history of cardiopulmonary/renal disease may require a more formal goal-directed resuscitation, guided by any of the various means of invasive hemodynamic monitoring.

E. Pediatric fluid resuscitation (infants and toddlers <20 kg)

1. The head and neck represent larger proportions of calculated TBSA than in adults (Fig. 33-1 and Table 33-1).

2. Careful fluid resuscitation is necessary to avoid:
  a. Pulmonary edema from excessive fluid administration
  b. Cerebral edema associated with hyponatremia

3. Formula for estimated fluid = **dextrose-based maintenance + 3 mL/kg/% TBSA LR over 24 hours**

TABLE 33-1 **General Body Differences: Children Versus Adults**

Factor	Difference
Size and shape	■ Less fat and connective tissue available for protection. ■ Energy is transferred and dispersed over a smaller body surface area. ■ Internal organs are in relatively close proximity, which predisposes to multiple organ injuries. ■ Solid organs are larger compared with the rest of the abdomen. ■ Rib cage is higher, affording less protection to abdominal organs. ■ The infant's head is disproportionately larger compared with the adult and subjected to a high incidence of shear injuries.
Skeleton	■ Incomplete ossification of bones causes them to be more pliable and thus less likely to fracture. As a result, pulmonary contusions and splenic lacerations often occur without rib fractures. ■ A different array of partial fractures (e.g., greenstick, torus, and buckle fractures). ■ Injuries to the growth plates during the various stages of childhood development result in a specific pattern of fractures.
Surface area	■ Large surface-area-to-weight ratio results in a greater predisposition to heat loss (three times greater) and hypothermia.
Psychological development	■ Children often regress to a previous developmental stage during stressful and anxiety-provoking situations.
Long-term effects of injury	■ Splenectomy in children places them at lifelong risk for overwhelming postsplenectomy infection (OPSI).

a. Maintenance volume is pro-rated over 24 hours.
b. One half of burn component in first 8 hours, and second half over ensuing 16 hours.
c. For example: A 3-year-old male weighing 20 kg with a 35% TBSA burn would require 2,100 cc LR and 1,500 cc D51/2NS with 40 mEq KCl/L over the first 24 hours following injury. The LR would be administered at 130 cc/hr for the first 8 hours and then at 65 cc/hr for the subsequent 16 hours, while the D51/2NS would run continuously at 60 cc/hr.
4. Goal is a well-perfused child with a urine output of 1.0 to 1.5 mL/kg/hour.

IV. INITIAL WOUND ASSESSMENT AND MANAGEMENT
A. Assessment
1. The TBSA of any burn is best estimated by **age-appropriate diagrams.** The rule of nines (Fig. 33-1) provides an initial approximation of burn size in adults. Further, for all individuals, the palmar surface of the entire hand (palm + digits) represents 1% TBSA and may be helpful in estimating the size of smaller burns.
2. Terminology for burn depth using "degree" has been replaced by the description of "thickness." Classification of depth at the time of admission is an estimate and may be inaccurate because severe burns tend to progress or evolve over the 12 to 72 hours following injury.
3. **Burn depth** (Fig. 33-2)
   a. Superficial (first degree, such as sunburn)
      i. Confined to epidermis with minimal tissue damage.
      ii. Mild erythema, pain resolving in 48 to 72 hours.
      iii. Epidermis may peel in small scales without scarring.
   b. Partial-thickness (second degree)
      i. Involves entire epidermis with variable layers of dermis.
       a) Superficial partial-thickness
        1) Painful, pink, edematous, and **blistered**
        2) Spontaneous healing in <2 to 3 weeks

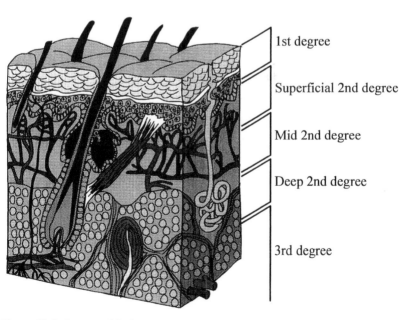

1st degree

Superficial 2nd degree

Mid 2nd degree

Deep 2nd degree

3rd degree

Figure 33-2. Burn wound depth.

   b) Deep partial-thickness
    1) Red or mottled red and white, often dry, **pinprick perceived as pressure rather than pain,** +/− blisters
    2) Prolonged healing without excision and grafting, usually with scarring

  c. Full-thickness (third degree)
   i. Entire epidermis and dermis destroyed
   ii. Relatively **painless,** leathery, waxy, or charred, sometimes with visible **thrombosed vessels**
   iii. Require excision and grafting for optimal outcome

B. Initial burn wound management
 1. Systemic prophylactic antibiotics are not indicated.
 2. In the emergency department (ED) before transport to a burn center:
  a. Wash gently with gauze soaked in saline.
  b. Remove any obviously loose skin.
  c. Apply topical agents (Section IV.B.4) only if anticipated delay in transfer, because removal of the agent at the burn center can prolong the initial assessment and is associated with increased pain.
  d. Irrigate debris from the eyes, as needed.
  e. Cover wounds with dry sterile dressings.
  f. Provide tetanus prophylaxis, as indicated.
 3. At the **burn center** or **definitive care hospital:**
  a. Burns <10% TBSA can be cleansed, locally debrided of all *loose* non-viable skin, and covered with a topical agent.
  b. Treat larger burns by placing the patient in a special gurney (usually located in the burn unit), which allows total exposure, overhead heating, rapid burn wound debridement by a specially trained team, cleansing using gentle irrigation, provision of adequate analgesia, and continuous monitoring of vital signs.
 4. Topical agents
  a. Silver sulfadiazine 1% cream (Silvadene, Hoechst Marion Roussel, Inc., Kansas City, Mo)
   i. Most common topical agent used on burn wounds.
   ii. Usually applied daily or twice daily in a thick layer, followed by wrapping loosely with sterile gauze.
   iii. Broad-spectrum, bacteriostatic, painless and usually soothing, with antifungal activity.
   iv. Transient neutropenia (sulfa effect) can occur—typically of no clinical consequence.
   v. Caution in pregnancy and very small infants (<2 months).
  b. Mafenide acetate cream or **5% solution** (Sulfamylon, Mylan Pharmaceuticals, Canonsburg, PA)
   i. Penetrates eschar, somewhat painful (cream >>solution)
   ii. Occasional, clinically inconsequential, mild metabolic acidosis (carbonic anhydrase inhibitor effect)
   iii. Broad-spectrum, bacteriostatic, no antifungal activity
  c. Bacitracin ointment
   i. Ointment (not cream) usually applied to smaller burns and surfaces difficult to cover with gauze (e.g., face)
   ii. May require several applications per day
   iii. Primarily bacteriostatic against gram-positive organisms
   iv. Neosporin, Polysporin, or gentamicin ointments can be substituted for broader bacterial coverage.
  d. Silver impregnated dressings (multiple formulations and material scaffolds)
   i. Left in place on the wound for 3 to 14 days, depending on the formulation and indication
   ii. Useful for outpatient burn management and donor site dressings

e. Silver nitrate 0.5% solution
    i. Broad-spectrum, bacteriostatic, antifungal activity
    ii. Costly, messy, electrolyte abnormalities (e.g., hyponatremia)
5. **Escharotomy**
    a. Circumferential **full-thickness** burns of the **trunk** or **extremities** can cause compartment syndrome.
    b. **Elevated airway pressures** in a circumferential torso burn mandate escharotomy, as do **diminished or absent distal pulses** in a circumferential extremity burn.
    c. Unless transport to definitive care is to be delayed or the patient deteriorates, escharotomies can typically wait to be done at the burn center.
    d. Technique (Fig. 33-3)

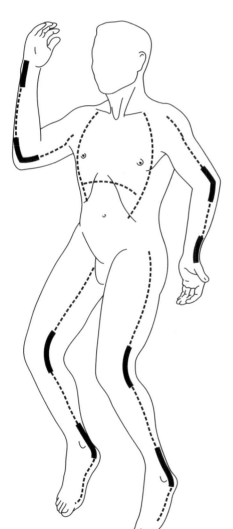

Figure 33-3. Preferred sites for escharotomy. (From Martin RR, Becker WK, Cioffi WG, et al. In: Wilson RF, ed. *Management of Trauma: Pitfalls and Practice.* Baltimore, MD: Williams & Wilkins, 1996, with permission.)

      i. In theory, bloodless and painless **(usually not the case).**

      ii. Provide adequate and appropriate analgesia and sedation.

      iii. Cleanse involved area

      iv. Perform with electrocautery, when available, or knife with topical hemostatic agents.

      v. Divide the eschar only, not the subcutaneous tissues or fascia.

      vi. Not a sterile procedure, which can be done in any clean medical treatment area.

      vii. Inadequate hemostasis with multiple escharotomies can result in significant blood loss, which can be troublesome if the patient is going to be transferred subsequent to the procedure.

V. INHALATION INJURY

A. Overview

1. Results from **direct thermal injury** (inhalation of superheated steam), or the inhalation of **toxic chemicals** in smoke, or a combination of both.
2. Injury to the proximal airway can cause rapid edema and obstruction.
3. Chemical irritants stimulate an intense inflammatory response in the more distal airways. The history of the environment of injury may be predictive of the extent of injury (e.g., closed space, incomplete combustion, etc.).
4. Inhalation injury is the **most frequent cause of death** in thermal injuries.

B. Evaluation

1. Consider present in all burn patients exposed to closed-space fires, until ruled out.
2. Signs and symptoms are outlined in Section III.B.
3. Obtain a **carboxyhemoglobin (COHb)** level with initial laboratory studies.
   - **a.** Carbon monoxide (CO) has 200 times the affinity for Hb than does O_2.
   - **b.** Elimination half-life ($t_{1/2}$) of CO breathing 100% O_2 is ~1 hour, while breathing room air it is ~4 hours.
   - **c.** COHb levels and clinical findings of CO poisoning:
     - **i.** <5%—normal
     - **ii.** <20%—usually asymptomatic
     - **iii.** 20% to 30%—headache, nausea/vomiting, loss of manual dexterity
     - **iv.** 30% to 40%—confusion, weakness, lethargy
     - **v.** 40% to 60%—coma
     - **vi.** >60%—death
   - **d.** Can occur as isolated CO poisoning. In the presence of thermal injury, an elevated COHb diagnoses an associated inhalation injury.
   - **e. A normal COHb level does not rule out inhalation injury.**
   - **f. Note:** Pulse oximetry (SpO_2) is inaccurate with CO poisoning.
4. Initial chest radiograph may be normal.
5. **Bronchoscopy**
   - **a.** An elective procedure that is delayed until the resuscitation is complete and the patient is stable.
   - **b.** If the patient is not intubated, thread an endotracheal tube onto the scope so that a definitive airway can be obtained if bronchoscopic findings warrant or the airway becomes threatened with instrumentation.
   - **c.** Positive findings include infraglottic erythema, edema, ulcerations, carbonaceous material, and/or mucosal sloughing.
   - **d.** Bronchoscopy has no material effect on outcome.

C. Treatment

1. Administer 100% oxygen to all patients until inhalation injury is excluded or the COHb is normal.
2. Early intubation and mechanical ventilation is recommended for symptomatic patients, as previously described.
3. Hyperbaric oxygen treatment is indicated for isolated CO poisoning with abnormal sensorium or ischemic chest pain. Those burn patients with CO

poisoning must be resuscitated and stable before any hyperbaric oxygen treatment.

VI. ELECTRICAL INJURY

A. Overview

1. Electrical injuries are uncommon and present a diagnostic challenge because of myriad clinical presentations. Small skin wounds can hide substantial underlying muscle and bony destruction.
   a. History of the event and voltage exposure are potentially crucial diagnostic factors.
2. Generally, electrical injuries are classified as low voltage ($<1,000$ volts) or high voltage ($\geq 1,000$ volts).
3. Severity of injury depends on the amperage of the current and the resistance of the tissue ($V = IR$).
4. The tissues with the greatest resistance tend to sustain the most heat damage. Tissue resistance in decreasing order is as follows.
   a. Bone $\rightarrow$ fat $\rightarrow$ tendon $\rightarrow$ skin $\rightarrow$ muscle $\rightarrow$ blood vessel $\rightarrow$ nerve.
      i. High voltage does not necessarily respect this hierarchy and usually destroys all tissues in its path.
   b. Wet skin has much less resistance than dry skin.
5. The pathway of current is unpredictable, but generally passes between two contact points: From the point of entry through the body to a grounded site (site with the lowest resistance). However, with high voltage, the pathway may be indiscriminate, exiting at multiple sites.
6. In general, alternating current (AC) is more dangerous than direct current (DC).
7. Electrical injuries may have associated serious traumatic injuries (e.g., fractures, dislocations, falls).

B. Low-voltage injury

1. Usually occurs in the home.
2. Cardiac **dysrhythmias** are common, particularly ventricular fibrillation.
3. Tetanic skeletal muscle contractions (AC household current) can cause fractures or dislocations and respiratory arrest.
4. Admit for telemetry monitoring if any EKG abnormalities are encountered. Otherwise analgesics and discharge are appropriate, unless burns are significant.
5. Wound management
   a. Topical antimicrobials and simple dressings.
   b. Excision and grafting, as warranted.
6. **Oral burns in children**
   a. Small children sucking on an electrical cord or plug.
   b. Can involve all oral structures, but most commonly the **lip.**
   c. Treatment includes:
      i. Hospitalization may be required because of feeding difficulties.
      ii. Feed by straw or syringe; rarely is nasogastric access required.
      iii. Delayed debridement.
      iv. Intraoral splint may be necessary.
      v. Tetanus prophylaxis.

C. High-voltage injury

1. The extent of tissue damage is typically underestimated because of the unpredictable path of injury. These are usually devastating injuries.
2. An associated flash-flame cutaneous burn is not uncommon and can distract from the more devastating electrical injury to the deeper and remote tissues.
3. The deep injury is characterized by myonecrosis, especially along deeper tissues adjacent to bone (high resistance area). Vessel thrombosis, compartment syndrome (both early and delayed), and nerve entrapment syndromes (both early and delayed) are common sequelae.
4. Fluid management
   a. Anticipate need for >4 mL/kg/% TBSA.

    b. If **myoglobinuria** present, ensure urine output >100 mL/hour via fluid loading and mannitol (rarely) if fluids are inadequate.

5. Wound management

    a. Extremity fasciotomy frequently required.

    b. Early, aggressive, and repetitive wound excisions and debridements.

    c. Because of the variable tissue necrosis, amputation of a devitalized extremity may be necessary (even in the presence of adequate blood supply).

6. General management

    a. Tetanus prophylaxis

    b. Effective pain management

    c. Topical antimicrobials to thermal injury only

    d. Anticipate the need for ventilatory support and probable organ dysfunction.

7. After initial resuscitation started, all patients with high-voltage injury should be transferred to a burn center.

VII. CHEMICAL BURNS

A. Overview

1. Occur from either acids or alkalis.

2. The extent of injury depends on the concentration of agent and duration of contact.

3. Tissue damage is frequently underestimated.

4. Alkali burns are generally more severe than acid burns (latter liquefies tissues and limits penetration).

B. Treatment

1. All providers should wear protective gowns, gloves, and eyewear/face shield.

2. Remove all garments and brush off any dry powder.

3. In the field and on arrival, **copiously irrigate with tepid tap water** for at least 15 minutes (avoid hypothermia).

4. Decontamination can occur in formal "decon" facilities at a hospital or in a simple shower. The critical element, thorough decontamination with copious water, is the most important initial treatment.

5. Irrigate the eyes and obtain an ophthalmology consult, as needed.

6. No specific antidote is available for most chemical burns (except hydrofluoric acid) and **neutralizers are contraindicated.**

C. Hydrofluoric acid (HF) burn

1. Highly toxic and painful.

2. Can cause hypocalcemia and dysrhythmias with systemic absorption.

3. Concentration >40% can be lethal if >2% TBSA is involved.

4. Treatment:

    a. Copious irrigation with water.

    b. Apply 2.5% calcium gluconate gel.

    c. Soft-tissue injection of calcium gluconate (1 g/10 mL) can be done in small areas for cases of persistent pain. Intra-arterial infusion of calcium gluconate may be indicated for selected finger and hand HF burns with limited tissue space for injection.

    d. Indications for intra-arterial infusion of calcium gluconate include severe pain, evidence of tissue necrosis, and pain not improving with calcium gluconate gel.

    e. Method for intra-arterial calcium gluconate infusion:

        i. Place a brachial artery catheter and perform angiogram to ensure adequacy of perfusion to involved fingers (a high brachial artery bifurcation is not uncommon).

        ii. Alternatively, a radial artery catheter can be used depending upon the digits involved. Check collateral circulation using Allen's test prior to catheter placement (recognizing the test is imperfect).

        iii. Infuse calcium gluconate (2 g) in D5W (100 mL) over 4 hours.

        iv. Repeat every 4 hours until pain is markedly decreased.

    f. Monitor serum electrolytes and treat abnormalities.

VIII. DEFINITIVE CARE OF THE BURN PATIENT

A. Burn wound

1. The depth of the burn wound may be obvious early. However, several days may be required to differentiate between superficial and deep partial-thickness wounds.
2. The best diagnostic tools are the eyes of a surgeon experienced in burn wound care.
3. Superficial (first degree) wounds require only cleansing and analgesia.
4. Superficial partial-thickness (second degree) wounds can heal spontaneously with cleansing, topical antibiotics (e.g., silver sulfadiazine), and analgesia.
   a. The appearance of epithelial "budding" is a useful predictor of primary healing, but is also associated with a transient increase in nocioception.
   b. Two or three weeks are usually required for epithelialization.
5. Deep partial-thickness (second degree) and full-thickness (third degree) wounds usually require excision and grafting to provide coverage and optimal healing.
6. Topical creams and ointments are applied once or twice daily with dressing changes, whereas solutions are applied to dressings every 4 to 8 hours.

B. Perioperative management

1. Perioperative antibiotic prophylaxis is indicated for excision and grafting procedures.
2. Counsel patients early of the eventuality of multiple skin grafts being harvested from varied areas, depending upon the extent of their injury.

C. Excision

1. **Small wounds** (<20% TBSA) typically can be excised and covered with a split-thickness autograft (STAG) as soon as the patient is stable.
2. **Larger wounds** (>20% TBSA) usually require staged excisions and placement of either temporary or permanent wound coverage.
3. A variety of dermatomes and free hand knives are available for excision.
4. **Tangential excision** (most common) attempts to remove only devitalized tissue and retain as many dermal elements as possible.
   a. Variable amounts of subcutaneous fat may be visible.
   b. Although fat can decrease the likelihood of graft success, it helps maintain cosmesis.
5. **Fascial excision** may be necessary in full-thickness burns with underlying fat necrosis.
   a. Although associated with less blood loss than tangential excision, the cosmetic outcome is typically inferior.

D. Wound coverage

1. Currently, the best permanent coverage for burn wounds is a STAG.
2. STAGs are typically harvested at 0.008 to 0.012 in. thick and can be variably meshed to increase coverage.
3. The graft must be secured to the wound, covered with a non-adherent dressing, and further dressed to protect from mechanical injury.
4. Protective positioning and splinting of the patient may be necessary.
5. Negative pressure wound dressings (e.g., V.A.C., KCI, and San Antonio, Texas) work well on burns.
6. The graft is usually inspected at 5 to 7 days (3 to 5 days with V.A.C.), unless signs of infection prompt an earlier evaluation.
7. **Temporary coverage** of the excised burn wound with cadaver skin, pigskin, or synthetic materials may be helpful in the following clinical circumstances:
   a. Inadequate autologous donor skin
   b. Uncertainty of the viability of the wound bed (i.e., potential need for further excisions)
   c. Need to reduce hypermetabolism resulting from the open wound
   d. To provide patient comfort
8. **Dermal substitutes,** which allow for the creation of a "neo-dermis" populated with autologous mesenchymal cells and extracellular matrix, are typically

reserved for larger burns. Integra (Integra LifeSciences, Plainsboro, NJ), Alloderm (Lifecell, Branchburg, NJ), and Dermagraft (Advanced Tissue Sciences, La Jolla, CA) are currently available, with Integra being the only one indicated for burns and most widely used.

   a. Allow for excision and coverage of the entire burn irrespective of available donor sites (except Alloderm).
   b. Employ epidermal autografts (0.006 to 0.008 in.) for definitive coverage, which allows earlier re-harvesting of potentially limited donor sites and subsequently earlier permanent coverage for a given burn.
   c. Require additional, staged operation(s), except for Alloderm that is designed to be immediately grafted on application.
   d. Successful use is associated with a learning curve and clinical results are invariably, user-dependent.
   e. Apparent improvements in functional and cosmetic outcomes are achieved with Integra.
9. Cultured epithelial autografts (CEAs: Epicel, Genzyme, Boston, MA), although fragile and very expensive, have been used to provide permanent coverage in massive burns where no autologous alternatives are available.

E. Critical care
1. Most critical care management parallels that of the trauma patient (Chapters 34 to 38).
2. Intensive care unit (ICU) issues specific to the burn patient include:
   a. The presence of inhalation injury and face/neck burns often requires a more prolonged approach to ventilator withdrawal and extubation than with other trauma patients.
   b. In major burns (>20% TBSA), the analgesia requirements for twice-daily dressing changes and sequential operative excisions are often high. Burns are painful.
   c. A warm environment will help prevent heat loss from wounds.
   d. The burn patient has a high metabolic rate even after the wounds are definitively covered, requiring ~2,000 kcal/m^2/day with a protein requirement of ≥2.0 g/kg/day.
   e. Enteral nutrition is superior to parenteral support in improving outcome.
   f. Fever is common in burn patients, but does not necessarily mean an infection exists.
      i. If fever is accompanied by thrombocytopenia, feeding intolerance/ileus, or hyperglycemia/increasing insulin requirements, the chance of a significant infection being the source of the fever is significantly increased.
   g. Ionized hypocalcaemia is common in burn patients, especially during the initial resuscitation.
   h. Patients with major burns may develop an inability to concentrate their urine and may have an obligatory increased urine output. This usually occurs in the post-resuscitation, critical care phase of their injury and can be misinterpreted as a parameter of adequate perfusion.

F. Burn wound sepsis
1. In general, significant bacterial colonization of the wound does not occur prior to 72 hours following injury. However, soon thereafter, colonization occurs with endogenous and endemic organisms.
2. The most common organisms recovered from burn wounds include *Staphylococcus* sp., B-hemolytic *streptococcus, Pseudomonas aeruginosa, Escherichia coli, Enterococcus* sp., and *Candida albicans.*
3. Invasive infection (vs. colonization) is best diagnosed by a burn wound biopsy and quantitative culture demonstrating >10^5 organisms/g of tissue.
   a. Early burn wound sepsis (first week) is usually caused by *S. aureus* (mortality ~5%).
   b. Later burn wound sepsis (7 to 10 days) is usually caused by *P. aeruginosa* (mortality ~20% to 30%).

c. *C. albicans* is another cause of later burn wound sepsis with a more insidious onset (high mortality ~30% to 50%).

4. The best **prevention and treatment** is the application of topical antibiotics combined with early excision and grafting of the wound. Prophylactic, systemic antibiotics are not effective because of the diminished/absent blood flow to the burn eschar. However, targeted antimicrobial therapy is indicated for burn wound sepsis suspected by clinical examination and diagnosed by wound biopsy with quantitative culture. Burn wound sepsis also mandates immediate excision, or even re-excision, if the patient is unstable.

G. Rehabilitation

1. Rehabilitation of the burn patient is one of the most challenging clinical issues in modern medicine because the process is life-long and the scars are permanent.

2. Rehabilitation should begin with admission and include the following components:

a. Early wound closure
b. Exercise
c. Positioning and splinting
d. Skin care
e. Thermoregulation
f. Psychological support
g. Restoration of function

3. Chapter 20 discusses rehabilitation after trauma.

AXIOMS

■ Patients sustaining burns in a closed space (e.g., building, mobile home, automobile, etc.) have an inhalation injury until proven otherwise.

■ Early intubation is wise for patients with significant orofacial burns or possible inhalation injury.

■ Burns often present as dramatic injuries; therefore, it is imperative to perform primary and secondary surveys to assess for concomitant non-thermal trauma.

■ After the initial resuscitation is started, burn patients meeting ABA criteria should be transferred to a dedicated burn center.

■ Singed nasal hairs are NOT associated with inhalation injury.

■ Document the time of burn injury and the amount of fluid infused before arrival at a hospital or burn center.

■ Formulas for fluid requirements are guides to resuscitation; adequate urine output is the best clinical measure of adequate volume resuscitation.

■ The initial calculation of TBSA, using the rule of nines, is designed to be an estimate of only partial- and full-thickness burns.

■ Definitive care of the deep partial- and full-thickness burn wound usually requires excision and grafting with STAG.

Suggested Readings

American Burn Association (www.ameriburn.org)
American Burn Association, National Burn Repository 2011, Version 7.0 (www.ameriburn.org/2011 NBRAnnualReport.pdf)
Greenhalgh DG, Saffle JR, Holmes JH 4th, et al. American Burn Association consensus conference to define sepsis and infection in burns: special report. *J Burn Care Res* 2007;28(6):776–790.
Sheridan RL. Burns. *Crit Care Med* 2002;30(suppl.):S500–S514.
UpToDate 19.3 (www.uptodate.com)

Priorities in the ICU Care of the Adult Trauma Patient

Philip S. Barie and Soumitra R. Eachempati

I. GOALS OF CARE

A. Fundamental goals of intensive care unit (ICU) management of the critically injured patient include early restoration and maintenance of tissue oxygenation, diagnosis and treatment of occult injuries, and prevention and treatment of infection and organ dysfunction.

B. Most early deaths from trauma occur from traumatic brain injury (TBI), exsanguination, or refractory shock, and are largely not preventable. Late deaths from multiple organ dysfunction syndrome (MODS) may be minimized by effective resuscitation, prevention or prompt recognition and treatment of hospital-acquired infection, identification and treatment of all injuries, and avoidance of error. Errors of surgical technique and critical care management may contribute to one-half of preventable trauma deaths.

C. Optimal trauma care in the ICU is provided by a multi-professional team of physicians, nurses, pharmacists, therapists, and others. An ICU environment where communication, patient safety, and infection control are innate to the culture creates conditions for the optimal care of the patient.

II. ICU ADMISSION CRITERIA.
The decision to admit the trauma patient to an ICU depends on the patient's age, injury severity, co-morbid conditions, and availability of both ICU beds and intermediate-level care ("step-down") beds (Table 34-1).

III. PHASES OF ICU CARE

A. Early phase (<24 hours). Primary concerns include shock, respiratory failure, intracranial hypertension, and the identification of occult injuries; diagnosis and treatment occur simultaneously.

1. Repetition of the primary survey. Repetition of the evaluation of the trauma patient is essential, beginning with the primary survey and followed by repeated secondary surveys.

a. Airway. The airway should be secured and positioned appropriately.

b. Breathing. Minute ventilation (V_E) must be adequate. The inspired oxygen concentration (FiO_2) must be adequate to maintain arterial oxygen saturation (SaO_2) above 90%.

c. Circulation. Intravenous access must be adequate for the administration of fluids, blood, and blood products sufficient to support the circulation, gas exchange, and hemostasis. If adequate peripheral venous access is unobtainable, insert a central venous catheter. If the circulation cannot be monitored adequately by heart rate, blood pressure, and urine output, assess acid–base status and consider non-invasive (e.g., esophageal Doppler probe, thoracic impedance or bioreactance, or echocardiography) or invasive hemodynamic monitoring.

d. Disability. The Glasgow Coma Scale (GCS) score is compared with initial observations for signs of neurologic deterioration or improvement. All limbs are re-inspected for deformity, abnormal or absent movement, abnormal sensation (if possible), and signs of vascular insufficiency. The level of sedation is assessed, and short-acting sedatives are given by titration to a validated sedation scale (e.g., Ramsay) to protect the patient from self-harm.

TABLE 34-1	Injuries and Post-injury Problems that Require ICU Admission

Injuries
- Multi-system trauma
- Severe TBI (GCS ≥8)
  - Lesser TBIs of anticoagulated patients (e.g., aspirin, warfarin)
- Cervical spinal cord injury
- Severe pulmonary contusion, flail chest
- Facial or neck trauma with threatened airway
- Repaired major vascular injuries
- Pelvic fracture with retroperitoneal hemorrhage or bony instability
- Blunt cardiac trauma with dysrhythmia or hypotension
- Crush injuries
- Severe burns (>20% TBSA, facial burns)
- Smoke inhalation
- Isolated high-grade solid organ injuries (grade III–V liver or spleen)

Problems
- Respiratory failure requiring mechanical ventilation
- Ongoing shock or hemodynamic instability
- Massive blood or fluid resuscitation
- Base deficit (>5)
- Hypothermia
- Seizures
- Pregnancy

Post-traumatic Injuries or Problems Suitable for Intermediate Care Monitoring[a]
- Isolated liver or spleen injuries (especially grade I–II)
- Uncomplicated blunt anterior chest trauma
- Isolated multiple rib fractures or pulmonary contusion with adequate oxygenation and ventilation
- Isolated thoracic spinal cord injury with stable hemodynamics
- Lesser TBI (GCS 9–14)
- Minor injuries with risk of alcohol withdrawal syndrome
- Isolated vascular injuries to the extremities

[a]Patients ≥65 years of age with co-morbidity or any hemodynamic instability should be considered for ICU admission.
ICU, intensive care unit; TBI, traumatic brain injury; GCS, Glasgow Coma Scale score; TBSA, total body surface area.

    e. Environmental. Core body temperature is determined and hypothermia (T <35°C) is treated or prevented.
  2. Repetition of the secondary survey. Examination of laboratory and radiologic data are reviewed to identify missed injuries, most often of the spinal column or spinal cord, bone or ligament injuries of the extremities, and injuries of the thoracic aorta, heart, or diaphragm. Seek abdominal compartment syndrome by urinary bladder pressure measurement in the appropriate clinical context.
B. Intermediate phase (24 to 72 hours). From 24 to 72 hours post-injury, all injuries should have been identified, but resuscitation may be ongoing. Management of respiratory failure and intracranial hypertension following TBI may be particularly active during the first 72 hours.
C. Late phase (>72 hours). Approximately one-half of critically injured patients remain in the ICU for more than 72 hours. Priorities are defined by injury severity, the prevention of complications, and management of complications that do arise. Prolonged ICU care carries risks of physical de-conditioning, hospital-acquired infection (Chapter 14), pressure ulcers, and organ dysfunction.

D. Recovery phase. In this phase (regardless of timing), patients are liberated from life support and prepared for the transition to lower levels of care and eventual hospital discharge. At this time, disabilities may become apparent, and physical therapy, assessment of long-term rehabilitation needs and potential and psychological support of patient and family are crucial. Approximately 4% of injured patients remain in the ICU for more than 28 days, but the chance of survival to hospital discharge is still >50%.

IV. **RESUSCITATION AND INITIAL MANAGEMENT.** To maximize chances for survival, treatment priorities must focus on resuscitation from shock (defined as O_2 delivery [DO_2]) inadequate to meet O_2 demand (O_2 consumption [VO_2]), including appropriate fluid resuscitation and rapid, definitive hemostasis. Inadequate oxygenation results in anaerobic metabolism and tissue acidosis. The depth and duration of shock leads to a cumulative oxygen "debt" that may not be "repayable" if profound or delayed. Traditional markers of "successful" resuscitation include normalization of blood pressure, heart rate, and urine output. However, occult, ongoing hypoperfusion and lactic acidosis (i.e., compensated shock) may persist despite normalization of vital signs. Prolonged hypoperfusion (and subsequent oxidant stress from re-perfusion) are associated with organ dysfunction and death.

A. Endpoints of resuscitation. When the traditional parameters remain abnormal (i.e., uncompensated shock), the need for additional resuscitation is clear. However, even after normalization, up to 85% of critically injured patients have evidence of hypoperfusion, whether metabolic acidosis, a persistent base deficit, or an elevated serum lactate concentration. Rapid recognition and reversal of this state are crucial to minimize the risk of organ dysfunction or death. Evidence-based guidelines for determining endpoints of resuscitation are provided in Table 34-2.

B. Hemostasis in resuscitation. Resuscitation from hemorrhagic shock is impossible without hemostasis. Withholding of fluid resuscitation may lead to exsanguination, whereas aggressive fluid resuscitation may raise blood pressure excessively or dilute clotting factors, leading to increased bleeding. Permissive hypotension may be beneficial until hemorrhage control occurs.

C. Classification of shock (Chapter 5)

1. Hypovolemic shock. Hypovolemia is the usual cause of hypotension or occult hypoperfusion in the early post-injury period, and may be caused by incomplete resuscitation, ongoing third-space fluid losses, or active hemorrhage. Failure to respond to volume replacement should stimulate a search for ongoing hemorrhage (the most likely cause) or other causes of shock.

2. Obstructive shock is a possible cause (e.g., cardiac tamponade, tension pneumothorax, abdominal compartment syndrome [ACS; abdominal hypertension from packing or over-resuscitation leading to decreased venous return], ventilation with high levels of positive end-expiratory pressure [PEEP], or rarely tension pneumopericardium) that should be sought.

3. Cardiogenic shock. Cardiogenic shock after trauma is usually caused by blunt myocardial injury, but the possibility of myocardial ischemia/infarction must be considered among older trauma patients. Blunt myocardial injury is excluded by an entirely normal electrocardiogram (ECG); with a normal ECG, cardiac enzyme determination is superfluous. Right ventricular function can be impaired by blunt myocardial injury, and is sensitive to volume repletion, followed by inotropic support if cardiac output is still inadequate. Cardiac valve injury is uncommon in patients surviving severe chest trauma, but may require immediate surgical repair. Suspect underlying valvular heart disease (e.g., aortic stenosis, mitral insufficiency) in older trauma patients with cardiogenic shock.

4. Neurogenic shock. Neurogenic shock can occur with spinal cord injury (or rarely with brain death). Affected spinal cord injury patients are usually paraplegic or quadriplegic. Autonomic dysfunction (loss of sympathetic tone) leads to vasodilation, a form of distributive shock (defined in the next paragraph). Once euvolemia is ensured with volume replacement, the treatment is primarily

TABLE 34-2	Guidelines for Endpoints of Resuscitation by the Eastern Association for the Surgery of Trauma

A. Recommendations Regarding Stratification of Physiologic Derangement

Level 1

1. Standard hemodynamic parameters do not quantify adequately the degree of physiologic derangement in trauma patients. The initial base deficit or lactate concentration can be used to stratify patients with regard to the need for ongoing fluid resuscitation, including red blood cell concentrates and other blood products, and the risks of organ dysfunction and death.

2. The ability of a patient to attain supranormal O_2 delivery parameters correlates with an improved chance for survival.

Level 2

1. The time to normalization of base deficit and lactate concentration is predictive of survival.

2. Persistently high or worsening base deficit may be an early indicator of complications (e.g., ongoing hemorrhage, abdominal compartment syndrome).

3. The predictive value of the base deficit may be limited by ethanol intoxication or a hyperchloremic metabolic acidosis, as well as administration of $NaHCO_3$.

Level 3

1. Right ventricular end diastolic volume index (RVEDVI) measurement may be a better indicator of adequate volume resuscitation (preload) than CVP or pulmonary artery occlusion pressure (PAOP).

2. Measurements of tissue (subcutaneous or muscle) O_2 or CO_2 concentration may identify patients who require additional resuscitation and are at risk for organ dysfunction and death.

3. Serum HCO_3 concentration may be substituted for base deficit.

B. Recommendations Regarding Improved Patient Outcomes

Level 1

1. There are insufficient data to formulate a Level 1 recommendation.

Level 2

1. The optimal algorithms for fluid resuscitation, blood product replacement, and the use of inotropes or vasopressors have not been determined.

(From Tisherman SA, Barie PS, Bokhari F, et al. Clinical practice guideline: Endpoints of resuscitation. *J Trauma* 2004;57:898–912.)

with a vasoconstrictor (e.g., phenylephrine). Hemodynamic instability may be prolonged, and vasopressor therapy may be required for days to weeks.

5. **Distributive shock.** Distributive shock is caused prototypically by sepsis and may develop late after injury. However, severely injured patients can demonstrate early a hyperdynamic state, similar to systemic inflammatory response syndrome (SIRS). A hyperdynamic circulation (cardiac index [CI] >3 $L/min/m^2$), hypotension, and low systemic vascular resistance (SVR <900 $dyne/s/cm^5$) are characteristic.

V. MONITORING AND DATA INTERPRETATION.
Additional monitoring is necessary to optimize DO_2 when clinical uncertainty exists, or when refractory hemodynamic instability or other factors confound the clinical assessment of the response to therapy. **Remember that such instability is due most commonly to ongoing blood loss.**

A. Blood testing. Blood sampling is essential for monitoring, but can be excessive. Blood removed for testing can exceed 70 mL/day.

1. Non-invasive hemodynamic monitoring, adoption of guidelines for diagnostic evaluation, and point-of-care (POC) testing can reduce blood testing while providing optimal patient care.

2. Glucose monitoring is the most prevalent example of POC testing, considering that targeted glycemic therapy to avoid excessive hyperglycemia reduces the risk of nosocomial infection, organ dysfunction, and death following trauma.

B. Blood gas monitoring. Blood gas analyzers measure directly the partial pressures of oxygen (pO_2) and carbon dioxide (pCO_2), and blood pH. SaO_2 is calculated from the pO_2, assuming a normal P_{50} (SaO_2 is 50% at a pO_2 of 26.6 mm Hg), and normal hemoglobin structure. Some analyzers incorporate co-oximetry to measure hemoglobin concentration directly. Bicarbonate and base excess are calculated from the pH and pCO_2.

C. Electrocardiography. ECG is standard; avoidance of tachycardia, especially in older patients, reduces morbidity. Tachycardia may be due to hypovolemia, hemorrhage, inadequate analgesia, or other causes. Tachycardia is inherently dangerous because of the risk of myocardial ischemia; however, routine ECG monitoring (four limb leads) is insensitive for detection of acute ST–T wave changes, which portends ischemia. A 12-lead ECG should be performed on patients suspected of myocardial ischemia, electrolyte abnormalities, blunt cardiac injury, or pericardial pathology.

  1. Perioperative mortality is decreased when beta-adrenergic blockade is started preoperatively before major elective general surgery in older patients, and recent data suggest the same to be true for elderly trauma and burns patients. Even if beta-blockade cannot be started before an emergency operation (e.g., uncorrected hypovolemia), it should be started as soon as possible thereafter, provided underlying hypovolemia, pain, or sepsis are controlled.

D. Pulse oximetry. Pulse oximetry is reasonably accurate over the range of SaO_2 between 70% and 100%, but less accurate below 70%. Pulsatile blood flow is essential for accurate pulse oximetry; reliable data can be obtained from the finger, earlobe, or forehead.

  1. Hypothermia, hypotension, hypovolemia, peripheral vascular disease, vasopressor therapy, ambient light, or motion artifact may cause inaccuracy.

  2. An elevated carboxyhemoglobin concentration will elevate S_pO_2 falsely because reflected light is absorbed at the same wavelength as oxyhemoglobin.

E. Temperature. The most reliable temperature measurement is core temperature obtained by an esophageal probe or pulmonary artery catheter (PAC) thermistor. Hypothermia may contribute to metabolic acidosis, vasoconstriction, myocardial dysfunction, arrhythmias, electrolyte imbalances, altered pharmacokinetics and drug metabolism, platelet dysfunction, and an increased risk of surgical site infection. Hypothermia may develop from exposure in the field, from disease (e.g., sepsis, hypothalamic injury), or under anesthesia. Induced, controlled hypothermia is an adjunct to several heart, brain, and spinal procedures and after cardiac arrest, but it is not beneficial after TBI or multi-system trauma.

  1. Fever. Fever (temperature exceeding the hypothalamic "set point") or hyperthermia (a reset hypothalamic set point) will increase heart rate, O_2 consumption, and insensible fluid loss. Postoperative fever is not invariably dangerous. Fever has salutary effects on host defenses, and in non-neurologically injured patients should not be suppressed unless the patient has symptomatic myocardial ischemia or other serious manifestations.

  a. One-half of episodes of postoperative fever are of non-infectious origin (Table 34-3); in the first 48 hours after surgery, the only consequential infectious causes of fever (other than an infection that prompted surgical intervention for source control) are surgical site infections caused by streptococci or clostridial organisms.

  b. Physical examination including inspection of ALL wounds is mandatory, but laboratory evaluation of fever is usually not helpful until after the third postoperative day. Thereafter, the differential diagnosis of postoperative fever is extensive (Tables 34-3 and 34-4).

  c. Suppress elevated temperature in TBI patients to <38°C when possible; this may improve outcomes.

  2. Hypothermia. Anticipate hypothermia in injured patients with exposure or shock, massive volume resuscitation, or prolonged surgery (Chapter 42). Patients who undergo damage control operations (see Chapter 6) are admitted to the ICU from a truncated operative procedure for secondary resuscitation, normalization of body temperature, and correction of coagulopathy. The crucial temperature of injured patients that influences mortality profoundly appears to

TABLE 34-3	**Non-infectious Causes of Fever in the ICU**

Acute respiratory distress syndrome (ARDS)
Adrenal insufficiency
Atelectasis
Blood transfusion
Cardiac arrest
Gastrointestinal hemorrhage
Ischemia/infarction
Hemorrhage/hematoma-parenchymal
Brain
Lung
Retroperitoneum
Soft tissue
Solid organ (liver, spleen)
Hyperthyroidism
Multiple trauma
Venous thromboembolic disease

be approximately 32°C, but substantial cardiac and hematologic morbidity is possible whenever the core body temperature is <35°C.

a. The major complications of hypothermia are platelet dysfunction (decreased adhesion due to inhibited thromboxane synthesis), impaired cardiac function (increased afterload due to systemic vasoconstriction), and dysrhythmias (altered myocardial sensitivity to endogenous catecholamines). Clotting

TABLE 34-4	**Infectious Causes of Fever in the ICU**

Blood stream infection
  Bacteremia
  Central line–associated blood stream infection
  Fungemia
Peritonitis/intra-abdominal abscess
  Anastomotic or suture line dehiscence
  Abscess of solid organ (e.g., liver, spleen)
  Biliary tract
    Acalculous cholecystitis
    Cholangitis
Pneumonia
  Empyema
Retroperitoneum
  Iliopsoas abscess
  Infected pancreatic necrosis
Sinusitis
Skin/soft tissue
  Hematoma
  Suppurative phlebitis
  Surgical site infection
  Traumatic wound infection
Urinary tract
  Cystitis
  Perinephric abscess
  Pyelonephritis

factor function, which is temperature-dependent, is reduced during hypothermia.

   b. Methods used for re-warming (Chapter 42) depend on the severity of hypothermia, ongoing hemorrhage and coagulopathy, hemodynamic stability, and availability of equipment and technical support. It is easier to keep a patient warm than to re-warm, as most methods are inefficient at transferring heat.

F. Capnography. Capnography measures the CO_2 concentration in expired gas, most reliably in ventilated patients. The peak CO_2 concentration occurs at end-exhalation (end-tidal CO_2 [$ETCO_2$]), at which time $ETCO_2$ approximates closely the alveolar gas concentration.

   1. Capnography can confirm successful airway intubation and monitor resuscitation and weaning from mechanical ventilation. Used with pulse oximetry, many patients can be liberated from mechanical ventilation without reliance on arterial blood gases or invasive hemodynamic monitoring.

   2. Capnography can provide other valuable information. An $ETCO_2$–$PaCO_2$ gradient >13 mm Hg after resuscitation is associated with increased trauma-related mortality. Gradually decreasing $ETCO_2$ is associated with hypovolemia, whereas a sudden decrease or even disappearance of $ETCO_2$ is observed with a low cardiac output (Q) state, disconnection from the ventilator, or pulmonary thromboembolism (Table 34-5). A gradual increase of $ETCO_2$ occurs with hypoventilation; the converse is also true.

TABLE 34-5   Changes in End-Tidal CO_2 ($ETCO_2$)

Increased $ETCO_2$
Decreased alveolar ventilation
  Reduced respiratory rate
  Reduced tidal volume
  Increased equipment dead space
Increased CO_2 production
  Fever
  Hypercatabolism
  Excess carbohydrate intake
Increased inspired CO_2 concentration
  CO_2 absorber exhausted
  Increased CO_2 in inspired gas
  Re-breathing of expired gas

Decreased $ETCO_2$
Increased alveolar ventilation
  Increased respiratory rate
  Increased tidal volume
Decreased CO_2 production
  Hypothermia
  Hypocatabolic state
Increased alveolar dead space
  Decreased cardiac output
  Pulmonary embolism (clot, air, fat)
  High positive end-expiratory pressure (PEEP)
Sampling error
  Air in sample line (no or diminished signal)
  Water in sample line (no or diminished signal)
  Inadequate tidal volume (no or diminished signal)
  Disconnection of monitor from tubing (no signal)
  Airway not in trachea (e.g., esophageal intubation) (no signal)

G. **Near-infrared spectroscopy.** Near-infrared spectroscopy (NIRS) is a non-invasive method to measure tissue pO_2 in close to real time. Analysis of the reflected light produces a measurement of tissue oxygenation (StO_2) in the skeletal muscle microcirculation. Skeletal muscle StO_2 correlates with DO_2I, base deficit, and serum lactate concentration in experimental and clinical hemorrhagic shock. Detection is most accurate for StO_2 >70%.

1. In a multi-center trial, an StO_2 >75% maintained during the first hour of monitoring indicated adequate tissue perfusion, with affected patients having an 88% MODS-free rate of survival. In contrast, StO_2 <75% in the first hour was manifested by 78% of patients who eventually developed MODS and 91% of those who died.

H. **Non-invasive cardiac output determination**

1. **Thoracic bioimpedance.** Thoracic bioimpedance derives information from electrodes placed on the anterior chest and neck to estimate Q by determining the left ventricular systolic time interval from time 1/m~ derivative bioimpedance signals. The main drawback of thoracic bioimpedance is sensitivity to any alteration of electrode contact or positioning on the patient.

2. **Esophageal Doppler monitor.** The esophageal Doppler monitor (EDM) device is a soft, 6 mm catheter that is placed non-invasively into the esophagus. A flow probe at the tip allows continuous monitoring of Q and stroke volume. The primary disadvantage of the EDM is that the waveform may be damped or lost entirely with only a slight positional change, rendering inaccurate readings.

VI. INVASIVE MONITORING

A. **Arterial catheterization.** Arterial blood pressure measurement is the simplest, most reproducible hemodynamic monitor. Although automated blood pressure cuffs are in common use in operating rooms and are suitable for periodic blood pressure measurement in stable patients, low or fluctuating blood pressure may mandate continuous monitoring via an indwelling catheter. Invasive blood pressure monitoring is indicated for prolonged operations (>4 hours), prolonged mechanical ventilation (>24 to 48 hours), unstable hemodynamics, vasopressor therapy, substantial blood loss, frequent blood sampling, or when precise blood pressure control is needed (e.g., TBI patients with low CPP, aortic dissection).

1. **Insertion technique.** Special-purpose thin-walled catheters maintain fidelity of the waveform and minimize luminal obstruction. The radial artery at the wrist is the most common site. Patency of the collateral circulation to the hand should be confirmed before cannulation at the wrist to minimize the possibility of catastrophic tissue loss.

a. In neonates, the umbilical artery may be catheterized; intestinal ischemia is a rare complication. The axillary artery is relatively free of plaque, well collateralized at the shoulder, and easy to cannulate percutaneously.

b. A risk with axillary catheterization is cerebral embolization when flushing the line. The superficial femoral artery is not preferred because of higher risks of distal embolization and infection. The dorsalis pedis artery is accessible, but should be avoided with peripheral vascular disease, hemodynamic instability, or lower extremity trauma. The brachial artery should be strictly avoided because collateral circulation at the elbow is poor; the risk of hand or forearm ischemia from thrombosis is high.

c. Peripheral vasoconstriction during vasopressor therapy may dampen the arterial waveform. A longer catheter placed at a more central location (e.g., axillary, femoral) may restore the fidelity of the tracing. Nosocomial infection of arterial catheters is unusual if basic tenets of infection control are honored and femoral artery catheterization is avoided.

B. **Central venous pressure monitoring.** The central venous pressure (CVP) is a function of circulating blood volume, venous tone, and right ventricular function. The CVP measures right ventricular filling pressure as an estimate of intravascular volume status; aside from extreme values (<6 mm Hg or >15 mm Hg), the absolute CVP is less helpful than the trend of CVP response to volume. Strict adherence to asepsis, full barrier precautions, and adherence to the principles of infection control are crucial to avoid central line–associated blood stream infection.

1. **Insertion technique.** Central venous access can be obtained using the basilic, femoral, external jugular, internal jugular, or subclavian veins.

   a. In the ICU, the internal jugular site is popular because of ease of accessibility, a high success rate of cannulation, and relatively few complications.

   b. The subclavian site is the most technically demanding, having the highest rate of pneumothorax (1.5% to 3.0%), but the lowest infection rate.

   c. The femoral vein site is least preferred in the ICU because of the highest complication rate, despite the relative ease of catheter placement. The risks of arterial puncture (9% to 15%), infection, and venous thromboembolism (VTE) are highest for femoral vein catheterization.

   d. Overall complications are comparable for internal jugular and subclavian vein cannulation (6% to 12%), and higher for femoral vein cannulation (13% to 19%).

2. Full barrier precautions are mandatory. The operator dons cap, mask, eye protection, and a sterile gown and gloves before preparing the patient's skin (2% chlorhexidine gluconate is associated with fewer infections than 10% povidone-iodine) and draping the patient completely with a full-bed drape.

C. **Pulmonary artery catheterization.** Data from PACs are used mainly to determine Q and preload, which is most commonly estimated by the PA occlusion pressure (PAOP). Other parameters calculated from Q include SVR and pulmonary vascular resistance (PVR), and right and left ventricular stroke work (RVSW, LVSW).

1. **Data interpretation.** Normally, PAOP approximates left atrial pressure, which in turn approximates left ventricular end-diastolic pressure (LVEDP), a reflection of left ventricular end-diastolic volume (LVEDV). The LVEDV represents preload, which is the actual target parameter.

   a. **Many factors cause PAOP to reflect LVEDV inaccurately,** including mitral stenosis, high levels of PEEP (>10 cm H_2O), and changes in left ventricular compliance (e.g., myocardial infarction, pericardial effusion, or increased afterload). Inaccurate readings may result from balloon overinflation, catheter malposition, alveolar pressure exceeding pulmonary venous pressure (PEEP ventilation), or pulmonary hypertension (which may make PAOP measurement difficult, if not hazardous). Elevated PAOP occurs in left-sided heart failure. Decreased PAOP occurs with hypovolemia or decreased preload.

   b. Mixed venous oxygen saturation ($S_{mv}O_2$) may be measured, although superior vena cava S_vO_2 via a CVP catheter may provide data of comparable utility. Causes of low $S_{mv}O_2$ include anemia, pulmonary disease, carboxyhemoglobinemia, low Q, and increased VO_2. The SaO_2: ($SaO_2 - S_{mv}O_2$) ratio determines the adequacy of DO_2. Ideally, the $P_{mv}O_2$ should be 35 to 40 mm Hg, with an $S_{mv}O_2$ of about 70%. Values of $P_{mv}O_2$ <30 mm Hg are critically low.

2. **Clinical use**

   a. Evidence is lacking that PAC use decreases morbidity or mortality. Some retrospective data even suggest that PAC use is associated with increased mortality.

   b. Ventilation of patients with acute respiratory distress syndrome (ARDS) on high levels of PEEP has been monitored commonly via PAC. The application of PEEP can decrease venous return markedly, and therefore Q, in a short time period; maintenance of Q is important to maintain ventilation–perfusion (V/Q) matching. However, the ARDS net investigators demonstrated no difference in outcome of patients with acute lung injury (ALI)/ARDS when managed by PAC or CVP. PACs may still be useful in select circumstances, such as cardiomyopathy, shock of various etiologies, oliguric acute kidney injury, or an unpredicted poor response to fluid therapy. Critically ill patients who require inotropic agents despite large-volume fluid resuscitation may also benefit from monitoring by PAC.

3. **Complications.** Complications common to PACs include infection (2% to 5%), hemo- or pneumothorax (2% to 5%), migration (5% to 10%), arrhythmia (10% to 15%), and hemorrhage (0.2%). Less frequent complications include catheter knotting, pulmonary infarction, cardiac or PA perforation, valvular injury, and endocarditis. A devastating complication is PA rupture, which occurs in fewer than 0.1% of cases, during insertion or during routine determination of PAOP, and is often fatal. Distal migration of the PAC within the PA increases the risk of rupture dramatically, and argues for routine daily bedside chest radiography for all patients with an indwelling PAC.

D. **Intracranial pressure (ICP) monitoring.** Monitoring of ICP is common monitoring in patients with severe TBI (GCS ≤ 8). In TBI, these devices facilitate "optimized" CPP above 60 mm Hg, although **no outcome himan** show a benefit for ICP monitoring in patients with TBI.

1. The intra-ventricular or "ventriculostomy" catheter can also drain cerebrospinal fluid (CSF) and thereby decrease elevated ICP. However, ventriculostomy is the most invasive method of ICP monitoring, and poses the highest infection risk (~8%). Despite the high risk of infection with ventriculostomy, neither prolonged antibiotic prophylaxis nor regular replacement of the catheter at 5- to 7-day intervals reduces the risk.

VII. MISSED INJURIES

A. However diligent the assessment in the ED, it is inevitable that some injuries will not be identified until the patient is in the ICU. An altered sensorium and the inability to make a complaint referable to the injury is a common reason, as is prior exigency of managing another life-threatening injury. Extremity fractures and dislocations are the most commonly missed injuries. The most serious missed injuries involve the spinal column, major cardiovascular structures, or hollow viscus.

B. Missed injuries are discovered by vigilance in the ICU, at a time when stabilization and treatment can still result in a good outcome. For patients with multiple severe injuries, repetition of the secondary survey upon ICU admission and serially thereafter is a prudent and relatively high-yield strategy.

VIII. PROPHYLAXIS

A. **Cardiovascular.** Beta-adrenergic blockade, begun preoperatively and continued for approximately 7 days thereafter, reduces the risk of perioperative myocardial infarction and death among elderly patients undergoing major non-cardiac surgery and in trauma patients. However, tachycardia is an important vital sign in the evaluation of the injured patient, particularly with respect to the presence of hypovolemia or pain. Blunting the heart rate response could be deleterious if recognition of such underlying conditions is impaired. Administration of beta-blockers to patients with severe TBI reduces mortality from injury by 50% to 70%, and can decrease catabolism in children with burns.

B. **Stress-related gastric mucosal hemorrhage**

1. Ischemia-reperfusion injury of the stomach is associated with disruption of the mucus blanket, back-diffusion of hydrogen ions, reduced buffering capacity, and ultimately gastric mucosal injury. Gastric mucosal injury may be exacerbated by lack of the trophic stimulus associated with enteral feeding. Mucosal injury has many manifestations, ranging from asymptomatic to overt upper gastrointestinal hemorrhage. The incidence has been reduced markedly by chemoprophylaxis and early nutritional support, to approximately 4% among critically ill patients. Patients at highest risk are those who receive mechanical ventilation for >48 hours, or who are coagulopathic. Trauma patients at increased risk include those with TBI or burns.

2. Agents for prophylactic use include H_2-histamine receptor antagonists, proton-pump inhibitors, and (rarely) sucralfate. Antacids are not recommended due to cumbersome administration and increased risk of pulmonary aspiration. H_2-antagonists appear to have a lower incidence of overt bleeding (but not

TABLE 34-6	Risk Factors for Venous Thromboembolism after Trauma: Analysis of 1,602 Episodes from the National Trauma Data Bank	
Parameter	**Odds ratio**	**95% confidence interval**
Univariate Analysis		
Age > 39 y	2.29	2.07–2.55
Pelvis fracture	2.93	2.01–4.27
Lower extremity fracture	3.16	2.85–3.51
Spinal cord injury with paralysis	3.39	2.41–4.77
TBI	2.59	2.31–2.90
Mechanical ventilation >3 d	10.62	9.32–12.11
Injury to major vein	7.93	5.83–10.78
Blood pressure <90 mm Hg on admission	1.95	1.62–2.34
Major surgical procedure	4.32	3.91–4.77
Multi-variable Analysis		
Age >39 y	2.01	1.74–2.32
Lower extremity fracture	1.92	1.64–2.26
TBI	1.24	1.05–1.46
Mechanical ventilation >3 d	8.08	6.86–9.52
Injury to major vein	3.56	2.22–5.72
Major surgical procedure	1.53	1.30–1.80

(From Knudson MM, Morabito D, Paiment GD, et al. Use of low molecular weight heparin in preventing thromboembolism in trauma patients. *J Trauma* 1996;41:446–459.)

occult bleeding) than sucralfate. No class I data support the use of proton-pump inhibitors for prophylaxis, despite widespread use.

  a. Concern that acid-reduction increased the risk of ventilator-associated pneumonia (VAP) compared with barrier protection (i.e., sucralfate) is unfounded.

C. Prophylaxis of venous thromboembolism (VTE). The VTE incidence is lower than previously estimated, perhaps reflecting the aggressive and successful use of prophylaxis. Risk factors include older age, major (Abbreviated Injury Score >3) lower extremity fracture, TBI, and major operative procedures. However, the most powerful predictors of VTE are prolonged mechanical ventilation (>3 days) and major venous injury. The striking association between VTE and prolonged ventilation (odds ratio >8) reflects prolonged bedrest, severity of injury, and a host of other factors (Table 34-6).

D. Metabolic prevention. Prevention of metabolic/nutritional complications is multi-factorial, including glycemic control, identification of adrenal insufficiency, and early, preferably enteral, nutritional support. These ostensible disparate aspects are linked through the hypophyseal–pituitary–adrenal (HPA) axis and other hormonal/metabolic pathways. For example, glycemic control by continuous infusion of insulin has been linked to a reduced incidence of surgical site infections and other nosocomial infections, and also to reduced organ dysfunction and mortality in the ICU. However, both glucocorticoid therapy and nutritional support (especially parenteral) can make glycemic control more difficult. Likewise, early enteral nutrition (e.g., <36 hours after injury) has been estimated to reduce the incidence of infection by more than 50%. By contrast, early parenteral nutrition (<8 days) is non-beneficial and may be detrimental.

  1. Glycemic control. An association with decreased infection and higher postoperative blood glucose concentrations has been made for trauma and major non-cardiac surgery. A recent meta-analysis suggests that the benefit of intensive insulin therapy accrues solely to surgical patients.

    a. The NICE-SUGAR multi-center trial of more than 6,000 patients conducted in Australia and New Zealand showed 3% excess mortality among patients treated with intensive insulin therapy (seeking glucose of 80 to 120 mg/dL), possibly due to the increased risk of hypoglycemia. There was no benefit observed in small subsets of surgical and trauma patients. Numerous methodologic differences make comparisons to the Leuven trial problematic.

b. A more modest reduction of serum glucose concentration (e.g., $\leq$150 mg/dL) appears to be equally beneficial with a lower incidence of hypoglycemia ($<$60 mg/dL).

c. A meta-analysis of 26 trials (13,567 patients) suggests that surgical patients benefit in particular from tight glycemic control, whereas a similar benefit is elusive to demonstrate for critically ill medical patients. Patients in surgical ICUs appeared to benefit from intensive insulin therapy (RR 0.63, 95% CI 0.44–0.91); patients in the other ICU settings did not (medical ICU: RR 1.0, 95% CI 0.78–1.28; mixed ICU: RR 0.99, 95% CI 0.86–1.12). The different targets of intensive insulin therapy (glucose level $\leq$110 mg/dL vs. $<$150 mg/dL) did not influence either mortality or the risk of hypoglycemia.

d. Avoidance of variability of the glucose concentration may be as important as the level itself. More moderate control may be beneficial if control is maintained as compared with a greater degree of control that is lost periodically.

2. Adrenal insufficiency. Adrenal insufficiency can be occult or develop under stress in a patient with initially normal HPA-axis responsiveness. Adrenal insufficiency is in the differential diagnosis of fever, hyponatremia, unexplained hypotension, and a host of other ICU-related maladies. Among the controversies are the true incidence of adrenal insufficiency in critical illness, the optimal method of diagnosis (random serum cortisol concentration vs. provocative testing), and the dose of the 1-25 C-terminal corticotropin analogue cosyntropin to use for provocation (1 mcg vs. 250 mcg).

a. The estimated incidence of adrenal insufficiency in critically ill patients varies widely, a function of the vigor and the criteria used for diagnosis. The simplest diagnostic method is simply based on a random serum cortisol concentration (diurnal variation is lost in critical illness), but accuracy is limited.

b. Manifestations of adrenal insufficiency may include fever, hyponatremia, refractory shock, or inability to wean the well-resuscitated patient from vasopressor therapy.

c. While provocative testing, comparing the difference between basal and 1-hour–stimulated cortisol concentrations in response to either 1 mcg or 250 mcg of cosyntropin (the former is probably more sensitive, but the latter dose is administered more widely), is often used, its value is limited. A recommended way to diagnose of adrenal insufficiency is when both basal and stimulated cortisol concentrations are $<$15 mcg/dL, refuted when both are $>$35 mcg/dL, and possible if the basal cortisol concentration is between 15 and 35 mcg/dL and the stimulated cortisol concentration exceeds the basal concentration by $<$9 mcg/dL.

d. Routine glucocorticoid therapy is not a part of the therapy of severe sepsis/septic shock. If insufficiency exists, hydrocortisone not exceed 300 mg/day is used with tapering when the patient is no longer vasopressor-dependent.

e. Etomidate, even a single dose, can alter steroid production for days to weeks but the clinical importance is uncertain outside existing adrenal dysfunction.

E. Ventilator "bundle." Care of the patient who requires mechanical ventilation (MV) is more than just providing O_2 and a bellows. Such critically ill patients are at risk of numerous complications, not all of which are related directly to ARF or MV. The patient at prolonged bedrest is at risk for deconditioning, VTE, and pressure ulcers. Sedatives and analgesics may impair the ability to protect the airway, increasing the risk of pulmonary aspiration of gastric contents. Over-sedation may be one component of prolonged MV, which is a definite risk factor for development of VAP. Prolonged MV ($>$48 hours) is itself a risk factor for development of stress-related gastric mucosal hemorrhage, a rare but serious complication ($>$50% associated mortality for overt bleeding).

1. Several "best practices" have been combined into a ventilator bundle of five maneuvers to optimize the outcomes of MV. Careful adherence can decrease the risk of prolonged MV.

a. Keep the head of the patient's bed up at least 30 degrees from level at all times unless contraindicated medically.

b. Administer prophylaxis against VTE.

c. Administer prophylaxis against stress-related gastric mucosal hemorrhage.

d. Perform a daily "sedation holiday" to assess for readiness to liberate from MV.

e. Provide decontamination of the oropharyngeal mucosa and accessible intraoral exterior surface of the artificial airway (i.e., endotracheal tube) several times daily with topical 0.12% chlorhexidine mouthwash.

IX. ORGAN SYSTEM SUPPORT

A. Cardiovascular. Cardiovascular support begins with adequate resuscitation and DO_2, which relates to fluid resuscitation, blood transfusion, MV support, and numerous other interventions. Specifically, cardiovascular support may consist of control of dysrhythmias, vasopressor support of refractory shock, management of hypertensive emergencies, and cardiopulmonary resuscitation (CPR).

1. Anti-dysrhythmic therapy

a. Atrial and supraventricular rhythm disturbances (Table 34-7). The most common dysrhythmia in the trauma setting is atrial fibrillation, which is caused usually by fluid overload (with atrial over-distension) or inflammation adjacent to the pericardium (e.g., pneumonia).

i. New-onset atrial fibrillation can usually be converted to sinus rhythm once the precipitant is controlled. Heart rate is controlled first, using a beta-blocker or calcium channel blocker (diltiazem by bolus and infusion is preferred because of its particular effectiveness in slowing conduction through the atrioventricular node). Digoxin (0.25 to 0.5 mg IV) is an alternative, but less used and slower onset. The goal should be a heart rate <100 beats/min (bpm), ideally <80 bpm if tolerated hemodynamically, especially if the patient has coronary artery disease.

ii. If needed, sinus rhythm may be restored with a bolus dose and infusion of amiodarone or procainamide. Long-term amiodarone toxicity (e.g., pulmonary fibrosis, hypothyroidism) is a non-issue with short-term control of dysrhythmias. The patient can be transitioned to short-term oral therapy while hospitalized until the stimulus (i.e., fluid overload) has been corrected. After sinus rhythm is restored, long-term therapy is seldom needed.

iii. If the rhythm is rapid, regular, QRS narrow (<0.12 msec) and cannot be diagnosed from an ECG rhythm strip, the ventricular response may be slowed transiently for diagnostic purposes with a bolus dose of adenosine 6 mg, which may be repeated twice in a dose of 12 mg. Re-entrant supraventricular tachycardia will terminate, and other supraventricular tachyarrhythmias will slow so they can be diagnosed. Transient (10 or less usually) bradyasystole may occur. Do not use adenosine if irregularity or wide QRS complexes exist or if the heart rate is over 250/min.

iv. Failure to restore sinus rhythm is unusual with new-onset atrial fibrillation and may require heparin anticoagulation after 48 hours to reduce the risk of embolism.

v. The usual causes of supraventricular tachycardia are the same as for atrial fibrillation in the trauma setting, with the addition of pulmonary embolism. The dysrhythmia can usually be terminated with a 10 to 15 mg diltiazem or 5 to 10 mg bolus of verapamil, but repetitive episodes may require a continuous infusion or be followed by oral therapy.

vi. With either atrial fibrillation or supraventricular tachycardia, a rapid ventricular rate (>140 bpm) may compromise diastolic filling to a degree

TABLE 34-7	ACLS Algorithm for Management of Adult Tachycardia

Assess clinical condition
Heart rate typically >150 bpm for tachyarrhythmia
Identify and treat underlying cause
    Maintain airway patency
    Ventilate patient as necessary
    Monitor cardiac rhythm, blood pressure, and oximetry
Oxygen if hypoxemic
Persistent tachyarrhythmia causing:
    Hypotension?
    Altered mental status?
    Shock?
    Ischemic chest discomfort?
    Acute heart failure?

YES	NO	
Synchronous cardioversion	Is QRS >0.12 s?	
Consider sedation		
Adenosine if regular narrow complex	YES	NO
	Obtain IV access and 12-lead ECG	
	Adenosine if regular and monomorphic	
	Consider expert consultation	
	Beta-blocker *OR*	*Consider* infusion
	Ca^{++}-channel blocker	of anti-arrhythmic

Doses for synchronized cardioversion;
    Narrow complex, regular 50–100 J
    Narrow complex, irregular 120–200 J biphasic, 200 J monophasic
    Wide complex, regular 100 J
Wide complex, irregular (defibrillate, NOT synchronous)
Doses for adenosine:
    6 mg once, followed by saline flush
    Repeat dose with 12 mg
Doses for anti-arrhythmic agents:
    Amiodarone
        150 mg over 10 min, followed by 1 mg/min for first 6 h. Repeat bolus if VT recurs.
    Procainamide
        20–50 mg/min until arrhythmia suppressed, hypotension or widened QRS >50% develops,
            or maximum dose 17 mg/kg. Maintenance infusion 1–4 mg/min. Avoid with prolonged QT
            or congestive heart failure.
Sotalol 100 mg (1.5 mg/kg) over 5 min. Avoid with prolonged QT.

that stroke volume is impaired, and decreased Q may lead to hypotension. Do synchronous electrical cardioversion for hemodynamically unstable atrial fibrillation or supraventricular tachycardia. Cardioversion after 72 hours should not be undertaken unless an echocardiogram excludes left atrial clot beforehand.

  b. Ventricular dysrhythmias. Ventricular rhythm disturbances are more complex to diagnose and manage, and generally more dangerous to the patient. Ischemia, hypoxemia, electrolyte abnormalities, and drug toxicity (the cause of the prolongation of the QT interval that precipitates the particular type of ventricular tachycardia called **torsades de pointes**). Unifocal ventricular premature contractions (VPCs) generally do not require therapy.

Multi-focal VPCs or couplet beats do, to avoid degeneration to ventricular tachycardia/fibrillation. Most complex ventricular arrhythmias can be suppressed with a bolus dose and infusion of amiodarone or lidocaine.

c. **Hypertensive emergencies**

   i. The postoperative and post-traumatic states are usually a hyperadrenergic, volume-overloaded state, in which some degree of hypertension is common. Aside from the autonomic hyperactivity and hypervolemia, pain, agitation, and increased ICP are all in the differential diagnosis of hypertension. Fortunately, **most episodes of hypertension in this setting are not dangerous, and do not require immediate specific anti-hypertensive therapy.** Making a diagnosis of the cause of hypertension is important, as diuresis, analgesia, or sedation may be the therapy that is needed. Moreover, treating hypertension associated with increased ICP is contraindicated if maintenance of CPP will be compromised.

   ii. Most cases of acute aortic dissection are associated with hypertension. The management is generally non-operative for Stanford Type B aortic dissections unless vascular insufficiency (e.g., visceral or lower extremity ischemia) is present. Treatment is with sedation, analgesia, beta-blockade (target heart rate <80 bpm) and a parenteral anti-hypertensive agent (target systolic blood pressure 100 to 110 mm Hg). Labetalol is an alternative agent that can aid heart rate and blood pressure control.

   iii. With the exception of fresh vascular suture lines, hemorrhage that is temporized by the use of temporary packing, or an aortic injury that is awaiting surgical repair, systolic hypertension <160 to 180 mm Hg does not require therapy to lower blood pressure immediately. In rare settings of ongoing bleeding, a target of systolic blood pressure of 100 mm Hg is common. Otherwise, only when organ function is threatened immediately (e.g., hypertensive nephropathy, acute myocardial infarction with active ischemia, suture line hemorrhage, aortic dissection, stroke) should blood pressure be lowered acutely.

   iv. Anti-hypertensive agents that are useful to decrease blood pressure immediately include nitroprusside, labetalol, and nicardipine, all of which are given by a titrated continuous infusion and are relatively easy to titrate. Although a potent vasodilator, hydralazine is also not recommended, as titration of the dose is difficult. Likewise, although nitroglycerin will decrease blood pressure by decreasing preload, it is not preferred as an anti-hypertensive agent unless the patient has an acute coronary syndrome or acute cardiogenic pulmonary edema.

d. **Cardiopulmonary resuscitation.** The 2010 American heart Association guidelines (Tables 34-8–34-10) detail these actions. The single rescuer should check the victim's responsiveness to voice and light touch; if no response, help should be summoned. Providing breaths to the patient is no longer emphasized. To prepare for CPR, place the patient supine on a hard surface, maintaining cervical immobilization unless the injury has been excluded. If the pulse is restored but the patient remains apneic, the airway should be secured. If the patient is pulseless, chest compressions and breaths are given at a rate of at least 100 compressions/min *without interruptions* short of electrical therapy. When the defibrillator is ready, the cardiac rhythm is checked for a rhythm likely to respond to shock, which if present is treated with a single shock followed immediately by five additional cycles of CPR.

   i. Electrical therapy. Early defibrillation is crucial for survival from sudden cardiac arrest. Ventricular fibrillation is treated effectively by defibrillation, but the probability of successful defibrillation decreases rapidly over time, and VF tends to deteriorate to asystole, which does not respond to defibrillation.

TABLE 34-8	Summary of Changes to 2010 Basic and Advanced Cardiac Life Support Guidelines

Cardiopulmonary Resuscitation Sequence
The sequence of BLS steps has changed from A–B–C (airway–breathing–circulation) to C–A–B
However, it is reasonable for inhospital providers to tailor the sequence to the likely cause of arrest

Chest Compression
Compression only (hands only) for the untrained lay rescuer
Compression of adequate depth (2.5 in. and rate, to allow complete chest recoil (BCLS and ACLS)
Minimization of the interval between stopping compression and delivery of a shock
Minimizing the pause between compressions and shock increases the likelihood of successful defibrillation

Ventilation
Avoid excessive ventilation, and aim for normal minute ventilation
Hypocarbic alkalosis is detrimental

Team Approach
Training should focus on building the team as each member arrives, or quick designation of roles when multiple trained rescuers are present
Improved outcomes are expected when an integrated team of trained rescuers provides resuscitation

a) Given that biphasic defibrillators may use one of two waveforms (neither of which appears to be superior), the initial energy dose is device-specific (120 joules [J] for a rectilinear biphasic waveform; 150 to 200 J for a biphasic truncated exponential waveform). Subsequent shocks are at the same or higher dose, regardless of waveform. There is no evidence that non-escalating or escalating energy shocks make any difference.

B. Acid–base and electrolyte disturbances. Anticipate acid–base and electrolyte imbalance in patients in shock or after massive transfusion. Electrolyte abnormalities come from dilution (e.g., hypomagnesemia, hyponatremia), diuresis (e.g., hypokalemia), therapeutic agents (e.g., hypernatremia), central nervous system injury (e.g., neurogenic diabetes insipidus causing hypernatremia, cerebral salt wasting or basilar skull fracture [syndrome of inappropriate antidiuretic hormone secretion] causing hyponatremia), acid–base disorders (acidosis-hyperkalemia, alkalosis-hypokalemia), or acute kidney injury (e.g., hyperkalemia). Rhabdomyolysis from fever, physical exhaustion, or crush injury may cause marked hyperphosphatemia, hypercalcemia, and hyperkalemia. Dilutional hypoalbuminemia, severe acute pancreatitis, or continuous RRT (using citrate anticoagulant) may cause hypocalcemia. Resuscitation with large volumes of 0.9% NaCl may cause or exacerbate a hyperchloremic metabolic acidosis. Protracted emesis or non-replaced large-volume losses from nasogastric drainage may cause a hypochloremic metabolic alkalosis. Protracted diarrhea, un-replaced ileostomy drainage, or high-volume enterocutaneous fistula may cause acidosis and hypokalemia. If hypokalemia occurs in this setting, it may be profound as acidosis is usually associated with hyperkalemia.

1. Acid–base disorders. Lactic acidosis is common and often multi-factorial, caused by shock, hypothermia, limb ischemia, or the metabolic response to trauma. Lactic acidosis that fails to normalize within the first 24 hours of ICU admission portends a high risk of death, especially among elderly patients. Most cases of persistent lactic acidosis in trauma are due to delayed or inadequate resuscitation or ongoing bleeding, and the treatment is control of hemorrhage and ongoing fluid resuscitation with transfusions of blood and blood products as indicated. Administration of $NaHCO_3$ is controversial but may be considered if the serum HCO_3 concentration is <15 mEq/L.

TABLE 34-9 | **Algorithm for Management of Pulseless Cardiac Arrest**

1. BLS algorithm-call for help, start CPR
2. Give oxygen
3. Attach monitor/defibrillator when available

Check rhythm—Shockable?

YES—ventricular tachycardia/fibrillation	NO—Asystole or pulseless electrical activity
Give one shock (recommended energy)	Resume CPR IMMEDIATELY—5 cycles
Biphasic 120–200 J	When IV or IO access is available, give vasopressor
	Epinephrine 1 mg—repeat every 3–5 min
Unknown 200 J	OR
Monophasic 360 J	
Resume CPR immediately thereafter—5 cycles	
Vasopressin 40 U may replace first or second dose of norepinephrine	
Consider atropine 1 mg for asystole or slow PEA rate	
Resume CPR immediately—5 cycles	
Check rhythm—Shockable? YES	Check rhythm—Shockable? YES
Continue CPR while defibrillator is charging	Give one shock (recommended energy) Biphasic 120–200 J
	Unknown 200 J
Give one shock as above, or higher energy if biphasic	
Resume CPR immediately thereafter—5 cycles	Monophasic 360 J
When IV or IO access is available, give vasopressor	Resume CPR immediately thereafter—5 cycles
Epinephrine 1 mg—repeat every 3–5 min	
OR	Check rhythm—Shockable? YES
Vasopressin 40 U may replace first or second dose of norepinephrine	Give one shock as above, or higher energy if biphasic
Resume CPR immediately thereafter—5 cycles	Give vasopressor again
	Resume CPR immediately thereafter—5 cycles
Consider advanced airway after second shock, but do not stop CPR	Consider advanced airway after second shock, but do not stop CPR
Continue cycle as long as rhythm remains shockable	Continue cycle as long as rhythm remains shockable
Consider anti-arrhythmic	Consider anti-arrhythmic
Amiodarone 300 mg once, then consider 150 mg once	Amiodarone 300 mg once, then consider 150 mg once
OR	OR
Lidocaine 1–1.5 mg/kg, repeat 0.5–0.75 mg/kg, max three doses	Lidocaine 1–1.5 mg/kg, repeat 0.5–0.75 mg/kg, max three doses
Consider Mg 1–2 g for torsades de pointes	Consider Mg 1–2 g for torsades de pointes
Check rhythm—Shockable? NO	

If asystole, resume CPR and give vasopressor again
If PEA, resume CPR and give vasopressor again
If pulse obtained, begin post-resuscitation care

1 cycle: 30 compressions then two breaths; 5 cycles ~2 min. Once advanced airway is placed, "cycles" of CPR are no longer given, rather give 8–10 breaths/min during continuous compressions. Check briefly for rhythm every 2 min.

TABLE 34-10	**Considerations for Good-Quality Cardiopulmonary Resuscitation**

Begin CPR
Give oxygen
Attach monitor/defibrillator
CALL for help
Push HARD and FAST (100/min; compress chest at least 2.5 in. in adults); release completely
Minimize interruptions in chest compressions
1 cycle: 30 compressions then 2 breaths; 5 cycles ~2 min (if no advanced airway)
Consider advanced airway after second shock
Secure airway and confirm placement
Avoid hyperventilation
Give vasopressor after second shock
Once advanced airway is placed, "cycles" of CPR are no longer given
Give 8–10 breaths/min during continuous compressions
Check briefly for rhythm every 2 min
Change compression personnel every 2 min, concurrent with rhythm check
Give anti-arrhythmic after third shock
Search for and correct possible underlying causes ("H" and "T")

H	T
Hypovolemia	Toxins
Hypoxia	Tamponade, cardiac
Hydrogen ion (acidosis)	Tension pneumothorax
Hypo/hyperkalemia	Thrombosis (coronary or pulmonary)
Hypoglycemia	Trauma
Hypothermia	

2. **Electrolyte disorders**
   a. **Hypokalemia.** The most common electrolyte disturbance of the injured patient is hypokalemia. Excessive renal losses of potassium occur as a result of diagnostic and therapeutic use of osmotic or loop diuretics, high doses of glucocorticoids (e.g., methylprednisolone in spinal cord injury), anti-fungal therapy with amphotericin B, or hyperaldosteronism due to hypovolemia. Alkalosis (or $NaHCO_3$ therapy), high catecholamine concentrations, and hypothermia can also cause intracellular shifting of potassium. Because trans-cellular shifts of potassium occur dynamically as acid–base status changes, and because total body potassium depletion cannot be estimated from the serum potassium concentration, monitor potassium administration closely.
   b. **Hyperkalemia.** Hyperkalemia may occur in patients with severe metabolic acidosis, large-volume blood transfusion, crush injury of skeletal muscle, rhabdomyolysis, or acute kidney injury. Hyperkalemia (>6.0 mEq/L) requires aggressive treatment to prevent cardiac arrest. Co-administered dextrose (50% dextrose in water, 50 mL, only if serum glucose <200 mg/dL) and regular insulin (10 U) will cause an intracellular shift of potassium. Next, use calcium salts (if the ECG is abnormal), $NaHCO_3$, or RRT. However, only RRT or ion-exchange resin (sodium polystyrene sulfonate, which removes 1 mEq K^+/g administered by mouth or per rectum) remove potassium perma-nently from the body.
   c. **Hypocalcemia.** Hypocalcemia occurs frequently in the severely injured patient, usually caused by a reduction in total calcium from dilution. Hypocalcemia can occur in patients with severe rhabdomyolysis or by acute respiratory alkalosis. Clinical manifestations of true (ionized) hypocalcemia are generally not evident until ionized calcium concentration is <0.7 mmol/L,

and include hypotension, impaired ventricular function, bradycardia, bronchospasm, laryngospasm, and impaired response to catecholamines. Treat hypocalcemia with an IV calcium salt (calcium gluconate is preferred) if the total calcium concentration is <8 mg/dL or the ionized calcium concentration is low (<0.7 mmol/L), or when hemodynamic instability or other complications of hypocalcemia occur.

d. **Hypomagnesemia.** Hypomagnesemia is also common in critically ill surgical patients and is commonly dilutional. Excessive renal or gastrointestinal losses and trans-cellular shifts (e.g., alkalosis) are other causes of hypomagnesemia. Complications of hypomagnesemia include hypocalcemia, refractory hypokalemia, skeletal muscle weakness, tetany, cardiac dysrhythmia, tremor, hyperreflexia, agitation, confusion, and seizures. Measurement of the serum magnesium concentration does not reflect the physiologically active ionized fraction (55%). A serum magnesium concentration <1 mEq/L is associated with hypokalemia and increased mortality and is one threshold for initiating aggressive therapy. Treat severe hypomagnesemia with IV MgSO$_4$ (2 to 4 g, 1 g = 8 mEq Mg^{+2}) administered slowly over 2 to 3 minutes with cardiac monitoring, followed by an optional continuous infusion (2 g/h for 5 hours followed by 1 g/h for 10 hours). Less severe degrees of hypomagnesemia can be treated as indicated by supplements added to intravenous fluid, or parenteral nutrition solution, or by enteral administration of Mg$_2$O$_4$.

C. **Pulmonary support.** The lung is the most common organ to fail in patients with severe injuries, the most common indication for care of the trauma patient in the ICU (Chapter 38).

1. **Etiology of acute respiratory failure.** The principal causes of acute respiratory failure (ARF) following injury are direct chest trauma, fluid overload, aspiration pneumonitis, ARDS, or cervical spinal cord injury. Pneumonia is the leading cause of ARF after the first 48 hours.

a. **Chest trauma.** Multiple rib fractures, or pulmonary contusion with or without flail chest, frequently cause ARF requiring MV. Rib fractures are challenging to manage because pain and splinting of the chest wall lead to hypoventilation; adequate analgesia may compromise spontaneous ventilation to the point that MV is required. Epidural analgesia can make management of the patient with multiple rib fractures simpler and safer, provided the torso does not need serial physical examinations to monitor injuries (e.g., splenic laceration) and that hemodynamics are stable.

i. Rarely, a major airway injury makes adequate gas exchange difficult because of massive air leakage. Signs suggestive of a major airway injury include subcutaneous emphysema, bronchopleural fistula (diagnosed usually by a large persistent air leak of inability to expand the lung with negative pressure administered via tube thoracostomy), pneumomediastinum, or hemoptysis. Most tracheal injuries in the neck occur at or above the fourth tracheal ring, whereas injuries in the mediastinum occur usually within 2.5 cm of the carina. The major airways are evaluated best by bronchoscopy. An air leak or pneumothorax that persists despite MV using minimal airway pressures is an indication for operative repair.

b. **Fluid overload.** Massive fluid resuscitation sometimes results in acute pulmonary edema, particularly with concomitant ALI/ARDS.

c. **Shock.** Any form of shock can cause ARF indirectly, as the work of breathing becomes excessive because of severe metabolic acidosis or inadequate DO$_2$ to the respiratory muscles.

d. **Aspiration of gastric contents.** Maxillofacial injury, impaired consciousness, nasogastric intubation, and endotracheal intubation are factors that predispose to aspiration. Hypoxemia results both from airway obstruction from aspiration of large particulates and from ALI secondary to acid aspiration. Two-thirds of patients develop only a sterile chemical pneumonitis and do not progress to late bacterial pneumonia. Reserve antibiotics for patients with microbiologic evidence of pneumonia.

TABLE 34-11	Protocol Summary for the Institution of Mechanical Ventilation for ALI/ARDS

Initial Ventilator Settings

Use a volume-controlled mode initially to ensure that V_T is delivered.

Use initial V_T 8 mL/kg; reduce by 1 mL/kg/2 h until 6 mL/kg is reached. Minimum V_T 4 mL/kg.

Set ventilator rate at 12–20 breaths/min.

Set maximum ventilator rate at 35 breaths/min.

Adjust ventilator subsequently based on goals of arterial pH (7.25–7.45); ventilator rate, and end-inspiratory plateau pressure (P_{plat}) (<30 cm H_2O).

Measure arterial pH upon admission to the ICU, each morning, and 15 min after each change in respiratory rate or V_T.

Manage alkalemia by decreasing ventilator rate by at least 2 breaths/min.

Manage mild acidemia (pH 7.15–7.25) by increasing ventilator rate until pH >7.25 or $PaCO_2$ <25 mm Hg up to 35 breaths/min. If ventilator rate >35 or $PaCO_2$ <25 mm Hg, give $NaHCO_3$.

Manage severe acidemia (pH <7.15) by increasing the ventilator rate up to 35 breaths/min. If ventilator rate >35 and pH <7.15, and $NaHCO_3$ has been given, increase V_T in increments of 1 mL/kg until pH >7.15. It may be necessary to exceed the target P_{plat} under these conditions.

Keep P_{plat} <30 cm H_2O. Measure P_{plat} at least every 8 h, and 5 min after each change in PEEP or V_T, and more frequently when changes in lung compliance are likely. Accurate measurement of P_{plat} requires a patient who is not moving or coughing.

If P_{plat} cannot be measured because of an air leak, substitute peak inspiratory pressure.

Set target ranges for PaO_2 at 55–80 mm Hg, or SaO_2 >88%. The combination of PEEP and FiO_2 is discretionary if FiO_2 <0.45.

When increasing PEEP above 10 cm H_2O, increase by 2–5 cm increments up to a maximum of 35 cm H_2O, until target ranges for PaO_2 are reached. Reduce PEEP to the previous level of PEEP if the change does not increase PaO_2 >5 mm Hg or if decreased DO_2 results from a decrease of Q.

Assess arterial oxygenation by blood gas determination or oximetry at least every 4 h.

If arterial oxygenation is below the target range, increase FiO_2 incrementally (up to 1.0), then PEEP (up to 35 cm H_2O within 30 min). Reassess every 15 min after each adjustment until target ranges for PaO_2 are regained. Brief periods of SaO_2 <88% (<5 min) may be tolerated. FiO_2 of 1.0 may be used transiently (<10 min) for arterial desaturation or during suctioning or bronchoscopy.

ALI, acute lung injury; ARDS, acute respiratory distress syndrome.
(Adapted from: Nathens AB, Johnson JL, Minei JP, et al, and the Inflammation and the Host Response to Injury Investigators. Inflammation and the Host Response to Injury, a large-scale collaborative project: Patient-oriented research core—Standard operating procedures for clinical care. I. Guidelines for mechanical ventilation of the trauma patient. *J Trauma* 2005;59:764–769.)

e. **Acute respiratory distress syndrome** (Table 34-11)
   i. **Definition.** In the setting of a precipitant, ARDS is characterized by severe hypoxemia (PaO_2:F_IO_2 <200), diffuse bilateral pulmonary infiltrates, a PAOP <18 mm Hg, and decreased lung compliance. A less severe form of lung injury, ALI, is defined by PaO_2:FIO_2 200 to 300.
   ii. **Causative factors.** Common causative factors for ARDS include sepsis, multiple long bone, or pelvis fractures causing fat microembolization, multiple transfusions (~10 U red blood cell [RBC] concentrates in <12 hours), pulmonary contusion, near-drowning, and acute pancreatitis.
   iii. **Pathophysiology.** Absent a direct lung injury (or with direct ALI, in the cases of lung contusion or pulmonary aspiration), a systemic inflammatory response to the underlying precipitant activates circulating phagocytes, causing adherence to endothelial cells and invasion of the interstitial space, where their activation and degranulation amplify the inflammatory response.

f. Spinal cord injury. Isolated high thoracic or cervical spinal cord injury can lead to ARF, as mechanical lung function is impaired consequent to denervation of respiratory muscles. About 30% of respiratory muscle power is lost from paralyzed accessory muscles with spinal cord injury at C_7, and 70% at C_5. Diaphragm impairment or paralysis occurs variably between C_3 and C_5, depending on the level of takeoff of the phrenic nerves. Although overt respiratory failure may not be evident within the first 24 hours, these patients are at high risk for decompensation as a result of progression of the spinal injury (ascension), deconditioning, or poor pulmonary toilet.

2. Mechanical ventilation. (See Chapter 38) MV may be required to manage ARF. New technology now provides several modes of MV that provide improved gas exchange, better patient comfort, and more rapid liberation from the ventilator. Non-invasive positive-pressure ventilation (NIPPV) permits some patients to be managed without endotracheal intubation. The most common indication for MV is to decrease the work of breathing. However, unless settings are chosen carefully to synchronize with the patient's own central respiratory drive, MV can cause an increase in work.

  a. Indications for mechanical ventilation. Nearly all ventilators can be set to allow full support of the patient, or periods of exercise, thus the physician determines MV settings for most patients. Controlled ventilation with suppression of spontaneous breathing leads rapidly to respiratory muscle atrophy. Assisted ventilation modes are preferred with machine-delivered breaths are triggered by the patient's own inspiratory efforts.

  i. Basic modes of assisted ventilation include assist-control ventilation (ACV), synchronized intermittent mandatory ventilation (SIMV), and pressure support ventilation (PSV). More advanced modes include pressure control ventilation (PCV), inverse-ratio ventilation (IRV), and airway pressure release ventilation (APRV). Regardless of the mode, all MV applies positive pressure to the airway, and modulates the interplay of mechanical support and the patients' own efforts.

3. Non-invasive ventilation. NIPPV is support delivered without an endotracheal airway, utilizing a nasal or face mask. Benefits of NIV include avoidance of endotracheal intubation and preservation of swallowing, feeding, speech, cough, and naso-oro-pharyngeal air warming and humidification. Non-intubated patients communicate more effectively, are more comfortable and require less sedation as a consequence, and can continue standard oral nutrition. NIPPV eliminates complications such as trauma during tube insertion or from an indwelling tube (particularly to the vocal cords or larynx [e.g., mucosal ulceration, fibrosis, or contracture of the arytenoids leading to impaired vocal cord approximation], aspiration, infection [e.g., VAP, sinusitis], and dysphagia after extubation).

  a. Contraindications. Successful NIPPV requires an awake, cooperative, patient, breathing patient with an intact cough reflex and ability to clear secretions. Relative contraindications include inadequate seal of the mask to the face, inability to cough, or inability to remove the mask quickly. Morbid obesity is also a relative contraindication secondary to decreased chest wall compliance and increased work of breathing arising from body habitus and the weight of the chest wall and abdominal viscera while the patient is supine.

  b. Complications. Focal skin necrosis may occur over the nasal bridge or over the zygoma, with an incidence of 7% to 10% among patients receiving full-face mask NIPPV. Other complications (incidence, 1% to 2% each) include conjunctivitis, gastric distention, aspiration, and pneumothorax. Most serious is failure to recognize when NIPPV is not providing a patient with adequate ventilation, oxygenation, or a patent airway.

4. Pressure support ventilation. Pressure support can assist spontaneous breathing during MV, either partially or fully, or can be used as a stand-alone mode for breathing patients not on MV.

5. Modes of mechanical ventilation—see Chapter 20

6. **Routine ventilator settings**
   a. Ventilator settings are based on the patient's ideal body mass and medical condition (Table 34-8). The normal lung (e.g., during general anesthesia) may be ventilated safely short term with V_T 8 to 10 mL/kg. Historically, critically ill patients with ALI/ARDS were ventilated with V_T 10 to 15 mL/kg, now considered excessive. Alveolar over-distention produces endothelial, epithelial, and basement membrane injuries associated with VILI.
   b. In patients with ALI/ARDS, V_T is reduced to ~6 mL/kg to achieve a P_{plat} <35 cm H_2O. Low V_T ventilation may lead to increased $PaCO_2$, which is termed **permissive hypercapnia.** If pH decreases below 7.20, V_E is increased or $NaHCO_3$ is administered.
   c. The set f depends on the mode. With ACV, the backup rate should be about 4 breaths/min less than the patient's spontaneous rate to ensure that the ventilator will continue to supply adequate V_E, should the patient hypoventilate or become apneic. With SIMV, the rate is typically high at first and then decreased gradually in accordance with patient tolerance.
   d. An inspiratory flow rate of 60 L/min is used with most patients during ACV and SIMV. With chronic airways obstruction, better gas exchange may be achieved at a flow rate of 100 L/min because increased E allows more complete emptying of trapped gas. If flow is insufficient, the patient will strain against pulmonary impedance and that of the ventilator, with a consequent increase in the work of breathing. In the ACV, SIMV, and PCV modes the patient must lower airway pressure below a preset threshold (usually minus1 to 2 cm H_2O) in order to trigger the ventilator to deliver a tidal breath.

7. **Liberation from mechanical ventilation.** Objective measures and proactive strategies can hasten the liberation of the patient from the ventilator. Each day of MV increases the need for sedation and the risk of VAP. Failure to separate readily from the ventilator may be due to disease- or therapy-related reasons (Table 34-12). Most clinical cases of failure are multi-factorial, but respiratory muscle fatigue is a common factor.
   a. There are four methods of weaning:
      i. Simplest is to perform spontaneous breathing trials each day with a T-piece circuit. Brief (5 to 10 minutes) trials can be increased in frequency and duration until the patient can breathe spontaneously for several hours.
      ii. An alternative is to perform a single daily T-piece trial of up to 2 hours; if successful, the patient is extubated; if not, the next attempt is made later that day or the following day.
      iii. SIMV and PSV can be combined. Assistance is decreased gradually by decreasing f or the amount of PS. When combined, f is set to zero before the level of pressure is decreased. Patients who breathe comfortably at PS 5 to 8 cm H_2O should be able to be extubated successfully. Approximately 10% to 20% of patients require re-intubation; their mortality is six-fold higher. Use of NIPPV after extubation may improve the likelihood of success.
      iv. Weaning from APRV is accomplished by manipulation of P_{high} and T_{high}. High pressure is decreased in increments of 2 to 3 cm H_2O down to about 15 cm H_2O, and T_{high} is lengthened progressively to 12 to 15 seconds in 1 to 2 seconds increments. Patients must be monitored carefully for signs of hypoventilation during the transition. The goal is to switch the patient to pure CPAP of 5 to 8 cm H_2O, at which point the patient may be extubated.

D. **Renal support.** AKI affects 10% to 25% of critically ill patients. The most common cause is renal hypoperfusion and related parenchymal dysfunction, referred to as acute tubular necrosis (ATN) (Table 34-13). One-third to one-half of cases of ATN occur during infection/sepsis, with the rest related to hypovolemia or toxin exposure. Patients with preexisting chronic kidney disease or diabetes mellitus are

TABLE 34-12	Differential Diagnosis of Failure to Separate from Mechanical Ventilation

Increased load on the respiratory system
Demand for increased minute ventilation
Increased CO_2 production
    Catabolic state
    Excess carbohydrate administered during nutritional support
Increased work of breathing
    Increased airflow resistance (e.g., bronchospasm, tracheal stenosis, tracheomalacia, glottic
        edema or dysfunction, mucus plugging)
Decreased thoracic compliance (muscle dysfunction due to nutritional or electrolyte causes,
    hypoxemia, hypercarbia, or possibly anemia)
Increased dead space ventilation
    Decreased cardiac output
    Pulmonary embolism
    Pulmonary hypertension
    Severe ALI
    Positive-pressure ventilation
Increased ventilatory drive
Muscle fatigue or failure
Stimulation of pulmonary J receptors
    Lung inflammation
    Lung parenchymal hemorrhage
    Central nervous system lesions
Psychological stress
    Inadequate analgesia or sedation
    Untreated agitation or delirium
    Acute alcohol or drug withdrawal

at particularly high risk for iodinated radiologic contrast-induced nephropathy. AKI seldom develops in isolation; coexistent respiratory failure ($\sim$67%), cardiac failure ($\sim$50%), or hepatic failure ($\sim$30%) are manifestations of MODS. In many series, more than one-half of patients who develop ARF will require acute RRT with consequent mortality >50%. The systemic pathophysiology of AKI (e.g., mental

TABLE 34-13	Indications for Initiation of Renal Replacement Therapy

Fluid and Electrolyte Abnormalities
Fluid overload
Hyperkalemia
Hypernatremia
Hyponatremia
Hypercalcemia
Hyperphosphatemia
Hyperuricemia
Metabolic acidosis
Metabolic alkalosis
Uremic Manifestations
Pericarditis
Uremic bleeding/platelet dysfunction
Encephalopathy
Nausea/vomiting

status changes, bleeding, pericarditis) increases the risk of developing non-renal complications. Because AKI is a systemic condition, there may be a limit to what can be achieved to improve organ dysfunction, and therefore AKI-related morbidity and mortality, by even optimized RRT. See Chapter 20 for AKI and RRT details.

E. Support of coagulation. Clotting factor deficiency and thrombocytopenia occur commonly in trauma patients with hemorrhagic shock requiring large-volume resuscitation (from consumption due to blood loss, or dilution due to use of crystalloid fluids), or massive TBI. Contributing factors include ongoing hemorrhage, shock, acidosis, hypothermia, and intraoperative blood salvage techniques. Coagulopathy may also occur with maternal-fetal hemorrhage, vitamin K deficiency, or due to drug therapy (e.g., aspirin, other antiplatelet agents, warfarin, or heparinoids).

F. Microvascular bleeding (also known as disseminated intravascular coagulation [DIC]) refers to bleeding in the setting of massive consumption of clotting factors and platelets (once surgical bleeding is controlled). Microvascular bleeding is non-surgical bleeding that appears as petechial hemorrhage, ecchymosis, or hematoma, and oozing from mucous membranes, puncture sites, and raw surfaces. It is not usually observed until the patient has received transfusion of RBC concentrates equal to 1 to 2 blood volumes. Current transfusion paradigms support the transfusion of units of RBC, fresh-frozen plasma (FFP), and platelets in a ratio approximating 1:1:1 during massive hemorrhage, with crystalloid relatively de-emphasized.

  1. Management. Normalization of body temperature (as discussed previously) is essential to ensure functional clotting factors and platelets. Ongoing occult bleeding that requires operative intervention (surgical bleeding) must be sought if the patient remains refractory to resuscitation. After the initial resuscitation, blood component therapy (Chapter 7) is given on the basis of identification of specific clotting defects in screening tests.

  a. Thrombocytopenia (most common) is treated with platelet concentrates, ideally to maintain the platelet count above $100,000/mm^3$ until active bleeding has ceased. The importance of platelet transfusions during massive hemorrhage cannot be over-stated.

  b. Prolongation of the prothrombin time (common) or aPTT (uncommon) is treated with FFP or prothrombin complex concentrates (less available but lower volume needed), and hypofibrinogenemia is treated with cryoprecipitate. Determination of the activity of specific clotting factors is seldom necessary unless there is refractory coagulopathy.

G. Neurologic support

  1. Increased ICP. TBI is a major cause of early mortality in blunt trauma patients admitted to the ICU. The fundamental goal in ICU management of the patient with severe TBI (after recognition and evacuation of intracranial mass lesions) is to prevent secondary brain injury from hypoperfusion, which may be due to increased ICP or decreased MAP, either of which results in reduced CPP. The uninjured brain can auto-regulate cerebral perfusion and preserve cerebral blood flow across a wide range of blood pressures, but one of the cardinal features of TBI is loss of auto-regulation. Other insults that are known to worsen neurologic injury include hypoxemia, hypercarbia (owing to cerebral vasodilation), and elevated body temperature (Chapter 17).

  a. Control of elevated ICP. The threshold for treatment of raised ICP is 20 to 25 mm Hg. Increased ICP is controlled most directly by the removal of CSF via an indwelling ventriculostomy. If a ventriculostomy is not used or venting of CSF is ineffective (e.g., massive brain swelling, obstructed catheter lumen), sequential use of sedation, hypertonic saline (usually 3% NaCl, up to 23.4%), neuromuscular blockade, mannitol, and barbiturates may be used to reduce refractory increased ICP. Hypertonic saline has supplanted mannitol because the latter crosses the blood–brain barrier and results in tachyphylaxis with repetitive use. Mannitol, 23.4% NaCl, or hyperventilation ($PaCO_2$ <25 mm Hg) may be used to interdict transtentorial herniation that usually manifests by marked anisocoria and pupillary non-reactivity (the "blown" pupil).

Marked hypocapnia ($PaCO_2$ <25 mm Hg) is best avoided for more than a few minutes unless therapy is guided by cerebral blood flow measurements or other indices of brain oxygenation (e.g., jugular venous oximetry). Tachyphylaxis develops rapidly, but decreased cerebral blood flow from cerebral vasoconstriction may cause secondary brain injury. High-dose barbiturate therapy (barbiturate coma) is reserved for patients with refractory intracranial hypertension.

b. Prevention of other secondary insults. Mean arterial pressure, SaO_2, $ETCO_2$, and core body temperature are monitored closely to avoid secondary brain injury. The goal is to maintain CPP >60 mm Hg, which is accomplished by a combination of low ICP and increased MAP. When ICP cannot be kept low, MAP must be supported pharmacologically to at least 90 mm Hg (depending on the resulting CPP). When volume expansion is unsuccessful in maintaining CPP, a vasopressor (usually phenylephrine) is employed. Antipyretics and other cooling techniques are used to keep core temperature <38°C and reduce cerebral DO_2.

2. Sedation and analgesia. Almost every critically ill patient requires analgesia and sedation; guidelines describe in detail the sustained use of these agents for indications such as prolonged mechanical ventilation or control of increased ICP.

a. A panoply of agents is available for use during bedside procedures and operations (Table 34-14). The choice of agent is made on several factors. Is the patient intubated? Are the patient's hemodynamics stable and normal? Does the procedure require general anesthesia, or will local anesthesia suffice? For how long must the anesthesia be effective? Will neuromuscular blockade be needed? If sedation is planned, will it be conscious sedation, or maintained at a deeper level? Will repetitive administration be required for multiple procedures? Will the agents require reversal, or will they be allowed to "wear off?" Does the need for repetitive neurologic examinations require use of either a short-acting or reversible agent? Will metabolism of the agents be impaired by abnormal organ function? Will the personnel available be able to manage the agent(s) chosen?

X. SPECIAL CONSIDERATIONS IN ICU CARE

A. Transport. The resources in personnel and portable monitoring equipment necessary for transport of a critically ill patient out of the ICU are substantial. Every "road trip" must be assessed not only from a risk–benefit perspective, but also from a risk–reward perspective.

1. Published guidelines for intra-hospital transport suggest that the ICU patient's respiratory therapist and nurse should accompany the patient out of the ICU for the duration of the transport. This may not be possible or could impact overall ICU capabilities. Physician accompaniment is a poor substitute, in that the physician is often junior, with limited familiarity with the patient's case, and limited skills for troubleshooting with infusion pumps, intravenous tubing, etc.

2. The incidence of transport-related mishaps is 5%, almost all of which are minor (e.g., tangled intravenous tubing, low battery). Even the sickest ICU patient can be transported safely if risk and benefits are weighed carefully, patients are stabilized insofar as possible before the transport is undertaken, and monitoring is continuous throughout.

B. The ICU as operating room (OR)

1. Preparation of the unit and staff. The staff of the ICU must be familiar with the use of the ICU as an OR. Experienced staff reduce the chance of procedure-related complications. Detailed protocols should be established that define roles and responsibilities, medications, monitoring equipment, disposable supplies, and surgical instruments needed for each procedure. All needed equipment (and reasonably anticipated needs) must be at the bedside prior to the start of the procedure. Communication is essential so that if additional nursing personnel will need to be at the bedside for the procedure, adequate

TABLE 34-14	Selected Agents for Analgesia, Anesthesia, and Sedation in the ICU	

Agent	Initial IV adult dose	Comments
Induction Agents		
Etomidate	6 mg or more	Maintains CO and BP. Reduces ICP but maintains CPP. Short $T_{1/2}$; use infusion for maintenance. Possible adrenal suppression.
Ketamine	1–2 mg/kg	Rapid-onset, short-duration agent. Can be given by continuous infusion for maintenance, and at lower dose for sedation without anesthesia. Transiently increases BP and HR. Raises ICP and intraocular pressure. Usually does not depress respiration. Generally safe in pregnancy and for neonates and children. Concurrent narcotics or barbiturates may prolong recovery. Anxiety, dis-orientation, dysphoria, and hallucinations during emergence, may be mitigated by a short-acting benzodiazepine. Atropine pretreatment can decrease secretions, but may increase incidence of dysphoria. Hepatic metabolism.
Propofol	1.5–2.5 mg/kg	Provides no analgesia. Potent amnestic effect. Causes apnea and loss of gag reflex. Can cause marked low BP. Infuse at 0.05–0.3 mg/kg/min for prolonged sedation. Minimal accumulation (hepatic insufficiency) facilitates rapid elimination. Account for 1 kcal/mL (lipid infusion) in nutrition prescription. Use of same vial >12 h associated with bacteremia. Safety for children still debated.
Intravenous Sedatives/Analgesics		
Midazolam	0.5–4.0 mg	Short $T_{1/2}$, but accumulates during infusion owing to active metabolites. Only benzodiazepine with potent amnestic effect. Can cause low BP and loss of airway. Primarily used for short-term sedation for ICU procedures. Renal elimination.
Diazepam	2.5–5.0 mg	Long $T_{1/2}$ limits use in ICU except for rare cases requiring very long-term sedation. Terminates seizure activity effectively. Hepatic elimination.
Lorazepam	1–4 mg	Effective anxiolytic. Preferred agent for continuous infusion of benzodiazepine (starting dose 1 mg/h). Can cause low BP, especially with hypovolemia, and paradoxical agitation. Hepatic elimination.
Morphine	2–10 mg	Analgesic and sedative effects. Can cause low BP, Q, and apnea. Tolerance and withdrawal possible after long-term use. Can be given as IV infusion or by PCA for analgesia or to facilitate prolonged mechanical ventilation or withdrawal of care. Hepatic elimination.
Hydromorphone	0.5–2.0 mg	Hydrated ketone of morphine with similar use and risk profiles. Approximately eight-fold more potent than morphine. Hepatic elimination.

(continued)

TABLE 34-14	Selected Agents for Analgesia, Anesthesia, and Sedation in the ICU (Continued)	

Agent	Initial IV adult dose	Comments
Fentanyl	50–100 mcg	Approximately 50-fold potency compared with morphine, but less likely to cause low BP in appropriate dosage (less histamine release). Versatile for ICU use given IV or by epidural infusion or PCA. Less potent than local anesthetics for epidural analgesia or abrogation of surgical stress response. Can cause truncal rigidity and apnea with inability to ventilate by hand (use neuromuscular blockade to facilitate intubation in that setting). Hepatic elimination.
Neuromuscular Blocking Agents (NBMAs)		
Atracurium	0.2–0.5 mg/kg	Short-acting non-depolarizing NMBAs (competitive inhibitors of Ach). Slow in onset compared with other agents in class. The drugs are similar, except atracurium causes histamine release and can cause high HR, low BP.
Cisatracurium	0.2–0.5 mg/kg	Cisatracurium, now used preferentially, requires IV infusion for prolonged effect. Effect potentiated by hypokalemia. Many drug interactions. Elimination by Hoffman elimination and ester hydrolysis, thus can be used for patients with renal/hepatic insufficiency
Mivacurium	0.15 mg/kg	Non-depolarizing NMBA with slow onset and moderate duration of action. Can be given by continuous infusion. Releases histamine; causes bronchospasm. Can cause decreased or increased HR and cardiac dysrhythmias. Faster onset/recovery in children ages 2–12 years. Enhanced blockade in pregnant patients given magnesium for pre-eclampsia.
Pancuronium	0.05–0.1 mg	Rapid onset, prolonged effect. Causes increased BP and HR. Induces neuromuscular blockade, but. should be converted, for example, to a maintenance cisatracurium infusion. Eliminated by kidneys and liver, accumulates in organ dysfunction with repeated doses.
Rocuronium	0.45–0.6 mg/kg	Intermediate onset and duration of effect. Onset and duration slightly longer in elderly patients. Metabolized by liver. Loading dose 0.45–0.6 mg/kg, followed by 10–12 mg/kg/min until desired level of blockade is achieved, then titrate to 4–16 mg/kg/min. Dose in obesity based on actual body weight. Physically incompatible with numerous medications used in the ICU; check product literature carefully. Elimination half-life averages 1.4 h.
Vecuronium	0.08–0.10 mg/kg	Non-depolarizing NMBA with rapid onset and short duration of action. Less potential for histamine release. Can cause malignant hyperthermia syndrome. Metabolized by liver.

(continued)

TABLE 34-14 Selected Agents for Analgesia, Anesthesia, and Sedation in the ICU (*Continued*)

Agent	Initial IV adult dose	Comments
Miscellaneous Agents		
Haloperidol	2–5 mg	Used for anxiolysis (often preferred to lorazepam), especially when respiratory depression is undesirable. Not FDA-approved for IV administration, but IV route is used commonly. Anti-dopaminergic properties contraindicate use in Parkinson disease. Can cause extrapyramidal effects. Hepatic elimination.
Ketorolac	0.5–1.0 mg/kg	Parenteral NSAID used in lieu of opioids or for opioid-sparing effect in combination. Interferes irreversibly with platelet function, and can cause incisional or GI hemorrhage and acute kidney injury. Use strictly limited to <5 days in postoperative period.
Reversal Agents		
Flumazenil	0.1–0.2 mg	Benzodiazepine antagonist. Rapid onset and short duration. Adverse effect of benzodiazepine can persist after drug wears off. Repeated doses of up to 0.8 mg can be used. Abrupt antagonism of chronic benzodiazepine use can precipitate seizures.
Naloxone	Up to 0.4 mg	Opioid antagonist. Rapid onset and short duration. Often diluted 0.4 mg/10 mL and titrated 0.04–0.08 mg at a time to reverse undesirable side effects while preserving analgesia. Repeated doses of up to 0.4 mg or continuous IV infusion can be used. Abrupt opioid antagonism can precipitate increased BP, increased HR, pulmonary edema, or myocardial infarction.
Edrophonium with Atropine	0.5–1.0 mg/kg 0.007–0.014 mg/kg	Edrophonium is an anticholinesterase inhibitor with anti-dysrhythmic properties. Rapid onset, short duration, therefore used usually with atropine, to counteract increased secretions, decreased HR, and bronchospasm. Does not reverse neuromuscular blockade caused by depolarizing agents. Renal and hepatic elimination (edrophonium). Atropine may cause fever.
Neostigmine with	0.5–2.0 mg	Cause salivation and severe low HR. May cause broncho- or laryngospasm. Renal metabolism.
Glycopyrrolate	0.1–0.2 mg	Does not reverse neuromuscular blockade caused by depolarizing agents. Give (same syringe) with glycopyrrolate (or atropine) to counteract low HR. May cause fever.

Ach, acetylcholine; BP, blood pressure; CO, cardiac output; CPP, cerebral perfusion pressure; ICP, intracranial pressure; FDA, U.S. Food and Drug Administration; GI, gastrointestinal; HR, heart rate; IV, intravenous; NMBA, neuromuscular blocking agent; NSAID, non-steroidal anti-inflammatory drug; PCA, patient-controlled analgesia; $T_{1/2}$, elimination half-life; TBI, traumatic brain injury; VO_2, oxygen consumption.

coverage for the other patients is assured. Consideration should also be given to whether an anesthesiologist or nurse anesthetist should be at the bedside for the procedure.

2. **Operations performed in the ICU.** Operations performed at the bedside will vary among ICUs based on specialty orientation and case mix. Among trauma patients, tracheostomy, thoracentesis and tube thoracostomy, paracentesis, cholecystostomy, percutaneous endoscopic gastrostomy, and laparotomy are among the operations and procedures that may be performed in the ICU.

   a. **Tracheostomy.** The most common indication for tracheostomy is ARF with prolonged MV, followed by airway "protection" for the patient who is obtunded or whose gag reflex is impaired or absent. The third most common indication is maxillofacial trauma.

      i. The optimal timing of tracheostomy remains unresolved. Proponents of early tracheostomy (generally within 7 days, as opposed to after 14 days) believe that pulmonary toilet is enhanced, leading to a lower incidence of VAP and shorter durations of MV and ICU length of stay.

   b. **Thoracentesis and tube thoracostomy.** Common bedside procedures on the thorax at the bedside include thoracentesis and tube thoracostomy. Thoracotomy is performed rarely and usually only for patients in extremis.

   c. **Paracentesis.** Ascites is common in critically ill patients, due to hepatic, renal, or cardiac failure, or anasarca with hypoalbuminemia. Occasionally, the presence of ascites warrants removal by paracentesis either for diagnosis or therapy. One therapeutic indication for paracentesis is decompression of abdominal compartment syndrome, with ascites due to massive fluid resuscitation. Rare but serious complications of paracentesis include abdominal wall or intraperitoneal hemorrhage, or bowel perforation. Hypotension may occur after large-volume paracentesis; restitution of intravascular fluid volume with crystalloid or colloid approximating the oncotic characteristics of the removed fluid is restorative.

   d. **Cholecystostomy.** Acute acalculous cholecystitis (AAC) is a manifestation of splanchnic ischemia-reperfusion injury relating to shock and resuscitation. Other risk factors include severe sepsis, diabetes mellitus, abdominal vasculitis, systemic lupus erythematosus, congestive heart failure, renal disease, total parenteral nutrition, and hypovolemia. Abdominal pain (if the patient can communicate), fever, leukocytosis, jaundice from cholestasis, and gallbladder ischemia are characteristic. AAC constitutes the majority of cases of AC in the ICU, but calculous disease is possible.

      i. The diagnosis of AAC may be difficult because most patients cannot communicate their symptoms. In addition, the gallbladder may be only one of several sources of sepsis. Consequently, the diagnosis is most frequently accomplished by ultrasound imaging of the gallbladder. Gallbladder wall thickness of >3.5 mm with pericholecystic fluid is diagnostic. Computed tomography is equally accurate for the same findings.

      ii. The usual treatment for AAC is percutaneous cholecystostomy, either at the bedside or in the interventional radiology suite.

   e. **Bedside laparotomy.** The OR is generally preferred for laparotomy, with optimized anesthetic administration, nursing, lighting, availability of instruments, and facilitated exposure. However, certain patients may be too unstable for transport or need immediate laparotomy in the ICU. The most urgent indication for bedside laparotomy is decompression of abdominal compartment syndrome. Other reasons for bedside laparotomy include changing of abdominal dressings, or treatment of diffuse abdominal infection (tertiary peritonitis).

XI. **REHABILITATION IN THE ICU.** Historically, bedrest and prolonged immobilization were common treatment, but are now understood to be detrimental. The deleterious effects of bedrest become apparent in several systems within 72 hours. Muscle strength decreases by as much as 1.5% per day during strict bedrest, with the greatest loss after the first week. Both the central and peripheral cardiovascular systems are altered, with increased heart rate and decreased stroke volume and cardiac size. Osteolysis also occurs, and on occasion can result in hypercalcemia. Pressure ulcers also occur with prolonged bedrest, with the incidence increasing dramatically after 7 days of critical illness. The critical illness polyneuropathy syndrome is a manifestation of MODS that is associated with sepsis and AKI, and causes profound muscle weakness that may persist for months in survivors. The cause is unknown, but neuromuscular blockade and aminoglycoside therapy are two proposed mechanisms. The diagnosis must be sought actively by performing bedside electromyography. There is no known therapy.

A. Basic mobilization in the ICU can counteract the effects of prolonged bedrest, and maintain or improve strength, functional ability, and endurance. Patients who are unstable need to be turned every 2 hours around the clock to avoid prolonged pressure on the occiput, calcanei, trochanters, pre-sacral tissue, and other pressure-sensitive areas. Particularly with prolonged ICU stays, initial interventions are passive, including an evaluation of positioning and the need for splinting devices to maintain joint integrity and to prevent skin breakdown. More stable patients are supported for their ability to roll, shift weight, grab, sit, and stand. The transition from a supine to sitting position can be especially challenging. Adequate pain control is mandatory to initiate mobilization.

1. MV is not a contraindication to rehabilitation. For patients breathing spontaneously, therapy can promote improved lung aeration, rib cage expansion, diaphragm capacity, and decreased accessory muscle use. Participation of medically tenuous patients will fluctuate session to session, with respiratory rate, heart rate, and SaO_2 indicating how well a patient is tolerating treatment. The impact of medications and pain on heart rate must also be considered.

2. Arousal level is also a frequent limitation. Elevating the head of the bed to stimulate the reticular activating system, repositioning, and olfactory and tactile stimulation are all used to enhance responsiveness. For the agitated patient, relaxation techniques, re-orientation, and decreased environmental stimulation may be attempted before pharmacologic treatment.

XII. END-OF-LIFE CARE. Recognition that injuries or the complications thereof (e.g., sepsis and MODS) may be non-survivable is crucial for effective, compassionate management. Patients (when they can participate) and their surrogates expect, and are entitled to, sufficient information about their diagnosis and prognosis to participate in decision making in a meaningful manner, including the right to forego additional treatment or to withdraw care, resulting in death.

A. Unfortunately, the majority of injured patients, young or old, still do not make known in advance their wishes for life-sustaining care, leaving trauma surgeons and surrogates to undertake what is believed to be in the best interest of the patient. The process is often laden with stress, given that the parties usually do not have a prior relationship, and surrogates may not be entirely reconciled (if not in denial) to the recent injury or newly acquired knowledge of the poor prognosis. In addition, caregivers may be struggling with the fact that the adverse outcome may sometimes be related to iatrogenesis, and a desire to "get the patient through."

B. Patients or surrogates should be asked if advance directives exist, whether living wills, durable powers of attorney for health care, or do-not-resuscitate (DNR) orders, depending on individual state laws. Patients with capacity must be offered the opportunity to designate a health care agent (proxy) by law. Patients who lack capacity but who have executed an advance directive may have designated a health care agent; if so, that person should be identified and engaged in dialogue as soon as possible.

1. The parameters under which limits on the provision of care may be set vary among jurisdictions, and clinicians must be aware of those applicable specifically to their practice locale. For example, not all jurisdictions use the same definition of "medical futility," or place the same weight on the living will. When end-of-life care planning is discussed, the patient's prognosis, religious preference, and functional limitations are all of paramount consideration. For example, some religious groups may refuse blood transfusion. Most hospitals have ethics committees to assist in end-of-life care planning, particularly when there are varying opinions or frank disputes among clinicians or between clinicians and surrogates.

2. When care is withdrawn, the clinician should be the patient's advocate, seeking to eliminate suffering during the process. Often, MV is withdrawn. If the patient is brain dead by definition there will be no spontaneous breathing efforts, but in other circumstances there may be agonal respirations. It is permissible to relieve suffering with opioid medications, even if so doing may hasten demise by exacerbating hemodynamic instability.

3. Palliative care is not just limited to the process of withdrawal of care, the dying patient only, or to just the patient himself or herself. Bereavement may accompany critical illness or injury regardless of the prognosis or outcome. Whereas the goals of critical care first and foremost are the saving of life, with the alleviation of suffering and improving the quality of life being secondary goals of considerable importance, for palliative care the hierarchy is reversed. Integration of critical care and palliative care brings these various (and sometimes conflicting) goals into concordance.

  a. Quality palliative care focus efforts in seven domains: Patient/family-centered decision making, communication within the care team and with patients/families, continuity of care, emotional support for families, spiritual support for families, symptom management and comfort care, and emotional and organizational support for ICU clinicians. Psychosocial support should be offered to patients and families within 24 hours of admission, perhaps by formal assessment by a multi-professional team consisting of physicians, nurses, social workers, clergy, and others. Within 72 hours of admission, a family meeting is recommended with a physician and nurse to develop the comprehensive care plan, and to document the plan in the medical record.

XIII. IDENTIFICATION AND CARE OF THE POTENTIAL ORGAN DONOR (see Chapter 41). Dying patients or their surrogates may be able to make the gift of life after death in the form of organ donation for orthotopic transplantation. The shortage of donor organs is so acute that to expand the donor pool, organs with marginal function may be considered for transplantation. For example, neither age nor blood stream infection represent absolute contraindications to organ donation.

XIV. PATIENT SAFETY AND SYSTEM MANAGEMENT

  A. The hazards of accidental injury by sharps (e.g., needles, scalpel blades) and the risks of blood-borne transmission of etiologic agents are real. Policies and procedures have been changed in all ORs to minimize the risk, which has been decreasing. In the OR, particular attention is paid to communication among team members, protocols for passing sharp instruments to and from the operative field and instrument table, and meticulous accounting of sharps throughout the operation. Similar attention to detail is mandatory if surgery at the bedside in the ICU will be made as safe as possible for the patient and the operating team. Sterile gowns, sterile double gloves, masks, caps, and eye protection should be used for any bedside procedure where the possibility exists of splashing blood or body fluids. The mattress must never be used as a "pin cushion" for needles. The period of highest risk to practitioners appears to be during clean-up in the aftermath of minor procedures, during which the accounting process for sharps may be haphazard. When drapes are collected for disposal at the end of the procedure (usually by the person who performed the procedure, who may have been working only with the patient's primary nurse), it is easy to overlook an unsecured sharp within the folds of a drape. Even if no injury occurs at the bedside, if a sharp is discarded inadvertently in the trash rather than the containers provided for the purpose, other hospital workers and sanitation workers are placed at risk.

B. Avoiding error

  1. Most inhospital trauma mortality occurs in the ICU during the first few days of admission because of TBI, respiratory failure, or refractory hemorrhagic shock; these deaths are largely not preventable. The remainder occurs late, usually because of MODS. Technical, monitoring, and management errors have been reported in up to one-half of preventable trauma deaths.

  2. Estimates of preventable death vary widely, indicating the variability of care inherent in trauma management and the need for standardized approaches. To reduce errors, institutions need effective means to identify errors and reduce error-associated deaths, which by their very infrequency may be difficult to characterize. Moreover, errors may occur for many reasons, including predisposing structural and systems factors, lack of knowledge, defective information processing, and errors of communication.

  3. Trauma-related errors may be characterized in four domains: Phase of trauma care, type of intervention, type of error, and cause of error.

  a. Errors characterized by the phase of trauma management may occur during initial assessment and resuscitation, secondary assessment, transport, initial intervention in the ED or OR, or in later phases of care in the ICU, on the ward, or even in the rehabilitation phase.

  b. Errors may occur in several clinical interventions in trauma care, including control of hemorrhage, airway management, hemodynamic resuscitation, management prioritization for unstable patients, performance of procedures, prophylaxis of potential complications, missed or delayed diagnoses, and others.

  c. Errors of intervention may be characterized as to a relationship to diagnosis, treatment, or prevention, and further as to an input error (e.g., lack of data), intention error (e.g., lack of knowledge or skill, including communication skill), or execution errors (e.g., technical flaw). Diagnostic errors, which are less common than treatment and prevention errors, are most common during the secondary trauma survey and in the ICU. Errors of hemorrhage control (the most prevalent trauma-related errors) are common during initial assessment and in the ICU, whereas errors related to procedures and prophylaxis are far more common in the ICU.

  d. The initial assessment, resuscitation, and intervention phases of trauma care are error prone. The majority of error-related deaths are intention errors that affect treatment; these types of errors are most amenable to remediation with protocols and algorithms. Interactive training approaches are used to facilitate learning through repetition and scenario management. By contrast, execution errors are addressed through technical training and ensuring through appropriate supervision that those performing tasks are competent and credentialed for the task. Input errors require the proper use and interpretation of diagnostic tests. Attention to detail, checklists, and supervision can reduce both execution and input errors. Regardless of the type of error-related problem or its effective remediation, learning from errors must occur in an environment of trust and transparency, working to improve process rather than assign blame or exact retribution.

Suggested Readings

Abdeen O, Mehta RL. Dialysis modalities in the intensive care unit. *Crit Care Clin* 2002;18:223–247.

Arbabi S, Campion EM, Hemmila MR, et al. Beta-blocker use is associated with improved outcomes in adult trauma patients. *J Trauma* 2007;62:56–61.

Barie PS, Hydo LJ, Shou J, et al. Decreasing magnitude of multiple organ dysfunction syndrome despite increasingly severe critical surgical illness: A 17-year longitudinal study. *J Trauma* 2008;65:1227–1235.

Chang A, Schyve PM, Croteau RJ, et al. The JCAHO patient safety event taxonomy: A standardized terminology and classification schema for near misses and adverse events. *Int J Qual Health Care* 2005;17:95–105.

Cook DJ, Rocker G, Giacommi M, et al. Understanding and changing attitudes toward withdrawal and withholding of life support in the intensive care unit. *Crit Care Med* 2006;34:S317–S323.

Eriksson EA, Christianson DA, Vanderkolk WE, et al. Tight blood glucose control in trauma patients: Who really benefits? *J Emerg Trauma Shock* 2011;4:359–364.

Field JM, Hazinski MF, Sayre MR, et al. Part 1: Executive Summary: 2010 American Heart Association guidelines for cardiopulmonary resuscitation and emergency cardiovascular care. *Circulation* 2010;122:S640–S656.

Griesdale DE, de Souza RJ, van Dam RM, et al. Intensive insulin therapy and mortality among critically ill patients: A meta-analysis including NICE-SUGAR study data. *CMAJ* 2009;180:821–827.

Mowrey NT, Gunter OL, Dossett LA, et al. Failure to achieve euglycemia despite aggressive insulin control signals abnormal physiologic response to trauma. *J Crit Care* 2011;26:295–302.

National Heart, Lung, and Blood Institute Acute Respiratory Distress Syndrome (ARDS) Clinical Trials Network, Wheeler AP, Bernard GR, et al. Pulmonary-artery versus central venous catheter to guide treatment of acute lung injury. *N Engl J Med* 2006;354:2213–2214.

Neumar RW, Otto CW, Link MS, et al. 2010 American Heart Association guidelines for cardiopulmonary resuscitation and emergency cardiovascular care science. Part 8. Adult advanced cardiovascular life support *Circulation* 2010;122:S729–S767.

NICE-SUGAR Study Investigators, Finfer S, Chittock DR, et al. Intensive versus conventional glucose control in critically ill patients. *N Engl J Med* 2009;360:1283–1297.

Tisherman SA, Barie P, Bokhari F, et al. Clinical practice guideline: Endpoints of resuscitation. *J Trauma* 2004;57:898–912.

35 Multiple Organ Dysfunction Syndrome

Philip A. Efron, Darwin N. Ang, Lyle L. Moldawer and Frederick A. Moore

I. INTRODUCTION

A. Multiple organ dysfunction syndrome (MODS) is defined as the dysfunction of at least two organ systems from an inflammatory insult, usually traumatic or infectious shock.

B. Up to half of all SICU patients will meet the criteria for MODS.

C. Mortality due to MODS is proportional to the number of affected organs and the duration of dysfunction.

D. The advent of mechanical ventilation, nutritional support, renal replacement therapy (RRT), and other support improved the rescue of these patients and prospective characterization of this syndrome.

E. In theory, organ function is recoverable, but patients can fail to return to baseline due to ongoing insults, some of which are iatrogenic (mechanical ventilation, transfusion are examples).

F. MODS after trauma often follows one of the two distinct patterns:
   1. Rapid single phase MODS due to massive trauma and tissue injury.
   2. Delayed MODS, usually due to moderate trauma and shock. This is followed by a secondary insult, often sepsis or an infection.

G. After trauma, patients who develop MODS are typically older and have a greater injury severity score (ISS) or present to the emergency department with hypotension (SBP <90 mm Hg). Also, patients who develop MODS after trauma are more likely to have early elevated base deficits (greater than 8 mEq/L) and failure to normalize lactate despite resuscitation. Finally, these patients are also more likely to receive blood transfusions. Increasing units of transfused packed red blood cells (PRBCs) correlate with an increased incidence of MODS.

II. FURTHER CLASSIFICATION/DEFINITIONS

A. Systemic inflammatory response syndrome (SIRS) (Table 35-1).

B. Sepsis
   1. SIRS due to an infection.
   2. Sepsis is the most common trigger or source of MODS in the surgical population.

III. MECHANISMS

A. MODS is thought to be due to inflammatory and immune dysregulation after an insult. These triggers include:
   1. Injury (trauma or operation)
   2. Burns
   3. Infection
   4. Ischemia/reperfusion
   5. Pancreatitis

B. Although any of the above factors can trigger the response, MODS is commonly induced by multiple or sustained insults (i.e., the "2-hit" hypothesis).

C. Some of these insults can be the treatments being used to preserve life, for example vasoconstrictors, transfusions, or mechanical ventilation. Other triggers include secondary events such as fat emboli.

TABLE 35-1 **Definition of SIRS**

Patient must have ≥ 2 of the following:
1. Body temperature $>38°C$ or $<36°C$
2. Heart rate >90 beats/min
3. Respiratory rate >20 breaths/min or $PaCO_2$ <32 mm Hg
4. White blood cell count $>12,000$ cells/mm^3 or $<4,000$ cells/mm^3 or $>10\%$ immature neutrophils

---

IV. PREDICTION/PROGNOSIS

A. There is no singular standard to identify MODS and no laboratory test has yet proven diagnostic or prognostic.

B. **Physiologic scoring systems** calculate the function of specific organs, determine a severity score and predict outcome. These include the multiple organ dysfunction (MOD) score, the sequential organ failure assessment (SOFA), the logistic organ dysfunction (LOD) systems score, the Marshal MOF score and the **Denver MOF** score (Table 35-2).

C. **The Acute Pathophysiology and Chronic Health Evaluation (APACHE II)** is the most common scoring system that reflects organ dysfunction and is based on

---

TABLE 35-2 **Multiple Organ Failure Score**

	Grade 0	Grade 1 Dysfunction	Grade 2 Dysfunction	Grade 3 Dysfunction
Pulmonary PaO_2/FiO_2 Ratio	>208	208 - 165	165 - 83	<83
Renal Creatinine (μmol/L)	<159	160–210	211–420	>420
Hepatic Total Bilirubin (μmol/L)	<34	34–68	69–137	>137
Cardiac Inotropes	No inotropes	Only one inotrope at a small dose*	Any inotrope at moderate dose or >1 agent, all at small doses*	Any inotrope at large dose or >2 agents at moderate doses*

*Inotrope doses (in ug/kg/min):

	Small	Moderate	Large
Milrinone	<0.3	0.4–0.7	>0.7
Vasopressin	<0.03	0.03–0.07	>0.07
Dopamine	<6	6–10	>10
Dobutamine	<6	6–10	>10
Epinephrine	<0.06	0.06–0.15	>0.15
Norepinephrine	<0.11	0.11–0.5	>05
Phenylephrine	<0.6	0.6–3	>3

Adapted from Moore, et al.

12 physiologic variables. The maximum score is 71; a score of 25 carries a 50% mortality.

D. Mortality exceeds 50% for patients with ≥3 organ dysfunction. MODS patients are more likely than non-MODS patients to develop complications. Correspondingly, it takes longer to liberate these patients from the ventilator.

E. The requirement for hemodialysis is also associated with increased mortality in these patients, with some surgical populations having up to a 50% mortality.

F. Most MODS patients who survive their hospital course will require prolonged rehabilitation, sometimes requiring transfer to a long-term acute care hospital. Up to 1/3 to 1/2 of older patients with significant organ failure die within months of discharge from the ICU.

G. Trauma patients who survive MODS have a higher overall mortality after discharge than the general population.

V. PATHOPHYSIOLOGY
A. Neurologic

1. Brain dysfunction during MODS is characterized by encephalopathy and a reduced level of consciousness.
2. Alterations in brain function are best considered MODS until disproven; start immediate efforts to isolate and treat any possible cause.
3. Lack of improvement after supportive measures and source control may require imaging (CT scan or MRI), functional (EEG) or invasive testing (lumbar puncture), or drug levels to exclude other etiologies of brain dysfunction.
4. Critical illness polyneuropathy is commonly found with sepsis and prolonged use of steroids or paralytic agents. Patients develop diffuse axonal motor and sensory neuropathy which may manifest as weakness and failure to wean from the ventilator.
5. **B. Pulmonary (see Chapter 38)** Patients with acute lung injury (ALI) and acute respiratory distress syndrome (ARDS) (Table 35-3) demonstrate lung injury associated with hypoxemia, non-cardiogenic pulmonary edema, decreased lung compliance, and increased capillary leakage.
6. The cause of ALI/ARDS can be direct (e.g., aspiration, pneumonia, chest trauma) or indirect (e.g., pancreatitis, ischemia/reperfusion of the intestines).
7. ALI/ARDS is divided into two phases:
   a. An initial *acute exudative phase*, characterized by acute onset hypoxemia and decreased compliance. This phase is refractory to supplemental O_2 but responsive to PEEP.
   b. A subsequent *fibroproliferative phase*, characterized by persistent hypoxemia, worsening compliance, pulmonary hypertension, and CO_2 retention. This phase is less responsive to PEEP. Pneumonia is the most common infection in MODS patients and is a major cause of subsequent morbidity and mortality.
8. COPD and other underlying pulmonary diseases are exacerbated by sepsis.

B. Cardiac

1. MODS can lead to overall myocardial dysfunction, regardless of the cause.
2. Underlying causes include repeated ischemic events, inflammatory mediators and altered splanchnic perfusion.

TABLE 35-3	Definition of Acute Lung Injury and Acute Respiratory Distress Syndrome

1. Bilateral pulmonary infiltrates on chest x-ray
2. Pulmonary capillary wedge pressure <18 mm Hg Or no clinical suspension
3. PaO_2/FiO_2 <300 mm Hg = ALI
4. PaO_2/FiO_2 <200 mm Hg = ARDS

TABLE 35-4	RIFLE Criteria	
	GFR criteria	**Urine output criteria**
Risk	↑ serum Cr × 1.5 or ↓ GFR >25%	Urine output <0.5 mL/kg/h for 6 h
Injury	↑ serum Cr × 2.0 or ↓ GFR >50%	Urine output <0.5 mL/kg/h for 12 h
Failure	↑ serum Cr × 3.0; or ↓ GFR >75% or serum Cr ≥4 mg/dL with >0.5 mg/dL ↑ serum Cr	Urine output <0.3 mL/kg/h for 24 h or anuria for 24 h
Loss	Persistent AKI or complete loss of renal function for >4 wks	
End-stage kidney disease	End-stage renal disease for >3 mos	

GFR, glomerular filtration rate; Cr, Creatinine. The classification system includes separate criteria based on creatinine and urine output and assessment is based on the worst possible value, if both are present.

3. MODS can induce right- or left-sided heart failure; echocardiography can detect this and aid therapy.

4. Persistently elevated lactate levels despite efforts to overcome cardiac dysfunction with adequate perfusion and delivery can indicate impaired distal mitochondrial function and correlate with poor outcome.

5. Demand cardiac ischemia is common in sepsis and usually self-limiting, especially after source control is obtained.

C. Renal (see Chapter 37)

1. More than half of ICU patients will develop acute kidney injury (AKI).

2. AKI is associated with an increased mortality; need for hemodialysis after an operation is associated with up to a 50% mortality during hospitalization.

3. Kidney failure can be due to multiple causes, including ischemia–reperfusion (e.g., hemorrhage) as well as efferent arteriole dilatation (e.g., sepsis).

4. AKI is under-recognized. Those patients with even small alterations in creatinine or urine output are at risk for renal injury or failure.

5. Renal failure can be staged by the risk, injury, failure, loss, end-stage kidney disease (RIFLE) criteria (Table 35-4). When using the RIFLE criteria, AKI should be both abrupt (within 1 to 7 days) and sustained (>24 hours).

6. Recent revisions to the RIFLE criteria by the AKI Network have generated the AKIN staging system (Table 35-5). The modifications are the following:

a. Risk, failure and injury have been altered to stages 1, 2, and 3, respectively. Any patient who receives acute RRT is also stage 3.

b. Diagnostic increments of serum creatinine occur during a period of no more than 48 hours (as compared to RIFLE's 7 days).

TABLE 35-5	AKIN Staging System	
Stage	**Serum creatinine increase from baseline**	**Urine output criteria**
1	≥0.3 mg/dL or ≥150–200%	<0.5 mL/kg/h for >6 h
2	>200–300%	<0.5 mL/kg/h for >12 h
3	>300% or acute RRT	<0.3 mL/kg/h for >24 h or anuria ≥12 h

    c. Diagnosis of AKI can be determined with a period of oliguria of at least 6 hours or a serum creatinine increase of $\geq$0.3 mg/dL from baseline. Appropriate volume resuscitation must be maintained as well as ascertaining that there is no urinary outlet obstruction prior to using urine output as a gauge for AKI. Also, realize that alterations in urine flow are less helpful as a diagnostic criterion due to the high incidence of nonoliguric AKI.

D. Hepatic (see Chapter 40)

    1. Hepatic injury and dysfunction is usually the result of inadequate perfusion. Liver injury in MODS often demonstrates a biphasic pattern, with initial alterations in INR and transaminases ("shock liver"). Subsequently, there is hepatic recovery, which may be followed by a more severe loss of liver function characterized by increasing bilirubin levels associated with cholestasis.

    2. With respect to the liver, MODS can manifest itself as a failure of hepatic function, including inadequate metabolic, synthetic, and detoxification functions. A lack of heme metabolism can produce jaundice.

E. Gastrointestinal/Nutrition

    1. The gastrointestinal system is both an instigator and a victim of MODS. Specifically, ischemia/reperfusion results in release of proinflammatory mediators by the intestine. Resultant gastrointestinal dysfunction due to MODS includes gastroesophageal reflux, gastroparesis, increased gastric pH, decreased splanchnic perfusion, decreased transit, increased colonization/permeability/translocation, and decreased immunity.

    2. MODS patients are typically catabolic and hypermetabolic. The metabolic response to injury and infection contributes to MODS pathophysiology. This includes nitrogen wasting, loss of muscle mass and muscle function, loss of visceral protein, decreased organ function, and dysfunctional immune response.

    3. Delays in nutritional supplementation induce worse outcomes; however, overfeeding can also increase morbidity and mortality. The ideal feeding pattern is still elusive.

    4. Abdominal compartment syndrome (ACS) is an early complication of severe trauma and resuscitation and will add to the MODS cascade.

F. Endocrine

    1. Most patients in MODS have insulin deficiency and resistance.

    2. Thyroid and adrenal insufficiency are under-recognized. Look for persistent hypotension after adequate volume or sodium/potassium changes to suspect adrenal insufficiency, especially in those on pretrauma supplementation. *Euthyroid Sick Syndrome,* an abnormal thyroid function, tests in the setting of nonthyroidal illness, often in the elderly and less obvious than typical hypothyroidism where bradycardia and malaise exist.

VI. TREATMENT

    A. The mainstay of treatment for MODS is rapid control of the cause. Without *source control,* organ dysfunction rapidly worsens and may result in death. Thus, rapid identification and serial assessment is required to optimize outcomes. Patients who survive the first 6 hours of hospitalization most likely survive to discharge, emphasizing the importance of early and adequate resuscitation of shock.

    B. *Source control* can include interventional or operative procedures. Failure or delay of source control, including inappropriate antibiotic selection, induces worse outcomes in all patient populations. Consultation with an intensivist is recommended for the treatment of the patient in septic shock.

    C. Typically, targeted resuscitation approaches are best. [See Chapter 44.]

    D. Attempts to blunt the SIRS response (e.g., anti-inflammatory agents) have not improved outcomes.

    E. Although blood products are life saving in hemorrhagic shock, transfusions outside that condition should be minimized as patient morbidity and mortality directly increase with the amount of product received. Given no extraneous circumstances (e.g., ST elevation MI, continued bleeding), a hemoglobin trigger of $\leq$7.0 g/dL is preferred threshold for transfusion.

TABLE 35-6	Example of PRBC Transfusion Criteria

- *Anemia*
    - *No acute cardiac disease and anemia*
        - Hct <19.5%: 2 units;
        - Hct >19.5% <22%: 1 unit
    - *Acute active cardiac disease*
        - Hct <22%: 3 units
        - Hct >22% <27%: 2 units
        - Hct >27% <30%: 1 unit
- *Active Bleeding*
- *Sudden unexplained HCT drop*
- *Low SvO$_2$*
- *Unstable on pressors with Hct <30% and SvO$_2$ <65%*
- *Traumatic Brain Injury (first 24 h of admission if part of a TBI protocol)*
- *Hemorrhagic shock (consider massive transfusion protocol)*

    1. Similarly, FFP is not routinely needed. Most procedures are safe, including intracranial interventions, at an INR <1.7. Do not arbitrarily correct an elevated INR, and if using FFP to correct a measured coagulopathy, choose the appropriate volume of FFP (10 to 15 mL/kg) (Tables 35-6 and 35-7).

  F. Activated Protein C cannot be recommended routinely or in clear subsets based on outcome data.

  G. Measures to support host immunity and prevent nosocomial infections include:

    1. Early enteral feeding.

    2. Discontinuation of antibiotics or narrowing the coverage spectrum of those drugs when possible.

    3. Removal of indwelling catheters as soon as possible, including endotracheal tubes, central lines, chest tubes, and bladder catheters.

    4. Early mobilization.

  H. Neurologic

    1. Maintaining adequate perfusion/delivery of oxygen to the brain is the primary goal, followed by anxiolytics for anxiety and analgesics for pain.

    2. Minimize the amount of drugs required to achieve the above goals, titrating to specific validated scoring systems, such as the Riker Sedation–Agitation Scale, FLACC score or pain scale.

    3. Removing neuromuscular blockade and sedation early improves strength and restores respiratory drive.

  I. Pulmonary

    1. Patients with MODS often require intubation and mechanical ventilation. Lung protective ventilation strategies should be utilized (Table 35-8).

TABLE 35-7	Example of FFP Transfusion Criteria

*Anticoagulants to be held; patient to receive 10–15mL/kg FFP
- Thrombotic thrombocytopenic purpura
- Congenital or acquired coagulation factor deficiencies for which no specific coagulation concentrates are available
- Warfarin anticoagulation-related ICH or TBI with INR ≥1.7
- Undergoing invasive procedure with INR ≥1.7
- Active bleeding or expanding ICH/TBI and INR ≥1.5
- Hemorrhagic shock (consider massive transfusion protocol)

TABLE 35-8	Ventilation Strategies for ALI/ARDS

1. PaO_2 >60 mm Hg
2. Tidal volume ≤8 mL/kg (ideal body weight)
3. Plateau pressure <30–35 cm H_2O
4. Minimum PEEP required to stent airways open (P_{flex})
5. Permissive hypercapnia (if tolerated), maintaining a pH ≥7.2

  a. Limit morbidity due to volutrauma/barotrauma (low tidal volume ventilation).
  b. Optimize gas exchange in the lung parenchyma while avoiding oxygen toxicity.
2. Adjuncts include Prostacyclin (e.g., epoprostenol), nitric oxide, high-frequency oscillatory ventilation, prone positioning, and extracorporeal membrane oxygenation. The effectiveness of adjunct therapies is still unclear; deploy each selectively as a rescue therapy.
3. Minimize the risk of ventilator-associated pneumonia (VAP); utilize ventilator bundles (Table 35-9).
4. The treatment of severe ARDS with a neuromuscular blocking agent (specifically, cisatracurium started within 48 hours and used for 48 hours) reduces barotrauma, improves P/F ratio, decreases the PEEP requirement, increases the number of ventilator-free days, and decreases mortality without increasing muscle weakness.
5. Steroids may play a role in the treatment of patients with chronic ARDS. In acute ARDS, steroids are not a routine therapy.
6. Early tracheostomy may facilitate ventilator support and accelerate liberation from the ventilator (in turn reducing the risk of VAP). However, patients with ALI/ARDS are susceptible to the complications of tracheostomy, requiring assessment of the risks and benefits for each patient. Those patients with CO_2 retention benefit the most since the tracheostomy bypasses the resistance of upper airway and oropharynx.
7. Pneumonia
  a. Prevention of pneumonia requires aggressive respiratory care to enhance lung volume and clear secretions.
  b. The clinical diagnosis of pneumonia is often unreliable.
  c. Overtreatment of the disease is associated with increased costs and bacterial resistance. Undertreatment in this patient population increases mortality.
  d. High risk patients should be treated empirically with invasive diagnostic techniques (including bronchoalveolar lavage) which allow earlier diagnosis as well as more rapid narrowing or discontinuation of antibiotic therapy.
  e. Guidelines for antibiotic therapy should be tailored to an ICU's particular antibiogram, considering the frequency of specific pathogens as well as the resistance patterns of those organisms.

TABLE 35-9	Example of Ventilator Bundle to Prevent Ventilator-associated Pneumonia

1. Proper infection control/handwashing
2. Patients head of bed raised ≥30 degrees
3. Chlorhexidine mouth wash twice daily
4. Oral care every 4 h
5. Endotracheal tubes with supraglottic suctioning
6. Turn patient every 2 h
7. Deep vein thrombosis prophylaxis
8. Daily sedation holiday and assessment for extubation
9. Peptic ulcer disease prophylaxis

J. Cardiac
1. The goal of therapy is to attain adequate perfusion as well maintain aerobic metabolism.
2. Measures of oxygen delivery and consumption (or lack thereof), such as mixed venous oxygen saturation, infrared measurements of tissue oxygen content, or serial lactate levels may be better indicators of appropriate circulatory function than simply blood pressure measurements.
3. Supranormal delivery of oxygen to tissues does not add benefit to the critically ill patient.
   End organ function, such as mentation or renal function, is also an important indirect measure of adequate cardiac function. Use an indwelling bladder catheter if urine output cannot be otherwise assessed accurately.
4. Cardiac dysfunction is best treated with appropriate pressors (norepinephrine) and inotropes (dobutamine). Acute right-sided heart failure should prompt seeking a cause, often acute pulmonary embolism.

K. Renal (see Chapter 37)
1. One of the most important treatments for renal dysfunction involves maintaining adequate intravascular volume.
2. Next, avoid the exacerbation of kidney injury by minimizing nephrotoxic agents.
3. Treat hyperkalemia based on symptoms, ECG findings, and the potassium level.
4. Indications for RRT include the "AEIOU" of hemodialysis: **A**cidosis (intractable), **E**lectrolyte disarray, **I**ntoxicants, **O**verload (fluid), and **U**remia (symptomatic).

L. Hepatic
1. Ensure adequate perfusion to the liver and intestinal tissue; attempt to minimize pressor use.
2. Although uncommon, acalculous cholecystitis is part of the differential diagnosis in the setting of hyperbilirubinemia. Image with ultrasound and operate if necessary, using percutaneous drainage in high risk patients.

M. Gastrointestinal/Nutrition
1. In general, enteral feeding is the preferred route of nutrition, based on outcome and cost. Enteral feeds should be started early, usually within 24 to 48 hours. Benefits of enteral nutrition include improved motility, mucosal immunity, and barrier function.
   a. Parenteral nutrition is better than no nutrition after several days of starvation, but parenteral nutrition can increase the risk of infection.
   b. If the patient is unable to achieve ≥60% of their targeted nutrition goal by the seventh day in the ICU, concurrent TPN should be considered.
2. Start enteral feeds when the patient is resuscitated and without abdominal distension. Feeding the ischemic or hypoperfused intestine or persistence in feeding with impaired gut motility can produce massive gut infarction. Similar to resuscitation and other treatments for MODS, the use of a standard protocol will result in the successful feeding of the most critically ill.
3. Specific nutritional goals and supplements are addressed in a separate chapter (see Chapter 8).
4. Although stress gastritis is uncommon in modern ICUs, especially with appropriate patient resuscitation, start prophylaxis early. H_2 antagonists are preferred over proton pump inhibitors (PPIs), which are associated with increased complications (pneumonia and *Clostridium difficile* infection). Stress ulcer prophylaxis is outlined in Table 35-10.
   a. Reasons to preferentially utilize a PPI include upper gastrointestinal bleeding or home use of a PPI.
5. Selective gut decontamination is not commonly practiced in the United States due to expense, labor, and concern of inducing resistant bacteria. Probiotics cannot be endorsed at this time as it may be detrimental in specific patient populations in MODS.
6. Post-pyloric feeding is typically recommended, but many patients tolerate gastric feeding. Regardless of the route, elevate the head of the bed >30 degrees and start the feeds at low rates (10 to 15 mL/hour).

TABLE 35-10	Guidelines for Stress Ulcer Prophylaxis

1. H_2 blocker is the agent of choice (GI route preferred, if the patient is able to take PO or PT)
2. Stress ulcer prophylaxis is indicated on admission when:
   a. Patient is on mechanical ventilation
   b. Patient has significant coagulopathy defined as INR >2.0 or platelet count <50.
   c. Consider for all Burn and Neurosurgical patients (Curling and Cushing ulcers)
3. Stress ulcer prophylaxis will be discontinued when possible.
   Exclusion criteria for discontinuation:
   ■ Active treatment for ulcer disease or GERD
   ■ Transplant patient
   ■ Gastrojejunal anastomosis (marginal ulcer)

    7. Diarrhea and abdominal distention are frequently encountered with tube feeds. Seek signs and symptoms of *C. difficile*, especially if the diarrhea is accompanied by signs of infection or in the setting of current/previous antibiotics use. Rapid technology (such as polymerase chain reaction [PCR] can help quickly detect *C. difficile*-associated diarrhea although a singular negative test will not exclude it.
      a. Diarrhea can generally be managed successfully in the ICU by slowing the infusion or altering the composition. Distension may be a sign of nonocclusive small bowel necrosis; however, with the use of more modest infusion goal rates (e.g., 60 mL/hour) and slower advancement rates (every 8 to 12 hours) for tube feeds, this complication is now uncommon.
  N. Abdominal compartment syndrome is a reversible cause of MODS. See Chapter 39 for details. Efforts to limit massive volume resuscitation, or at least prevent over-resuscitation, should be implemented. Bladder pressures should be routinely monitored in this population.
  O. Endocrine
    1. Insulin is a powerful anabolic hormone. Glucose control is best achieved with standardized protocols for checking blood glucose levels regularly and titrated insulin. Often, this may require insulin drips for continuous therapy. Hypoglycemia and hyperglycemia are both dangerous. Therefore, previous recommendations for tight glucose control have been relaxed. Glucose levels <150 mg/dL (without hypoglycemia) are optimal, although levels between 150 and 180 mg/dL are acceptable and utilized in some ICUs.
    2. There is no data demonstrating benefit or harm with thyroid hormone replacement in patients with *Euthyroid Sick Syndrome*. In patients who are considered adrenal insufficient, balanced steroid replacement is needed. Steroid therapy is not without risk, and the benefits of therapy should outweigh the risk. Determining true adrenal insufficiency in critically ill patients is difficult as many of the standard tests are unreliable in this patient population. A random cortisol level of <10 to 15 μg/dL in the setting of MODS is often considered adrenal insufficiency and treated, especially if the patient is symptomatic (e.g., refractory hypotension).
      a. Do not perform cosyntropin stimulation tests during septic shock. Rather, patients who are unresponsive to vasoconstrictive medications after appropriate volume resuscitation should receive empiric steroid therapy. Hydrocortisone is recommended for its simultaneous mineralocorticoid effects; use of additional mineral-corticoids is no longer recommended. Hydrocortisone 200 to 300 mg/day, as a drip or in divided doses.
    3. At this time, growth hormone is contraindicated.

AXIOMS

■ Early identification and intervention for insults that can induce MODS are vital to prevent mortality and morbidity.
■ Once MODS is present, source control, appropriate resuscitation and support of failing organs, nutritional support and prevention of iatrogenic injury (e.g., utilization of ARDS

ventilation strategies), or further insult (e.g., appropriate use of blood products) are the current therapies.

Suggested Readings

Bihorac A, Delano MJ, Schold JD, et al. Incidence, clinical predictors, genomics, and outcome of acute kidney injury among trauma patients. *Ann Surg* 2010;252:158–165.

Buchman TG. Multiple organ dysfunction and failure. In: Cameron JL, et al. eds. *Current Surgical Therapy.* 10th ed. Philadephia, PA: Elsevier Mosby; 2011:1149–1153.

Efron PA, Coopersmith CM. In: Rabinovici R, et al. eds. *Trauma, Critical Care and Surgical Emergencies.* London: Informa UK; 2010:362–368.

Elhassan EA, Schrier RW. Acute kidney injury. In: Vincent J-L, et al. eds. *Textbook of Critical Care.* 6th ed. Philadelphia, PA: Elsevier Saunders; 2011:883–893.

Mizock BA. The multiple organ dysfunction syndrome. *Dis Mon* 2009;55:476–526.

Moore FA, Moore EE. Postinjury multiple organ failure.*Trauma.* 5th ed. New York, NY: McGraw-Hill; 2004:1397–1423.

Papazian L, Forel JM, Gacouin A, et al. Neuromuscular blockers in early acute respiratory distress syndrome. *N Engl J Med* 2010;363:1107–1116.

Reinhart K, Bloos F. Pathophysiology of sepsis and multiple organ dysfunction. In: Vincent J-L, et al. eds. *Textbook of Critical Care.* 6th ed. Philadelphia, PA: Elsevier Saunders; 2011:983–991.

36 Cardiovascular Disease and Monitoring

Mayur Narayan and Thomas M. Scalea

I. INTRODUCTION

Cardiovascular monitoring can help guide optimal therapy by ensuring adequate oxygen delivery to tissues while allowing for assessment and manipulation of cardiac contractility.

Hemorrhage is the most common etiology of shock after injury. Patients with blood loss or those undergoing surgery may also develop cardiac dysfunction. Critically ill patients at risk for development of systemic inflammation from trauma or sepsis will require monitoring to guide supportive measures and limit organ dysfunction. Shock and hypoperfusion can be occult or compensated, yet just as deadly and require more aggressive monitoring. Specific injuries require targeting specific endpoints, such as maintenance of cerebral or spinal cord perfusion pressures.

II. ELECTROCARDIOGRAPHY.
Electrocardiogram (ECG) is a static depiction of the electrical events of the heart. The basic tools are a 12-lead ECG coupled with continuous monitoring of one or two leads allows early detection of heart rate (HR) or ischemic changes, transient abnormal beats, and dysrhythmias. Inadequate electrode–skin contact, electrical interference within the equipment, patient motion or shivering, may produce artifacts and an inaccurate HR.

A. Heart rate monitoring
1. The most practical clinical estimate of HR is the pulse rate palpated in an extremity.
2. More accurate determination of HR can be assessed by:
   a. Observing the arterial pressure waveform of an invasive arterial catheter
   b. Observing ventricular contractions during echocardiography
   c. Observing changes in pressures using a pulmonary artery catheter (PAC)
   d. Auscultation for cardiac sounds alone is often unreliable in the ED and ICU, especially when HR is rapid or with excessive ambient noise.
      Note: The pulse rate *typically* equals the mechanical HR. **However, do not assume this to be true.** Exceptions to this rule include irregular ventricular contractions, states of poor peripheral perfusion, or cardiac pump dysfunction. It is important to recognize the patient with an electrical heart rate on the monitor but without corresponding cardiac activity and perfusion (electromechanical dissociation).

B. Ischemia monitoring
ECG changes suggestive of myocardial ischemia may occur without associated symptoms or signs. Early detection allows management of myocardial ischemia. The precordial leads are the most sensitive for detection of myocardial ischemia, particularly V_1, aVf, and V_5. V_5 is the most sensitive lead, detecting 75% of ischemic events. Lead II is most sensitive for P wave evaluation and inferior wall ischemia. *Simultaneous monitoring of leads II and V_5 is recommended.*

1. ST changes
Elevation of the ST segment 1 mm or more in the clinical setting of acute ischemic chest pain represents acute myocardial injury before it evolves into irreversible infarction; it is an indication for thrombolysis or percutaneous revascularization. A down sloping depression more often represents ischemia than a horizontal or up sloping segment. In patients with Q waves, ST segment elevation may be related to wall motion abnormalities. In patients without Q waves, leads with ST segment

TABLE 36-1	Common Dysrhythmias
Atrioventricular	Supraventricular
Atrioventricular junctional rhythm	Sinus bradycardia
Atrioventricular nodal re-entrant tachycardia	Sinus tachycardia
Accelerated atrioventricular junctional rhythm	Sinus arrest
Wolff–Parkinson–White syndrome	Sick sinus syndrome
Ventricular	Sinus node re-entrant tachycardia
Ventricular tachycardia	Atrial flutter
Ventricular flutter	Atrial fibrillation
Ventricular fibrillation	Multifocal atrial tachycardia
	Ectopic atrial tachycardia
	Atrial re-entrant tachycardia

elevations are specific indicators of the location of ischemia. T wave inversions and new Q waves are suggestive of either recent or evolving MI. Other causes of ST elevation include pericarditis and coronary vasospasm.

ST segment depression occurs when coronary perfusion drops below a critical value but before injury (latter causes ST elevation).

C. Dysrhythmia monitoring

Continuous ECG monitoring identifies changes in cardiac rhythm. Dysrhythmias are divided into tachydysrhythmia (ventricular rate >100 bpm) or bradydysrhythmia (ventricular rate <60 bpm). The origin of the electrical impulse can be sinoatrial (SA), atrial, atrioventricular (AV), or ventricular. The presence of P waves suggests SA node origin and is best observed in lead II. Lack of P waves or abnormal P wave morphology indicates an origin other than the SA node, and an associated QRS complex widening may help localize the source to the AV junction or the ventricles (QRS >0.14 msec is usually from a ventricular source).

A full rhythm strip can determine the rhythm and reveal ectopic or multifocal patterns exist. Conduction sequence analysis determines whether the conduction pattern is normal, delayed, blocked, or aberrant. These identifying points facilitate appropriate treatment selection. Table 36-1 outlines common dysrhythmias.

D. Arterial pressure monitoring

Measurement of arterial blood pressure quantifies the hydraulic pressure head supplying the cardiovascular system. Depending on the method used, there can be great measurement variability. The mean arterial pressure (MAP) is the mean blood pressure during the cardiac cycle and estimates end organ perfusion. It is calculated by $MAP \approx DP + 1/3(SP - DP)$, where DP is diastolic pressure and SP is systolic pressure. MAP is highest in the ascending aorta, and drops until the peripheral arteriolar bed is reached.

1. Noninvasive arterial pressure monitoring

Noninvasive techniques utilize a cuff that is connected to a sphygmomanometer that occludes a peripheral artery to the point of no-flow. Measurements that occur at the time of arterial occlusion and return of flow correlate with arterial blood pressure.

a. Palpation

Systolic arterial blood pressure can be estimated, based on measuring the pressure required to compress the brachial artery. This is often used when a stethoscope is not readily available or when background noise precludes auscultation. The cuff should be inflated to a level about 30 mm Hg above the pressure at which the pulse disappears. Next, release the pressure *slowly* until the return of a regular palpable pulse. This pressure is a rough estimate of systolic arterial pressure.

b. Auscultation

Using a stethoscope for auscultation gives the clinician the ability to measure diastolic pressure in addition to a more accurate systolic pressure. Releasing the cuff pressure allows return of pulsatile flow producing Korotkoff sounds. These sounds can be grouped into phases ranging from 1 to 5 according to AHA guidelines. Phase 1 is when sounds are first heard and corresponds with systolic arterial blood pressure. Phase 5 is when the sounds disappear corresponding to diastolic pressure.

c. **Automated intermittent devices: Oscillometry**

Automated noninvasive blood pressure provides regular and repeated pressure measurements using oscillometry. As the occluding cuff is slowly deflated, the return of arterial pulsations results in a counter pressure onto the cuff. With continued cuff deflation and progressive increase in arterial pulsations, the oscillation amplitude increases. The pressure is the point of rapid increase in oscillation amplitude, while the mean pressure is the point of maximum oscillation amplitude. With some devices, diastolic pressure is taken to be the point of rapid decrease in oscillation amplitude while with other manufacturers, the diastolic pressure is a derived value based on the systolic and mean pressure measurements. **In the hypotensive patient (SBP <80 mm Hg), the automated intermittent devices may falsely _overestimate_ actual blood pressure.** In these situations, manual techniques or an invasive arterial line are better.

d. **Future of continuous automated technology**

i. **Photoplethysmography**

Photoplethysmography relies on infrared light transmission to monitor the volume in a finger. An inflatable cuff maintains the finger at a constant volume, and continuous arterial pressure is measured as the counter pressure required to maintain constant finger volume. Measurements of pressure with this technique are sensitive to misapplication of the finger cuff, contributing to errors and limiting the reliability of the device.

ii. **Arterial tonometry**

This technique utilizes a surface pressure transducer applied onto the skin directly over an artery, to measure transmitted arterial pressure directly generating a continuous waveform and pressure measurement. In normotensive and hypertensive patients, tonometric pressures and waveforms usually correlate with the intra-arterial measurements. The reliability of the measurements is limited during rapid or large changes in blood pressure.

2. **Invasive arterial pressure monitoring**

Intra-arterial cannulation with continuous blood pressure transduction is the common method for arterial blood pressure monitoring in critically ill patients (Table 36-2).

TABLE 36-2	**Indications for Invasive Intra-Arterial Blood Pressure Monitoring**

Patient-related indications
- Shock states
- Significant coronary artery disease
- Myocardial pump dysfunction
- Significant cerebrovascular disease
- Significant pulmonary disease, COPD, PE, pulmonary hypertension, ARDS, pneumonia
- Severe renal, acid–base, electrolyte, or metabolic disorders
- Severe burns

Procedure-related indications
- Major procedures involving large fluid shifts or blood loss
- Anticipated deliberate hypotension, hypothermia, or hemodilution
- Procedures with high risk for spinal cord ischemia
- Liver, heart, or lung transplantation
- Aortic cross clamp or other major vascular procedures

a. Intra-arterial site selection

i. Sites commonly used include the radial, femoral, and axillary arteries. Typically, the radial artery of the *non-dominant* hand is utilized.

ii. Alternate sites can be chosen based upon several criteria:

a) The artery should be large enough to accurately reflect systemic blood pressure.

b) The chosen site should be free of infection.

c) There should be sufficient collateral flow to prevent distal ischemia.

d) The limb should be free of injury (e.g., proximal or distal fracture, crush, etc.).

iii. Allen's test is often done prior to cannulation of the radial artery to assess adequacy of perfusion and collateral flow. The radial and ulnar arteries are compressed. The patient's fist is clenched until it blanches. The patient's hand then relaxed and the pressure on the ulnar artery is released. If the hand becomes hyperemic, collateral ulnar flow is considered adequate for radial artery cannulation. Cold, ischemic digits are an absolute contraindication to radial arterial cannulation. Large pre-operative trials note that this test has limited utility, though avoiding cannulation when collateral flow is absent is wise. If short term cannulation (hours to day) is planned, clinically important occlusion is rare.

b. Complications of intra-arterial pressure monitoring

i. Mechanical

a) Thrombosis is the most common mechanical complication. Partial or complete radial artery occlusion occurs in more than 25% of patients after prolonged (>1 day) radial artery cannulation. Necrosis requiring amputation is rare. Remove any arterial cannula as soon as evidence of ischemia, infection, or embolic events is seen.

ii. Pseudoaneurysm/AV Fistula

a) Improper technique of catheter insertion may result in pseudoaneurysm or arterio-venous fistula formation. These risks are greatest with *multiple passes* through an artery and if the posterior wall of the artery is punctured.

iii. Infection

a) Sterile insertion technique, catheter care, and dressing protocols limit the incidence of infection. As catheter infections increase over time, routine monitoring of insertion sites for infection will minimize infective complications.

III. CENTRAL VENOUS PRESSURE MONITORING (CVP)

A. Indications

1. Estimation of intravascular volume can help guide fluid therapy. Some indications for CVP monitoring include hemorrhage, sepsis, and cardiovascular dysfunction, especially during the perioperative period, fluid resuscitation, or blood transfusion.

2. Central lines can be used for resuscitation if large bore, peripheral IV access is not attainable. A large diameter catheter should be used. Standard CVP lines (long length and narrow lumen) have resistance to flow.

3. Ultrasound guidance for puncture and insertion is recommended.

4. Attempts and insertions in the subclavian region and neck require a post-procedure chest x-ray.

B. Site selection

1. Subclavian vein

a. Preferred access site in trauma patients is the left subclavian vein because of the ease of insertion compared to the right. Also, choose a side with an existing chest tube to limit any later needed therapies.

b. Subclavian access offers less blood stream infections and better neck mobility.

c. Relative contraindications

i. Coagulopathic or thrombocytopenic patient

a) Inadvertent arterial puncture is more difficult to compress externally because the bony clavicle overlies the subclavian artery, and the pliable pleura and lung do not offer effective counter pressure.

ii. Agitated patients or those having active chest compressions during CPR are poor candidates because of the high risk for iatrogenic pneumothorax.

2. Internal jugular vein

a. These sites are associated with the least risk of arterial puncture. Arteries can easily be compressed externally, and pneumothorax is less common compared to the subclavian approach.

b. May be difficult to place in patients who have cervical immobilization ongoing. An assistant should immobilize the neck during the procedure.

c. Ultrasound is recommended to help identify vascular relationships and assist with insertion.

d. Contamination of the catheter site and dressing in patients with tracheostomy or copious secretions is more likely with internal jugular vein catheters. Use a different site in these patients when possible.

3. Femoral vein

a. Useful in the acutely injured or unstable patient because of ease of insertion and access. However, central venous pressure cannot be monitored from this site.

b. The least ideal site for prolonged use because of increased risk of lower extremity deep venous thrombosis and catheter-related blood stream infections.

c. Avoid catheterization of the ipsilateral femoral or subclavian vein in the patient with a same side injured extremity. Venous return from the injured extremity may be limited by the catheter, causing swelling and pain, thrombosis, increasing compartment pressures, and lowering tissue perfusion and healing.

C. Interpretation

1. CVP provides an estimate of right atrial volume or cardiac preload, and is normally 0 to 10 mm Hg. The typical CVP waveform consists of three waves ("a," "c," and "v") and two descents ("x" and "y"). Venous tone and overall status of intravascular volume will influence CVP measurement. Outside of extremes, CVP *trends* are better indicators of volume status than an absolute number—CVP values that increase to volume boluses confirm the therapy. Targeting a CVP of 8 to 12 mm Hg is common but not always ideal. A CVP <6 mm Hg is virtually always a sign of volume need; one over 16 mm Hg is almost always seen with adequate or increased volume.

2. Effect of mechanical ventilation and positive end-expiratory pressure (PEEP)

a. In the spontaneously ventilating patient, inspiration decreases intrathoracic pressure and CVP. Expiration increases intrathoracic pressure and CVP. For patients on mechanical ventilation, ventilator cycles increase intrathoracic pressure and CVP, while it falls during expiration.

b. CVP measurements are obtained at the same point of the respiratory cycle. To avoid the influence of intrathoracic pressure, CVP is measured at end-exhalation in both spontaneously and mechanically ventilated patients. When PEEP is applied, increased intrathoracic pressure at end-expiration reflects the CVP.

c. Pathologic central venous pressure waveforms

i. "a" wave, indicating the venous pressure during atrial contraction, is magnified in conditions of resistance to right atrial outflow. A giant or "cannon a" wave is seen when the atrium contracts against a closed tricuspid valve or with increased resistance to right atrial emptying as seen in tricuspid stenosis. Right ventricular failure, pulmonary stenosis, or pulmonary hypertension may cause the "a" wave to be accentuated. The "a" wave is absent during atrial fibrillation. In tricuspid regurgitation, the "c" and "v" waves are combined to form a large regurgitant CV wave, obliterating the normal "x" descent.

d. Overall, the CVP provides an estimate of the pressure of blood in the thoracic vena cava, but may be a poor indicator of intravascular volume in some patients.

TABLE 36-3	Major Indications for Pulmonary Artery Catheter Use in Trauma

- Guide resuscitation in hemodynamically unstable patients not responding predictably to conventional fluid/pressor management
- Conditions in which CVP is a poor guide to LVEDV : Left ventricular dysfunction, valvular heart disease, pulmonary hypertension, extra-cardiac causes of diastolic dysfunction
- Improve clinical decision-making in complicated cases of severe acute respiratory distress syndrome, progressive oliguria/anuria, myocardial injury, congestive heart failure, or major thermal injury
- To establish futility of care

IV. PULMONARY ARTERY CATHETER MONITORING (PAC)

The PAC directly measures three key parameters not available with other invasive monitoring devices (Tables 36-3 and 36-4). PACs are multi-lumen catheters, approximately 80 to 120 cm in length, introduced into the pulmonary artery through a central vein. Lumen opening at 25 to 30 cm from the tip allows measurement of CVP and central delivery of drugs, while the distal lumen opens at the tip.

A. Indications

CVP and right atrial pressure do not accurately estimate left atrial pressure or left ventricular preload. Patients who require precise knowledge of cardiac performance may benefit from a PAC (Table 36-3). Measurements can then be used to calculate hemodynamic parameters and guide therapy (Tables 36-4 and 36-5). PAC should be used *selectively* to help assess cardiac function in critically ill patients. It is particularly useful in the elderly population with significant cardiac disease. Routine use of the PAC has not been shown to improve outcomes.

B. Insertion

Utilizing sterile technique, the catheter is passed through an introducer placed in a central vein. The left subclavian vein and right internal jugular vein are the preferred access points for ease of advancing the PAC. With the balloon deflated, the catheter is passed to a distance of 12 to 15 cm beyond the introduction tip. At this point the flotation balloon is inflated, and the PAC is carefully advanced while simultaneously observing the pressure waveforms. The initial CVP waveform leads to the right atrial pressure waveform. Upon reaching the right ventricle, there is an abrupt and obvious high spiking pressure waveform of 20 to 30 mm Hg, representing the systolic right ventricular pressure, with a diastolic pressure that is unchanged from the CVP. This waveform leads to the pulmonary artery waveform with its characteristic step-up in diastolic pressure and a clear dicrotic notch. Finally, as the inflated balloon reaches a pulmonary arterial wedge, the waveform flattens as it loses its systolic and diastolic variations. After briefly observing the wedge waveform, the balloon should be deflated to confirm the reappearance of the pulmonary artery waveform.

C. Pulmonary artery wedge pressure (PAWP)

Inflation of the balloon at the tip of a correctly positioned PAC seals the surrounding artery and creates a continuous, stationary column of blood between the tip of the

TABLE 36-4	Values Derived from PAC

Parameters	Formula	Normal values
Cardiac index	CO/BSA	3–4 L/min/m^2
Pulmonary vascular resistance index	[(MPaP − PaWP) × 80]/CI	200–400 dyn m^2/cm^5
Stroke volume	CO/HR	55–100 mL
Stroke index	CO/(HR × BSA)	35–70 mL/m^2
Systemic vascular resistance index	[(MPaP − cVP) × 80]/CI	1,600–2,400 dyn s m^2/cm^5

TABLE 36-5	Hemodynamic Profiles Based on Variables		
	PAWP	**CO**	**SVR**
Hypovolemia	Low	Low	High
Fluid overload	High	High	Low
Septic shock	Low	High	Low
Left heart failure	High	Low	High
Pulm HTN	Low	Low	Normal

catheter and the left atrium. This is the *wedge pressure* and is a measure of the filling pressure of the left ventricle, and indirectly of the volume.

D. Cardiac output

The PAC uses a thermodilution method to determine cardiac output (CO), with the injection of a bolus of cold solution. 10 mL of cold fluid is injected into the right atrial port. The rate of blood flow determines the resultant temperature change, sensed by a thermistor at the tip of the catheter. The device then calculates a CO by integration of the change in temperature over time, where the area under the temperature–time curve is inversely proportional to the CO.

V. CONTINUOUS MONITORING PACS

A. Continuous mixed venous oximetry

Newer generation PACs can continuously monitor mixed venous oxygen saturation using fiberoptic bundles and an optical transducer in the tip of the catheter. Oxyhemoglobin relative to total hemoglobin is determined as red blood cells flow past the catheter tip. Mixed venous oxygen saturation is calculated using the Fick equation, measuring oxygen extraction. A reduction in mixed venous oxygen saturation may suggest an uncompensated increase in oxygen demand or poor delivery, that is, occult shock. Ideally, central venous saturation should be 70% or above—use volume and pressors as first steps, then blood or dobutamine as those fail.

B. Continuous cardiac output

Continuous cardiac output (CCO cont.) PACs use a heating filament to deliver thermal pulses, instead of traditional injections of cold solution. This allows the thermodilution technique for measurement of CO.

C. Right ventricular end-diastolic volume index and right ventricular ejection fraction

The right ventricular function catheter calculates the right ventricular end-diastolic volume index (RVEDVI) as the estimation of preload right ventricular ejection fraction and contractility. Temperature changes between baseline and residual temperatures in successive heartbeats are computer analyzed to generate the ejection fraction. The RVEDVI may be a better measure of right ventricular preload than CVP or PAWP. When the RVEDVI is 130 mL/m^2 or less, volume administration usually increases the cardiac index.

D. Potential drawbacks

1. Calibration of the measurements and troubleshooting of dysfunctional catheters
2. Reliability of the displayed measurements
3. Poor signal quality of the device may lead to inaccurate readings
4. Response to fluctuating readings may result in inappropriate therapy
5. Added cost of the modified catheters (may be up to twice the cost of traditional PACs).
6. Decreased use has led to decreased familiarity with what displayed measurements actually mean.

VI. NONINVASIVE CARDIOVASCULAR MONITORING

A. Esophageal Doppler monitoring (EDM)

The EDM uses a probe placed in the distal third of the esophagus to measure blood velocity in the descending aorta through the esophageal wall. Ultrasound waves are analyzed to measure the velocity of blood flow and preload, afterload, and contractility. CO is calculated assuming that 70% of CO flows through the descending aorta. There is a good correlation with other estimates of CO, and an analysis of velocity–time profile gives qualitative information on inotropic state and filling volumes. Proper positioning is critical to achieve accurate results, and subsequent probe movement out of position is difficult to prevent. This technique may better predict preload than either PAWP or CVP. This method is poorly tolerated by awake patients, limiting its use.

B. Echocardiography

Two-dimensional echocardiography can identify valvular abnormalities, structural abnormalities, ventricular filling and ejection fraction, contractility, and presence of pericardial effusion and tamponade. Newer modalities allow ultrasound to guide resuscitation.

Three techniques of echocardiography are described below.

1. Transthoracic echocardiography (TTE)

TTE examines parasternal, apical, subcostal, and suprasternal windows. Most areas of the heart can be accessed, but views of the mitral valve, aorta, and atria may be limited. Examination may be suboptimal in patients with obesity, emphysema, other hyperinflation states, recent surgical incisions, or those who are mechanically ventilated. It is relatively rapid but requires skilled operators to perform and interpret.

2. Transesophageal echocardiography (TEE)

In TEE, an acoustic transducer is mounted at the tip of a modified endoscope. It requires sedation/topical anesthesia and a skilled operator and is useful in the ICU when TTE fails. TEE is superior to TTE in diagnosis of left atrial disease such as thrombus or endocarditis and can identify aortic dissection. Intraoperative use permits real-time assessment of left ventricular performance. Currently disposable TEE devices are available and popular for continuous monitoring in the ICU.

3. Ultrasound (FREE)

The focused rapid echocardiographic examination (FREE) is a transthoracic examination incorporating hemodynamic information from the echo exam with the patient's clinical scenario to generate treatment recommendations about the use of fluid, inotropic agents, and vasopressors. The views obtained during the test are those of the standard TTE and include parasternal long axis, parasternal short axis, and apical four-chamber and subxiphoid windows. IVC diameter and diameter change with respiration can be determined. Unlike TEE or TTE, the FREE is increasingly being adapted by surgical intensivists as a relatively simple and quick bedside study not requiring skilled operators who may be unavailable, especially after hours.

C. Pulse contour analysis

Arterial pulse contour analysis measures stroke volume on a beat-to-beat basis from the arterial pulse pressure waveform. There are several theoretical advantages of this technique compared to thermodilution. It is noninvasive using already placed arterial catheters. In addition, the clinician can monitor changes in stroke volume and cardiac output on an almost continuous basis.

1. FloTrac/Vigileo™

The FloTrac system provides accurate reliable and continuous measurements, as well as calculations of systemic vascular resistance and stroke volume variation. The system uses an existing arterial line. A built-in analysis algorithm that performs the calibration based on patient demographics and waveform analysis.

2. PiCCO™

The PiCCO system measures cardiac output through pulse contour analysis of the arterial waveform by a transpulmonary thermodilution technique using a CVA line. It requires external calibration. Measurements are based on beat-to-beat signals, not averaged readings. Global end-diastolic volume measurements of all four heart chambers and intrathoracic blood volume are used as a measure of preload. The cardiac function index reflects global contractility and is the ratio of flow to preload.

3. LiDCO Plus™

The LiDCO™ plus system uses bolus lithium dilution cardiac output measurement. A small dose of lithium chloride is injected via a central or peripheral venous line. The resulting arterial lithium concentration–time curve is recorded by withdrawing blood past a lithium sensor attached to the patient's existing arterial line. Similar to the FloTrac system, it uses an analysis of pulse contour from an arterial line to determine stroke volume and CO.

a. The major difference between these technologies is in the method of calibration for contour analysis. Patients with aortic valve regurgitation, aortic reconstruction, those being treated with an intra-aortic balloon pump and those with pronounced peripheral arterial vasoconstriction are relative contraindications to using this system. These conditions affect the software of the device and may skew results.

D. Noninvasive and continuous hemoglobin monitoring (SpHb®)

Noninvasive and continuous hemoglobin (SpHb®) monitoring may correlate with invasive laboratory hemoglobin testing and may be beneficial in the operating room and ICU. This device has potential for real-time assessment of hemoglobin. A few centers around the country are testing its efficacy.

Suggested Readings

American Society of Anesthesiologists Task Force on Pulmonary Artery Catheterization: practice guidelines for pulmonary artery catheterization: An updated report by the anesthesiology 2003;99:988–1014.

Bellomo R, Uchino S. Cardiovascular monitoring tools: use and misuse. *Curr Opin Crit Care* 2003;9(3):225–229.

Chiu, William. Cardiovascular monitoring. In: Wilson WC, Grande CM, Hoyt DB, eds. *Trauma: Critical Care.* New York, NY: Informa Healthcare USA, Inc; 2007:155–170.

Davis JW, Davis IC, Bennink LD, et al. Are automatic blood pressure measurements accurate in trauma patients? *J Trauma* 2003;55:860–863.

Goedje O, Höke K, Goetz AE, et al. Reliability of a new algorithm for continuous cardiac output determination by pulse-contour analysis during hemodynamic instability. *Crit Care Med* 2002;30(1):52–58.

Madan AK, UyBarreta VV, Aliabadi-Wahle S, et al. Esophageal Doppler ultrasound monitor versus pulmonary artery catheter in the hemodynamic management of critically ill surgical patients. *J Trauma* 1999;46:607–612.

Marik PE. Pulmonary artery catheterization and esophageal Doppler monitoring in the ICU. *Chest* 1999;116:1085–1091.

Nakano KJM, Waxman K. Pulmonary artery catheterization. In: Shoemaker WC, Velmahos GC, Demetriades D, eds. *Procedures and Monitoring for the Critically Ill.* Philadelphia, PA: W.B. Saunders Company; 2002:24.

Reuter DA, Felbinger TW, Schmidt C, et al. Stroke volume variations for assessment of cardiac responsiveness to volume loading in mechanically ventilated patients after cardiac surgery. *Intensive Care Med* 2002;28(4):392–398.

Richard C, Warszawski J, Anguel N, et al. Early use of the pulmonary artery catheter and outcomes in patients with shock and acute respiratory distress syndrome. *JAMA* 2003;290:2713–2720.

Sakka SG, Meiere-Hellmann A, Reinhart K. Assessment of cardiac preload and extravascular lung water by single transpulmonary thermodilution. *Intensive Care Med* 2000;26(2):180–187.

Sandham JD, Hull RD, Brant RF, et al. A randomized, controlled trial of the use of pulmonary artery catheters in high-risk surgical patients. *N Engl J Med* 2003;348:5–14.

Scalea TM, Simon HM, Duncan AO, et al. Geriatric blunt multiple trauma: Improved survival with early invasive monitoring. *J Trauma* 1990;30:129–136

Velmahos GC, Wo CC, Demetriades D, et al. Invasive and non-invasive physiological monitoring of blunt trauma patients in the early period after emergency admission. *Int Surg* 1999;84:354–360.

Wang K, Asinger RW, Marriott HJL. ST-Elevation in conditions other than acute myocardial infarction. *N Engl J Med* 2003;349:2128–2135.

Wilkins RG. Radial artery cannulation and ischemic damage: a review. *Anaesthesia* 1985;40:896–899.

37 Acute Kidney Injury

Feihu Zhou and John A. Kellum

I. INTRODUCTION

Acute kidney injury (AKI) is common in critically ill trauma patients and increases mortality. Most often, AKI is part of multiple organ failure and may arise from injuries or sepsis.

The terms acute kidney injury (AKI) and acute renal failure are not synonymous. The term renal failure is reserved for patients who have lost renal function to the point that life can no longer be sustained without intervention, whereas AKI describes patients with earlier or milder forms of acute renal dysfunction and those with overt failure.

II. DEFINITION AND CLASSIFICATION

International consensus criteria for AKI use the RIFLE criteria to describe three levels of renal impairment (risk, injury, failure) and two clinical outcomes (loss and end-stage kidney disease, see Figure 37-1). The RIFLE classification system includes separate criteria for serum creatinine (SCrt) and urine output. The criteria which lead to the worst classification define the stage of AKI.

A. Note that RIFLE-F is present even if the increase in SCrt is <3-fold, so long as the new SCrt is >4.0 mg/dL in the setting of an acute increase of at least 0.5 mg/dL. The shape the figure denotes the fact that more patients (high sensitivity) will be included in the mild category, including some without actually having kidney damage (less specificity). In contrast, at the bottom the criteria are strict and therefore specific, but some patients will be missed.

III. EPIDEMIOLOGY

AKI occurs in 6.3% to 27% of critically ill trauma patients, with mortality ranging from 22% to 95.3%.

A. Severity of illness. Increased severity of AKI is associated with a step-wise increase in the risk of death. Hospital mortality rates for ICU patients with AKI are approximately: R—9%, I—11%, F—26% compared to 6% for ICU patients without AKI.

  1. The incidence and the attributed morbidity and mortality of AKI associated with trauma vary widely. For example, in burn patients, the occurrence rate of AKI is 22.5% while it is 9.2% in patients with traumatic brain injury.

B. Injury severity scores and associated organ failure: In 2010, a matched cohort study utilizing data derived from the National Trauma Data Bank (NTDB, 2007) revealed that of the 94,795 severely injured trauma patients (Injury Severity Score ≥9), 10,478 (11.1%) patients developed at least one complication. The cumulative incidence of renal failure was 1.3% and the crude mortality was 29.3%. Renal failure is one of four complications (cardiovascular, acute respiratory distress syndrome, renal failure, and sepsis) associated with increased mortality (relative risk increase 24%). Plurad et al. reported that although incidence of renal failure was 1.1%, the mortality with renal failure was much higher than the overall mortality in ICU trauma patients (50% vs. 15.4%). Renal failure is associated with a longer duration of mechanical ventilation and stay in ICU, an increased cost of care, and increase in risk of death (>7-fold.)

C. Etiology. Causes of trauma-associated AKI are often multifactorial.

  1. Early-onset AKI is more likely to be directly attributable to trauma (e.g., shock, direct kidney trauma, rhabdomyolysis, exposure to radiocontrast media, early

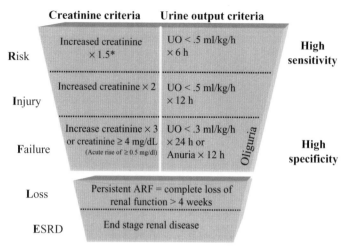

Figure 37-1. RIFLE criteria for Acute Kidney Injury. The classification system includes separate criteria for creatinine and urine output. A patient can fulfill the criteria through changes in SCrt or changes in urine output, or both. The criteria that lead to the most severe stage should be used. Note that the F stage of RIFLE is present even if the increase in SCrt is under 3-fold as long as the new SCrt is greater than 4.0 mg/dL (350 μmol/L) in the setting of an acute increase of at least 0.5 mg/dL (44 μmol/L). The shape of the figure denotes the fact that more patients (high sensitivity) will be included in the mild category, including some without actually having kidney damage (less specificity). In contrast, at the bottom of the figure the criteria are strict and therefore specific, but some patients will be missed. Abbreviations: AKI, acute kidney injury; ESRD, end-stage renal disease; RIFLE, Risk, injury, failure, loss and end-stage renal disease. Permission obtained from BioMed Central © Bellomo et al. *Crit Care* 2004;8:R204–R212.

intra-abdominal hypertension); whereas delayed-onset AKI is more likely associated with complications such as sepsis and multiple organ dysfunction syndrome (MODS).

2. In some series, AKI in trauma patients is most often due to crush injuries and rhabdomyolysis, whereas in other reports shock was the most common cause of AKI.

3. Abdominal trauma and use of furosemide are independent risk factors for AKI.

4. Renal abnormalities seen on autopsy include death or damage of tubular epithelial cells. Overall, risk factors for trauma-induced AKI include the following:
   a. Severity and duration of shock
   b. Sepsis
   c. Increasing age, especially age >62 years
   d. Greater severity of illness as per APACHE III or SOFA scores
   e. Pre-existing chronic kidney disease
   f. Prior admission to a non-ICU ward in the hospital
   g. Preexisting cardiovascular disease
   h. Emergent surgery
   i. Need for mechanical ventilation
   j. Nephrotoxin use including aminoglycoside antibiotics and radiologic contrast agents
   k. Abdominal injuries—abdominal compartment syndrome

D. Patient susceptibility. Advanced age is a major determinant of susceptibility to trauma-associated AKI. Once corrected for exposure, AKI frequency and outcomes appear similar for men and women.

E. Mechanisms of kidney injury. Traditionally, mechanisms of azotemia are divided into pre-, intra- and postrenal. This categorization is not a classification system for AKI. Both pre- and postrenal insults will result in parenchymal (intrarenal) injury if not treated promptly.

  1. Prerenal. The driving force for glomerular filtration is the pressure gradient from the glomerulus to Bowman's space. Glomerular pressure is dependent on renal blood flow (RBF) and is controlled by combined resistances of renal afferent and efferent arterioles.

  a. Prerenal mechanisms of AKI result in hypoperfusion of the kidney and may be from a number of different causes. Decreased GFR in the face of reduced RBF is an adaptive response. Severe volume depletion or hypotension in the face of a structurally intact nephron will result in decreased GFR and may fulfill the diagnostic criteria for AKI.

  b. Hypovolemia may result from losses from internal or external hemorrhage, gastrointestinal (GI) and cutaneous sources (e.g., burns).

  c. Hypotension is an important risk factor for AKI, especially in trauma. During this initial phase, renal autoregulatory mechanisms attempt to maintain GFR and RBF by altering the vascular tone of the afferent and efferent arterioles of the glomerulus. Treatment with fluid resuscitation is important but many patients will also require vasoactive therapy once volume is restored to maintain arterial blood pressure. Despite a common belief among many practitioners, norepinephrine does not increase the risk of AKI compared to dopamine; in animal models with sepsis, RBF increases with norepinephrine. If volume and blood pressure restoration does not occur, the worsening ischemia results in tubular cell injury resulting in intrinsic AKI.

  d. Elevated intra-abdominal pressure may also produce AKI, notably abdominal compartment syndrome (see Chapter 39). As intra-abdominal pressures rises, RBF becomes compromised. Surgical decompression is the only definitive therapy and best done before irreversible end-organ damage occurs.

  2. Intrinsic AKI. The duration and magnitude of shock correlates with the risk of AKI. However, injury to the kidney can arise from distant damage. For example, myonecrosis is a common cause of AKI in which remote tissue damage causes inflammation and cell damage in the kidney. Rhabdomyolysis-induced injury results from ischemia/reperfusion and inflammation by neutrophils that infiltrate damage muscle, as well as excess myoglobin from skeletal muscle injury, which may obstruct the renal tubules.

  a. A variety of damage-associated molecular patterns (DAMPs) will induce activation of dendritic cells within the renal parenchyma. Part of the reason that the kidney is so sensitive to these insults is that the kidney filters the blood and many small molecules are concentrated in the tubular fluid, where they may induce inflammation.

  3. Postrenal. This results from obstruction of the outflow tracts of the kidneys. The obstruction can occur at any point in urine flow between the proximal tubules and the external urethral meatus.

  a. Distal obstruction at the bladder neck, bilateral ureteric obstruction, or unilateral ureteric obstruction may occur from multiple causes. For trauma patients, postrenal injury may be caused by obstruction from clots, benign strictures, edema, inadvertent surgical ligature, or external compression.

  b. During the early stages of obstruction (hours to days), continued glomerular filtration leads to increased intraluminal pressure upstream to the site of obstruction. As a result, there is gradual distention of the proximal ureters, renal pelvis, and calyces and a fall in GFR.

  c. Urinary output may vary in postrenal failure from anuria and oliguria to polyuria. Anuric patients commonly have an obstruction at the bladder level or below. Because postrenal causes are usually reversible if diagnosed promptly, it is imperative to exclude them.

  d. Recovery of renal function is inversely proportional to the duration of the obstruction.

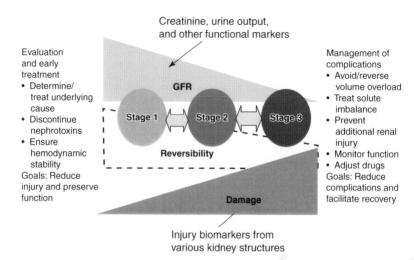

Figure 37-2. Evaluation and management principles for AKI. Early imperatives are shown on the left and later imperatives on the right. GFR, glomerular filtration rate.

  e. Specific gravity and urine sodium are variable. Serum BUN and creatinine levels will be elevated and the BUN–creatinine ratio will be normal (1:20) or elevated.
  f. Renal ultrasonography can assess for hydronephrosis and avoids the contrast dye used for CT. Early on, the negative predictive value of ultrasound may be low.

IV. TREATMENT

Management of AKI in the trauma and acute surgical patient is divided into two phases:
A. Early care, where the focus on determining the cause and reversing injury is paramount.
B. Later care, where managing the complications of AKI and facilitating recovery take precedence (Fig. 37-2).
C. Management of early AKI. Initial management of AKI integrates diagnosis and general management principles. Some forms of AKI require specific therapy and are reversible if treated promptly.
  1. Allergic interstitial nephritis often responds to removal of the inciting antigen, typically a drug.
  2. Urinary tract obstruction can usually be relieved before permanent damage occurs but only if identified.
  3. Abdominal compartment syndrome rarely causes permanent renal failure if decompression is performed promptly.
  4. Part of the diagnostic workup for AKI may include a trial of volume therapy. For example, although hypovolemia is usually apparent by physical examination it may be difficult to ascertain in some cases without invasive hemodynamic monitoring or use of fluid challenge.
D. Diagnostic workup. The following tests may be useful in determining the cause of AKI.
  1. Physical examination. Assess volume status; look for rashes or evidence of allergic reactions; assess for sites of infection; examine the abdomen and pelvis to seek obstruction or abdominal hypertension.
  2. Review medication list. Look for: Intravenous or intra-arterial radiocontrast given within the prior 2 to 4 days; antimicrobials, especially aminoglycosides and

amphotericin; sulfa containing drugs (including most loop diuretics) in anyone with a history of sulfa allergy; drugs that reduce renal plasma flow (calcineurin inhibitors, ACE inhibitors, and nonsteroidal anti-inflammatory agents).

3. **Urinalysis.** Blood may indicate trauma to the urinary tract. Heme-positive but RBC negative suggests myoglobinuria. Pyuria can indicate infection or allergic interstitial nephritis (eosinophils may also be present). Active urine sediment (very rare) with RBC casts is diagnostic of vasculitis or glomerulonephritis. Muddy brown casts suggest renal tubular cell sloughing and may be due to a variety of injuries.

4. **Urine electrolytes.** When renal tubular function is intact, the kidney will respond to a reduction in cardiac output by increasing sodium reabsorption such that urine sodium will be very low. If the cause of an increased SCrt is hypovolemia AND renal tubular function is intact, the urine sodium should be less than 20 mmol/L.

   a. A more sensitive and specific test is to calculate the fractional excretion of sodium (FENa). A FENa <1 means that the kidney is behaving as though its perfusion is compromised.

   $$FENa = (P_{Cr} \times U_{Na})/(P_{Na} \times U_{Cr}) \times 100$$

   Contrary to popular belief the FENa does not establish a diagnosis. A low FENa has been documented in cases of intrarenal AKI especially due to sepsis. A high FENa does not rule out hypovolemia if renal tubular function is impaired (e.g., established AKI, diuretics).

5. **Renal ultrasound.** This is used to look for hydronephrosis, diagnostic of obstruction. The absence of hydronephrosis, especially early on, does not exclude obstruction. The other purpose for renal ultrasound is to evaluate kidney structure (a CT scan is superior for this purpose). Kidney size is important in evaluating a patient who presents with an elevated SCrt. Small kidneys are indicative of chronic kidney disease.

6. **Hemodynamic assessment.** Low urine output is an early sign of hypovolemia but it is also indicative of AKI due to any cause or obstruction.

7. While hypovolemia is commonly the cause of decreased urine output, do not simply "give fluids" for all with oliguria. It is best to assess fluid status first (see Chapter on Initial Resuscitation).

8. **Sepsis workup.** If any suspicion or when an AKI cause cannot be identified, begin a workup for sepsis (see Sepsis Chapter).

E. **Management of established AKI.** Once AKI has been established, the treatment priorities shift toward management of the complications of AKI and facilitating recovery.

1. **Avoid/reverse volume overload.** Patients with AKI frequently have oliguria that is not fluid responsive. The practice of continuing fluid loading in a patient in positive fluid balance will lead to complications (delayed wound healing, pulmonary edema, atrial distension and arrhythmias, impaired gut function) and will not benefit the kidney. Each liter of normal saline (0.9% NaCl) has 9 g of sodium. Diuretics can aid management of volume overload but can produce renal injury and many are ototoxic. Diuretics are not a solution to imprudent use of fluids.

2. **Consider renal support.** Timing of renal support (e.g., dialysis, hemofiltration) is controversial. Many clinicians believe that renal support is often initiated too late, and national trends favor earlier initiation of therapy. In general, patients should be started on renal support (assuming they are candidates for organ support) prior to the development of complications.

   a. Most patients in RIFLE-failure (stage 3) are candidates for renal support if it has not been started already.

   b. Subclavian venous access should be avoided if possible to reduce the risk of stenosis, which will hamper permanent dialysis access.

3. **Adjust drugs.** Many drugs are eliminated by the kidneys and drug selection and dosing should be adjusted to the patient's renal function.

4. Monitor functional recovery and plan for follow-up. Monitor renal function frequently and plan for long-term follow-up. Many patients will require long-term management by a qualified practitioner.

V. PROGNOSIS. Hospital mortality rates for patients with severe AKI approach 50%; of those who survive, less than half will make a complete recovery of renal function.
   A. Age is the major determinant of recovery with those >65 years of age having a far greater chance of needing chronic dialysis.
   B. Even less severe AKI may not resolve and lead to permanent dysfunction.
   C. Prompt recognition and supportive treatment is the only effective therapy.
   D. Some suggest that continuous renal replacement therapy (as opposed to intermittent dialysis) leads to better long-term outcomes, but no randomized clinical trial has established this relationship.

AXIOMS

■ AKI is common in trauma patients and best avoided rather than treated.
■ Seek AKI in ill trauma patients and others at risk by measuring SCrt and urine output in all patients at risk.
■ Early-onset AKI is more likely to be directly attributable to trauma, whereas delayed-onset AKI is more likely associated with sepsis.
■ Discontinue all unnecessary nephrotoxic agents in high risk patients and in those with AKI.
■ Maintaining optimal circulating blood volume is key in limiting AKI, but watch for volume overload, especially once AKI sets in.
■ Do not wait for complications to start renal replacement therapy—consult early.

Suggested Readings

Bellomo R, Ronco C, Kellum JA, et al. Acute renal failure—definition, outcome measures, animal models, fluid therapy and information technology needs: the second international consensus conference of the Acute Dialysis Quality Initiative (ADQI) group. *Crit Care* 2004;8(4):204–212.
Bagshaw SM, George C, Gibney RT, et al. A multi-center evaluation of early acute kidney injury in critically ill trauma patients. *Ren Fail* 2008;30(6):581–589.
Brandt MM, Falvo AJ, Rubinfeld IS, et al. Renal dysfunction in trauma: even a little costs a lot. *J Trauma* 2007;62(6):1362–1364.
de Abreu KL, Silva Júnior GB, Barreto AG, et al. Acute kidney injury after trauma: Prevalence, clinical characteristics and RIFLE classification. *Indian J Crit Care Med* 2010;14(3):121–128.
Gomes E, Antunes R, Dias C, et al. Acute kidney injury in severe trauma assessed by RIFLE criteria: a common feature without implications on mortality? *Scand J Trauma Resusc Emerg Med* 2010;18:1.
Ingraham AM, Xiong W, Hemmila MR, et al. The attributable mortality and length of stay of trauma-related complications: a matched cohort study. *Ann Surg* 2010;252(2):358–362.
Mehta RL, Kellum JA, Shah SV, et al. Acute kidney injury network: report of an initiative to improve outcomes in acute kidney injury. *Crit Care* 2007;11(2):R31.
Plurad D, Brown C, Chan L, et al. Emergency department hypotension is not an independent risk factor for post-traumatic acute renal dysfunction. *J Trauma* 2006;61(5):1120–1127.
Sabry A, El-Din AB, El-Hadidy AM, et al. Markers of tubular and glomerular injury in predicting acute renal injury outcome in thermal burn patients: a prospective study. *Ren Fail* 2009;31(6):457–463.
Vanholder R, Sever MS, Erek E, et al. Rhabdomyolysis. *J Am Soc Nephrol* 2000;11(8):1553–1561.

38 Acute Respiratory Failure and Mechanical Ventilation

Cory J. Vatsass and Lena M. Napolitano

I. **INTRODUCTION.** Acute respiratory failure (ARF) is gas exchange dysfunction including oxygenation and/or carbon dioxide elimination. Common etiologies in trauma and acute care surgery patients include pulmonary contusion, pneumonia, atelectasis, aspiration, pulmonary edema, acute lung injury (ALI) and acute respiratory distress syndrome (ARDS), and pulmonary embolus (Table 38-1). Mechanical ventilation and noninvasive ventilation (NIV) are the primary therapies for treatment of ARF.

II. **CLASSIFICATION AND EPIDEMIOLOGY.** ARF is classified as either hypoxemic or hypercapnic. Severe hypoxemic ARF raises the concern for ALI or ARDS.

   A. *Hypoxemic respiratory failure* (Type I), defined as arterial partial pressure of oxygen (PaO_2) <60 mm Hg on room air, is the most common form of respiratory failure and a threat to organ function.

   B. *Hypercapnic respiratory failure* (Type II), defined as arterial partial pressure of carbon dioxide ($PaCO_2$) of >50 mm Hg on room air.

   C. *ALI and ARDS* (Definitions in Table 38-2) are syndromes of acute hypoxemic respiratory failure that arise from **direct** (pulmonary) or **indirect** (extrapulmonary) insults (Table 38-3) that induce pulmonary inflammation, damage the cells of the alveolar-capillary membrane, and lead to severe ARF. A new definition for ARDS (Berlin definition, Table 38-4) classifies ARDS into mild, moderate, and severe categories, and includes specific amounts of positive end-expiratory pressure (PEEP) at which the PaO_2/FiO_2 ratio is calculated.

      1. ALI has an estimated crude incidence of 78.9 per 100,000 person-years, with a potential national annual incidence of 190,600 cases resulting in 74,000 deaths. The inhospital mortality rate is 38.5%; the mortality rate increases with age. The rate of ARDS in trauma is decreased with the use of protective ventilator strategies. ARDS and ALI both have pathologic changes and diffuse alveolar damage (DAD) that includes alveolar flooding, characteristic hyaline membranes; this creates the impaired gas exchange and barrier functions of the endothelial and epithelial layers of the alveolar-capillary membrane (Fig. 38-1). Parenchymal injury is not a "diffuse" process, rather has regionalization of the inflammation, injury, and subsequent mechanical abnormalities. This heterogeneity can impact the mechanical ventilation strategy since there is preferential delivery of ventilatory breaths to pulmonary regions with higher compliance and lower resistance (i.e., the more normal regions) rather than to diseased parenchyma resulting in potential regional over distention and ventilation/perfusion mismatch. ARDS stages include *exudative, proliferative,* and *fibrotic* phases.

III. **TREATMENT—NONINVASIVE VENTILATION (NIV)**

   A. NIV provides positive pressure ventilator support without the need for an invasive (tracheal placed) airway. NIV is a first-line therapy in ARF due to chronic obstructive pulmonary disease (COPD) exacerbation and can decrease mortality, need for intubation, complications, and length of hospital stay. Similarly, NIV is an effective and safe treatment of adult patients with ARF due to acute cardiogenic pulmonary edema.

TABLE 38-1	Common Etiologies of Acute Respiratory Failure and Need for Mechanical Ventilation

- Apnea or respiratory arrest
- Tachypnea (respiratory rate >30 breaths/min) or bradypnea
- Vital capacity <15 mL/kg, <1.0 L or <30% predicted
- Minute ventilation >10 L/min
- Hypoxemia
- Hypercarbia
- Exacerbation chronic obstructive pulmonary disease
- Respiratory muscle fatigue
- Neuromuscular diseases
- Obtundation or coma
- ALI
- ARDS

TABLE 38-2	The American–European Consensus Conference (AECC) Definition of ALI and ARDS Developed in 1994
ALI criteria	Timing: Acute onset Oxygenation: PaO_2/FiO_2 ≤300 mm Hg (regardless of PEEP level) Chest radiograph: Bilateral infiltrates seen on frontal chest radiograph Pulmonary artery wedge: ≤18 mm Hg when measured or no clinical evidence of left atrial hypertension
ARDS criteria	Same as ALI except: Oxygenation: PaO_2/FiO_2 ≤200 mm Hg (regardless of PEEP level)

TABLE 38-3	Clinical Disorders Associated with the Development of ALI/ARDS

Clinical Disorders Associated with the Development of ALI/ARDS

DIRECT insult PULMONARY	INDIRECT insult EXTRA-PULMONARY
Common	Common
■ Aspiration pneumonia ■ Pneumonia	■ Sepsis ■ Severe trauma ■ Shock
Less common	Less common
■ Inhalation injury ■ Pulmonary contusions ■ Fat emboli ■ Near drowning ■ Reperfusion injury	■ Acute pancreatitis ■ Cardiopulmonary bypass ■ Transfusion-related TRALI ■ Disseminated intravascular coagulation ■ Burns ■ Head injury ■ Drug overdose

Atabai K, Matttiay MA. *Thorax*. 2000.
Frutos-Vivar F, et al. *Curr Opin Crit Care*. 2004.

TABLE 38-4   **New Proposed ARDS Definition – "Berlin" Definition**

	Mild	Moderate	Severe
Timing	Acute onset within 1 wk of a known clinical risk factor or new/worsening respiratory symptoms		
Hypoxemia	PaO$_2$/FiO$_2$ 201–300 with PEEP/CPAP $\geq$5	PaO$_2$/FiO$_2$ 101–200 with PEEP $\geq$5	PaO$_2$/FiO$_2$ $\leq$100 with PEEP $\geq$5
Origin of edema	Respiratory failure not fully explained by cardiac failure or fluid overload[b]		
Radiologic abnormalities	Bilateral opacities[a]	Bilateral opacities[a]	Opacities involving 3 + quadrants[a]

[a]Not fully explained by effusions, nodules, masses, or lobar/lung; use training set of CXRs.
[b]Need objective assessment if no risk factor present (see table).
The ARDS Definition Task Force. *JAMA* 2012;307(23):2526.

B. NIV as a weaning strategy for intubated patients with ARF uses early extubation with immediate application of NIV. A recent systematic review notes NIV decreased mortality, ventilator-associated pneumonia (VAP), and ICU and hospital length of stay, and total duration of mechanical ventilation.

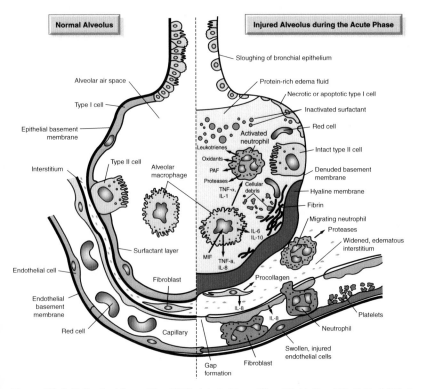

Figure 38-1. Pathophysiology of the ARDS. Adapted from: Ware LB, Matthay MA. *N Engl J Med* 2000;342(18):1334.

C. The role of NIV in the treatment of ARF for severe asthma exacerbations is less clear, where it must be used with caution and carefully monitored.

D. NIV can also be used to treat ARF from other conditions such as severe pneumonia, obesity hypoventilation and to improve respiratory outcome in post-surgical patients.

IV. TREATMENT—INTUBATION (SEE CHAPTER 3).

If NIV fails or is not possible/indicated, endotracheal intubation is required, with the orotracheal route preferred. The optimal intubating conditions require a combination of short- and rapid-acting sedatives with a neuromuscular blocking agent, often etomidate and succinylcholine. The approach is discussed in detail elsewhere.

A. After insertion and clinical confirmation with auscultation and capnography, obtain a chest radiograph to confirm position; the target tip placement of the tube above the carina and below the glottis is followed by securing a standard tube at 23 cm in men and 21 cm in women, measured at the incisors. Assure the cuff pressure is adequate and not overinflated. Sedation is required for endotracheal tube and MV tolerance, and intravenous infusions of short-acting opioids and sedatives are used commonly. If volume and hemodynamic status is normalized, a continuous propofol infusion can be used and allows both sedation and rapid recovery with cessation. A sedation scale will aid finding best response to dose of any regimen.

B. Benzodiazepines may increase delirium, especially in the elderly and in those with organ dysfunction or failure.

V. TREATMENT—VAP PREVENTION

A. Implement aggressive actions to prevent VAP immediately after intubation and initiation of mechanical ventilation. The key components of the ventilator bundle for VAP prevention are as follows:
   1. Elevation of the head of the bed (at least 30 degrees)
   2. Daily "sedation vacations" and assessment of readiness to extubate
   3. Daily oral care with chlorhexidine
   4. Peptic ulcer disease prophylaxis
   5. Deep venous thrombosis prophylaxis

B. Other evidence-based strategies for prevention can be considered in ICUs with a high prevalence of VAP, including continuous aspiration of subglottic secretions (CASS) tubes, silver-coated endotracheal tubes, and selective oral decontamination (SOD) or digestive tract decontamination (SDD).

VI. TREATMENT—MECHANICAL VENTILATION (MV)

A. The goals are adequate oxygenation and alveolar ventilation, reduced work of breathing and minimizing ventilator-induced lung injury (VILI).

B. The treatment for hypoxemic ARF (Type I) is to improve oxygenation and reverse/prevent tissue hypoxia by achieving adequate oxygen delivery to tissues; seek arterial oxygen saturation >90% on the lowest FiO_2 concentration possible. The treatment of failure to ventilate, that is, hypercapnic ARF (Type II), is to increase alveolar ventilation by achieving adequate minute ventilation.

C. MV can lead to additional lung injury, that is, VILI. VILI mechanisms include barotrauma, diffuse alveolar injury resulting from overdistension (volutrauma), injury caused by repeated cycles of recruitment/de-recruitment (atelectrauma) (Fig. 38-2) and the most subtle form of injury related to the release of local mediators in the lung (biotrauma) (Fig. 38-3).

D. Variables that can be adjusted for MV include:
   1. Mode of ventilation
   2. Tidal volume (Vt)
   3. Respiratory rate (RR)
   4. Supplemental oxygen (FiO_2)
   5. Inspiration/expiration ratio (I:E)
   6. Inspiratory flow rate
   7. PEEP
   8. Trigger sensitivity (effort required to trigger the ventilator to deliver a breath)

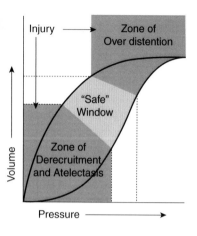

Figure 38-2. Pathogenesis of ventilator-associated and ventilator-induced lung injury. (Adapted from: Belperio JA, Keane MP, Lynch JP 3rd, et al. The role of cytokines during the pathogenesis of ventilator-associated and ventilator-induced lung injury. *Semin Respir Crit Care Med* 2006;27(4):350–364.)

9. Rise time (determines speed of rise of flow or pressure in each breath)

10. Temperature and humidity of inspired air

E. Oxygen uptake via the lungs depends on both PaO_2 (FiO_2, alveolar pressure) and ventilation–perfusion matching (reversing atelectasis, reduce intrapulmonary shunting). To improve oxygenation, use these strategies:

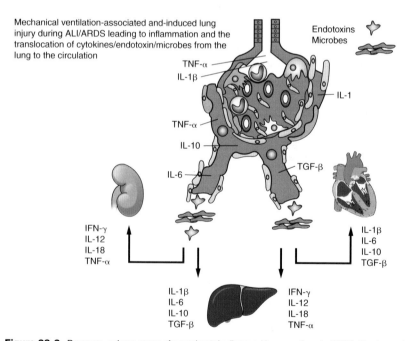

Figure 38-3. Pressure–volume curve of a moderately diseased lung, such as in ARDS. Two hazard zones exist: Over distention and derecruitment/atelectasis. Higher end-expiratory pressures and small tidal volumes are needed to stay in the "Safe" window. High-frequency oscillatory ventilation may have a larger margin of safety in keeping the lung open within the desired target range and avoiding alveolar over distention. (Adapted with permission from: Imai Y, Slutsky AS. High-frequency oscillatory ventilation and ventilator-induced lung injury. *Crit Care Med* 2005;33(3 Suppl):S129–S134.)

1. Increase FiO_2. Be wary since prolonged, high levels (FiO_2 >50%) are associated with oxygen toxicity and absorptive atelectasis.
2. Increase mean alveolar pressure by increasing mean airway pressure (increase PEEP or increase I:E ratio, increase inspiratory time), recruitment maneuver with PEEP (i.e., 30 cm H_2O PEEP for 30 seconds, 40 cm H_2O PEEP for 40 seconds, or pressure control RM with high PEEP 40, low PEEP 20, I:E 1:1 for 2 minutes).
3. Ventilation is largely dependent on alveolar ventilation. Alveolar ventilation = respiratory rate × (tidal volume −.dead space). To improve CO_2 elimination, increase minute ventilation (increase tidal volume or respiratory rate).

VII. MODES OF MECHANICAL VENTILATION

A. Controlled MV is used initially to ensure adequate alveolar ventilation, arterial oxygenation, reduce work of breathing, and reduce further lung damage. Early conversion to spontaneous breathing modalities during MV is best whenever possible.
B. Mechanical positive pressure ventilation can be delivered via a volume or pressure target.
C. No single mode of MV for ARF is superior in terms of clinical outcomes.
1. **Volume modes.** Tidal volume is set and airway pressure is variable. The airway pressure will be based upon the rate of delivery of the tidal volume, pulmonary compliance (plateau pressure), and airway resistance (peak pressure). This variability in airway pressure may result in barotrauma if high peak airway pressures occur.
   a. **Controlled mechanical ventilation mode (CMV).** Set respiratory rate and tidal volume to achieve exact minute ventilation; does not allow patient interaction. CMV may result in diaphragmatic inactivity, promoting atrophy, and contractility dysfunction, so it is not commonly used.
   b. **Assist-control (AC) ventilation mode.** A patient- or time-triggered, flow-limited, and volume-cycled. The tidal volume of each delivered breath is the same, whether triggered by the ventilator or the patient. The ventilator delivers breaths in coordination with the respiratory effort of the patient. If a patient triggering event does not occur in a set time interval, then the ventilator will deliver a breath similar to control mode. This allows for patient participation with regards to breath initiation. AC is associated with low work of breathing, as every breath is supported and tidal volume is guaranteed.
   c. **Synchronous intermittent mandatory ventilation mode (SIMV).** The ventilator delivers both mandatory (set rate, tidal volume) breaths delivered in coordination with the respiratory effort of the patient and pressure support (set pressure) breaths to support spontaneous breathing. Most SIMV modes will default to a control-mode setting in the event that the patient does not trigger the ventilator in a certain time window around the preset respiratory rate. Synchronization of the tidal volume delivery and native inspiratory effort attempts to limit barotrauma.
2. **Pressure modes.** Airway pressure is set and tidal volume is variable. The tidal volume will be affected by any factor that changes the airway pressure, including thoracic compliance and pulmonary resistance, and by the inspiratory time. As the lung inflates, the inspiratory flow tapers which results in a more homogenous gas distribution throughout the lungs. Since tidal volume is variable in pressure control modes, a sudden decrease in pulmonary compliance can cause a rapid reduction in tidal volume and minute ventilation resulting in acute respiratory acidosis, and this mode necessitates close monitoring of the minute ventilation and possible intrinsic- or auto-PEEP (Fig. 38-4).
   a. **Pressure-control (PC) ventilation.** Set an inspiratory pressure and inspiratory time rather than tidal volume and inspiratory flow rate. Tidal volume is dependent on set pressure, inspiratory time, and patient's compliance/resistance. In patients with hypoxemic ARF or ARDS, changing from

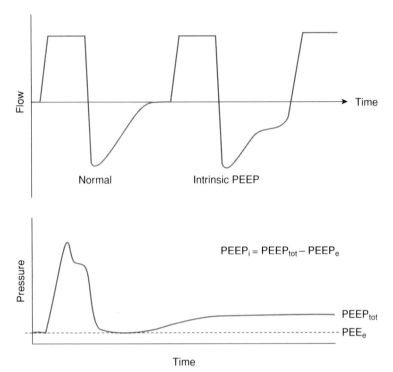

Figure 38-4. Intrinsic- or Auto-PEEP. Examination of the flow–time curve from the ventilator gives an indication that there is intrinsic PEEP but does not give an indication of the magnitude. The patient does not need to be apneic. A quantitative measurement of intrinsic PEEP can be obtained in an apneic patient by using the expiratory pause hold control on the ventilator. This allows equilibration of pressures between the alveoli and the ventilator allowing the total PEEP to be measured. The value for total PEEP can be read from the PEEP display. Intrinsic PEEP = Total PEEP − Set PEEP.

a volume control mode to pressure control mode may result in lower peak airway pressures.

b. Pressure support ventilation (PSV). Breaths are assisted by a set inspiratory pressure, which is delivered until inspiratory flow drops below a predetermined threshold (e.g., 25% of peak flow). Respiratory rate and tidal volume are determined by the patient. Can be a stand-alone mode or with SIMV (PSV only with spontaneous breaths). Apnea alarms are required to ensure patient safety. Some ventilators may have a set back-up IMV rate should spontaneous respirations cease. PSV has been advocated to limit barotrauma and decrease the work of breathing. PSV is also used at low levels (5 cm H_2O) during spontaneous breathing trials.

c. Pressure-regulated volume control (PRVC) or volume control plus (VC+). Automatically adjusts inspiratory pressure in response to dynamic changes in patient mechanics to guarantee a set tidal volume in a pressure-control breath. Constant pressure is applied throughout inspiration (like pressure control), but the ventilator will adjust the inspiratory pressure with each breath (compensating for changes in airway resistance and compliance) to deliver a set tidal volume. PRVC is a patient- or time-triggered, pressure-limited, time-cycled mode.

d. Airway pressure-release ventilation (APRV). This is an inverse-ratio pressure mode of MV that alternates between High PEEP (generally set

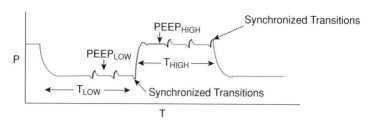

Figure 38-5. Bi-level ventilation uses two pressure levels (PEEP-low and PEEP-high) for two time periods (Time-low and Time-high), with spontaneous breathing at PEEP-low or PEEP-high.

between 25 and 30 cm H_2O) and Low PEEP (usually 0 cm H_2O), with a longer inspiratory time (Time-high), I:E commonly 7:1 to 10:1, and a very short expiratory time or "release" (Time-low). APRV achieves high mean airway pressures resulting in improved alveolar recruitment without high plateau pressures. Tidal volume is determined by the difference between high/low PEEP. Spontaneous breathing can occur, and APRV is well tolerated both hemodynamically and in terms of patient comfort.

e. Bi-level or biphasic ventilation. Similar to APRV, mandatory breaths are pressure-controlled and spontaneous breathing can occur at Time-high or Time-low (Fig. 38-5). Spontaneous breaths may be pressure-supported. Compared to APRV, Bi-level Time-low is generally longer, which allows for more spontaneous breaths during Time-low.

VIII. ADVANCED MODES OF MECHANICAL VENTILATION IN THE ICU

A. Newer modes of MV are focused on improving the patient–ventilator interface, resulting in decreased ventilator dyssynchrony and improved patient comfort, allowing greater time in spontaneous breathing.

1. Proportional assist ventilation (PAV). During PAV, the airway pressure is proportional to the instantaneous effort of the patient and is amplified according to the respiratory mechanics (pulmonary compliance and airway resistance) and the chosen level of assistance (0% to 100%) for the respiratory muscles.

a. A recent advance is the development of PAV+, a mode that provides intermittent automated measurements of the compliance and resistance, which are used by the ventilator to adjust the specific support for the patient. No studies have yet documented improved outcome using PAV.

2. Adaptive support ventilation (ASV). This mode can deliver both controlled (like pressure-control) and assisted (like pressure support) pressure cycles related to a minute ventilation target set by the clinician and based on automated measurements of the patient's respiratory mechanics.

3. Neurally adjusted ventilatory assist (NAVA). Like PAV, the level of ventilator assistance is proportional to the patient's effort, but the signal is a diaphragmatic electromyogram signal from diaphragmatic contraction obtained from electrodes on an esophageal catheter. A benefit of NAVA is improvement in patient–ventilator synchrony and reduced work of breathing by ensuring the respiratory muscles are supported throughout inspiration when compared with other commonly used MV modes. NAVA is not yet in widespread use, and the patient groups most likely to benefit are undefined.

4. SmartCare. This closed loop system provides automated adaptation of the level of PSV and initiates an automated weaning protocol to decrease the level of PSV and initiate spontaneous breathing trials when a low level of PSV is attained. The first multicenter study comparing automated weaning to standard of care ($n = 144$) documented a reduced the total duration of mechanical ventilation, weaning duration and proportion of patients requiring NIV after extubation.

IX. MECHANICAL VENTILATION STRATEGIES FOR ALI AND ARDS

A. Many recent advances have been made in developing protective MV strategies for patients with ALI and ARDS. These include low tidal volume ventilation, permissive hypercapnia, open lung strategy, and high-frequency oscillatory ventilation (HFOV). The initial strategy for management of ALI/ARDS should include the use of low tidal volume ventilation (6 mL/kg) with adequate PEEP.

B. Low tidal volume ventilation. Alveolar stretch from high tidal volumes can create VILI through stimulation of an alveolar and systemic inflammatory response. High tidal volumes may increase plateau pressures and may increase mortality. The ARDS Network trial documented that low tidal volume (6 mL/kg) versus high tidal volume (12 mL/kg) ventilation in ARDS patients was associated with lower mortality (31% vs. 40%; $p = 0.007$) and more ventilator-free days in the low tidal volume group. The *"Guidelines for Mechanical Ventilation of the Trauma Patient"* standardized clinical management in trauma patients to ensure that a low tidal volume, lung-protective strategy is used for patients with ALI/ARDS. This also provides guidelines for the PEEP and weaning of mechanical ventilation (Table 38-5).

C. Permissive hypercapnia. Low tidal volume ventilation to reduce volutrauma can decrease minute ventilation, leading to hypercapnia and acute respiratory acidosis. Permissive hypercapnia accepts deliberate hypoventilation to reduce alveolar over distension and pressures in ARDS patients with severe hypoxemia. Resultant hypercarbia and respiratory acidosis is managed medically with sodium bicarbonate or tromethamine (THAM). Tidal volume is gradually reduced to allow a slow increase in $PaCO_2$. Hypercapnia should not be used in the initial management of patients with TBI because of the effect on cerebral blood flow.

D. Open lung strategy. Combining the use of low tidal volume strategies, PEEP at levels above the lower inflection point, and permissive hypercapnia is called an "open-lung approach." Depletion of surfactant and low levels of PEEP lead to cyclic atelectasis with repeated collapsing and opening of the remaining function alveoli in ARDS patients. Cyclic opening and closing of alveoli can lead to leukocyte activation, VILI, and loss of functional residual lung capacity (FRC). Increased levels of PEEP lead to recruitment of collapsed alveoli, reducing ventilation–perfusion mismatch, improved arterial oxygenation, and increased FRC.

1. By maintaining end-expiratory pressure, alveoli that are unstable and prone to collapse will remain open. The optimal PEEP level is difficult to determine but evidence suggests that maximal recruitment and lung volume maintenance occurs when the PEEP is set at a level just above the inflection point (Pflex) on the pressure–volume curve in ARDS patients. A recent meta-analysis confirmed that higher versus lower levels of PEEP was associated with improved survival among patients with ARDS. Despite the use of increased PEEP, it has been demonstrated that decreasing plateau pressures (Pplat) results in a lower mortality in ARDS patients (Fig 38-6).

E. High-frequency oscillatory ventilation (HFOV). HFOV delivers small tidal volumes at frequencies of 3 to 15 Hz to maintain adequate minute ventilation. Oxygenation is manipulated by adjusting mean airway pressure similar to the use of PEEP in conventional mechanical ventilation. Ventilation and carbon dioxide elimination is controlled by changing the tidal volume, by amplitude or power, or by adjusting the frequency. Increasing the amplitude or decreasing the frequency will cause an increase in carbon dioxide elimination. Amplitude or power is set to achieve appropriate chest wall movement and adequate CO_2 elimination.

1. HFOV was initially used as a rescue strategy when other modes of mechanical ventilation had failed. A recent meta-analysis concluded that HFOV in adults with ARDS is a safe and may improve outcome (RR 0.77, 95% CI 0.61–0.98) compared to conventional MV.

2. HFOV is an option in patients with bronchopleural fistulae or tracheobronchial injuries to maintain low mean airway pressures in an effort to resolve air leaks within the tracheobronchial system.

TABLE 38-5	Pocket Card Summary of Mechanical Ventilation of the Trauma Patient

Mechanical Ventilation Protocol-Inflammation and the Host Response to Injury

In patients with ALI or established ARDS (PaO_2/FiO_2 ≤300 or PaO_2/FiO_2 ≤200, respectively, with bilateral pulmonary infiltrates) aim for the following within 24 h of meeting criteria:

1. Initial tidal volumes may be set at 8 mL/kg PBW; tidal volumes should be reduced by 1 mL/kg at intervals of <2 h until the tidal volume = 6 mL/kg. Tidal volume calculations are based on PBW as follows:
   For males: PBW (kg) = 50 + 2.3 {height (in) − 60}
   For females: PBW (kg) = 45.5 + 2.3 {height (in.) − 60}.

2. PaO_2 55–80 mm Hg or SpO_2 88%–95% FiO_2/PEEP ratio should be ≤5 and PEEP must be ≤35 cm H_2O.

3. Arterial pH 7.25–7.45 with RR <35 and $PaCO_2$ ≥25. HCO_3 infusion may be given if necessary. If pH <7.15 then Vt may be increased by 1 mL/kg to pH ≥ 7.15 and target plateau pressures (see below) may be exceeded.

4. Plateau pressures (PP) ≤30 cm H_2O, reduce Vt to no less than 4 mL/kg. If Vt <6 mL/kg and PP <25 then increase Vt until PP = 25–30 or Vt = 6 mL/kg.

Patients not meeting ALI/ARDS criteria can be ventilated using the mode, rate, and tidal volume chosen at the treating physician's discretion.

Patients should undergo a daily assessment of their readiness for a spontaneous breathing trial (SBT):

(a) Resolution or stabilization of the underlying disease process; (b) no residual effects of neuromuscular blockade; (c) exhibiting respiratory efforts; (d) hemodynamically stable; (e) FiO_2 ≤0.5 and PEEP ≤8 cm H_2O; (f) PaO_2 >70 mm Hg; (g) Ve <15 L/min; (h) arterial pH between 7.30 and 7.50; (i) ICP <20 cm H_2O. If not ready for an SBT, then return to a comfortable, nonfatiguing mode of ventilator support and reassess daily.

If ready, then the patient should receive **a trial of spontaneous breathing (SBT) on CPAP for 30–90 min. Criteria for failure of an SBT:**

(a) RR >35 for ≥5 min; (b) SpO_2 <90% for ≥30 s; (c) HR >140 or increase or decrease of 20% from baseline; (d) SBP >180 mm Hg or <90 mm Hg; (e) sustained evidence of respiratory distress; (f) cardiac instability or dysrhythmias; (g) arterial pH ≤7.32; (h) ICP ≥20 cm H_2O. If any criteria are met, the CPAP trial is terminated and the patient returned to a nonfatiguing mode of support and rested overnight. Repeat CPAP in the morning.

If patient completes CPAP trial, the following criteria should be assessed to determine readiness for extubation and patient extubated if possible:

(a) Does not require suctioning more than q4h; (b) good spontaneous cough; (c) endotracheal tube cuff leak; (d) no recent upper airway obstruction or stridor; (e) no recent reintubation for bronchial hygiene.

From: Nathens AB, et al. Inflammation and the host response to injury, a large-scale collaborative project: Patient-oriented research core–standard operating procedures for clinical care. I. Guidelines for mechanical ventilation of the trauma patient. *J Trauma* 2005;59(3):764–769.

3. Theoretically, HFOV is an ideal lung-protective method, and may have a larger margin of safety in keeping the lung open within the desired target range of alveolar over distintion in heterogeneously injured ARDS lungs, but outcome benefits are unproven, with two ongoing trials (OSCILLATE and OSCAR).

4. Although the exact severity threshold at which to initiate a trial of HFOV remains unclear, an emerging approach includes the following severity criteria:
   a. FiO_2 >0.60 and SpO_2 <88% on CMV with PEEP >15 cm H_2O, or
   b. Plateau pressures >30 cm H_2O, or
   c. Mean airway pressure 24 cm H_2O, or APRV with High pressure 35 cm H_2O

F. **Airway pressure-release ventilation (APRV).** APRV is a pressure-limited, time-cycled mode of mechanical ventilation that allows the patient unrestricted spontaneous breathing during application of continuous positive airway pressure

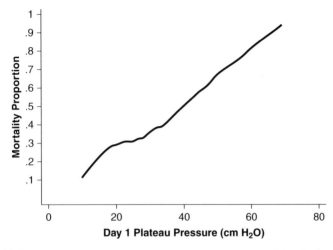

Figure 38-6. Relationship between mortality and day 1 plateau pressures. Adapted with permission from Hager DN, Krishnan JA, Hayden DL, et al. Tidal volume reduction in patients with acute lung injury when plateau pressures are not high. *Am J Respir Crit Care Med* 2005;172(10):1241–1245.

(CPAP) with a very short release time, resulting in open lung MV. APRV has two settings of pressure. The high pressure setting allows spontaneous breathing and accounts for 80% to 95% of the cycle time creating an open lung. The remainder of the cycle allows for a periodic pressure release to the low pressure setting to allow for ventilation and carbon dioxide clearance while preventing alveolar collapse. APRV is used when patients are able to spontaneously breathe, yet high mean airway pressure is required for alveolar recruitment for severe hypoxemia.

X. ADJUNCTS TO MECHANICAL VENTILATION IN ARDS AND SEVERE HYPOXEMIA

  A. In patients with severe life-threatening hypoxemia, fluid management, recruitment maneuvers, neuromuscular blockade, prone position, inhaled nitric oxide, and extracorporeal membrane oxygenation (ECMO) can aid.

    1. Recruitment maneuvers. Alveolar recruitment is aimed at improving pulmonary gas exchange, preventing VILI, atelectasis, and atelectrauma. Recruitment maneuvers (RMs) can increase alveolar FRC and PEEP can then maintain the alveoli to prevent collapse. Recruitment refers to the dynamic process of reopening unstable airless alveoli through an intentional transient increase in transpulmonary pressure, accomplished via many methods.

      a. A common method for RMs is to provide sustained inflation with 30 cm H_2O PEEP for 30 seconds or 40 cm H_2O PEEP for 40 seconds; alternatively, the use of a pressure control RM with high PEEP 40, low PEEP 20, I:E 1:1 for 2 minutes is effective. The optimal methods of RMs (sustained inflation versus incremental PEEP) and optimal pressure, duration and frequency of RMs have not been tested in large clinical trials.

      b. Transient hypotension and desaturation during RMs is common but is self-limited without sequelae. Given the uncertain benefit and lack of information regarding impact on clinical outcomes, use RMs only in patients with life-threatening hypoxemia.

    2. Fluid management. After initial volume restoration, a conservative fluid management strategy can improve lung function and oxygenation and decreased duration of MV and ICU stay, though mortality may not be altered. Diuretic therapy may aid severe hypoxemia (PaO_2/FiO_2 ratio <100). A careful assessment of adequacy of perfusion and cardiac performance should be completed before initiation of diuretic therapy, and re-assessment continued while diuresis is ongoing.

3. **Neuromuscular blockade.** A multicenter, double-blind trial of 340 patients with severe ARDS confirmed that early administration of a neuromuscular blocking agent (cisatracurium) improved 90-day survival and increased time off mechanical ventilation without increasing muscle weakness compared to placebo. Enthusiasm for this approach is tempered with concern for critical illness polyneuropathy.

4. **Inhaled nitric oxide (NO).** Nitric oxide is a selective pulmonary vasodilator leading to decreased pulmonary vascular resistance, pulmonary arterial pressure, and right ventricular afterload. Low-dose inhaled NO improves short-term oxygenation in ALI and ARDS patients without affecting duration of mechanical ventilatory support or mortality. Inhaled NO is a salvage therapy in patients who continue to have life-threatening hypoxemia despite optimization of all other treatment strategies.

5. **Prone positioning.** Changes in patient positioning can have a dramatic effect on oxygenation and ventilation in severe ARDS and severe hypoxemia. Prone position can improve the distribution of perfusion to ventilated lung regions, decreasing intrapulmonary shunt and improving oxygenation. Recent meta-analyses in ARDS patients documented decreased mortality with prone positioning, with an absolute mortality reduction of 10% in severely hypoxemic ARDS patients.

6. **Extracorporeal membrane oxygenation (ECMO).** ECMO is considered in patients with severe ARDS and hypoxemia with reversible lung disease who have failed other rescue strategies. ECMO provides oxygenation, ventilation with total extracorporeal CO_2 clearance, minimizes barotrauma with complete lung rest, and is accomplished via veno-venous ECMO support, until the endogenous lung function improves.

   a. ECMO potential complications include bleeding (including intracranial hemorrhage), coagulopathy, thrombosis, and mechanical complications.

   b. Of 1,473 adults with severe ARDS, ECMO was associated with a 50% survival to discharge.

   c. Patients with severe ARDS and hypoxemia should be referred to an ARDS center with ECMO experience to achieve the best outcomes possible.

   d. Adult patients are cannulated percutaneously with 21–31 French venous catheters for drainage of deoxygenated blood and infusion and oxygenated blood. Anticoagulation is necessary, and heparin continuous infusion is common, and monitored with ACT or PTT studies.

XI. INCREMENTAL APPROACH TO THE MANAGEMENT OF SEVERE ARDS

A. Development of ICU protocols reduces undesirable variability, mandates best evidence practice, promotes action and timeliness, and facilitates multi-disciplinary communication.

B. An evidence-based algorithm (Fig 38-7) for management of critically ill patients with severe ARDS/severe hypoxemia is provided.

C. In ARDS patients, initial low tidal volume ventilation should be initiated, set at 6 to 8 mL/kg of predicted body weight (PBW); tidal volumes should be reduced by 1 mL/kg at intervals of 2 hours until the tidal volume is set at 6 mL/kg. Goal: SpO_2 88% to 95%, PO_2 55 to 80 mm Hg, plateau pressures <30 cm H_2O while using lowest FiO_2 possible.

D. If no improvement, recruitment maneuvers should be considered. If oxygenation improves during recruitment maneuvers, the PEEP should be increased until optimal PEEP is achieved.

E. If no improvement, evaluate for a possible intracardiac shunt or pulmonary hypertension using a pulmonary artery catheter placement or transthoracic or transesophageal echocardiogram. Inhaled nitric oxide can improve oxygenation, and adding prone positioning is wise.

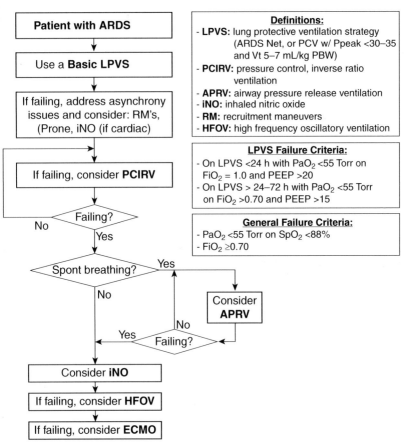

Figure 38-7. ARDS mechanical ventilation algorithm, including rescue strategies, used at the University of Michigan.

    F. After these measures, transfer all patients with persistent severe hypoxemia to an ARDS Referral Center, with experience in other ARDS treatment modalities, including rescue strategies, APRV, HFOV and ECMO. (Fig. 38-8).

XII. WEANING AND LIBERATION FROM MECHANICAL VENTILATION

    A. Mechanical ventilation has potential risks best avoided by liberation from mechanical ventilation once adequate lung recovery has occurred.

    B. Nearly half of the time spent with mechanical ventilation is spent weaning the patient.

    C. Perform a daily spontaneous awakening trial (SAT) followed by a spontaneous breathing trial (SBT) in all patients on MV (Table 38-5). A randomized multicenter trial that compared this "wake up and breathe" protocol (paired SAT/SBT) versus usual care plus a daily SBT in the control cohort confirmed that SAT/SBT resulted in improved outcomes with reduced mortality, increased ventilator-free days and reduced ICU, and hospital length of stay.

    D. Continuous protocols for weaning from mechanical ventilation directed by respiratory therapists are associated with shorter duration of ventilation and ICU length

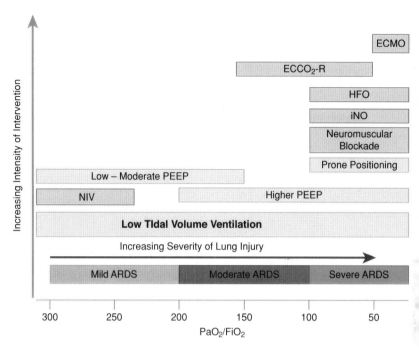

Figure 38-8. Increasing intensity of treatment intervention for increasing severity of ARDS, with all treatment strategies available at ARDS referral center, including ECMO.

of stay. Patients who fail a SAT/SBT trial are returned to their previous ventilator settings and re-screened for another SAT/SBT trial in 24 hours. Identify any cause for the SAT/SBT failure, notably altered mental status, anxiety, pain, secretions, muscle weakness, atelectasis, hypoxemia, or hypercarbia.

E. Assess patients who complete a paired SAT/SBT trial (CPAP with low pressure support [5 cm H_2O] or automatic tube compensation, or T-piece) to determine readiness for extubation. At the completion of the SAT/SBT trial, the rapid shallow breathing index (RSBI), the ratio of respiratory frequency to tidal volume (f/Vt, respiratory rate × tidal volumes in liters), is calculated and an arterial blood gas is obtained to evaluate for hypercarbia. For example, a patient who has a respiratory rate of 25 breaths/min and a tidal volume of 250 mL/breath has an RSBI of (25 breaths/min)/(.25 L) = 100 breaths/min/L. RSBI <105 is associated with 80% wean success; RSBI ≥105 is associated with 95% wean failure.

F. Before considering extubation, assess a patient to ensure the following: (a) Does not require tracheal suctioning more than every 4 hours; (b) has a good spontaneous cough; (c) has an endotracheal tube cuff leak; (d) no recent upper airway obstruction or stridor; (e) did not need recent reintubation for bronchial hygiene.

G. If failure to wean and/or extubate persist despite efforts to achieve these endpoints, other steps may be required before successfully liberating the patient from MV. Some patients require prolonged and more gradual ventilator weaning, which may be best facilitated by tracheostomy placement. In addition, data from observational studies shows that up to 60% of ventilator-dependent patients who are discharged from the ICU can be successfully weaned when they are transferred to specialized units dedicated to ventilator weaning.

XIII. TRACHEOSTOMY

A. Some patients benefit from early tracheostomy, especially those with traumatic brain injury and those who will require prolonged mechanical ventilation (i.e., ARDS patients) for patient comfort.

1. Previous studies suggested that tracheostomy was superior to prolonged intubation for VAP prevention. However, 2 recent, large, prospective, randomized, clinical trials have found no difference in VAP or any other outcomes measures in comparing early (6–8 days) with late (13–15 days) tracheostomy in 419 patients or comparing early (4 days) with late (after 10 days) tracheostomy in 909 patients in the TracMan trial. Early tracheostomy should not be performed for VAP prevention but may be considered for other reasons, such as difficult airway and difficult-to-wean patients, particularly for patient comfort.

AXIOMS

- ARF is classified as either hypoxemic (Type I) or hypercapnic (Type II).
- Think of ALI when severe hypoxemic ARF exists (PaO_2/FiO_2 ratio <300) or ARDS (PaO_2/FiO_2 ratio <200).
- NIV is a good start for patients with ARF due to COPD or pulmonary edema.
- Following intubation for ARF, use all strategies to prevent VAP.
- In ALI/ARDS, use low tidal volume ventilation (6 mL/kg) with adequate PEEP.
- Weaning of mechanical ventilation should be initiated to allow spontaneous breathing as soon as possible.
- Early tracheostomy should not be performed for VAP prevention, but may be considered for other reasons, such as difficult airway, severe traumatic brain injury for airway protection, and difficult-to-wean patients.
- Perform a paired daily spontaneous awakening trial (SAT) and spontaneous breathing trial (SBT) in all patients on MV, since it is associated with reduced mortality and length of stay, and reduced ventilation duration.

Suggested Readings

Boldrini R, Fasano L, Nava S. Noninvasive mechanical ventilation. *Curr Opin Crit Care* 2011. [Epub ahead of print]

Burns KE, Adhikari NK, Keenan SP, et al. Noninvasive positive pressure ventilation as a weaning strategy for intubated adults with respiratory failure. *Cochrane Database Syst Rev* 2010;(8):CD004127.

Dickinson S, Park PK, Napolitano LM. Prone-positioning therapy in ARDS. *Crit Care Clin* 2011;27(3):511–523.

Fan E, Wilcox ME, Brower RG, et al. Recruitment maneuvers for acute lung injury: a systematic review. *Am J Respir Crit Care Med* 2008;178(11):1156–1163.

Girard TD, Kress JP, Fuchs BD, et al. Efficacy and safety of a paired sedation and ventilator weaning protocol for mechanically ventilated patients in intensive care (Awakening and Breathing Controlled trial): a randomised controlled trial. *Lancet* 2008;371(9607):126–134.

Muscedere J, Dodek P, Keenan S, et al. Comprehensive evidence-based clinical practice guidelines for ventilator-associated pneumonia: prevention. *J Crit Care* 2008;23(1):126–137.

Napolitano LM, Park PK, Raghavendran K, et al. Nonventilatory strategies for patients with life-threatening 2009 H1N1 influenza and severe respiratory failure. *Crit Care Med* 2010;38(4 Suppl):e74–e90.

Nathens AB, Johnson JL, Minei JP, et al. Inflammation and the host response to injury, a large-scale collaborative project: Patient-oriented research core–standard operating procedures for clinical care. I. Guidelines for mechanical ventilation of the trauma patient. *J Trauma* 2005;59(3):764–769.

National Heart, Lung, and Blood Institute Acute Respiratory Distress Syndrome (ARDS) Clinical Trials Network, Wiedemann HP, Wheeler AP, et al. Comparison of two fluid-management strategies in acute lung injury. *N Engl J Med* 2006;354(24):2564–2575.

Park PK, Napolitano LM, Bartlett RH. Extracorporeal membrane oxygenation in adult acute respiratory distress syndrome. *Crit Care Clin* 2011;27(3):627–646.

Raghavendran K, Napolitano LM. ALI and ARDS: Challenges and advances. *Crit Care Clin* 2011; 27(3):xiii–xiv.

Singer BD, Corbridge TC. Basic invasive mechanical ventilation. *South Med J* 2009;102(12):1238–1245.

The Acute Respiratory Distress Syndrome Network. Ventilation with lower tidal volumes as compared with traditional tidal volumes for acute lung injury and the acute respiratory distress syndrome. *N Engl J Med* 2000;342:1301–1308.

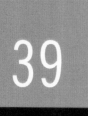

39

Abdominal Compartment Syndrome, Open Abdomen, Enterocutaneous Fistulae

James F. Whelan, Michel B. Aboutanos and Rao R. Ivatury

I. ABDOMINAL COMPARTEMENT SYNDROME (ACS)

A. Introduction

Abdominal compartment syndrome (ACS) is a clinical condition in which intra-abdominal hypertension (IAH) leads to impaired end-organ perfusion. If left untreated or unrecognized, this hypoperfusion will lead to gut ischemia, renal insufficiency, and multiple organ dysfunction syndrome. IAH also causes elevation of the diaphragm with resultant respiratory embarrassment and decreased cardiac return to the heart leading to decreased cardiac output and further deterioration in end-organ perfusion. Onset can be insidious or fulminant; clinicians must be astute in making the diagnosis. Mortality of ACS ranges from 42% to 68% after detection and treatment and 100% in those not undergoing decompression. Reduced rates of morbidity and mortality depend on early and aggressive detection and management.

B. Clinical scenarios

The most common inciting event in the development of ACS is major abdominal trauma. ACS has also been reported after ruptured abdominal aortic aneurysm repair, intraperitoneal hemorrhage, pancreatitis, ileus, intestinal obstruction, post-operative bowel edema, pneumoperitoneum (e.g., secondary to barotrauma), septic shock, overzealous resuscitation, neoplasm, and liver transplantation.

C. Classification

Two types of ACS have now been described, **primary** and **secondary.** The following are the definitions from a consensus conference of the **World Society of Abdominal Compartment Syndrome (WSACS):**

1. **Primary ACS** is caused by a condition associated with injury or disease in the abdominopelvic region that frequently requires surgical or interventional radiologic intervention, or a condition that develops following abdominal surgery such as abdominal organ injuries requiring surgical repair or damage control surgery. Visceral edema from third space losses and ongoing bleeding (surgical and disseminated intravascular coagulopathy) are important factors in the development of primary ACS.

2. **Secondary ACS** is caused by conditions that do not originate from the abdomen such as sepsis with associated capillary leak, major burns, major soft tissue and skeletal trauma, or other conditions requiring massive fluid resuscitation. The chief mechanism appears to be fluid sequestration within the viscera due to reperfusion injury and increased capillary permeability. **Any patient undergoing massive resuscitation (>10L crystalloid or >10 units of packed red blood cells [PRBCs]) is at risk for the development of IAH and ACS.**

3. **Recurrent ACS** is a condition in which ACS develops following prophylactic or therapeutic surgical or medical treatment of primary or secondary ACS (e.g., persistence of ACS after decompressive laparotomy) or development of a new ACS episode following definitive closure of the abdominal wall after the previous utilization of a temporary abdominal wall closure.

D. Clinical manifestations

Diagnosis of ACS should be considered in any trauma or ICU patient with oliguria and abdominal distension or any patient requiring massive resuscitation. Physical examination will not always reveal a distended firm abdomen and is not a reliable marker for IAH or the development of ACS. Liberal use of bladder pressure measurements is recommended.

1. **Pulmonary** effects occur via elevation of the diaphragm, which results in decreased thoracic compliance and elevated peak airway pressures (>40 to 60 cm H_2O). The end results are hypoxia, hypercapnia, and respiratory acidosis.

2. **Cardiac** manifestations occur due to elevated thoracic pressure, which causes falsely elevated filling pressures (central venous pressure [CVP] and pulmonary capillary wedge pressure [PCWP]), decreased venous return to the heart, and decreased cardiac compliance. The end result is low cardiac output and decreased end-organ perfusion.

3. **Renal** effects result from direct parenchymal and caval compression, and decreased cardiac output causing decreased renal blood flow, depressed glomerular filtration rate (GFR) and oliguria.

4. **Gastrointestinal (GI)** effects occur from hypoperfusion of the splanchnic beds (direct compression and decreased cardiac output leading to bacterial translocation and increased septic complications.

E. Diagnosis

Intra-abdominal pressure (IAP) measurements are essential to the diagnosis of IAH and ACS.

1. **Bladder pressure** measurement is the standard for estimation of IAP and can be performed at the bedside with the use of the arterial line pressure transducer. *Technique:*
   a. **Cross-clamp** the Foley catheter drainage tubing just distal to the aspiration port.
   b. **Inject** 50 to 100 cc of sterile saline into the bladder with a catheter-tipped syringe via the Foley catheter and reconnect to the drainage tubing.
   c. **Connect** a 16 gauge needle to the arterial line pressure tubing; flush and insert into the aspiration port.
   d. **Zero** the system at the symphysis pubis while the patient is supine.

2. **IAH** is defined by a sustained increase in IAP of 12 mm Hg or more, recorded by a minimum of three standardized measurements conducted 4 to 6 hours apart, with or without a low abdominal perfusion pressure (APP) <60 mm Hg.
   Key Definition: APP = MAP (mean arterial pressure) − IAP (intra-abdominal pressure)

3. **ACS** is defined as a sustained increase in IAP of 15 to 20 mm Hg or more with or without APP <60 mm Hg and single or multiple organ dysfunction or failure.

F. Treatment

The current state-of-the-art management of IAH/ACS according to WSACS recommendations is based upon four general principles:

1. **Serial monitoring** of IAP. The critical IAP that leads to IAH and ACS varies from patient to patient. The current recommendation is to serially measure APP and to maintain it above 50 to 60 mm Hg in patients with IAH/ACS.

2. **Optimization** of systemic perfusion and organ function should be achieved via judicious and balanced fluid resuscitation.

3. Institution of specific **medical procedures** to reduce IAP
   Non-operative medical management strategies currently play a vital role in both the reduction of IAP and the prevention of organ dysfunction due to IAH. The medical management of IAP may include:
   a. Improvement in abdominal wall compliance via body positioning (such as limiting head elevation to <20 mm Hg), sedation and analgesia to decrease thoracoabdominal muscle tone, and brief use of neuromuscular blockade mainly for mild (12 to 15 mm Hg) to moderate (16 to 20 mm Hg) IAH.
   b. Evacuate intraluminal contents via nasogastric/colonic decompression and the use of prokinetic motility agents.
   c. Evacuate abdominal fluid collections via **percutaneous decompression.** This is most useful for increased IAH and secondary ACS where elevated IAP is mainly due to fluid sequestration within the viscera.

d. Correcting positive fluid balance which may include restrictive/judicial fluid resuscitation, diuresis, or continuous venovenous hemofiltration/ultrafiltration.

4. Prompt **surgical decompression** for refractory IAH.

  a. **Decompressive celiotomy** has long been the standard of care for the treatment of ACS. Currently, it is considered a life-saving intervention when a patient's IAH has become refractory to medical procedures noted above. **This is a surgical emergency** and should be undertaken with the utmost urgency once medical management has been optimized. In combination with the clinical scenario described above, most see IAH measures of >20 mm Hg as indicative of the need for decompressive celiotomy.

  i. **Preoperative preparation:** In addition to ensuring that the patient is adequately resuscitated and the blood bank has additional blood products on hold, anesthesia should be carefully appraised of the situation. Decompression results in the release of numerous toxic metabolites and acids into the systemic circulation which can lead to profound cardiac depression and hypotension. Therefore, alerting the anesthesia team of the risks of **reperfusion syndrome** before incising the fascia and releasing the IAP is an important step. Loading the patient with 2 to 4 amps of sodium bicarbonate just prior to or during decompression may also temper any associated hemodynamic instability.

  ii. **Operative facilities:** There may be temptation to perform decompression at the bedside, but this should be generally avoided in case ongoing bleeding or missed injury is discovered. Most ICUs are not the appropriate place to handle such problems.

  b. **Minimally Invasive Therapies:** Minimally invasive techniques for abdominal decompression have been employed with success in small series. In general, these therapies are most applicable for patients with secondary rather than primary IAH leading to ACS. The most often employed technique in this category is the subcutaneous release of the linea alba.

II. OPEN ABDOMEN:

It is now widely accepted to leave the abdomen open and use temporary closure techniques after laparotomy in face of significant visceral edema, especially when further fluid sequestration is expected. This prophylactic approach has resulted in a reduction in the occurrence of ACS.

Management of the open abdomen is of the utmost importance in the prevention of devastating complications, especially in those instances where the abdomen remains open for an extended amount of time. *The key concept here is expedient coverage of all exposed bowels.* A variety of techniques have been employed for abdominal closure and are generally institution-specific.

A. Temporary closure

  1. Vacuum-assisted closure devices (wound VACs). In addition to increasing the volume of the abdominal cavity, negative pressure dressings evacuate edema fluid, serum, inflammatory mediators, and blood. Originally described by Barker and colleagues, a negative pressure dressing can easily be constructed utilizing plastic drapes, surgical towels, and closed suction drains. Commercially available negative pressure products are also now available. Delays in fascial closure up to 1 month may be achieved by a running skin closure over a vacuum sponge with incremental fascial approximation as edema subsides. Recent data suggest that prolonged application of vacuum-assisted dressings is safe, increases the rate of fascial closure at first hospitalization, and reduces need for later abdominal wall reconstruction.

  2. Prosthetic coverage. Prosthetic use for bowel coverage represents an inexpensive option. Coverage with plastic intravenous solution containers (Bogota bags), fluid warmer drapes, x-ray cassette covers, woven Vicryl mesh, fascial zippers and velcro devices have all been described with varying degrees of success and **with the main risk being fistula formation.** These products are often attached to the fascial edges preventing further retraction and allow the application of tension making future fascial closure easier. IV bags, sterile x-ray cassette covers or fluid warmer drapes sewn to the skin are generally cheapest and usually adequate if early takeback is anticipated. **Absorbable mesh** (i.e., Vicryl mesh) has a number of advantages in this scenario. It can be placed safely in a contaminated field. It can accept STSG when granulation tissue is present or the fascia can safely be closed over it if that option should become available. **Biologic mesh** is a viable option because of its ability to be placed in a contaminated field, but many feel this option has limited application as a temporary bowel coverage because of the expense of these products.

B. Permanent closure

1. **Primary closure** of the fascia closure is the preferred technique. When visceral edema has sufficiently resolved, fascial closure should be performed. If primary closure cannot be performed by post-operative days 7 to 10, it will generally not occur because the abdomen becomes "socked-in" and later, staged reconstruction will be necessary. When primary closure is employed we recommend leaving the skin open thereby preventing wound infections, and using delayed primary closure of the skin.

2. **Split-thickness skin** graft is used if primary fascial closure cannot be performed. This technique should be employed at the first appearance of granulation tissue. Allowing exposed bowel to granulate is extremely fistulogenic. This procedure will generally permit the bowel edema to resolve and adhesions to subside.

3. **Skin mobilization and closure** can be used in patients with excessive skin. Flaps can be mobilized on either side of the laparotomy wound and closed in the middle. This will avoid skin grafting and looks better cosmetically. Care must be taken to avoid devascularizing the skin flaps.

4. **Delayed abdominal wall reconstruction.** When the skin graft can easily be lifted off the underlying bowel (the pinch test), generally 6 to 9 months following grafting, abdominal wall reconstruction is possible. Rectus sheath advancement (components separation techniques) or permanent prosthetic placement is usually necessary due to loss of abdominal domain.

III. COMPLICATIONS

Complications from prolonged open abdomen increase mortality, morbidity, and cost up to 10 fold. Complications include:

A. **Intra-abdominal abscess formation** requiring repeated wash outs and delay abdominal closure, especially in the "socked-in" or "frozen" abdomen where abscess drainage may not be feasible.

B. **Hernia development** is an expected result when the STSG technique or skin only closures are employed. Interval repair of the subsequent abdominal wall hernia can be done at 6 to 9 months. At this point, reconstruction can be accomplished through excision of the split-thickness skin graft, complete adhesiolysis between the small-bowel mat and the parietal peritoneum, followed by anterior abdominal wall component separation technique.

C. **An enterocutaneous fistula** is a communication between the gastrointestinal tract and the skin. A hole in the exposed bowel in the middle of an open abdomen is a special problem—a so-called *enteroatmospheric (or exposed) fistula*. Continuous exposure of the abdominal viscera to succus entericus causes ongoing peritonitis, with inflamed bowel loops that predispose to the development of additional fistulas in the gastrointestinal tract. The results are a complex wound, severe catabolism from uncontrolled sepsis, and high mortality.

Principles of Enteroatmospheric Fistula Management:

1. **Prevention.** Regardless of the method chosen for temporary abdominal closure, protect any exposed abdominal viscera. Limit access to the wound to one or two experienced care providers who know the wound intimately. Free access to the wound for all members of the surgical and nursing team almost guarantees fistula formation.

2. **Attempts to close a fistula** in the midst of an open abdomen are usually unsuccessful. In selected patients, fibrin glue and acellular dermal matrix can seal a small enteroatmospheric fistula.

3. **Control the fistula effluent.** If the fistula occurs in an open abdomen that has not yet granulated into a "frozen" visceral block, continued contamination will occur and predispose to sepsis. Exteriorization of the fistula and proximal diversion are the best solutions, but are often not possible because of massive edema and foreshortening of the mesentery. Other options include sealing the rest of the abdomen to isolate the fistula and treat it as a stoma; creating a "floating stoma" as described by Subramanian and colleagues. This consists of suturing the edges of the fistula to the plastic silo used for temporary coverage, creating a controlled stoma over which a stoma bag can be applied. Often these choices do not work well and there is no choice but daily dressings and manual removal of enteric contents until the visceral block is fixed.

Once this is accomplished, the open abdominal wound is essentially a carpet of granulation tissue, ongoing peritoneal contamination is not a major issue, but control of the effluent and protection of the adjacent skin remain difficult problems. Recently, reports have described successful use of vacuum-assisted wound management in the control of fistula effluent with eventual healing of the fistula. Another alternative is to use wound drainage bags, which require the expertise of wound management teams. If these measures are unsuccessful, covering the exposed bowel with a skin graft or mobilized skin flaps becomes primary. This is crucial to avoid the development of more fistulas from exposed bowel.

4. **Cover the fistula with well-vascularized tissue.** Occasionally, an open abdomen and fistula can be managed by soft tissue cover with fascia or even skin as previously discussed, combined with fistula intubation to create a drainage tract. In this situation, intubation of a fistula at the time of soft tissue coverage is important to establish an effective drainage tract. The fistula can then heal because it is covered by well-perfused soft tissue.

5. **Nutritional support.** The combination of open abdomen and fistulae is catabolic and the patient needs to be supported by aggressive nutrition. If the fistula allows (distal fistula) enteral nutrition may be allowed by well-placed feeding tubes. Otherwise, total parenteral nutrition (TPN) may be necessary.

6. **Resect chronic fistula when patient is fit and infection free.** Patients with enteroatmospheric fistulas are generally ill with a hostile abdomen. Definitive resection of the involved bowel segment must be delayed for many months. These procedures often require extensive planning and complex abdominal wall reconstruction.

AXIOMS

■ ACS should be suspected in any trauma or burn patient with abdominal distension and oliguria despite normal or elevated central filling pressures.

■ As with any compartment syndrome, measurement of compartment (bladder) pressure is instrumental in establishing the diagnosis and should be routinely monitored in patients at risk.

■ Patients with IAP >15 mm Hg and signs of physiologic compromise should be decompressed.

■ Non-operative medical management strategies currently play a vital role in both the reduction of IAP and the prevention of organ dysfunction due to IAH.

■ Skin closure over exposed viscera, when possible, is the best temporary dressing and prevention of the fistulas is the key.

■ Once established, the fistulas are best managed by meticulous wound care and nutritional support.

■ Enteroatmospheric fistula in the midst of the open abdomen is a difficult problem that demands attention to detail, innovativeness and patience on the part of the surgical team.

Suggested Readings

Balogh Z, Moore FA, Moore EE, et al. Secondary abdominal compartment syndrome: a potential threat for all trauma clinicians. *Injury* 2007;38:272–279.

Cheatham ML, Malbrain ML, Kirkpatrick A, et al. Results from the International Conference of Experts on Intra-abdominal Hypertension and Abdominal Compartment Syndrome. II. Recommendations. *Intensive Care Med* 2007;33:951–962.

Draus JM Jr, Huss SA, Harty NJ, et al. Enterocutaneous fistula: are treatments improving? *Surgery* 2006;140(4):570–576.

Duchesne JC, Howell MP, Eriksen C, et al. Linea alba fasciotomy: a novel alternative in trauma patients with secondary abdominal compartment syndrome. *Am Surg* 2010;76:312–316.

Eddy V, Nun C, Morris JA Jr. Abdominal compartment syndrome: The Nashville experience. *Surg Clin North Am* 1997;77:801–812.

Evenson AR, Fischer JE. Current management of enterocutaneous fistula. *J Gastrointest Surg* 2006;10(3):455–464.

Fabian TC, Croce MA, Pritchard FE, et al. Planned ventral hernia: Staged management for acute abdominal wall defects. *Ann Surg* 1994;219:643–650.

Ivatury RR, Diebel LN, Porter JM, et al. Intra-abdominal hypertension and the abdominal compartment syndrome. *Surg Clin North Am* 1997;77:783–800.

Jamshidi R, Schecter WP. Biological dressings for the management of enteric fistulas in the open abdomen: a preliminary report. *Arch Surg* 2007;142(8):793–796.

Maxwell RA, Fabian TC, Croce MA, et al. Secondary abdominal compartment syndrome: An underappreciated manifestation of severe hemorrhagic shock. *J Trauma* 1994;47:955–1003.

Miller PR, Thompson JT, Faler BJ, et al. Late fascial closure in lieu of ventral hernia: the next step in open abdomen management. *J Trauma* 2002;53:843–849.

Ouellet JF, Ball CG. Recurrent abdominal compartment syndrome induced by high negative pressure abdominal closure dressing. *J Trauma* 2011;71(3):785–786.

Schecter WP, Ivatury RR, Rotondo MF, et al. Open abdomen after trauma and abdominal sepsis: a strategy for management. *J Am Coll Surg* 2006;203(3):390–396.

40

Liver Failure

Deanna Blisard

I. ACUTE LIVER FAILURE

A. Introduction

1. Fulminant hepatic failure (FHF) is synonymous with acute liver failure (ALF).
2. Approximately 2,000 cases of ALF occur in the United States per year.
3. ALF is the rapid deterioration of liver function, which results in altered mental status and coagulopathy in previously normal individuals.
4. Loss of hepatic function can quickly lead to multiorgan failure and death.

B. Definition

1. Most widely accepted definition of ALF is the presence of coagulation abnormalities and any degree of encephalopathy in a patient without preexisting cirrhosis, with an illness of <26 weeks duration.
2. Classified according to length of illness:
   a. Hyperacute: <7 days
   b. Acute: 7 to 21 days
   c. Subacute: >21 days and <26 weeks
3. Length of illness has no prognostic significance distinct from cause of the illness.

C. Etiology

1. Major indicator of prognosis; also dictates specific management options.
2. Viral—hepatitis A, hepatitis B, herpes, cytomegalovirus, Epstein–Barr virus.
3. Vascular—Budd–Chiari syndrome, right heart failure, shock liver.
4. Metabolic—Wilson's disease, HELLP syndrome, acute fatty liver of pregnancy, tyrosinemia.
5. Drugs and toxins—acetaminophen, Amanita phalloides, Bacillus cereus toxin, herbal remedies.
6. Miscellaneous/indeterminate—malignant infiltration, autoimmune hepatitis, severe sepsis.

D. Acetaminophen

1. Acetaminophen toxicity is the leading cause of ALF in the United States, accounting for 40% of cases.
2. Suspected when evidence of excessive ingestion, usually as a suicidal attempt or ingestion of supratherapeutic quantities of pain medications.
3. Dose related toxin, most ingestions that lead to ALF exceeding 10 g/day.
4. Acetaminophen overdose leads to the accumulation of N-acetyl-p-benzoquinone imine, a metabolite normally conjugated by glutathione that is toxic to hepatocytes.
   a. Acetaminophen levels should be drawn on all patients presenting with ALF, and the agent N-acetylcysteine (NAC) started.
   b. Excessive ingestion of acetaminophen leads to depletion of glutathione stores, and NAC augments glutathione levels.
   c. NAC should be started as early as possible, but can be useful even 48 hours or more after ingestion.
   d. The oral dosing is 140 mg/kg diluted to 5% solution, followed by 70 mg/kg by mouth q4h × 17 doses.
   e. The intravenous dosing is a loading dose of 150 mg/kg in 5% dextrose over 15 minutes, followed by maintenance dosing of 50 mg/kg over 4 hours, followed by 100 mg/kg administered over 16 hours.

E. Presentation of ALF

1. Presenting symptoms are often nonspecific. ALF patients are heterogeneous but share the common disease process of acute hepatocyte necrosis and its sequelae.
2. Symptoms include fatigue, malaise, anorexia, nausea, abdominal pain, fever, and jaundice.
3. Often these symptoms progress to severe coagulopathy and encephalopathy and/or coma.

F. Initial treatment

1. Regular monitoring including frequent vital signs, blood glucose, and neurologic status.
2. Initial laboratory testing should include:
   a. Complete blood count
   b. Biochemical panel, including renal function, liver function tests
   c. Hematologic panel
   d. Immunologic panel
   e. Hepatitis panel
   f. Toxic drug screens
   g. Arterial blood gas and lactate levels to assess metabolic disturbances.
3. Radiographic tests include:
   a. Chest x-ray
   b. Abdominal ultrasound with Doppler studies to evaluate hepatic and portal venous flow patterns
   c. Triphasic CT scan to evaluate hepatic parenchyma for tumors, ischemia/necrosis, and fatty infiltration.
4. Clinical deterioration can be rapid, and any worsening in the clinical condition should prompt referral to a transplant center.
5. Patients who present in full ALF often have severe metabolic acidosis, hypoglycemia, coagulopathy, and encephalopathy/coma.
   a. Stabilization includes volume resuscitation, mechanical ventilation, and hemodynamic support.

G. Hepatic encephalopathy (HE) and intracranial hypertension (ICH)

1. Definition
   a. Hallmark feature of ALF.
   b. Prognosis is inversely correlated with the degree of encephalopathy.
   c. Most serious complication of ALF is cerebral edema and ICH, affecting 50% to 80% of patients with severe ALF (grade III or IV coma).
2. Presentation
   a. HE can vary from subtle changes in affect, insomnia, or difficulties with concentration (grade I) to deep coma (grade IV). Table 40-1 illustrates encephalopathy grades.
   b. Grades I and II encephalopathy seldom have signs of cerebral edema.
   c. Progression to grade III portends 25% to 35% increased risk of edema; 65% to 75% or more in patients reaching grade IV HE.
   d. ICH presents with signs of systemic hypertension, bradycardia, abnormal papillary signs, aggravation of HE, epileptiform activity, and decerebrate posturing.
3. Pathophysiology
   a. Two theories for ICH in ALF:
      i. Brain edema due to osmotic astrocyte swelling secondary to ammonia-induced accumulation of glutamine or
      ii. Alteration of cerebral blood flow (CBF) regulation with increased intracranial blood volume.
      iii. Typical course of grade III/IV HE includes reduction in CBF along with a reduction in cerebral metabolic rate early, followed by gradual cerebral vasodilatation due to loss of autoregulation.
      iv. Preterminal phase shows marked reduction in CBF resulting from cerebral edema, with cerebral herniation as the end result.
4. Testing and monitoring

TABLE 40-1   **Stages of Encephalopathy in Acute Liver Failure**

Stage	Mental status	Tremor	EEG
I	Euphoria, occasional depression, fluctuant mild confusion, slowness of mentation and affect, untidy, slurred speech	Slight	Usually normal
II	Accentuation of stage I, drowsiness, inappropriate behavior, able to maintain sphincter control	Present (easily elicited)	Abnormal, generalized slowing
III	Sleeps most of the time but is arousable, incoherent speech, marked confusion	Usually present if patient cooperative	Always abnormal
IV	Not arousable, may or may not respond to painful stimuli	Usually absent	Always abnormal

    a. Most accurate method to diagnose ICH is intracranial pressure (ICP) monitoring.
      i. Advantages not yet demonstrated by a randomized study.
      ii. ICP monitoring may be helpful to establish the presence of ICH and guide specific therapy.
      iii. ICP transducers can be in the brain parenchyma, epidural, or subdural spaces; epidural devices have lower complication rates (3.8%) versus subdural bolts (20%) or parenchymal monitors (22%).
      iv. Epidural transducers may be the safest choice to monitor ICP even though they are less precise than the other devices.
      v. The use of recombinant factor VIIa (rFVIIa) appears to minimize the associated risk of hemorrhage when placing these monitors. A single dose of 40 μg/kg is recommended prior to placement.
    b. Transcranial Doppler (TCD) is a noninvasive measurement of the systolic flow velocity of the middle cerebral artery.
      i. Normal systolic velocity is less than 120 cm/second.
      ii. Attenuation of the diastolic flow signal may signal ICH and decreased cerebral perfusion.
      iii. A pulsatility index (systolic velocity − diastolic velocity/systolic velocity) greater than 1.6 is a poor prognostic sign.
    c. Arterio-jugulovenous oxygen difference ($AVjDO_2$) changes in response to changes in CBF, which is a reflection of the ratio of the flow to metabolism.
      i. Catheter is placed in the internal jugular vein toward the base of the skull.
      ii. A normal $AVjDO_2$ is 5 to 6 mL/100 mL.
      iii. A narrow $AVjDO_2$ difference is suggestive of cerebral hyperemia.
      iv. A widened $AVjDO_2$ is suggestive of cerebral ischemia.
  5. Treatment
    a. Treatment of elevated ICPs involves decreasing brain volume or decreasing the CBF and intracranial blood volume.
    b. Mannitol works by increasing blood osmolarity, thereby inducing fluid movement from the brain to the vascular space.
      i. Mannitol (0.5 to 1 g/kg IV) repeated once or twice as needed is recommended, not exceeding serum osmolality of 320 mOsm/L.
      ii. Efficacy is affected by acute renal failure.
    c. Hypertonic saline works similarly to mannitol.
      i. Recent controlled trial of 3% hypertonic saline to maintain serum sodium levels of 145 to 155 mEq/L suggested induction and maintenance of hypernatremia can be used to prevent a rise in ICP values.
      ii. A survival benefit was not demonstrated in this trial.

  d. Hyperventilation, indomethacin, thiopental, and induced hypothermia reduce ICP through vasoconstriction of cerebral blood vessels, thereby decreasing CBF.

  i. The American Association for the Study of Liver Diseases (AASLD) position paper on the management of ALF does not support prophylactic hyperventilation; hyperventilation may be used temporarily to acutely lower ICP and prevent impending herniation.

  ii. Indomethacin induces cerebral vasoconstriction through inhibition of the endothelial cyclooxygenase pathway, alterations in extracellular pH, and reduction in cerebral temperature. Studies are small and need further evaluation before widespread use.

  iii. Thiopental induces cerebral vasoconstriction possibly by inhibition of nitric oxide synthase, thought to be important in the pathogenesis of increased ICP in ALF.

  a) Continuous infusions are started and titrated based upon the EEG (5 to 10 second EEG burst suppression), ICP, and hemodynamics.

  b) Systemic hypotension limits use of thiopental, and pressors or inotropes may be needed to maintain adequate mean arterial pressures.

H. Cardiovascular

1. Presentation

  a. The prodrome of ALF includes nausea, vomiting, and loss of appetite, and patients may present with profound dehydration.

  b. Systemic vasodilatation, low systemic vascular resistance, hypotension, and a compensatory increase in cardiac output are the notable clinical cardiovascular sequelae.

  c. Abnormal oxygen transport and utilization is also present.

  d. Oxygen delivery is adequate but decrease in tissue oxygen uptake results in tissue hypoxia and lactic acidosis.

2. Monitoring

  a. Low systemic vascular resistance can result in hypotension even in the volume-resuscitated patient, and a pulmonary artery catheter is used to assess volume status and guide further management.

  b. An arterial line is needed to titrate vasoactive medications.

3. Treatment

  a. Volume resuscitate initially with primarily colloid and complement with crystalloid solutions.

  b. Inotropes or pressor support may be required to maintain a mean arterial pressure of at least 80 mm Hg (without an ICP monitor, ICP is usually assumed to be 20 mm Hg, giving a cerebral perfusion pressure of 60 mm Hg).

  c. Norepinephrine and dopamine are generally used to maintain vital organ perfusion.

  d. Vasopressin is generally avoided unless significant systemic hypotension is present.

I. Respiratory

1. Presentation

  a. Patients often hyperventilate; a respiratory alkalosis develops before a metabolic acidosis is present as the liver failure progresses.

  b. Mortality in ALF escalates with the presence of pulmonary edema and ARDS, with ARDS present in up to one-third of patients.

  c. Ventilation–perfusion mismatch may develop acutely and worsen as the liver function deteriorates further, and hypoxia can contribute to neurologic injury.

2. Treatment

  a. Positive end-expiratory pressure (PEEP) may compromise cardiac output and oxygen delivery, resulting in increased ICP and hepatic congestion.

  b. Most appropriate intervention is increased FiO_2.

  c. Those patients with ARDS can undergo liver transplantation, but risk of death is high.

J. *Gastrointestinal/metabolic*

1. Presentation

a. Upper GI (UGI) bleeding is often stress related.

b. Metabolic derangements common in ALF include alkalosis or acidosis, hypoglycemia, hypophosphatemia, and hypokalemia.

c. Hypoglycemia can be seen in up to 45% of ALF patients and indicates significant hepatic necrosis, leading to defective glycogenolysis, gluconeogenesis, and insulin metabolism.

2. Treatment

a. Histamine-2 receptors blocking agents and proton pump inhibitors for GI prophylaxis.

b. Hypoglycemia is treated with continuous glucose infusions, often D10 or D20 solutions.

c. Electrolytes should be replaced, and followed frequently.

d. Early enteral nutrition when feasible.

K. Renal failure

1. Presentation

a. Reported incidence from 40% to 85%.

b. Often multifactorial, common causes include:

i. Prerenal azotemia

ii. Renal ischemia

iii. Acute tubular necrosis

iv. Hepatorenal syndrome

2. Treatment

a. Avoid nephrotoxins and maintain adequate intravascular volume to maintain renal function.

b. Continuous venovenous hemodialysis (CVVHD) is the preferred mode when needed.

i. Intermittent hemodialysis has been associated with increased ICP and decreased CPP.

ii. CVVHD is usually better tolerated and may impart beneficial effects on ICP.

L. Hematologic

1. Presentation

a. The liver is responsible for the synthesis of several clotting factors.

b. Primary hematologic derangements common to ALF include platelet dysfunction and thrombocytopenia, reduced fibrinogen, and a prolonged prothrombin time.

c. Clinically significant bleeding occurs in <10% of patients with ALF.

2. Treatment

a. Correction of the prothrombin time (PT) is not routinely done unless there is bleeding or procedures are planned, as the PT is a prognostic indicator as well as a way to monitor worsening of the liver injury.

b. Complete correction of clotting abnormalities is usually not achievable, and can lead to volume overload, oxygenation issues, and exacerbation of ICH.

M. Infection

1. Presentation

a. The liver is the site of complement synthesis. Low levels are reported in ALF.

b. Reduced complement has been associated with impaired opsonization and sepsis.

c. The most common pathogens include:

i. Staphylococcal species

ii. Streptococcal species

iii. Gram negative rods

iv. Fungal (particularly *Candida albicans*)—occur in up to one-third of ALF patients with risk factors of renal failure and prolonged antibiotic therapy.

d. Common sites of infection include pneumonia (50%), bacteremia (20%) and urinary tract infections (25%).

2. Treatment

a. Prophylactic antibiotics reduce incidence of infection, but no survival benefit shown; thus, not recommended.

b. Surveillance includes chest x-ray and pan cultures.

N. Transplantation and prognosis
1. Only definitive therapy for patients with massive hepatic necrosis without regeneration of hepatocytes is orthotopic liver transplantation (OLT).
2. Overall survival rates in ALF have improved from 15% in pretransplant era to >60% with transplantation.
3. Delays in listing patients can lead to probability of complications precluding transplant.
4. Contraindications include:
   a. Extrahepatic malignancy
   b. Uncontrolled sepsis
   c. Irreversible brain damage
   d. Unresponsive cerebral edema with sustained elevation of ICP >50 mm Hg and decrease in CPP (<40 mm Hg).
5. Current prognostic scoring systems neither adequately predict outcome nor determine candidacy for liver transplantation.

II. PORTAL HYPERTENSION (PH)
A. Introduction
1. PH is defined as a portal pressure gradient between the portal vein and hepatic veins (hepatic venous pressure gradient) of greater than 5 mm Hg.
2. PH can be classified as prehepatic (e.g., portal or splenic vein thrombosis), intrahepatic (e.g., cirrhosis, parenchymal disease), or post-hepatic (e.g., hepatic vein stenosis, Budd–Chiari syndrome, cardiac disease).
3. Common clinical manifestation of PH and cirrhosis include gastrointestinal (GI) bleeding, ascites, and encephalopathy (Table 40-2).
4. Other manifestations include hepatorenal syndrome, coagulopathy, and malnourishment/deconditioning.
5. Sepsis and infections are also common.
B. OLT as a definitive therapy for end-stage liver disease (ESLD) has changed the care of these patients.
1. Over 6,000 liver transplants are performed annually in the United States. Average 1-, 5-, and 10-year patient and graft survival rates are 88.4%, 73.8%, 60% and 84.3%, 68.4%, 54.1%, respectively.
2. Most common disease indications for OLT in adults are alcoholic liver disease and hepatitis C (30% to 40%). Other disease states include hepatocellular carcinoma, cholestatic liver diseases (Primary Biliary Cirrhosis [PBC], Primary Sclerosing Cholangitis [PSC]), metabolic diseases (hemochromatosis, alpha-1-antitrypsin deficiency), and non-alcoholic steatohepatitis (NASH).
3. Management of the patient with hepatic decompensation is directed toward stabilization, support, and ensures viability for transplant candidacy.
4. Care of these patients is multidisciplinary, including the critical care team, transplant surgeons, hepatologists, nephrologists, and ancillary support services.
C. Upper GI (UGI) bleeding

TABLE 40-2	Child's Classification		
	1 point	**2 points**	**3 points**
Serum albumin (g/dL)	>3.5	2.8–3.5	<2.8
Total bilirubin (mg/dL)	<2	2–3	>3
INR	<1.7	1.7–2.2	>2.2
Ascites	None	Medically managed	Poorly controlled
Encephalopathy	None	Medically managed	Poorly controlled

Child's A: <7 points, B: 7–9 points, C: ≥10 points.

1. Description
   a. Portal-mesenteric venous systems are low-pressure venous beds that drain the entire GI tract. This system is separate from the systemic venous system, and portal hypertension results in the formation of varices or shunts (collaterals).
   b. Most commonly occur in the distal esophagus, umbilicus ("caput medusae"), splenic area, and in the rectum.
   c. Congestion of the GI mucosa can lead to portal hypertensive gastropathy (PHG).
   d. Spontaneous splenorenal shunts are natural shunts occurring between the splenic and left renal veins.
2. Prevalence
   a. The prevalence of esophageal varices (EV) in ESLD is 24% to 81%, and UGI bleeding from EV accounts for 60% to 90% bleeding in cirrhotic patients.
   b. Risk of bleeding from EV is not wholly dependent on elevated portal pressures, but also related to the size of the varices (larger the varices, greater risk of hemorrhage). Also important are the patient's fluid status, respiratory cycle, meal ingestion, presence of esophagitis, and Valsalva maneuvers.
   c. Presence of red color signs (red streaks or wheals) in distal esophagus on endoscopy has been shown to be an independent risk factor for variceal bleeding.
   d. Gastric varices (GV) are present in 20% of patients, and frequently found with EV. GV are found in the fundus or along of lesser curvature, with the former accounting for the majority of bleeding. GV bleeding is less frequent but more severe than EV.
   e. PHG is a dilation of capillaries and venules in the gastric mucosa, and characterized by gastric mucosal changes (usually a mosaic pattern) endoscopically.
3. Mortality
   a. The mortality with EV hemorrhage ranges from 30% to 50%; mortality greatest within the first 6 weeks of the bleed or in those with advanced liver disease.
4. Management
   a. The initial management of an UGI bleed is the same as that for a trauma victim; follow the "ABCs."
      i. The patient's airway must be secured, especially when presenting with hematemesis. This facilitates endoscopy as well as reduces the risk of aspiration pneumonia.
      ii. Hemodynamic monitoring is usually best performed by central venous catheters, along with an arterial line. A bladder catheter is placed to monitor urine output in response to resuscitation.
      iii. Correction of coagulopathy and thrombocytopenia.
   b. A nasogastric tube is placed to confirm that the UGI tract is the source of bleeding and also to decompress the stomach. This must be accomplished gently and carefully in the patient with esophageal varices.
   c. The first line of therapy is pharmacologic with vasoactive drugs.
      i. Octreotide (a somatostatin analog) is the most commonly used agent in the United States. Somatostatin has been shown to decrease portal pressure.
      ii. Vasopressin is a potent vasoconstricting agent with added benefit of splanchnic vasoconstriction. However, vasopressin can cause a reduction in cardiac output, and proper monitoring is necessary.
      iii. Terlipressin is a semi-synthetic vasopressin analog widely used in Europe, but not yet available in the United States.
      iv. Patients are also routinely placed on proton pump inhibitors (via intravenous drip) and prophylactic broad-spectrum antibiotics.
5. Endoscopic management
   a. Esophagogastroduodenoscopy (EGD) is performed as soon as possible to determine the source of bleeding, as well as the primary therapeutic modality.
      i. Sclerotherapy involves the injection of agents (e.g., ethanolamine oleate, sodium tetradecyl sulfate, absolute alcohol) around or into a varix.

      ii. Band ligation is the most common modality; involves endoscopic placement of a rubber band around a varix, leading to eventual thrombosis.

      iii. Over 90% of cases are effectively controlled with endoscopic and/or pharmacologic treatments.

      iv. GV are best treated with obliteration using endoscopic injection with cyanoacrylate, not band ligation.

      v. Refractory bleeding can be controlled with balloon tamponade with a Sengstaken–Blakemore or Minnesota tube, which are multiluminal nasogastric tubes with esophageal and gastric balloons. Balloon tamponade can be used for 24 hours; effective in controlling bleeding in 80% to 100% of cases, allowing stabilization and more definitive treatment. Rebleeding occurs in up to 50% of patients when balloons are deflated without subsequent definitive treatment.

6. Interventional radiology management

    a. The development of the Transjugular Intrahepatic Portosystemic Shunt (TIPS) is the preferred next line of treatment.

    b. TIPS is placed by interventional radiology under local anesthesia and involves a transjugular approach in which one of the hepatic veins is cannulated followed by the accession of a branch of the portal vein using a Rosch needle.

    c. The tract is then widened after which a covered metal stent is placed, providing immediate reduction in portal pressures and relief of bleeding in over 90% of cases.

    d. Complications include procedural-related bleeding (e.g., perforation of the portal vein), worsening of encephalopathy, renal failure, congestive heart failure, infection, and liver failure.

7. Surgical management

    a. Esophageal transection effectively controls bleeding; rarely used today with the success of TIPS.

    b. Gastric devascularization is indicated for patients with portomesenteric thrombosis.

    c. Surgical shunts still play a role in the treatment of variceal hemorrhage, most commonly in an elective setting and targeted toward prophylaxis from recurrent bleeding.

      i. Selective shunts (e.g., distal splenorenal shunt, DSRS) are preferred over non-selective shunts (e.g., portacaval or mesocaval shunts); hepatic flow is preserved and avoids dissection in the hepatic hilum.

      ii. Visceral angiography is critical to detail the porto-mesenteric venous system and diagnose porto-mesenteric venous thrombosis.

D. Ascites

1. Pathophysiology leading to ascites formation in cirrhotics includes portal hypertension, development of systemic vasodilatation, and activation of the renin–angiotensin–aldosterone pathway.

2. Development of refractory ascites has a <50% 1-year survival. Hyponatremia commonly accompanies ascites and is a poor prognostic indicator for patients waiting for OLT.

3. Primary treatment is with diuretics—furosemide and aldactone.

4. Patients with symptomatic or tense ascites are treated with large volume paracentesis.

    a. Ascites fluid is usually sent for cell count, gram stain, and cultures.

    b. Ascites is often replaced with intravenous salt-poor albumin (SPA) infusion IV.

5. TIPS is considered for patients refractory to medical treatment and requiring frequent drainage.

6. Spontaneous bacterial peritonitis (SBP) is a common complication, diagnosed when either ascitic neutrophil count >250/mm^3 or total WBC >500/mm^3, or a positive culture.

    a. Gram-positive infections are most common, followed by gram-negative infections, and broad-spectrum antibiotics should be administered.

    b. SBP is associated with higher rates of sepsis post-transplantation.

E. Encephalopathy

1. HE is a common indication for admission to the ICU. Inability to protect the airway is the main concern with severe encephalopathy, and intubation is often needed.
2. Standard therapy is with oral lactulose with or without neomycin. Lactulose is given every hour via nasogastric tube until the patient has a bowel movement, and titrated after that for 3 to 4 loose BMs.
3. Xifaxan (rifaximin) is an alternative to neomycin and has been shown to effectively reduce the occurrence and risk of hospitalization from HE.
4. The common precipitating factors include GI bleed, new or worsened portal vein thrombosis, or infection, and these causes must be found and treated on admission.

F. Hepatorenal syndrome

1. Characterized by the development of renal insufficiency or failure in the absence of intrinsic kidney disease.
2. Clinical criteria for diagnosis include:
   a. Absence of pre- and post-renal azotemia and other causes of renal impairment (e.g., acute tubular necrosis, nephrotoxicity)
   b. Lack of improvement after withdrawal of diuretics and administration of volume
   c. Oliguria
   d. Urine sodium <10 mEq/L
   e. Urine osmolality greater than plasma osmolality
   f. Hyponatremia (<130 mEq/L)
3. Two types of HRS exist:
   a. Type I HRS is rapid and progressive, with doubling of the serum creatinine to greater than 2.5 mg/dL in less than 2 weeks. Survival of Type I HRS is <50% after 1 month.
   b. Type II HRS is slower in progression with a median survival of 6 months.
4. Management
   a. The first line of treatment is adequate hydration, stopping diuretics, and avoiding nephrotoxic substances (e.g., drugs, IV dye).
   b. The use of midodrine (usually 10 mg PO TID), octreotide (100 mcg SQ TID), and albumin has been shown to improve survival and renal function in HRS patients.
   c. The use of renal replacement therapy (RRT) is instituted when clinically indicated.
   d. OLT is the definitive treatment for HRS. Since renal failure significantly increases mortality after transplantation, an increasing number of patients undergo combined liver and kidney transplantation.

AXIOMS

- Loss of hepatic function can quickly lead to multiorgan failure and death.
- Patients who present in full ALF often have severe metabolic acidosis, hypoglycemia, coagulopathy, and encephalopathy/coma.
- Most serious complication of ALF is cerebral edema and ICH.
- Only definitive therapy for patients with massive hepatic necrosis without regeneration of hepatocytes is OLT.
- EGD is performed as soon as possible in the cirrhotic patient to determine the source of bleeding, as well as the primary therapeutic modality.

Suggested Readings

Bosch J, Abraldes JG, Berzigotti A, et al. The clinical use of HVPG measurements in chronic liver disease. *Nat Rev Gastroenterol Hepatol* 2009;6:573–582.

Charlton M. Nonalcoholic fatty liver disease: A review of current understanding and future impact. *Clin Gastroenterol Hepatol* 2004;2:1048–1058.

Costa G, Cruz RJ, Abu-Elmagd KM. Surgical shunt versus TIPS for treatment of variceal hemorrhage in the current era of liver and multivisceral transplantation. *Surg Clin North Am* 2010;90:891–905.

Detry O, Roover AD, Honore P, et al. Brain edema and intracranial hypertension in fulminant hepatic failure: Pathophysiology and management. *World J Gastroenterol* 2006;12(46): 7405–7412.

Garcia-Tsao G, Bosch J. Management of varices and variceal hemorrhage in cirrhosis. *N Engl J Med* 2010;362:823–832.

Jain R. Acute liver failure: current management and future prospects. *J Hepatol* 2005;42:S115–S123.

Mehta G, Abraldes JG, Bosch J. Developments and controversies in the management of oesophageal and gastric varices. *Gut* 2010;59:701–705.

Polson J, Lee WM. AASLD position paper: the management of acute liver failure. *Hepatology* 2005;41:1179–1197.

Raghavan M, Marik PE. Therapy of intracranial hypertension in patients with fulminant hepatic failure. *Neurocrit Care* 2006;4:179–189.

Rahman T, Hodgson H. Clinical management of acute hepatic failure. *Intensive Care Med* 2001;27:467–476.

Saito C, Zwingmann C, Jaeschke H. Novel mechanisms of protection against acetaminophen hepatotoxicity in mice by glutathione and N-acetylcysteine. *Hepatology* 2010;51:246–254.

Sass DA, Chopra KB. Portal hypertension and variceal hemorrhage. *Med Clin North Am* 2009;93:837–853.

Sass D, Shakil O. Fulminant hepatic failure. *Gastroenterol Clin North Am* 2003;32:1195–1211.

Sass D, Shakil O. Fulminant hepatic failure. *Liver Transpl* 2005;11(6):594–605.

Stravitz RT, Kramer A, Davern T, et al. Intensive care of patients with acute liver failure: recommendations of the U.S. Acute Liver Failure Study Group. *Crit Care Med* 2007;35(11):2498–2508.

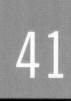

41 Support of the Organ Donor

Patrick K. Kim, Matthew V. Benns, Patrick M. Reilly and
C. William Schwab

I. **INTRODUCTION.** Organ availability is the major limitation to increasing the benefit of organ transplantation. In the United States, the number of people awaiting organ transplantation has doubled over 10 years, whereas the organ supply has only increased by one-third. Thus, median waiting times for transplants have increased **and more people die waiting for organs than ever receive an organ transplant.**

A. Organs that can be transplanted include the heart, lung, liver, kidney, pancreas, and small bowel. Other tissues that can be transplanted include bone, bone marrow, cartilage, cornea, fascia, heart valves, and skin.

B. Trauma, especially severe head injury, is the second most common source of organ donors (after stroke) and provides more organs per donor. Currently one-third of available organs for transplant come from patients sustaining lethal injury. All professionals involved with trauma care must be knowledgeable of and involved with the organ procurement approaches. One large challenge for increasing the pool of donor organs is the high refusal rate by the public to proceed with donation (only 15% to 20% of the potential donor pool proceeds to donation). Enhanced strategies to increase the percentage of actual donors play a critical role in securing organ availability.

C. The failure to procure potential organs is multifactorial and includes family refusal, the lack of awareness by the treating physician, and the inadequate resuscitation of the potential organ donor (Table 41.1). According to the Federal Conditions of Participation of the Centers for Medicare and Medicaid Services, hospitals must contact their local organ procurement organization (OPO) in a timely manner if a patient is expected to die. The trauma practitioner plays the key role in identifying potential donors, contacting the OPO, and maintaining normal physiologic in the potential donor.

1. The OPO should be notified early in the evaluation of **all** potential donors. Once involved, the OPO and transplant team, *not the ED or trauma staff*, should assess the suitability of a potential donor. In addition, the OPO is skilled in approaching the family of potential donors and can be a resource in the diagnosis and mechanics of the confirmation of brain death. When the OPO provides the *initial* approach to the family regarding organ donation, families are more likely to proceed to organ donation than contact started by physicians or staff involved in the care of the potential donor.

II. **POTENTIAL ORGAN DONORS.** The legal framework for modern organ transplantation is largely based on two Uniform Acts and their subsequent revisions: The Uniform Anatomical Gift Act of 1968 and The Uniform Determination of Death Act of 1981. These acts provided:

(a) An individual with the legal right to donate organs or tissue after death and

(b) included a neurologic basis for the definition of death: "An individual who has sustained either (1) irreversible cessation of circulatory and respiratory functions, or (2) irreversible cessation of all functions of the entire brain, including the brainstem, is dead." The majority of current organ donors are comprised of patients who have been declared dead on the basis of their neurologic function. However, an increasing proportion of donors are declared dead on the basis definitions of circulatory and respiratory arrest.

TABLE 41-1 Failure to Donate: Causes and Remedial Strategies

Causes	Remedial strategies
1. Failure to recognize potential organ donors	■ Provide continuous education ■ Develop a hospital-based organ donation team (social workers, ministers, OPO, ICU staff)

2. Family refusal
  – Family approached about organ donation by the primary care team (perceived conflict of interest)
  – Family informed of death and approached about organ donation at the same time (perceived conflict of interest)
  – Low acceptability of organ donation by minorities
	■ Primary service informs family of death
	■ OPO approaches family
	■ Temporally separate the discussion of death and the request for donation
	■ OPO should approach the family regarding donation
	■ Understand cultural diversity

3. Failure to expedite diagnosis of brain death	■ Create clear guidelines for the diagnosis of brain death
4. Failure to maintain organ homeostasis	■ Optimize organ perfusion (volume first followed by pressors as needed) ■ Use lung protective ventilatory strategies ■ Anticipate and treat endocrine abnormalities

OPO, organ procurement organization; ICU, intensive care unit.

A. All patients identified to have a fatal disease process are potential organ/tissue donors, even if they have severe pre-existing disease in one or more organ systems. Exceptions to donation include:
   1. Viral infections: Human immunodeficiency virus (HIV) infection, human T-cell leukemia–lymphoma virus, systemic viral infections (e.g., measles, rabies, adenovirus, enterovirus, parvovirus), and herpetic meningo-encephalitis
   2. Viral hepatitis: Hepatitis-positive patients, however, can donate to hepatitis-positive recipients
   3. Tuberculosis
   4. Untreated septicemia: The presence of bacteremia or fungemia, is not an absolute contraindication. Patients who receive organs from infected donors do not do worse than those who receive organs from non-infected donors
   5. Extracranial malignancies: Exceptions include non-melanoma skin cancers
   6. Intravenous drug abuse
   7. Known prion-related diseases

III. DETERMINATION OF BRAIN DEATH (Table 41-2). The majority of trauma patients who proceed to organ donation will do so because of lethal brain injury. It is therefore essential that the trauma team and practitioner have knowledge of the process to establish brain death.
   A. Brain death is a clinical diagnosis. The practical steps and technical determination of brain death may vary between institutions, but the usual criteria are as follows:
      1. Documentation of coma
      2. No motor response to painful stimuli
      3. No brainstem reflexes
         a. Pupils are nonreactive to a bright light
         b. Ocular movements are absent; there is no response to head turning or tympanic caloric testing with ice water
         c. Corneal, laryngeal, and tracheal reflexes are absent

TABLE 41-2	Steps in the Organ Donation Process (Brain Injured Patients)

1. Determine severity of head trauma.
2. Determine the likelihood of reversing the patient's disease process.
3. Notify the OPO.
4. Inform the family of the patient's condition and prognosis.
5. Optimize organ function, perfusion, and oxygen transport. Maintain homeostasis.
6. Determine irreversibility of brain injury. Perform first brain death clinical examination.
7. Family approached by OPO regarding the possibility of organ donation.
8. Second brain death clinical examination, laboratory evaluations, and secondary investigational studies (e.g., nuclear medicine flow study).
9. Consent.
10. Donation laboratory studies, echocardiogram, and bronchoscopy (if needed).
11. Organ procurement.

  4. Apnea: The absence of respiratory movements with an increase in $PaCO_2$ >60 mm Hg in the setting of Normal PaO_2 (Table 41-3)
  5. No increase in heart rate following intravenous administration of 2 mg atropine
  6. The brain death examination should be completed at least twice at different time intervals (traditionally 2 to 12 hours apart) by two different *qualified* physicians who are not part of the transplant team.
  B. A number of tests can aid in confirming clinical brain death. They are useful when a complete clinical evaluation cannot be done (i.e., in the setting of uremia or encephalopathy, the presence of central nervous system [CNS] depressants, or the inability to assess pupillary response secondary to ocular trauma). The tests include electroencephalography (EEG), cerebral angiography, transcranial Doppler ultrasonography, nuclear medicine or xenon flow studies, and somatosensory-evoked potentials. EEG, Doppler studies, and evoked potentials can be difficult to interpret and lack specificity for brain death. Although angiography is an option, it requires an invasive procedure. For these reasons, most centers currently utilize brain flow studies for additional confirmation of brain death.

TABLE 41-3	Apnea Test

1. Prerequisites
   - Core temperature >36.5°C
   - Systolic blood pressure (SBP) >90 mm Hg
   - Euvolemia
   - Normal $PaCO_2$
   - Normal PaO_2
   - No paralytics, sedation, or drug intoxication
   - Normal electrolyte and acid–base status
2. Pre-oxygenate with 100% FiO_2 for 20 minutes
3. Normalize $PaCO_2$ and draw a baseline ABG
4. Connect pulse oximeter and disconnect ventilator
5. Deliver 100% oxygen, 8–12 L/min, into the trachea
6. Look closely for respiratory movements
7. Measure arterial PO_2, PCO_2, and pH after 5 and 10 minutes and reconnect to the ventilator
   - If respiratory movements are absent and $PaCO_2$ increases to ≥60 mm Hg, apnea is present and the diagnosis of brain death is supported
   - If respiratory effort is seen, the diagnosis of brain death is not supported
8. Abort the test if:
   - Hemodynamic instability (i.e., decrease in SBP <90 mm Hg) or ventricular arrhythmia
   - Oxygen desaturation (<90%)

TABLE 41-4   Steps in the Donation after Cardiac Death Process

a. Determine severity and likelihood of reversing patient's disease process
b. Notify the OPO
c. Inform the family of the patient's condition and prognosis
d. Optimize organ function, perfusion, and oxygen transport. Maintain homeostasis.
e. Have OPO approach family regarding the possibility of organ donation.
f. Obtain consent
g. Perform donation laboratory studies, echocardiogram, and bronchoscopy (if needed).
h. Assess likelihood of patient expiration within time constraints upon withdrawal of care.
i. Patient taken to operating room with procurement team on standby.
j. Patient is extubated and supportive care is withdrawn. Sedatives and pain medication may be administered as appropriate if consent is obtained.
k. Patient is closely monitored for up to 1 h
l. If asystole occurs for a period of 5 min (actual time may vary by institution), patient is declared dead and procurement immediately commences
m. If patient does not progress to full asystolic period within 1 h of withdrawal, donation process is aborted.

C. The diagnosis of brain death also requires the *exclusion* of confounding factors, which include:
   1. Drug intoxication or poisoning (i.e., barbiturates)
   2. Hypothermia (core temperature must be at least 32°C)
   3. Severe electrolyte and acid–base abnormalities
   4. Severe endocrine disturbances
   5. Hemodynamic instability (systolic blood pressure <90 mm Hg)
D. After two clinical examinations (with additional confirmatory tests as needed) have corroborated lack of brain activity, the patient is declared dead. At some locations, a single clinical examination and cerebral blood flow study are sufficient to declare brain death in a patient with an obviously devastating brain insult (injury or stroke).

IV. DONATION AFTER CARDIAC DEATH (Table 41-4).

Donation after cardiac death (DCD) donors are patients who have been declared dead via cessation of cardiac and respiratory functions. Although the concept remains controversial, these donors are becoming more frequent potential donors.
A. DCD donors most commonly have severe and irreversible neurologic injury but do not meet criteria for brain death declaration. Patients with high spinal cord injury, end stage musculoskeletal disease, or pulmonary disease may be candidates.
B. Given the inherent drawbacks with warm ischemia time associated with the procurement, DCD is commonly limited to liver and kidney procurement. However, other solid organs such as pancreas, lungs, and heart have been transplanted from DCD donors. With properly selected donors and procurement techniques, outcomes from DCD donors are equivalent to those of brain dead donors.
C. In 2007, the JCAHO implemented its first accreditation standard for DCD. In addition, the Organ Procurement and Transplantation Network (OPTN) and United Network for Organ Sharing (UNOS) developed "model elements" to aid in the development of institution specific DCD protocols.
   1. Once a patient has been identified as a possible donor, the OPO is notified and the family is approached for consent to withdraw life-sustaining measures.
   2. Timing of withdrawal coordinated with the transplant procurement team is generally conducted in the operating room.
   3. A patient is declared dead after a period of asystole generally lasting 5 minutes, although the period could be as short as 2 minutes at some institutions.
   4. Once life support is withdrawn, the general time window for procurement is approximately 30 minutes for the liver and 60 minutes for kidneys. If a patient

TABLE 41-5 University of Wisconsin Donation After Cardiac Death Evaluation Tool

Criteria	Assigned points
Spontaneous respirations after 10 min	
Rate >12	1
Rate <12	3
Tidal Volume >200 mL	1
Tidal Volume <200 mL	3
NIF >20	1
NIF <20	3
No spontaneous respirations	9
BMI	
<25	1
25–39	2
>30	3
Vasopressors	
No vasopressors	1
1 vasopressor	2
>1 vasopressor	3
Patient age	
0–30	1
31–50	2
>51	3
Intubation method	
Endotracheal tube	3
Tracheostomy	1
Oxygenation after 10 min	
02 sat >90%	1
02 sat 80–89%	2
02 sat <79%	3

8–12 points: High risk for continuing to breathe after extubation
13–18 points: Moderate risk for continuing to breathe after extubation
19–24 points: Low risk for continuing to breathe after extubation

does not proceed to asystole within this time limit, the donation process is abandoned.

5. Pharmacologic agents to aid in donor management such as heparin may be administered during the withdrawal process with explicit consent. Similarly, placing a femoral catheter prior to expiration is accepted with consent.

6. **No member of the organ recovery team** or OPO staff may participate in the guidance or administration of pre-declaration care or the declaration of death.

7. OPO policy ensures that no donation-related expenses are passed to the donor family.

D. Potential DCD donors should undergo an assessment to predict whether they will expire within the time constraints upon withdrawal of care. Use a tool like the University of Wisconsin Donation after Cardiac Death Evaluation for this purpose (Table 41-5).

V. CARE OF THE POTENTIAL ORGAN DONOR (Table 41-6).

The physiologic effects of brain death are profound and challenging for the practitioner. Progression from brain death to somatic death results in the loss of 10% to 20% of potential donors. Without aggressive management, cardio-pulmonary arrest generally follows brain death within a short time period. The use of standardized guidelines improves the hemodynamic stability of potential donors and optimizes organ retrieval and graft outcome.

TABLE 41-6   **Physiologic Goals in the Organ Donor**

Cardiovascular
– Systolic blood pressure >100 mm Hg, mean arterial pressure ≥60 mm Hg
– Central venous pressure 6–10 mm Hg
– Pulmonary capillary wedge pressure 8–12 mm Hg
– Left ventricular ejection fraction ≥45%
– Inotropic support—dopamine (ideally <10 μg/kg/min)
– Consider vasopressin and other endocrine support

Pulmonary
– Arterial O_2 saturation ≥95%
– Fio_2 ≤60%
– PIP ≤30 mm H_2O
– PEEP—5–7.5 cm H_2O or the minimum necessary to attain PaO_2 >80 mm Hg

Fluid and electrolyte management
– Avoid hypernatremia and hypokalemia
– Urinary output ≥1.0 mL/kg/h, less than 200 cc/h
– Treat underlying cause of acidosis, if needed add sodium bicarbonate to intravenous fluids

Hormonal Support
– 1 amp dextrose 50%
– methylprednisolone 15 mg/kg q24h
– insulin 20 U IV push
– levothyroxine 20 μg IV push, followed by 5–10 μg/h infusion
– vasopressin (0.5–4.0 units/h).

Hematologic
– Hematocrit ≥30%
– Platelets ≥80,000
– INR ≤2
– Blood products should be cytomegalovirus seronegative and transfused through leukocyte filters.

PIP, peak inspiratory pressure; PEEP, positive end-expiratory pressure.

A. Cardiovascular support. The effects of brain death on the cardiovascular system are secondary to progressive rostral to caudal ischemia of the brain and spinal cord. Initially, ischemia at the medullary level provokes a sympathetic surge to maintain cerebral perfusion pressure. As the spinal cord becomes progressively ischemic, there is a deactivation of the sympathetic nervous system. A state of profound vasodilation develops with associated low levels of circulating catecholamines. Brain ischemia is also associated with sub-endocardial myocyte necrosis and cardiac dysfunction. These events can lead to a period of hemodynamic instability. *Cardiac arrest in the donor is more common in the setting of hypotension; anticipate and manage this instability.*

1. **Maintain euvolemia and adequate perfusion pressures.** Approximately 30% of donor referrals for cardiac transplantation are unsuitable secondary to poor hemodynamic function. The goals of cardiovascular management are to maintain blood pressure and cardiac output to ensure adequate organ perfusion. This is obtained initially by restoration of intravascular volume.

   a. Use lactated ringers or half-normal saline with added bicarbonate for volume expansion to avoid hypernatremia.
   b. If the patient is anemic, transfuse packed red blood cells to a goal hematocrit of 30%. More liberal blood transfusions are not supported by data.
   c. Maintain urine output at >0.5mL/kg/hour.
   d. With consent, place arterial and venous monitoring devices to aid in resuscitation.

2. **Vasopressors.** If hemodynamic instability persists despite adequate volume resuscitation, start vasopressors. Dopamine or dobutamine are the preferred initial vasoactive agents given the pump dysfunction and minimal vasoconstriction.
   a. If you need more than 10 μg/kg/min of dopamine or dobutamine exceeds more than 10 μg/kg/min, add an addition agent. Arginine vasopressin, a hormone normally secreted by the posterior pituitary gland, is often chosen in these situations.
      i. Vasopressin at low doses (0.01 to 0.04 units/min) enhances the vascular sensitivity to catecholamines such that lower doses of vasoconstrictive agents may suffice for hemodynamic stability. Higher doses may be necessary if diabetes insipidus develops.
3. More than 70% of donors can maintain hemodynamic stability by a combination of volume resuscitation and a low dose of vasopressors. Importantly, patients who require higher doses of multiple pressors for support are *not* precluded from organ donation.
4. **Dysrhythmias.** Rhythm disturbances and conduction abnormalities are common. Correct any underlying fluid and electrolyte disturbances. Often the dysrhythmias are resistant to standard treatment. In the absence of hypotension, bradydysrhythmias require no treatment. With brain herniation, bradyarrhythmias are often secondary to vagus nerve disruption and standard treatment with atropine is generally ineffective. In these cases, use isoproterenol or epinephrine if bradycardia is associated with hypotension. Ventricular dysrhythmias generally respond to standard therapy with lidocaine or amiodarone. If cardiac arrest occurs, use standard ACLS protocols. Transient cardiac arrest is not a contraindication to solid organ donation.
5. **Echocardiogram.** Obtain an echocardiogram in all patients considered for cardiac donation to assess cardiac function. An echocardiogram can also detect structural problems that might preclude donation.
6. **Coronary Angiography.** Patients under the age of 35 considered for cardiac donation generally do not require angiography. Male donors aged 35 to 45 or female donors aged 35 to 50 should undergo angiography if there are >3 risk factors for coronary artery disease or there is a history of cocaine use. Angiography is recommended for potential cardiac donors over the age of 45 for men and over the age of 50 for women.

B. **Pulmonary Support.** Insult to the CNS can cause neurogenic pulmonary edema through incompletely understood mechanisms involving changes in pulmonary capillary hydrostatic pressure and increased permeability. Potential donors may also have initial lung injury, respiratory complications, or excess lung water from fluid administration. All of these elements contribute to the low rate of lung procurement in potential donors (~20%).
   1. **"Pulmonary toilet":** Start simple measures to prevent accumulation of secretions and atelectasis: Frequent suctioning, turning and repositioning, bronchoscopy, and the use of inhaled albuterol may help.
   2. **Ventilator settings:** The use of a "lung protective" low tidal volume ventilator strategy can increase the number and success of potential lung donors compared to traditional ventilator settings. (See Chapter 38.)
   3. **Avoid excessive volume resuscitation:** The use of excessive amount of intravenous fluids can impair pulmonary function and affect the suitability of the lungs for organ donation. Colloids such as albumin or plasma (if coagulopathy) are recommended as the fluid of choice for resuscitation with potential lung donors. The use of a pulmonary artery catheter can aid in guiding volume resuscitation with a goal pulmonary capillary wedge pressure of 8 to 12 mm Hg. In the event of over-resuscitation, diuresis may help salvage potentially usable lungs.

C. **Fluid and electrolyte therapy.**
   1. **Diabetes insipidus.** Diabetes insipidus (DI), with concomitant loss of free water, occurs frequently in brain-dead patients. The clinical diagnosis is confirmed by the presence of increased urinary output (>200 cc/h), low urinary osmolality, and hypernatremia. Desmopressin acetate (DDAVP 0.3 mg/kg IV infusion) or

vasopressin (0.5 to 4.0 units/h) may be required. Adequate volume replacement is essential.

2. **Hypernatremia.** Monitor serum electrolytes and aggressively correct any abnormalities. Use lactated Ringer's or half-normal saline to keep the sodium level less than 150 mmol/L. Ongoing hypernatremia in the donor is associated with poor graft outcome in liver transplantation.

3. **Hyperglycemia.** Avoid profound hyperglycemia, with its resultant osmotic diuresis. Glycemic control (80 to 150 mg/dL) with an insulin infusion and hourly blood sugar monitoring is ideal.

4. **Acidosis.** Add sodium bicarbonate (50 mmol/L) as needed to correct acidosis and normalize pH.

5. **Alternative colloids.** Avoid hydroxyethyl starch since it may induce renal tubular cell injury.

   Endocrine support. Start hormone replacement therapy for potential donors who remain hypotensive after volume infusion. Potential cardiac donors with an ejection fraction <45% on initial echocardiogram should also receive hormonal resuscitation. Often, hypothalamic–pituitary–adrenal dysfunction exists in the setting of brain death. Low levels of thyroid hormone, cortisol or vasopressin may contribute to cardiovascular lability. Exogenous hormonal replacement therapy can decrease the need for vasoactive support in unstable donors and is associated with an increase in the number of organs suitable for transplantation. See Table 41-5.

   Hematologic support. Disorders of blood coagulation are common in the setting of traumatized or necrotic brain tissue. Coagulopathy may be exacerbated by ongoing hemorrhage, massive transfusion, acidosis, hypothermia, or consumption of coagulant factors. Give blood products to target a hematocrit of >30%, to maintain a platelet count of greater than 80,000/mm^3, and to correct an INR to less than 2. Blood products should be cytomegalovirus seronegative and transfused through leukocyte filters.

   Temperature regulation. The potential organ donor will frequently have a loss of hypothalamic thermoregulation and adaptive warming mechanisms such as shivering. This is exacerbated by large volume fluid shifts from aggressive resuscitation or diuresis. Resulting hypothermia can contribute to cardiac dysfunction, dysrhythmias, and coagulopathy. Use warmed fluids, blood products, and inhaled gasses coupled with external warming devices and insulating blankets to maintain normal body temperature.

D. **Antibiotic prophylaxis.** Patients identified as organ donors are often given a broad spectrum antibiotic(s) if not already receiving antibiotic therapy.

AXIOMS

- Trauma victims are a large potential population of organ donors.
- Early notification and involvement of the OPO increases organ donation.
- Brain death from trauma is a common source of organ donation and has strict criteria for determination and confirmation.
- Preservation of organ homeostasis increases the chances for a successful function of each transplanted organ.
- Restoration and maintenance of normal physiology with pulmonary support, targeted resuscitation, reversal of coagulopathy, anti-dysrhythmic and vasoactive drugs plus hormonal supplementation are key to optimization of care.

Suggested Readings

Evans RW, Orians CE, Ascher NL. The potential supply of organ donors. *JAMA* 1992;267(2):239–246.

Gram HJ, Meinhold H, Bickel U, et al. Acute endocrine failure after brain death? *Transplantation* 1992;54(5):851–857.

Grenvik A, Darby JM, Broznick BA. Organ transplantation: an overview of problems and concerns. In: Civetta JM, ed. *Critical Care*. Philadelphia, PA: JB Lippincott; 1992:803–813.

Jenkins DH, Reilly PM, Schwab CW. Improving the approach to organ donation: a review. *World J Surg* 1999;23:644–649.

Kennedy AP, West JC, Kelley SE, et al. Utilization of trauma-related deaths for organ and tissue harvesting. *J Trauma* 1992;33(4):516–520.

Lewis J, Peltier J, Nelson H, et al. Development of the University of Wisconsin donation after cardiac death evaluation tool. *Prog Transplant* 2003;13(4):265–273.

Mascia L, Pasero P, Slutsky AS, et al. Effect of a lung protective strategy for organ donors on eligibility and availability of lungs for transplantation: A randomized controlled trial. *JAMA* 2010;304(23):2620–2627.

Recommendations of the Secretary's Advisory Committee on Organ Transplantation: Critical Pathway for the Organ Donor. Retrieved from http://www.organdonor.gov/pdf/acotapp3.pdf.

Steinbrock R. Persepctive: Organ Donation after Cardiac Death. *N Engl J Med* 2007;357:209–213.

Wood KE, Becker BN, McCartney JG, et al. Care of the potential organ donor. *N Engl J Med* 2004;351:2730–2739.

www.unos.org

42

Accidental and Therapeutic Hypothermia, Cold Injury, and Drowning

Samuel A. Tisherman

I. **INTRODUCTION.** Accidental hypothermia occurs in up to half the victims of major trauma and is associated with increased morbidity and mortality. Hypothermia in trauma patients occurs secondary to injury, environmental exposure, shock, fluid resuscitation, anesthesia, and alcohol or drug intoxication; it must be differentiated from exposure hypothermia or from hypothermia secondary to medical conditions (e.g., thyroid or adrenal insufficiency). Uncontrolled, accidental hypothermia differs from controlled, therapeutic hypothermia (as used in cardiac surgery or after cardiac arrest).

A. **Classification of hypothermia.** Hypothermia is classified primarily by the patient's core temperature:

1. **Mild:** 32°C to 35°C—physiologic findings subtle
2. **Moderate:** 28°C to 32°C—signs and symptoms present, but variable
3. **Severe:** Below 28°C—central nervous system (CNS) and hemodynamic alterations impending or present (often extreme)

B. **Core temperature must be measured.** This requires probes able to measure low temperatures. Rectal, bladder catheter, central venous, and esophageal thermistors offer the best temperature data. Rectal probes are preferred because of their safety and ease of insertion.

II. **PHYSIOLOGY OF HYPOTHERMIA**

A. **Maintenance of temperature** within a narrow range despite widely varying environmental temperatures is critical for humans. The normal response to a cold environment is to simultaneously minimize heat loss and increase heat production.

1. **Heat loss** occurs via radiation, conduction, convection, and evaporation. Hypothermic patients can also minimize heat loss by behavioral responses (moving to a warmer environment), use of warm clothing, and cutaneous vasoconstriction.

2. **Increased physical activity, shivering, increased feeding, and nonshivering thermogenesis can increase heat production.** Shivering causes an increase in oxygen consumption for which the patient may not be able to physiologically compensate, vasodilation that may cause more heat loss, and metabolic acidosis. Thus, shivering may be detrimental and fail to increase temperature. When and how to stop shivering is controversial and no singular agent is ideal, although opioids or neuromuscular blockers are used.

B. **Clinical effects of hypothermia.** A progression of changes occurs in all physiologic parameters as temperature decreases, with subtle and inconsistent findings seen with mild hypothermia and more predictable abnormalities seen with severe hypothermia.

1. **Metabolic.** The body initially attempts to conserve body heat via increased metabolic activity and shivering during mild hypothermia. These responses are lost as hypothermia progresses, with an eventual decrease in metabolism.

2. **Respiratory.** Tachypnea may be seen initially, but with further cooling the respiratory rate slows, eventually leading to apnea. Arterial oxygenation is usually maintained, but tissue oxygenation may be impaired due to intense vasoconstriction and leftward shift in the hemoglobin dissociation curve, leading to decreased release of oxygen. Hypothermia alters the measured arterial pH, PCO_2, and PO_2, tempting some to suggest "correcting" blood gas values for the patient's

temperature before treating the values since blood gas analyzers typically warm the sample to 37°C. This is unnecessary as there is no proven benefit in using the corrected values.

3. **Hemodynamic.** Tachycardia is common early with mild hypothermia, but bradycardia is seen with more severe hypothermia. On the electrocardiogram (ECG), prolonged PR, QRS, and QT intervals; J (Osborn) waves; sinus bradycardia; atrial flutter or fibrillation; and ventricular arrhythmias may be seen with moderate to severe hypothermia. Below 28°C, there is a high risk of ventricular fibrillation (VF), heart block, or asystole. Pulses often are not palpable because of vasoconstriction even if cardiac function continues and tissue perfusion is adequate for that temperature level. In addition to the changes in cardiac rhythm, vasodilation occurs with mild hypothermia and shivering, causing further heat loss and predisposing the patient to hypotension. Vasoconstriction occurs as the temperature decreases.

4. **Neurologic.** Changes with mild to moderate hypothermia include apathy, confusion, or loss of coordination. *An abnormal sensorium in a trauma patient at risk for hypothermia should not be attributed solely to hypothermia.* Traumatic brain injury, hypovolemic shock, and alcohol or drug intoxication need to be considered. With severe hypothermia, coma occurs, often with electroencephalogram silence, although normal neurologic recovery is still possible.

5. **Coagulation.** One of the most frequent findings is thrombocytopenia due to platelet sequestration. This is complicated by abnormal platelet function, leading to prolonged bleeding times. Impairment of the coagulation cascade occurs secondary to decreased enzyme function. Increased plasma fibrinolytic activity also may occur. In addition to hypothermia, the use of massive transfusions for associated blood loss from trauma can cause dilution of platelets and clotting factors, and a metabolic acidosis. Finally, the tissue trauma can alter coagulation changes in trauma patients. Accurately measuring coagulation function in hypothermic patients is problematic because the standard laboratory instruments warm the blood to 37°C.

6. **Renal.** Hypothermia decreases the ability of the kidney to reabsorb fluid and electrolytes, leading to an initial inappropriate "cold" diuresis, increasing the risk of hypotension. As temperature decreases further, urine output decreases. Consequently, urine output has limited utility as a marker of adequate organ perfusion in hypothermic patients. Rhabdomyolysis is another concern in those patients who may have been immobile for a prolonged period of time.

III. ACCIDENTAL HYPOTHERMIA IN TRAUMA

A. **Predisposition to hypothermia.** In trauma patients, the incidence and severity of hypothermia correlate directly with injury severity. Between 21% and 50% of severely injured trauma patients become hypothermic. This is due to:

1. **Exposure** in the field with inadequate or wet clothing.
2. **Blood loss** and shock.
3. **Common standard treatments,** including infusion of cool fluids, removal of all clothing, and opening of body cavities.
4. **Limited ability to produce heat** because of trauma and hemorrhagic shock; administration of analgesic, sedative, and anesthetic agents; or alcohol and other drugs taken by the patient. For example, general anesthesia may decrease heat production by 20%.

B. **Hypothermic trauma patients have higher mortality** than their counterparts even when other factors that affect mortality are taken into account. As a result of severe trauma and resuscitation attempts, the patient is often hypothermic, coagulopathic, and acidotic (the "triad of death"). The "damage control" abbreviated laparotomy (rapid control of active arterial bleeding, rapid control of contamination, packing the abdomen, rewarming in the intensive care unit [ICU], and delayed definitive procedures) can break the cycle of bleeding, transfusion, worsening coagulopathy, worsening hypothermia, and more bleeding.

IV. TREATMENT

A. Prevention. Awareness of the existence of or potential for hypothermia in trauma patients is the key first step. Measures to prevent hypothermia should be initiated in the field and continued in the emergency department (ED), operating room (OR), and ICU. These include:

1. **Warming the environment** in the transport vehicle, ED, OR, and ICU. Room temperature is a critical determinant of cooling because it dictates the rate of heat loss by radiation, convection, and evaporation from skin and operative sites.
2. Use of warm, humidified oxygen.
3. Infusion of warmed intravenous fluids and blood. Countercurrent fluid warmers are particularly effective.
4. Minimization of exposure. Covering the patient with a blanket or heat trapping/generating garment can decrease heat loss.
5. Active warming can be accomplished by using a heating blanket, radiant heat lamps or other heating devices.

B. Standard treatment. This begins with standard resuscitation efforts (outlined in Table 42-1 and Fig. 42-1).

1. **Airway and breathing.** Hypothermic patients who maintain a patent airway and spontaneous ventilation generally do not require immediate intubation. Endotracheal intubation is indicated for apneic patients and those with profound obtundation or impaired protective reflexes.
2. **Circulation.** External chest compressions should be initiated in all patients with VF or asystole. If a severely hypothermic patient has no pulse but is breathing spontaneously and has evidence of an organized cardiac rhythm on the ECG,

---

TABLE 42-1   **Treatment of Hypothermia**

General
1. Handle the patient gently.
2. Prevent further heat loss.
3. Evaluate ABCs:
   A—Airway
   B—Breathing
   C—Circulation
4. For the patient in coma, consider empiric treatments:
   D50
   Naloxone
   Thiamine

Options for treatment
1. Passive external rewarming:
   Insulating blanket
   Warm room
2. Active external rewarming:
   Heating blankets (Bair Hugger®)
   Heating lamps
   Immersion
3. Active internal rewarming:
   Warm IV fluids
   Warm, humidified oxygen
   Gastric, colonic, bladder lavage
   Peritoneal, pleural, mediastinal lavage
   Specially designed central venous catheter
   Continuous arteriovenous rewarming
   Hemodialysis
   Cardiopulmonary bypass

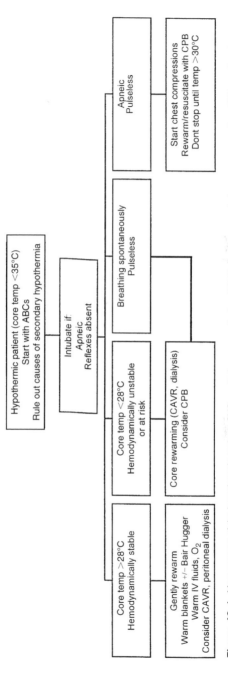

Figure 42-1. Management of the hypothermic patient. CVC, central venous catheter; CAVR, continuous arteriovenous rewarming; CPB, cardiopulmonary bypass.

cardiac output should be sufficient to maintain the viability of vital organs and no closed chest massage is indicated. In these patients and those with a pulse but with hypotension or evidence of end-organ dysfunction, infusion of warm (39°C to 40°C) fluids coupled with rapid core rewarming is the primary treatment.

3. For severely hypothermic patients in VF, up to three electrical countershocks should be attempted. If unsuccessful, the patient should have ongoing cardiopulmonary resuscitation (CPR) and be warmed prior to further defibrillation attempts. Cardiopulmonary bypass (CPB) may be indicated for both circulatory support and rewarming. Antiarrhythmic agents tend to be ineffectual while the patient remains hypothermic. Hypovolemia, caused by capillary leak, cold diuresis, and injuries, needs to be corrected.

4. **Neurologic.** Other causes of coma, such as intracranial injury, hypoglycemia, electrolyte abnormalities, or drug overdose should be sought and treated (e.g., with dextrose 50%, naloxone, or flumazenil). In addition, spinal immobilization must be provided if circumstances suggest any risk of torso or head injury.

C. **Procedures, patient handling, and VF.** As the core temperature decreases to 28°C and below, the risk of spontaneous VF increases. This risk may be enhanced by physical stimuli. Only those necessary procedures should be performed. Naso- and orogastric tubes, urinary bladder catheters, central venous catheters, and dramatic physical repositioning or movement of the patient are rarely lifesaving in the initial phases of resuscitation and should be withheld until the core temperature increases to at least 32°C. Above this temperature, risk of VF is negligible. Conversely, **intubation in apneic patients or those unable to maintain airway patency** should not be withheld, but it should be done with care. Topical anesthesia should be considered.

D. **Drug therapy.** Nonessential drugs should be avoided in hypothermic patients because of unpredictable metabolism, which may lead to toxicity as the patient rewarms.

E. **Signs of irreversibility.** Hypothermic patients may appear dead. Nonetheless, resuscitative efforts should start and not cease until moderate to severe hypothermia is reversed (i.e., the patient is nearly normothermic). The only exceptions are for those patients who have sustained injuries incompatible with life or when hypothermia is the natural result of the poikilothermic state created with prolonged cardiac arrest in initially normothermic patients. Initial metabolic parameters such as a pH <6.8 or a potassium >7.0 mEq/L are *relative* markers of irreversibility.

V. **REWARMING.** In hypothermic trauma patients, after the primary survey has been completed and the ABCs have been addressed, rewarming should be initiated. The average warming rates of commonly used rewarming techniques are listed in Table 42-2.

A. **Mild hypothermia (32°C to 35°C).** Patients with mild hypothermia can be treated with passive, external rewarming methods such as insulating blankets, or active, external rewarming methods such as heating blankets or convective air warmers (Bair Hugger®, Augustine Medical, Inc., Eden Prairie, Minnesota).

B. **Moderate hypothermia (28°C to 32°C).** External rewarming alone of moderately to severely hypothermic patients may lead to "afterdrop," a decrease in core temperature during rewarming attempts due to cold peripheral blood flowing to the core as peripheral vasodilation occurs. Patients with moderate hypothermia need more active, internal rewarming methods (e.g., warm IV fluids and warm inspired gas). Gastric, colonic, bladder, peritoneal, pleural, or mediastinal lavage; or hemodialysis may be indicated. Specialized central venous catheters that allow temperature-controlled saline to circulate through balloons positioned around the catheter can be used. Continuous arteriovenous rewarming (CAVR) uses a heparin-bonded extracorporeal circuit with a countercurrent warming device attached to cannulas placed in the femoral artery and vein. Venovenous rewarming also can be used in a similar fashion by adding a roller pump.

TABLE 42-2	Rewarming Rates
Passive external rewarming	0.5–2.0°C/h
Shivering	3–4°C/h
Heated O_2	1.0–2.5°C/h
Peritoneal lavage/dialysis	1.0–2.5°C/h
Continuous arteriovenous rewarming	2–3°C/h
Cardiopulmonary bypass	10°C/h

C. **Severe hypothermia (<28°C).** The severely hypothermic patient is at high risk of cardiac arrest. Use of CPB, initiated via the femoral vessels, jugular vein or the chest, is the treatment of choice since CPB is the most efficient rewarming method and can support circulation. If hemodynamics are adequate and dysrhythmias have not occurred, active, internal rewarming is appropriate with CPB available should the patient deteriorate.

VI. SPECIAL SITUATIONS
A. **Exposure hypothermia** (without trauma) causes approximately 100,000 deaths worldwide each year. To enhance survival, three things are essential: Recognition of patients who are at risk, accurate identification of the condition using core temperature measurements, and early initiation of appropriate therapy.
   1. **Risk factors**
      a. Extremes of age (the elderly and neonates/infants)
      b. Alcohol, sedative, or illicit drug use
      c. Concomitant neurologic disease or injury, especially stroke and spinal cord lesions and psychiatric illnesses.
      d. Dermal disruption, including burns
      e. Certain medications, including adrenergic blockers, antipsychotics, and antidepressants
      f. Endocrinologic diseases such as diabetes, hypothyroidism and hypoadrenalism
      g. Submersion
   2. **The cause of hypothermia may not be exposure alone.** Clinical clues that there is an underlying cause of hypothermia include absence of bradycardia; inability to increase temperature with routine measures; and abnormal mental status, stupor, or coma after rewarming to >32°C in the absence of previous cardiac arrest.
B. **Drowning (or submersion injury)** is defined as suffocation from submersion in a liquid medium; it is a common cause of accidental death, particularly in children and adolescents/young adults. Risk factors for submersion injuries include hypothermia, inability to swim, diving accidents, alcohol and drug ingestion, and exhaustion. Submersion rapidly leads to hypothermia, which may increase risk of drowning, but may also provide critical cerebral protection if asphyxiation or cardiac arrest occur.
   1. **Pulmonary failure** is common after submersion unless aspiration is prevented by laryngospasm. Freshwater aspiration causes pulmonary damage because of washout of surfactant and reflex mechanisms that cause increased airway resistance. Saltwater aspiration causes pulmonary damage via an osmotic gradient leading to shifts of protein-rich fluid into the alveoli. The fluid shifts caused by both types of aspiration generally do not cause profound serum electrolyte imbalances. Water contaminants add to the damage from either type of aspiration.
   2. **CNS damage** due to cerebral hypoxia is found in 12% to 27% of survivors. Cold water temperature can decrease brain temperature to protective levels before cardiac arrest occurs. Mild hypothermia for 12 to 24 hours can improve neurologic outcome and survival after normothermic cardiac arrest. It may be

advantageous to continue mild hypothermia after resuscitation of the submersion victim if comatose.

3. **Since diving into water is common in submersion victims, cervical spine injury may** exist and needs to be considered.

4. **Shock** is uncommon after submersion alone. Its presence should prompt a search for other causes.

5. **Treatment** is based as above, beginning with airway, breathing and circulation assessment. Ventilatory support (non-invasive positive pressure or with intubation) may be needed despite minimal chest radiography findings initially. There is no role for prophylactic antibiotics or steroids.

6. **Victims of submersion in cold water** may appear dead. If the patient has been immersed for <1 hour, resuscitative efforts are indicated at least until the core temperature is >30°C.

C. **Frostbite**

1. **Pathophysiology.** The local complications of hypothermia to external organs (digits, appendages such as the nose or ear, etc.) is termed frostbite, which involves tissue freezing and microvascular occlusion leading to cellular ischemia and death. The extent of tissue injury varies from hyperemia and edema to vesicle formation to full-thickness necrosis.

2. **Treatment.** Limiting cold exposure is the best way to minimize progression of injury. Affected extremities should be rapidly rewarmed by immersion in warm water (38°C to 41°C). The extremity should be elevated to minimize edema. Tetanus toxoid should be administered. Escharotomy may be needed if vascular compromise occurs. Surgical debridement or amputation should be delayed until clear demarcation has occurred, unless wound sepsis has intervened.

VII. THERAPEUTIC HYPOTHERMIA

A. **Animal studies** suggest a protective role for *controlled or therapeutic* hypothermia during hemorrhagic shock. In theory, hypothermia may protect organs that are ischemic or are vulnerable to ischemia (especially the brain and heart) and improve outcomes. The mechanisms of the beneficial effects of hypothermia include decreased metabolic demands, altering oxidant injury, changing inflammatory responses, and other potential mechanisms. Clinical studies regarding therapeutic hypothermia during hemorrhagic shock are lacking still and wide spread use not recommended outside of research. Until these studies are conducted, rapid rewarming of trauma patients is recommended, particularly if they are coagulopathic.

B. **Cardiac arrest.** Some patients who suffer a non-traumatic cardiac arrest and have successful restoration of spontaneous circulation remain comatose. For those comatose survivors of cardiac arrest, particularly out-of-hospital with an initial rhythm of VF or ventricular tachycardia (VT), the American Heart Association and its international counterparts recommend therapeutic hypothermia at 33°C to 34°C for 12 to 24 hours. In other settings (non-VF/VT or in-hospital arrest), therapeutic hypothermia should be considered although evidence is less robust. For trauma patients who remain comatose (without traumatic brain injury) after resuscitation from a cardiac arrest, therapeutic hypothermia is a consideration if there are no contraindications (e.g., coagulopathy, ongoing bleeding).

C. **Neurologic trauma.** While pre-clinical data are encouraging, clinical studies have not clearly demonstrated benefit of therapeutic hypothermia in these patients. However, *hyperthermia is clearly detrimental* in these situations. Active temperature control to maintain normothermia seems prudent.

AXIOMS

- All trauma patients are at risk for developing accidental hypothermia—look for it using a low-reading rectal probe and make sure that you actively prevent it from occurring (warm fluids, blankets, warming lights).
- Moderately and severely hypothermic patients need **active** core rewarming.

- Severely hypothermic patients may present with cardiac arrest. Unless obvious injuries incompatible with life are present, patients should not be declared dead until they have been rewarmed.
- Drowning victims are at high risk of pulmonary complications, as well as anoxic neurologic damage. Treatment is mainly supportive.

Suggested Readings

Delaney KA, Vassallo SU, Larkin GL, et al. Rewarming rates in urban patients with hypothermia: prediction of underlying infection. *Acad Emerg Med* 2006;13:913.

Gentilello LM, Jurkovich GJ, Stark MS, et al. Is hypothermia in the victim of major trauma protective or harmful? *Ann Surg* 1997;226:439–447.

Gregory JS, Flancbaum L, Townsend MC, et al. Incidence and timing of hypothermia in trauma patients undergoing operations. *J Trauma* 1991;31:795–800.

Jurkovich GJ, Greiser WB, Luterman A, et al. Hypothermia in trauma victims: An ominous predictor of survival. *J Trauma* 1987;27:1019–1024.

Laniewicz M, Lyn-Kew K, Silbergleit R. Rapid endovascular warming for profound hypothermia. *Ann Emerg Med* 2008;51:160.

Martini WZ, Pusateri AE, Uscilowicz JM, et al. Independent contributions of hypothermia and acidosis to coagulopathy in swine. *J Trauma* 2005;58:1002–1010.

Morita S, Seiji M, Inokuchi S, et al. The efficacy of rewarming with a portable and percutaneous cardiopulmonary bypass system in accidental deep hypothermia patients with hemodynamic instability. *J Trauma* 2008;65:1391.

Peberdy MA, Callaway CW, Neumar RW, et al. Part 9: post-cardiac arrest care: 2010 American Heart Association Guidelines for Cardiopulmonary Resuscitation and Emergency Cardiovascular Care. *Circulation* 2010;122(suppl 3):S768–S786.

Sabharwal R, Johns EJ, Egginton S. The influence of acute hypothermia on renal function of anaesthetized euthermic and acclimatized rats. *Exp Physiol* 2004;89(4):455–463.

Splittgerber FH, Talbert JG, Sweezer WP, et al. Partial cardiopulmonary bypass for core rewarming in profound accidental hypothermia. *Am Surg* 1986;52:407–412.

Tisherman SA. Hypothermia and injury. *Curr Opin Crit Care* 2004;10:512–519.

Wang HE, Callaway CW, Peitzman AB, et al. Admission hypothermia and outcome after major trauma. *Crit Care Med* 2005;33:1296–1301.

Wu X, Kochanek PM, Cochran K, et al. Mild hypothermia improves survival after prolonged, traumatic hemorrhagic shock in pigs. *J Trauma* 2005;59(2):291–299.

43

Introduction to Emergency General Surgery: Evaluation of the Acute Abdomen

Grace S. Rozycki and David V. Feliciano

Over the past several years, the acute care surgeon has emerged as the surgeon who provides care for patients whose lives are immediately threatened by surgical disease. These patients may present at any time of day or night, include almost any age, have the potential for complex medical histories, may deteriorate quickly, have minimal opportunity for preoperative work up, and therefore, are more prone to complications. Emergency general surgery covers a wide range of diseases. The acute abdomen includes many time-dependent diseases for which the principles of rapid assessment, diagnosis and treatment will lead to optimal outcomes. When assessing the patient with a potential acute abdominal condition, it is key to gather a focused history and physical examination, order the targeted tests and radiologic examinations, and then make a presumptive diagnosis or plan. If the diagnosis can be made with reasonable certainty, the second critical decision is to decide if an operation is indicated and, if so, then the third decision is optimal timing of the operation. If an obvious diagnosis cannot be reached through the usual mechanisms, then an alternative goal is to choose extended observation or to perform an emergent operation.

PAIN

The visceral layer of the peritoneum is supplied by autonomic nerves, whereas the parietal peritoneum is supplied by somatic innervation from the spinal cord. Consequently, as pain fibers enter the spinal cord ipsilaterally, the pain localizes to that side versus that of visceral pain which is perceived to arise in the midline because sensory input enters the spinal cord bilaterally. Visceral pain is dull or crampy while parietal pain is sharp and usually persistent. Referred pain is felt at a site different from its origin and is sharp and persistent. An example is right shoulder pain from right-sided residual pneumoperitoneum. The complexity of pain is illustrated with appendicitis as the pain is initially poorly localized in the periumbilical area and, as the inflammatory process progresses, the irritation of the parietal peritoneum results in a change in the character of the pain to be sharper and more localized to the right lower quadrant of the abdomen.

HISTORY

The etiologies of acute abdominal pain stem from intraperitoneal or extraperitoneal processes and include esophageal, gastrointestinal, vascular, gynecologic, urologic, and non-abdominal causes. The history should focus on the onset, character, location of the pain, prior symptoms, associated illnesses including medications, and previous abdominal surgery. A characterization of the *onset and character* of the pain is critical to help narrow the differential diagnosis. For example, if the patient recalls almost precisely when sudden and severe abdominal pain occurred, it is often due to a perforated hollow viscus or mesenteric ischemia. A more gradual onset of pain is more likely to occur with inflammatory conditions (pancreatitis, appendicitis, colitis) or a bowel obstruction.

The *location* of the abdominal pain may also narrow the differential diagnosis. Figure 43-1 shows the location of pain by abdominal quadrant for some common diseases. Localizing the pain to a specific area often helps to limit the differential and to determine what, if any, investigational studies need to be performed. The localization of abdominal pain by quadrant is not a precise indicator as the pain may be diffuse, occur in adjacent quadrants, or change location as the disease progresses. Of note, acute abdominal gynecologic

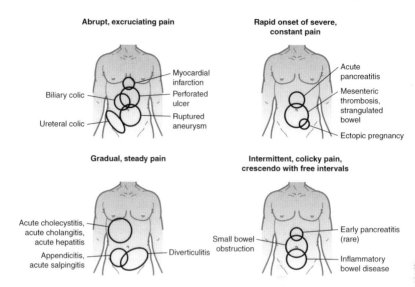

Figure 43-1. The location and character of pain are helpful in the differential diagnosis of the acute abdomen.

problems (including ectopic pregnancy) usually cause pain in the lower quadrants, while pneumonia and myocardial infarction may be associated with pain in the upper quadrants (Table 43-1).

For the immunocompromised patient, the differential diagnosis of acute abdominal pain is similar to that for the immunocompetent patient, but also includes infectious processes (especially cytomegalovirus and Epstein–Barr viruses), neutropenic enterocolitis, and bowel perforation secondary to lymphoma, CMV, sarcoma, mycobacteria, or pseudomembranous colitis.

PHYSICAL EXAMINATION

Inspection of the patient may yield important information to support a diagnosis. For example, jaundice may indicate hepatobiliary disease, restlessness may indicate colic (renal, hepatobiliary) and resistance to mobility may be consistent with peritonitis. The vital signs yield important information about the patient's response to the disease process; for example, hypotension, fever, and tachycardia are consistent with dehydration or possible septic shock, often compensated but still dangerous.

A well-organized and systematic approach to the abdominal examination decreases the likelihood of omitting important steps or making a premature diagnosis. To differentiate tense muscles in the abdominal wall from peritonitis, ask the patient to bend their knees and place a pillow underneath them. Before beginning the examination, review with the patient the initial location of the abdominal pain and ask the patient to point to the area of maximal pain. Standing at the patient's right side, the abdominal examination consists of the following steps:

1. *Inspect* for distension, pulsations, bulges, masses, discolorations, hematomas, or previous scars. A flank hematoma (Grey Turner's sign) or periumbilical hematoma (Cullen's sign) may indicate a retroperitoneal or intraperitoneal hematoma, respectively. Included in this step is the observation of respiratory movement including the use of the abdominal wall muscles.

2. *Auscultate* for the presence and character of bowel sounds or bruits. The presence of active, high-pitched bowel sounds may indicate a mechanical small bowel obstruction.

TABLE 43-1   **Causes of Abdominal Pain**

Gastrointestinal	**Urologic**
Stomach/Esophagus	Kidney stone
Peptic ulcer disease	Urinary tract infection/acute cystitis
Gastritis/esophagitis	Acute pyelonephritis
Gastroesophageal reflux	Ruptured bladder
Boerhaave's syndrome	Acute epididymitis
Mallory–Weiss syndrome	Testicular torsion
Small Bowel	Renal infarct
Gastroenteritis	**Gynecologic**
Crohn's disease	Ovarian torsion
Meckel's diverticulitis	Ectopic pregnancy
Small-bowel obstruction	Ovulation
Large Bowel	Ovarian cyst
Appendicitis	Pelvic inflammatory disease
Large-bowel obstruction	Tubo-ovarian abscess
Diverticulitis	Endometriosis
Ulcerative colitis	**Vascular**
Other	Abdominal aortic aneurysm
Perforated viscus	Acute mesenteric ischemia
Hernia	Aortic dissection
Cancer	Mesenteric venous thrombosis
Hepatobiliary/Pancreatic	**Other**
Cholecystitis	Pneumonia
Acute pancreatitis	Myocardial infarction
Cholangitis	Diabetes mellitus
Hepatitis	Porphyria
Hepatic abscess	Sickle-cell anemia
Sphincter of Oddi dysfunction	Henoch–Schonlein purpura
Hepatic tumor	Muscular contusion/hematoma
Splenic	Familial Mediterranean fever
Splenic infarct	Retroperitoneal hemorrhage
Splenic rupture	

3. *Percuss* and *palpate* the abdomen to elicit signs of tenderness, peritonitis, and organomegaly. Percussion can be used to determine the presence of peritonitis, ascites, distended bowel, or hepatomegaly. Palpation should start from the opposite quadrant of maximal pain. Rebound tenderness is elicited when the examiner's hands are quickly released from the patient's abdomen. The information obtained with this maneuver is usually similar to that obtained from deep palpation, and, therefore, does not add much to the results of the physical examination. Figure 43-1 shows some common signs on abdominal examination that are relevant to the evaluation of the patient with an acute surgical abdomen.

4. A rectal examination (males and females) and a pelvic examination in women are often omitted but helpful in many. The rectal examination can detect pelvis masses or tenderness, prostate size and tenderness, fecal impaction, or bleeding. Tenderness along the right rectal vault may suggest appendicitis or a pelvic abscess. A bimanual examination should be performed to confirm gynecologic causes of pain such as pelvic inflammatory disease, ovarian mass, tubo-ovarian abscess, or ectopic pregnancy (Table 43-2).

5. Serial abdominal examinations, preferably by the same examiner, are often needed to follow changes in the severity and location of abdominal tenderness. The use of pain scales can aid in following the patient and limiting variation.

TABLE 43-2	Common Abdominal Examination Signs	
Sign	**Description**	**Diagnosis/Condition**
Grey Turner's Sign	Local areas of discoloration around umbilicus and flanks	Acute hemorrhagic pancreatitis
Iliopsoas Sign	Elevation and extension of leg against resistance causes pain	Appendicitis with retrocecal abscess
Murphy's Sign	Pain caused by inspiration while applying pressure to right upper abdomen	Acute cholecystitis
Obturator Sign	Flexion and external rotation of right thigh while supine creates hypogastric pain	Pelvic abscess or inflammatory mass in pelvis
Rovsing's Sign	Pain at McBurney's point when compressing the left lower abdomen	Acute appendicitis

ADJUNCTIVE DIAGNOSTIC TESTS

These tests include laboratory, imaging, and procedures. Although they may be helpful in evaluation of the patient with acute abdominal pain, they are considered supplementary to the history and physical examination, not a replacement for them. Further, they should be carefully selected to yield the maximum amount of diagnostic information, avoid iatrogenic complications, and minimize the delay in the definitive treatment of the patient.

LABORATORY TESTS

The most commonly used laboratory tests include hemoglobin/hematocrit, white blood cell count (WBC) with differential, electrolytes, blood urea nitrogen (BUN), creatinine, glucose, amylase, lipase, total and direct bilirubin, alkaline phosphatase, serum aminotransferase, urinalysis, and urine human chorionic gonadotropin. None are required in all settings, but these are the common core labs, especially when the presentation is indistinct.

1. A high *hematocrit* may accompany dehydration, while a low *hemoglobin* in a patient with abdominal pain prompts consideration of acute or subacute bleeding, including both intra-abdominal or retroperitoneal hemorrhage.
2. A high or rising *WBC* is consistent with inflammation and infection; most patients with an acute abdomen have a leukocytosis or bandemia. A WBC rarely diagnoses an infection or inflammatory event, and a normal WBC cannot exclude either condition (though it may become less likely if present).
3. The serum *electrolytes, BUN, and creatinine* assess for more profound dehydration, third space losses, vomiting (as indicated by hypochloremic, hypokalemic, metabolic alkalosis) diarrhea, or a metabolic derangement. (Dehydration is consistent with a BUN/Cr ratio $\geq 20:1$) Another way to assess the patient's metabolic state is to use the anion gap which is $Na - (Cl + HCO_3) = 3$ to 11 mEq/L. High anion gap acidosis may be due to lactic acidosis, ketoacidosis, end-stage renal failure, or chemical overdoses.
4. An elevated serum *amylase or lipase* indicates pancreatitis, small-bowel infarction or perforation, and renal insufficiency or failure. The degree of elevation of these laboratory values often does not correspond to the disease severity.
5. Elevated transaminases (Aspartate aminotransferase [AST] and Alanine aminotransferase [ALT]) indicate hepatocellular dysfunction or injury including viral hepatitis, abscess, ischemia, acetaminophen poisoning. An elevated alkaline phosphatase is more consistent with a bile flow obstruction such as with a common bile duct stone, cholangitis, or primary sclerosing cholangitis. The *Gamma-Glutamyl Transferase* (GGTP) level isolates the increased alkaline phosphatase as originating from the biliary tree. An elevated INR or decreased albumin level can indicate long-standing liver disease such as cirrhosis,

important in the event that a patient needs an operation. Neither is sensitive for liver disease, but when abnormal portends a worse prognosis.

6. A high *lactate* level may indicate intestinal ischemia or infarction.

7. *Urinalysis* helps identify diseases of the kidney or urinary bladder and urinary tract infection. Urine with pyuria and a positive nitrite or the presence of leukocyte esterase indicates a urinary tract infection, acute pyelonephritis, or cystitis. Occasionally, urinalysis may show a positive leukocyte esterase without pyuria (or modest pyuria) indicating an intra-abdominal inflammatory process such as appendicitis.

8. All women of child-bearing age should have a pregnancy test (urine or serum, latter if any concerns for early ectopic pregnancy) to eliminate or confirm any gestational etiology.

IMAGING STUDIES

Plain Radiographs

The abdominal series consists of an upright chest film and flat and upright abdominal films. Subdiaphragmatic air detected on an upright chest x-ray may indicate a perforated viscus. This finding together with a history of sudden abdominal pain and a markedly tender or rigid abdomen obviates the need for further imaging studies and should be followed by immediate laparotomy. The presence of "gas" in the portovenous system usually indicates intestinal ischemia or an infectious process as the gas is produced by bacteria.

Plain films may also show calcifications such as appendicolith, gallstones, or renal calculi, although each of these is uncommonly seen. Occasionally, pancreatic and vascular calcifications may be visualized. Flat and upright abdominal films show bowel gas patterns and can be helpful in determining partial or complete obstruction of the small bowel or colon by the presence or absence of gas in the rectosigmoid area. These films are particularly helpful as they require no contrast agents, can be performed at the patient's bedside, and are easily repeatable. Plain abdominal films are also helpful in diagnosis of sigmoid or cecal volvulus and toxic megacolon in the patient with a history of inflammatory bowel disease. Pneumatosis intestinalis is an ominous sign as it indicates bowel ischemia. Edema of the bowel wall may indicate an inflammatory process such as *Clostridium difficile* colitis or inflammatory bowel disease, while "thumbprinting" may be consistent with mesenteric ischemia.

Ultrasound

Abdominal ultrasonography is the preferred imaging study for the evaluation of the patient with abdominal pain in the right upper quadrant. It is accurate (>95%) for the detection of gallstones and the other pathologic signs associated with biliary tract disease, such as pericholecystic fluid, thickened gallbladder wall, and sludge. Further, ultrasound can detect dilatation of the extra- and intrahepatic bile ducts and common bile duct stones. Ultrasound also accurately detects free abdominal fluid and measures the diameter of the abdominal aorta. For example, a patient with acute abdominal pain radiating to the back and ultrasound detects an 8 cm abdominal aorta with free fluid, a diagnosis of a ruptured abdominal aortic aneurysm is likely. Ultrasound is portable, noninvasive, rapid, and easily repeatable making it particularly advantageous for patients who are hypotensive and cannot be safely transported to the radiology suite. In addition, it uses no ionizing radiation making it particularly safe for the pregnant patient. Transvaginal ultrasound improves detection of pelvic pathology such as an ovarian cyst, torsion, or ectopic pregnancy. The accuracy of ultrasound is obviously user-dependent. When combined with the history and physical examination, a focused ultrasound of the abdomen is a helpful diagnostic maneuver.

Computed Tomography (CT)

Improvements in technology have revolutionized the speed and accuracy of CT. If the patient can tolerate the oral contrast, it is helpful to differentiate the bowel from other intra-abdominal organs or abscesses; however, non-contrast scans are nearly as accurate and easier to obtain and better tolerated in most patients. Intravenous contrast CT can aid in detection of retroperitoneal pathology and some vascular abnormalities. For example, venous thrombosis of the pelvic and femoral veins may be visualized in a patient who is otherwise asymptomatic. CT is accurate in detection of an abdominal aortic aneurysm in a hemodynamically normal patient. The disadvantages of CT include ionizing radiation, need for a nephrotoxic contrast agent, and the need to transport the patient to the radiology suite.

Scintigraphy (Radioisotope Imaging)

1. Biliary scintigraphy is useful to assess the biliary tree and function of the gallbladder. Nonvisualization of the gallbladder at 2 hours after the injection of the iminodiacetic acid-based compound is consistent with cystic duct obstruction. False-positives may occur in patients who are malnourished or receiving total parenteral nutrition.
2. As 99mTc-pertechnetate is taken up by the mucus secreting cells of the gastric mucosa and ectopic gastric tissue, scintigraphy with this agent can be used to detect a Meckel's diverticulum. Although this test is accurate in children, it is less so in adults as ectopic gastric mucosa occurs less frequently. If this test does not demonstrate a Meckel's diverticulum, then further work-up may include a barium study or an angiogram.

Angiography

This test may be useful for the diagnosis of mesenteric ischemia or for the treatment of a gastrointestinal bleed. Patients with mesenteric ischemia have abdominal pain out of proportion to the physical findings of absent or mild tenderness, often with a WBC $>20,000/mm^3$ and some may have a metabolic acidosis. Although angiography identifies the site of occlusion, usually the superior mesenteric artery, it is not mandatory that it be done as surgery offers the best chance of successful treatment. Occasionally, access to an intra-abdominal bleeding site may be particularly difficult, and angiography offers a method to localize the bleeding and embolize it.

PROCEDURES

1. Colonoscopy and sigmoidoscopy may be helpful in assessment of the bowel mucosa for ischemia, pseudomembranes, or for localizing a bleeding site in the lower gastrointestinal tract. If the patient has signs and symptoms of a toxic megacolon, **do not do endoscopy.**
2. Diagnostic peritoneal lavage (DPL) is an invasive but sensitive bedside test. The indications for DPL in the patient with an acute abdomen are suspected perforated or ischemic bowel or intra-abdominal hemorrhage. The test is useful to evaluate critically ill patients when the risk of transport is high. The effluent is sent for analysis with particular attention to the presence of fecal matter, bacteria, or an abnormal WBC count.
3. *Laparoscopy.* With advances in equipment, this technique has found indications in the patient with an acute abdomen. Part of its appeal is that it can be used for both diagnosis and treatment. For example, laparoscopy may be used to repair a perforated pyloric channel ulcer or perform an appendectomy. Diagnostic laparoscopy is most useful in young women with abdominal pain whose differential diagnosis also includes gynecologic diseases.

AXIOMS

- The key to diagnosing the source of acute abdominal pain is the history and examination; testing is ancillary to this and best done targeted.
- Those with clear evidence on history and examination of peritonitis and any signs of perforation, shock, or organ failure (including gut death) need an immediate operation, not more testing.
- Serial examinations are needed in those patients without a clear cause for their pain and when no signs of compensated shock or organ dysfunction exist.
- The emergency physicians and inpatient physicians should notify their surgical colleagues early when any concern of acute abdomen exists and before reaching diagnostic certainty, allowing for a coordinated plan of care.

Suggested Readings

Diaz JJ, Miller RS, May AK, et al. Acute care surgery: a functioning program and fellowship training. *J Trauma* 2007;141:310–316.

Earley AS, Pryor JP, Kim PK, et al. An acute care surgery model improves outcomes in patients with appendicitis. *Ann Surg* 2006;244:498–504.

Evers BM. Small intestine. In: Townsend CM, Beauchamp RD, Evers BM, Matsox KL, eds. *Sabiston Textbook of Surgery.* 18th ed. Philadelphia, PA: Saunders; 2008:1323.

Halstead WS. The training of the surgeon. *Johns Hopkins Hosp Bull* 1904;15:267–275.

Hameed SM, Brenneman FD, Ball CG, et al. General surgery 2.0: The emergency of acute care surgery in Canada. *Can J Surg* 2010;53:79–83.

Jurkovich GJ. Acute care surgery: The trauma surgeons' perspective. *Surgery* 2007;141:293–296.

Marino PL. *The ICU Book.* 3rd ed. Philadelphia, PA: Lippincott Williams & Wilkins; 2007:539.

Postier RG, Squires RA. Acute abdomen. In: Townsend CM, Beauchamp RD, Evers BM, Mattox KL, eds. *Sabiston Textbook of Surgery.* 18th ed. Philadelphia, PA: Saunders; 2008:1187.

Preparation, Initial Resuscitation, and Management of the Patient for Emergency Operation

Ali Y. Mejaddam and George C. Velmahos

INTRODUCTION

Initial evaluation of a patient is directed largely at determining the need for operative intervention, based on physical examination findings and relevant diagnostic tests. The assessment of the operative risk according to patient age, co-morbidities, and physiologic condition upon presentation plays a major role on the decision to operate. This chapter reviews the pertinent components of preoperative evaluation and preparation for an urgent operation for trauma or emergency surgical disease.

I. **FLUID RESUSCITATION.** The three most common reasons for hypovolemia and the need for fluid resuscitation are hemorrhage, sepsis, and loss of fluid through vomiting or diarrhea. The optimal method for clinical assessment of hypovolemia and appropriate endpoints of fluid resuscitation are debated.

   A. **Clinical assessment.** Hemorrhage is one of the leading causes of mortality following trauma, accounting for approximately 50% of deaths in the first 24 hours after injury. The most important element in the management of hemorrhagic shock, defined as inadequate end-tissue perfusion due to blood loss, is to recognize the presence and origin of bleeding early with prompt control of the hemorrhage. Overt clinical signs may be initially absent and the compensatory mechanisms may mask blood loss up to the point of cardiovascular collapse.

   1. Hypotension in the setting of trauma is often arbitrarily defined as a systolic blood pressure below 90 mm Hg. The sensitivity and specificity of this cut-off point as an indicator of severe hemorrhage is poor. Elderly patients, who normally have a higher baseline blood pressure, may be in shock long before the systolic blood pressure falls to 90 mm Hg. On the other end, pediatric patients and many adults have normal perfusion 90 mm Hg or lower. Some suggest that a threshold of 110 mm Hg be used in trauma patients, since this is a more sensitive mortality predictor though it will be non-specific.

   2. Similar to blood pressure, heart rate is an inaccurate indicator of severe bleeding. Often, the heart rate will increase in the absence of bleeding, because of other adrenergic inputs, such as anxiety, fear, or pain. More dangerously, heart rate may remain normal – or even decrease – in the face of major blood loss; beta blockers, high spinal cord injury, or simply advanced age are the most common reasons. Failure to mount a tachycardic response after bleeding in trauma patients is an ominous sign. For the stated reasons, the clinical assessment of hypovolemia cannot rely upon any single factor, but is rather made on the basis of multiple signs and symptoms. The measurement of metabolic markers, notably elevated serum lactate (over 3.0) and arterial blood gas analysis (looking for base deficit) can help the clinician detect occult hypovolemia or shock.

   B. **Method of resuscitation**

   1. If hypovolemia is caused by unchecked bleeding, the physician must balance the need for aggressive versus limited fluid resuscitation. New thought suggests delayed resuscitation, also known as "permissive" hypotension, in the context of uncontrolled hemorrhage The suggested mechanism for worse outcomes with early, aggressive resuscitation is that increased blood pressure and dilution of clotting factors disrupts clots and augments bleeding and mortality. Of note, most of the supporting data is derived from models of vascular injury, which does not

comprehensively address the pathophysiology of blunt trauma. Also, hypotensive episodes have a detrimental effect in traumatic brain injury, making the optimal endpoint of blood pressure in this setting less clear; the exact blood pressure targets are unknown during the early pre-resuscitation phase.

  2. In non-trauma bleeding patients, who may have multiple co-morbidities, be older, and tolerate poorly an ongoing metabolic deficit with delayed resuscitation. Overall, it seems that this relatively new concept is applicable in selected cases, most commonly the patient with penetrating torso injury or ruptured abdominal aortic aneurysm. At the other end of the spectrum lies the patient who is in septic shock, with relative hypovolemia resulting from the increase in the intravascular space from vasodilatation compounded by loss of fluid through capillary leak. The urgent need for resuscitation is often overlooked in these patients, allowing prolonged periods of cellular hypoperfusion. The approach to shock and early therapies, including physiologic targets, is discussed in detail elsewhere (see the chapter Sepsis and Septic Shock). The Society of Critical Care Medicine has created guidelines to aid with care as part of the Surviving Sepsis Campaign. Adherence to these guidelines can decrease morbidity and mortality. Fluid resuscitation plays an important role among septic patients but also early provision of appropriate antibiotics is essential; delay in such therapy is associated with a time-dependent increase in mortality.

C. Resuscitative fluids. In multiple studies colloids failed to show a decrease in mortality compared to crystalloid resuscitation in critically ill patients. The lack of improved benefit and increased costs of colloids do not justify their continued use in routine care.

  1. Hypertonic saline permits resuscitation with smaller volumes and has been suggested to have anti-inflammatory effects. Despite this, prospective studies have failed to show a difference in mortality between hypertonic and isotonic fluid resuscitation.

  2. At this point, isotonic crystalloids remain the mainstay of sepsis-related fluid resuscitation. Large volume saline infusions can create metabolic acidosis and while similarly large Ringer's lactate can create a mild alkalosis.

D. Blood and blood products. Blood transfusion is key in patients who are hypovolemic from severe hemorrhage. In such patients, massive blood transfusion protocols improve survival and have been adopted by most hospitals treating trauma patients. In a significant departure from past practices – which typically called for administration of fresh frozen plasma (FFP) after the sixth unit of blood transfusion and at 3:1 FFP to packed red blood cell ratio – the newer protocols recommend early and aggressive administration of blood and blood products with a 1:1:1 ratio of FFP to platelets to packed red blood cells. According to non-randomized studies, this method decreases coagulopathy and mortality in severely injured patients who require massive transfusion (greater than 10 units of red blood cells in 24 hours), yet the topic remains controversial. If the prediction for the need of massive blood transfusion is correct, avoiding coagulopathy by starting early FFP infusion seems to be a prudent strategy. But when the patient does not require massive transfusion and no more than 6 units of blood are required, early and aggressive use of FFP may result in a higher incidence of adult respiratory distress syndrome and multiple organ dysfunction syndrome.

E. Vasopressors and inotropes may be required in addition to resuscitation with crystalloids and blood products in the treatment of shock. Pharmacologic agents that enhance vascular and cardiac contractility may be needed. By using these agents, volume overload from excessive fluid administration can be avoided. However, the risks of contracting vessels, depriving peripheral tissue blood supply, and increasing cardiac work are substantial and should be weighed in the difficult decisions to balance fluid resuscitation versus vasopressors.

  1. Vasopressors are generally indicated when signs of end-organ dysfunction arise in the setting of a mean arterial pressure (MAP) below 60 mm Hg or a decrease of more than 30 mm Hg from baseline systolic pressure. In an attempt to identify superior vasopressors, a recent Cochrane review by Havel et al* reported no difference in mortality between norepinephrine and dopamine, the two most commonly used vasopressors. The most commonly used inotrope, dobutamine, acts mainly through beta-1-adrenergic receptors to increase cardiac contractility. Its use is predominantly reserved for patients with cardiac dysfunction as evidenced by low cardiac output despite adequate MAP and fluid resuscitation.

II. PREOPERATIVE ANTIBIOTICS

A. Systemic antimicrobial prophylaxis prior to surgery decrease postoperative infections, particularly of the wound. Provide parenteral antibiotics with both aerobic and anaerobic coverage within one hour of surgical incision. For longer procedures or during major resuscitation, repeat a dose at appropriate intervals, usually three hours for abdominal surgery. Cease prophylaxis within 24 hours of end of surgery in the absence of signs of infection. In trauma, prolonged antibiotics do not help even in the presence of severe injuries or major colonic contamination.

In sepsis, antibiotics should be continued for longer periods of time and after the septic focus is surgically controlled. There are no universally accepted guidelines for the duration or type of antibiotics in these situations. Generally, antibiotics may be discontinued following clinical improvement as evidenced by return of white blood cell count and temperature curve to normal.

B. For specific diseases, such as fulminant *Clostridium difficile* colitis, give oral metronidazole or vancomycin.

III. REVERSAL OF ANTICOAGULATION

A. Coumadin. The use of warfarin or antiplatelet drugs as prophylaxis against thromboembolic disease is common, and many patients in need of urgent surgery are at an increased risk of perioperative bleeding. The risk of bleeding needs to be weighed against the risk of thromboembolic events. While no consensus exists regarding modification of anticoagulation for elective surgery, cessation and reversal of anticoagulation is often required when urgent surgical procedures are necessary.

1. Cessation of warfarin therapy is best five days before surgery to achieve an international normalized ratio (INR) below 1.5.

2. In emergency surgery patients, correct the INR with vitamin K and FFP. Dosing of FFP is mainly empiric and necessitates regular monitoring of INR, as no dose-dependent relationship of reversal of INR with FFP exists. Ideally, the INR should be below 1.6; however, the likelihood of bleeding is low with an INR below 2.0. The precise INR target is not concrete for all patients and depends on the type of patient, type of procedure, sense of urgency, and initial indication for anticoagulation.

3. Prothrombin complex concentrates (PCCs) contain varying amounts of Factor II, VII, IX, X, and proteins C and S, which can help replenish vitamin-K–dependent clotting factors caused by warfarin use. PCCs can be given without delay, unlike FFP which requires blood typing and thawing. PCC is given intravenously over a period of less than five minutes. Currently, there are limited outcome data to evaluate the clinical superiority of PCCs over FFP.

4. Following the emergency procedure, there is typically a postoperative period over which the restarting of Coumadin is dangerous. During this period the patient is "bridged" by heparin until Coumadin can be restarted. The methods of bridging vary. Low-molecular-weight heparins (notably enoxaparin 1 mg/kg twice daily) are a common choice for bridging therapy, but clinical judgment remains necessary to determine appropriate dosing regimens as supporting evidence is limited.

B. Antiplatelet agents. The reversal of antiplatelet therapy, including aspirin and clopidogrel, includes cessation of the therapy and administration of platelets. Despite

---

*Havel C, Arrich J, Heidrun L, et al. Vasopressors for hypotensive shock. *Cochrane Database of Systematic Reviews*. 2011;8.

no current supportive outcome data, one to two sets of platelets are often given for this purpose. If antiplatelet therapy is given for secondary prevention of cardiovascular and cerebrovascular disease, serious thromboembolic risks are associated with the cessation of these medications. If alert, the patient needs to be involved in the decision-making process for such modifications.

IV. OTHER ISSUES
A. Informed consent
1. Informed consent can be obtained only when the patient understands the benefits, risks, and alternatives to the procedure .It is imperative that the physician determines if the patient has the capacity to understand the suggested treatments. If not, for example in minors or mentally handicapped persons, a health care proxy should be identified and sought for consent.
2. In emergency surgical practice, patients are commonly unable to be part of the informed consent process. At times, a health care proxy may have not been identified within the time limitations of an emergency. Under these circumstances the surgeon may act independently, trying to do what a reasonable person would want done. If prior wishes are known, however, this takes precedence. In the rare cases of refusal of life-saving interventions despite a reasonable assumption of successful outcome, seek help assessing capacity from psychiatric and social support personnel.
B. Advanced directive.
In appropriate situations, the issue of advanced directives should be raised. Many with pre-existing condition or later in life have expressed their desire about resuscitation and other advanced interventions. Address "Do-not-resuscitate (DNR) orders" prior to surgery; according to statements by the American College of Surgeons, DNR orders should neither be suspended implicitly nor followed explicitly. For example, short-lived insults amenable to resuscitation may cause a potentially preventable death if one follows orders explicitly.
C. Operative checklist.
Checklists standardize management, increase safety and reduced mortality and complications. An appropriate list of items on the checklist should include a review of necessary equipment, preoperative medications, marking of operative site, and presentation of staff roles. Many institutions have now adopted operative safety checklists. Although more easily used under elective than emergency conditions, every effort should be made to adhere to the practice unless the extra time compromises the likelihood for optimal outcome.

AXIOMS

- The standard and commonly used hemodynamic parameters for assessment of stability can often be misleading.
- Crystalloid fluids are the standard resuscitation fluid, augmented by blood and blood products, as needed.
- Delayed resuscitation can optimize care in actively bleeding penetrating trauma patients.
- Targeting resuscitative outcomes and recognizing shock early improves outcomes in patients with sepsis of surgical origin.
- Prophylactic and empiric antibiotics are crucial and should be given early and before operation.

Suggested Readings

Bickell WH, Wall MJ Jr, Pepe PE, et al. Immediate versus delayed fluid resuscitation for hypotensive patients with penetrating torso injuries. *N Engl J Med* 1994;331(17):1105–1109.

Brasel KJ, Guse C, Gentilello LM, et al. Heart rate: is it truly a vital sign? *J Trauma* 2007;62(4):812–817.

Demetriades D, Chan LS, Bhasin P, et al. Relative bradycardia in patients with traumatic hypotension. *J Trauma* 1998;45(3):534–539.

Frazee LA, Bourguet CC, Gutierrez W, et al. Retrospective evaluation of a method to predict fresh-frozen plasma dosage in anticoagulated patients. *Am J Ther* 2008;15(2):111–118.

Havel C, Arrich J, Losert H, et al. Vasopressors for hypotensive shock. *Cochrane Database Syst Rev* 2011;5:CD003709.

Kauvar DS, Lefering R, Wade CE. Impact of hemorrhage on trauma outcome: an overview of epidemiology, clinical presentations, and therapeutic considerations. *J Trauma* 2006;60(6 Suppl):S3–S11.

Korte W, Cattaneo M, Chassot PG, et al. Peri-operative management of antiplatelet therapy in patients with coronary artery disease. *Thromb Haemost* 2011;105(5):743–749.

Kumar A, Roberts D, Wood KE, et al. Duration of hypotension before initiation of effective antimicrobial therapy is the critical determinant of survival in human septic shock. *Crit Care Med* 2006;34(6):1589–1596.

Levy MM, Dellinger RP, Townsend SR, et al. The Surviving Sepsis Campaign: results of an international guideline-based performance improvement program targeting severe sepsis. *Intensive Care Med* 2010;36(2):222–231.

Malato A, Saccullo G, Lo Coco L, et al. Patients requiring interruption of long-term oral anticoagulant therapy: the use of fixed sub-therapeutic doses of low-molecular-weight heparin. *J Thromb Haemost* 2010;8(1):107–113.

Perel P, Roberts I. Colloids versus crystalloids for fluid resuscitation in critically ill patients. *Cochrane Database Syst Rev* 2011;3:CD000567.

Rivers E, Nguyen B, Havstad S, et al. Early goal-directed therapy in the treatment of severe sepsis and septic shock. *N Engl J Med* 2001;345(19):1368–1377.

Statement of the American College of Surgeons on Advance Directives by Patients. "Do Not Resuscitate" in the operating room. *Bull Am Coll Surg* 1994;79(9):29.

Thachil J, Gatt A, Martlew V. Management of surgical patients receiving anticoagulation and antiplatelet agents. *Br J Surg* 2008;95(12):1437–1448.

Weed HG. Antimicrobial prophylaxis in the surgical patient. *Med Clin North Am* 2003;87(1):59–75.

Acute Abdomen in ICU Patients

Matthew R. Rosengart

I. INTRODUCTION

Intra-abdominal pathology necessitating surgical intervention occurs in approximately 4% of patients admitted to the intensive care unit (ICU). The number of patients requiring surgical evaluation is several fold higher. The most common etiologies necessitating surgical intervention in ICU patients are bowel perforation, bowel ischemia, cholecystitis, bowel obstruction, and cecal/sigmoid volvulus. An emerging indication for operation in ICU patients is fulminant antibiotic associated colitis from *Clostridium difficile* infection. Distinguishing those in need of surgical intervention from the total population evaluated is difficult; many of the characteristics accompanying critical illness, such as mechanical ventilation, narcotics and sedatives, and distracting pathology (e.g., stroke), confound the ability to obtain an accurate historical and physical examination. Thus, diagnosis relies heavily upon ancillary laboratory and radiologic studies. At times, even these can be difficult to obtain in the critically ill patient with tenuous physiology that limits the diagnostic armamentarium that can be brought to the bedside. Nevertheless, timely diagnosis is essential, as any delay, in either diagnosis or treatment, is associated with a poor outcome.

The goals of this chapter are to provide a systematic approach for the evaluation of the acute abdomen in critically ill patients. Particular difficulties in both diagnosis and treatment are emphasized, as are alternative strategies to facilitate achieving both endpoints. The reader is referred to specific citations for a more comprehensive review.

II. EVALUATION

A. History. Many aspects of either critical illness or the ICU environment make obtaining accurate data from the historical examination difficult. Comorbidities, such as dementia or delirium consequent to the admission diagnosis (e.g., traumatic brain injury or sepsis), are common. In fact, 70% or more of ICU patients experience delirium during their ICU course. Many interventions (e.g., mechanical ventilation, surgery) and pathology (e.g., orthopedic trauma, traumatic brain injury) necessitate sedation, narcotic analgesics, or paralysis in the course of treatment.

Acknowledging these limitations during an exhaustive attempt to acquire all historical data is essential. If feasible, temporarily discontinuing any sedating agent may enable an objective examination. For the alert patient, a pen and pad or electronic tablet may facilitate communication. Although tedious and conveying small volumes of data, any information may prove decisive for either continued observation or surgical exploration. The ICU nurse, present continuously at the patient bedside, is an invaluable source of information. All available family members, prior caregivers, or other close associates should be interviewed for any salient information that might facilitate a diagnosis (Table 45-1).

Questions to be posed are similar for all patients undergoing surgical evaluation of the acute abdomen. The aspects prompting a surgical evaluation are critically important: Right upper quadrant pain versus cardiovascular collapse. Is this the primary impetus for admission, or did it develop during the treatment of other pathology? A thorough understanding of past medical and surgical issues establishes the context in which to interpret the current signs and symptoms and generate a priority list of the risks of particular surgical diseases. It is here that the time invested in interviewing family members is rewarded. Determination of the duration of the

TABLE 45-1 Leading Causes for Abdominal Operative Exploration in Intensive Care Unit Patients and Characteristic Findings

Diagnosis	History/physical examination	Laboratory	Radiology	DPL/laparoscopy
Ulcer perforation (gastric/duodenal)	Acute onset upper abdominal pain followed by diffuse pain/diffuse peritonitis	Leukocytosis	X-ray: Free air; CT: Duodenal edema, ascites, free air	DPL: WBC > 200/mm³, >50% PMN DL: Suppurative ascites Visualization of perforation
Colon perforation	Lower quadrant abdominal pain/focal peritonitis	Leukocytosis	X-ray: Free air; CT: Free air, ascites, colonic edema, mesenteric stranding, diverticula	DPL: WBC > 200/mm³, >50% PMN DL: Suppurative ascites Visualization of perforation
Bowel ischemia (small bowel)	History of atrial fibrillation, vascular disease/severe, diffuse abdominal pain; tenderness may not be pronounced, hemocult positive	Leukocytosis common. Lactate elevation and acidosis may also be present	X-ray: Free air, thumbprinting; CT: Thumbprinting, pneumatosis, ascites, mesenteric atherosclerosis	DPL: WBC > 200/mm³, >50% PMN DL: Suppurative ascites Visualization of necrotic bowel
Cholecystitis	Right upper quadrant pain/right upper quadrant tenderness (Murphy's sign)	Leukocytosis; may have elevated liver function tests	U/S: Thickened gallbladder wall (>3 mm), cholelithiasis, right upper quadrant pain	DPL: Normal in absence of inflammation DL: Inflamed gallbladder
Bowel obstruction	Prior abdominal surgery, vomiting, obstipation/abdominal distention, tympany, tenderness typically mild without ischemia	Leukocytosis may be present	X-ray: Air fluid levels, distended bowel, air may be in rectum if obstruction is partial CT: Same, may identify a transition point	DPL: Normal in absence of ischemia DL: Dilated loops of bowel
Sigmoid volvulus	History of constipation/abdominal distention, tenderness	Leukocytosis, acidosis if intestinal ischemia present	X-ray: "Omega loop" CT: Volvulus identified	DPL: Normal in absence of intestinal ischemia DL: Volvulus visualized
C. difficile colitis	History of prior antibiotic use; pain typically diffuse and accompanied with diarrhea	Leukocytosis positive stool assay for toxin A and/or B	X-ray: Non-specific CT: Thickened, inflamed colon, ascites	DPL: Unknown DL: Diffusely inflamed and edematous colon

DL, diagnostic laparoscopy; DPL, diagnostic peritoneal lavage; PMN, polymorphonuclear.

signs or symptoms that prompted the evaluation indicates the acuity of the process, as it relates to rapidity with which a diagnosis needs to be made and definitive treatment instituted. The details of the abdominal pain are important: Time of onset and aspects of duration, intensity, location, radiation, nature, exacerbating and mitigating circumstances if available. The gastrointestinal review of systems may generate useful data: Intolerance of tube feeds, nausea, emesis, hematemesis, melena, or hematochezia. Compromise of other subsystems, including the development of renal failure, acute lung injury, or hemodynamic instability, should raise concern of a catastrophic intra-abdominal process.

Finally, if time permits, identifying the medical decision-maker for this patient and advanced directives can simplify the decision process and ensure that the process of care achieves the patient's wishes. These discussions should include aspects of quality and function of life in addition to those of life and death. However, emergency intervention should never be delayed awaiting informed consent.

B. Physical examination. Many of the conditions hindering a historical examination render the abdominal examination unreliable: Altered level of consciousness, either iatrogenic (e.g., narcotics) or because of concomitant pathology (e.g., stroke, trauma). Hence, there is a lack of sensitivity for subtle findings, and even signs of abdominal catastrophe may be obfuscated. Medications such as steroids and immunosuppressants may mask the signs of peritoneal irritation. In this context, alternate endpoints and surrogate markers of tenderness (facial grimacing and localization) are utilized, though this compromises specificity. Physiologic changes such as tachycardia or hypertension during the examination may also serve as surrogate markers of tenderness.

The physical evaluation commences with a review of vital signs: Heart rate, blood pressure, and urine output (Table 45-1). The frequency with which physiologic and biochemical data are recorded enables trends in these parameters to be tracked, which can elucidate the temporal sequence of events. For example, the detailed records can be reviewed to assess when oliguria ensured, when the ventilatory requirements increased, or when vasopressors were instituted. The combination of these data, lends insight into whether this process is acute, subacute, or has taken place over a period of hours or days.

A thorough abdominal examination should follow. The presence and location of abdominal scars should be noted and correlated with the details of the past surgical history. The presence, character, and location of tenderness should be elicited. Temporally related events (e.g., cardiac catheterization, ruptured abdominal aneurysms) and precipitating or alleviating factors (e.g., movement, meals, emesis) may narrow the differential (e.g., mesenteric ischemia, biliary colic). Peritonitis, in particular involuntary guarding, is suggestive of surgical pathology. Distension and tympany, although non-specific, suggest obstruction or ileus. A rectal examination should be performed to check for masses, distal passage of stool and presence of blood. Melena or hematochezia suggest mucosal injury (e.g., ischemia). The nature and volume of nasogastric aspirate (e.g., bloody vs. bilious) may provide insight. Hernias should be identified and characterized as reducible, incarcerated, or strangulated.

Extra-abdominal findings may provide additional corroboration of a particular diagnosis. Signs of peripheral vascular disease support a diagnosis of mesenteric ischemia/infarction. The lacelike livedo reticularis is an uncommon sign seen in cholesterol embolism, as might occur after cardiac catheterization. Similarly, atrial fibrillation may underlie distal embolization to the mesenteric circulation and bowel infarction. Alternatively, the absence of particular signs (e.g., scaphoid abdomen, absence of distension, and emesis) may reasonably exclude specific pathology.

C. Laboratory. Attempt to tailor labs specific to the differential diagnosis, although the paucity of historical and physical data usually translate into the acquisition of a broad amount of biochemical data: A complete blood count (CBC) with cell differential, electrolytes, liver function tests, amylase, lipase, urinalysis, arterial blood gas with lactate (Table 45-1).

Complete blood count

Leukocytosis, a sign of inflammation, may be suggestive of an abdominal problem. However, its absence does not exclude surgical abdominal disease. Indeed, in a cohort of elderly patients (>80 years), fever and leukocytosis were absent in 33% of cases of acute surgical disease. In the absence of leukocytosis or leukopenia, a significant "left shift" (a large proportion of neutrophils or immature band forms) may be indicative of acute intra-abdominal pathology.

Metabolic profile

Electrolyte abnormalities such an elevated or rising creatinine or low bicarbonate indicate poor perfusion and the development of shock. Similarly, acute kidney injury and a rising blood urea nitrogen or creatinine may be early and sensitive signs of serious intra-abdominal catastrophe. Although sensitive to the presence of ischemia and shock, these signs lack specificity in identification of the etiology. Hyperbilirubinemia may indicate hepatic or gallbladder disease, although may also occur with sepsis not of hepatobiliary origin. Similarly, an elevated total amylase is not specific to acute pancreatitis. In a study of patients presenting with an acute abdomen, 50% of patients had hyperamylasemia but did not have pancreatitis. This study highlights the value of fractionating serum amylase in determining the source (i.e., salivary, intestinal, pancreatic), and thus, facilitating diagnosis. Serum lactate is produced through anaerobic metabolism and thus is elevated during shock or organ-specific ischemia (mesenteric thromboembolism). In one study, it was elevated above the reference level in 100% of patients with mesenteric ischemia and 50% of patients with bowel obstruction. However, a similar study of patients with mesenteric ischemia observed a normal lactate (<2 mmol/L) level in 24%. Base deficit (the amount of base needed to normalize 1 L of blood to pH = 7.4 under standard conditions) is obtained from an arterial blood gas analysis. An abnormal base deficit (>2.0 mmol/L) provides similar information about tissue hypoperfusion as lactate concentration, although some data suggest that they compliment each other. It is the author's practice to obtain both measurements. As aforementioned, the temporal trends of lactate and base deficit tend to proffer a wealth of prognostic information. In a study of critically ill surgical patients a persistent lactate elevation was more predictive of poor outcome than a persistently elevated base deficit.

III. DIAGNOSTIC ADJUNCTS

The physiologic status of the patient may preclude transportation for diagnostic studies. Transportation typically involves a transition to more portable versions of complicated equipment such as ventilators and continuous infusions, as well as, significant physical manipulation of the patient, which may be intolerable. This tenuousness is more typical of patients requiring inotropic/vasopressor support or maximal ventilatory support. The location to which the patient is transported creates a potentially hazardous environment to which it is difficult to summon qualified help immediately, to access the patient, and that lacks essential emergency equipment. In light of these dangers, the information to be gained from any diagnostic test and the extent to which this information may alter management must be interpreted in the context of the potential harm to the patient. In certain circumstances, one is limited to that which can be brought to the bedside: Surgeon, portable x-ray and ultrasound, or diagnostic peritoneal lavage.

A. Plain radiographs. A supine and upright/decubitus (three views) abdominal radiograph is easy to obtain and may identify free air or evidence supporting the diagnosis of small or large bowel obstruction. In the setting of a critically ill patient, these data may be sufficient to warrant operative exploration. More subtle signs of thumbprinting and pneumatosis represent bowel ischemia. Three views of the abdomen provide superior information than a single abdominal x-ray. However, by contrast to other radiographic tests, the sensitivity of plain radiographs is low. In known cases of bowel infarction, the abdominal films are normal in 25% and characteristic findings such as pneumatosis or thumbprinting are present in less than 40%.

B. CT scan. CT is the mainstay of the diagnostic evaluation of abdominal disease, although certain limitations render the benefit:risk ratio lower in the ICU patient population. CT possesses unparalleled resolution of intra-abdominal viscera and organ structures and enables the identification of fluid collections, the stranding of inflammation, and small amounts of pneumoperitoneum. The Hounsfield units provide an estimate of the density of fluid, and thus can distinguish ascites from blood or exudate. Liver and spleen hematomas are well characterized by CT, and thus elucidate the source of hemoperitoneum due to trauma. Similarly, the presence and extent of inflammatory diseases such as diverticulitis or appendicitis can be determined and quantified, enabling determination of the need for operative or nonoperative therapeutic intervention. CT has been used with variable success to identify features of mesenteric ischemia including bowel thickening, pneumatosis intestinalis (i.e., air in bowel wall), or atherosclerosis and vascular thrombus. However, even with dynamic contrast the sensitivity to mesenteric ischemia/infarction is 64%.

The disadvantages of CT include the inherent risks of transporting a critically ill patient out of the ICU. Some data suggest that ancillary CT imaging may delay surgical intervention in cases of clinically likely intra-abdominal pathology. The need to administer oral and intravenous contrast carries the risks of intolerance, emesis with aspiration, and acute kidney injury. In one randomized controlled trial, orally administered N-acetylcysteine (600 mg PO BID) the day prior to and of CT imaging combined with hydration decreased the rise in creatinine in patients with chronic renal insufficiency receiving intravenous contrast. This regimen has been the practice at our institution. Similar results have been obtained with infusion of 1 L of isotonic sodium bicarbonate. Although CT can be performed without contrast, this may limit image quality, the data rendered, and thus the utility of the study. While fluid collections and free air can be seen, it may be difficult to characterize a collection as an abscess in the absence of the rim enhancement afforded by intravenous contrast. Observing a pooling of extraluminal contrast facilitates visualizing a contained perforation. Thus, if an enhanced CT will enable determining the appropriate management of a critically ill patient, contrast should be administered.

C. Abdominal ultrasound. Ultrasound (US) can be performed at the bedside and does not carry the risks of radiation and intravenous contrast inherent to CT. However the images and thus data obtained depend upon the experience of the sonographer and characteristics of the patient. Obesity, subcutaneous air, and bandages hinder the acquisition of good sonographic windows. Ultrasound provides little information regarding hollow viscera. Nonetheless, ultrasound provides excellent imaging of the hepatobiliary system. Intra- and extrahepatic biliary dilatation can be well visualized. Pericholecystic fluid, gallbladder wall thickening, and a sonographic Murphy's sign are nearly diagnostic of acute cholecystitis. US is sensitive to ascites and intra-abdominal fluid collections (e.g., abscess). The Focal Abdominal Sonography for Trauma (FAST) has become the principle modality for evaluation of the abdomen in the acutely injured patient and is sensitive to hemoperitoneum exceeding approximately 150 mL.

D. Diagnostic peritoneal lavage (DPL). Translated from the field of trauma to the arena of the general surgeon, DPL attempts to determine the need for abdominal exploration. It has become particularly useful in the diagnostic management of the patient deemed too ill for transportation and for whom a non-therapeutic laparotomy would be intolerable (Table 45-1). Unlike trauma, emphasis is upon the concentration of leukocytes, rather than blood, in the lavage effluent. However, the leukocyte (cells/mm^3) threshold to optimize sensitivity and specificity for pathology requiring operative intervention remains controversial. In one study of general surgery patients, a WBC count greater than or equal to 200 cells/mm^3 was associated with a 99% probability of peritonitis. One retrospective study indicated that DPL is 100% sensitive and 88% specific in identifying abdominal pathology requiring operation in non-trauma patients. Their conclusion was that a negative DPL excludes intra-abdominal pathology but a positive DPL does not necessarily denote the presence of surgical disease. It has been the practice of our institution to use a threshold of 200 cells/mm^3. The procedure for performing a DPL and the criteria for a positive test in the context of trauma are outlined in the trauma section of this manual.

E. Bedside laparoscopy. Diagnostic laparoscopy (DL) is an extension of the DPL, whereby pneumoperitoneum is created and laparoscopic visualization of the abdominal viscera is performed at the bedside. By contrast to DPL, DL enables the manipulation and direct visualization of the viscera. Uncomplicated procedures, such as enterectomy, can be performed, thereby sparing a critically ill patient the stress of transportation to and an operation in the operating room. Multiple studies have demonstrated the feasibility and safety of performing DL in the ICU. An exploration of the stomach, small bowel, colon, liver, and gallbladder can be performed with a camera port and two additional ports. Use of a 30- or 45-degree angled laparoscopic camera facilitates inspection of nearly the entire abdomen. More recently, authors have described a technique for minilaparoscopy using a 3.3 mm laparoscope and 3 mm instruments with success. In the aforementioned study, when compared to DPL, bedside laparoscopy seemed to be more specific than DPL.

However, DL typically requires general endotracheal anesthesia, and thus is limited to the critically ill patient, who is already mechanically ventilated. The pneumoperitoneum may decrease renal blood flow and venous return and induce unfavorable hemodynamics; thus it is relatively contraindicated in the severely ill patient (i.e., high vasopressor use). Unfortunately, it is this very population for whom DL may provide the greatest benefit. The procedure itself requires the availability and portability of appropriate sterile instrumentation, videoscopic monitors and gas insufflation equipment. Depending on the individual institutional commitment, the ease and availability of these procedures will be variable.

IV. SURGICAL EXPLORATION

Refinements in diagnostic capabilities have allowed a more selective application of laparotomy, reducing the number of non-therapeutic laparotomies without increasing morbidity and mortality. In light of the compelling evidence that delay in surgical consultation and intervention is associated with worse outcome, preparation should occur concomitantly with diagnostic evaluation.

A. Preoperative preparation. Preoperative preparation includes a full laboratory analysis including electrolytes, CBC, and coagulation factors. Many patients will have either coagulopathy or electrolyte imbalances that will necessitate correction. Accomplishing this preoperatively may be difficult and cause undue, life-threatening delay; many derangements can be readily addressed by the anesthesia team. Hence, a type and screen and a type and cross should be obtained if transfusion is anticipated. Remember that it will take at least a half an hour to obtain type specific blood. An EKG and a CXR are helpful but should not delay emergency surgery. Active fluid resuscitation is critical prior to anesthetic induction; a patient in profound shock who is intravascularly volume depleted may arrest upon receipt of anesthetic agents. In tenuous patients, it is our practice to have the resuscitation team accompany the patient to the operating room. If possible, informed consent should be obtained from the patient or relative; however, delays awaiting consent, particularly in the context of emergent surgery, are inexcusable,

B. Preoperative OR. The patient should be positioned supine with both arms abducted and available to the anesthesia staff for intravenous or intra-arterial access. Modifications in this positioning (e.g., lithotomy) should be tailored to the anticipated pathology. Although the need for lithotomy is best determined preoperatively, perineal and anorectal access can be achieved by "frogging" the legs under the sterile drapes.

After positioning, the necessary monitoring and resuscitation lines, including invasive arterial cannulas and central venous access should be placed. Sequential compression devices for DVT prophylaxis should be placed prior to the induction of general anesthesia. All patients require bladder catheterization and gastric intubation. Empiric broad-spectrum antibiotics should be administered. In the absence of a known drug allergy, a second-generation cephalosporin (cefoxitin, cefotetan) or penicillin (ampicillin/sulbactam) provides excellent coverage for both integument and enteric organisms. A combination of ciprofloxacin and metronidazole is a reasonable alternative in the penicillin/cephalosporin-sensitive patient. Suspicion of nosocomial organisms should prompt broadening coverage to include non-lactose fermenting gram-negative rods (pseudomonas, acinetobacter), methicillin-resistant staphylococcus aureus (MRSA), enterococcus, or yeast. A long duration (>72 hours) of hospitalization or prior antibiotic usage increases the likelihood of these nosocomial organisms. The patient's skin should be prepped from the nipple line to the pubis. The prep may be modified to include the bilateral groins or chest if clinically indicated. Ensure that adequate help, illumination, and suction are available.

C. **Operative.** The goals of the operation remain the same for each patient: Control hemorrhage and contamination and treat the source pathology. However, the techniques to achieve these goals may be modified by the clinical/physiologic status of the patient. Most patients should be explored through a midline laparotomy. Ensure that exposure is ideal so as not to compromise surgical technique. An "indecisive" periumbilical midline incision is a reasonable initial approach that enables one to determine whether the pathology is in the upper or lower abdomen and avoid an overly lengthy incision. Alternatively, the incision may be tailored to a preoperative diagnosis (e.g., a right or left upper quadrant incision two fingerbreadths below the costal margin for procedures on the liver/gallbladder or spleen, respectively). These regional incisions only provide exposure to a portion of the abdomen; thus, if the pathology resides outside this area, a much larger incision will be necessary. Likewise, although the appendix is typically removed through an incision in the right lower quadrant, a vertical lower midline incision will also serve well for this purpose and enable access to other abdominal quadrants.

Upon laparotomy, definitive care should be provided to any obvious pathology. Typically, the pathology threatening the patient is obvious. Sources of enteric contamination may be temporarily controlled with clamps or oversewing until the remaining peritoneal viscera have been thoroughly evaluated and all pathology identified. Non-viable bowel is resected. Doppler interrogation of the mesenteric vessels or fluorescein dye with woods lamp illumination may more objectively define the adequacy of perfusion to marginally perfused bowel. The utilization of the GIA staplers has markedly facilitated the process of resection. The vascular EndoGIA™ stapler can markedly reduce the time needed for mesenteric division.

The decision to pursue versus postpone intestinal reconstruction depends predominantly on the stability of the patient. Hypothermia, hypotension, coagulopathy or the need for blood transfusion are signs that reconstruction should be delayed. Borrowing from the field of trauma, "damage control laparotomy" has been applied to critically ill acute surgical patients. In essence, it entails addressing that pathology posing an immediate threat to life and the postponement of all else until full resuscitation and acceptable physiology are attained in the ICU. Divided bowel is returned to the peritoneal cavity in discontinuity, coagulopathic hemorrhage is packed, and temporary abdominal closure applied with the plan to re-explore and restore intestinal continuity when homeostasis (i.e., hypothermia, hypotension, acidosis, coagulopathy addressed) has been achieved. In addition, compromised bowel may be re-examined at the second laparotomy to ensure an anastomosis involving viable bowel.

A variety of temporary closure methods of the abdomen are available: Sterile IV bag (Bogota Bag), skin-only closure, and vacuum assisted techniques. These dressings reduce, but do not eliminate, the likelihood of developing abdominal compartment syndrome. They permit the drainage of intra-abdominal fluid, which has been suggested to reduce the inflammatory response. Disadvantages include the need for sedation to prevent evisceration, although this has been debated, committal to a second operation, and with time, fascial retraction, increasing the likelihood of incisional hernia formation.

D. **Postoperative.** Once the operation has been completed and the acute pathology addressed, efforts focus on resuscitation and subsystem support. Endpoints of resuscitation (i.e., markers of adequate tissue perfusion) include conventional parameters (e.g., heart rate, blood pressure, urine output), global parameters (e.g., lactate, base deficit, SvO_2), and regional measures (e.g., mucosal pH, capnometry, and near infrared spectroscopy).

V. OUTCOMES
As ICU care continues to improve, the outcomes for emergency abdominal surgery in critically ill patients should improve. However, critical care should compliment, rather

than supplant, the expeditious involvement of a surgeon and prompt, definitive operative intervention. The frail state of this patient population limits the capacity to endure and recover from the stress of surgery. The overall mortality rate in the entire population remains high, approximately 38%, which correlates with organ system failure index (OSFI) and APACHE scores; the greater degree of preoperative physiologic derangement, the higher the mortality. In one observational study, a high OSFI and APACHE score was associated with a mortality of 89%, but if both scores were low, only 5% died. Diagnostic delay, if present, continues to be independently associated with a higher mortality.

AXIOMS

■ The evaluation and management of the acute abdomen in the ICU patient is challenging. Although the approach is similar to that of the non-critically ill patient, the amount and sources of data are limited.

■ Often both the historical and physical examinations are obfuscated by the illness itself, and thus unreliable.

■ Diagnostic studies, such as CT, may provide definitive information, but their value must be weighed against the potential risks of transportation and the study itself (e.g., contrast nephropathy).

■ At operation decisions need to be made regarding definitive reconstruction, creation of stomas or abbreviated "damage-control".

■ Although mortality still remains high, no single factor carries a greater potential to optimize outcome than the rapid involvement of a surgeon and the expeditious provision of definitive operative care.

Suggested Readings

Alverdy JC, Saunders J, Chamberlin WH, et al. Diagnostic peritoneal lavage in intra-abdominal sepsis. *Am Surg* 1988;54(7):456–459.

Bailey RL, Laws HL. Diagnostic peritoneal lavage in evaluation of acute abdominal disease. *South Med J* 1990;83(4):422–424.

Dallal RM, Harbrecht BG, Boujoukas AJ, et al. Fulminant Clostridium difficile: an underappreciated and increasing cause of death and complications. *Ann Surg* 2002;235(3):363–372.

Eltarawy IG, Etman YM, Zenati M, et al. Acute mesenteric ischemia: the importance of early surgical consultation. *Am Surg* 2009;75(3):212–219.

Gagné DJ, Malay MB, Hogle NJ, et al. Bedside diagnostic minilaparoscopy in the intensive care patient. *Surgery* 2002;131(5):491–496.

Gajic O, Urrutia LE, Sewani H, et al. Acute abdomen in the medical intensive care unit. *Crit Care Med* 2002;30(6):1187–1190.

Husain FA, Martin MJ, Mullenix PS, et al. Serum lactate and base deficit as predictors of mortality and morbidity. *Am J Surg* 2003;185(5):485–491.

Kollef MH, Allen BT. Determinants of outcome for patients in the medical intensive care unit requiring abdominal surgery: a prospective, single-center study. *Chest* 1994;106(6):1822–1828.

Lange H, Jackel R. Usefulness of plasma lactate concentration in the diagnosis of acute abdominal disease. *Eur J Surg* 1994;160(6–7):381–384.

Larson FA, Haller CC, Delcore R, et al. Diagnostic peritoneal lavage in acute peritonitis. *Am J Surg* 1992;164(5):449–452.

Martin MJ, FitzSullivan E, Salim A, et al. Discordance between lactate and base deficit in the surgical intensive care unit: which one do you trust? *Am J Surg* 2006;191(5):625–630.

McNicoll L, Pisani MA, Zhang Y, et al. Delirium in the intensive care unit: occurrence and clinical course in older patients. *J Am Geriatr Soc* 2003;51(5):591–598.

Merten GJ, Burgess WP, Gray LV, et al. Prevention of contrast-induced nephropathy with sodium bicarbonate: a randomized controlled trial. *JAMA* 2004;291(19):2328–2334.

Oldenburg WA, Lau LL, Rodenberg TJ, et al. Acute mesenteric ischemia: a clinical review. *Arch Intern Med* 2004;164(10):1054–1062.

Pace BW, Bank S, Wise L, et al. Amylase isoenzymes in the acute abdomen: an adjunct in those patients with elevated total amylase. *Am J Gastroenterol* 1985;80(11):898–901.

Rivers E, Nguyen B, Havstad S, et al. Early goal-directed therapy in the treatment of severe sepsis and septic shock. *N Engl J Med* 2001;345(19):1368–1377.

Taourel PG, Deneuville M, Pradel JA, et al. Acute mesenteric ischemia: diagnosis with contrast-enhanced CT. *Radiology* 1996;199(3):632–636.

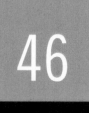

46 Bowel Obstruction

Vishal Bansal and Raul Coimbra

INTRODUCTION

Bowel obstruction is a common indication for surgical consultation. The source of obstruction may be within the lumen of the bowel itself (i.e., neoplasm), the result of pathology external to the bowel (i.e., adhesions), or secondary to anatomic abnormalities (i.e., hernia). Although symptoms may be similar, it is important to establish whether the small or large intestine is obstructed since the differential diagnosis of bowel obstruction, management, and treatment vary according to anatomic location. A careful H&P, coupled with select radiologic imaging is often sufficient to distinguish large bowel from small bowel obstruction.

I. DEFINITIONS

  A. **Partial bowel obstruction**—bowel lumen is narrowed but permits passage of some air and fluid as evidenced by flatus or distal gas radiographically.

  B. **Complete bowel obstruction**—lumen is totally occluded and does not allow passage of air or fluid as evidenced by a lack of flatus or distal gas radiographically.

  C. **Simple bowel obstruction**—lumen is partially or completely obstructed without compromise of intestinal blood flow.

  D. **Complicated bowel obstruction**—blood flow to a portion of bowel is compromised, either from increased intraluminal pressure interrupting venous outflow, or interruption of mesenteric flow by twisting or entrapment.

  E. **Closed loop obstruction**—outflow of bowel contents obstructed at both ends of bowel preventing prograde and retrograde decompression which leads to more rapid distension and increased likelihood of bowel ischemia.

  F. **Volvulus**—a segment of intestine twists about its mesentery.

II. INITIAL EVALUATION

  A. Patients who present with bowel obstruction typically require intravascular volume repletion. Depending on the duration of symptoms and level of obstruction, patients will present with severe volume depletion. Concurrent with diagnostic evaluation, early fluid resuscitation should be instituted.

  1. Initial resuscitation begins with isotonic fluids.

  2. The frequently present potassium deficiency is corrected with potassium chloride after restoration of intravascular volume, usually noted by the return of adequate urine output.

  3. Treatment with sodium bicarbonate is only a temporizing measure that should be avoided.

  B. Adjuncts to resuscitation, including nasogastric decompression and bladder catheter placement, are beneficial in all but the mildest cases of bowel obstruction. Invasive monitoring may be indicated in patients with cardiac, pulmonary, or renal insufficiency.

  C. Evaluation for the possibility of a complicated obstruction should take first priority in the patient with bowel obstruction. These patients require few if any imaging studies and treatment centers on rapid resuscitation and prompt exploratory laparotomy. Although there are no specific findings or diagnostic tests which confirm or exclude strangulating obstruction, the following findings are worrisome for this diagnosis and should prompt consideration for urgent intervention.

1. **Physical findings**—fever, severe continuous abdominal pain, tachycardia, rebound tenderness, and abdominal rigidity.
2. **Laboratory findings**—acidosis, leukocytosis.
3. **Radiologic findings of complicated obstruction**—Pneumatosis intestinalis, portal venous gas, or pneumoperitoneum suggest that necrosis has already occurred. Thumbprinting, loss of mucosal pattern, and bowel wall gas are also ominous findings that usually warrant surgical exploration.

III. SMALL BOWEL OBSTRUCTION
A. Etiology

1. **Adhesions.** Post-operative adhesions account for 70% of SBOs. A history of a previous intra-abdominal operation is suggestive. A history of other pathology (without previous abdominal operation) such as perforated peptic ulcer disease, diverticulitis, pelvic inflammatory disease, or a history of radiation may cause peritoneal scarring and omental adhesions which serve as a nidus for SBO.
2. **Hernias.** Incarcerated hernias are the second most common etiology of SBO; and the most common cause in patients without previous abdominal surgery. Inguinal, umbilical, ventral, or femoral hernias are readily identifiable on physical examination. Computed tomography (CT) may help diagnose partial incarcerations (Spigelian or Richter's hernia), paraesophageal, or internal hernial defects.
3. **Neoplasms.** Neoplasms (most often benign in small bowel) can serve as an obstructing lesion or as an anatomic lead point for an intussusception. Suspicion for a neoplasm is best detected on CT, small bowel follow through or occasionally capsule endoscopy.
4. **Crohn's disease.** A known history of inflammatory bowel disease coupled with CT or endoscopic imaging is usually diagnostic. Etiology may be from acute exacerbation, chronic stricture, intra-abdominal abscess, or enteric fistula.
5. **Intussusception.** A viral prodrome often with mesenteric lymphadenopathy, Meckel's diverticulum, or intestinal neoplasm may lead to intussusception. CT shows a "target" sign representing the proximal small bowel intussusceptum telescoping within the intussuscipiens.
6. **Gallstone ileus.** Commonly occurs in elderly and infirmed patients, more commonly female, with undiagnosed chronic cholecystitis causing a cholo-enteric fistula. Plain abdominal x-rays may reveal a stone in the right lower quadrant. CT may demonstrate pneumobilia or an obstructing gallstone at the ileocecal valve.
7. **Foreign bodies.** Foreign objects and migrating bezoars are most often seen in the pediatric or psychiatric population. History and imaging is diagnostic.

B. Presentation and initial assessment. The most important determination to make during the initial assessment is if the patient has findings consistent with bowel strangulation, gangrenous/ischemic bowel, or peritonitis. Patients with these findings should undergo immediate exploration without further diagnostic modalities.

1. The clinical presentation is an important clue to etiology and management. Patients usually present with colicky abdominal pain, distension, nausea, and vomiting with obstipation. In proximal obstruction, vomiting can be severe and patients may not be distended. Often, especially with adhesive disease, patients have had previous similar episodes.
2. History should address previous operative procedures or abdominal pathology given the likelihood of adhesions as the cause. In the absence of this history, adhesive disease is not likely and other etiologies must be considered. Other past medical history such as hernia, Crohn's disease, history of radiation, and recent viral illness should be elicited. The adult patient presenting with a bowel obstruction in the absence of previous abdominal surgery or hernia on examination generally has an anatomic cause for the obstruction which will require surgery.
3. Physical examination should be focused to detect findings of peritonitis or devitalized small bowel. Additionally, observe previous surgical scars or hernias. No other diagnostic modality should be undertaken if peritonitis has been documented; these patients should be explored expeditiously. In patients without peritoneal signs, degree of distension and severity or absence of abdominal pain is

important to document and follow serially. The patient with complete bowel obstruction or closed loop obstruction should undergo early operation. Patients with incomplete bowel obstruction without signs of peritonitis may be admitted for serial examination.

C. Laboratory abnormalities. Most laboratory values are non-specific and often normal, even in the face of a closed loop obstruction or bowel ischemia. A complete blood count (CBC) and an electrolyte panel may be helpful in management.

  1. CBC. Follow the white blood cell count in patients managed non-operatively. An initially high or rising leukocytosis should be cause of concern for ischemic bowel and exploration should be considered. Importantly, a normal CBC does not preclude bowel ischemia.

  2. Electrolyte panel. Electrolyte abnormalities may be significant, especially hypokalemia, in proximal SBO with intense vomiting. A rising serum creatinine may be a result of dehydration.

D. Radiographic evaluation. Radiographic evaluation may help delineate the anatomic location and degree of obstruction. An acute abdominal x-ray (AXR) may be the only study required, especially if adhesive disease is the etiology of the SBO. Abdominal CT often may help direct management.

  1. AXR. Plain abdominal x-ray films include a supine and an upright view in addition to a plain chest film. The presence of dilated loops of small bowel ("stack of coins") and air–fluid levels on the upright view is suggestive of an SBO (Fig. 46-1).

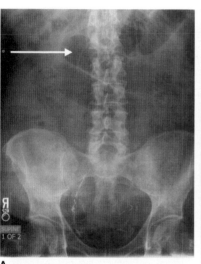

A

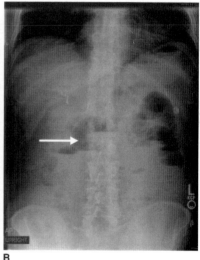

B

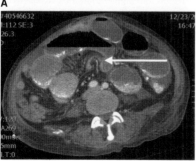

C

Figure 46-1. Abdominal imaging showing a high grade small bowel obstruction. **A:** Supine abdominal x-ray. Notice the several loops of distended bowel (*arrow*). **B:** An upright film with the arrow marking a fluid meniscus sign within the bowel. **C:** The corresponding CT imaging. The arrow demonstrates a clear transition point with proximal small bowel dilation and distal small bowel collapse.

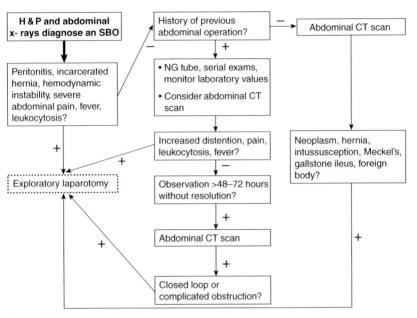

Figure 46-2. Suggested algorithm for management of an SBO.

The presence of air in the colon and rectum should have little consequence directing management unless serial AXRs show migration or an increase in colorectal air.

2. **CT.** Intravenous contrast improves accuracy by delineating vasculature, mesentery, and bowel wall. Oral contrast may exacerbate abdominal pain or increase vomiting and should be used cautiously or preferably not at all. CT imaging may show a distinct "transition point" with dilated proximal bowel and decompressed bowel distally. Imaging may also reveal a "target sign" suggestive of intussusception. CT findings suggestive of a closed loop obstruction include "mesenteric swirling" or a distinctly enlarged U- or C-shaped segment of bowel. Significant ascites, pneumatosis intestinalis or portal venous gas are suggestive of severe intestinal ischemia or necrosis.

E. **Treatment (Fig. 46-2)**
   1. **Adhesions.** Patients without signs of strangulation or complete obstruction can be managed non-operatively if post-surgical abdominal adhesions are the likely etiology. In these patients, non-operative management with nasogastric decompression and appropriate fluid resuscitation succeeds in 70% to 75%. Physical examination, radiologic imaging and laboratory values can help delineate complete versus partial obstruction or strangulation. However ischemic bowel may be present without significant laboratory abnormalities. Clinical intuition and experience cannot be overlooked.
      a. Non-operative management consists of nasogastric decompression, serial abdominal examinations, and daily laboratory values. Vital signs, urine output (Foley catheter), and nasogastric output are carefully recorded.
      b. Isotonic IV fluid resuscitation and correction of electrolyte abnormalities is initiated. Significant hypovolemia secondary to sequestration of fluid within dilated bowel is common. An elevated serum creatinine or elevated BUN/creatinine ratio may be indicative of dehydration severity.

c. Increasing abdominal pain, peritonitis, distension, fever, leukocytosis, or persistent acidosis may indicate strangulation and exploration is indicated.

d. Duration of non-operative SBO management is controversial. 80% of patients with non-operative management resolve their SBO within 48 hours (when due to adhesive disease). Patients with continued abdominal distention and lack of bowel function have little chance of resolving after 72 hours and operative management often becomes necessary.

2. Non-adhesive causes. Outside of adhesive disease, SBO does not usually resolve without operative exploration. The operative approach varies according to causative etiology. An initial laparoscopic approach may be a helpful adjunct for diagnosis and in some instances for definitive operative repair.

a. The operative approach for an incarcerated hernia varies depending on type and location of the hernia. Inguinal or femoral hernias are best approached through an inguinal incision whereas umbilical or incisional hernias are best approached directly over the hernia site. Patients with peritonitis or suspected bowel necrosis should undergo prompt laparotomy.

b. Intestinal neoplasms can cause direct obstruction of the lumen or be a lead point for intussusception. In these cases, en bloc resection of the affected bowel with primary anastomosis is optimal. In select cases of severe intra-abdominal disease, such as diffuse metastases, the obstruction may be best relieved by bypass or diversion.

c. SBO from intussusception is usually resected en bloc. SBO caused by intussusception that resolves should be evaluated for neoplastic disease through either a small bowel follow through or capsule endoscopy.

d. Meckel's diverticulum can either be resected with a small portion of proximal and distal bowel or by diverticulectomy.

e. Gallstone ileus is best approached through an enterotomy proximal to where the gallstone is impacted in the ileum, milk the gallstone to this site and extract the gallstone. A cholecystectomy with takedown of the cholo-duodenal fistula should not be performed at the time of initial operation.

f. Bowel inflammation (Crohn's, radiation enteritis) is usually self-limiting and treated medically. Chronic strictures may require operative resection or strictureplasty (see Chapter 52).

IV. LARGE BOWEL OBSTRUCTION. Unlike an SBO, a large bowel obstruction (LBO) is rarely caused by adhesive disease. Therefore, proximal decompression and observation is unlikely to be therapeutic without operative intervention. LBO may occur gradually as with tumor, or progress acutely as with volvulus. As in SBO, LBO can cause severely dilated and ischemic bowel leading to perforation. The cecum is usually the site of perforation given the larger luminal radius, the thinnest wall and accordingly greatest wall tension (Law of Laplace). Patients with impending perforation usually have cecal distention >12 cm in diameter.

A. Etiology

1. Neoplasm. A malignant tumor narrowing the colonic lumen is the leading cause of LBO. LBO occurs most commonly from a tumor in the sigmoid colon (75%) the transverse colon, splenic flexure or left colon; obstruction from right sided malignancies occur less commonly because of the wider diameter of the colonic lumen. Rectal cancers or occasionally large anal cancers can also be a cause. Patients may report a history of gradually narrowing stools, or blood per rectum. Chronic obstipation is frequently encountered.

2. Volvulus. Sigmoid volvulus can be characterized by an "omega loop" sign or a "coffee bean" sign on plain abdominal x-ray. Patients are often elderly with a large, redundant sigmoid colon. Recurrence rates are 50% to 90% if simple endoscopic decompression is performed without surgical resection. Cecal volvulus occurs secondary to congenital non-fixation of the right colon resulting in torsion and a closed loop obstruction (cecal bascule). The small bowel can also be dilated and is sometimes included within the torsion.

3. **Diverticulitis.** Both acute and chronic diverticulitis can cause LBO from inflammation or stricture, respectively. Differentiating from malignant causes may not be obvious during initial presentation. Endoscopy for tissue biopsy and CT may be helpful.

4. **Inflammatory bowel disease (IBD)** (see Chapter 52). Both Crohn's and ulcerative colitis may cause LBO. Medical therapy may help with acute obstructive inflammation. Chronic obstruction may be secondary to stricture. Malignancy must be excluded.

5. **Foreign body.** Foreign objects such as sex toys can cause both obstruction and acute rectal perforation. The obstructed object may need to be retracted under a general anesthetic or occasionally by laparotomy and colotomy for proximal removal.

6. **Colonic pseudo-obstruction (Ogilvie's syndrome).** Generally occurs in hospitalized or immobilized patients. Narcotic use, prolonged bed rest, electrolyte abnormalities, and other medications contribute. These patients rarely require operative intervention. Gastrografin enemas or endoscopy help exclude mechanical obstruction.

7. **Fecal impaction.** Commonly occurs in elderly or institutionalized patients. Patients often require manual disimpaction since enemas or laxatives are rarely helpful in the acute setting. Evaluation for underlying malignancy is important.

B. **Presentation and initial assessment.** Complete LBO is an operative emergency. Delay may lead to ongoing colonic dilation with ischemia or perforation.

1. Patients often present with nausea and abdominal discomfort as well as obstipation for several days. Timing of obstructive symptoms is important as is quality and location of accompanying symptoms such as pain or hematochezia. History should also address previous colonic endoscopy, episodes of diverticulitis, or history of IBD.

2. Physical examination should determine degree of distension and assess for peritonitis. The presence of peritonitis mandates prompt laparotomy without need for extensive radiographic evaluation. A rectal examination may allow digital palpation of anal or low rectal tumors.

C. **Radiographic and adjunct evaluation.** An AXR can be diagnostic, as in cases of sigmoid volvulus, as well as evaluate the severity of obstruction (Fig. 46-3). CT may help distinguish the obstructed segment of colon. In cases of malignancy, CT may also determine tumor size or distal metastasis. Contrast enemas have limited value with adequate CT unless differentiating pseudo-obstruction from anatomic obstruction is a concern. Endoscopy is important for tissue diagnosis and assessing for malignancy. In a stable patient, without evidence of bowel ischemia, endoscopic decompression is the first line therapy for sigmoid volvulus.

D. **Treatment (Fig. 46-4)**

1. LBO is unlikely to resolve without operative intervention. Patients with complete obstructive symptoms or with evidence of peritonitis, perforation or ischemic bowel need urgent laparotomy. Partial obstruction, or near complete obstruction may undergo further imaging or endoscopy to determine exact anatomic location of the obstruction or to obtain tissue for pathology.

2. Colonic preparation is usually ineffective and can increase colonic distention in LBO. Lack of colonic preparation should not preclude primary anastomosis in suitable cases of partial obstruction with minimal to moderate proximal dilation. Some have recommended on table colonic lavage, particularly with inspissated feces proximal to a long standing obstruction. However, the benefit of on-table lavage is not well supported.

3. Endoscopic decompression is the first line therapy for a sigmoid volvulus without signs of colonic ischemia. However, a 40% to 50% recurrence rate is expected within the first year. In the face of severe or recurrent sigmoid volvulus, operative intervention is the treatment of choice with sigmoidectomy and Hartmann's pouch. In cases without significant proximal colonic dilation, a primary anastomosis can be safely performed.

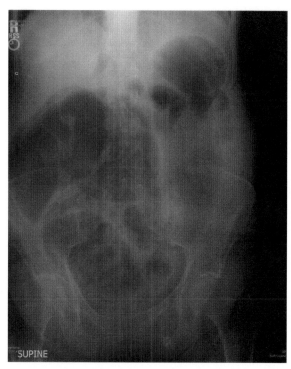

Figure 46-3. Supine abdominal x-ray showing a large bowel obstruction secondary to a large rectal cancer. Notice the proximal sigmoid colon has both large amounts of stool and air.

4. LBO from diverticulitis or diverticular stricture should undergo resection. In acute diverticulitis, the most conservative and well-supported option is sigmoidectomy with descending end colostomy (Hartmann's procedure). A single-stage operation with intraoperative colonic lavage and primary anastomosis has been reported in selected patients. Chronic diverticular stricture can usually be resected with a primary anastomosis.

5. LBOs from malignancy should be resected.
   a. The extent of the resection is determined by tumor location and size. Masses at the hepatic flexure should undergo an extended right hemicolectomy with primary anastomosis. Tumors at the transverse colon, splenic flexure, descending or sigmoid colon undergo wide segmental resection. The decision for primary anastomosis versus proximal colostomy depends on the severity of proximal colonic dilation and degree of fecal impaction. Proximal colostomy with mucous fistula or a blind distal pouch is a safe option.
   b. Rectal tumors that are partially obstructing should undergo neoadjuvant chemoradiation therapy for the goal of decreasing tumor burden and a future low anterior resection with primary anastomosis. Obstructing rectal tumors fixed to surrounding tissue are difficult to resect primarily. These patients should undergo proximal diversion with chemoradiation if appropriate. Endoluminal stents placed for obstructing rectal tumors may provide a temporary solution and allow elective resection at a later date. Large tumor burden with metastatic disease and significant local invasion should undergo proximal diversion for purposes of palliation.

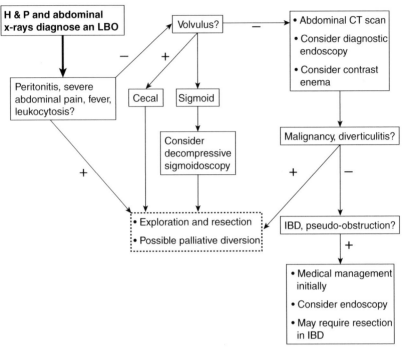

Figure 46-4. Suggested algorithm for management of an LBO.

6. Pseudo-obstruction rarely requires operative intervention. Endoscopic colonoscopy may be helpful to decompress severe dilation. Neostigmine has been also shown to induce colonic motility and relieve the pseudo-obstruction. Mechanical obstruction from tumor must be excluded which can be accomplished by a contrast enema.

AXIOMS

- Concurrent with diagnostic evaluation of the patient with a bowel obstruction, early fluid resuscitation should be instituted.
- Early in the course of evaluation, the obstruction should be differentiated as small bowel obstruction or LBO. Etiology and management differ.
- Small bowel obstruction is most commonly due to adhesive disease.
- The adult patient presenting with small bowel obstruction without previous surgery or evidence of a hernia has an anatomic cause for the obstruction and generally requires prompt operation.
- The most common causes for large bowel obstruction are cancer and diverticular disease.

Suggested Readings

Beck DE, Opelka FG, Bailey HR, et al. Incidence of small-bowel obstruction and adhesiolysis after open colorectal and general surgery. *Dis Colon Rectum* 1999;42:241–248.

Coufal NG, Kansagra AP, Doucet J, et al. Gastric trichobezoar causing intermittent small bowel obstruction: report of a case and review of the literature. *Case Report Med* 2011;2011:217570.

Dalal KM, Gollub MJ, Miner TJ, et al. Management of patients with malignant bowel obstruction and stage IV colorectal cancer. *J Palliat Med* 2011;14:822–828.

Ellis H, Moran BJ, Thompson JN, et al. Adhesion-related hospital readmissions after abdominal and pelvic surgery: a retrospective cohort study. *Lancet* 1999;353:1476–1480.

Ellozy SH, Harris MT, Bauer JJ, et al. Early postoperative small-bowel obstruction: a prospective evaluation in 242 consecutive abdominal operations. *Dis Colon Rectum* 2002;45:1214–1217.

Kahi CJ, Rex DK. Bowel obstruction and pseudo-obstruction. *Gastroenterol Clin North Am* 2003;32:1229–1247.

Nauta RJ. Advanced abdominal imaging is not required to exclude strangulation if complete small bowel obstructions undergo prompt laparotomy. *J Am Coll Surg* 2005;200:904–911.

Oren D, Atamanalp SS, Aydinli B, et al. An algorithm for the management of sigmoid colon volvulus and the safety of primary resection: experience with 827 cases. *Dis Colon Rectum* 2007;50:489–497.

Ponec RJ, Saunders MD, Kimmey MB. Neostigmine for the treatment of acute colonic pseudo-obstruction. *N Engl J Med* 1999;341:137–141.

Sarr MG, Bulkley GB, Zuidema GD. Preoperative recognition of intestinal strangulation obstruction. Prospective evaluation of diagnostic capability. *Am J Surg* 1983;145:176–182.

Sheedy SP, Earnest F 4th, Fletcher JG, et al. CT of small-bowel ischemia associated with obstruction in emergency department patients: diagnostic performance evaluation. *Radiology* 2006;241:729–736.

Strodel WE, Brothers T. Colonoscopic decompression of pseudo-obstruction and volvulus. *Surg Clin North Am* 1989;69:1327–1335.

Szomstein S, Lo Menzo E, Simpfendorfer C, et al. Laparoscopic lysis of adhesions. *World J Surg* 2006;30:535–540.

Zielinski MD, Eiken PW, Bannon MP, et al. Small bowel obstruction-who needs an operation? A multivariate prediction model. *World J Surg* 2010;34:910–919.

47 Gastrointestinal Bleeding

Kent Zettel and A. James Moser

I. GASTROINTESTINAL BLEEDING

A. Overview.

Blood loss into the gastrointestinal (GI) tract from either proximal to the ligament of Treitz (upper GI bleed) or distal (lower GI bleed) is a consequence of many potential causes and has wide array of symptoms, ranging from asymptomatic hemoccult positive stools, recurrent intermittent blood loss, to hemorrhagic shock. For the purpose of this chapter, a general view of gastrointestinal bleeding will focus on the sources of active gastrointestinal bleeding.

B. Statistics.

Due to the advent of proton-pump inhibitors and H2 inhibitors, the incidence of peptic ulcer bleeding is decreasing, with most of these episodes associated with NSAID use and in the elderly (68% of cases of peptic ulcer are seen in those over the age of 60 years). More recent estimates place the incidence of upper GI bleeding at 89 per 100,000 population annually, with the decrease in incidence found only in those less than 70 years of age. Gastrointestinal bleeding is more common in men, who use NSAIDs and aspirin-related products, and the elderly, who are at an increased risk of death.

C. Initial patient history and physical evaluation

1. Due to the multiple etiologies of GI bleeding, seek information on risk factors and comorbid conditions. Keep an open mind for rare causes of GI bleeding, as atypical bleeding sources may present in the manner of typical etiologies.

2. The symptoms of GI hemorrhage range from an asymptomatic positive fecal occult blood test to hypovolemic shock with cardiovascular collapse. The severity of vomiting in upper GIB ranges from frank blood (hematemesis) to coffee ground emesis (hemoglobin degraded by gastric acid). The most common presentation in the hospital setting for lower GIB is hematochezia (gross blood seen either on toilet paper or mixed with stool), although it may also present as melena, anemia, abdominal pain, or hemodynamic instability.

3. Key questions include presence of abdominal pain, weight loss, change in bowel habits, vomiting blood, blood per rectum, color of vomit or feces, and clots in their vomitus or feces.

4. Evaluate for medications that interfere with the clotting cascade: Aspirin, novel anti-platelet agents such as clopidogrel, dabigatran, NSAID, enoxaparin, heparin, warfarin.

5. Past medical history:

   a. Ask about bleeding-specific diseases. Prior GIB, portal hypertension due to liver disease or Budd–Chiari, alcohol abuse causing gastritis, *Helicobacter pylori* infection or treatment for known peptic ulcer disease (PUD), factor VIII deficiency, Von Willebrand disease.

   b. Next, seek general diseases that may cause bleeding. Prior operations, GI cancers such as colorectal cancer, gastrointestinal stromal tumors (GISTs), abdominal aortic aneurysm surgery, inflammatory bowel disease (IBD), radiation enteritis, pancreatitis (pseudocysts causing pseudoaneurysm and hemosuccus pancreaticus, splenic vein thrombosis causing sinistral portal hypertensive gastropathy), esophageal varices.

    c. Check for significant comorbidities that may impair resuscitation or be exacerbated by resuscitation. Renal failure, congestive heart failure, myocardial infarction, underlying coagulopathy, transfusion reactions.

6. Family history. Cancer (colon, pancreatic, gastric).

7. Physical examination. Pay particular attention to the following:

    a. Vital signs and orthostatic vital sign assessment to detect hypovolemia or shock.

    b. Scleral icterus may identify underlying hepatic dysfunction, while pale conjunctivae demonstrate the degree of anemia.

    c. Look for jugular venous distension and sternal evaluation for prior sternotomy scar to evaluate for signs of cardiac failure, murmurs from an underlying cardiomyopathy, previous infarction, rhythm, or prior cardiac surgery.

    d. Abdominal examination with the focus of

        i. Signs of liver disease: Hepatomegaly, jaundice, caput medusa, liver masses (primary or metastatic disease).

        ii. Splenomegaly: Coagulopathy or portal hypertension.

        iii. Scars indicating previous operations.

        iv. Focal tenderness or masses: Perforation, strictures, or cancer.

    e. Asterixis suggests encephalopathy and potential end-stage liver disease, while agitation or depressed sensorium, may be from shock.

    f. Rectal examination is targeted for a mass, tenderness, hemorrhoids, presence of stool or blood (overt or by guaiac testing), hemorrhoids, or fissures.

8. Young and athletic individuals can tolerate more severe stress than their counterparts before demonstrating signs of shock, which may be more abrupt.

D. Causes of gastrointestinal bleeding

1. The most common cause of melena (digested blood per rectum) is an upper GI source (five times more common than a lower GI source).

2. Population-specific sources of gastrointestinal bleeding include the following:

    a. Young patients. IBD, Meckel's diverticulum, HIV/CMV infection.

    b. Middle-aged patients. IBD, polyps, cancer, hemorrhoids, ulcers, varices, diverticulosis.

    c. Older patients. Same as the middle-aged patient but also including AVM and ischemia.

3. Use the history to help identify the cause (i.e., history of surgery and anticoagulation with anastomotic bleeding; an alcoholic with esophageal variceal bleeding; excessive NSAID use leading to an ulcer; or recent weight loss, pain, and thin stools that may indicate the presence of a bleeding colon cancer).

4. Use the output to judge the location of the bleeding.

    a. Hematemesis or coffee ground emesis imply an upper source or one that is proximal to the Ligament of Treitz.

    b. Hematochezia and clots per rectum imply a lower source or a very brisk upper source.

    c. Melena is black, tarry stool that is usually from an upper source. Fifty cubic centimeters of blood can produce this color and it is foul smelling (unlike the stool from a patient taking bismuth compounds that may have a similar black color).

    d. Note that left colon bleeding is usually red; right colon bleeding typically produces melena, unless brisk.

5. To determine the cause of a bleed, consider site specific pathology in combination with the four main categories of pathology: Vascular lesions, inflammation, cancer, and specific anatomic lesions.

    a. Vascular lesions: Dieulafoy lesions, AVMs, varices.

    b. Inflammation: IBD.

    c. Cancer: Colon cancer, gastric cancer, polyps.

    d. Anatomic lesions: Diverticulosis, Meckel's diverticulum.

E. Upper gastrointestinal bleeding sources

  1. Esophagus. The most common are varices, Mallory–Weiss tear at the gastroesophageal junction (most will stop spontaneously), erosive esophagitis, cancer, Boerhaave's syndrome.

  2. Stomach. A highly vascular organ with seven named arteries and perfused via many collaterals.

  a. Gastric ulcers. Associated with aspirin, NSAID use or abuse, *H. pylori* infection, and gastric hypersecretion.

  b. Type I is a single ulcer, usually on the lesser cure. Type II (gastric body ulcer in combination to a duodenal ulcer) and type III (prepyloric gastric ulcer) peptic ulcers are associated with increased gastric acid secretion. Type IV ulcers are juxtaesophageal.

  c. Other causes. Bleeding from pseudoaneurysm due to pancreatic pseudocyst, lymphoma, cancer, polyp, GIST, Dieulafoy's lesion, sinistral portal hypertensive gastropathy due to varices caused by splenic vein thrombosis, post-surgical marginal ulceration.

  3. Duodenum

  a. Ulcers here cause 50% of upper GIB; most are in the duodenal bulb and if posterior involve the gastroduodenal artery.
  A rare cause of duodenal ulcers is from hypergastrinemia from Zollinger–Ellison syndrome, which is associated with multiple duodenal ulcers, distal duodenal or proximal jejunal ulcers and ulcers recalcitrant to medical therapy.

  b. Other causes include cancer, diverticulum, hemobilia, aortoenteric fistula (after an abdominal aortic aneurysm repair).

F. Lower sources of GIB.

  1. Most (80%) will stop spontaneously, but 25% will recur. Most present in the elderly (>65 years) with medical comorbidities, making the patient less able to tolerate the consequences of major bleeding. Bleeding from a lower source is more likely to present as bright red blood per rectum. Brisk GI bleeding from an upper gastrointestinal source can also present with bloody stool and is often associated with hemodynamic compromise. About 10% of lower GIBs will have no identifiable source, and up to 40% of lower GIBs have more than one potential source.

  2. Small bowel

  a. Meckel's diverticulum (omphalomesenteric remnant). These are located within 2 ft of the ileocecal valve in the ileum and may contain acid-secreting gastric mucosa. The gastric mucosa is the target of technetium-99m during a "Meckel's scan."

  b. Other causes include intussusception, sprue, IBD, AVMs associated with radiation enteritis, cancer, entero-enteral fistula, melanoma, lymphoma, infection, ischemia, small bowel diverticula, Zollinger–Ellison syndrome causing jejunal ulcers, aortoenteric fistulae.

  3. Large bowel

  a. Diverticulosis. 30% to 50% of diverticular bleeding is massive; 25% of bleeds will recur after the initial spontaneous resolution.

  b. AVM cause 20% to 30% of massive lower GIB cases. These are detected later in life (age 60 years or older) when ectatic and dilated vessels become thin-walled. The right colon is more often affected and they are usually multiple.

  c. IBD. The majority of ulcerative colitis patients and one- third of Crohn's patients will present with a GIB.

  d. Cancer. Hemorrhage can arise from colonic polyps or cancers.

  4. Rectum/perianal disease including fistulae, fissures, hemorrhoids (with or without associated liver disease), and rectal prolapse. Many patients have a previous history, and an external examination with anoscopy may be helpful.

II. INITIAL RESUSCITATION AND DEVELOPMENT OF A TREATMENT PLAN

A. Initial resuscitation.

  1. Check the ABCs, start two large-bore (16 gauge preferred) IVs, and resuscitate initially with 1 to 2 L of crystalloid.

TABLE 47-1	The Glasgow-Blatchford Score Assess the Likelihood That a Patient with an UGIB will Require Intervention. A Score of 0 Identifies Low Risk Patients Who Can be Managed in an Outpatient Setting

Risk factor	Score
BUN	
≥6.5–<8.0	2
≥8.0–<10.0	3
≥10.0–<25	4
≥25	6
Hemoglobin (men, women) (g/dL)	
≥12.0–<13, men; ≥10.0–<12.0, women	1
≥10.0–<12.0, men	3
<10.0, men; <10.0, women	6
Systolic blood pressure (mm Hg)	
100–109	1
90–99	2
<90	3
Other	
Pulse ≥100 beats/min	1
Presentation with melena	1
Presentation with syncope	2
Hepatic disease	2
Cardiac failure	2

    a. Recognize that if vital signs are initially profoundly abnormal or fail to respond to first fluid infusions, the patient is likely to need transfusion. Failure to respond to resuscitation also raises the likelihood that operative intervention will be required.

    b. Determine the degree of shock and integrate into the decision making process (i.e., class III shock in an 80-year-old woman will need a far more aggressive plan than a 20-year-old with blood visible upon wiping).

    c. Large bore central venous catheters may be indicated for unstable patients or when peripheral access is limited.

B. Develop a treatment plan

    1. Risk-stratify the patient: Determine degree of anemia which can be tolerated and the best setting in which to resuscitate the patient. Several scoring systems have been developed to identify high-risk patients who will benefit from urgent intervention. Scoring systems for upper GIB include the Blatchford score (Table 47-1) and the Rockall score (Table 47-2).

    a. The Blatchford score (Table 47-1) stratifies the risk that a patient will require intervention for GI bleeding. Patients with Blatchford score of zero may be discharged without endoscopic therapy and treated in outpatient setting.

    b. The Rockall score (Tables 47-2 and 47-3) evaluates the risk of mortality of a patient with GI bleeding. Although this is a good predictor of mortality, it does not adequately assess the risk of need for intervention.

    2. Location. Unstable patients, elderly patients, or patients with signs of massive hemorrhage should be transferred to the ICU. Other relatively more stable patients may be best managed in a monitored floor setting.

    3. Laboratory evaluation. There are no set action thresholds but the following are reasonable goals:

    a. Hemoglobin should be maintained ≥7 g/dL. A hemoglobin level ≥10 g/dL in a patient with active acute coronary syndrome is appropriate.

TABLE 47-2	The Rockall Score is a Screening Evaluation to Assess the Risk of Mortality of a Patient with an UGIB. The Full Score Requires Endoscopy. The Maximum Score Prior to Endoscopy is 7, and After Endoscopic Findings, the Maximum Score is 11. The Pre-endoscopy Rockall Score is a Poor Predictor of Need for Endoscopic Therapy in Upper GIB. The Glasgow-Blatchford is a Better Predictor of the Need for Endoscopic Therapy.

Risk factor	Score
Age (y)	
<60	0
60–79	1
≥80	2
Shock	
No shock, SBP >100 mm Hg, HR <100 beats/min	0
Tachycardia (HR ≥100 beats/min)	1
Hypotension (SBP <100 mm Hg)	2
Comorbidities	
None	0
Cardiac failure, ischemic heart disease, any major comorbidity	2
Renal failure, liver failure, disseminated malignancy	3
Diagnosis	
Mallory–Weiss	0
All other diagnoses	1
Malignancy of upper GI tract	2
Stigmata of recent hemorrhage	
None	0
Blood in upper GI tract, adherent clot, or spurting vessel	2

b. Do not wait for a specific hemoglobin or hematocrit value before transfusing the patient who is rapidly exsanguinating. Also, operate or intervene early on these unstable patients.

c. An initial hemoglobin and hematocrit evaluation can be falsely elevated due to isovolemic blood loss with intravascular volume depletion, making serial hemoglobin evaluation important.

TABLE 47-3	Mortality Associated with Rockall Score Calculated Prior to Endoscopy and Afterward, as Well as Mortality Associated with Rebleeding After Endoscopic Treatment

Rockall score	Pre-endoscopic mortality	Post-endoscopic mortality	Mortality of rebleeding
0	0.2%	0%	—
1	2.4%	0%	—
2	5.6%	0.2%	—
3	11.0%	2.9%	10%
4	24.6%	5.3%	15.8%
5	39.6%	10.8%	22.9%
6	48.9%	17.3%	33.3%
7	50.0%	27.0%	43.4%
8	NA	41.1%	52.5%

d. Frequent blood draws should include serial hemoglobin/hematocrit every 4 to 6 hours as needed, platelets, coagulation profile, and (if needed) a thromboelastogram or fibrinogen level.

e. If bleeding continues despite resuscitation and therapeutic interventions, consider an underlying coagulopathy that may require a hematology consult and specific labs to be drawn. The most common cause for coagulopathy is ongoing hemorrhage and resuscitation.

f. With UGIB, an elevated BUN is commonly seen; a low MCV denotes chronic blood loss; and an elevated creatinine or cardiac enzymes identify end-organ complications that will complicate resuscitation.

4. Transfusion support

a. For larger bleeds or massive bleeds, see Chapter 7 on the massive transfusion protocol (used for those patients with an expected PRBC transfusion of greater than 10 units in 24 hours). Call the blood bank to ensure they have a specimen for a type and cross. Stay 4 units ahead and get platelets and fresh frozen plasma (FFP) ready.

b. A patient may continue to have melena and hemoccult positive stools days after the bleeding source.

c. Massive transfusion may lead to hypothermia; this is best avoided since it further impairs coagulation. Warming blankets and warmed intravenous (IV) fluids are important.

5. Chart the amount of blood products transfused to keep track of the overall scale of the resuscitation and to watch for massive transfusion syndrome or dilutional coagulopathy.

6. Interaction with other teams.

a. Upper or lower endoscopy (or both) may be required acutely and the appropriate consultant should be involved in the care of the patient immediately.

b. In all cases of massive blood loss and for unstable patients, a surgeon must be consulted immediately. A small proportion of patients may be too unstable for diagnostic testing and should be resuscitated and taken promptly to the operating room (OR). For such a patient the OR and anesthesia must be notified immediately.

7. Family. Due to the potential mortality and morbidity, the physician in charge should contact the family. Pertinent details of a history should be obtained, especially if the patient is unresponsive or intubated at the time of admission. Explain the potential need for an invasive procedure (esophagogastroduodenoscopy [EGD], colonoscopy, surgery) and get the best contact number to facilitate care.

8. The last aspect of a plan is repeated examinations and close monitoring of vital signs and lab values. Anticipating problems is far better than reacting to a decompensating patient.

III. DIAGNOSTIC TESTS

A. Diagnostic modalities that involve mobilizing the patient form the safe environment of the ICU should be limited in the critical patient with gastrointestinal hemorrhage

B. Primary modalities to determine the location of bleeding.

1. Nasogastric tube (NGT). A nasogastric lavage with 250 cc of normal sterile saline may return clots, red blood, or coffee grounds indicating an upper GIB. If it is bilious, then the pylorus is open allowing adequate sampling of the duodenal contents. The false negative rate is 25% of NG aspiration for an upper source. The usefulness of this is equivocal.

2. Esophagogastroduodenoscopy (EGD)

a. This may be both a diagnostic and therapeutic procedure. Bleeding varices may be banded or bleeding ulcers can be clipped, injected with epinephrine or coagulated with a heater probe. Based on the appearance of the ulcer or vessel, prognostic information about the rate of rebleeding can be provided.

3. Colonoscopy. Depending on the hospital and consulting GI team, a colonoscopy may be a diagnostic and therapeutic test for a lower GIB. As blood may function as a cathartic, a bowel preparation may not be necessary. In the face of a massive lower GI bleed, utility of colonoscopy may be limited due to poor visibility.

4. Anoscopy or proctoscopy. For patients with suspected perianal or rectal disease hemorrhoids, fistulas or low cancers may be seen.

5. Bleeding scan. This detects bleeding at a rate >0.5 cc/min. This test will find a source 45% of the time. The advantages are the low rate of bleeding needed to get a positive scan and that it requires no contrast. The disadvantages are that it is not therapeutic and that the patient leaves the ICU setting for an extended period. It also poorly localizes the lesion to a specific source (due to peristalsis) which in the face of pending surgery may limit its usefulness. It is not suitable for unstable patients.

6. Angiogram. Detects bleeding at a rate >1 cc/min. Similar to a bleeding scan, the patient must leave the ICU, but this test may be both diagnostic and therapeutic. It can provide good localization and a bleeding vessel may be coiled or vasopressin may be injected. Disadvantages include the administration of contrast, especially with an elderly patient with abnormal renal function, the risk of bowel infarction with coiling or vasopressin, and the patient leaving the ICU.

C. Other diagnostic tests

1. Endoscopic retrograde cholangiopancreatography (ERCP) for diagnosis of hemobilia or other biliary or pancreatic lesions.

2. Enteroclysis looking for small-bowel polyps or signs of Crohn's such as a stricture or fistula.

3. Capsule endoscopy. This is a good study for occult GI bleeding, with sensitivity of 95% and specificity of 75%. Capsule endoscopy is relatively contraindicated in patients with pacemakers and implanted cardiac defibrillators.

4. Meckel's scan.

IV. TREATMENT MODALITIES FOR GASTROINTESTINAL HEMORRHAGE

A. General Considerations

1. Most GIB will stop spontaneously. When developing a plan, the bleeding site should be localized and the risk of rebleeding determined. The algorithm for an upper GIB (Figs. 47-1 and 47-2) is different from that for a lower GIB (Fig. 47-3).

2. Procedures can be performed without mobilizing the patient, such as EGD, colonoscopy, anoscopy, or proctoscopy, are preferred in the critical patient with tenuous hemodynamic status.

3. Protection of the airway is paramount. Do not start any procedure if a patient has a tenuous airway. Such patients should be intubated to perform the necessary diagnostic and therapeutic procedures.

4. Correction of coagulopathy should be performed but do not delay endoscopic intervention; the exception is the patient on supratherapeutic anticoagulant therapy where reversal can improve conditions. Although reversal targets of an INR of <1.5 are preferred, levels of up to 2.5 are safe in patients prior to endoscopic therapy, and should not delay the evaluation.

   a. Elevated INR in those with cirrhosis does not correlate to bleeding risk and should not delay endoscopic therapy.

   b. Use of thermocoagulation is safe in patients with INR up to 2.5.

5. Delay endoscopy in patients with acute coronary syndrome or suspected perforation.

6. Even after initial endoscopic application of hemostasis, the ulcer may rebleed. There are a number of features that may predict rebleeding, including: Size >2 cm, active bleeding (especially arterial rather than venous oozing) at time of endoscopy (20%), visible non-bleeding vessel (15%), adherent clot (5%), vessel size >2 mm, ulcer location at the posterior lesser curvature of gastric wall or posterior duodenal wall.

7. Non-variceal upper GI bleeding treated with injection alone is associated with the highest repeat EGD rates due to rebleeding compared to that of thermal monotherapy and combination thermal/injection therapy. In a meta-analysis, hemostasis is better with hemoclip (86.5%), or hemoclip with injection (88.5%) than with

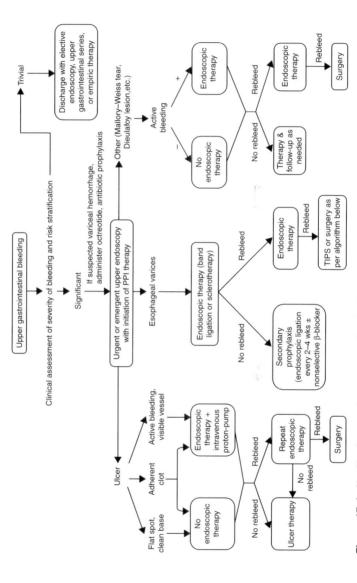

Figure 47-1. Algorithm for managing upper gastrointestinal hemorrhage.

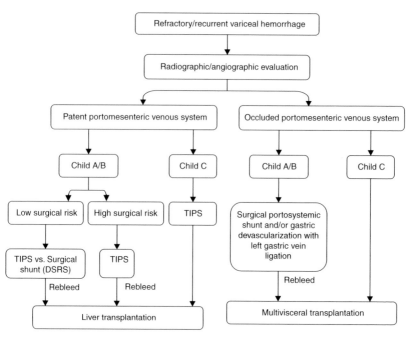

Figure 47-2. Algorithm for managing refractory variceal hemorrhage.

injection alone (75.4%). There is no difference between hemoclip and thermo-coagulation in regard to definitive hemostasis (81.2% vs. 81.5%, respectively), surgery, or mortality. Hemoclip failure occurs more commonly at the posterior duodenal wall, posterior gastric body wall, and the lesser curvature of the stomach.

8. A surgeon should perform the endoscopy or be present at the time of the endoscopy for a massive bleed or with an unstable patient for pre-operative planning purposes should the endoscopic therapeutic approach fail.

9. Hold any anticoagulation, reversing with vitamin K, plasma, prothrombin complexes, and platelets if needed. Newer antiplatelet agents (dabigatran and rivaroxaban) do not have specific reversal agents but are also shorter acting.

B. Non-variceal upper GI bleeding (Fig. 47-2).

1. For upper GIB, risk stratification should be performed early, using scales as described above, and upper endoscopy should be performed within the first 24 hours of admission.

2. Upper endoscopy is indicated for all lesions, including high-risk lesions.

   a. All blood must be aspirated and clots removed to allow full visual inspection of the target region.

   b. Injection therapy (epinephrine) should not be used alone.

   c. Clips or thermocoagulation, or sclerosant either alone or in combination with injection therapy are recommended.

3. A second look with endoscopy should be performed in instances of rebleeding. Do not do routine second look endoscopy however.

4. Start high-dose proton-pump inhibitor therapy as this may permit healing, but should not delay endoscopy. Continue it after endoscopic hemostasis, as this decreases both risk of rebleeding and mortality in patients with high-risk

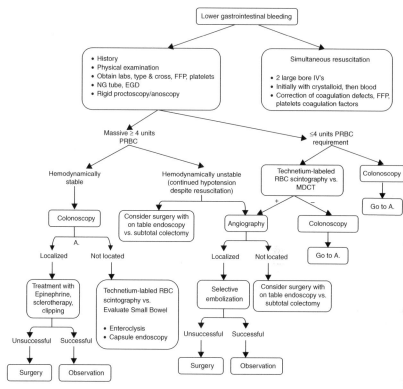

Figure 47-3. Algorithm for managing lower gastrointestinal hemorrhage.

stigmata. IV protonix is given as an 80 mg bolus and then continued as an 8 mg/h continuous infusion.

5. High-risk patients should remain hospitalized for 72 hours after endoscopic-applied hemostasis. Low risk patients may be discharged soon after endoscopy.

6. Perform endoscopic *H. Pylori* testing for all bleeding gastric ulcer patients, and treat if present with confirmation of eradication. Negative *H. Pylori* endoscopic testing should be repeated through alternative means such as stool antigen test or serum analysis.

7. Patients on cardiovascular prophylaxis should restart aspirin within 7 days (when cardiovascular risks outweigh risk of GI bleeding). Aspirin plus a proton-pump inhibitor is preferred over clopidogrel alone in the setting of recent UGI bleed.

8. With the advancement of endoscopic therapy, surgical therapy for peptic ulcer bleeding includes failure of endoscopic therapy and interventional radiology (if available) to stop bleeding and early elective/planned surgery to prevent further life-threatening rebleeding in high-risk patients.

9. Operation. If the patient is at high risk of rebleeding, has failed non-operative therapy, or may not tolerate rebleeding, operative intervention may be the best option. In such circumstances, a definitive surgical procedure is preferable to a test with a low probability of localizing the lesion (Chapters 51 and 52). Some commonly performed procedures are as follows.

10. Operative strategies for peptic ulcers include:
    a. There is much controversy over the appropriate surgical approach in regard to minimal versus definitive approach. Several prospective randomized

controlled trials have shown that definitive therapy has decreased risk of rebleeding, with similar overall mortality. Due to the advances of endoscopic therapy of bleeding peptic ulcers, those patients who require surgical therapy have more comorbidity, with higher surgical risk. As such, in the emergent setting, plication or resection of the ulcer has taken precedence over higher risk acid-reducing ("definitive") operations, which are less often necessary in the era of PPI therapy and *H. pylori* treatment. Definitive approaches can be entertained in early elective/planned operations.

b. Ulcerectomy or plication of peptic ulcer should be treated with concomitant life-long acid-suppression therapy. Gastric ulcers should be biopsied or excised.

c. Vagotomy and antrectomy is the preferred procedure for persistent gastric ulcers despite PPI therapy. The antrectomy removes the gastrin secreting cells of the stomach. This may be closed through either Billroth I, Billroth II or Roux-en-Y gastrojejunostomy.

d. Vagotomy and drainage with oversewing of the ulcer is another option. This includes a truncal vagotomy with pyloroplasty to close the defect without narrowing the gastric outlet.

11. Operative strategies for duodenal ulcers include:

a. A longitudinal incision is made across the pylorus to expose the ulcer bed after two traction sutures are placed on the pylorus to aid visualization.

b. The gastroduodenal artery is the artery most likely to bleed as a result of a posterior duodenal bulb ulcer. The GDA is oversewn with three stitches, superior, inferior, and medial to the ulcer, with 2-0 or a heavier suture (see Fig. 47-4) to occlude the GDA proximal and distal to the ulcer and prevent back-bleeding from the transverse pancreatic artery.

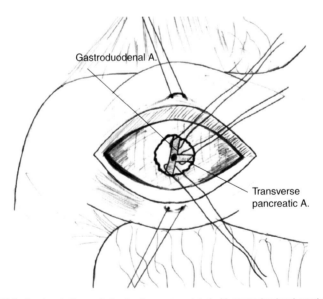

Figure 47-4. An ulcer in the posterior duodenum associated with gastroduodenal arterial bleeding needs to be oversewn with three stitches, superior, inferior, and medial to the ulcer. The superior and inferior sutures ligate the proximal and distal gastroduodenal artery, while the medial suture ligates the transverse pancreatic branch.

    c. The common bile duct should be clearly identified to ensure it is not inadvertently occluded with these suture ligatures.

    d. Vagotomy and pyloroplasty should be performed in those patients who have failed acid suppression therapy. Truncal vagotomy is preferred in the acute setting in a hemodynamically stable patient. The pyloroplasty is performed by closing the longitudinal incision transversely in a Heineke–Mikulicz fashion.

12. Angiography is an alternative to surgery and reserved for high-risk patients who cannot tolerate an operation.

C. Variceal upper GI bleeding (Fig. 47-1 and 47-2).

  1. 6-week mortality with each episode of hemorrhage is 15% to 20%, with 0% with Child's A cirrhosis to 30% in patients with Child's C cirrhosis.

  2. With volume resuscitation in the patient with underlying liver disease, keep a systolic BP lower than 90 mm Hg and tachycardia at baseline due to circulatory dysfunction and hyperdynamic circulation. The goal in these cases is a systolic BP of 90 to 100 mm Hg and pulse of 100 beats/min.

    a. Studies demonstrate that vigorous volume resuscitation can enhance variceal bleeding.

    b. There is no benefit to using colloids, including albumin, in the management of variceal bleeding.

  3. Arterial lactate is a poor measurement of systemic perfusion in cirrhotics due to delayed hepatic clearance leading to baseline abnormal levels.

  4. Start octreotide early in patients with suspected variceal hemorrhage.

    a. Start before endoscopy.

    b. Continue for 2 to 5 days.

    c. Dose—IV Octreotide is given as 50 mcg bolus, followed by 50 mcg/h continuous infusion. Repeat the bolus in the first hour if hemorrhage is uncontrolled.

    d. Vasopressin, even with nitrates, should not be used in the management of variceal hemorrhage due to the improved safety profiles of octreotide, somatostatin, and terlipressin.

  5. Perform endoscopy within the first 12 hours of bleeding from esophageal varices, with treatment either by sclerotherapy or endoscopic band ligation.

    a. Endoscopic band ligation is the procedure of choice.

    b. Endoscopic therapy should be attempted one more time if first attempt failed with preference given to endoscopic band ligation.

  6. Give antibiotic prophylaxis to all patients with variceal bleeding

    a. Norfloxacin 400 mg BID for 5 to 7 days or until discharge.

    b. Ceftriaxone 1 g daily for 5 to 7 days or until discharge.

  7. Sengstaken–Blakemore tubes should be used only in instances of massive hemorrhage with ongoing shock not amendable to IV fluid resuscitation. This should be left in place for no longer than 24 hours as a bridge for definitive therapy (Transjugular Intrahepatic Portosystemic Shunt [TIPS] or endoscopic intervention) due to associated complications of aspiration, URI, esophageal wall laceration/perforation, and pressure necrosis of the nose.

  8. Refractory variceal bleeding can be treated with either TIPS or surgical shunt, such as the splenorenal shunt.

    a. TIPS and distal splenorenal shunt are equivalent in efficacy in Child A and B cirrhotics in control of variceal bleeding, although TIPS has a higher re-intervention rate. The choice depends on availability of the surgeon and facilities for monitoring and to re-intervene when needed.

  9. Start prophylaxis against variceal hemorrhage with β-blocker + nitrate therapy before discharge

    a. Non-selective β-blocker dose should be adjusted to the maximal dose tolerated by the patient without inducing side-effects or until HR is approximately 55 beats/min

    b. Propranolol dose is initiated at 20 mg PO daily

    c. Nadolol dose is initiated at 40 mg PO daily

    d. Isosorbide mononitrate (in addition to a β-blocker) is initiated at 10 mg every night, and increased to a maximum of 20 mg BID as tolerated with maintenance systolic BP >95 mm Hg.

  10. PPI therapy is a popular choice to promote ulcer healing, although there is no evidence that it prevents post-banding ulcer bleeding.

  11. Portal hypertensive gastropathy usually presents with slow hemorrhage resulting in anemia. This is treated with iron supplementation and non-selective β-blockers. Portosystemic shunt therapy is used for recurrent hemorrhage requiring blood transfusion.

  12. Gastric varices are better treated with endoscopic obscuration with tissue adhesives such as N-butyl-2-cyanoacrylate than endoscopic band ligation.

  13. When gastroesophageal varices are seen with normal liver function and normal liver parenchyma or when portovenous thrombosis is suspected, do an angiographic evaluation or CT of abdomen and pelvis with portovenous phase.

  14. Varices secondary to pre-hepatic causes (portovenous thrombosis) can occur in advanced cirrhosis and in patients with hypercoagulable state.

    a. Obtain a hypercoagulable work-up, including testing for protein C, protein S, antithrombin III, total homocysteine levels, factor V Leiden, prothrombin and Jak-2 mutations, anticardiolipin, lupus anticoagulant, and antiphospholipid antibodies.

    b. A surgical shunt is necessary in instances of refractory variceal bleeding in association with portovenous thrombosis, as TIPS is unhelpful as it bypasses the portal system beyond the obstruction.

D. Lower GI bleeding (Fig. 47-3).

  1. Hemodynamic stabilization is the priority in managing lower GI bleeds. Once stabilized, localization of the source of bleeding is the next priority. Once the etiology has been determined, the treatment can then be provided. Angiography, bleeding scans, colonoscopy, and capsule endoscopy all aid in localizing the etiology.

  2. When hemodynamic stability cannot be achieved, emergent laparotomy is performed to both identify and treat the offending source.

    a. Criteria for emergent subtotal colectomy include >4 to 6 units of PRBC in 24 hours with continued hemodynamic instability, inability to stabilize the patient by other interventions, or inability to localize by other interventions despite continued bleeding.

    b. Reserve subtotal colectomy for those patients who meet these criteria, as it is associated with a 25% to 33% mortality compared to 7% in those who undergo segmental colectomy once bleeding has been localized.

    c. Segmental resection should only be performed once the inciting lesion has been identified as "blind" segmental resection is associated with 57% mortality and high risk of rebleeding.

  3. Place an NGT with gastric lavage in the initial evaluation of a lower GI bleed to identify an upper GIB source masquerading as a lower GIB.

  4. Perform colonoscopy early in the diagnostic work-up of the hemodynamically stable patient. The diagnostic yield of this procedure is higher when performed early in the evaluation of lower GIB.

  5. When cancer is discovered in the work-up of gastrointestinal bleeding, an oncologic resection should be performed, if possible.

AXIOMS

- Most GIB will stop spontaneously.
- The patient with active GIB must have a protected airway (intubate if needed) and be adequately volume resuscitated.
- Give blood early if vital signs are deranged or do not respond quickly to crystalloid.
- Start octreotide early in those with variceal bleeds and any hemodynamic signs of moderate/severe blood loss.
- Massive upper GIB may present with hematochezia.

- Angiography/embolization and endoscopic interventions have made the need for operative control of bleeding less common.
- Make every effort to localize the source of GIM early and prior to operation; but in the uncommon circumstance of the hemodynamically unstable patient who responds poorly to volume resuscitation, operate early to control hemorrhage.

Suggested Readings

Abe N, Takeuchi H, Yanagida O, et al. Surgical indications and procedures for bleeding peptic ulcer. *Dig Endosc* 2010;22:S35–S37.

ASGE Standards of Practice Committee, Fisher L, Krinsky ML, et al. The role of endoscopy in the management of obscure GI bleeding. *Gastrointest Endosc* 2010;72:471–479.

Barkun AN, Bardou M, Kuipers EJ, et al. International consensus recommendations on the management of patients with nonvariceal upper gastrointestinal bleeding. *Ann Intern Med* 2010;152(2):101–113.

Chung IK, Kim EJ, Lee MS, et al. Endoscopic factors predisposing to rebleeding following endoscopic hemostasis in bleeding peptic ulcers. *Endoscopy* 2001;33:969–975.

Costa G, Cruz RJ Jr, Abu-Elmagd KM. Surgical shunt versus TIPS for treatment of variceal hemorrhage in the current era of liver and multivisceral transplantation. *Surg Clin North Am* 2010;90(4):891–905.

Enestvedt BK, Granlnek IM, Mattek N, et al. Endoscopic therapy for peptic ulcer hemorrhage: practice variations in a multi-center U.S. consortium. *Dig Dis Sci* 2010;55(9):2568–2576.

Farner R, Lichliter W, Juhn J, et al. Total colectomy versus limited colonic resection for acute lower gastrointestinal bleeding. *Am J Surg* 1999;178:587–591.

Fireman Z, Friedman S. Diagnostic yield of capsule endoscopy in obscure gastrointestinal bleeding. *Digestion* 2004;70:201–206.

Garcia-Tsao G, Bosch J. Management of varices and variceal hemorrhage in cirrhosis. *N Engl J Med* 2010;362(9):823–832.

Gralnek IM, Barkun AN, Bardou M. Management of acute bleeding from a peptic ulcer. *N Engl J Med* 2008;359:928–937.

Henderson JM, Boyer TD, Kutner MH, et al. Distal splenorenal shunt versus transjugular intrahepatic portal systematic shunt for variceal bleeding: a randomized trial. *Gastroenterology* 2006;130(6):1643–1651.

Lanas A, García-Rodríguez LA, Polo-Tomás M, et al. Time trends and impact of upper and lower gastrointestinal bleeding and perforation in clinical practice. *Am J Gastroenterol* 2009;104:1633–1641; advance online publication, May 5, 2009.

Lee J, Costantini TW, Coimbra R. Acute lower GI bleeding for the acute care surgeon: current diagnosis and management. *Scand J Surg* 2009;98(3):135–142.

Rockall TA, Logan RF, Devlin HB, et al. Risk assessment after acute upper gastrointestinal haemorrhage. *Gut* 1996;38:316–321.

Stanley AJ, Ashley D, Dalton HR, et al. Outpatient management of patients with low-risk upper-gastrointestinal haemorrhage: multicentre validation and prospective evaluation. *Lancet* 2009;373:42–47.

Sung JJ, Tsoi KK, Lai LH, et al. Endoscopic clipping versus injection and thermo-coagulation in the treatment of non-variceal upper gastrointestinal bleeding: a meta-analysis. *Gut* 2007;56(10):1364–1373. Epub 2007 Jun 12.

48 Acute Pancreatitis

Ari K. Leppäniemi

I. **INTRODUCTION.** The annual incidence of acute pancreatitis varies between 7 and 102/100,000 population, depending on the prevalence of gallstone disease and the level of alcohol consumption. Of patients admitted for acute abdominal pain, acute pancreatitis is responsible for 3% to 4%. About 80% of the patients have the edematous or mild form of the disease that usually resolves with symptomatic treatment in a few days. The severe form, necrotizing or hemorrhagic pancreatitis, is a life-threatening condition with hospital mortality rates of 10% to 20%.

   A. The management of severe acute pancreatitis (SAP) is resource-intensive and is associated with lengthy hospital and ICU stays, multiple interventions, and high costs. Once identified, the management of SAP follows the same principles – with some additional procedures for gallstone- induced pancreatitis – regardless of the etiology.

II. **ETIOLOGY AND PATHOGENESIS**

   A. Excessive **alcohol consumption** and **gallstone** disease (passage of gallstones into the common bile duct) account for 70% to 80% of cases of acute pancreatitis. However, only a small minority of patients with symptomatic gallstone disease develop acute pancreatitis.

   B. Rare causes of acute pancreatitis include hypercalcemia, hypertriglyceridemia, trauma, certain drugs, infections, postoperative conditions (e.g., cardiac surgery), endoscopic retrograde cholangiopancreatography (ERCP), developmental anomalies (e.g., pancreas divisum), tumors, hereditary and autoimmune diseases. In about 10% of the cases, the etiology remains unknown.

   C. The pathogenesis of acute pancreatitis involves several steps: First, a triggering factor is needed to initiate the pancreatic acinar cell injury. Second, pancreatic proenzymes (zymogens) become activated intracellularly, resulting in acinar cell injury. This is followed by local inflammation of the pancreas resulting in activation of several inflammatory cells and release of inflammatory mediators. If this inflammation cannot be controlled locally, a systemic inflammatory response syndrome (SIRS) develops. A frequent complication of SIRS is the development of multiple organ dysfunction syndrome (MODS) characterized by impairment of the respiratory, cardiovascular, renal, hepatic, hematologic, gastrointestinal, or central nervous system.

   1. Recently, increased intra-abdominal pressure (IAP) and the development of abdominal compartment syndrome (ACS) have been recognized as a contributor to the development of early MODS in SAP.

   2. If the patient survives the initial inflammatory insult, a second phase usually follows 2 to 4 weeks later with the appearance of local infection, sepsis or other complications. Infection of the pancreatic and peripancreatic necrosis occurs in 20% to 40% of patients with SAP, and is associated with worsening MODS. Local complications, such as the development of pancreatic abscesses or pseudocysts, especially after non-operative management, can develop even at a later stage, 4 to 6 weeks after the initial symptoms.

III. **CLINICAL PRESENTATION AND DIAGNOSIS**

   A. **History.** Seek history of any previous episodes of acute pancreatitis and causes along with recent abdominal trauma, surgical or endoscopic procedures, new drugs, infections, and family history of acute pancreatitis. The history of alcohol abuse can be difficult to demonstrate and often patients underestimate the amount of alcohol consumed. Acute pancreatitis can also be the first manifestation of a gallstone disease.

1. A typical patient complains of sudden pain in the epigastrium, often radiating into the back and feeling like a belt around the upper abdomen. The pain is more constant than colicky, and the patient may ask for strong analgesics. Nausea and vomiting are frequently seen. Fever is common in manifest disease and in patients with accompanying cholangitis.

2. Some patients with alcohol-induced pancreatitis have altered sensorium and cannot give an appropriate history. Interview family members or relatives to form a reliable picture of the events leading to the acute condition.

B. Physical examination.

1. Assess the vital signs and airway adequacy to guide initial care. *Start crystalloid fluid resuscitation immediately if any shock* (overt hypotension) exists, and consider occult or compensated shock when vital signs seem "close to normal" (mild tachycardia or low normal systolic blood pressure).

2. Look for abdominal distension (caused by ileus, ascites, visceral edema), and possible discolorations around the umbilicus (Cullen's sign) or in the flanks (Grey-Turner's sign). Palpation may reveal local (epigastric) or generalized tenderness, and ascites. Also, absence of bowel sounds suggests ileus.

C. Laboratory data. Serum amylase or lipase levels can be used to diagnose acute pancreatitis, but the amylase levels may have returned to normal if several days have passed from the onset of symptoms. C-reactive protein level (CRP) elevations lag 24 to 48 hours behind and can be completely normal in the initial phase of even a severe form of the disease.

1. Blood count, liver function tests, electrolyte, glucose, and renal function should be assessed in all to identify illness severity. In those who appear ill, arterial blood gas analysis and serum lactate measurements can aid detection of cellular hypoperfusion. Triglyceride levels should be measured, if suspected to be the cause.

D. Imaging

1. Except for those patients with potential gut obstruction or perforation, plain abdominal radiographs are not needed. **Chest radiographs** are used if any respiratory symptoms exist to evaluate for concomitant infection or edema.

2. **Abdominal CT** is the best imaging test. Oral contrast can be used, but intravenous contrast material should be used with caution and only after confirming adequate circulating volume and urine output. A non-contrast scan provides much information and detects virtually all severe forms of acute pancreatitis.

   a. If necrotizing pancreatitis is suspected, a later abdominal CT with intravenous contrast can be done once volume restoration and renal function are restored. If infection and necrosis are suspected (recurring CRP increase, persistent fever, worsening organ dysfunctions), gas bubbles seen in CT scan are diagnostic (Fig. 48-1).

3. **Ultrasonography** is useful to identify gallstones and a dilated common bile duct (when duct stones or cholangitis are suspected).

4. **Magnetic resonance cholangiopancreatogram (MRCP)** is helpful to confirm that a common bile duct stone has passed through to the duodenum, thus saving an unnecessary ERCP examination.

5. **ERCP** is indicated when ultrasonography reveals dilated common bile duct and there is a suspicion of a persistent stone or the patient has signs of cholangitis. Endoscopic sphincterotomy with clearance of the common duct from stones and/or drainage of pus (in cholangitis) is justified, even if does not affect the natural course of the pancreatitis itself.

E. Differential diagnosis. The most common differential diagnoses include perforated peptic ulcer, biliary colic, acute cholecystitis, ruptured abdominal aortic aneurysm, reflux esophagitis, acute mesenteric ischemia, intestinal obstruction, acute hepatitis, inferior myocardial infarction, basal pneumonia. It is important to differentiate between secondary (perforation) peritonitis usually requiring urgent surgery from acute pancreatitis (where early surgery is usually harmful).

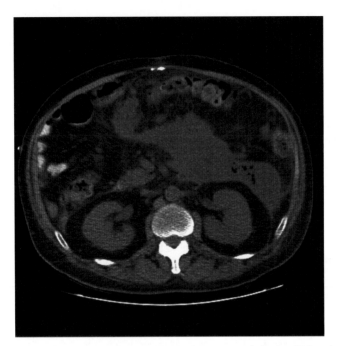

Figure 48-1. CT scan with gas bubbles near the tail of the pancreas indicative of infected necrosis.

IV. TREATMENT/MANAGEMENT STRATEGIES
A. Mild acute pancreatitis
1. Treatment of mild or edematous pancreatitis is supportive and consists of fluid resuscitation, analgesia, anti-emetics, and sometimes the management of accompanying delirium tremens in patients with alcohol-induced pancreatitis. Monitor urine output and titrate volume to vital signs and that output.
2. Nasogastric tube insertion is not routinely indicated, but is helpful in patients with dilated stomach and/or paralytic ileus.
3. Start oral feeding as soon as it is tolerated.
4. Seek signs of progressive disease (worsening symptoms or lack of improvement, elevated CRP, organ dysfunctions).
5. In patients with mild biliary pancreatitis, laparoscopic cholecystectomy can be performed during same admission to prevent recurrent biliary pancreatitis.

B. Severe acute pancreatitis (SAP)
1. **Initial and ICU phase.** Those with hemodynamic problems, CT necrosis, or organ dysfunctions (e.g., decreased renal function, pulmonary edema, or altered sensorium) can develop severe disease and should be admitted to the ICU and monitored. Historically, Ranson's criteria consisting of 11 variables measure at the time of presentation or after 48 hours have been used to identify patients at risk for the severe form of the disease. The principles and treatment goals in the initial phase include:
   a. Endotracheal intubation and sedation as needed
   b. Aggressive fluid resuscitation initially, more conservative after the initial phase, especially if signs of increased IAP noted
   c. Goals: Mean arterial pressure (MAP) >65 mm Hg (higher if IAP is elevated, then abdominal perfusion pressure (APP) = MAP − IAP should be >60 mm Hg), SvO_2 >65% or $ScvO_2$ >70%, normal lactate and base excess, adequate cardiac index, normal creatinine, urine output >1 mL/kg/min, normoglycemia

d. IAP monitoring using a bladder manometer at least every 4 to 6 hours, goal <20 mm Hg; if elevated, using non-operative management first: Empty stomach, reduce fluid resuscitation, remove excessive fluids with diuretics or with dialysis (CVVH/UF), bowel function (prokinetics or laxatives), percutaneous drainage of excessive ascites. If insufficient, consider surgical decompression of the abdomen (see later)

e. Early (first working day) endoscopic sphincterotomy for biliary stasis and cholangitis

f. Infection prophylaxis: Early enteral feeding within 24 hours (try nasogastric tube first; if unsuccessful, insert a nasojejunal feeding tube)

g. Prophylactic antibiotics are not recommended unless manifest infection (cultures)

h. Parenteral nutrition (note triglyceride levels) only as supportive or if enteral nutrition fails

i. Stress ulcer and thrombosis prophylaxis as per institutional ICU protocols

j. Analgesia: Most commonly with titrated and continuous opioids

k. Multivitamins and thiamine are given to those with long standing alcohol abuse coupled with benzodiazepine sedation to avoid withdrawal

l. Daily measurement of one of the organ dysfunction scores (SOFA, MODS) to monitor progress

m. Look for complications requiring surgical intervention: ACS, intra-abdominal hemorrhage, intestinal necrosis or perforation, infected necrosis

2. Surgical interventions

a. Abdominal compartment syndrome (ACS)—see Chapter 20

The incidence of intra-abdominal hypertension (IAH) in patients with acute pancreatitis admitted to ICU is about 60%, and the incidence of the clinical syndrome of ACS comprising of IAP ≥20 mm Hg and a new-onset organ dysfunction is up to 27%. Although adequate fluid resuscitation is important in the early phase of SAP, avoid excessive volumes. Prevention and management of gastric dilatation with a nasogastric tube and percutaneous drainage of excessive pancreatic ascites are useful adjuncts to non-operative management. Short-term use of neuromuscular blockers may also be considered. Removal of fluid by extracorporeal techniques is effective in rapidly removing excess fluid. When non-surgical interventions fail to change the progressive deterioration of organ dysfunctions in the presence of fulminant ACS, consider surgical decompression with midline laparotomy, where all abdominal wall layers are divided through a vertical midline incision extending from the xiphoid to the pubis with a few centimeters of fascia left intact at both ends to facilitate subsequent closure or late reconstruction. An alternative method utilizes a bilateral subcostal incision few centimeters below the costal margins. A less invasive technique is the subcutaneous linea alba fasciotomy (SLAF) where the fascia alone is divided through three short horizontal skin incisions leaving the peritoneum intact.

  i. The aim of surgical decompression is to achieve adequate APP of >60 mm Hg.

  ii. Opening the abdomen to reduce IAP may subsequently create enteric fistulas and giant ventral hernias.

  iii. A recently described method of vacuum-assisted wound closure combined with mesh-mediated fascial traction seems to increase the fascial closure rate up to 90% (Fig. 48-2 and Fig. 48-3).

b. Infected pancreatic or peripancreatic necrosis

Perform surgical or radiologic drainage and debridement in patients with infected necrosis and clinical signs and symptoms of sepsis. Sterile necrosis should be treated non-operatively. Whenever possible, operative necrosectomy and/or drainage should be delayed at least 2 to 3 weeks to allow for demarcation of the necrotic pancreas.

Although minimally invasive necrosectomy is feasible in some patients, open necrosectomy is still the most used approach. Open necrosectomy is

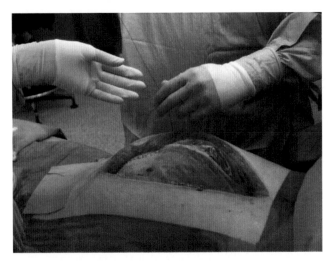

Figure 48-2. Mesh-mediated vacuum-assisted wound closure.

usually performed through a bilateral subcostal incision followed by exposure of the lesser sac through the gastrocolic ligament. Using blunt finger dissection the peripancreatic area is cleared from necrotic fat tissue. Occasionally, the disease process has eroded through the body of the pancreas, in which case the tail can be removed by careful blunt dissection avoiding splenectomy (Fig. 48-4). Attempt to close the main pancreatic duct at the proximal pancreatic stump.

　　i. Following removal of all necrotic tissue (may require mobilization of the left or right colonic flexures), the area is irrigated with warm saline and hemostatic sutures are placed as needed. Several large sized drains are inserted in the area of removed necrosis and irrigation is commenced through one

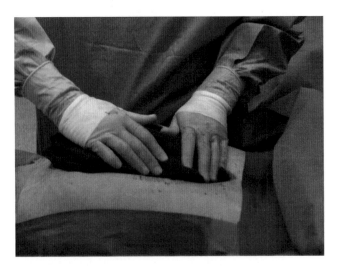

Figure 48-3. Mesh-mediated vacuum-assisted wound closure.

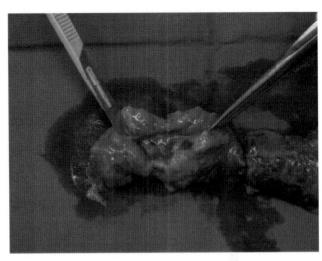

Figure 48-4. Necrotic pancreas removed with distal pancreatectomy.

of the drains if the secretion is copious, thick and pus-like. Unless there is a risk for ACS, the abdominal incision is closed in layers.

   ii. The step-up approach of percutaneous drainage followed by, minimally invasive retroperitoneal necrosectomy has lower rate of incisional hernias and new-onset diabetes compared to fully open approaches.

  c. Extra-pancreatic complications

   i. Bleeding is a rare complication in SAP but requires prompt surgical intervention or angiographic embolization.

   ii. In patients with clear evidence of necrosis or perforation of the colon, early surgical intervention and removal of the affected segment is justified. Primary colonic anastomosis is risky and a temporary colostomy is a better option.

  d. Biliary surgery after SAP

   In patients with mild gallstone pancreatitis, laparoscopic cholecystectomy performed during same admission results in a shorter hospital length of stay with no apparent impact on the technical difficulty of the procedure or perioperative complication rate. In SAP, delay cholecystectomy until the inflammatory response resolves and clinical recovery.

AXIOMS

■ Seek signs of SAP early—shock (obvious or compensated), organ dysfunction including renal and respiratory failure, altered sensorium, radiographic necrosis, or metabolic derangement. Most patients will not have SAP, but those who do have high mortality and morbidity.

■ Early volume restoration is key to resuscitation, but not to excess—latter may create ACS later.

■ Monitor bladder pressure to detect ACS and treat if >20 mm Hg.

■ Titrate opioids to need and level of awareness to optimize outcomes—"one size does **not** fit all."

■ Feed by mouth or tube as early as possible for all forms of acute pancreatitis to limit infectious complications.

■ In patients with SAP, look for signs of infected necrosis usually 2 to 4 weeks into the course of the disease, if the patient's condition becomes worse.

Suggested Readings

Aboulian A, Chan T, Yaghoubian A, et al. Early cholecystectomy safely decreases hospital stay in patients with mild gallstone pancreatitis. A randomized prospective study. *Ann Surg* 2010;251:615–619.

Al-Omran M, Albalawi ZH, Tashkandi ME, et al. Enteral versus parenteral nutrition for acute pancreatitis. *Cochrane Database Syst Rev* 2010;(1):CD002837.

Bradley El III, Dexter ND. Management of severe acute pancreatitis. A surgical Odyssey. *Ann Surg* 2010;251:6–17.

Hegazi R, Raina A, Graham T, et al. Early jejunal feeding initiation and clinical outcomes in patients with severe acute pancreatitis. *JPEN J Parenter Enteral Nutr* 2011;35:91–96.

Mentula P, Hienonen P, Kemppainen E, et al. Surgical decompression for abdominal compartment syndrome in severe acute pancreatitis. *Arch Surg* 2010;145:764–769.

Petrov MS, van Santvoort HC, Besselink MGH, et al. Enteral nutrition and the risk of mortality and infectious complications in patients with severe acute pancreatitis. A meta-analysis of randomized trials. *Arch Surg* 2008;143:1111–1117.

Rosas JM, Soto SN, Aracil JS, et al. Intra-abdominal pressure as a marker of severity in acute pancreatitis. *Surgery* 2007;141:173–178.

Simchuk EJ, Traverso LW, Nukui Y, et al. Computed tomography severity index is a predictor of outcomes for severe pancreatitis. *Am J Surg* 2000;179:352–355.

Tonsi AF, Bacchion M, Crippa S, et al. Acute pancreatitis at the beginning of the 21st century: The state of the art. *World J Gastroenterol* 2009;15:2945–2959.

van Santvoort, Besselink MG, Bakker OJ, et al. A step-up approach or open necrosectomy for necrotizing pancreatitis. *N Engl J Med* 2010;362:1491–1502.

49 Biliary Tract Disease

Benjamin Braslow

I. ACUTE CHOLECYSTITIS

A. Acute cholecystitis is a syndrome of right upper quadrant (RUQ) pain, fever, and leukocytosis associated with an acute inflammation of the gallbladder. Ninety percent of cholecystitis is calculous in origin resulting from persistent obstruction of the gallbladder outlet by an impacted stone. This obstruction results in gallbladder distension, sub-serosal edema, mucosal sloughing, venous and lymphatic congestion, and localized ischemia. The natural history of acute cholecystitis depends on relief of the obstruction, development and extent of secondary bacterial invasion, age of the patient, and comorbidities. Most attacks resolve spontaneously without surgery or other specific therapy. Some progress to free perforation with local abscess formation or generalized peritonitis. Other complications include sepsis, empyema (suppurative cholecystitis), gallstone ileus, and cholecystic–enteric fistula. Repeated episodes of acute inflammation lead to chronic cholecystitis where the gallbladder wall becomes thick, fibrotic, and often contracted.

B. The cause of acute cholecystitis is speculative; most result from stagnation of bile secondary to stone impaction and subsequent infection. The edema and inflammation can play a role in elevating the gallbladder wall away from the impacted stone, thus resulting in disimpaction and spontaneous drainage. Failure of spontaneous disimpaction results in continued cystic duct obstruction, gallbladder ischemia, and increased inflammatory that necessitates operative intervention.

C. Clinical presentation
Acute cholecystitis presents with severe pain below the right costal margin. The pain frequently radiates to the back, the right scapula, or the right clavicular area. Majority of patients will recount a previous attack of biliary colic at first indistinguishable from the present illness. This new pain, however, does not mitigate and in fact worsens with time and is often associated with nausea, emesis, anorexia, or low grade fever (38 to 38.5°C). Mild icterus is present in about 10% of cases. High fever with chills is uncommon and suggests the possibility of cholangitis. Likewise, severe jaundice suggests the presence of common bile duct (CBD) stones, cholangitis, or obstruction of the common hepatic duct by severe pericholecystic inflammation associated with an impacted large stone in Hartmann's pouch, which mechanically obstructs the bile duct **(Mirizzi's syndrome).**

  1. Physical examination reveals RUQ tenderness to palpation. A RUQ mass is palpable in one-third of patients. Murphy's sign is accentuated tenderness and pain with a deep breath during palpation in the right subcostal region.

  2. The white blood cell count (WBC) is usually elevated to 12,000 to 15,000/mm^3 but normal counts are not uncommon. A high WBC (>20,000/mm^3) should suggest further complications of cholecystitis such as gangrene, perforation, or cholangitis. A mild elevation of the serum bilirubin (2 to 4 mg/dL) is common presumably a result of secondary inflammation of the CBD; higher values usually indicate the presence of CBD stones. Mild elevations in alkaline phosphatase, transaminases, amylase, or lipase may also be present. However, dramatic elevations in any of these laboratory values suggest the presence of complications.

D. Imaging

  1. Ultrasound is the initial diagnostic modality to identify cholecystitis with ~95% specificity and sensitivity. Ultrasound findings most suggestive of acute cholecystitis include gallbladder distension, gallbladder wall thickening (>4 mm), pericholecystic fluid, an impacted stone, biliary sludge, or positive sonographic Murphy's sign. Comorbid factors (e.g., ascites) decrease the specificity of this test.

2. When ultrasound is equivocal, technically not possible, or negative in a patient with high clinical suspicion for cholecystitis, the patency of the cystic duct can be assessed with cholescintigraphy. Intravenous administration of gamma-emitting Tc-labeled hydroxyl iminodiacetic acid (HIDA) or diisopropyl iminodiacetic acid (DISIDA), is rapidly taken up by hepatocytes and secreted into the bile.

   a. The scan is considered normal when radionucleotide is detected in the gallbladder, CBD, and small bowel within 30 to 60 minutes.

   b. An abnormal or "positive scan" is defined as the non-visualization of the gallbladder with preserved excretion into the CBD or small bowel. HIDA scanning has a high sensitivity and specificity (100% and 95%, respectively), and a diagnostic accuracy rate approaching 98% in patients with clinical evidence of acute calculous cholecystitis.

   c. A false-positive scan, defined as the absence of isotope in the gallbladder, is seen in patients who have fasted for more than 5 days, that is, critically ill patients or those receiving total parenteral nutrition (TPN). In this population, false-positive rates are high. Augmentation with morphine (which increases sphincter of Oddi and common duct pressure) is used if the gallbladder has not visualized after 60 minutes to decrease false-positive scans.

3. In most cases, the use of computed tomography (CT) in uncomplicated acute cholecystitis is limited unless other abdominal pathology is suspected or concern for gallbladder perforation, abscess, or enteric fistula. CT is less sensitive than US in the detection of gallstones.

4. Magnetic resonance imaging (MRI), although accurate in detection of cholecystitis, has a limited role in acute cases. Magnetic resonance cholangiopancreatography (MRCP) is an excellent modality for detection of CBD stones that complicate acute cholecystitis (see later).

E. Management

Patients with acute cholecystitis should be admitted. Initial therapy includes intravenous hydration, pain relief, and correction of any electrolyte disorders.

1. The need for antibiotic treatment in uncomplicated acute cholecystitis remains unproven, yet the practice in the United States has been to provide patients with antibiotic prophylaxis. Despite the low incidence of positive bile cultures assayed from patients with acute cholecystitis, broad spectrum intravenous antibiotics are given to most patients for an episode of cholecystitis.

2. The most common pathogens include *Escherichia coli*, Enterococcus, Klebsiella, and Enterobacter. Suggested regimens of antibiotics include: (1) Metronidazole plus a third generation cephalosporin or a fluoroquinolone or aztreonam, (2) piperacillin/tazobactam, (3) ampicillin/sulbactam, (4) ticarcillin–clavulanate, or (5) imipenem.

3. Patients with elevated liver function test results (specifically serum total bilirubin or alkaline phosphatase) or dilated bile ducts (>6 mm) on ultrasound should be further evaluated for the presence of CBD stones (see section later).

4. The definitive therapy for acute cholecystitis is cholecystectomy. Cholecystectomy (open or laparoscopic) has low complication rates: <0.2% mortality, <5% major morbidity, and a bile duct injury rate of ~0.4%. Laparoscopic cholecystectomy has become the preferred operation in most patients; reduces hospital LOS and hastens recovery time and return to normal activity.

   a. Conversion to open cholecystectomy is an important option to ensure patient safety. In laparoscopic cases with extensive inflammation, adhesions or bleeding that can make dissection of Calot's triangle and recognition of the biliary anatomy hazardous, conversion to an open cholecystectomy or tube cholecystectomy is recommended.

   b. Conversion is also advocated for persistent bleeding or intraoperative injury to a duct (other than the cystic duct) or bowel. Conversion should not be considered a complication or failure of laparoscopic surgery, rather a judicious surgical decision in a complicated case to avoid further problems. Predictors of conversion include male gender, history of biliary disease, delay in surgery of more than 48 hours, marked leukocytosis (>18,000/mm^3), obesity, adhesions, and inability to demonstrate the biliary anatomy.

5. The timing of cholecystectomy is variable. Ten to twenty percent of patients require immediate operation (for hemodynamic instability or generalized peritonitis). These findings suggest gangrene and perforation of the gallbladder; delays in operation increase morbidity and mortality. In the remaining 80% to 90%, the timing of operation remains controversial. In the past, delayed cholecystectomy, 6 to 12 weeks after resolution of symptoms, was preferred for acute cholecystitis. Current practice is early cholecystectomy for acute cholecystitis. Early cholecystectomy (within 72 hours) whether performed laparoscopically or open, results in reduced overall hospital LOS, decreased costs and no difference in complications. More importantly, 23% of people awaiting delayed cholecystectomy require urgent operation because of recurrent or worsening symptoms.

6. Emergent cholecystectomy in high-risk patients with acute cholecystitis, (severe comorbid conditions, i.e., advanced cardiopulmonary disease) carries mortality near 50%. Percutaneous gallbladder drainage (cholecystostomy) is the treatment of choice. The procedure is routinely performed by interventional techniques using fluoroscopic or ultrasound guidance. The preferred route for tube insertion is transhepatic, which takes advantage of a stabilized gallbladder during insertion and decreases peritoneal leakage. The transhepatic route is also preferred over the transperitoneal route in the setting of ascites to promote tract maturation. The procedure is well tolerated with less than 5% morbidity (i.e., catheter dislodgement, bleeding, liver hematoma, bile leakage, etc.). If the percutaneous method is not available, a small right subcostal incision permitting visualization of the fundus is made under local anesthesia. The gallbladder is then aspirated, decompressed, and a mushroom tip-catheter inserted and secured with a purse string suture. The catheter is exteriorized away from the costal margin, and secured to the skin.

    a. The optimal timing of removal of tube cholecystostomy is debated. In the majority of patients with a transhepatic cholecystostomy, a 2-week period was sufficient for the tract to mature, while a minimum of 3 weeks were needed for the transperitoneal route. Tube cholecystography should be performed after resolution of the cholecystitis. If contrast flows into the duodenum and no stones are identified the cholecystostomy tube can be removed. Patients with gallstones should undergo an interval cholecystectomy after recovery from their acute illness as approximately 80% will have recurrent symptoms or further complications. The laparoscopic approach to interval cholecystectomy is successful in the majority of patients.

7. Complications

    Complications of acute cholecystitis are common and often require surgical intervention. These include empyema, emphysematous cholecystitis, perforation and cholecystenteric fistula.

    a. **Empyema of the gallbladder** (suppurative cholecystitis), describes an inflamed and infected gallbladder containing frank pus. The patient is septic and toxic, with high fever (39 to 40°C), chills, and an elevated WBC (15,000/mm^3 or greater). Severe sepsis with hemodynamic instability and multi-system organ failure may be present or develop rapidly without prompt diagnosis and treatment. Treatment consists of fluid resuscitation, administration of broad-spectrum antibiotics (including anaerobic coverage), and emergent cholecystectomy or cholecystostomy.

    b. **Emphysematous cholecystitis** is characterized by bubbles of gas from anaerobic infection appearing in the gallbladder lumen, its wall, the pericholecystic space, and, on occasion, the bile ducts. Clostridia species are the most common identified organism, but other potential gas forming anaerobes require antibiotic coverage as well. Males outnumber females (3:1) and 20% of patients are diabetic. The disease is often *not* associated with gallstones.

Patients present with severe pain, are toxic in appearance, with high fever and a significant leukocytosis. Abdominal x-rays or CT usually demonstrate air within gallbladder. Broad-spectrum antibiotics, including an anti-clostridial agent are given; fluid resuscitation and emergent cholecystectomy are indicated. Cholecystostomy can be used in unstable patients.

  c. **Perforation** occurs when gallbladder wall ischemia progresses to gangrene. Perforation may occur early (within 3 days) or late (2 weeks or later) after the onset of acute cholecystitis. This occurs in <10% of cases and may be localized or free perforation. Localized perforation results in the formation of a pericholecystic abscesses as the omentum walls off the contamination limiting it to the RUQ. In these cases, cholecystectomy (open or laparoscopic) with abscess drainage can be performed safely after resuscitation and antibiotic therapy. Again, in those critically ill patients, cholecystostomy or percutaneous abscess drainage can be used to temporize the situation.

  d. **Cholecystenteric fistula** occurs in 1% to 2% of patients with acute cholecystitis. The inflamed gallbladder becomes adherent to a neighboring hollow viscus and as necrosis develops, penetration into the adjacent lumen occurs and fistula formation follows. The duodenum (~20%) and the hepatic flexure of the colon (~80%) are the most common sites, but fistulas to the stomach are also reported. After the fistula forms, the episode of acute cholecystitis resolves as the gallbladder spontaneously decompresses. Rarely, patients vomit gallstones or develop steatorrhea, but in most cases the acute attack subsides and the cholecystenteric fistula remains clinically undetected. If a large gallstone passes into the small intestine, a mechanical bowel obstruction may result, which is termed *gallstone ileus*. This occurs in 10% to 15% of patients; patients present with signs and symptoms of small bowel obstruction. The pain may be episodic as the stone temporarily impacts at one site in the intestinal lumen then dislodges and is carried distally by peristalsis where it obstructs again. The terminal ileum is the usual final site of stone impaction. Often abdominal plain films will show dilated small bowel loops with air–fluid levels, pneumobilia and a calcified gallstone in the right lower quadrant.

  i. The initial management of gallstone ileus includes removal of the obstructing stone, via a *proximal* enterotomy in a segment of non-edematous small bowel.

    There is no debate over the need to emergently relieve the obstruction. However, if and when the cholecystenteric fistula should be addressed is debated. The traditional approach favored treating only the obstruction at the urgent operation and if symptomatic, the gallbladder removed after an interval of recovery. This may still be the safest approach. The cholecystenteric fistula does not require definitive treatment at exploration for small bowel obstruction. This approach is based on evidence that the majority of cholecystenteric fistula will close spontaneously with a less than 5% recurrence rate of gallstone ileus. Recently, several studies suggest a one-stage procedure consisting of enterolithotomy, cholecystectomy, and fistula excision, either with open or a laparoscopic approach.

II. ACUTE ACALCULOUS CHOLECYSTITIS

  A. Acute acalculous cholecystitis accounts for 5% to 10% of patients with acute cholecystitis. The disease often has a more fulminant course than acute calculous cholecystitis, often progressing to empyema, or gangrene with perforation. There is a strong association with clinical illnesses and conditions including recent non-biliary surgery, major trauma or burns, sepsis/shock, immunosuppression, TPN, diabetes mellitus, prolonged mechanical ventilation, narcotic administration, or multiple connective tissue/rheumatologic disorders.

  B. Patients are usually critically ill, and in an intensive care unit. The diagnosis usually follows a workup for unexplained fever, leukocytosis, sepsis, vague abdominal discomfort, or distension. The conditions associated with acalculous cholecystitis lead to gallbladder stasis and ischemia, which result in a local inflammatory response in the gallbladder wall. Secondary infection with enteric pathogens, *E. coli, Enterococcus faecalis,* klebsiella, pseudomonas, proteus species, or bacteroides follows and antibiotic therapy should be directed against these organisms initially.

C. Signs and symptoms are similar to those of calculous cholecystitis with RUQ tenderness, fever, elevated WBC count, and elevated liver enzymes. Up to 20% of patients are jaundiced secondary to partial biliary obstruction induced by inflammation extending into the CBD. This finding is in sharp contrast to calculous acute cholecystitis in which jaundice is uncommon. Often the diagnosis is delayed, as symptoms are difficult to detect in critically ill patients, those receiving narcotics or with an altered mental status. This in part, accounts for the increased morbidity and mortality (up to 40%).

D. As in acute calculous cholecystitis, ultrasonography is the investigation of choice. Ultrasonographic features suggestive of acalculous cholecystitis include absence of gallstones or sludge, thickening of the gallbladder wall (>5 mm) with pericholecystic fluid, a positive Murphy's sign induced by the ultrasound probe in a conscious patient, emphysematous cholecystitis with gas bubbles present in the fundus of the gallbladder (Champagne Sign), and occasionally, failure to visualize the gallbladder secondary to surrounding inflammation. The reported accuracy of HIDA scans in these patients is variable, with a sensitivity of 70% to 80% and a specificity of 90% to 100%. Again, failure to opacify the gallbladder is the most sensitive and specific finding. Leakage of tracer into the pericholecystic space suggests perforation.

E. Emergency cholecystectomy is the treatment once the diagnosis is established or highly suspected. Both open and laparoscopic techniques have been utilized. The gallbladder is often encased in an inflammatory mass, which makes the laparoscopic approach more complicated and creates a higher risk of bile duct or vascular injury. The incidence of complications such as gangrene, perforation, or empyema exceeds 50%; cholecystectomy rather than cholecystostomy is usually required in this setting. However, in patients too ill to travel from the ICU, percutaneous cholecystostomy may be a temporizing maneuver.

F. In cases treated with percutaneous cholecystectomy in which the patient recovers and the underlying problem causing the cholecystitis resolves, subsequent cholecystectomy is generally unnecessary. A recent series of 50 patients reported that only 24% with acalculous cholecystitis required cholecystectomy at a mean follow-up period of 12 months.

III. ACUTE CHOLECYSTITIS IN PREGNANCY

Acute cholecystitis, caused by gallstones is the second most common non-obstetrical cause of acute abdomen during pregnancy (after appendicitis). The incidence of cholelithiasis in pregnant woman undergoing routine obstetric ultrasound examinations is 3.5% to 10%. The progesterone-induced smooth muscle relaxation of the gallbladder promotes stasis of bile and increases the risk of cholelithiasis and subsequently of acute cholecystitis. In addition, elevated levels of estrogen increase the lithogenicity, which further increases stone formation and the risk of cholecystitis.

A. The symptomatology of acute cholecystitis is similar in pregnant and non-pregnant women. The differential must include HELLP syndrome (hemolysis, elevated liver enzyme values, low platelet count during pregnancy) and pre-eclampsia. Both LFT's (specifically alkaline phosphatase) and serum amylase values may be elevated as a result of the pregnancy and not indicate a pathologic condition. Ultrasound remains the best diagnostic procedure.

B. The current recommendation is to perform laparoscopic cholecystectomy in the first, second, and early in the third trimester. Surgery has become the primary treatment over non-operative management because: (1) It can be done safely with minimal effect on mother and fetus, (2) recurrence rate during pregnancy is high (44% to 92%), depending on the trimester of initial presentation, (3) safer anesthetics and medications, (4) shorter hospital length of stay, and (5) avoidance of complications such as perforation, sepsis, or peritonitis. In addition, early surgery avoids the risk of gallstone pancreatitis which occurs in up to 13% of those with symptomatic gallstones and results in fetal loss in 10% to 20%. Non-operative management is associated with higher incidence of spontaneous abortion, preterm labor, and preterm delivery than among those undergoing cholecystectomy.

C. The laparoscopic procedure is modified by using an open supraumbilical technique (Hasson technique) for trocar insertion, reverse Trendelenburg positioning with the left side down to expose the RUQ and preserve vena cava blood flow, low-pressure pneumoperitoneum, and if possible laparoscopic ultrasound (LUS) to detect CBD stones. Transvaginal ultrasound for fetal assessment is ideal during laparoscopy.

1. There is an increased incidence of common duct stones during pregnancy and controversy over intraoperative cholangiography (IOC) exists between limited use of IOC and those who recommend it for every patient at the time of cholecystectomy. The use of IOC in the pregnant patient depends on trimester and gestational age and the suspicion of choledocholithiasis on the basis of clinical, biochemical, or ultrasonic evidence. IOC is safe in the second and third trimester because organogenesis is complete and small doses of radiation are delivered. Shielding the uterus further reduces the risk of radiation exposure. Alternative methods to investigate the CBD without radiation exposure during the first trimester and at the time of surgery include intraoperative ultrasonography, transcystic duct choledochoscopy, and endoscopic papillotomy performed under ultrasonographic guidance.

IV. COMMON BILE DUCT STONES

A. Choledocholithiasis presents with a wide clinical spectrum from asymptomatic, incidentally found CBD stones to acute cholangitis/biliary sepsis. Primary CBD stones are calculi that originate in the bile duct. These stones often result from impaired drainage of the CBD secondary to stricture or mass effect on the CBD or ampulla of Vater. These stones are caused by stasis within the CBD and consist of calcium bilirubinate. They are soft, brown, and form a "cast" of the bile duct.

B. Operative intervention must include clearance of the duct, as well as a drainage procedure. More commonly, CBD stones are secondary stones. These stones are formed within the gallbladder and migrate to the CBD. Secondary stones are predominately cholesterol stones formed by an imbalance of the three main components of bile: Bile salts, lecithin, and cholesterol. Cholesterol stones are often yellow, multiple, and faceted. The management of CBD stones is varied and dependent upon the timing of diagnosis and the patient's presenting symptoms.

C. Presentation and initial management

1. Most commonly, patients present with symptoms of cholecystitis, biliary colic, pancreatitis, jaundice, or cholangitis (7% cholecystitis, 16% biliary colic, 20% pancreatitis, 45% with jaundice, and CBD stones). The classic presentation of cholangitis is abdominal pain, fever, and jaundice—Charcot's triad. Some patients may progress to sepsis with shock and altered mental status—Reynolds' pentad. Preoperative blood work may reveal elevations of alkaline phosphatase, glutamic oxaloacetic transaminase, lactate dehydrogenase, or bilirubin. If one of these values is elevated, CBD stones are present in 20% of patients with cholelithiasis. If two of these values are elevated, choledocholithiasis will be present 40% of the time. However, normal serum liver enzymes do not assure a clear common duct. Five to twelve percent of patients with normal enzymes and minimal to no symptoms will have CBD stones.

2. Initial management depends on presenting symptoms. Most patients admitted will be dehydrated from inanition and/or vomiting, therefore, intravenous fluids should be administered. Placement of a nasogastric tube may be necessary for nausea and vomiting. If symptoms of infection, such as fever and leukocytosis are present, antibiotics should be administered.

3. Patients with cholangitis require resuscitation, hemodynamic monitoring, and aggressive workup. The most commonly found pathogens in patients with cholangitis are *E. coli*, Klebsiella spp., Enterobacter spp., and Enterococcus spp. Anaerobes are found in 3% of bile cultures. Broad spectrum antibiotic therapy should be promptly initiated. Penicillin derivatives such as piperacillin–tazobactam, ampicillin–sulbactam, or ticarcillin–clavulanic acid offer excellent coverage.

Second and third generation cephalosporins with metronidazole also provide adequate therapy to treat the most common pathogens and anaerobes. If a patient has a history of vancomycin resistant enterococcus (VRE), combination therapy with linezolid should be instituted. Once the patient has been stabilized, imaging studies and therapeutic interventions can proceed.

D. Diagnosis

Ultrasound, endoscopic retrograde cholangiopancreatography (ERCP), MRCP, and endoscopic ultrasound (EUS) are frequently used prior to operation and intraoperative cholangiogram remains an important operative technique. An NIH consensus statement found that MRCP, ERCP, and EUS were comparable in their sensitivities, specificities, and accuracy rates for the detection of CBD stones.

1. Ultrasound

Ultrasonography is excellent for detection of biliary stones and CBD dilation. The sensitivity of ultrasound for detection of intrahepatic and extrahepatic duct dilation is high (96%), comparable to ERCP 96%. The sensitivity of ultrasonography for detection of CBD stones is lower than EUS and ERCP, (25% and 63%) but highly specific(95%).

2. Magnetic resonance cholangiopancreatography (MRCP)

MRCP is reliable in the detection of CBD stones. The sensitivity, specificity, and accuracy of MRCP are 90%, 95%, and 95%, respectively. There is also excellent intraobserver agreement in the diagnosis of CBD stones. MRCP has fewer potential complications and is and less costly than ERCP. However, it does not offer a therapeutic option.

3. Endoscopic retrograde cholangiopancreatography (ERCP)

ERCP is highly specific for detection of CBD stones; sensitivity is between 90% and 95%. The advantage of ERCP is the ability to perform therapeutic removal of stones at the time of diagnosis. The disadvantage is the associated morbidity and mortality of the procedure. The 30-day morbidity of ERCP has been reported as high as 15.9%. Procedure related mortality rates of 1% are also reported. Approximately 61% of patients undergoing ERCP are found to have no CBD stones. Thus, ERCP is best reserved for patients for whom there is a high probability of CBD stones or CBD stones have been documented by other studies.

4. Endoscopic ultrasound (EUS)

Reported sensitivity between 94% and 98% and specificity is 99% for CBD stones. In some centers, EUS has been used in conjunction with upper GI endoscopy to avoid radiation exposure and other risks of ERCP.

5. Intraoperative evaluation for CBD stones

a. Intraoperative cholangiography (IOC)

IOC should be performed during laparoscopic cholecystectomy if CBD stones are suspected, a history of pancreatitis, jaundice, or abnormal liver function tests, the CBD is dilated, or any difficulty in defining anatomy in the OR. Some centers perform routine IOC with an incidence of CBD stones between 10% and 14%. The sensitivity and specificity of IOC are 98% and 94%, respectively.

6. Laparoscopic ultrasound (LUS)

LUS is an attractive alternative to IOC; however, most surgeons have little experience with this technique. Studies have shown that LUS is more sensitive than IOC and as accurate and specific as IOC.

E. Treatment of common bile duct stones

If CBD stones are identified preoperatively, there are several options for management.

1. ERCP/ES followed by laparoscopic cholecystectomy

For centers without experience in laparoscopic CBD exploration, patients can undergo ERCP with endoscopic sphincterotomy (ES). ERCP with ES will be successful in clearing the CBD in 90%. Laparoscopic cholecystectomy should follow successful endoscopic clearance of the CBD. If ERCP with ES is unsuccessful, the CBD must be surgically cleared. Laparoscopic CBD exploration (LCBDE) or open CBD exploration are the options and should be performed by experienced surgeons. LCBDE has been shown to have a 100% success rate in salvaging failed preoperative ERCP/ES. Open common duct explorations are occasionally necessary. Contraindications for open or laparoscopic CBD exploration include portal hypertension, severe periportal inflammation, or a CBD smaller than 5 mm. Choledochotomy should be avoided on a small CBD because of the high incidence of post-surgical stricture.

   a. Other indications for open CBD exploration include the presence of primary duct stones and impacted stone(s) at the ampulla of Vater. The presence of primary duct stones requires a drainage procedure, such as choledochoduo-denostomy or choledochojejunostomy. Stones impacted at the ampulla of Vater require sphincterotomy or sphincteroplasty. Elderly or debilitated patients with CBD stones can be treated by ERCP/ES without cholecystectomy. Studies have shown that 75% to 84% of patients remain symptom-free with up to 70 months of follow-up.

F. Treatment of acute cholangitis

   1. Once the patient with acute cholangitis is stabilized, emergent or urgent decompression of the biliary tree is indicated. Endoscopic management is associated with less morbidity and mortality than surgical decompression. ES can be successfully performed in 97%. ES both drains the duct and promotes clearance of stones. If stones cannot be removed, a stent can be placed across the obstruction. Stents can also relieve obstruction caused by malignant and benign strictures.

   2. As an alternative, percutaneous transhepatic cholangiography (PTC) and placement of a percutaneous transhepatic biliary drain can also decompress an obstructed biliary tree. PTC is performed if endoscopy is unavailable, unsuccessful or not feasible because of patient anatomy (prior surgery, such as Billroth II or Roux-en-Y anatomy).

   Rarely surgical decompression is required. This can be done by laparoscopic or open techniques depending on surgeon preference and patient condition. Patient status also determines if simple drainage by choledochotomy and T-tube is performed or full exploration with duct clearance.

V. GALLSTONE PANCREATITIS

Most cases of *acute* pancreatitis in North America are the result of gallstones migrating into the CBD and passing through the ampulla of Vater. The resultant pancreatic duct obstruction causes pancreatic and peripancreatic inflammation and at times severe systemic illness. Initial management focuses on supportive care, severity staging, and surgical or endoscopic management of patients.

A. Incidence

The risk of developing pancreatitis in patients with asymptomatic gallstones is 3% to 4% and approximately equal in both sexes. Cholecystectomy reduces the incidence of gallstone pancreatitis. Smaller sized gallstones (<5 mm) and "mulberry" shaped stones are factors.

B. Etiology

Gallstones and alcohol are the most common etiologies for acute pancreatitis. Approximately 10% to 20% of gallstone pancreatitis cases are the result of passage of a single gallstone; in many patients no stones are identified. If gallbladder imaging reveals no evidence of stones, acute bile duct dilation and elevated liver function tests are strongly indicative of the diagnosis. It is prudent to consider all other causes of acute pancreatitis in the differential (i.e., alcohol, post-ERCP, hyperlipidemia, drugs, viral infections, collagen vascular disease, hypercalcemia, etc.), but in some cases of pancreatitis with no apparent cause, further evaluation of the bile is necessary. Bile crystals and biliary sludge can precipitate acute pancreatitis and are too small to be seen with conventional imaging. In some patients, microscopic examination of the bile is necessary.

C. Pathophysiology

The "common channel" theory of gallstone pancreatitis suggests that the reflux of bile into the pancreatic duct via this common anatomic channel incites an acute inflammatory process and pancreatitis. Other studies suggest that transient pancreatic duct hypertension without the influence of bile salt contamination is the inciting event. This pancreatic duct hypertension is more likely to occur in patients with a common biliopancreatic channel. However, the pancreatic and peripancreatic autodigestion appears to result from the activated secreted pancreatic enzymes: Amylase, lipase, and ribonuclease.

D. Presentation

1. Most patients with acute gallstone pancreatitis present with severe epigastric pain which may radiate to the back, with nausea, vomiting, and significant abdominal distension. Fever usually develops within the first 48 to 72 hours. The pain of acute pancreatitis is sudden in onset and may mimic severe biliary colic or acute peritonitis. Jaundice indicates bile duct obstruction from pancreatic edema or persistent obstruction of the biliary tree.

2. Approximately 85% to 95% of patients develop a mild form of pancreatitis with resolution of symptoms in 3 to 5 days. A small percentage of patients evolve into the severe, necrotizing pancreatitis. Profound ileus, third space fluid accumulation, hemodynamic instability, and multisystem organ failure are common complications of necrotizing pancreatitis. Flank ecchymoses (Grey Turner's sign) or periumbilical ecchymoses (Cullen's sign) are indicators of retroperitoneal hemorrhage. Acute hemorrhagic pancreatitis is the most severe form of pancreatitis and is highly morbid.

E. Laboratory findings

1. Most patients have a marked elevation of amylase and lipase; however, the absolute level of amylase elevation does not correlate with the severity of the pancreatitis. In most patients, amylase elevations will resolve within 3 to 5 days following the initial attack. Persistent elevations beyond this time frame are suspicious for more severe ongoing pancreatitis, pancreatic ductal obstruction, or pseudocyst development.

2. The systemic inflammatory response associated with severe pancreatitis and subsequent third spacing results in dehydration and abnormal serum electrolyte values. Hemoglobin and hematocrit are initially elevated, as are BUN and creatinine from intravascular volume depletion. Serum glucose likewise can be elevated and is an indicator of severe pancreatic parenchymal injury and systemic stress.

3. Mild gallstone pancreatitis is associated with transient elevations of the liver function tests, including bilirubin (direct and indirect) and transaminases. These values usually normalize shortly after resolution of the abdominal pain. Persistent elevation of bilirubin, especially within the first 24 to 48 hours, suggests an impacted stone. Mild elevations of the bilirubin are often seen in patients with pancreatic edema causing partial common duct obstruction and usually do not require any decompression unless associated with signs of biliary sepsis.

4. Severe pancreatitis can be associated with hypertriglyceridemia, as well as hypocalcemia and hypoalbuminemia. Severe pancreatitis may be associated with hemorrhage, disseminated intravascular coagulation (DIC) syndrome, manifested as thrombocytopenia, elevated levels of fibrin split products, and decreased fibrinogen levels.

5. Measurement of serum C-reactive protein (CRP) has been proposed as a sensitive predictor of pancreatitis severity. CRP values are useful after 48 hours following onset of symptoms. The absolute value predictive of severe pancreatitis has varied between numerous studies; however, the Santorini Consensus Conference in 1999 recommended a "cut-off" value of greater than 15 mg/dL as a strong indicator of progression to severe necrotizing pancreatitis.

6. Serum phospholipase A_2 (PLA_2) is a serum isoenzyme associated with acute pancreatitis. Marked increases in the PLA_2 level are considered to be evidence of systemic inflammation associated with multiple organ failure.

F. Diagnostic imaging

1. In acute pancreatitis, the etiology and severity of the pancreatitis is determined by imaging studies performed early in the clinical course. An ultrasound of the abdomen is obtained to assess for gallstones and bile duct dilation. CT or MRI allows assessment of the extent of pancreatic necrosis and peripancreatic inflammatory change, which is important in prognosis. Intravenous (IV) contrast administration is preferred to non-contrast studies to assess the degree of enhancement

and estimate the area of necrosis. Evidence of gas within the peripancreatic fluid collections can be a sign of superinfection.

2. Most centers obtain contrast enhanced CT on admission and again between the third and tenth day if necessary to assess for pancreatic necrosis or other complications. Each patient should be evaluated for hydrational status and any evidence of renal insufficiency before receiving intravenous iodinated contrast.

3. MRI is another useful study to evaluate the severity of acute pancreatitis. Gadolinium has less nephrotoxicity than iodinated dyes, which makes its use more attractive in patients with contrast dye allergy or renal insufficiency. MRI also allows assessment of the biliary and pancreatic ductal systems as well as surrounding vasculature. Its high sensitivity (>90%) for detecting CBD stones can be helpful in determining those patients who may need ductal drainage.

G. Severity assessment of gallstone pancreatitis

The severity of acute pancreatitis of any etiology is based on the systemic inflammatory response, the extent of pancreatic necrosis, and the presence of associated organ failure.

A number of assessment scoring tools are available. Ranson's criteria identified eleven prognostic indicators and have been further modified to better characterize gallstone pancreatitis. The Glasgow Score is based on nine severity assessment criteria.

H. Treatment

The initial treatment for gallstone pancreatitis includes admission, hemodynamic monitoring, volume and electrolyte resuscitation, and pain control. Management is then based upon the clinical course, severity of systemic response and follows that prescribed for the management of acute pancreatitis from any cause. The use of protease inhibitors or octreotide has not been found to be beneficial. Prophylactic antibiotics are not recommended for routine cases.

Those patients with mild gallstone pancreatitis usually resolve their acute symptoms within 3 to 5 hospital days. Once the acute abdominal pain has resolved, a low fat diet can be started. This is not predicated upon the normalization of pancreatic enzymes, which may take several days longer.

Cholecystectomy is recommended on the initial admission to prevent any future attacks of pancreatitis, as approximately 25% to 50% will experience a recurrent bout of gallstone pancreatitis within 3 months. The surgical goal is removal of the gallbladder and evaluation and clearance of the biliary tree. See above section on CBD stones.

In cases of severe gallstone pancreatitis, early ERCP and stone extraction has been debated. The current recommendation is that emergency endoscopic procedures should be performed in those patients who are categorized as moderate to severe pancreatitis with evidence of persistent bile duct obstruction and in cases complicated by cholangitis. In those patients in whom ERCP and duct clearance is unsuccessful, transhepatic cholangiocatheter insertion for decompression or, in rare cases, open cholecystectomy and T-tube placement will enable duct decompression.

Patients who progress to severe necrotizing pancreatitis often require an extensive ICU and hospital course. Mortality is high, ranging from 15% to 20%. Certain patient populations, the elderly or severely debilitated patient, present unique challenges and higher risks. ERCP and sphincterotomy may serve as definitive therapy in this high-risk groups. The pregnant patient who presents with gallstone pancreatitis will benefit from elective laparoscopic cholecystectomy and IOC during the second trimester of pregnancy. Patients who present after the second trimester are usually managed expectantly until cholecystectomy can be performed following delivery of the fetus.

I. Outcomes

Approximately 85% to 95% of patients with acute gallstone pancreatitis develop only mild, self-limited pancreatitis and are ultimately offered cholecystectomy as definitive treatment. Mortality in this low-risk group ranges between 1% and 3%. In 10% to 20% of patients who develop severe acute pancreatitis, mortality remains high.

AXIOMS

- 90% of cholecystitis is calculous in origin and results from a persistent obstruction of the gallbladder outlet by an impacted stone. Upon diagnosis, most patients are initiated on antibiotic therapy.
- Ultrasound is the first line diagnostic modality to identify cholecystitis with ~95% specificity and sensitivity. When equivocal or unobtainable, HIDA scan is the definitive test.
- The definitive treatment for cholecystitis is cholecystectomy during index admission. This is usually achievable via the laparoscopic approach but a low clinical threshold to convert to open procedure in complicated cases is recommended.
- Patients too unstable to undergo cholecystectomy should have percutaneous drainage procedure performed as temporizing measure. In acalculous cholecystitis this can often be definitive therapy.
- Laparoscopic cholecystectomy is feasible and recommended over non-operative management for treatment of acute cholecystitis during pregnancy in the first, second, and early third trimester.
- Treatment of CBD stones depends on experience of surgeon and health center resources with laparoscopic CBD exploration reserved for centers with significant laparoscopic resources. ERCP with ES +/− stent placement prior to laparoscopic cholecystectomy is recommended for cases of CBD stones and cholangitis.
- Gallstones are the most common etiology for acute pancreatitis in North America. The current recommendation is that emergency endoscopic procedures should be performed in those patients who are categorized as moderate to severe pancreatitis with evidence of persistent bile duct obstruction.
- Cholecystectomy during index admission for gallstone pancreatitis is recommended to prevent possibility of recurrent attacks.

Suggested Readings

Caddy GR, Tham TCK. Symptoms, diagnosis, and endoscopic management of common bile duct stones. *Best Pract Res Clin Gastroenterol* 2006;20(6):1085–1101.

Christensen M, Matzen P, Schulze S, et al. Complications of ERCP: A prospective study. *Gastrointest Endosc* 2004;60:721.

Curet MJ. Special problems in laparoscopic surgery: previous abdominal surgery, obesity, and pregnancy. *Surg Clin North Am* 2000;80:1093–1110.

Curet MJ. Management of Common bile duct stones. In: Cameron JL, ed. *Current Surgical Therapy*. 10th ed. Philadelphia, PA: Mosby; 2011:342–345.

Date RS, Kaushal M, Ramesh A. A review of the management of gallstone disease and its complications in pregnancy. *Am J Surg* 2008;196(4):599.

Helou H, Gadacz TR. Gallstone ileus. In: Cameron JL, ed. *Current Surgical Therapy*. 10th ed. Philadelphia, PA: Mosby; 2011:370–373.

Hungness ES, Soper NJ. Management of common bile duct stones. In: Yeo CJ, Dempsey DT, Klein AS, Pemberton JH, Peters JH, eds. *Shackelford's Surgery of the Alimentary Tract*. Philadelphia, PA: Saunders; 2007:1590–1596.

Jonnalagadda S, Strasberg SM. Acute cholangitis. In: Cameron JL, ed. *Current Surgical Therapy*. 10th ed. Philadelphia, PA: Mosby; 2011:345–348.

Soffer D, Blackbourne LH, Schulman CI, et al. Is there an optimal time for laparoscopic cholecystectomy in acute cholecystitis? *Surg Endosc* 2007;21:805.

Van Arendonk KJ, Duncan MD. Acute cholecystitis. In: Cameron JL, ed. *Current Surgical Therapy*. 10th ed. Philadelphia, PA: Mosby; 2011:338–342.

Wang AJ, Wang TE, Lin CC, et al. Clinical predictors of severe gallbladder complications in acute acalculous cholecystitis. *World J Gastroenterol* 2003;9:2821.

Appendicitis

Daniel N. Holena and C. William Schwab

I. GENERAL. Appendicitis is the most common surgical emergency. Physicians evaluating abdominal pain must have a clear understanding of the presentation, differential diagnosis, and management of appendicitis. Appendicitis has no single set of symptoms, signs, or physical findings consistently portray its clinical presentation. Recognizing both classic and unusual presentations of appendicitis will limit delays and complications.

II. INCIDENCE
  A. Approximately 250,000 people a year in the United States develop appendicitis
  B. More frequent in males (1.4:1)
  C. Most common in the second and third decades of life although it may occur at any age
  D. Appendicitis has a lifetime incidence of 7% in the United States (lifetime risk 8.6% in males vs. 6.7% in females). Prompt diagnosis and treatment of appendicitis is especially important in females, as the risk of infertility in a female with ruptured appendicitis increases five-fold

III. ETIOLOGY. The cause of acute appendicitis is occlusion of the appendiceal lumen 90% of the time. This may be secondary to:
  A. Fecalith
  B. Lymphoid hyperplasia
  C. Malignancy
  D. Parasitic infection
  E. Idiopathic
  F. Foreign body

IV. CLINICAL MANIFESTATIONS
  A. The "classical" presentation of appendicitis is ***present only 50% of the time.*** This presentation includes anorexia and periumbilical pain which subsequently localizes to the right lower quadrant, often associated with nausea and vomiting. Physical examination will reveal tenderness to palpation in the right lower quadrant at McBurney's point (two-third the distance from the umbilicus to the right anterior superior iliac spine).
  B. The diagnosis of appendicitis must be made as quickly as possible, as the rate of rupture increases after the first 24 hours of symptoms.
  C. A long list of clinical entities (Table 50-1) have presentations that overlap with appendicitis and make diagnosis a challenge.

V. EVALUATION. The history and physical examination are important in differentiation of appendicitis from other ailments.
  A. Key points from the history include:
    1. Onset of pain. The time to presentation from initial onset of pain is important since it may alter management decisions. If the symptoms have been present for more than 3 days, perform a CT to seek perforation with abscess or phlegmon. Patients who present earlier and with diagnostic uncertainty after examination and imaging should either be admitted and followed by serial examinations or

TABLE 50-1	Differential Diagnosis of Acute Appendicitis

Inflammatory conditions
Acute mesenteric adenitis
Acute gastroenteritis
Acute epididymitis
Meckel's diverticulitis
Crohn's disease
Peptic ulcer disease
Urinary tract infection
Yersinia infection

Gynecologic conditions
Pelvic inflammatory disease
Ruptured ovarian follicle
Ruptured ectopic pregnancy

Mechanical problems
Testicular torsion
Intussusception
Ovarian torsion

taken to the operating room for diagnostic laparoscopy, with possible appendectomy.

2. **Quality of pain.** Early in the course of the classical presentation of appendicitis, the pain is typically poorly localized, constant, and dull in nature (visceral pain). As the inflammatory process becomes transmural and the parietal peritoneum becomes involved, the quality may change to a sharper and more localized pain that is exacerbated by movement, urination, defecation, cough, sneezing, and palpation.

3. **Localization.** The initial pain is usually periumbilical in location. This pain tends to progress to pain localized in the right lower quadrant over the next several hours as the appendiceal lumen becomes increasingly distended and irritates the parietal peritoneum. Less than 50% of patients present with this "classic" history.

4. **Children and elderly.** It may be more difficult to elicit a complete history and physical examination in young children. The elderly may have a vague abdominal pain or no pain at all. **In either age extreme, fever of unknown origin or septic shock can be the sole presentation.**

5. **Relief of pain.** Traditional surgical teaching indicates that spontaneous relief of pain in a patient who has continued abdominal pain from appendicitis for over 24 hours indicates rupture. This should be soon followed by generalized peritonitis and more diffuse pain, malaise and systemic signs of peritonitis.

6. **Anorexia** is common with appendicitis, but this finding does not have the sensitivity or specificity to assure or exclude the diagnosis.

B. **Physical examination.** Many factors of the physical examination may help clarify the diagnosis of acute appendicitis. *All examination findings are fallible* and must be used in conjunction with the history and testing.

1. **Fever.** Appendicitis is often associated with low grade pyrexia (less than 38.5°C (101°F). If the fever is greater than 39.4°C (103°F), alternative diagnoses or a ruptured appendix are more likely present.

2. **Tenderness at McBurney's point.** Physical examination findings will be dictated by the anatomic location of the inflamed appendix. If the appendix is located in the typical anterior location, the patient has tenderness in the right lower quadrant. If the appendix is retrocecal, the patient may have minimal anterior abdominal tenderness. Once the appendix has ruptured, abdominal findings are more diffuse, less localized.

3. **Rectal examination.** For most patients, this has little utility. On rare occasions, tenderness may suggest appendicitis if the tip is in the pelvis. In cases of delayed presentation, rectal examination may elicit a mass and tenderness indicating an abscess or phlegmon.

4. **Psoas sign.** Performed with patient laying on the left side and the examiner slowly extends the right thigh. If extension produces pain, this suggests a retrocecal appendix.

5. **Rovsing's sign.** Pain in the right lower quadrant when *left* lower quadrant is palpated. Suggests localized peritoneal process in the right lower quadrant.

6. **Obturator sign.** Performed with patient laying supine while the examiner internally rotates the patient's flexed thigh and knee. Pain in hypogastric region suggests irritation of the obturator muscle by a low lying pelvic appendix.

Use of opioids for pain control in patients with suspected appendicitis is safe and does not increase errors of diagnosis or management. *The key is titration and continuing the search for the cause while relieving pain*—not just relieving pain alone.

C. **Laboratory evaluation.** Because of the acute onset of appendicitis, few laboratory tests are needed in patients with acute appendicitis.

1. White blood cell counts are commonly obtained but have limit utility in individual patients. Some patients may have mild leukocytosis ranging from 10,000 to 15,000/mm³; usually associated with a left shift in the differential. Leukocytosis much greater than these values may be suggestive of a perforated appendix. A normal white blood cell count does not rule out the diagnosis of appendicitis.

2. Urinalysis is also important to exclude urinary tract infection as the cause of the symptoms. On the other hand, it is not uncommon to find pyuria or microscopic hematuria with acute appendicitis secondary to the inflamed appendix sitting on the ureter or bladder; typically without bacteriuria.

VI. **IMAGING STUDIES.** Abdominal and pelvic CT with PO and IV contrast represents the current common practice in the diagnosis of appendicitis, but other radiographic studies may be performed as part of the workup for undifferentiated abdominal pain. Oral contrast may be omitted in those with active vomiting; conversely, in the very thin, dual contrast is often key to detect appendicitis because of limited fat planes.

A. **Plain film radiography.** May be useful in the initial evaluation of abdominal pain to exclude another etiology, but is neither sensitive nor specific for the diagnosis of appendicitis. Visualization of a fecalith is the sole specific finding but rare (15% of cases).

B. **Sonography.** Ultrasound is inexpensive and rapid. Disadvantages include operator dependence and limitations due to body habitus, particularly in obese patients. Sonographic evidence of appendicitis includes:

1. Non-compressibility of the appendix

2. Appendiceal diameter >7 mm

3. Visualization of fecalith

4. Periappendiceal fluid

Ultrasound is 78% sensitive (95% CI: 67% to 86%) and 83% specific (95% CI: 76% to 88%) for the diagnosis of acute appendicitis. Transvaginal ultrasonography may help detect pelvic pathology in female patients or pregnant women.

C. **Helical computed tomography.** Oral and IV contrast is generally given if not contraindicated. Rectal contrast is not necessary. IV-contrasted CT in all but the thinnest patients retains much of the diagnostic utility of dual contrast scans and is easier to perform. CT should not delay treatment in the patient whose history and physical clearly suggests appendicitis.

1. CT signs of appendicitis include:

   a. Dilation of the appendix >7 mm

   b. Appendiceal wall thickness ≥2 mm, often with concentric thickening of the wall

   c. Periappendiceal stranding

   d. Visualization of a fecalith (~50% of cases)

   e. Abscess or extraluminal gas in the case of perforation

   f. Periappendiceal or pericecal fluid

   CT is 91% sensitive (95% CI: 84% to 95%) and 90% specific (95% CI: 85% to 94%) for the diagnosis of appendicitis; CT may also be useful in clarifying other causes of abdominal pain; early and frequent use has reduced the negative laparotomy rate.

D. Diagnostic laparoscopy. When the diagnosis of appendicitis remains uncertain after appropriate workup, diagnostic laparoscopy is an option. This is especially useful in women, where alternative diagnoses are abundant. Appendectomy is often performed in these patients even when the appendix appears normal so that a recurrence of symptoms does not raise the question of appendicitis again. In addition, 5% of "grossly normal" appendices have microscopic pathology.

VII. OPERATIVE INDICATIONS

A. Because of the complications and prolonged morbidity of rupture, once appendicitis is certain or strongly suspected, promptly operate. Recent literature supports a negative appendectomy rate of up to 10% as acceptable. This has declined over the past decades with the increased use of CT.

B. Once perforation exists with physiologic compromise, diffuse peritonitis, or free air, an urgent operation is best.

VIII. TREATMENT. Antibiotic therapy should be directed against aerobic gram-negative organisms and anaerobic organisms.

A. Uncomplicated appendicitis. *Uncomplicated a*cute appendicitis may be approached either by laparoscopy or open technique. The choice of technique is dictated by the comfort level and preference of the surgeon and patient. One technique has not been consistently shown to have superior outcomes to the other. For uncomplicated appendicitis, the duration of antibiotic therapy is no more than 24 hours.

  1. Laparoscopic appendectomy (LA) confers a slightly lower LOS and decreased length of return to activity, although the cost and duration of the operation is often greater. A recent Cochrane review concluded: (1) wounds infections are less common after laparoscopic appendectomy than open appendectomy (OA), (OR 0.43); (2) risk of intra-abdominal abscess was higher with LA (OR 1.87); (3) hospital length of stay is shorter with LA; (4) return to normal activities and work was shorter after LA; (5) cost of operation was higher with LA; (6) with earlier return to work, costs outside of work were less with LA. Laparoscopy may be useful as both a diagnostic and therapeutic technique in patients with unclear diagnoses.

  2. For an open technique, an incision is made transversely (Rockey-Davis) or obliquely (McBurney's) in the right lower quadrant at McBurney's point.

  3. In either operative approach, if appendicitis is not found, search to find another cause. Many surgical maneuvers assure complete visualization of the distal small bowel, right colon, pelvis and at times the right upper quadrant. These should include at least 2 to 3 ft of the terminal ileum proximal from the ileocecal valve, examination of the ovaries in women and visualization of the entire right colon, gallbladder, distal stomach, and proximal duodenum as necessary. Except in cases of suspected inflammatory bowel disease, an appendectomy is performed to eliminate the future diagnosis of appendicitis.

  4. In uncommon situations, antibiotics and bowel rest may be used to manage uncomplicated appendicitis in up to 68% of cases. However, this approach is complicated by a 12% progression rate and up to 26% recurrence rate at 1 year. Surgical intervention for acute appendicitis remains the accepted practice in the United States.

B. Complicated appendicitis. Up to 25% of cases of acute appendicitis will present with perforation. Those with a delayed course and with a right lower quadrant mass often have a phlegmon.

  1. Patients with ruptured appendicitis who have generalized peritonitis or shock require resuscitation, broad spectrum antibiotics and then be taken to the operating room for surgical source control.

  2. Patients with ruptured appendicitis but without generalized peritonitis may present in a delayed fashion. If small abscesses or a phlegmon are present, initial management with IV antibiotics and hydration is possible. Operating in the setting of phlegmon increases the risk of iatrogenic injury to adjacent viscera and difficulty of the operation.

3. If a well-localized abscess exists, this can be treated with antibiotics and subsequent percutaneous CT or ultrasound guided drainage of the abscess. Obtain a culture of fluid and secure the percutaneous drain.

4. A complex abscess may not be amenable to percutaneous intervention and require planned operative drainage. Operative drainage of a complex abscess should involve appendectomy at time of drainage *only* if easily accessible.

5. Delayed removal of the appendix after initial non-operative management of complicated appendicitis (interval appendectomy) is controversial. Up to 15% of patients will have recurrent disease. Of patients who undergo interval appendectomy, unexpected pathology is discovered in up to 12% of specimens. The decision for interval appendectomy is made after careful consideration of host, environment, and disease conditions.

6. The antimicrobial regimen for perforated appendicitis should cover common aerobic and anaerobic organisms. Multiple effective single agent (ertapenem, meropenem, piperacillin/tazobactam) and combination ([cefazolin, cefuroxime, or levaquin] + [clindamycin or flagyl]) regimens exist, all acceptable. Limit the duration of antibiotics to 4 to 7 days except in the case of inadequate source control or treatment failure. Discontinue antibiotics when the patient is without clinical evidence of infection (afebrile with normal white blood cell count). Each case requires individual scrutiny and constant clinical review.

C. **Incidental appendectomy.** Appendectomy at the time of another abdominal operation is controversial. Proponents argue that the procedure is safe, eliminates the risk of future appendicitis, and reveals pathology in ~3% of cases. Despite this, removal of the normal appendix incurs some risk of complications, increases operative time, and increases costs associated with the procedure. In general, the risk of appendicitis declines with age, so incidental appendectomy is withheld in elderly patients.

Relative indications for incidental appendectomy include:

1. The patient is a child about to receive chemotherapy
2. The patient is about to travel to a location where there is no access to medical care
3. In an individual who is unable to respond appropriately to abdominal pain
4. The patient has Crohn's disease and a cecum that is free of disease
5. Patients in whom the appendix is not in the normal anatomic position (e.g., RUQ, LLQ, intestinal malrotation, etc.)

D. **Appendicitis in pregnancy.** Acute appendicitis has an incidence of 0.15 to 2.10 per 1,000 pregnancies carried to term; appendectomy is the most common non-obstetrical surgical procedure performed during pregnancy. Normal physiologic changes that occur throughout pregnancy may make the diagnosis more difficult, and prompt diagnosis is critical as perforated appendicitis is associated with a four-fold increase in fetal loss when compared to uncomplicated appendicitis.

1. **Evaluation** begins with a history and physical as for the non-pregnant patient. Symptoms of appendicitis may be confused with other common pregnancy related abdominal complaints. Diagnosis is hampered by cephalad displacement of the appendix as gestation progresses, and pain may be present at any location in the right abdomen.

2. **Laboratory evaluation.** Is similar to that of non-pregnant patients with the caveat that mild leukocytosis is a common normal finding in pregnancy, further limiting that test utility.

3. **Imaging studies.** May help make the diagnosis of appendicitis in pregnant patients and avoid fetal risks associated with non-therapeutic surgical intervention.

   a. Ultrasound is preferred but operator dependent and less sensitive and specific than CT for the diagnosis of appendicitis in pregnancy; given the absent risk of ionization radiation, it is a common first test.

b. CT has excellent sensitivity and specificity for the determination of appendicitis in pregnancy. The dose of radiation provided by one CT of the abdomen and pelvis is less than 50 mGy, below the threshold for harmful effects to the fetus—but theoretical risks still exist. Where possible, avoid CT in the *first* trimester during which time the fetus is most sensitive to ionizing radiation.

c. MRI is an alternative to CT and ultrasound when available.

4. Surgical options. Laparoscopy is safe in the first two trimesters; beyond this, the gravid uterus may preclude adequate visualization. In the open technique, incision should be made over the point of maximal tenderness to account for the variable position of the appendix during pregnancy. There is no difference in the fetal risk profile of the two approaches.

5. Antibiotics should be targeted at aerobic gram-negative organisms and anaerobic organisms with attention to drug safety in pregnancy. Acceptable options include second generation cephalosporins + metronidazole or clindamycin.

6. Obstetrical considerations. Obstetrical consultation and monitoring, including documentation of fetal heart tones before, during, and after the procedure, are key.

AXIOMS

- Appendicitis is usually diagnosed by careful history and physical examination.
- Abdominal findings will be dictated by location of the appendix. A retrocecal appendix may not produce anterior peritoneal irritation.
- Prompt diagnosis and treatment of appendicitis is important in all, especially women.
- Based on surgeon comfort and ability and patient input, either laparoscopic appendectomy or open appendectomy is appropriate.

Suggested Readings

Albright JB, Fakhre GP, Nields WW, et al. Incidental appendectomy: 18-year pathologic survey and cost effectiveness in the nonmanaged-care setting. *J Am Coll Surg* 2007;205(2):298–306.

Gilo NB, Amini D, Landy HJ. Appendicitis and cholecystitis in pregnancy. *Clin Obstet Gynecol* 2009;52(4):586–596.

Humes DJ, Simpson J. Acute appendicitis. *Br Med J* 2006;333(7567):530–531.

Ingraham AM, et al. Effect of delay to operation on outcomes in adults with acute appendicitis. *Arch Surg* 2010;145(9):886–892.

Parks NA, Schroeppel TJ. Update on imaging for acute appendicitis. *Surg Clin North Am* 2011;91(1):141–154.

Ranji SR, Goldman LE, Simel DL, et al. Do opiates affect the clinical evaluation of patients with acute abdominal pain? *JAMA* 2006;296(14):1764–1774.

Sakorafas GH, et al. Conservative treatment of acute appendicitis: Heresy or an effective and acceptable alternative to surgery? *Eur J Gastroenterol Hepatol* 2011;23(2):121–127.

Sauerland S, Jaschinski T, Neugebauer EAM. Laparoscopic versus open surgery for suspected appendicitis. *Cochrane Database Syst Rev* 2010;(10):CD001546.

Schwartz SI, Brunicardi FC. *Schwartz's Principles of Surgery.* New York, NY: McGraw-Hill, Medical Pub. Division; 2010.

Simpson J, Scholefield JH. Acute appendicitis. *Surgery* 2008;26(3):108–112.

Solomkin JS, Mazuski JE, Bradley JS, et al. Diagnosis and management of complicated intra-abdominal infection in adults and children: Guidelines by the Surgical Infection Society and the Infectious Diseases Society of America. *Clin Infect Dis* 2010;50(2):133–164.

51 Esophagus, Stomach, and Duodenum

Louis H. Alarcon, Ryan M. Levy and James D. Luketich

The focus of the chapter is non-traumatic diseases that cause inflammation, perforation, or obstruction of the upper gastrointestinal tract, often requiring operative intervention. A key principle is the importance of prompt recognition of the patient who requires immediate surgical intervention, rather than expending time and effort on diagnosis of the specific pathology in this patient. Delayed management is associated with increased morbidity and mortality. The evaluation and management of gastrointestinal bleeding is discussed in Chapter 47.

I. ESOPHAGEAL PERFORATION

A. **Clinical presentation.** Perforation of the esophagus is seen in many clinical scenarios.

1. **Boerhaave's syndrome** is post-emetic esophageal perforation. This may occur in patients with previously normal esophageal function or patients with underlying esophageal pathology or motor disorders. The pathophysiology involves a violent episode of vomiting or retching that results in a rapid increase in intraluminal pressure within the esophagus. Most commonly, the perforation is seen in the lower third of the esophagus.

2. The esophagus can be perforated during upper endoscopy.

   a. Typically, when encountered in a patient with normal esophageal function, perforation occurs in the cervical esophagus. This is a result of failure to navigate the cricopharyngeus muscle that guards the upper portion of the esophagus. Aggressive blind passage through this region of the esophagus can result in passage of the endoscope through the pyriform sinus. The increasing use of side-viewing endoscopic ultrasound and transesophageal echocardiography probes that are larger and more difficult to pass places this anatomic region at increased risk for injury.

   b. Perforation can occur in patients with esophageal pathology during upper endoscopy.

      i. In patients with **Zenker's diverticulum,** failure to negotiate past the hypertensive cricopharyngeus can lead to perforation of the pyriform sinus, as described previously. In addition, inadvertent forcible passage of the scope within Zenker's diverticulum can lead to perforation of the diverticulum.

      ii. Perforation during endoscopy for obstructing malignancies can occur proximal to the obstruction or within the obstructing lesion.

      iii. Perforation can occur when attempting to pass the endoscope across a tortuous or strictured cervical esophagus or hypopharynx, such as those seen in patients with a history of head and neck cancer or irradiation.

      iv. On occasion, perforation occurs with endoscopic interventional procedures. Patients with achalasia who are being treated with esophageal dilation or botulinum injection can suffer from distal esophageal perforation. Perforation can be seen in the setting of laser therapy, sclerotherapy, or photodynamic therapy, or retrieval of foreign objects. In addition, the foreign object itself may perforate the esophagus.

3. Perforation of the esophagus may occur perioperatively. Manipulation of the esophagus, particularly in procedures such as fundoplication or Heller myotomy, can result in delayed presentation of esophageal perforation.

4. Perforation can occur with ingestion of caustic materials. The esophagus is particularly susceptible to ingestion of alkali but relatively immune to ingestion of

acidic material. Lye ingestion is the most common caustic agent causing perforation, while standard household bleach does not cause significant alkali injury. Ingestion of lye can lead to both acute and subacute full-thickness necrosis and subsequent perforation of the entire length of the esophagus. Those who survive the acute event are at risk for recalcitrant stricture. In addition, there is increased long-term risk of malignancy (squamous cell carcinomas).

  5. Tumor necrosis can extend the full thickness of the esophageal wall and cause spontaneous or post-treatment perforation. This is a particular concern after photodynamic therapy ablation of an obstructing esophageal malignancy or external beam radiation therapy in the setting of an esophageal stent.

  6. Perforation after penetrating or blunt trauma can occur anywhere along the entire length of the esophagus depending on the path of the offending agent. The cervical esophagus is particularly prone to injuries sustained from knife or gunshot wounds in the neck. Esophageal perforation secondary to blunt trauma associated with motor vehicle accidents is less common.

B. Evaluation

  1. Clinically, the patient may present with neck, chest, or abdominal pain. The patient may have an acute abdomen or be moribund. The physical examination may reveal neck or upper body crepitus secondary to subcutaneous emphysema. The patient with associated mediastinitis, empyema, or frank peritonitis may be hemodynamically unstable.

  2. Common initial tests include an electrocardiogram, complete blood count with differential, coagulation profile, and electrolyte assay although none are diagnostic. It is wise to type and screen in preparation for surgery.

  3. Imaging

  a. A chest radiograph (CXR) is the first radiographic examination. This may reveal an associated pleural effusion, hydropneumothorax, or pneumoperitoneum.

  b. CT of the chest and abdomen is usually next, with oral contrast when possible. This may reveal pneumomediastinum, pneumoperitoneum, or extraluminal contrast.

  c. Esophagogram with water-soluble contrast followed by thin dilute barium to identify the location of the perforation is frequently used to guide management as well. The esophagogram may be used in lieu of CT or as an adjunct. The contrast esophagogram may demonstrate whether the leak is uncontained, contained, or drains spontaneously back into the lumen of the esophagus. Special care should be taken when an associated obstruction is suspected to prevent aspiration of the water-soluble contrast. In patients with suspected esophageal obstruction, do not use gastrografin or water-soluble contrast, which leads to severe chemical pneumonitis if aspirated.

  4. In stable patients with contained leaks being managed nonoperatively, avoid endoscopy and the risk of worsening any perforation. Insufflation during endoscopy may blow out a contained leak and necessitate surgery.

C. Management begins with resuscitative measures. Securing the airway, if necessary, along with volume resuscitation and broad-spectrum antibiotics against enteric organisms and anaerobes. A urinary catheter aids assessment of volume repletion and renal function.

  1. In a patient who is hemodynamically stable, follow the imaging sequence above (CXR, CT, contrast esophagogram).

  2. In a stable patient, if the leak is contained or drains spontaneously back into the esophagus, nonoperative management with IV fluids and antibiotics may be sufficient. Such management is predicated on a nontoxic patient physiology and **complete** drainage of any associated fluid collections, such as pleural effusions. These patients should be kept fasted initially and have serial radiographs over the next 48 to 72 hours. A repeat CT is important to ensure that no new, undrained fluid collections have developed; if they occur, they **must** be drained or operative intervention planned. A repeat contrast esophagogram should also be obtained; if no leak or perforation, liquids by mouth may be started. If the patient deteriorates during nonoperative management, operate.

3. Surgery for esophageal perforation is classified into four broad categories: Repair, resection, diversion, or wide drainage. Regardless of the type of surgical intervention, upper endoscopy at the time of surgery assesses mucosal viability and the integrity of the repair.

  a. If the patient is stable, attempt primary repair regardless of time of presentation and debride nonviable and necrotic tissue. A two-layer repair (mucosa to mucosa and muscle to muscle) over a 42 Fr bougie or a gastroscope is recommended. It may help to buttress the repair with soft tissue such as intercostal muscle, serratus muscle, omentum, or pericardial fat. Place drains in the proximity of the repair. If the viability or quality of the esophageal tissue is marginal, repair over a T-tube (size 14 F), in addition to placement of periesophageal drains. Often, a decompressive gastrostomy tube and a feeding jejunostomy tube are good early options.

  i. Perforation in the setting of dilation or botulinum toxin injection for achalasia may be repaired primarily. Typically, the perforation occurs at the site of or just above the hypertensive lower esophageal sphincter. A Heller myotomy needs to be performed 180 degrees away from the site of perforation. The myotomy needs to be at least 6 cm long and extend to the very proximal gastric cardia. In addition, a partial fundoplication (Toupet or Dor fundoplication) should be performed in conjunction with the repair and myotomy.

  b. In patients with esophageal malignancy, end-stage achalasia, or caustic injury with esophageal necrosis, do an esophagectomy if the patient is stable. Drainage of the mediastinum with large-bore chest tubes or soft drains (e.g., Jackson-Pratt drain) is needed if there is extensive soilage.

  c. Diversion is a good option in patients where repair or resection is not possible either because of anatomic considerations (e.g., locally unresectable esophageal cancer) or who are unstable. In addition, as with caustic injuries, the final proximal and distal extent of the necrotic injury may not be readily apparent. In particular, this is an issue when there is necrosis of the stomach that may need to be utilized as the conduit for reconstruction. Diversion can be accomplished via a lateral cervical esophagostomy. However, it is preferable to dissect and mobilize the intrathoracic esophagus and then create an end cervical esophagostomy below the clavicle via a left-neck approach. This allows for easier management of the stoma appliance. In addition, it allows for a longer segment of proximal esophagus for potential future reconstruction. A gastrostomy and/or jejunostomy tube should be placed. Wide drainage with large-bore tubes should be placed at the site of perforation.

  d. In a patient who is in extremis, emergent operation is required. Wide debridement and drainage may be the only option. This maneuver may allow the patient to stabilize enough to undergo repair or resection at a later date. A nasogastric tube should be placed with the tip in the distal esophagus to allow drainage of saliva within the esophagus. Place a decompressive gastrostomy tube to prevent reflux of gastric contents and a feeding jejunostomy placed for enteral access.

  i. Debridement and drainage are appropriate and sufficient for perforation of the cervical esophagus. In these patients, be concerned about extension of soilage from the cervical area into the mediastinum. Drainage of the mediastinum in these cases can be accomplished through the cervical incision. Rarely, video-assisted thoracoscopy or even thoracotomy may be necessary to fully drain the superior mediastinum. Figure 51-1 describes an algorithm for the management of esophageal perforation.

II. ESOPHAGEAL OBSTRUCTION
A. Presentation

  1. Obstruction of the esophagus can occur in the setting of primary esophageal pathology, such as malignancy, benign strictures, or esophageal dysmotility such as achalasia. In addition, obstruction of the esophagus can occur in patients with

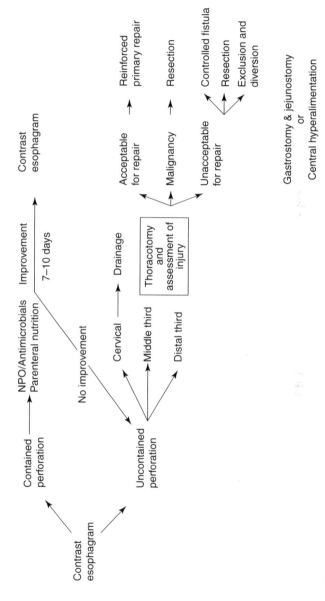

Figure 51-1. Algorithm for management of esophageal perforation. (From Bufkin BL, Miller JI Jr, Mansour KA. Esophageal perforation: Emphasis on management. *Ann Thorac Surg* 1996;61:1447–1451, with permission.)

a normal esophagus, often in children or those with psychiatric illness where ingestion of foreign objects is common. Another common group includes adult patients who have failed to masticate a large food bolus (e.g., meat).

2. Obstruction of the esophagus can cause respiratory compromise secondary to aspiration of retained saliva. Obstruction associated with a chronic process is often coupled with a dilated esophagus. The dilated esophagus may have a pool of retained saliva and food debris, which may lead to an acute obstruction of the narrowed lumen. Clinically, a patient with an obstructed esophagus may present with substernal pain, especially in a patient without previous esophageal pathology. Hypersalivation and aspiration may occur. In severe cases, a totally obstructed esophagus may present with respiratory compromise or inability to protect the airway.

3. Obstruction of the esophagus can occur at multiple points along the esophagus. In an otherwise normal esophagus, three areas are narrowed in caliber and are the usual sites where food or a foreign body can lodge: The cricopharyngeus, mid-esophagus (where the aortic arch indents the esophagus), or the lower esophageal sphincter.

B. Evaluation and management

1. Seek key historical features noted above. In patients with a history of a known obstructing lesion, such as malignancy, achalasia, or stricture, there may be a large volume of pooled secretions and food debris. In patients with foreign body ingestion, it is important to determine whether sharp objects that may perforate the esophagus are present.

2. Assess the airway and intubate if any concerns for aspiration exist.

3. In patients who are stable, do a contrast esophagogram. The risk of aspiration during the study must be assessed, notably by evidence of pooling or any airway difficulty present. If there is any doubt about the risk of aspiration, forego the study. Contrast esophagogram may demonstrate a previously undiagnosed esophageal lesion, identify the level of obstruction, and also exclude perforation of the esophagus. Use dilute barium for this esophagogram.

4. Flexible endoscopy under general anesthesia is recommended next or when the esophagram cannot be safely done. Once the impacted food or foreign body is retrieved, do a more thorough assessment of the esophagus. Biopsy any suspicious lesions. Endoscopic dilation can relieve stricture or malignancy. In patients with achalasia, a delayed and elective Heller myotomy is best, reserving dilation and botulinum toxin injection for those who are not a candidate for myotomy.

   a. Endoscopy under general anesthesia will decrease risk of inadvertent aspiration.

   i. Large-volume lavage of the esophagus with a large-bore tube may be necessary to irrigate the impacted material.

   ii. When flexible esophagoscopy is unsuccessful, rigid esophagoscopy under general anesthesia may be necessary. Avoid inadvertent perforation during rigid esophagoscopy.

III. CHEMICAL BURNS/CORROSIVE INJURIES

A. Acidic or alkali ingestion can result in a burn to the esophagus, stomach, and duodenum. Alkali is the more common agent, notably lye (but not household bleach, which does not cause important injury). Ingestion occurs most often in children and is accidental. In adults, ingestion is often part of a suicide attempt. Although the site of injury can be anywhere in the esophagus, the lower esophagus is often more injured due to a greater contact time with the offending agent. Burns of the mouth, pharynx, epiglottis, or larynx may complicate the presentation and result in respiratory compromise.

B. Conservative management consists of intravenous fluid resuscitation, nothing by mouth, and pain control.

C. Immediate esophagoscopy is not indicated unless perforation is suspected or the patient demonstrates evidence of shock. Esophagoscopy is recommended after 48 hours. The scope is passed to the first area of burn. If severe injury is encountered, do not pass the scope further. Perform a complete endoscopy in the setting of minor burns or erythema. Repeat endoscopy is indicated 3 to 4 weeks later. A contrast esophagogram can detect delayed strictures.

D. Surgical intervention is seldom necessary unless a full-thickness injury occurs. This may necessitate esophagectomy or esophageal exclusion and diversion.

E. The role of steroids in the treatment of corrosive esophageal injuries is controversial. No evidence supports the routine use of steroids in this setting. Careful endoscopic dilation of the stricture may begin 4 weeks after caustic ingestion. This may need to be repeated.

IV. PEPTIC ULCER DISEASE (PUD)

A. General

1. Historically, the pathogenesis of PUD was attributed to an imbalance between the toxicity of the gastric acid and pepsin and the mucosal defense mechanisms of the stomach and duodenum. The discovery of bacterium *Helicobacter pylori* in association with most gastric and duodenal ulcers changed thinking on ulcer disease.

2. Peptic ulcers present as either acute or chronic focal defects in the gastric or duodenal mucosa. Acute complications from this disease process result from the erosion into the surrounding deeper layers of the submucosa and muscularis propria with erosion into blood vessels (hemorrhage) or full-thickness intestinal wall damage (perforation). Over time, the inflammatory process may lead to scarring and compromise of the intestinal lumen (obstruction). The evaluation and management of gastrointestinal bleeding is covered in Chapter 47.

B. Incidence

1. Peptic ulcer continues to be a common diagnosis; however, the rate of elective surgery for PUD has declined steadily over the past 3 decades. Meanwhile, the rate of emergency ulcer surgery has increased.

2. The estimated incidence of PUD is between 1,500 and 3,000 cases per 100,000 people per year. The overall prevalence of PUD in the United States is about 2%, with a current lifetime risk of 10%.

3. During the natural course of their disease, patients with PUD carry a lifetime risk of hemorrhage (15% to 20%), perforation (5%), and obstruction (2%) if left untreated.

C. Risk factors

1. *H. pylori* infection is found in more than 90% of duodenal ulcers and 75% of gastric ulcers. As much as 50% of the adult population in the United States has *H. pylori* colonization. However, only 15% to 20% of those patients colonized will develop PUD in their lifetime.

2. Approximately, 15% to 20% of peptic ulcers are associated with NSAID use. Complications of PUD are more common in patients taking NSAIDs.

3. Physiologic stressors that increase PUD risk are trauma, shock, severe head injuries, sepsis, and surgery.

4. In critically ill patients, the most important risk factors for stress-induced gastritis are respiratory failure and coagulopathy.

5. Uremia.

6. Cigarette smoking. People who smoke are twice as likely to develop PUD compared with nonsmokers.

7. Zollinger–Ellison syndrome.

D. Pathogenesis/etiology

1. Peptic ulcers are caused by an imbalance in either the action of peptic acid or a compromise of the mucosal defense mechanisms or both.

2. *H. pylori* infection plays a major role in the weakening of mucosal defenses and subsequent ulcer development. Furthermore, the inflammation and local alkalinization that accompanies *H. pylori* infection decreases antral somatostatin secretion (antral D-cells) and disrupts the inhibitory control of gastrin release (antral G-cells). The result is a hypergastrinemic state promoting parietal cell hypertrophy and hypersecretion of gastric acid.

3. NSAID use is believed to compromise normal mucosal defense mechanisms.

4. Duodenal ulcerations are most commonly found in the first portion of the duodenum and are associated with acid hypersecretion.

5. Gastric ulcerations may or may not be associated with peptic acid hypersecretion and are classified further based on their anatomical features.

    a. Type 1 gastric ulcer (most common) is typically located near the incisura on the lesser curvature and is associated with normal or decreased acid secretion.

    b. Type 2 gastric ulcer is stomach body ulceration in combination with a duodenal ulcer and is associated with acid hypersecretion.

    c. Type 3 gastric ulcer is pre-pyloric and associated with increased acid secretion.

    d. Type 4 gastric ulcer occurs at the gastroesophageal (GE) junction and acid secretion is normal or below normal.

E. Clinical manifestations

1. Epigastric pain is a cardinal feature of PUD for >90% of patients and is typically described as a burning, stabbing, or gnawing discomfort. Ingestion of food or antacids may temporarily alleviate symptoms for those with duodenal ulcers and may exacerbate symptoms for those with gastric ulceration.

2. Other symptoms may include nausea, vomiting, and anorexia.

3. Upper GI bleeding from peptic ulcer can present with hematemesis (coffee ground emesis), melena, guaiac positive stools, or symptoms of hypotension secondary to hemorrhage (often near-syncope or syncope) (Chapter 47).

4. Perforation complicates PUD in up to 10% of patients. Perforated peptic ulcers typically present with sudden onset of severe abdominal pain and findings of generalized peritonitis on examination. Patients may also exhibit fever, tachycardia, or leukocytosis.

F. Diagnostic modalities

1. In suspected perforation with obvious clinical signs of peritonitis, upright or left lateral decubitus abdominal plain films can assess for free air in the abdomen (80% to 85% of cases). In those patients with less dramatic presentations, abdominal CT may be warranted.

2. It is imperative to quickly diagnose a perforated peptic ulcer. The outcome is improved if surgery is performed within 6 hours of presentation, whereas a delay in treatment beyond 12 hours following perforation is associated with an increase in both morbidity and mortality.

3. In non-emergent presentations of PUD, esophagogastroduodenoscopy (EGD) is the preferred diagnostic modality, allowing both visualization of the ulcer disease and biopsy (*H. pylori* can be confirmed on biopsy). Alternatively, (with less sensitivity), upper gastrointestinal contrast radiograph may demonstrate retention of contrast in the ulcer.

G. Operative indications

1. Medical treatment of *H. pylori* infection and the use of proton pump inhibitors (PPIs) have reduced the need for elective surgery in the treatment of PUD. Emergent surgery for PUD is indicated for the treatment of life-threatening complications: Perforation and bleeding.

2. Signs of peritonitis on examination and free air on plain abdominal x-ray necessitate emergent surgical exploration. Treatment begins with fluid resuscitation, nasogastric decompression, acid suppression, and empiric antibiotic therapy to cover enteric gram-negative rods, anaerobes, and fungus, followed by immediate surgery.

3. Bleeding (Chapter 47).

4. Obstruction (Section V).

5. Intractability. With current therapy against *H. pylori* and PPI use, surgery for intractable ulcer disease is uncommon.

H. Surgical management

1. The goal of treatment of PUD is to decrease acid production; historically, this was accomplished through disruption of the nerve supply to the parietal cell mass of the stomach. In the case of complete truncal vagotomy, a concomitant drainage procedure (pyloromyotomy or pyloroplasty) or gastrectomy is essential.

The majority of peptic ulcers are adequately treated by one of the three operations: Highly selective vagotomy (HSV), truncal vagotomy and drainage procedure (V + D), or vagotomy and antrectomy/distal gastrectomy (V + A). Following antrectomy or distal gastrectomy, intestinal continuity can be reestablished with either a Billroth I gastroduodenostomy or a Billroth II loop gastrojejunostomy. In the modern era of PPI and treatment of *H. pylori* infection, these operations are infrequently performed in the emergent setting.

2. **Perforation**

   a. Duodenal and pyloric channel perforations are the most common sites of peptic ulcer perforation. The most often used technique for perforated duodenal ulcer is a patch repair with an omental pedicle (Graham patch or omentopexy). In this procedure, the ulcer is not closed primarily, but instead a pedicle of vascularized omentum is sutured over the perforation with interrupted sutures. These repairs may open or laparoscopic (if the patient is not unstable). Always follow repair with *H. pylori* eradication (see later) to decrease the incidence of recurrent ulcer disease.

   b. Historically, repair of a perforated duodenal ulcer was accompanied by a definitive ulcer operation, either a vagotomy and pyloroplasty or omental patch repair and a parietal cell vagotomy. With our current understanding of the pathogenesis of peptic ulcers, definitive ulcer surgery is no longer necessary in most cases.

   c. A definitive ulcer operation (HSV or V + D) is best in the rare patient with perforated duodenal ulcer who is hemodynamically stable, has minimal intra-abdominal contamination, and is either known to be *H. pylori* negative, has failed previous medical therapy, or is non-compliant with PPI therapy.

   d. A challenging clinical scenario is the perforated giant duodenal ulcer. With a duodenal ulcer perforation >2 cm, there is an increased risk of failure with omental patch repair. In this setting, recommendations for repair include controlled tube duodenostomy, jejunal pedicled graft, jejunal serosal patch, or partial gastrectomy.

   e. In the case of a perforated gastric ulcer, either ulcer excision and repair of the defect, or biopsy and omental patch is the most expeditious approach in the emergency setting. Histologic investigation of the ulcer site is essential because gastric cancer may present with perforation.

   f. For perforated gastric ulcers on the greater curvature, antrum, or body of the stomach, simple wedge excision with a linear stapler simultaneously obtains tissue for biopsy and closes the perforation. Ulcers along the lesser curvature of the stomach are challenging because of their proximity to the left gastric artery and the GE junction. For distal lesser curve ulcers, distal gastrectomy offers comparable outcomes to patch or simple excision. Perforated ulcers located near the GE junction may be treated with a subtotal gastrectomy to include the ulcer with a Roux-en-Y esophagogastrojejunostomy.

3. *H. pylori* eradication with a triple combination of twice daily PPI, clarithromycin, and amoxicillin for 14 days, or a quadruple regimen of twice daily PPI, bismuth subsalicylate, metronidazole, and tetracycline for 14 days is best.

4. Stop any NSAID, and add a PPI if antacid surgery is not performed.

I. **Outcomes**

1. Emergent surgery for peptic ulcer perforation carries a mortality risk of 6% to 30%. Risk factors for increased mortality include evidence of shock on admission, delayed laparotomy >12 hours, concurrent medical illness, age, cirrhosis, immunocompromised state, high American Society of Anesthesiologists (ASA) class, hypoalbuminemia on admission, or elevated serum creatinine.

2. Overall, complications from gastric ulceration carry a higher mortality rate when compared to duodenal ulcers because of the increased prevalence of gastric ulcers in the elderly population and the ubiquitous use of NSAIDs in this population.

3. Successful eradication of *H. pylori* infection fundamentally changes the natural history of ulcer disease and nearly eliminates recurrence.

4. Incidence of ulcer recurrence after antisecretory surgery is comparable between HSV and V + D (5% to 15%) and superior with V + A (<2%). However, V + A carries higher risk of morbidity and mortality, especially if attempted in unstable patients.

J. Complications

1. Dumping syndrome occurs in 5% to 10% of patients after pyloroplasty or distal gastrectomy. Clinically significant diarrhea occurs in 5% to 10% of patients after truncal vagotomy. Other complications include gastric stasis, bile reflux gastritis, marginal ulceration, cholelithiasis, weight loss, anemia, and osteopenia.

2. A complete truncal vagotomy carries a risk of esophageal perforation.

V. GASTRIC OUTLET OBSTRUCTION

A. General.
Gastric obstruction results from the fibrotic narrowing of the pyloric channel, mechanical twisting of the stomach, or impaction of undigestible matter or objects. Search for a malignancy, especially in older patients.

B. Incidence

1. Gastric outlet obstruction secondary to PUD represents about 5% of ulcer-related complications with operations for obstruction totaling about 2,000 per year in the United States.

2. The incidence of malignancy in patients presenting with gastric outlet obstruction is >50%.

3. Obstruction from gastric volvulus, bezoars, and foreign objects is uncommon.

C. Risk factors

1. Chronic PUD or other inflammatory processes of the upper GI tract increases obstruction risk. Gastric cancer is seen more often in those patients with a family history, a diet high in nitrates, history of gastric adenomas, hereditary non-polyposis colorectal cancer (HNPCC), *H. pylori*, tobacco use, and a >10 year history from prior gastrectomy or gastrojejunostomy.

2. A large paraesophageal hiatal hernia or diaphragmatic defect from another cause (congenital or traumatic) may lead to gastric volvulus. The majority (80%) of cases of gastric volvulus occur in adults with peak incidence in the fifth decade of life. The remaining 20% occur in infants under 1 year of age.

D. Etiology

1. The chronic inflammation of PUD may lead to pyloric channel stenosis. This promotes gastric stasis and increased gastric pH resulting in increased gastrin production and excess acid production. The resulting acute inflammation compounds preexisting chronic fibrosis and leads to gastric outlet obstruction. Other less common inflammatory causes of outlet obstruction include Crohn's disease, pancreatitis, cholecystitis, corrosive stricture, sarcoidosis, tuberculosis, and amyloidosis.

2. Malignancies may result in gastric obstruction including gastric adenocarcinoma, pancreatic adenocarcinoma, or lymphoma.

3. Mechanical obstruction from gastric volvulus. Twisting of the stomach usually occurs in association with a large hiatal or paraesophageal hernia. Organoaxial volvulus is an anterior and superior rotation of the greater curvature over the long axis of the stomach. Mesoaxial volvulus is the rotation of a very lax and floppy distal stomach and duodenum over the shorter transverse axis of the stomach and occurs in one-third of cases of gastric volvulus. This is more common secondary to ligamentous laxity around the crura.

4. Bezoars are concretions of undigestible material that accumulate in the stomach. Phytobezoars are composed of vegetable matter (classically citrus fruits and persimmons) and are associated with altered gastric emptying. Trichobezoars consist of a mass of ingested hair and other fibers. Other less common causes include medications (pharmacobezoar) and chemical ingestion (shellac).

E. Clinical manifestations

1. Patients typically present with nonbilious vomiting or regurgitation of undigested food and have pain or discomfort.

2. Hypochloremic metabolic alkalosis.

3. If the condition is long-standing, the patient may report weight loss.

4. Gastric volvulus may present with sudden, severe pain in the upper abdomen or lower chest with radiation to the back and shoulders, and is accompanied by nonproductive retching. Pressure on the adjacent thoracic organs may result in dyspnea, palpitations, or dysphagia. The initial diagnosis on these patients may erroneously be thought to be cardiac ischemia. Chest film reveals a gas-filled viscus in the lower chest and a nasogastric tube may be difficult or impossible to pass. (In this setting, be aware of the possible diagnosis and do not attempt to force the NG tube. Perforation may result.) Gastric infarction results in a moribund state.

5. Large bezoars may elicit sensations of epigastric fullness and early satiety.

F. Diagnostic modalities

1. The etiology of the gastric outlet obstruction is confirmed by endoscopy. Do biopsies to seek malignancy, although the sensitivity in the setting of gastric obstruction is poor (<40%). Thus, a benign pathologic report does not eliminate the possibility of cancer.

2. The diagnosis of volvulus is made on clinical findings and confirmed by plain chest x-ray; however, if the diagnosis is unclear, an upper GI contrast study is diagnostic.

G. Operative indications

1. Obstruction due to complicated PUD is often initially treated with conservative management (nasogastric suction, fasting, gastric acid suppression, and IV fluids) for 3 to 5 days; however, most patients will ultimately require a definitive surgical procedure.

2. Gastric obstruction from malignant tumors requires operative resection or gastric bypass for palliation.

3. Obstruction from volvulus carries a risk of strangulation; prompt surgical intervention is necessary.

H. Treatment

1. Initial management includes correction of volume and electrolyte abnormalities.

2. Nonoperative management of obstructing PUD with endoscopic pneumatic dilation may temporarily alleviate symptoms and allow an elective surgical procedure in poor surgical candidates.

3. The choice of procedure for gastric outlet obstruction secondary to PUD is either resection of the obstructed antrum and pylorus, or bypass. Because a gastrojejunal bypass is ulcerogenic, resection is preferred as long as the proximal duodenum can be safely divided and closed. Otherwise, bypass procedures are preferred to the morbidity associated with a potential duodenal stump leak. Patients treated with gastrojejunostomy require acid reduction in the form of vagotomy or lifelong PPI.

4. Surgical resection (preferably with 5 cm margins) and lymphadenectomy is optimal for palliation and potential cure for gastric adenocarcinoma causing gastric outlet obstruction. Reconstruction is determined by the location of the lesion and degree of gastric resection that is needed. Obstructing pancreatic cancer may be palliated with loop gastrojejunostomy.

5. Gastric volvulus is a surgical emergency. Initial decompression with a nasogastric tube is accompanied by resuscitation. The volvulized stomach is reduced via an open or laparoscopic approach and appropriate gastric resection (partial or subtotal) performed if necrosis is present. Closure and repair of diaphragmatic defects with gastropexy or gastrostomy tube placement can prevent recurrence.

6. Uncomplicated phytobezoar can usually be managed medically with repeated doses of cellulase (or less commonly, papain and acetylcysteine). Persistent phytobezoar can be managed with endoscopic fragmentation and removal. Trichobezoars and obstructing phytobezoars are surgically removed through a gastrotomy.

I. Outcomes

1. Long-term results of endoscopic dilation for obstructing PUD are poor. Short-term alleviation of symptoms is attained in 83% to 100% of patients. However, only one-third of patients have lasting improvement (>3 months). Operation for gastric outlet obstruction secondary to peptic ulcer has a 5% mortality.

2. Mortality for gastric volvulus may be as high as 30% to 50%, mandating early recognition and prompt surgical correction. The need for gastric resection increases morbidity and mortality.

J. Complications

1. Sequelae of gastric resection (Section IV).
2. Gastric volvulus may result in ulceration, perforation, hemorrhage, pancreatic necrosis, or omental avulsion. Rarely, the rotation of the stomach may also disrupt the splenic vasculature and result in hemorrhage or splenic rupture.

VI. DIVERTICULAR DISEASE OF THE DUODENUM

A. General. Diverticula may occur anywhere in the gastrointestinal tract. It is either described as being acquired as in the small bowel or colon or congenital as in Meckel's diverticulum (Chapter 52). Congenital diverticula tend to be true diverticula in that they incorporate all layers of the intestine, whereas acquired diverticula tend to be "false" diverticula in that they only contain mucosa and submucosa.

B. Duodenal diverticula

1. **Incidence**
   a. Duodenal diverticula are a relatively common entity with a prevalence measured by autopsy reports of about 9% of the population.
   b. They are most commonly found between the sixth and eighth decades of life.
   c. Approximately 75% of duodenal diverticula are periampullary and located within 2 cm of the ampulla.

2. **Etiology.** The exact pathophysiology of duodenal diverticula remains unclear; however, it appears that they occur secondary to a combination of:
   a. Disordered duodenal motility.
   b. Advancing age.
   c. Weakness of duodenal musculature.
   d. Congenital defects contribute to their origin.
   e. Traction diverticula may occur near the first part of the duodenum secondary to scarring from PUD.

3. **Clinical manifestations**
   a. Duodenal diverticula are usually asymptomatic and do not require treatment. The symptoms that occur may be secondary to compression of the pancreaticobiliary tree and include jaundice or pancreatitis.
   b. There has been an association made between periampullary duodenal diverticula, bacterobilia, and common bile duct stones.
   c. Patients may also present with upper GI bleeding from the diverticula, anemia, and signs of diverticulitis, perforation, or ulceration.

4. **Diagnostic modalities**
   a. Use upper endoscopy to evaluate the cause of bleeding in upper GI tract; it may help treat bleeding as well.
   b. Endoscopic retrograde cholangiopancreatography (ERCP) can evaluate the biliopancreatic tree and relieve jaundice.
   c. Upper GI contrast study.
   d. CT scan with oral contrast can occasionally detect these lesions.

5. **Operative indications**
   a. Observe asymptomatic patients.
   b. Operate if hemorrhage cannot be controlled by endoscopy.
   c. Operate on all with perforation.

6. **Treatment**
   a. Patients with evidence of upper or brisk lower GI bleeding should have an upper endoscopy (Chapter 47). Diverticulectomy is generally not recommended in patients presenting with pancreaticobiliary symptoms.
   b. The surgical management of perforated duodenal diverticuli is similar to perforated duodenal ulcers discussed previously.

VII. FOREIGN BODY INGESTION AND RETENTION

A. Ingestion of foreign bodies

1. Incidence

a. The majority of foreign body ingestions occur in children with a peak incidence between the ages of 6 and 36 months.

b. In adults, the majority of foreign body ingestions occurs in those with intellectual disabilities, psychiatric disorders, illegal smuggling of drugs in ingested condoms, or are incarcerated and seeking secondary gain.

c. Food bolus impaction, especially if underlying esophageal pathology is present.

2. Clinical manifestations

a. History

i. In an alert older child or adult, the patient may report the item that was ingested and the amount of time passed since ingestion.

ii. Ask about the size, shape, and sharpness of the object.

iii. Prior history of dysphagia is important, for many esophageal impactions occur at sites of underlying esophageal pathology.

b. Physical examination

i. Usually examination is normal, but subcutaneous emphysema, new-onset pleural effusion, abdominal distension, evidence of gross blood per rectum, or peritonitis may signify complications of ingestion.

3. Diagnostic modalities

a. Radiographs give pertinent information as to the location of the object, and presence of mediastinal or intraperitoneal free air. Anteroposterior and lateral radiographs of the neck, chest, and abdomen help identify radiopaque objects; they do not detect radiolucent objects such as fish bones, wood, plastic, and most glass.

b. Oral contrast examinations increase risk of aspiration if foreign body impaction and obstruction are present.

c. In a patient who has no visible object on radiography and is asymptomatic, no further treatment is necessary.

4. Operative indications

a. Any object in oropharynx or esophagus that is not able to be removed endoscopically

b. Any evidence of perforation or obstruction

c. Narcotic packets that have not passed and have shown signs of rupture or obstruction

5. Treatment. The management of foreign body ingestion varies depending on the location of the foreign body at time of diagnosis as well as its type and size.

a. Stomach. The majority of objects entering the stomach will pass through the rest of the gastrointestinal tract without problems.

i. For objects >10 cm (e.g., toothbrushes), that are unlikely to pass the duodenal sweep, do endoscopic removal.

ii. Retrieve sharp objects endoscopically only if it can be accomplished safely. Otherwise, follow the patient with serial plain radiographs and physical examination to make sure that the object progresses. Any nausea, vomiting, fever, abdominal pain, or GI bleeding warrants operative intervention.

iii. Blunt objects that do not pass the stomach and pylorus in 3 to 4 weeks should be removed endoscopically.

iv. Batteries may produce injury by multiple mechanisms; electrical discharge and mucosal burn, pressure necrosis with larger batteries, mercuric oxide toxicity, or caustic injury from leakage. The patient at highest risk for these complications is younger than 4 years with ingestion of cylindrical or larger (>18 mm) lithium batteries. Liquefaction and perforation may occur as quickly as 2 hours if lodged in the esophagus; these must be removed promptly. Batteries that have passed beyond the esophagus do not require intervention unless symptomatic, large diameter (>2 cm), or remain in the stomach greater than 48 hours.

v. If endoscopic retrieval fails, patients can be managed conservatively for symptoms to develop prior to operative intervention. The majority of all objects, including sharp ones, will pass without complications.

b. Illicit drug packets. Illicit drugs such as heroin or cocaine are occasionally smuggled by people ingesting latex condoms or plastic bags filled with the drugs. Try to avoid rupturing these bags, since lethal overdose can result. Usually, the asymptomatic patient is best observed, and surgery reserved for those with evidence of obstruction or systemic signs of rupture.

AXIOMS

- In the stable patient, primarily repair esophageal perforation.
- In the patient in extremis from esophageal perforation, wide debridement and drainage followed by delayed repair or resection is best.
- Total obstruction of the esophagus may present with respiratory compromise and inability to protect the airway.
- *H. pylori* infection is associated with more than 90% of duodenal ulcers and 75% of gastric ulcers.
- Perforation complicates up to 10% of PUD.
- Gastric volvulus is a surgical emergency.

Suggested Readings

Behrman SW. Management of complicated PUD. *Arch Surg* 2005;140:201–208.

Brunicardi FC, Andersen DK, Billiar TR, et al. *Schwartz's Principles of Surgery*. 9th ed. New York, NY: McGraw-Hill; 2009.

Bufkin BL, Miller JI Jr, Mansour KA. Esophageal perforation: Emphasis on management. *Ann Thorac Surg* 1996;61:1447–1451

Cameron JL, Cameron AM, eds. *Current Surgical Therapy*. 10th ed. Philadelphia, PA: Mosby; 2011.

Cohen H. Peptic ulcer and *Helicobacter pylori*. *Gastroenterol Clin North Am* 2000;29:775–789.

Eisen GM, Baron TH, Dominitz JA, et al. Guideline for the management of ingested foreign bodies. *Gastrointest Endosc* 2002;55:802–806.

Lai AT, Chow TL, Lee DT, et al. Risk factors predicting the development of complications after foreign body ingestion. *Br J Surg* 2003;90:1531–1535.

Lee CW, Sarosi GA Jr. Emergency ulcer surgery. *Surg Clin North Am* 2011;91:1001–1013.

Millat B, Fingerhut A, Borie F. Surgical treatment of complicated duodenal ulcers: Controlled trials. *World J Surg* 2000;24:299–306.

Napolitano L. Refractory peptic ulcer disease. *Gastroenterol Clin North Am* 2009;38:267–288.

Neel D, Davis EG, Farmer R, et al. Aggressive operative treatment for emetogenic rupture yields superior results. *Am Surg* 2010;76:865–868.

Svanes C. Trends in perforated peptic ulcer: Incidence, etiology, treatment, and prognosis. *World J Surg* 2000;24:277–283.

Wang YR, Richter JE, Dempsey DT. Trends and outcomes of hospitalizations for peptic ulcer disease in the United States, 1993 to 2006. *Ann Surg* 2010;251:51–58.

Weiland ST, Schurr MJ. Conservative management of ingested foreign bodies. *J Gastrointest Surg* 2002;6:496–500.

Wu JT, Mattox KL, Wall MJ, Jr. Esophageal perforations: new perspectives and treatment paradigms. *J Trauma* 2007;63:1173–1184.

Zittel TT, Jehle EC, Becker HD. Surgical management of PUD today—Indication, technique and outcome. *Langenbecks Arch Surg* 2000;385:84–96.

Inflammatory Diseases of the Intestines

Sean P. Whelan, Vaishali D. Schuchert and Brian S. Zuckerbraun

INFLAMMATORY DISEASES OF THE STOMACH AND SMALL INTESTINE

I. GASTRODUODENAL PERFORATION

Perforation of the stomach or duodenum can be secondary to trauma, neoplasm, foreign body ingestion, or iatrogenic perforation from diagnostic or therapeutic procedures. The most common cause of gastroduodenal perforation is ulcer disease, with an incidence between 2% and 10% in patients with ulcers. For more details regarding peptic ulcer disease refer to Chapter 51. In this section we will focus on other common causes of perforation including marginal ulcer and iatrogenic perforation.

A. Marginal ulcer

A perforated marginal (perianastomotic) ulcer occurs in a patient who has surgically altered anatomy by previous gastrojejunostomy or other gastric anastomosis. With increasing numbers of patients undergoing bariatric surgery, understanding short- and long-term complications is key. Elective surgery is occasionally performed for intractable ulcers (not responding to maximal medical therapy after 3 months.) Emergency surgery may be necessary in the case of perforated marginal ulcers.

1. Incidence

a. The reported incidence of marginal ulcer after Roux-en-Y gastric bypass (RYGB) varies from 1% to 16%, with a median time of presentation 18 months after RYGB. Gastric partition without transection (commonly performed in open gastric bypass) has a higher incidence of marginal ulcer than with transection of the stomach.

2. Pathophysiology

a. Smoking, excessive alcohol intake, NSAID, and steroid use increase risk for the development of marginal ulcers. Ulceration is most commonly on the jejunal side of the anastomosis, suggesting acid exposure from the stomach as a causative factor. Neither prophylactic acid suppression nor vagotomy reduces the rate of marginal ulcers after RYGB.

3. Management

a. Goals of an emergency operation for perforated marginal ulcer are the same as in any upper gastrointestinal perforation: Close the defect, ensure adequate drainage, and manage sepsis. Alternate enteral access for postoperative nutritional support may be required, generally jejunostomy.

b. A large ulcer or abscess may require resection. Anastomosis in the face of frank purulence or shock should be deferred until the patient has recovered. Laparoscopic repair of perforated marginal ulcer is an option in stable patients without abscess.

B. Iatrogenic perforation

With more liberal use of esophagoduodenoscopy for diagnostic and therapeutic purposes, iatrogenic injury is an increasingly common cause of gastroduodenal perforation. Endoscopic retrograde cholangiopancreatography (ERCP) carries a risk of perforation between 0.5% and 2%. Perforation is described rarely following placement of inferior vena cava filters or biliary stents.

1. Management

a. Microperforation secondary to a wire or sphincterotomy during ERCP often may be managed non-operatively. If needed, the standard therapy for free duodenal wall rupture has traditionally been surgical repair. Advances in endoscopic techniques now allow possible closure of a duodenal perforation endoscopically if recognized immediately and the defect is small.

b. Intravenous antibiotics and close observation are mandatory.

c. If surgical repair of an iatrogenic gastric or duodenal perforation is indicated (size, ongoing leak), the patient's hemodynamic status guides surgical management. Repair of the defect, peritoneal lavage, and placement of drains can be done by laparoscopy or laparotomy.

  i. The patient with peritonitis and in shock should be managed with laparotomy with antifungal therapy added to broad antibiotic therapy.

  ii. A repaired gastric defect may not require extraluminal drains, but a duodenal perforation should be drained widely after repair.

  iii. Proximal decompression in either case is achieved adequately with a well-positioned nasogastric tube on sump suction.

  iv. We do not recommend lateral duodenostomy, but favor placement of closed suction drains in Morison's pouch to provide egress for potential duodenal leak in the form of a controlled fistula.

  v. Create surgical enteral access for postoperative nutritional support.

II. CROHN'S DISEASE OF THE SMALL BOWEL

A. Introduction. Crohn's disease is the most common primary surgical disease of the small intestine. It is an inflammatory process which can affect any portion of the alimentary tract from mouth to anus, but most commonly affects the terminal ileum. Up to 55% of patients with Crohn's disease have ileocolic disease, 30% have isolated small bowel disease, and 15% to 30% have disease involving only the colon or anorectum.

B. Pathophysiology

1. Unlike ulcerative colitis, Crohn's disease is transmural and often discontinuous. Grossly, the affected bowel is characterized by creeping fat and a thickened bowel wall and mesentery. Cobblestoning of the mucosa is characteristic but is not pathognomonic of Crohn's disease.

2. Crohn's disease is associated with a greater degree of extraintestinal manifestations as compared to ulcerative colitis, with up to 25% of patients having at least one extra-intestinal manifestation of disease (Table 52-1).

C. Etiology/risk factors

1. The incidence of Crohn's disease is highest in North America and Northern Europe. Males and females appear to be affected equally.

2. Peak incidence is in the third decade of life with a smaller peak in the sixth decade of life.

D. Management

1. No cure is known for Crohn's disease; the goals of treatment are amelioration of symptoms and improvement in quality of life. Fifty percent to 70% of patients with Crohn's disease will require an operation at some point, but surgery is reserved for refractory cases or in those with complications.

2. Initiate prophylaxis for all hospitalized patients against venous embolism since inflammatory bowel disease (IBD) is a risk factor for development of deep venous thrombosis.

3. Clinical patterns of Crohn's disease are *stricturing, perforating,* and *inflammatory.* Fibrosis and stenosis of discontinuous segments of bowel are the hallmark of the stricturing pattern. Repeated episodes eventually lead to strictures that no longer respond to medical therapy and ultimately require surgery. Abscess and fistulae characterize the perforating pattern. The inflammatory pattern tends to produce a more diffuse distribution, generally treated medically.

E. Treatment of inflammatory Crohn's disease

1. First line therapy for mild symptoms is 5-ASA (Pentasa, Asacol).

2. For a severe acute episode, or "Crohn's flare," corticosteroids are the usual treatment to induce remission. Budesonide is often used to induce remission

TABLE 52-1	Extraintestinal Manifestations of Crohn's Disease (from Schuchert et al.)	
Eyes	Uveitis
	Iritis
	Episcleritis
	Conjunctivitis
Skin	Erythema nodosum
	Erythema multiforme
	Pyoderma gangrenosum
Blood	Deep venous thrombosis/pulmonary embolism
	Hemolytic anemia
	Thrombocytosis
Liver and pancreas	Sclerosing cholangitis
	Triaditis
	Pancreatitis
Joints and bones	Ankylosing spondylitis
	Arthritis
	Spondyloarthropathy
	Osteoporosis
	Clubbing
Kidney	Nephrotic syndrome
	Amyloidosis
Nervous system	Seizure
	Stroke
	Myopathy
	Peripheral neuropathy
	Headache

because of less systemic absorption and more tolerable side effects compared to prednisone.

3. Antibiotics, typically metronidazole, may be used as adjunctive therapy.

4. Infliximab, a monoclonal antibody against TNF-alpha, is used for the treatment of severe active Crohn's disease resistant to conventional therapy. Infliximab is effective as an induction agent, up to 70% patients responding within 1 to 2 weeks from a single infusion.

5. Following successful induction therapy, the goal of treatment becomes maintenance of remission. Steroids are ineffective as maintenance therapy. The two most common agents used for maintenance of remission are azathioprine and 6-mercaptopurine. Patients must be monitored closely for complications which include bone marrow suppression, hepatotoxicity, and pancreatitis.

F. Treatment of perforating Crohn's disease

1. The primary goal of treatment for abscess or fistula is control of sepsis. Image-guided drainage of an abdominal abscess with parenteral antibiotics is the mainstay of therapy.

2. Nutritional and metabolic support are essential.

3. The three most important types of fistulae are enterocutaneous, enteroenteral, and enterovesical.

   a. Enterocutaneous fistulae (ECF) occur in 4% of patients with Crohn's disease. Medical management should be initiated with antibiotics, nutritional support, and infliximab, the latter associated with greater than 60% response rate for closure.

  b. Enteroenteric fistulae in themselves do not mandate operation. Surgery is indicated if the fistulae are associated with an acute inflammatory exacerbation refractory to medical management, abdominal mass, hemorrhage, or uncorrectable malnutrition.

  c. Enterovesical fistula is characterized by chronic or recurrent urinary tract infection (88%), pneumaturia (88%), fecaluria (38%), and hematuria (63%). Do operative repair of enterovesical fistulae to prevent injury to the kidneys from recurrent urinary tract infections.

G. Diagnostic imaging
  1. Radiographs with oral contrast and small bowel follow-through help determine length of bowel and location of disease, identify fistulae, and evaluate strictures.
  2. CT identifies masses, fluid collections, and bowel wall thickening.
  3. Colonoscopy may help establish the presence and extent of disease.

H. Preoperative workup
  1. Assess and optimize the nutritional status prior to surgery.
  2. A bowel prep should be performed if possible.
  3. Consult with the stoma care nursing team for preoperative counseling and marking potential stoma sites is helpful.
  4. Seek any history of recent corticosteroid use to determine whether perioperative steroid replacement or stress dosing is needed. Perioperative corticosteroid use increases postoperative complications, so a rapid taper postoperatively should be a goal when possible.
  5. Other immunosuppressive medications may be safely discontinued preoperatively.

I. Operative indications
  1. Surgical therapy of Crohn's disease is aimed at treatment of complications, relief of symptoms, and optimization of quality of life. Urgent operation may be necessary for free perforation (rare), acute hemorrhage, or uncontrolled sepsis from abscesses not amenable to percutaneous drainage.
  2. Less urgent operation is indicated for enterovesical fistula or acute Crohn's flare, obstruction, or fistula refractory to medical management.

J. Operative approach
  1. Whether elective or emergent, open or laparoscopic, certain basic principles apply to the surgical management of Crohn's disease.
    a. Resect only the segment causing complications and only to grossly (not microscopically) negative margins; minimize length of resected intestine.
    b. Stricturoplasty is a good option when dealing with obstruction.
    c. Consider bypass a last resort because of the risk of bleeding, perforation, and future malignancy in the bypassed portion, although it may be the only viable option with duodenal disease.
    d. In high-risk patients (high-dose steroids, profound malnutrition) endostomy or protective loop ileostomy for a distal anastomosis is advisable.
    e. Perform an appendectomy when safe to avoid future diagnostic dilemma (base of the appendix and adjacent cecum should be free of active Crohn's disease).
  2. In the patient with peritoneal contamination or shock, primary anastomosis is associated with a high leak rate; here, a damage control approach is prudent. This includes resection of bowel to grossly negative margins, peritoneal lavage, and planned re-operation 24 to 48 hours later.
  3. Stricturoplasty may be more appropriate than resection in the patient with concern for short gut. A Heineke–Mikulicz-type stricturoplasty is typically used for strictures less than 10 to 12 cm in length. For longer strictures, up to 25 cm in length, a Finney-type stricturoplasty is preferred.
  4. Selected patients are candidates for laparoscopic surgery for Crohn's disease. Length of stay, morbidity, and overall cost in the first 3 postoperative months are lower in patients undergoing a minimally invasive surgical approach.
    a. Diagnosis
      i. Most patients presenting with severe colitis from IBD already have that underlying diagnosis. In those who do not, it is important to consider alternative diagnoses such as infectious or ischemic colitis. In patients with a

diagnosis of IBD, consider cytomegalovirus (CMV) or *Clostridium difficile* infection.

ii. Plain films of the abdomen can evaluate for perforation, disease, extent, or toxic megacolon; CT is more accurate for these findings.

iii. Colonoscopy assesses the severity and the extent of mucosal inflammation and ulceration. Biopsy and inspection may help diagnose ischemic colitis, Crohn's colitis, CMV infection, *C. difficile,* or other infectious colitides.

b. Management

i. Medical management parallels that noted in small bowel IBD (see earlier).

c. Operative indications

i. Failure of medical therapy, clinical deterioration, perforation, or toxic megacolon requires operative intervention.

ii. Patients will generally undergo a subtotal abdominal colectomy, end-ileostomy, and creation of a Hartmann's pouch. Total proctocolectomy is usually avoided in the acute setting if a restorative procedure is possible in the future.

iii. Early consultation with a stoma therapist will help guide management and enhance patient understanding.

III. ENTEROCUTANEOUS FISTULA

A. General. The management of (ECF is challenging. Fistulae are often complicated by sepsis, fluid and electrolyte abnormalities, malnutrition, and complex wound management issues; mortality ranges from 10% to 20%. ECF develop as a result of technical factors from a previous operation, factors related to healing and tissue integrity inherent to the patient, and factors related to specific disease processes.

B. Pathophysiology

1. The majority of ECF occur as a complication of an abdominal operation, often from anastomotic leak, unrecognized enterotomy, incorporation of bowel in the fascial closure, or ischemia. Risk factors include emergency abdominal procedures, contaminated operations, severe malnutrition, steroid use, radiation, or chemotherapy. Serum albumin levels less than 3.0 g/dL is a risk factor for the development of ECF.

C. Clinical manifestation

1. ECF classically presents as a wound infection following abdominal surgery. Wound drainage with the appearance and odor of enteric contents is diagnostic. Evaluate the underlying fascial integrity since ongoing leakage of enteric contents may lead to fascial dehiscence and evisceration. Conversely, ECF is in the differential diagnosis of a patient presenting with fascial dehiscence or evisceration.

2. In general, the more proximal the fistula, the more pronounced the electrolyte abnormalities, fluid losses, and malnutrition. Distal fistulae may essentially function as an ileostomy or colostomy without fluid, electrolyte, or nutritional abnormalities.

D. Diagnostic imaging

1. Upper GI contrast study or CT with oral contrast may demonstrate an ECF along with possible obstruction, abscess, potential foreign body, or loss of domain (large ventral defect). A chronic fistula tract can be injected with oral contrast to locate the site of communication with the intestinal tract (fistulogram).

E. Management

1. The primary goal of treatment of an ECF is source control and control of sepsis. Uncontrolled sepsis is the major cause of mortality in patients with ECF. Correction of fluid and electrolyte imbalances, nutritional support, and skin care are essential adjuncts.

2. In the absence of sepsis, a trial of medical management may eliminate the need for operation. In those who still require operation, the additional time allows the fistula tract to mature and inflammation to subside.

3. Image-guided drainage of abdominal abscesses usually precludes the need for early operation.

4. Consultation should be made to the wound and ostomy care nursing team to assist with the complex wound management that most of these patients will have.

5. Negative pressure vacuum dressings may promote healing. Creative skin grafting around the fistula may simplify wound care and provide patient comfort while the fistula matures or closes.

6. Adequate nutritional support is essential while awaiting spontaneous closure of an ECF; however, neither parenteral nor enteral nutrition induce closure of an ECF. Protein and caloric requirements may be double their baseline requirements. Providing as little as 10% to 20% of nutritional needs enterally helps maintain gut mucosal integrity and immunologic function. Parenteral nutrition may sometimes be used to supplement enteral feeding for profoundly malnourished patients or patients who cannot tolerate full enteral feeds.

7. Closure rate of an ECF is 10% to 40% with conservative management. The use of octreotide as adjunctive therapy may decrease fistula output, but does not impact frequency of spontaneous closure.
   a. An ECF that persists 6 to 8 weeks after resolution of sepsis and correction of nutritional deficits is unlikely to close spontaneously, especially if the output is high (>500 mL/day).
   b. Factors associated with failure of an ECF to close include high output fistula, ongoing malnutrition, distal bowel obstruction, short fistula tract, abscess, foreign body (including mesh), malignancy, radiation, and steroids.

F. Operative approach

1. Early surgical intervention may be necessary in septic patients with uncontrolled leakage of enteric contents into the abdomen or abscesses not amenable to percutaneous drainage. A limited bowel prep should be performed when possible preoperatively.

2. Fully mobilize the bowel to allow proper identification of involved segments, ensure patency of the length of the bowel, and to perform segmental resection of the fistulae with tension-free anastomosis.

3. Closure of the abdominal wall and distancing the repair from the incision should be routine. Surgical enteral access for postoperative nutritional support should be secured.

IV. SMALL BOWEL DIVERTICULAR DISEASE

General. Small bowel diverticulosis is an uncommon entity and less than 4% of all small bowel diverticuli will become symptomatic in a person's lifetime. Because the clinical presentation may be dramatic with bleeding, perforation, or acute inflammation, the acute care surgeon should be prepared to manage complications that may arise from these diverticula. There are two types of small bowel diverticula: False diverticula are acquired defects with herniation of mucosa and submucosa along the mesenteric side of the bowel where vessels penetrate the bowel wall. True diverticula are congenital anomalies arising in the anti-mesenteric side of the distal ileum (Meckel's diverticulum).

A. Duodenal diverticula

1. Incidence/etiology

a. A duodenal diverticulum typically presents during or after the fifth decade of life as a solitary outpouching along the mesenteric side of the duodenal wall. It is the most common (45% to 79%) small bowel diverticulum.

b. The majority (61% to 75%) are located in the periampullary area, or within 2 cm of the ampulla of Vater. The inherent defects in the muscularis propria caused by the penetration of the pancreatic and biliary ducts predispose to the development of these false diverticula.

2. Clinical manifestations

a. Patients present with symptoms related to biliary or pancreatic ductal obstruction including cholangitis, jaundice, or pancreatitis.

b. Patients with duodenal diverticula have a higher incidence of choledocholithiasis with pigment and bilirubinate stones.

c. Duodenal diverticula are part of the differential diagnosis for patients with pancreatitis of unclear etiology.

3. Diagnosis

  a. Diagnosis is by upper endoscopy, contrast radiography, or CT with oral contrast. They are found in 10% to 20% of patients undergoing ERCP.

4. Management

  a. Less than 1% require treatment. Asymptomatic or incidentally found duodenal diverticuli should not be resected. The patient should be informed of the incidental finding and potential sequelae.

  b. Choledocholithiasis in association with a duodenal diverticulum should be managed conventionally as in patients without duodenal diverticula.

  c. Inflammation, perforation into the retroperitoneum or peritoneal cavity; and hemorrhage occurs less frequently but may necessitate surgery acutely.

5. Operative approach

  a. The surgical approach begins with a complete Kocher maneuver and identification of the pancreaticobiliary structures and their relationship to the diverticulum. Diverticulectomy with primary closure is the procedure of choice when the ductal structures are not involved and when there is no retroperitoneal contamination.

   i. For duodenal diverticula distal to the ampulla, options include diverticulectomy with jejunal serosal patch repair or segmental resection with end-to-end anastomosis.

   ii. Roux-en-Y biliary bypass may be necessary when the ampulla is involved.

B. Jejunoileal diverticula

1. Incidence/epidemiology

  a. Jejunoileal diverticula occur in 1% to 3% of the general population, comprising only 25% of all small bowel diverticula. However, these are the most likely to be symptomatic.

  b. They are often multiple, with 80% occurring in the jejunum, 15% in the ileum, and 5% along the full length.

  c. Patients typically present at age 50 years or older.

2. Clinical manifestations

  a. Patients may present with perforation, obstruction, hemorrhage, or inflammation causing peritonitis.

  b. More commonly, the symptoms are related to the intestinal dysmotility, that is the underlying pathophysiology for the development of these acquired diverticula. Signs and symptoms related to stasis and malabsorption include abdominal pain, steatorrhea, megaloblastic anemia, or neuropathy.

  c. Small bowel follow-through radiography establishes the diagnosis.

3. Diagnosis

  a. CT with oral contrast has the added benefit of assessment of inflammation or subtle signs of perforation and the anatomic relationship of diverticula to surrounding structures.

  b. Diagnosis is often made at laparoscopy or laparotomy.

4. Management

  a. In patients with malabsorption due to bacterial overgrowth, medical therapy with metronidazole and amoxicillin-clavulanate plus nutritional support with vitamin supplementation is successful in 75% of cases.

5. Operative indications

  a. Surgical intervention is indicated in patients in whom medical therapy fails.

  b. Segmental resection of the involved diverticula is the treatment of choice for symptomatic diverticula.

  c. Diverticula encountered incidentally during laparoscopy or laparotomy should not be excised.

C. Meckel's diverticulum

1. Incidence

  a. Meckel's diverticula, true diverticula on the antimesenteric side of the bowel, are the most common congenital anomaly of the small bowel and account for 25% of all small bowel diverticula.

2. Pathogenesis

a. Failure of the vitelline (omphalomesenteric) duct to obliterate may manifest as an ileo-umbilical fistula, vitelline duct cyst, but most commonly as a Meckel's diverticulum.

b. The defining features of a Meckel's diverticulum are described by the "rule of two": 2% of the population, 2 in. long, within 2 ft of the ileocecal valve, and two types of heterotopic mucosa. It typically presents within the first 2 years of life but may present in the adult.

c. Half of Meckel's diverticula contain heterotopic mucosa with 75% being gastric mucosa and 15% pancreatic.

3. Clinical manifestations

a. The most common cause of lower gastrointestinal bleeding in pediatric patients. Acid secretion from heterotopic mucosa within the diverticulum leads to ulcer formation on the opposite side of the bowel wall that may bleed.

b. The most common presentation of a symptomatic Meckel's diverticulum in adults is bowel obstruction secondary to intussusception, volvulus, or incarceration within an inguinal hernia (Littre's hernia).

c. Meckel's diverticulitis occurs in 25% of symptomatic patients and is often found at laparoscopy for what is initially thought to be appendicitis.

4. Diagnosis

a. A "Meckel's scan," used to identify uptake of radioisotope by gastric mucosa, may be helpful in the workup of GI bleeding but plays no role in the workup of an acute abdomen. Patients presenting with obstruction or diverticulitis are often diagnosed intraoperatively.

5. Management

a. In cases of obstruction or localized inflammation, stapled diverticulectomy or wedge excision with primary closure is adequate. With significant inflammation or with a wide-based diverticulum, segmental bowel resection is preferred. With hemorrhage, segmental resection is necessary to include the bleeding ulcer on the opposing bowel wall. Appendectomy should be performed to avoid future diagnostic dilemma.

b. Incidentally found Meckel's diverticula in children should be removed.

c. Relative indications for removal include evidence of heterotopic tissue, signs of prior diverticulitis, or the presence of a mesodiverticular band. The initial indication for operation and implications for future planning should also be considered. Most surgeons do not favor removing a Meckel's diverticulum found incidentally in an adult patient.

INFLAMMATORY DISEASES OF THE COLON

I. COLONIC DIVERTICULITIS

A. General

1. Colonic *diverticulosis* refers to the presence of diverticulum in the colon in the absence of inflammation, while *diverticulitis* refers to the presence of inflammation and infection associated with a diverticulum.

2. Colonic diverticulosis is common in the Western population and incidence increases with age. Diverticulosis is rarely seen in individuals younger than age 30, but the prevalence increases to 40% by the age of 60 years and 60% to 80% by 80 years of age.

3. Diverticula generally involve the sigmoid and left colon. With increasing age, prevalence of diverticulosis that extends more proximally in the colon increases.

4. Between 10% and 25% of patients with diverticulosis develop diverticulitis.

B. Pathophysiology

1. Colonic diverticula are pulsion or false diverticula, acquired as the mucosa and submucosa "herniate" through the colonic wall where the vasa recta penetrate the circular muscle layer. Diverticula tend to occur on either side of the mesenteric tenia or on the mesenteric border of the two antimesenteric teniae.

C. Etiology
    1. Diverticulosis
        a. Several hypotheses to explain development of diverticulosis include generation of high intracolonic pressures due to disordered colonic motility and the role of low dietary fiber.
        b. Additional risk factors include increasing age, geographic factors, cigarette smoking, nonsteroidal anti-inflammatory use, obesity, decreased physical activity, and caffeine ingestion.
    2. Diverticulitis
        a. The etiology is thought to be similar to the development of acute appendicitis, in which obstruction of the diverticulum leads to bacterial overgrowth, distension, and tissue ischemia. This results in localized inflammation possibly leading to contained perforation with peridiverticular abscess or free intraperitoneal perforation with peritonitis. The inflammatory process may fistulize into adjacent structures such as the bladder. The most common cultured isolates are anaerobic bacteria followed by gram-negative aerobes. *Enterococcus* is the most common gram-positive aerobe.

D. Symptoms/clinical manifestations
    1. The symptoms of diverticulitis range from mild abdominal pain to peritonitis and sepsis. The most common symptom complex during acute diverticulitis involves left lower quadrant pain and fever. Patients often describe a change in bowel habits with mild diarrhea. Bleeding per rectum is usually not associated with diverticulitis and would suggest other etiologies of colitis. Nausea or vomiting may be present due to associated ileus, an obstruction related to phlegmon, or inflammatory stricture.
    2. Physical examination most often reveals tenderness in the LLQ, at times with an associated mass. Laboratory evaluation often demonstrates a leukocytosis, but no laboratory tests are confirmatory.
    3. When associated with colovesical fistula, symptoms are marked by cystitis, pneumaturia, pyuria, or fecaluria. Similarly, colovaginal or uterine fistulae may present with vaginal discharge, passage of air or stool per vagina.

E. Differential diagnosis
    1. The differential diagnosis for patients with diverticulitis includes appendicitis, bowel obstruction, IBDs, ischemic colitis, colorectal cancer, gynecologic disease, and irritable bowel syndrome.

F. Diagnostic imaging
    1. Diverticulitis is a clinical diagnosis, but if there is suspicion for complications, CT can determine the diagnosis of diverticulitis, complications, or detect other causes. CT severity scoring also correlates with recurrence in patients who are managed non-operatively. The Hinchey classification system (Table 52-2) is the most accepted for prognosis.
    2. Contrast enema may diagnose diverticulosis or strictures associated with diverticulitis, but these should not be used in acute diverticulitis due to risk of perforation. When done, use water-soluble contrast, not barium.
    3. Following the initial presentation of diverticulitis, endoscopy is import later to exclude an underlying malignancy. Colonoscopy is most often performed at least 6 weeks after the episode of diverticulitis due to concerns of exacerbating or creating microperforations.

TABLE 52-2	Hinchey Stages of Diverticulitis

Stage 1: Small, pericolonic or mesenteric abscess
Stage II: Pelvic or distant intra-abdominal abscess
Stage III: Purulent peritonitis
Stage IV: Feculent peritonitis

G. Management

1. Uncomplicated diverticulitis is treated with antibiotic therapy. Although the ideal regimen has not been determined, antibiotics should have activity against anaerobes and aerobic gram negatives and gram positives, good tissue penetration, minimal toxicity, and clinical efficacy. Common regimens include ciprofloxacin and metronidazole or amoxicillin/clavulanate and ciprofloxacin orally.

2. Patients with minimal symptoms and mild examination findings are often treated as outpatients; however, patients with more severe tenderness, fever, systemic symptoms, or inability to tolerate oral intake should be hospitalized for IV fluids, antibiotics, and CT scan.

3. Patients with uncomplicated disease (Hinchey stages 0 or I) are generally treated with bowel rest and transitioned to an oral regimen following clinical improvement.

4. Diverticular abscesses are present in about 15% of patients with diverticulitis and can be in the following locations:
   a. Mesocolic or pericolic (Hinchey stage I)
   b. Pelvic or retroperitoneal (Hinchey stage II)

5. Large abscesses (usually greater than 4 cm) are treated with percutaneous drainage if accessible. Transabdominal drainage is preferable; however, transgluteal, transperineal, transvaginal, and transrectal drainage are alternatives.

H. Operative indications

1. Free perforation with purulent or feculent peritonitis (Hinchey stage III or IV).
   a. Only 1% of patients will develop free perforation, and it is the initial attack of diverticulitis in 70% of patients.
   b. The standard treatment is Hartmann's procedure (resection of the perforated segment of colon, closed distal end left intraperitoneally, and end descending colostomy).
   c. There is increased advocacy for alternative approaches, including exploratory laparoscopy to determine the extent of disease and contamination, and if this reveals only purulent peritonitis, then proceeding with a laparoscopic peritoneal washout and placement of a drain. If feculent peritonitis is encountered then a Hartmann's procedure is performed.

2. Diverticular abscess
   a. Decision made on case-by-case basis for urgent or elective operation, usually guided by clinical condition and ability to achieve percutaneous drainage.

3. Repeated bouts of uncomplicated diverticulitis
   a. Controversial traditional teaching was to operate after two or more bouts. Recent data have shown 70% of patients with free perforation have no prior episodes. Young age (<50 years) is similarly no longer an indication for colon resection after the first bout of diverticulitis. There are no clear frequency-based guidelines currently to guide elective operations.
   b. On the other hand, colon resection is recommended after the first bout of diverticulitis in the immunosuppressed patient or the patient with a bout of complicated diverticulitis (abscess requiring drainage, fistula).

4. Colovesical fistulae
   a. Often require surgical treatment although urgent operation is rarely required as the fistula usually decompresses the infection.

5. Diverticular stricture
   a. Repeated attacks can result in stricture that causes obstruction. The management of obstruction is covered in more detail in Chapter 46.

II. INFECTIOUS COLITIDES

These include *C. difficile*, *Campylobacter*, *Salmonella*, *Yersinia*, *Shigella*, and *Escherichia coli*. In addition, CMV can result in colitis, particularly in immunosuppressed patients. Additional infections include amebic colitis from *Entamoeba histolytica* and toxic megacolon in Chagas disease from *Trypanosoma cruzi*. This section will focus on *Clostridium difficile*–associated disease (CDAD) as this bacterium is the leading culprit in nosocomial infectious colitis.

TABLE 52-3 Risk Factors for *Clostridium difficile* Colitis (from Schuchert et al.)

Antibiotics
Advanced age
Hospitalization
Long-term care facilities
Immunosuppression
Postoperative
Proton pump inhibitors
Elemental diet
Inflammatory bowel disease

A. *Clostridium difficile*–associated disease (CDAD):

1. **General.** CDAD affects over 3 million patients annually, causing 15% to 35% of antibiotic-associated diarrhea, and 70% of cases of antibiotic-associated colitis. *C. difficile* colitis has a high morbidity (30% to 80%) and mortality (4% to 10%), a high recurrence (25% of patients), and an increasing incidence of fulminant disease.

2. **Pathophysiology**
   a. CDAD is acquired through the oral ingestion of *C. difficile* spores that are resistant to gastric acidity. Colonization occurs in 31% of hospitalized patients receiving antibiotics and 56% of these develop symptomatic disease.
   b. With colonization, the depletion of competitive flora by antibiotic therapy allows *C. difficile* to overgrow and produce exotoxins. This is usually limited to the colon resulting in diarrhea, but in the subset of patients with severe, complicated disease; the consequences of toxemia become systemic. Major risk factors include antibiotic exposure, hospitalization, and advanced age (Table 52-3).

3. **Clinical manifestation**
   a. The most common clinical presentation is diarrhea associated with a history of antibiotic use (either a few days after the antibiotic is started up to 12 weeks after they are stopped). Patients may have diarrhea associated with cramps, fever, leukocytosis, fecal leukocytes, abdominal pain usually localized to lower quadrants, or hypoalbuminemia due to protein losses in stool.
   b. On rare occasion, diarrhea may be absent—this is usually in a toxic patient with an ileus.

4. **Diagnosis**
   a. Includes the clinical findings listed above as well as a stool test positive for *C. difficile* toxins or toxigenic *C. difficile*.
   b. Visual or pathologic evidence of pseudomembranous colitis.
   c. CT is a useful adjunct but is less sensitive than stool toxin assays and rarely diagnostic. Most severe CDAD will show a pancolitis and moderate ascites.

5. **Management**
   a. Standard hospital isolation precautions to reduce the spread must be instituted, and antibiotics previously employed should be discontinued if possible.
   b. Mild or moderate disease: Use oral metronidazole 500 mg three times per day or 250 mg four times per day for 10 to 14 days.
   c. Severe disease manifests with fever, leukocytosis (15 to 20,000 cells/mm^3), cramps and diarrhea but without hypotension, ileus, or megacolon. This is treated with oral vancomycin (125 mg four times per day) for 10 to 14 days.
   d. Recurrent disease: First recurrence—either drug regimen is adequate. Two or more recurrences—course of vancomycin with taper over time.
   e. Patients unable to tolerate oral antibiotics: Metronidazole 500 mg IV every 8 hours—achieves therapeutic concentrations in the colon via biliary secretion but only in patients with diarrhea. Vancomycin IV is ineffective, as it does not reach the intestinal lumen.

6. Operative indications and approach

a. Surgical treatment improves outcomes in severe complicated CDAD—for example, those patients admitted to intensive care units with organ failure, or the need for vasoactive agents or ventilatory assistance.

b. The common approach for severe complicated, "fulminant," CDAD is total abdominal colectomy.

c. We believe that fulminant CDAD in the majority of many patients can be treated operatively with creation of loop ileostomy and intraoperative colonic lavage, followed by antegrade vancomycin flushes via the ileostomy. However, this is a new approach and unvalidated.

B. Bacterial enterocolitis

A number of bacterial infections can cause enterocolitis. These include *E. coli, Campylobacter, Salmonella, Yersinia,* or *Shigella.* The most common symptom is diarrhea, and the care is mainly supportive. Treatment with antibiotics, typically fluoroquinolones, can hasten recovery. Although these infections can be serious, they usually do not require surgical consultation or treatment.

C. Cytomegalovirus (CMV) colitis

In an immunocompetent host, the CMV virus remains in a chronic latent state in host cells, with viral proliferation prevented by host cell–mediated immunity. CMV colitis is generally limited to patients with immunodeficiency and is seen in 2% to 16% of patients with solid organ transplants and 3% to 5% of patients with HIV/AIDS. Another at risk population includes patients with ulcerative colitis, with 9% to 27% case rates.

1. Clinical manifestations

a. CMV colitis causes a painful vasculitis that manifests as peritonitis on examination. Also, if left untreated, it may lead to ischemia and transmural necrosis, resulting in perforation and peritonitis.

2. Diagnosis

a. This can be difficult to discern from other forms of colitis. Ulcers can develop and erode into blood vessels causing profuse bloody diarrhea.

b. Inflammatory polyps may develop which, rarely, may cause obstruction.

c. Colonoscopy and biopsy diagnose CMV infection. Culture may be positive, but testing for viral antigens using immunofluorescent antibodies increases the sensitivity.

3. Management

a. Due to the common finding of peritonitis on examination, exploratory laparotomy and surgical resection is common. With increased awareness of CMV infection in immunocompromised patients and treatment with antivirals, the need for operation is now rare.

b. First line antiviral therapy is ganciclovir, with foscarnet used as a second line agent in most cases.

c. In patients with ulcerative colitis, CMV colitis can result in toxic megacolon if therapy is initiated late in the course; and colectomy may be necessary.

III. ISCHEMIC COLITIS

A. General. Ischemic colitis is the most common form of gastrointestinal ischemia. There are numerous etiologies for ischemic colitis, but all result in decreased blood supply that is injurious to the colon. Ischemic colitis can range from limited injury to the colonic mucosa to full thickness injury with colonic necrosis and the development of sepsis. The diagnosis of ischemic colitis is challenging and often the exact etiology is not determined.

B. Pathophysiology

1. Blood flow to the colon can be decreased secondary to changes in perfusion that affect the systemic vasculature or local changes in blood flown in the mesenteric vasculature. The etiologies are often classified as occlusive or non-occlusive.

a. Occlusive: Embolic phenomena, thrombosis, atherosclerosis, or small vessel disease.

b. Non-occlusive: Shock states, medication effects, or colonic obstructions.

2. Specific clinical situations that can precipitate ischemic colitis include aortic surgery (limits flow to the IMA) and angiographic embolization to treat gastrointestinal bleeding.

C. Clinical manifestations

1. The onset is characterized by sudden, crampy abdominal pain that is poorly localized. Subsequently, patients will often pass bloody or maroon stools; a manifestation of mucosal ischemia. The quantity is usually not significant, and if bleeding is more substantial, other etiologies should be suspected. Pain can be more localized if transmural necrosis leads to inflammation of the parietal peritoneum.

2. The majority of patients who develop ischemic colitis in non-hospitalized settings present with normal hemodynamics and mild abdominal tenderness. In the case of transmural necrosis, peritonitis will be present, and hemodynamic instability may be present.

3. Laboratory evaluations are non-specific and underwhelming until severe disease is present. Patients may have an elevated white blood cell count or a metabolic acidosis or elevated lactate levels.

D. Diagnosis. Diagnosis is made by history and physical examination in combination with radiologic studies and colonoscopic inspection.

1. Plain films of the abdomen may demonstrate thickened colon wall or "thumbprinting," or less commonly, pneumatosis coli. Usually, no specific findings exist.

2. Avoid contrast enemas in the acute setting.

3. CT with IV contrast or CT angiography allows visualization of the mesenteric vasculature. Findings of ischemic colitis are non-specific and include colon thickening and ascites.

4. Colonoscopy is the most sensitive and specific test. It may show submucosal hemorrhage and allows biopsy to help differentiate inflammatory, ischemic, or infectious causes of colitis. If the mucosa appears gray-green or black, this suggests more advanced ischemia and possibly transmural ischemia.

E. Management

1. In the absence of signs of colonic gangrene or perforation, ischemic colitis is managed non-operatively.

a. Use bowel rest with intravenous fluid resuscitation; if a significant ileus or bowel distention is present, a nasogastric tube is placed to suction.

b. Cardiac function is optimized and drugs that can impair mesenteric blood flow (vasoconstrictors) are limited if possible.

c. Broad-spectrum antibiotics are started in most patients to cover the usual colonic flora, although there is little data to support this practice.

d. Avoid bowel preps or enemas as they may worsen ischemia.

2. If transmural necrosis, infarction, or perforation is suspected, prompt operative exploration is indicated. The ischemic colon is resected to areas with normal mucosa.

a. If ischemia involves multiple segments, a subtotal colectomy is needed. As a general rule, performing an anastomosis in the setting of resection for colonic ischemia is ill-advised; because of concern for the blood supply of the remaining bowel, a proximal stoma (ileostomy or colostomy) is safer.

IV. ACUTE PRESENTATION OF COLONIC INFLAMMATORY BOWEL DISEASE SEE EARLIER (UNDER SMALL BOWEL CROHN'S DISEASE) for general information.

AXIOMS

■ Acute inflammatory processes of the intestinal tract may require urgent operation but often are managed well medically.

■ Resist the temptation to do too much in the operating room during an emergency operation. The primary goals of the operation must remain the focus.

- Crohn's disease is the most common primary surgical disease of the small intestine.
- The primary goal of treatment of an enterocutaneous fistula is source control and control of sepsis.

Suggested Readings

Alamili M, Gogenur I, Rosenberg J. Acute complicated diverticulitis managed by laparoscopic lavage. *Dis Colon Rectum* 2009;52:1345–1349.

Dallal RM, Harbrecht BG, Boujoukas AJ, et al. Fulminant clostridium difficile: an underappreciated and increasing cause of death and complications. *Ann Surg* 2002;235:363–372.

Graham DY, Fischbach L. Helicobacter pylori treatment in the era of increasing antibiotic resistance. *Gut* 2010;59:1143–1153.

Lundell L, Dent J, Bennett J, et al. Endoscopic assessment of esophagitis: clinical and functional correlates and further validation of Los Angeles classification. *Gut* 1999;45:172–178.

Neal MD, Alverdy JC, Hall DE, et al. Diverting loop ileostomy and colonic lavage: an alternative to total abdominal colectomy for the treatment of severe, complicated C. difficile associated disease. *Ann Surg* 2011;254:423–429.

Ng EK, Larn YH, Sung JJ, et al. Eradication of H pylori prevents recurrence of ulcer after simple closure of duodenal ulcer perforation. *Ann Surg* 2000;231:153.

Poley JW, Steyerberg EW, Kuipers EJ, et al. Ingestion of acid and alkaline agents: outcome and prognostic value of early upper endoscopy. *Gastrointest Endosc* 2004;60:372–377.

Rafferty J, Shellito P, Hyman NH, et al. Practice parameters for sigmoid diverticulitis. *Dis Colon Rectum* 2006;49:939–944.

Schuchert M, Schuchert V, Zuckerbraun B. Inflammatory conditions of the gastrointestinal tract. In: Britt LD, Peitzman AB, Jurkovich JJ, Barie P, eds. *Acute Care Surgery.* Wolters/Kluwer; 2012.

Similis C, Purkayastha S, Yamamoto T, et al. A meta-analysis comparing conventional end-to-end anastomosis vs other anastomotic configurations after resection in Crohn's disease. *Dis Colon Rectum* 2007;50:1674.

Talamini G, Tommasi M, Amdei V, et al. Risk factors of peptic ulcer in 4943 patients. *J Clin Gastroenterol* 2008;42:373–380.

53

Acute Anorectal Pain

Frederick J. Denstman

I. INTRODUCTION

A. The most common causes of anal pain are fissure, hemorrhoidal thrombosis, and infection. Most patients afflicted by one of these lesions presents with a chief complaint of "rectal pain." The key first step in the history taking process is garnering a more precise description of the pain and its location.

B. Most etiologies of anal pain can be diagnosed on the history coupled with a simple examination, which generally consists of inspection and palpation. Anal pain should never be dismissed as being due to hemorrhoids without a diligent exam.

C. Only a few simple instruments are required for the diagnosis and treatment of most acute cases of anorectal pain. Many colon and rectal surgeons employ a proctology table which allows examination in the prone jackknife position. Although ideal, these tables are seldom available in most emergency departments, and a standard examination table with a decubitus positioned patient is adequate. A good examination light is imperative and this need be little more than the light provided by a 60 W light bulb. Although anoscopes and rigid sigmoidoscopes should be available in the emergency room and acute care clinic, it should be stressed that in most patients with severe anal or rectal pain, endoscopy is usually unnecessary for arrival at the correct diagnosis and often causes avoidable discomfort for the patient.

D. Lidocaine ointment 5% is an excellent topical agent. For infiltration, lidocaine 0.5% with epinephrine is an excellent choice for local anesthesia. Some practitioners will mix this with bicarbonate solution to decrease the acidity of the lidocaine and therefore the pain of injection. Bupivacaine 0.25% can also be mixed with the lidocaine or used alone or after initial anesthesia to extend the duration of relief.

E. To deliver the local anesthesia, a $1\frac{1}{2}$ cc or 3 cc syringe with a 21 or 22 gauge needle with which to draw up local anesthesia is adequate. A 27 or 30 gauge needle is sufficient to inject the local anesthesia; injection with a 25 gauge needle is painful. A larger gauge needle, such as a 16 gauge, is excellent for aspiration of a suspected site of abscess.

II. ANATOMY

A. The rectum and anus are specialized segments of the gastrointestinal tract. The rectum functions primarily as a reservoir for stool. The rectosigmoid junction is marked by the merging of the taenia coli into the complete layer of longitudinal muscularis propria of the rectum. This junction is easily defined during laparotomy but can only be estimated during endoscopy. The distance between anal verge and rectosigmoid junction varies over a fairly wide range from patient to patient, from approximately 12 to 16 cm.

B. The surgical rectum ends at the level of the puborectalis muscle, which marks the hiatus through the levator ani muscles. This hiatus is palpable during digital rectal examination as the **anorectal ring.** The anal canal begins at the anorectal ring and extends to the anal verge. It is embraced by the anal sphincter muscles. The **dentate line (pectinate line) is** the line between mucosa and skin and is located several centimeters proximally within the canal. The skin immediately distal to this line is the anoderm. The anoderm is a modified squamous epithelium, containing no accessory glands. The anoderm is exquisitely sensitive to pain, whereas the anal mucosa is relatively insensitive. The **anal** verge marks the junction between the

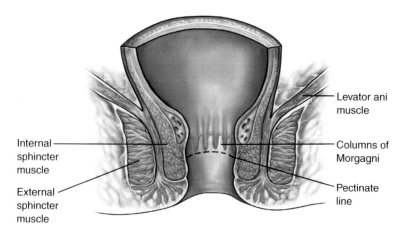

Figure 53-1. Anatomy of the anal canal. (From http://www.lww.com/webapp/wcs/stores/servlet/product_Fischer's-Mastery-of-Surgery_11851_-1_12551_Prod-9781608317400)

anoderm and normal skin. This is easily identified by the appearance of hair-bearing skin.

C. **Hemorrhoids** are normal anatomic structures surrounding the anus. This collection of arteries and veins forms an anal cushion and is thought to participate in the mechanism of fecal continence. The vessels proximal to the dentate line or mucocutaneous border and covered by mucosa are called **internal hemorrhoids.** Those vessels distal to the dentate line and covered by anoderm are called **external hemorrhoids.** These vessels are supported by surrounding connective tissue. Degeneration of this supporting connective tissue seems to be a common pathway to the development of hemorrhoidal disease.

III. FISSURE-IN-ANO

A. **Anal fissure** is the most common cause of acute anal pain. When asked to describe the pain from a fissure, most patients will use terms such as "sharp," "cutting," or "it feels like something tore." The pain usually is brought on by a bowel movement, but often the pain becomes most severe immediately following the movement and persists for 5 to 10 minutes. Occasionally it is constant or increased by sitting.

B. When asked, most patients will describe minor anal bleeding, usually on the toilet tissue, streaking the outside of the stool or occasionally dripping into the bowl. Patients will occasionally ascribe the pain to a swelling, but unlike the swelling described for hemorrhoids or abscesses, this swelling is usually chronic and small. The swelling is in fact not the exact site of the pain but is a sentinel skin tag. A sentinel tag is a small, firm mound of anoderm, which is adjacent but distal to the actual fissure. The tag itself is not painful. Removing the tag alone will not cure the pain, and in fact may make the fissure worse.

C. Fissures are typically classified as either acute or chronic, although many patients will have features of both. The typical **acute fissure** occurs following some excessive wear and tear on the anoderm, which is the sensitive ring of skin that extends from the dentate line to the anal verge. This is usually a hard, forceful bowel movement, although multiple loose stools over a short period of time (e.g., following colonoscopy bowel prep) can have an equally harmful effect. Patients with irritable bowel syndrome are prone to multiple, acute anal fissures. In an otherwise normal anal canal, an acute fissure will heal in a day or two. These acute fissures are usually superficial, narrow and linear, resembling a paper cut.

D. In patients with **chronic fissure,** the fissure fails to heal. Excessively high tone in the internal anal sphincter muscle is the accepted etiology of the chronic fissure, and this is thought to act by decreasing blood flow to the anoderm. As the fissure matures, it becomes deeper and wider, eventually exposing the fibers of the internal sphincter muscle. The classic picture of the chronic fissure is completed by the development of a sentinel tag and an adjacent enlarged anal papillae, although these two additional features need not be present for the diagnosis.

E. Many patients seem to have a subacute syndrome, with overlapping features of both acute and chronic fissure. Their pain is characterized by good weeks and bad weeks. The fissure becomes relatively asymptomatic as it covered by a thin layer of immature scar, only to be split open again by a difficult bowel movement. This pattern of alternating severe pain and relief persists over a course of months. Even though these patients may present with acute pain, these fissures are best treated as chronic fissures.

F. Occasionally the fissures become infected. This usually occurs as a result of incomplete healing of the fissure, such that a hood of skin forms over the fissure and traps stool particles beneath. These lesions are more practically treated as infections than fissures in the acute setting (*vide infra*).

G. Diagnosis. In most cases, a careful history suggests the diagnosis, which can be verified on physical examination. Typical anal fissures are located in either the posterior or anterior midline. Since fissures reside in the anoderm, the most superficial aspect of the anal canal, an anoscope is usually not required to make this diagnosis, and insertion of an examining finger or anoscope may be painful and unnecessary. The anoderm can usually be well visualized by simply spreading the buttocks apart.

1. The acute fissure is usually superficial and linear. The classic chronic fissure is a tear-drop shaped ulceration of the anoderm, with an associated "sentinel tag" on its distal end and a hypertrophied papilla on its proximal end. The transversely oriented fibers of the internal sphincter may or may not be visible within the bed of the chronic fissure. The sphincter is not visible in an acute fissure. As stated, patients can sometimes manifest features of both acute and chronic fissures.

2. Once a typical midline fissure is visualized, no further immediate diagnostic maneuvers are required. If no fissure is visualized, proceed with a gentle digital examination. If the examination fails to evoke tenderness, anoscopy can be performed. If anoscopy is negative, assume the patient had an acute fissure, which has healed. If digital examination is tender in the absence of a visible fissure, rule this out as a diagnostic consideration and move down the list of differential diagnoses.

3. If the fissure is located well off the midline, this is referred to as an **atypical fissure,** and this must be noted as such because it may have special diagnostic and therapeutic significance.

H. Treatment. By definition, an acute fissure should heal after the precipitating problems with bowel habit are corrected. This is usually a matter of prescribing a better diet for the patient, including more fiber, water or a bulk laxative. Constipating medications, such as narcotics, should be avoided when possible. An antidiarrheal medication may be helpful in patients with chronic loose stools.

1. To treat the acute pain, topical anesthetic in the form of 5% lidocaine ointment is helpful. The patient places one inch of the ointment into the anal canal by fingertip about 5 minutes before a bowel movement. This will usually provide good pain relief while waiting for the fissure to heal.

2. With proper diet, most acute fissures, and even some chronic fissures will heal. However if healing does not occur within 3 to 4 weeks of good conservative management, additional treatment may be required. The standard for treatment of chronic fissure is a partial, lateral internal sphincterotomy. This surgical treatment has the advantage of a rapid and lasting relief of symptoms in 95% of patients.

3. Several topical medications are potential alternatives to sphincterotomy. These include injectable botulinum toxin and ointment formulations of 0.2% nitroglycerin, 2% diltiazem, or 0.3% nifedipine applied twice daily. These treatments avoid division of the internal sphincter but tend to be disappointing because they are temporary or incomplete.

I. Atypical fissure. Fissures located well off the midline are called **atypical fissures.** Occasionally patients with diarrhea will develop multiple, very superficial fissures related to excessive bowel movements and wiping. This type of atypical fissure usually will heal spontaneously.

1. **Solitary atypical fissures that do not heal quickly are a reason for concern.** The differential diagnosis includes squamous cell carcinoma of the anus, Crohn's disease, and syphilis. Many patients with Crohn's will already carry a diagnosis. Even for the undiagnosed Crohn's patient, there will usually be other signs or symptoms of the disease. However, there are rare patients whose initial presentation consists only of a painful, persistent atypical fissure. Squamous cell carcinoma of the anus can present as a small fissure. These early cancers tend to be extremely painful. As the disease progresses, the lesion takes on the more typical appearance of an ulcerated, hard mass. Diagnosis requires biopsy. At their earliest presentation these cancers are difficult to diagnose and may resemble typical fissures.

IV. HEMORRHOIDS
- **A.** Thrombosis of external hemorrhoids
    1. External hemorrhoid thrombosis is a common cause of anal pain. It is caused by clot formation within the portion of the hemorrhoid covered by skin. The patient complains of a painful swelling, usually of acute onset. The pain is constant and the swelling is tender. This can occur without any obvious cause, or may follow straining, multiple loose stools, etc.
    2. Thrombosis runs a typical course of severe pain peaking over a 48- to 72-hour period. In time the clot begins to soften as it is resorbed, and the pain decreases. The swelling may persist for weeks and often leaves behind a soft, nontender skin tag.
    3. If the swelling is severe, pain is caused by stretching of the overlying skin which can become ischemic or may even develop superficial gangrene. With gangrene, the skin may necrose, allowing the clot to extrude spontaneously, which brings on relief of pain. Prior to the spontaneous extrusion of the clot, the pain will be at its most severe. Clot evacuation generally is incomplete leading to prolonged bloody drainage. Patients generally find this distressing.
- **B.** Thrombosis of internal hemorrhoids
    1. Internal hemorrhoids rarely thrombose. In patients with severe, circumferential, irreducible (stage 4) prolapse, patients may experience severe pain which is sometimes described as a "hemorrhoidal crisis." These patients frequently have a combination of internal and external hemorrhoid thrombosis. This is usually seen in patients who have ignored symptomatic hemorrhoids over a period of years.
    2. Prolapse of hemorrhoids without thrombosis can cause discomfort, or a dull ache, but this is typically a chronic complaint.
- **C.** Etiology
    1. Hemorrhoids are a collection of arteries and veins lining the anal canal, present at birth. These vessels are supported by connective tissue. If the connective tissue degenerates, the vessels lose support and fixation, leading to toruosity, dilatation. The internal hemorrhoids then tend to prolapse into the anal canal. The blood within the external hemorrhoids tends to clot or thrombose.
    2. In some cases, there is a hereditary trait for hemorrhoids to become symptomatic at an earlier age.
    3. Pregnancy causes a general engorgement of hemorrhoids which can present as limited or diffuse thrombosis and enlargement.
- **D.** Diagnosis
    1. Many patients with acute anal pain will present with a chief complaint of "hemorrhoids." It is up to the doctor to confirm this diagnosis. *Diagnosis requires direct inspection. History alone is never sufficient to rule out other causes of anal pain.* External hemorrhoid thrombosis is almost always visible by simple inspection alone. Insertion of an anoscope is not necessary to visualize the blue-tinged swelling in a lateral position. Midline swelling is usually not due to hemorrhoids. This needs to be distinguished from an abscess, which is typically erythematous, fluctuant, etc.

2. Internal hemorrhoids do not cause pain without severe prolapse, so this also should not require insertion of an instrument.

3. Severe hemorrhoidal prolapse should be distinguished from complete rectal prolapse. Severe internal hemorrhoid prolapse is generally a collection of discrete nodular swellings separated by radial clefts. Complete rectal prolapse is a single, donut shaped swelling of circumferential, mucosal rings.

4. In the absence of thrombosis or severe prolapse, anal pain should not be ascribed to hemorrhoids. In this case, pain is more likely related to infection or fissure.

E. Treatment. In the acute setting of the first 24 to 48 hours, the best treatment for a simple thrombosed hemorrhoid is surgical excision.

1. This is best done in prone jackknife position, although it can be done in lateral position as well. The skin overlying the hemorrhoid is infiltrated with **0.5% lidocaine with 1:200,000 epinephrine.** An unhurried injection through a 30 gauge needle will decrease the discomfort from this injection. Both the overlying skin and underlying subcutaneous tissue should be infiltrated.

2. Using a fine, sharp scissors (Metzenbaum or iris scissors) an ellipse of overlying skin will expose the underlying thrombus, which can then be excised as well. Since multiple small clots are generally encountered, simple "lancing" or incision of the hemorrhoid is usually inadequate and should be avoided.

3. Excision may also avoid a recurrence of future thrombosis in the hemorrhoid. **Do not excise the anoderm;** keep the excision well lateral in the hair-bearing region only. Involving the anoderm will lead to more postoperative pain and perhaps the development of a chronic fissure.

4. Since the hemorrhoid is thrombosed, little bleeding is encountered, especially if local anesthesia contains epinephrine. Silver nitrate can be applied for nuisance bleeding. Traditionally, this small wound is left open and heals nicely, although suturing the wound closed with chromic catgut or some other absorbable material is an option.

5. **Bupivacaine** can be injected to prolong the duration of anesthesia. The patient is advised to take two to three sitz baths or tub baths a day, for 2 to 3 days, or until minor bleeding on a clean pad or gauze stops. Provide a prescription for an opioid for 24 to 48 hours.

6. If the hemorrhoid has been present for longer than 48 to 72 hours, and is beginning to soften or hurt less, excision will generally not be necessary. If the hemorrhoid has already necrosed and begun to drain, no operation is required, although occasionally there is a role for minor debridement of the gangrenous tissue or assistance with complete evacuation of the clot. This requires local anesthesia.

F. Complicated hemorrhoid disease. Patients may present with multiple discrete areas of external thrombosis. They may develop a more involved process with nearly circumferential or confluent areas of thrombosis and extensive edema. These patients may also have irreducible, circumferential prolapse of the internal hemorrhoids (grade 4 prolapse). The internal hemorrhoids can then begin to thrombose. This can further progress to the development of gangrenous changes in the skin and anal mucosa. This is sometimes referred to as *"hemorrhoidal crisis."*

1. These more severe expressions of hemorrhoidal disease cannot be treated by the acute care physician in a simple outpatient setting. These patients are probably best served by referral to colon and rectal surgeon.

V. PERIANAL INFECTIONS

A. Perianal and ischiorectal abscesses are common causes of perianal pain. The pain is usually severe, constant, and tends to increase with time. Most abscesses develop over the course of a day or two; occasionally, a more chronic presentation is noted.

B. Patients will usually describe a tender swelling. Unlike fissures, the pain is usually not strongly associated with bowel movements. When present, the symptoms of fever and malaise can suggest abscess, but fever is often absent.

C. Etiology. Most perianal suppurative disease begins in the cryptoglandular space. The infection migrates along the course of the anal gland's ducts. These ducts travel to various anatomic spaces around the anus, and the abscess evolves where these ducts terminate.

1. Anal fissures probably are responsible for many perianal infections. In this case, the fissure is a direct portal for bacterial invasion into the underlying subcutaneous or intersphincteric space. These patients will usually describe a typical fissure type history which precedes the development of the constantly tender swelling.

2. Although only a small percentage of abscesses are caused by Crohn's disease, it is important to consider this in patients with an abscess. All patients with abscesses should be questioned about chronic diarrhea and abdominal pain, the presence of which should at least raise the suspicion of inflammatory bowel disease. However, it is not necessary to perform an involved work-up for Crohn's disease in most patients, unless there are other Crohn's symptoms.

D. Diagnosis. The perianal infection generally is apparent on simple inspection as a raised, erythematous swelling near the anal verge. The swelling is usually quite tender and often fluctuant.

1. Abscesses deep in the ischiorectal or posterior anal spaces may be less obvious on inspection, lacking the erythematous skin changes, but can be identified by a tender area of induration and swelling. The swelling is sometimes subtle when palpated through the skin, but generally obvious on palpation through the anal mucosa during digital examination.

2. Abscesses confined to the intersphincteric space are less common and more difficult to identify. These tend to be small with only subtle amounts of swelling palpable on digital examination. These patients will give a history more suggestive of fissure, with pain strongly associated with bowel movements, but on physical examination no fissure is seen. There may be a complete absence of physical findings, other than tenderness.

3. Imaging studies have little role in patients with perianal infection. These infections are usually readily apparent on physical examination, and the use of CT scans, ultrasound and MRI should be reserved for the experienced surgeon who is unable to arrive at a diagnosis on physical examination.

E. Treatment. The treatment for an abscess is operative drainage. There is no indication for allowing an abscess to "mature" or "ripen." Furthermore, antibiotics are not a substitute for drainage.

1. Most abscesses are superficial and easily drained with simple instruments and techniques. The deeper infections may require consultation with a surgeon and examination under anesthesia and drainage in the operating room.

2. For the majority of patients, the overlying skin is anesthetized with 0.5% lidocaine and epinephrine. The skin is then incised with the number 11 scalpel blade, allowing drainage of the pus. A generous disk of skin, at least 5 mm in diameter, should be excised to allow ongoing drainage of the pus, and to prevent premature closure of the skin, which leads to rapid recurrence of the infection.

3. If the abscess is deep and not easily demonstrated by simple inspection or palpation, a trial aspiration with the larger 16 gauge needle may be employed as a localizing maneuver.

4. The routine practice of packing perianal wounds should be abandoned. If the drainage incision is adequate, packing is not needed to maintain drainage, and in fact packing may impede drainage. More importantly, packing and unpacking is a needlessly painful procedure for the patient. One exception to this would be to control bleeding and this should be a rare occurrence if meddlesome probing is avoided during the initial I and D procedure.

5. Probing into the abscess cavity should be avoided. This can lead to creation of false openings into the anal canal as well as unnecessary bleeding from the depth of the wound.

6. In some cases, drainage of an abscess is a definitive therapy leading to a complete resolution of the suppurative process. Unfortunately, more than 50% of patients will develop a recurrent abscess or form an anal fistula, indicating the presence of a persistent internal opening within the anal canal. Follow-up is required and is most appropriately performed by a colon and rectal surgeon experienced in the treatment of anal fistulae.

7. Although antibiotics are not appropriate as primary treatment of an abscess, they may be added as an adjunct to drainage in patients who are immunocompromised or those with cellulitis surrounding a well-drained abscess cavity. The resolution of erythema within a few minutes of the incision and drainage procedure is a good sign that antibiotics will not be required. If needed, antibiotic therapy should be directed toward gram-negative and anaerobic organisms.

VI. PILONIDAL DISEASE

A. Pilonidal disease typically presents during puberty or young adulthood. It is more common among young men. Presentation is similar to most abscess processes. The patient is more likely to describe this in relation to the tailbone as opposed to the anus.

B. Etiology. Pilonidal disease is believed to be initiated by the ingrowth of hair follicles. It is most common in hirsute males, although occasionally seen in women with little hair. The process is encouraged by the presence of a deep gluteal cleft. It is believed to begin as one or a series of midline sinuses. Skin flora migrate down the sinus tracts and cause midline abscess formation, and frequently extend bilaterally. Hair shafts frequently migrate down the sinus tracts and on occasion rather large hair plugs are trapped within the abscess cavity.

C. Diagnosis. Pilonidal abscess is easily diagnosed as a tender, erythematous midline swelling. The lesions generally originate superior to the coccyx, although extension of the primary process toward the coccyx is not unusual. Careful scrutiny will usually reveal one or more sinuses with protruding hair shafts. Pilonidal disease must be distinguished from posterior midline perianal abscess, which is treated differently.

D. Treatment for pilonidal abscess is drainage, often performed in the emergency department or clinic setting.

1. With the patient placed in either prone jackknife or Sims position, the skin overlying the abscess is infiltrated with local anesthesia. The abscess is then incised with a number 11 scalpel blade. Following this a disk of skin should be excised to enhance adequate drainage. Hair plugs should be removed if present.

2. Packing is not indicated except to control bleeding. The overlying skin may be several millimeters thick and require a fairly deep incision to initiate the drainage. An exploratory needle aspiration may be helpful.

3. Antibiotics may be used as an adjunct in immunocompromised patients or in cases with extensive cellulitis.

4. With pilonidal disease, abscess recurrence is the rule rather than the exception. Referral to a surgeon for follow-up is required. Definitive treatment of pilonidal disease is controversial.

VII. FOURNIER'S (PERINEAL) GANGRENE

A. Fournier's gangrene is a surgical emergency. These patients generally present with fever, leukocytosis, and other systemic signs of infection. This is a disease which tends to afflict diabetics and immunocompromised adults.

B. These patients will complain of severe, diffuse perineal and perianal pain. Although urinary retention is associated with any form of perianal pain, it is common with Fournier's gangrene. There may be an antecedent history of trauma. These patients are often brought in by ambulance because the pain prohibits them from walking.

C. Fournier's gangrene is a necrotizing infection of the deep perianal or perineal fascia. The portal of entry can be any form of perianal infection, but breaks in the perineal, vaginal, or scrotal skin are often the source of infection. Blunt trauma can be the initiator. In many cases the first site of bacterial entry is never identified.

D. Diagnosis. The classic finding is crepitance on palpation of the exquisitely tender perineal skin or a blackened area of ischemic skin in the perineum, perianum, scrotum, or vaginal labia. A worrisome clue to the diagnosis of Fournier's gangrene is a gray, watery discharge from an abscess cavity, or the presence of gray subcutaneous tissue at the base of the abscess. Although imaging studies are usually not necessary to make this diagnosis, the presence of gas in the soft tissues can be seen on plain x-ray or CT films. Systemic signs – fever, tachycardia, tachypnea, chills – are often seen.

E. Fournier's gangrene is a potentially life-threatening disease and requires prompt attention, with both immediate broad spectrum antibiotics and surgical evaluation.

　1. Once resuscitated, these patients must be treated in the operating room with aggressive, wide surgical debridement.

　2. Although not necessary in all cases, many patients will require fecal diversion at some point in the course of their disease.

F. Hidradenitis suppurativa is an infection of apocrine sweat glands that can involve the perianal, perivaginal, and groin skin. This disease tends to mimic perianal abscess and fistula disease, except that it never communicates with an internal anal opening. These patients tend to present with chronic, recurrent, bilateral, and superficial skin abscesses that communicate with each other through strictly subcutaneous sinuses. Often these abscesses must be drained. Antibiotics may play a role in the treatment as well.

VIII. RECTAL PAIN FOLLOWING THE TREATMENT OF HEMORRHOIDS

A. Barron ligation is a common and time-proven treatment for prolapsing internal hemorrhoids. With this technique a small rubber band is applied to a small section of mucosa at the apex of a prolapsing internal hemorrhoid. The band strangulates this small disk of mucosa which then sloughs in 2 to 3 days, leading to the formation of a small ulcer and ultimately a small scar. The scar leads to fixation of the hemorrhoid so it no longer prolapses into the anal canal during bowel movements, and is therefore less likely to bleed.

　　The properly applied rubber band should be placed at least 2 cm above the dentate line where there are no somatic pain receptors; ideally, the patient should have no pain following proper application of the band. However, three different types of discomfort may be experienced and need to be differentiated.

　1. The most common discomfort is a vague pressure or sense of tenesmus that is noted soon after band application. This is due to the physical presence of a small mass in the anal canal which visceral receptors interpret as a stool bolus. This is usually a mild discomfort and generally passes within 24 hours, requiring no treatment beyond reassurance of the patient.

　2. The second most common discomfort is a severe, sharp pain which the patient feels very soon or immediately with application of the band. This occurs when the band is applied too far distally, i.e., at the level of somatic skin sensation. This should hopefully be recognized by the doctor applying the band and remedied by either removing or repositioning the band more proximally.

　3. The third type of discomfort is rare but must be recognized and treated aggressively. This presents in a delayed fashion as severe rectal pain, perhaps a day or two after the procedure, frequently accompanied by urinary retention, fever, or other signs of sepsis. This pain results from infection and possibly necrosis, extending from the anal mucosa to deeper layers of the rectum and ultimately into the pelvis. Recognition of this entity requires institution of broad spectrum parenteral antibiotics and possible debridement of the rectal wall. Left untreated, this rectal sepsis can lead to death. Consultation with an experienced surgeon is required.

B. Procedure for prolapsing hemorrhoids (PPH). PPH is relatively new method of treating prolapsing internal hemorrhoids. The PPH device is a modified form of the intraluminal circular stapling device employed for creating low anterior anastomoses. The PPH device excises a ring of anal mucosa and then reanastomoses it, causing fixation of the mucosa. This then prevents prolapse of the internal hemorrhoids. It is analogous to Barron ligation but creates a circumferential fixation as opposed to scarring down one hemorrhoid at a time.

　1. Similar to the rubber banding technique, this device ideally should cause no sensation. However, this is not always the case and discomfort is common. The acute care physician should be aware of two different types of discomfort following the PPH procedure.

　　a. The most common discomfort is best described as severe tenesmus, or a very strong and false urge to defecate. This can be distressing enough for the

patient to request narcotic pain relief. It can persist for days or weeks after surgery.
   b. A rare but much more serious pain can occur as a symptom of pelvic sepsis, similar to the situation of infection developing after Barron ligation. These patients present with various other symptoms and signs of systemic sepsis, and again must be treated aggressively with parenteral antibiotics and require surgical consultation.

IX. PELVIC FLOOR PAIN
   A. Levator pain. The floor of the pelvis is formed primarily by the levator and puborectalis muscles. A separate hiatus exists for the ostia of the gastrointestinal and genitourinary systems. Pain in the levator muscle or any organ traveling through its hiatus is frequently perceived as a rectal pain.
   1. Levator spasm can present with a constant feeling of fullness or pain. The patient frequently compares this to the sensation of sitting on a ball. This pain tends to be chronic and is unlikely to be a presenting symptom in the emergency department. Consultation with a specialist is recommended.
   2. Proctalgia fugax is a severe, acute pain that frequently will awaken a patient from sleep. It is typically self-limited, lasting only minutes, but can be quite alarming to the patient with its first presentation and may trigger a visit to the emergency department. This is a poorly understood entity and is thought to be an acute spasm of some portion of the levator muscle. These patients are almost always pain free by the time they present to the physician and the sudden onset and brief duration of this rectal pain is pathognomonic of this disorder. There is a complete absence of visible physical findings. The main treatment of proctalgia fugax is to make the diagnosis and then reassure the patient that the pain, no matter how distressing, is a form of muscle cramp, is not a serious health problem, but may be prone to recurrence.
   B. Uterine pain. Lesions arising from the uterus or uterine adnexa can present with pain radiating to the rectum. The gynecologic origin of this pain may at least be suspected by the history. A gentle but thorough digital examination which includes manipulation of the uterine cervix should also suggest the extrarectal origin of this pain. This should then be followed by a bimanual pelvic examination.
   C. Prostatic pain. Men frequently describe pain arising in the prostate gland as rectal pain. This will most likely be prostatitis, with the finding of a tender, soft prostate gland on digital rectal examination. This pain usually responds to antibiotic therapy directed against the usual urinary pathogens. A more problematic entity is prostadynia, a pain in the prostate not necessarily caused by acute infection. This is a chronic disorder, more appropriately treated by a urologist on a nonurgent basis.

AXIOMS

■ Careful history and simple examination will diagnose most causes of anal pain.
■ Imaging studies are seldom helpful, and are no substitute for physical exam, which is mandatory.
■ An anal fissure which is off the midline, an *atypical fissure,* may be a squamous cell carcinoma.
■ The treatment for a perianal abscess is operative drainage. A 5 mm disc of skin should be excised to ensure adequate drainage. Antibiotics are not a substitute for drainage.
■ Referral to a colon and rectal surgeon is required when the diagnosis is unclear or follow-up is required.

Suggested Readings
Philips RKS, ed. *A Companion to Specialist Surgical Practice: Colorectal Surgery.* Saunders; 2009.
Sands L, Sands DR. *Ambulatory Colorectal Surgery.* USA: Informa Healthcare; 2009.
Wolf B, Pemberton JH, Wexner SD, et al. *The ASCRS Textbook of Colon and Rectal Surgery.* Springer; 2007.

54 Soft Tissue Infection

David Morris and Babak Sarani

I. **INTRODUCTION.** Soft tissue infections are common, with most responding to antibiotic therapy. Some infections cause systemic symptoms and require inpatient treatment or surgical debridement. This chapter describes the basic anatomic structure of the soft tissue, common etiologies of soft tissue infections, and principles of treatment. Special attention will be paid to necrotizing soft tissue infections (NSTIs), as these infections are increasing in incidence, difficult to diagnose, treat, and require *urgent* surgical exploration and debridement.

II. **ANATOMY.** Each of the anatomical layers of the body wall can be infected from the superficial epidermis to the deep muscle and can behave in a very distinct fashion. In some cases, multiple layers are infected; the more layers and when deeper layer are involved generally denotes more serious illness with systemic manifestations. Although these infections are generally referred to as "soft tissue infections," a patient may have an infection of the skin (erysipelas, cellulitis), subcutaneous tissue (necrotizing cellulitis or adipositis), fascia (necrotizing fasciitis), or the muscle (necrotizing myositis) or multiple layers. The skin is made up of the epidermis and dermis; beneath are other tissues that are not skin but part of the soft tissue.

A. **Epidermis.** The epidermis is the most superficial skin layer of stratified squamous epithelium cells arising from the deeper basal lamina. The cells are gradually filled with keratin as they are pushed upward. The keratinized cell layer performs a barrier function, limiting water loss, preventing entry of microbes, and regulating temperature.

B. **Dermis.** The dermis is located deep to the epidermis and is attached to it via hemidesmosomes. The dermis houses blood vessels, which nourish the epidermis via the basal cell layer. It also contains the sensory nerves and skin appendages: Sweat glands and hair follicles. In addition, the dermis provides tensile strength to the skin with type I collagen comprising the major structural protein responsible for tensile strength.

C. **Subcutaneous tissue.** Deep to the dermis is the subcutaneous tissue. This tissue varies in thickness and cellular composition in different areas of the body and generally consists of adipocytes, fibroblasts, macrophages, blood and lymph vessels, fibrous anchoring bands, nerves, and occasional skeletal muscle (e.g., platysma), glandular tissue (salivary glands, breast tissue), and bursae. The subcutaneous tissue provides cushioning for the deeper tissues and acts as insulation to help regulate internal body temperature.

D. **Investing fascia.** Deep to the subcutaneous tissue is a layer of investing fascia that covers the skeletal muscle. This fibrous layer surrounds muscles, nerves, and vascular structures. It consists of collagen fibers that provide tensile strength.

E. **Muscle.** The skeletal muscle is invested by the fascia and is connected to the bony skeleton. It is generally well vascularized and is largely resistant to infection, except in circumstances described below.

III. **RISK FACTORS.** Any patient may develop a soft tissue infection, with or without skin disruption. Cellulitis is a frequent complication of even minor wounds encountered. Patients at risk for NSTI generally are immunocompromised from a variety of causes that include diabetes mellitus, malignancy, HIV, and use of immunosuppressive

TABLE 54-1	Organisms Isolated in Type I (Polymicrobial) Necrotizing Soft Tissue Infections	
Organism	**Percent of isolates n = (162) (Anaya and Dellinger, 2007)**	**Percent of isolates n = (272) (Anaya et al., 2005)**
Streptococcus	19	17
S. aureus	16	22
Klebsiella	10	
E. coli	7	
Gram Negatives		18
Anaerobes	7	18
Clostridia sp.	Rare	Rare

medications such as corticosteroids, infliximab, antitumor chemotherapy, or antirejection drugs. Patients with chronic skin conditions such as psoriasis may also be predisposed to these infections due to the breakdown of the barrier function of the epidermis. In addition, other factors that contribute to local tissue ischemia, such as peripheral vascular disease and cigarette smoking, may increase the risk of NSTI. Recent reports describe otherwise healthy young patients with none of the above risk factors developing an aggressive NSTI, often caused by methicillin-resistant *Staphylococcus aureus* (MRSA). The microbiologic factors contributing to these infections will be discussed.

IV. NECROTIZING SOFT TISSUE INFECTIONS (NSTIs). NSTIs are known by many names, including necrotizing fasciitis, gas gangrene, Fournier's gangrene, Meleney's ulcer, and in the popular media as "flesh-eating bacterial infections." They are rapidly progressing and may result in significant tissue loss or death, if not treated aggressively.

A. Types. Several different classification systems have been developed in an attempt to uniformly describe NSTIs consistently from. One widely used schema is based on the microbiology of the infection.

  1. Type I infections are the most common, comprising 55% to 75% of all NSTIs, and are polymicrobial in nature. Tissue isolates demonstrate an average of four organisms in most wounds. The most commonly isolated bacteria are gram-positive cocci, gram-negative rods, and anaerobes (Table 54-1). These infections tend to occur in immunocompromised (including diabetic) and obese patients.

  2. Type II infections are monomicrobial in nature. Classically, the causative organism was group A Streptococcus (GAS) but MRSA is becoming more prevalent. These infections tend to occur in relatively young and healthy patients, although they can also cluster in intravenous drug users.

B. Pathophysiology. Microbial invasion of the subcutaneous tissues from an external source most often occurs after trauma; the most common internal source is direct spread from a perforated colon, rectum, anus, or urogenital organ. One less common route of entry is in-dwelling vascular or enteral catheters. The inciting event may be unknown in as many as 50% of cases.

  The bacteria then proliferate in the subcutaneous tissues, producing endo- and exotoxins that cause tissue ischemia and liquefactive necrosis. As the innate immune cascade develops, systemic illness can occur. The infection may spread rapidly – as fast as 1 in./h with little overlying skin change.

  The seriousness of a given infectious process depends heavily on the presence or absence of endo- and exotoxins elaborated by the microbes involved. *Clostridia* species produce α-toxin, which leads to extensive tissue necrosis locally and hypotension and shock systemically. *S. aureus* and *Streptococci* produce a wide variety of virulence factors including the surface proteins M-1 and M-3, exotoxins A, B, C, streptolysin O, and superantigen. M-1 and M-3 allow the microbe to escape phagocytosis. Exotoxins A and B cause a loss of endothelial integrity with tissue

TABLE 54-2	Laboratory Risk Indicator for Necrotizing Fasciitis (Wong et al., 2004)	
Variable		**Score**
C-reactive protein		
■ <150		0
■ ≥150		4
WBC (cells/mm³)		
■ <15		0
■ 15–25		1
■ >25		2
Hemoglobin (g/dL)		
■ >13.5		0
■ 11–13.5		1
■ <11		2
Sodium (mmol/L)		
■ ≥135		0
■ <135		2
Creatinine (μg/L)		
■ ≤141		0
■ >141		2
Glucose (mmol/L)		
■ ≤10		0
■ >10		1

A score of 6 or higher is associated with NSTI. The probability of NSTI increases as the score increases above 6.

edema and increased oxygen diffusion distance. CD4 cells and macrophages are stimulated by these toxins to produce tumor necrosis factor-α, interleukin-1, and interleukin-6, which may lead to systemic inflammatory response syndrome (SIRS), sepsis, septic shock, multiorgan system dysfunction, or death. *S. aureus* strains can produce Panton–Valentine leukocidin (PVL) which is a pore-forming exotoxin that results in destruction of leukocytes. PVL has been identified in the majority of community-acquired methicillin-resistant strains of *S. aureus* and leads to necrotizing skin infections. The various bacteria also produce superantigens which lead to complement activation and stimulation of the bradykinin–kallikrein system and coagulation cascade. The end result is local tissue ischemia, which creates a favorable environment for further bacterial proliferation and spread. The lack of perfusion therefore prevents effective delivery of antibiotics, making surgical debridement *absolutely necessary* to eradicate the infection.

V. DIAGNOSIS

A. Presentation. The patient with a superficial soft tissue infection will generally present with pain, erythema, and swelling of the involved overlying skin. Occasionally, the erythema may be seen to spread in a linear "streaking" pattern that corresponds to the lymphatic drainage of the infected area. This is a more serious sign, and may warrant inpatient treatment with intravenous antibiotics.

A patient with an NSTI often presents similarly, and the differentiation from a less serious infection may be difficult *early* in the disease process. If a patient presents with pain that is out of proportion to the physical findings, or if the patient presents with tense edema, bullae, crepitus, anesthesia, or discoloration of the affected skin, or signs of systemic toxicity such as hypotension, tachycardia, fever, or organ dysfunction, NSTI is strongly considered. Unfortunately, these signs occur later in the disease process and are indicative of well-established infection. In many cases, the progression from what appears to be a minor infection to full blown septic shock may be rapid. Delay in appropriate treatment, especially surgical exploration, may be fatal.

B. Laboratory. Laboratory findings are typically nonspecific although an elevated white blood cell count, sodium level <135 mmol/L, or blood urea nitrogen (BUN) >15 mg/dL on admission to the hospital often accompanies a necrotizing infection as compared to a non-necrotizing infection. Creatine phosphokinase levels may be elevated if muscle necrosis is present.

C. Imaging. A variety of imaging modalities may be used in the work up of NSTI, with the caveat that *any imaging technique that results in delay of definitive treatment, especially surgical debridement, should be avoided.* Plain radiographs may show subcutaneous gas, although the frequency of this finding is only roughly 15%. Modern computed tomography is readily available and efficient; this technique detects gas in the tissues and can delineate the extent of involvement. CT may be especially useful if there is suspicion that the source of the infection originated from a perforated intra-abdominal organ or structure. **Magnetic** resonance imaging is sensitive for signs of infection, including soft tissue gas and *edema but these studies are often unavailable or time-consuming. In addition, the MRI suite precludes the ability to intervene* in critically ill or acute deteriorating patients.

D. Surgical biopsy. If there is any suspicion that an NSTI may be present, *the diagnostic test is a surgical incision for direct visualization of the tissues. This can be done at* the bedside with local anesthesia. Worrisome findings include "dishwater" fluid in the tissues without a discrete abscess pocket, foul smelling fluid, minimal bleeding, and loss of tissue plane integrity along the fascial planes. Tissue samples should be sent for culture and Gram stain, although if the findings on exploration are at all worrisome, transfer to the operating room for wide exploration and definitive debridement is indicated, at times before the results of the biopsy are available. The Gram stain and culture in these circumstances may guide antibiotic therapy but should not delay initiation of broad spectrum antimicrobials or surgery.

VI. TREATMENT

A. Surgical. The mainstay of therapy for NSTI is early surgical debridement. Failure to do so results in dramatic increases in mortality. Wong and colleagues reported a nine-fold increase in mortality if the *adequate* debridement was delayed >24 hours from the time of hospital admission.

The extent of the skin excision should contain the area of erythema at a minimum, and often requires excision of much more otherwise normal appearing skin to expose healthy, bleeding tissues. Serial debridements should be expected, as full eradication is rare with a single debridement. The surgeon should not be dissuaded from performing an adequate resection, including amputation of involved extremities if a joint is involved or the rate of spread is rapid, to gain control of the infection. Amputation may be needed in up to 20% of infections. Consultation with another surgeon experienced in managing NSTI is helpful when available.

NSTI of the perineum, scrotum, and perianal soft tissues (Fournier's gangrene) may be encountered. In addition to full debridement of the infected soft tissue, consider a diverting colostomy especially in cases with perineal body or perianal involvement to assure proper wound hygiene and care. Scrotal debridement may result in exposure of the testicles and require that they be wrapped in saline-soaked gauze or even protected in soft tissue pockets in the medial thighs. It is rarely necessary to remove the testicles since they are usually not involved with the infectious process.

B. Wound care. As with any infected wound, frequent examination and dressing changes are critical to successful treatment. The patient may need several returns to the operating room for dressing changes that can be done most easily and comfortably. Negative pressure occlusive dressings are frequently employed and allow excellent control of wound exudate and overall wound hygiene. The ultimate goal for these wounds is shrinkage of size, diffuse granulation, and eventual skin grafting after the systemic effects of the illness have subsided and the wound beds are clean.

C. Antibiotics. Antibiotic therapy should be considered as a necessary *adjunctive* (to surgical debridement) treatment for NSTIs. Timely administration of an antibiotic regimen with appropriate antimicrobial coverage can help prevent bacterial spread and systemic sepsis. Traditionally, NSTI were treated with high-dose penicillin and clindamycin for broad gram-positive and gram-negative coverage. These medications are particularly effective against *Clostridia* species, as a synergistic effect occurs.

Due to the relative low rate of infection with *Clostridia* species and the emergence of resistant strains of Staphylococcus and Streptococcus, current recommendations for antibiotic therapy include vancomycin, linezolid, or daptomycin. High-dose intravenous penicillin is the agent of choice for treatment of GAS. Fluoroquinolones have excellent soft tissue penetration and are an option for the penicillin-allergic patient. Clindamycin has the added advantage of inhibition of M protein and exotoxin synthesis by GAS however, many MRSA strains are resistant.

Antibiotic therapy should be continued until no further surgical debridement is necessary or the patient no longer shows signs of systemic illness.

In the typical case, broad spectrum antibiotics are initiated and then the cultures or biopsies allow narrowing therapies.

D. IVIG. IV immune globulin treatment (IVIG) may be considered, although it is not FDA-approved for treatment of NSTI. Theoretically, immunoglobulin G isotypes can bind the elaborated exotoxins and limit the body's immune response to these molecules. The use of IVIG remains controversial and should only be considered in patients who are critically ill and are known to be infected with either *Staph* or *Strep* species.

VII. HYPERBARIC OXYGEN (HBO) THERAPY. HBO therapy can inhibit anaerobic infections. This therapy may be considered in patients who are known or suspected to have anaerobic pathogens, especially clostridial infection. Studies examining the use of HBO in human NSTIs have yielded conflicting results. One key limitation of this therapy is that the patient is required to enter and remain in a relatively austere environment for extended intervals, a challenge in critically ill patients.

VIII. OUTCOMES

A. Mortality. Even with appropriate therapy, mortality rates for NSTI range from 14% to 40% based on the type of infection and location. Typically, patients with Type II infection with toxic shock syndrome and those with Fournier's gangrene have higher mortality rates, most likely due to the concomitant organ dysfunction and larger areas of debridement with these infections. The most important factor that influences mortality is the time to definitive and appropriate surgical debridement.

IX. MORBIDITY. Patients who survive NSTI may have many complications, including nosocomial infection (76%), ventilator-dependent respiratory failure and adult respiratory distress syndrome (29%), acute renal failure (32%), seizure (5%), stroke (4%), cardiac arrest (3%), and heart failure (2%).

AXIOMS

- Think about necrotizing infections any time you evaluate a patient with risk factors, profound pain, or systemic manifestations with the skin infection.
- Exhaustive workups should be avoided.
- CT scan of all affected areas is helpful to confirm the diagnosis and show anatomical extent of the infection.
- Early, aggressive surgical debridement and directed antimicrobial therapy are the mainstays of care.
- Prolonged and complicated hospital courses are common and require ongoing care.
- Morbidity and mortality remain high even in ideal conditions.

Suggested Readings

Anaya DA, Dellinger EP. Necrotizing soft-tissue infection: Diagnosis and management. *Clin Infect Dis* 2007;44(5):705–710.

Anaya DA, McMahon K, Nathens AB, et al. Predictors of mortality and limb loss in necrotizing soft tissue infections. *Arch Surg* 2005;140(2):151–157; discussion 158.

Darenberg J, Luca-Harari B, Jasir A, et al. Molecular and clinical characteristics of invasive group A streptococcal infection in Sweden. *Clin Infect Dis* 2007;45(4):450–458.

Elliott DC, Kufera JA, Myers RA. Necrotizing soft tissue infections. risk factors for mortality and strategies for management. *Ann Surg* 1996;224(5):672–683.

Freischlag JA, Ajalat G, Busuttil RW. Treatment of necrotizing soft tissue infections. The need for a new approach. *Am J Surg* 1985;149(6):751–755.

Hackett SP, Stevens DL. Streptococcal toxic shock syndrome: Synthesis of tumor necrosis factor and interleukin-1 by monocytes stimulated with pyrogenic exotoxin A and streptolysin O. *J Infect Dis* 1992;165(5):879–885.

Laucks SS 2nd. Fournier's gangrene. *Surg Clin North Am* 1994;74(6):1339–1352.

Melles DC, van Leeuwen WB, Boelens HA, et al. Panton-valentine leukocidin genes in staphylococcus aureus. *Emerg Infect Dis* 2006;12(7):1174–1175.

Miller LG, Perdreau-Remington F, Rieg G, et al. Necrotizing fasciitis caused by community-associated methicillin-resistant Staphylococcus aureus in Los Angeles. *N Engl J Med* 2005;352(14):1445–1453.

Wall DB, de Virgilio C, Black S, et al. Objective criteria may assist in distinguishing necrotizing fasciitis from nonnecrotizing soft tissue infection. *Am J Surg* 2000;179(1):17–21.

Wong CH, Chang HC, Pasupathy S, et al. Necrotizing fasciitis: Clinical presentation, microbiology, and determinants of mortality. *J Bone Joint Surg Am* 2003;85-A(8):1454–1460.

Wong CH, Khin LW, Heng KS, et al. The LRINEC (laboratory risk indicator for necrotizing fasciitis) score: A tool for distinguishing necrotizing fasciitis from other soft tissue infections. *Crit Care Med* 2004; 32:1535–1541.

Vascular Emergencies

Syed M. Faisal Alam and Christopher H. Byrne

I. INTRODUCTION

The acute care surgeon is often called to evaluate and manage patients in the emergency department who have a vascular etiology for their complaints. Prompt recognition and treatment of the vascular pathology can diminish the morbidity and mortality associated with these vascular surgery conditions.

II. RUPTURED AORTIC ANEURYSM

A. Introduction. An aneurysm is a permanent localized dilatation of a vessel that creates a 50% (1.5 times) or greater increase in its expected normal diameter.

  1. Abdominal aortic aneurysm (AAA) is the most common form of true aneurysm. The most common location is below the renal artery. Thoracoabdominal aneurysms are less common and a larger treatment challenge.

  2. It is estimated that 200,000 new AAA cases are diagnosed each year with more than 50,000 repairs done.

  3. The incidence of detected AAA has tripled since 1970; the age-specific death rate from aneurysm rupture has also increased.

  4. In the USA there are an estimated 15,000 deaths annually due to AAA, making it the 13th leading cause of death.

  5. Rupture of an AAA is often a lethal event. The best way to reduce mortality is to identify and treat the lesion before rupture occurs.

  a. Two randomized control trials, the Aneurysm Detection and Management (ADAM) trial and the UK Small Aneurysm Trial, support a threshold of 5.5 cm or greater to trigger elective repair.

  b. A rapid increase in size (0.7 cm in 6 months or 1 cm in 1 year) should also be electively repaired.

  c. Of note, women rupture more often and some advocate repair at a threshold size of 5 cm or greater.

B. Diagnosis

  1. Risk factors for AAAs (Table 55-1)

  2. History and physical examination

  a. The classic manifestations of ruptured AAA consist of diffuse back/flank or abdominal pain, shock, and a pulsatile abdominal mass. Classic presentations are not common—often, one or more feature is absent.

  b. The presence of aneurysm is known only in 25% to 33% of patients before rupture.

  c. Pain, most commonly occurs on the left side since the left posterolateral wall, is the most common site of rupture.

  d. The duration of symptoms may vary from a few minutes to up to 24 hours. Although free aneurysm rupture is a catastrophic event, the hematoma can be contained for prolonged periods.

  3. Imaging modalities

  CT scan

  CT is most commonly used modality for diagnosis of AAA. The preferred way to diagnose and plan any operation is a CT angiogram with fine cuts; this is often not possible in unstable patients or in patients with abnormal renal function.

TABLE 55-1	Independent Risk Factors for Detecting an Unknown 4 cm Diameter or Larger AAA during US Screening	
Risk factor	**Odds ratio[a]**	**95% CI**
Increased risk		
Smoking history	5.1	4.1–6.2
Family history of AAA	1.9	1.6–2.3
Older age (per 7-y interval)	1.7	1.6–1.8
Coronary artery disease	1.5	1.4–1.7
High cholesterol	1.4	1.3–1.6
COPD	1.2	1.1–1.4
Height (per 7 cm interval)	1.2	1.1–1.3
Decreased risk		
Abdominal imaging within 5 y	0.8	0.7–0.9
Deep venous thrombosis	0.7	0.5–0.8
Diabetes mellitus	0.5	0.5–0.6
Black race	0.5	0.4–0.7
Female gender	0.2	0.1–0.5

From Lederle FA, Johnson GR, Wilson SE, et al. The aneurysm detection and management study screening program: validation cohort and final results. Aneurysm Detection and Management Veterans Affairs Cooperative Study Investigators. *Arch Intern Med* 2000;160:1425
AAA, abdominal aortic aneurysm; CI, confidence interval; COPD, chronic obstructive pulmonary disease.
[a]Odds ratio indicates relative risk in comparison to patients without that risk factor.

Ultrasound (US)

Abdominal US is a useful bedside tool in trained hands. US is user dependent. It is not useful for the suprarenal aorta and is unreliable for defining relationship between aortic aneurysm and renal arteries. Examination is limited to presence of AAA and presence of free fluid.

MRA or traditional angiogram

There is no role of either of the modalities in diagnosis of ruptured AAA.

C. Treatment

1. Urgent operation is required in the setting of a presumed ruptured AAA.
2. Standard adjuncts for management include large-bore IVs, central venous access, airway control, permissive hypotension, and foley catheter. Immediate availability of blood products is mandatory as part of operative planning.
3. Permissive hypotension involves controlled resuscitation of patients to an SBP of 80 to 90 mm Hg for temporarily adequate end organ perfusion but not to exceed 100 mm Hg.
4. Skin preparation and draping include chest, abdomen, and thighs prior to induction.

Operative strategies

5. **Open repair**
   a. Midline incision (retroperitoneal approach also well described).
   b. Recognition of retroperitoneal staining demands supraceliac control via opening gastrohepatic ligament, exposure of aorta by dividing crus of diaphragm. A nasogastric tube allows identification and protection of the esophagus.
   c. Mobilize duodenum to the right
   d. Proximal and distal aortic control.
   e. Open aneurysm, oversew lumbar branches.
   f. Graft sewn in place; rapid repair with a tube graft if possible.
      i. The shortest operation with least systemic physiologic insult is key to improved outcomes.
      ii. Iliac aneurysms up to 3 to 4 cm diameter can be repaired in a delayed fashion unless they are the source of rupture.

    g. Inferior mesenteric artery (IMA) perfusion

        i. Safety of IMA ligation based on collateral pathways—patients with underlying celiac or superior mesenteric artery (SMA) occlusive lesions, previous bowel resection, significant pelvic occlusive disease and patients with hypotension in the perioperative period are at risk.

        ii. Presence of back-bleeding of the IMA in addition to normal appearing colon would indicate ability to ligate the IMA.

        iii. Ligation is performed from within aneurysm sac to prevent ligation of branches of IMA.

    h. Aneurysm sac closed over repair, retroperitoneum closed, and abdomen closed.

  6. Endovascular repair

    a. An area under investigation in vascular surgery.

    b. Recent studies suggest improved outcomes in centers with endovascular ruptured AAA programs.

D. Outcomes

  1. Eighty to ninety percent of patients with ruptured AAA die before reaching a hospital.

  2. Mortality of patients reaching the operating room is about 50%.

  3. Patients need to be monitored in the ICU postoperatively. Appropriate restoration of volume and use of blood and blood products – including platelets and FFP – optimizes outcomes.

  4. Bowel ischemia is a common postoperative problem.

  5. Endovascular repair has better perioperative morbidity and mortality compared to open repair.

III. VISCERAL ANEURYSMS

A. Introduction

  1. Visceral arterial aneurysms are an uncommon but important vascular disease. Nearly 22% of these aneurysms present as surgical emergencies including about 9% resulting in death. The major visceral vessels involved with these aneurysms in decreasing order of frequency are the splenic, hepatic, SMA, and celiac arteries.

B. Presentation

  1. Most are asymptomatic and diagnosed as an incidental finding

  2. If symptomatic

    a. Pain is the most common symptom

    b. Palpable mass depending on the size and location of the aneurysm

    c. Hemorrhage

        i. Intra-abdominal

        ii. GI bleeding

        iii. Hemobilia

C. Diagnosis

  1. Most patients with rupture are diagnosed either in the operating room during exploration or with a pre-op contrast enhanced CT scan. Patients with non-ruptured but symptomatic aneurysms are diagnosed with a combination of CTA, US, and angiography.

D. Affected vessels

  1. Splenic artery

    a. Sixty percent of all reported visceral aneurysms.

    b. Associated with grand multiparas, medial fibrodysplasia, portal hypertension, and pancreatitis.

    c. Vague abdominal discomfort.

    d. Double rupture phenomenon (initial bleeding contained in the lesser sac followed by free intraperitoneal hemorrhage).

    e. Rupture not associated with pregnancy has 25% mortality.

    f. Rupture associated with pregnancy has 70% maternal and 75% fetal mortality.

Treatment options

g. Aneurysm resection with interposition graft or primary anastomosis

h. Percutaneous transcatheter embolization

i. Endovascular stent graft exclusion of splenic artery aneurysm

j. Splenectomy, excision of the aneurysm

2. Hepatic artery

a. Twenty percent of all visceral aneurysms.

b. Most are false aneurysms.

c. Secondary to trauma to the liver, biliary tract procedures. Seventeen percent of hepatic artery aneurysms are related to liver transplant.

d. Most are asymptomatic but may cause right upper quadrant pain and epigastric pain.

e. Large aneurysms of hepatic artery may cause obstructive jaundice.

f. Rupture carries 35% mortality.

g. May cause hemobilia or free intraperitoneal hemorrhage.

Treatment options

h. Common hepatic artery aneurysms are generally treated with aneurysmectomy or aneurysm exclusion.

i. Percutaneous transcatheter obliteration of hepatic artery aneurysms with balloons, coils, or thrombogenic particulate matter is an endovascular alternative.

3. SMA

a. Aneurysm of the proximal SMA is the third most common visceral aneurysm accounting for 5% of these lesions.

b. SMA aneurysms are related to medial degeneration, periarterial inflammation, and trauma.

c. Aneurysm rupture or dissection is rare.

d. May occlude and cause hemodynamic instability from intestinal ischemia.

e. Mycotic aneurysm secondary to bacterial endocarditis is well described.

Treatment options

f. Ligation and aneurysmorrhaphy is the most common means of managing these lesions.

g. Aneurysmectomy or simple ligation of vessels entering or exiting the SMA aneurysm may necessitate intestinal revascularization by means of aortomesenteric bypass.

h. Endovascular treatment has appeal for certain SMA aneurysms (saccular) or in high risk patients.

  i. Stent graft.

  ii. Obliteration by coils.

4. Celiac artery

a. Celiac artery aneurysm accounts for 4% of visceral aneurysms.

b. Secondary to medial degeneration.

c. Usually saccular in nature affecting the distal trunk.

d. Rupture in 13% of the aneurysms with mortality up to 50%.

e. May cause life-threatening intra-abdominal hemorrhage, rarely may cause GI bleeding.

Treatment options

f. Aneurysmectomy with arterial reconstruction is the preferred surgical therapy.

g. Endovascular therapy of celiac artery is usually not appropriate because of the need to occlude the hepatic, splenic, and left gastric arteries.

IV. AORTIC DISSECTION

A. Introduction

1. Acute aortic dissection is the most common aortic catastrophe with an incidence of 5 to 30 cases per million population each year.

2. May have a dramatic presentation and catastrophic outcome in the absence of prompt diagnosis and treatment.

3. Dissection and aneurysm are frequently misused terms. Dissections may arise in the setting of an aneurysm. Dissecting aneurysm as a term should be confined to this particular setting.

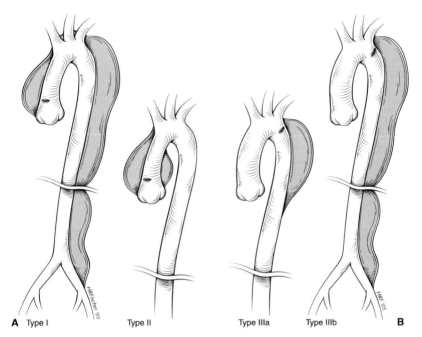

Figure 55-1. The Stanford and DeBakey classifications for aortic dissections. (From Kaiser L, Kron I, Spray T. *Mastery of Cardiothoracic Surgery.* 2nd edition, Lippincott, Williams & Wilkins, 2007.)

B. Pathophysiology

1. The process of aortic dissection is dynamic; dissection can occur anywhere along the course of the aorta creating a wide range of clinical manifestations.
2. The pathognomonic lesion is an intimal tear followed by blood surging typically antegrade and cleaving the intimal and medial layers of the aortic wall longitudinally. Thus creating separation of layers of the aortic wall into a "true lumen" and "false lumen."
3. Typically one or more tears in the intimal septum allow communication between the true and false lumens.

C. Classification (Fig. 55-1)

1. **Chronicity**
   a. Acute <14 days
   b. Chronic >14 days
2. **DeBakey classification**
   a. Type I—ascending aorta and variable extent of descending
   b. Type II—limited to ascending aorta
   c. Type III
      i. IIIa—descending aorta without extension to the abdomen
      ii. IIIb—descending aorta with extension to the abdomen
3. **Stanford classification**
   a. Type A—proximal to takeoff of left subclavian artery
   b. Type B—distal to takeoff of left subclavian artery

D. Diagnosis

1. **History and physical examination**
   a. Severe tearing anterior chest (Stanford A) or back and or abdominal pain (Stanford B) of abrupt onset.

  b. Most patients have hypertension at presentation.
  c. Discrepancy in pulse examination or BP examination in the extremities is seen but not invariable.

2. Radiography
  a. CT angiogram—most commonly used modality and shows the intimal flap.
  b. MR angiogram—generally not used because of urgent nature of the presentation.
  c. Transesophageal echocardiogram—good for emergent evaluation of proximal dissection.
  d. Arteriography—more difficult because it requires imaging of both true and false lumens. Rarely used to establish diagnosis; however used frequently in management with endovascular stent graft repair.
  e. CXR—may show enlarged aortic knob, mediastinal widening, left pleural effusion, displacement of left main stem bronchus in proximal dissection with aneurysmal changes.

E. Management
1. Stanford Type A
  a. Urgent operative intervention with replacement of the ascending aorta is generally warranted.

2. Stanford Type B
  a. Medical management
    i. ICU monitoring, central venous access, indwelling urinary catheter to monitor output.
    ii. Arterial line blood pressure monitoring (extremity with highest BP should be used).
    iii. Blood pressure and heart rate control to decrease wall stress. IV beta-blockers such as esmolol and labetalol (titrated to HR of 60 to 80 bpm with an SBP of 100 to 110 mm Hg). Vasodilators such as nitroprusside, calcium channel blockers, and ACE inhibitors are used as necessary.
    iv. Follow up CT scan to assess aortic expansion in the acute phase.
    v. Long-term anti-hypertensives, preferably beta-blockers, are used.
    vi. Routine CT scan in chronic phase to assess aneurysmal degeneration.
  b. Surgical management
    i. Acute surgical intervention reserved for patients with malperfusion syndrome
    ii. Lower extremity ischemia
    iii. Acute renal failure
    iv. Mesenteric ischemia
    v. Paralysis
    vi. Surgical management may also be warranted for aneurysmal degeneration or impending rupture
  c. Surgical options
    i. Open repair
      a) Graft replacement
      b) Open fenestration
      c) Glue aortoplasty
    ii. Endovascular repair
      a) Stent graft to obliterate the entry point and the false lumen
      b) Fenestration
      c) Intravascular ultrasound is a good adjunct to identify intimal tears and branching points during endovascular repair

F. Outcomes
  1. Stanford A dissections carry a mortality rate of 20% to 30% in expert hands.
  2. Stanford B dissections have a more favorable outcome because of the paradigm shift in the management of this disease, specifically with rapidly evolving endovascular techniques, better ICU monitoring and blood pressure control. In most series 85% to 100% success rate is reported.

V. AORTOENTERIC FISTULA (AEF)

A. Introduction

1. Patients with AEF may present with life-threatening hemorrhage. The majority of these cases result from prior aortic surgery due to the loss of retroperitoneal plane between the aorta and the duodenum. Occurs in 1% to 2% of patients following open AAA repairs. Approximately 0.4% of patients with reconstructions will develop a fistula.

B. Etiology

1. **Primary:** Majority associated with AAA
2. **Secondary:** Occur in the presence of previous vascular surgery with prosthetic material; average time to formation after primary intervention is 5 years
   a. Graft enteric fistula—75%
   b. Graft enteric erosion—25%

C. Symptoms

1. **GI bleeding**
   a. "Herald bleed" but present without hemodynamic compromise
   b. Unstable with large volume blood loss
2. **Graft infection**
   a. One-half of patients will grow out an organism—most commonly mixed flora with *Streptococcus, Escherichia coli,* and *Staphylococcus aureus.*
3. Pain
4. Fever

D. Site of bowel involvement

1. Duodenum—75%
2. Small bowel—19%
3. Colon—6%

E. Diagnosis

1. Patient with a history of aortic reconstruction presenting with a GI bleed has an AEF until proven otherwise.
2. EGD—use a pediatric colonoscope needed to view entire duodenum.
   a. Findings suggestive of AEF include compression of duodenum by extrinsic mass, ulceration, active bleeding, and visualization of bile-stained graft material.
3. CT scan—findings are subtle but sensitivity (94%) and specificity (85%) suggest rival EGD as first line test for AEF.
4. UGI
5. Aortography
6. Nuclear scan
7. Colonoscopy

F. Treatment

1. Extra-anatomic bypass and excision of graft with debridement of aorta and surrounding tissues
2. Reconstruction with autogenous graft material from common femoral veins.
3. Homograft replacement of aorta
4. *In situ* rifampin-soaked prosthetic reconstruction

G. Outcome

1. Twenty percent to fifty percent mortality.
2. Extra-anatomic bypass in this setting results in amputation rates as high as 30%

VI. MESENTERIC ISCHEMIA

A. Introduction

1. Presentation is characterized by subjective complaints of pain and a relative paucity of physical findings; *acute mesenteric ischemia can lead to mortality rates as high as 60% to 80%.* The diagnosis of acute mesenteric ischemia remains challenging and mortality rates remain high. Rapid diagnosis and intervention are essential to optimize outcome; *the high mortality is related directly to delay in diagnosis and treatment.*

B. Etiology
   1. **Arterial embolism**—40% to 50% of cases. Most emboli originate from the heart, frequently in the setting of atrial fibrillation. The SMA is more frequently involved because of the gentler angle relative to the other visceral vessels (most arterial emboli lodge at first branch point of SMA).
   2. **Arterial thrombosis**—25% to 30% of cases; generally in setting of advanced atherosclerosis and chronic mesenteric ischemia; most commonly at origin of SMA.
   3. **Non-occlusive**—20% of cases; poorly understood; low cardiac output and vasoconstriction in setting of critically ill patient; most likely to affect watershed regions of bowel.
   4. **Venous thrombosis**—10% of cases; may be secondary to underlying hypercoagulable state, malignancy, sepsis, portal hypertension, or pancreatitis; usually segmental; most commonly involves SMV; slower onset than embolic or thrombotic. Clinical presentations are often indolent and non-specific.

C. Diagnosis
   1. **History and physical examination**
      a. Patients with embolic events generally have an acute onset of diffuse pain that may be followed by diarrhea (perhaps bloody).
      b. Patients with thrombotic events may have a more insidious onset of symptoms, as they are more likely to have a well-developed collateral system due to chronic atherosclerosis.
      c. "Pain out of proportion to examination" is the common feature; patients may have evidence of volume depletion, hemodynamic instability, tachypnea.
   2. **Radiography**
      a. Plain films have a limited role; unenhanced CT helps exclude other causes of abdominal pain; CT angiography has become the modality of choice.
      b. Preoperative angiogram can be helpful but should not delay definitive intervention.
      c. Chronic occlusion may demonstrate well-formed collateral vessels.
   3. **Laboratory tests**
      a. Metabolic acidosis; elevated lactate; increased base deficit; leukocytosis; may have evidence of dehydration (elevated BUN/creatinine ratio).

D. Treatment
The key is early recognition and diagnosis with prompt restoration of mesenteric blood flow. While traditionally done via surgical exploration, newer endovascular techniques also aid. Both are appropriate options in well-selected patients. Initial management in all patients involves fluid resuscitation and anticoagulation.
   1. **Operative**
      a. Exploratory laparotomy with exposure of the superior mesenteric vessels is the basic approach, with transverse arteriotomy and thrombectomy in the setting of an otherwise normal vessel.
      b. Do mesenteric bypass if flow is not restored or if severe underlying vessel disease exists.
         i. Retrograde iliac—SMA bypass with C loop to prevent kinking
         ii. Antegrade supraceliac aorta—SMA, celiac bypass
         iii. Autogenous graft if bowel contamination present
      c. Assess intestinal viability (e.g., Wood's lamp, Doppler of distal vessels) in conjunction with resection of non-viable bowel.
      d. Often, a second-look assessment of bowel should be performed in 24 to 48 hours.
   2. **Endovascular**
      a. Reports of success in endovascular techniques, but these do not allow assessment of bowel viability.
      b. Thrombolytics are generally not indicated, as mesenteric flow must be reestablished as the first priority.

3. Treatment of non-occlusive mesenteric ischemia
   a. Correct any low cardiac output state to improve mesenteric perfusion. Use angiographic vasodilators to relieve vasospasm in patients who do not respond to resuscitation alone.
4. Treatment for mesenteric venous thrombosis
   a. Anticoagulation, bowel rest, and resuscitation. Questionable role for thrombolytic agents.
E. Outcomes
   1. Survival is 50% if diagnosis is made within 24 hours of onset of symptoms; mortality exceeds 70% if diagnosis is delayed.
   2. Thrombolytics have been used in select patients with anecdotal success.
   3. Prognosis for acute mesenteric ischemia is worse than for those patients with chronic ischemia.

VII. ACUTE LOWER EXTREMITY ISCHEMIA
A. Clinical manifestations. The six P's
   1. Pain (the most common presenting symptom)
   2. Pallor
   3. Paresthesias
   4. Paralysis
   5. Pulselessness
   6. Poikilothermia
B. Diagnosis
   1. Physical examination is key
      a. Complete pulse examination including non-affected limb
      b. Ankle/brachial index (systolic BP in both areas—<0.8 is abnormal)
      c. Motor and sensory examinations indicate severity of ischemia and dictate the treatment.
         i. Ischemia criteria (Table 55-2)
C. Etiology
   1. Thrombotic (85%)
      a. Arises in setting of advanced underlying atherosclerotic disease.
      b. Overall, bypass graft thrombosis is the most common cause of acute limb ischemia.
   2. Embolic (15%)
      a. More likely in younger and those patients without prior cardiac or vascular history. After restoration of flow, seek the source, which may include cardiac echocardiography (evaluate for valvular vegetation), CTA chest, abdomen and pelvis (possible aortic aneurysm), or lower extremity duplex to assess for iliac, femoral, or popliteal aneurysms.
   3. The differential diagnosis of acute limb ischemia includes several less common etiologies that should be evaluated including but not limited to aortic dissection, popliteal aneurysm, adventitial cystic disease, and popliteal artery entrapment syndrome.
D. Treatment
   1. Restore any circulating volume deficit, and then institute heparin to prevent propagation of clot or further embolus from the source.
   2. Urgent operative intervention is warranted in patients with neurologic deficits, especially any loss of motor function.
      a. The level of exploration is often dictated by level of vascular occlusion or can be based on remote embolization with over the wire Fogarty embolectomy catheters and endovascular techniques.
      b. Additional procedures may be required to restore adequate blood flow to foot, such as endarterectomy or bypass.
   3. Thrombolysis
      a. Appropriate for those patients presenting with acute onset of symptoms (<14 days from occurrence), thromboemboli not accessible to embolectomy

TABLE 55-2 Classification of Acute Limb Ischemia—Rutherford Criteria

| Category | Description/Prognosis | Findings | | Doppler signals | |
		Sensory loss	Muscle weakness	Arterial	Venous
I. Viable	Not immediately threatened	None	None	Audible	Audible
II. Threatened					
a. Marginally	Salvageable if promptly treated	Minimal (toes) or none	None	Inaudible	Audible
b. Immediately	Salvageable with immediate revascularization	More than toes, associated with rest pain	Mild, moderate	Inaudible	Audible
III. Irreversible	Major tissue loss or permanent nerve damage inevitable	Profound, anesthetic	Profound, paralysis (rigor)	Inaudible	Inaudible

From Rutherford RB, Baker JD, Ernst C, et al. Recommended standards for reports dealing with lower extremity ischemia: revised version. *J Vasc Surg* 1997;26:517–538.

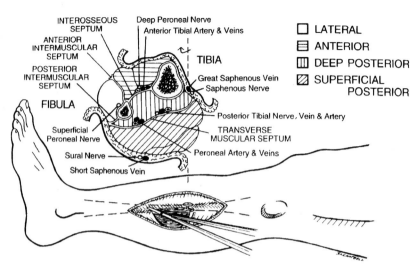

Figure 55-2. Surgical approach for four-compartment fasciotomy in the lower leg. (From Ombrellaro MP, Steven SL. Compartment syndrome: A collective review. In: Maull KI, Cleveland HC, Feliciano DV, et al, eds. Advances in Trauma and Critical Care. St. Louis, Mo: Mosby—Year Book; 1995;10:100, with permission.)

catheters, and cases in which lysis may improve the outflow or uncover outflow for a bypass graft.
  b. Chemical thrombolysis (tPA or other agents).
  c. Mechanical thrombolysis.
  4. Reperfusion injury
      a. Reperfusion of the extremity may result in the release of toxic oxygen metabolites which can result in local edema leading to compartment syndrome and systemic metabolic derangements.
      b. If prolonged ischemia exists, do a prophylactic fasciotomy prior to revascularization. Be sure to release of all four compartments (Fig. 55-2).
      c. Aggressive hydration, mannitol, and possible alkalinization of urine can aid prevent precipitation of myoglobin and renal failure.
  E. Outcome
    1. Amputation rates from 10% to 30% and mortality as high as 15% at 30 days.
    2. Monitor extremities frequently postoperatively for changes in sensation or compartment pressures.

AXIOMS

■ A patient with a pulsatile mass and abdominal pain has a ruptured AAA until proven otherwise.
■ Ascending aortic dissection is a surgical emergency. Dissection of the descending aorta is generally managed medically with antihypertensive medications.
■ GI bleeding in a patient with prior aortic surgery is an AEF until proven otherwise.
■ Pain out of proportion to examination suggests mesenteric ischemia, the majority of which are the result of embolic or thrombotic events requiring operative intervention.
■ Acute lower extremity ischemia most often arises in setting of prior lower extremity bypass. Look for compartment syndrome before and after reperfusion.

Suggested Readings
Boley SJ, Feinstein FR, Sammartano R. New concepts in the management of emboli of the superior mesenteric artery. *Surg Gynecol Obstet* 1981;153(4):561–569.

Crawford ES, Saleh SA, Babb JW III, et al. Infrarenal abdominal aortic aneurysm: Factors influencing survival after operation performed over a 25-year period. *Ann Surg* 1981;193(6):699–709

Donaldson MC, Rosenberg JM, Bucknam CA. Factors affecting survival after ruptured abdominal aortic aneurysms. *J Vasc Surg* 1985;2(4):564–570.

Dormandy J, Heeck L, Vig S. Acute limb ischemia. *Semin Vasc Surg* 1999;12(2):148–153.

Gabelmann A, Gorich J, Merkle EM. Endovascular treatment of visceral artery aneurysms. *J Endovasc Ther* 2002;9(1):38–47.

Hagan PG, Nienaber CA, Isselbacher EM, et al. The International Registry of Acute Aortic Dissection (IRAD): New insights into an old disease. *JAMA* 2000;283(7):897–903.

Lederle FA, Simel DL. The rational clinical examination: Does this patient have abdominal aortic aneurysm? *JAMA* 1999;281(1):77–82.

O'Hara PJ, Hertzer NR, Beven EG, et al. Surgical management of infected abdominal aortic grafts: Review of a 25-year experience. *J Vasc Surg* 1986;3(5):725–731.

Oldenburg WA, Lau LL, Rodenberg TJ, et al. Acute mesenteric ischemia: A clinical review. *Arch Intern Med* 2004;164(10):1054–1062.

Pipinos II, Carr JA, Haithcock BE. Secondary aortoenteric fistula. *Ann Vasc Surg* 2000;14(6):688–696.

Zelenock GB, Strodel WE, Knol JA, et al. A prospective study of clinically and endoscopically documented colonic ischemia in 100 patients undergoing aortic reconstructive surgery with aggressive colonic and direct pelvic revascularization, compared with historic controls. *Surgery* 1989;106(4):771–779.

I. INTRODUCTION

A. Hernia repairs are one of the most common operations performed.

B. An estimated 20 million hernia repairs occur each year worldwide. Of those, 5% to 15% are repaired emergently.

C. About 10% of hernia repairs are for recurrence.

D. Hernias site frequency (highest to lowest) is inguinal, umbilical, epigastric, incisional, femoral, and finally other rare types of hernias.

II. ABDOMINAL WALL ANATOMY

A. Hernias occur in areas of weakness or openings within the fascia, often where nerves, blood vessels, or gonadal structures penetrate the fascia.

B. The abdominal wall is created by layers of muscle and fascia.

  1. The rectus muscle is in the midline and surrounded by the anterior and posterior fascia (Fig. 56-1).

    a. The external oblique contributes to the anterior rectus fascia while the internal oblique splits and contributes to both the anterior and posterior fascia superiorly.

    b. At the level of the arcuate line, the entire internal oblique fascia courses anteriorly.

    c. The transversus abdominis contributes to the posterior sheath to the level of the arcuate line.

    d. Only the peritoneum covers the posterior rectus muscle caudad to the arcuate line.

  2. The inguinal canal contains the ilioinguinal nerve, the genital branch of the genitofemoral nerve and the round ligament in females or the spermatic cord in males (Fig. 56-2).

    a. The roof of the canal is internal oblique and transversus abdominis muscles.

    b. The floor is created by the inguinal ligament.

    c. Anteriorly, the canal is formed by the external oblique aponeurosis

    d. Posteriorly, the canal is formed by transversalis fascia and the conjoint tendon.

    e. The superficial or external inguinal ring is formed by the external oblique fascia.

    f. The deep or internal inguinal ring is located approximately halfway between the anterior superior iliac spine and the pubic tubercle. The deep ring is created by the transversalis fascia.

III. PRESENTATION OF HERNIAS

A. Symptoms. Can range from none to sepsis from obstruction with strangulation.

  1. Most hernias present as a bulge on the abdominal wall with associated discomfort or pain. The bulge can be accentuated by having the patient increase intra-abdominal pressure through a Valsalva maneuver.

  2. Patients with incarceration or strangulation may have findings of bowel obstruction, including nausea, vomiting, abdominal pain, distension, constipation, or obstipation.

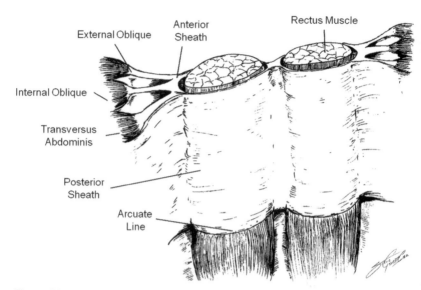

Figure 56-1. Anterior abdominal wall anatomy. The anterior rectus sheath is comprised of fascia from the external oblique and the anterior leaflet of the internal oblique. The posterior rectus sheath is comprised of fascia from the transverses abdominis and the posterior leaflet of the internal oblique.

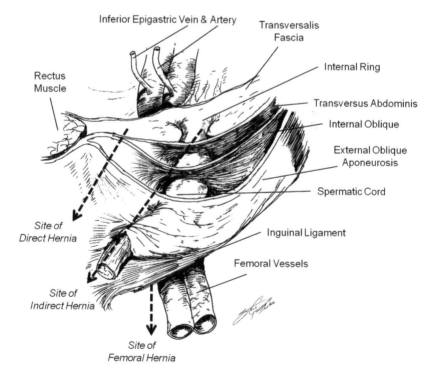

Figure 56-2. Inguinal anatomy and location of groin hernias. Sites of direct, indirect, and femoral hernias are shown.

3. Look for a hernia in any patient with a suspected bowel obstruction , as this is the most common cause of obstruction worldwide and the second most common cause of obstruction in the United States (after adhesive disease).

4. If strangulation and bowel necrosis is present, patients may be toxic appearing, febrile, and have peritonitis.

IV. DIAGNOSIS

A. History and physical examination is diagnostic for most types of hernias. Examine patients both standing and supine, as the defect may become more obvious in one of the positions. Evaluate the entire abdomen, as some patients have multiple hernias.

B. Radiologic studies. If the patient history is consistent with a hernia, but a defect is not appreciated on physical examination, various radiologic modalities can be beneficial.

  1. Plain films of the abdomen are useful when bowel obstruction is suspected; otherwise have little role.

  2. Computed tomography is useful when a patient presents with abdominal pain and multiple causes are suspected. This modality gives the benefit of being able to evaluate other intra-abdominal organs and etiologies for abdominal pain.

  3. Ultrasound can aid, especially in distinguishing scrotal hernias from hydroceles.

V. COMPLICATIONS

A. There are three main complications of all types of hernias: Incarceration, obstruction, and strangulation.

  1. Incarceration occurs when abdominal contents are present within a hernia sac and cannot be reduced back into the abdomen.

    a. The risk of incarceration is approximately 4 per 1,000 patients per year for groin hernias.

    b. Obstruction occurs when intestine is present within the hernia sac and leads to a mechanical blockage. This may present as an acute or chronic obstruction, and partial or complete obstruction.

  2. Strangulation occurs when a hernia is incarcerated *and* the blood supply becomes compromised leading to ischemia and necrosis of the incarcerated organ.

    a. The pathogenesis of strangulation is incarceration leading to bowel wall edema followed by venous congestion which further increases the edema, eventually resulting in arterial compromise. This ultimately results in bowel ischemia, necrosis, and perforation.

    b. Strangulation often requires bowel resection and is associated with increased morbidity and mortality.

VI. MANAGEMENT

A. Most hernias can be repaired electively. Incarcerated hernias should be repaired emergently if they cannot be reduced or if strangulation is suspected.

B. Patients with major medical comorbidities may receive nonoperative management. The risk and benefit of operation versus observation must be carefully considered. The signs and symptoms of incarceration and strangulation must be explained. The morbidity and mortality associated with an emergent repair is higher, especially if the incarcerated bowel becomes necrotic.

C. Recent data suggests that asymptomatic inguinal hernias in patients under 50 years old may be treated with "watchful waiting," as the risk of incarceration is as low (1.8 per 1,000 patients per year in that population.)

D. For patients who present with incarcerated hernias, attempt gentle manual reduction.

  1. If the hernia can be reduced, the repair can happen then or on an elective basis.

  2. If a patient has local signs of ischemic intestine such as cellulitis, or abdominal findings consistent with strangulation such as peritonitis, **do not try** reduction. An infarcted segment of intestine may go unrecognized when reduced into the peritoneal cavity or preperitoneal space (*reduction en-masse*). Emergent surgical intervention is required.

VII. SPECIFIC HERNIAS
A. Inguinal hernia
1. **Incidence.** Lifetime risk of inguinal hernias for men is approximately 27% compared to 3% for females. There is also a slight right-sided predominance of inguinal hernias.
2. **Anatomy.** There are two basic types of inguinal hernias: Direct and indirect (Fig. 56-2).
   a. Indirect inguinal hernias are more common and may extend down into the scrotum. These hernias are lateral to the inferior epigastric vessels and enter the inguinal canal through the deep ring.
   b. Direct inguinal hernias are medial to the inferior epigastric vessels and enter through a weakening in the floor of the inguinal canal.
3. **Treatment.** Regardless of the type of inguinal hernia, most are repaired today with a mesh repair.
   a. Lichtenstein repair is the most common open repair. This repair is a tension-free repair performed with mesh.
   b. Laparoscopic repair has the advantage of being able to assess for and repair bilateral and femoral hernias through a single, three-incision approach.
   c. In general, the operative time is less for open repairs but the incidence of postoperative hematoma and pain is higher. In the event of a recurrence, many surgeons repair through a different approach than the first repair.
   d. In the event of bowel ischemia, resection may be carried out through a groin incision. However, if the bowel cannot be adequately inspected through this incision, one must be prepared to convert to a midline laparotomy or laparoscopy.

B. Femoral hernia
1. **Incidence.** Femoral hernias are more common (7×) in females. (However, indirect inguinal hernia is the most common groin hernia in females.) They account for less than 5% of hernias. Up to 40% of femoral hernias present as emergencies.
2. **Anatomy.** Femoral hernias are bound by the inguinal ligament anteriorly, pectineal ligament posteriorly, lacunar ligament medially, and the femoral vein laterally (Fig. 56-2).
3. **Presentation.** Femoral hernias may present as a bulge inferior to the inguinal ligament, but are often asymptomatic until obstruction occurs.
4. **Treatment.** Femoral hernias may be approached via an infra-inguinal incision, trans-inguinal approach, or laparoscopically. Similar to inguinal hernias, if the bowel cannot be appropriately inspected, be prepared to convert to laparotomy.

C. Umbilical hernia
1. **Causes.** Any comorbidity that increases intra-abdominal pressure contributes to the development of umbilical hernias, specifically obesity, pregnancy, COPD, and physical strain.
2. **Treatment.** Most umbilical hernias require surgical repair.
   a. In pediatric patients many defects spontaneously close; therefore, they are generally not repaired until 5 years of age unless they are large or incarcerated. If umbilical hernias do not spontaneously resolve, the defects are usually amendable to primary repair without mesh.
   b. Most umbilical hernias in adults should be repaired with mesh. In patients with defects greater than 3 cm or in obese patients, many surgeons opt for laparoscopic repair with mesh.
   c. Cirrhosis presents a difficult problem, as many of these patients will persistently leak ascites after the repair and can develop spontaneous bacterial peritonitis. These patients need aggressive medical management of their ascites both pre- and postoperatively.

D. Incisional hernia
1. **Incidence.** Incisional hernias develop in 13% to 20% of patients who undergo midline laparotomy, and in more than one-fourth of the patients who have a postoperative wound infection. Wound infection is the most consistent factor in development of wound dehiscence or incisional hernia.

2. **Treatment.** Most incisional hernias are repaired with mesh, generally as an underlay. Many mesh products are available, but the principle is the same for all repairs: Cover the defect and have the mesh overlap several centimeters of healthy fascia. Close the fascia primarily whenever possible.
   a. Recurrence rates after repair of incisional hernias range from 10% to 50% depending on the type of repair.
   b. Recent data suggest that recurrence rates for laparoscopic mesh repairs are comparable to open mesh repair for incisional hernia; that is, still higher than we would like. Laparoscopic incisional hernia repair can be difficult in the re-operative abdomen due to adhesions.

E. **Peristomal hernia**
   1. **Presentation.** Peristomal hernias present as a bulge adjacent to a stoma. Patients may complain of poorly fitting ostomy appliances, pain, or obstructive symptoms.
   2. **Treatment.** Primary repair of peristomal hernias often results in recurrence. Many studies have shown that the most successful operation is relocation of the stoma and closure of the initial fascial defect.

F. **Spigelian hernia**
   1. **Anatomy.** Spigelian hernias generally occur along the semilunar line (or line of Spiegel) between the level of the umbilicus and the anterior superior iliac spine (Fig. 56-3).
      a. This is due to the absence of the posterior rectus sheath at this level and the increased width of the Spigelian fascia.
      b. This type of hernia is difficult to diagnose on physical examination because the hernia often passes through the transversalis fascia only and dissects between

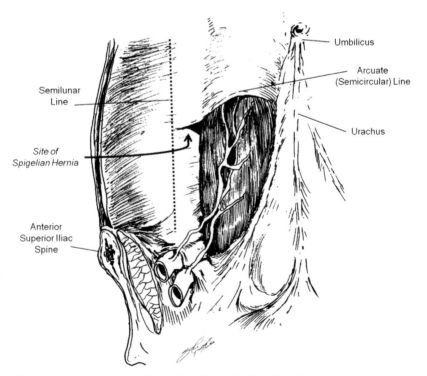

Figure 56-3. Spigelian hernia. The semilunar line is the site of Spigelian hernias.

muscle planes still deep to external oblique muscle, and a bulge may not be palpable.

2. **Diagnosis.** Discomfort in the area of the line of Spiegel should alert the clinician. CT scan is helpful to detect a Spigelian hernia.

3. **Treatment.** Open repair is difficult because the hernia cannot always be palpated. Due to this, laparoscopy is ideal for repairing Spigelian hernias. A mesh underlay is generally used.

G. Obturator hernia

1. **Anatomy.** The obturator foramen is bound by the rami and pubic bones and is covered with the obturator membrane. The obturator canal runs through the membrane carrying the obturator nerve, artery, and vein. Hernias occur due to laxity of the pelvic floor (Fig. 56-4).

2. **Presentation.** Most commonly patients with obturator hernias are elderly, multiparous women, often after weight loss.

  a. Obturator hernias are difficult to diagnose on examination, and many patients present with bowel obstruction.

  b. Hip and medial thigh pain with external rotation and extension of the hip (Howship–Romberg sign) may help establish the diagnosis.

  c. Patients occasionally present with a mass on the medial thigh.

3. **Treatment.** Generally, obturator hernias are diagnosed at laparotomy performed for intestinal obstruction. Most defects can be repaired primarily.

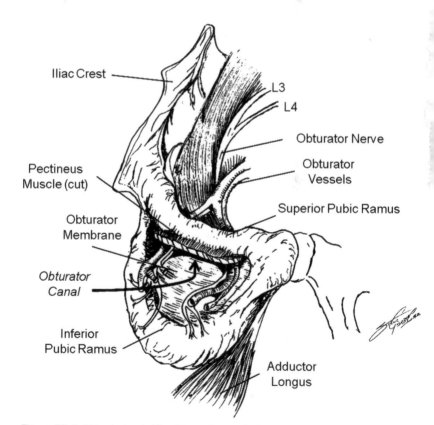

Figure 56-4. Obturator hernia. The obturator foramen is shown with its boundaries.

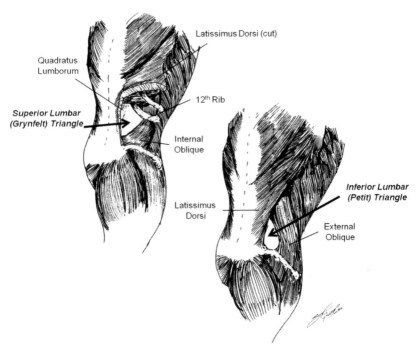

Figure 56-5. Lumbar hernia. The superior triangle (Grynfeltt triangle) and the inferior triangle (Petit triangle) are shown with their borders.

Intestinal resection is often necessary with this type of hernia due to the high rate of incarceration.

H. Lumbar hernia

  1. Anatomy. Most lumbar hernias occur in one of two locations: The superior and inferior lumbar triangles (Fig. 56-5).

  a. The superior triangle, also known as *Grynfeltt triangle*, is bound by the twelfth rib superiorly, the quadratus lumborum medially, and the internal oblique muscle laterally.

  b. The inferior triangle, or *petit triangle*, is defined by the iliac crest inferiorly, by the latissimus dorsi posteriorly, and by the external oblique anteriorly.

  2. Diagnosis. Patients often present with a bulge in the flank and complain of vague flank pain.

  a. CT may help to differentiate a hernia from a lipoma or other mass.

  3. Treatment. Lumbar hernias can be approached via direct posterior approach or anterior retroperitoneal approach. Small hernias may be primarily repaired while larger defects may require mesh or myocutaneous flap for closure. Laparoscopic approach to lumbar hernias has been described as well. Recurrence rates are high.

I. Internal hernia

  1. Internal hernias are usually the result of a previous operation where a defect in the peritoneum, mesentery, or omentum was created and not closed.

  a. Some operations, such as gastric bypass procedures are at high risk of internal hernias due to the rearrangement of normal anatomy.

  b. On occasion, congenital anomalies are diagnosed in adulthood, such as malrotation, and may be the cause of an internal hernia.

2. **Presentation.** Patients with internal hernias may complain of intermittent abdominal pain from bowel sliding in and out of the defect. Patients may also present with signs of bowel obstruction or peritonitis.

3. Any patient with suspected internal hernia should undergo emergent laparotomy or laparoscopy, as the risk of strangulation is high.

J. Richter's hernia is herniation with incarceration of only the anti-mesenteric portion of the bowel wall through an abdominal wall hernia. A Richter's hernia may occur with any abdominal wall or inguinal hernia. Diagnosis may be difficult as the patient will not have signs of a bowel obstruction, yet intestinal wall is at risk. Because of difficulty in diagnosis, bowel necrosis or perforation often results.

K. Planned ventral hernia and the open abdomen

1. With the advent of damage control surgery for trauma and other abdominal catastrophes, more patients are being treated with open abdomen. There are numerous techniques to assist with the closure of the open abdomen, but regardless of the technique used, some patients are left with a planned ventral hernia. Several techniques are used for abdominal wall reconstruction, with varying recurrence rates.

2. Some surgeons advocate using mesh alone, with no division of the fascial components. This often results in recurrence or laxity of the mesh that resembles a hernia.

3. Component separation is a technique that utilizes the layers of the abdominal wall for reconstruction (Fig. 56-6).

    a. This technique involves the release of the external oblique fascia just lateral to the rectus abdominis.

    b. Several centimeters of length are gained to aid in closure of the fascia in the midline.

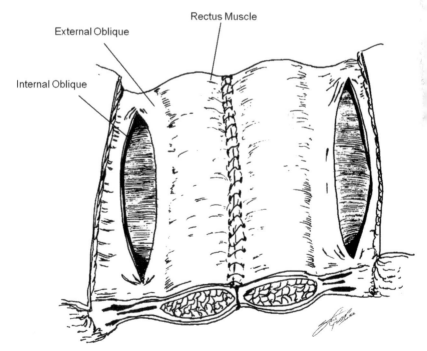

Figure 56-6. Component separation. The external oblique fascia is released just lateral to the rectus abdominis muscle.

    c. In extremely large defects, as often seen with open abdomen, the standard component technique may not be sufficient for closure without a prosthetic adjunct.

4. The modified component separation technique may be used to reconstruct the abdominal wall without the use of prosthetics. This is important as many of these repairs are complicated by enterotomies and procedures are often combined with ostomy reversal. The modified component separation technique essentially doubles the length obtained from the standard component separation (Fig. 56-7).

    a. The modified component separation begins similar to the standard components with anterior release of the external oblique (Fig. 56-7A).

    b. The posterior sheath is dissected from the rectus muscle.

    c. The anterior portion of the internal oblique fascia is then divided down to the level of the arcuate line, which frees the anterior sheath and muscle from the posterior sheath (Fig. 56-7B).

    d. Finally, the medial border of the posterior sheath is sutured to the lateral border of the anterior sheath, and the anterior fascia is closed in the midline (Fig. 56-7C).

    e. Recent studies have shown that this modification produces excellent long-term outcomes with very low recurrence rates.

5. Any of these techniques of abdominal wall reconstruction may be used with the adjunct of mesh.

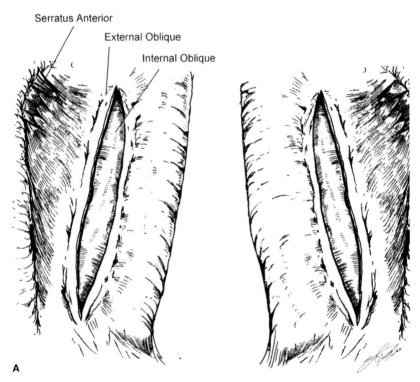

Serratus Anterior

External Oblique

Internal Oblique

A

Figure 56-7. Modified components separation. **(A)** The external oblique fascia is divided and the posterior rectus sheath is mobilized from the rectus muscle. **(continued)**

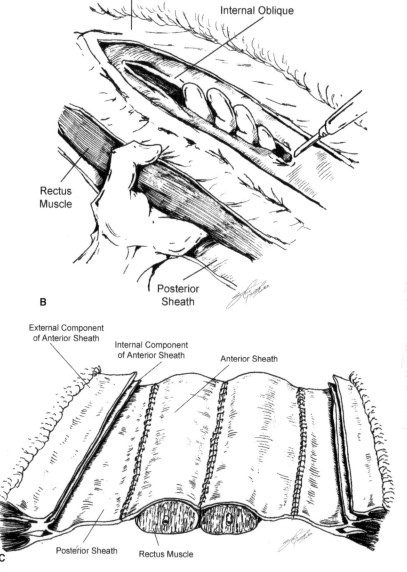

Figure 56-7. (Continued) (B) The internal oblique component of the anterior rectus sheath is divided down to the arcuate line. **(C)** Completed repair, suturing the medial border of the posterior sheath to the lateral border of the anterior sheath, with approximation of the medial portion of the anterior sheath in the midline.

AXIOMS

- Hernias are common and repairs frequently needed, both elective and emergent.
- Most hernias can be diagnosed with careful history and physical examination; imaging usually not required.
- Incarcerated hernias are surgical emergencies and bowel must be inspected for viability.
- Nonoperative management with close observation is a reasonable option in patients with major comorbidities or minimal symptoms.
- For incarcerated inguinal hernias, a traditional groin approach is accepted; if the bowel is unable to be adequately inspected, convert to laparotomy or laparoscopy.

Suggested Readings

Cameron JL, et al. *Current Surgical Therapy.* 6th ed. Mosby; 1998.
Dabbas N, Adams K, Pearson K, et al. Frequency of abdominal wall hernias: is classical teaching out of date? *JRSM Short Rep* 2011;2:5–10.
Derici H, Unalp HR, Bozdag AD, et al. Factors affecting morbidity and mortality in incarcerated abdominal wall hernias. *Hernia* 2007;11(4):341–346.
DiCocco JM, Magnotti LJ, Emmett KP, et al. Long-term follow-up of abdominal wall reconstruction after planned ventral hernia: a 15-year experience. *J Am Coll Surg* 2010;210(5):686–698.
Fitzgibbons RJ, Giobbie-Hurder A, Gibbs JO, et al. Watchful waiting vs repair of inguinal hernia in minimally symptomatic men. *JAMA* 2006;295(3):285–292.
Kingsnorth A, LeBlanc K. Hernias: inguinal and incisional. *Lancet* 2003;362:1561–1571.
Kurt N, Oncel M, Ozkan Z, et al. Risk and outcome of bowel resection in patients with incarcerated groin hernias: Retrospective study. *World J Surg* 2003;27:741–743.
Mittal T, Kumar V, Khullar R, et al. Diagnosis and management of Spigelian hernia: A review of the literature and our experience. *J Minimal Access Surgery* 2008;4(4):95–98.
Ohana G, Manevwitch I, Weil R, et al. Inguinal hernia: challenging the traditional indication for surgery in asymptomatic patients. *Hernia* 2004;8(2):117–120.
Ramirez OM, Ruas E, Dellon AL. "Components separation" method for closure of abdominal-wall defects: an anatomic and clinical study. *Plast Reconstr Surg* 1990;86:519–526.
Van den Heuvel B, Dwars BJ, Klassen DR, et al. Is surgical repair of an asymptomatic groin hernia appropriate? A review. *Hernia* 2011;15(3):251–259.

57 Obstetric and Gynecologic Emergencies

Glenn Updike

INTRODUCTION

A wide variety of emergent obstetric and gynecologic issues lead women to seek care. This chapter outlines the pathophysiology, diagnosis, and management of the common obstetric and gynecologic conditions encountered by surgeons and emergency physicians.

ECTOPIC PREGNANCY

I. INTRODUCTION. Ectopic pregnancies are those pregnancies that occur outside of the fundus of the uterus. While most ectopic pregnancies are in the fallopian tube, extrauterine pregnancies may also occur in the cervix, abdomen, cornua of the uterus, ovary, or in a previous cesarean scar. Rarely, an ectopic pregnancy may co-exist with a normal intrauterine pregnancy (a heterotopic pregnancy). Ectopic pregnancy can result in maternal morbidity or death. Prompt diagnosis and appropriate management, whether medical or surgical, is critical to prevent hemorrhage and its complications.

II. INCIDENCE AND EPIDEMIOLOGY
A. Approximately 20 per 1,000 pregnancies.
B. Most commonly occurs in the fallopian tube (98%).
C. Risk factors include:
   1. Previous ectopic pregnancy. In a patient with a prior ectopic pregnancy, subsequent ectopic pregnancy occurs in 8% to 15%.
   2. A history of tubal surgery including tubal ligation. Nearly 50% of pregnancies are ectopic in location after having tubal ligation.
   3. Previously documented tubal pathology
   4. *In utero* diethylstilbestrol exposure
   5. Previous pelvic inflammatory disease (PID) or ruptured appendicitis
   6. Infertility
   7. Increasing number of lifetime sexual partners
   8. Cigarette smoking

III. DIAGNOSIS OF TUBAL ECTOPIC PREGNANCY
A. The triad of a missed menstrual cycle, vaginal bleeding, and abdominal pain raises the suspicion for ectopic pregnancy.
B. The most common symptom is abdominal pain (greater than 95% of patients).
C. Physical examination may reveal abdominal tenderness or an adnexal mass. Rebound tenderness or guarding may be present.
D. Screen by using a urine pregnancy test.
E. When ectopic pregnancy is suspected, the patient should have a pelvic ultrasound by a sonographer experienced in gynecologic ultrasound.
F. The absence of an intrauterine gestational sac on transvaginal ultrasound with a corresponding serum hCG of greater than 1,500 mIU/mL should raise the suspicion for ectopic pregnancy.
G. An adnexal mass may be visualized by ultrasound with ectopic pregnancy. An adnexal gestational sac, yolk sac, and embryo may be visualized. There may be evidence of free fluid (blood) in the abdomen with ectopic pregnancy. The classic description of a tubal ectopic pregnancy on ultrasound includes a hyperechoic ring with surrounding vascular flow on Doppler, the so-called "ring of fire."

H. If there is no extrauterine or intrauterine pregnancy visualized, order a serum quantitative hCG; if that serum hCG is less than 1,500 mIU/mL, repeat in 48 hours in the otherwise stable patient.

I. In a normal pregnancy, the serum quantitative hCG should approximately double every 48 hours. In rare circumstances, the 48 hour increase in serum hCG may be as low as 35%.

J. If the serum quantitative hCG is rising abnormally but it is unclear by ultrasound whether the pregnancy is extra- or intrauterine, a diagnostic dilation and curettage may be performed to assess for the presence of villi. The absence of villi and intermediate trophoblast cells on pathologic examination suggests the presence of an ectopic pregnancy. Additionally, following dilation and curettage the hCG should decline substantially within 24 hours with an intrauterine pregnancy, but will not decline significantly in the setting of an extrauterine pregnancy.

IV. MANAGEMENT OF TUBAL ECTOPIC PREGNANCY

A. Expectant management
1. Reserved only for highly specialized circumstances.
2. Patients should be highly compliant with a documented falling quantitative serum hCG that is less than 1,000 mIU/mL.

B. Medical management
1. Also reserved for specialized circumstances in the compliant patient.
2. Absolute contraindications to medical management include:
   a. Poor compliance
   b. Hemodynamic instability
   c. Medical contraindications to methotrexate therapy
3. Relative contraindications to medical management include:
   a. Adnexal mass greater than 3.5 cm
   b. Presence of embryonic cardiac activity
   c. High quantitative hCG level. Success of single-dose therapy is lower in tubal ectopic pregnancies with a quantitative hCG level greater than 5,000 mIU/mL.
4. Therapy consists of the administration of methotrexate delivered as a single dose of 50 mg/m^2.
5. The serum hCG is assessed on days 4 and 7 after administration.
6. If the serum hCG has not fallen by at least 15% between days 4 and 7, the patient may be given a second dose of methotrexate or offered surgical management after reassessment.
7. If the serum hCG decreases by 15% between days 4 and 7, the serum quantitative hCG should be assessed at weekly intervals until it is less than 20 mIU/mL.
8. Multi-dose treatment protocols for methotrexate are available for select patient with risk factors for failure of the single-dose regimen.

C. Surgical management
1. This remains the traditional management of ectopic pregnancy.
2. Laparoscopic approach is favored in most cases except in the setting of hemodynamic instability.
3. Options for surgical management include salpingostomy (the tubal pregnancy is removed through an incision in the fallopian tube) and salpingectomy (complete removal of the fallopian tube).
4. Patients undergoing salpingostomy must have serial assessment of the quantitative hCG post-operatively to ensure complete resolution of the pregnancy.
5. The relative benefits of salpingostomy as compared to salpingectomy with regard to future fertility are unclear.

MISCARRIAGE

I. INTRODUCTION. Spontaneous abortion is defined as loss of the pregnancy prior to 20 weeks of gestation. When women experience bleeding during pregnancy, they often present to the emergency department for initial care. The term *threatened abortion* is used when there is vaginal bleeding in the first half of pregnancy and the cervical os is closed. A *missed abortion* is a pregnancy in which there is embryonic demise or lack of progression of the pregnancy in the setting of a closed cervical os. *Inevitable abortion* is used to describe pregnancies in the first 20 weeks in which the cervix has begun to dilate or there is gross rupture of fetal membranes, but the pregnancy has not yet been expelled. *Incomplete abortion* refers to pregnancies in which the cervix has dilated and delivery of the fetus or placenta has begun, but products of conception remain in the uterus. This may be accompanied by heavy bleeding. *Complete abortion* refers to the passage of all products of conception and subsequent closure of the cervix.

II. EPIDEMIOLOGY AND PATHOPHYSIOLOGY
   A. Fifteen percent of pregnancies end in spontaneous abortion.
   B. Risk factors include advanced maternal age, previous miscarriage, and assisted reproductive technology.
   C. Sixty percent of spontaneous abortions in the first trimester are the result of chromosomal anomalies.

III. DIAGNOSIS
   A. Patients may present with vaginal bleeding or cramping.
   B. Physical examination may reveal blood in the vaginal vault. The cervix may appear dilated and the uterus is usually enlarged.
   C. Gestational age by ultrasound may be inconsistent with the last menstrual period. Also, ultrasound may show an empty gestational sac or an embryo without a cardiac activity. On transvaginal ultrasound, cardiac activity should be noted in the embryo when the crown rump length is 5 mm, or by 5 to 6 weeks' gestation.
   D. A failed first trimester pregnancy is also likely when on transvaginal ultrasound, the mean gestational sac diameter exceeds 8 mm without visible yolk sac or when the mean gestational sac diameter exceeds 16 mm and without visible embryo.
   E. Always assess for concomitant ectopic pregnancy with ultrasound.

IV. MANAGEMENT
   A. No therapy is effective in the prevention of miscarriage during threatened abortion. Pelvic rest and limitation of activity does not decrease the chance of spontaneous abortion.
   B. Patients who are not bleeding heavily, are hemodynamically stable, and not in excessive pain can be managed expectantly.
   C. Medical management with drugs such as misoprostol and mifepristone can aid resolution of early pregnancy failure.
   D. Dilation and curettage is the treatment for patients who are bleeding heavily, are hemodynamically unstable, or unwilling to undergo expectant or medical management.
   E. All patients who have bleeding during pregnancy should have a blood type and antibody screen. In patients who are Rh negative and bleeding during the first trimester, administer anti-D immune globulin.

THIRD TRIMESTER BLEEDING

   I. INTRODUCTION. During the third trimester, uterine blood flow has increased to over 500 cc/min. As such, a variety of pathologic states involving the placenta and uterus can result in massive blood loss in a short period of time. Prompt recognition and appropriate resuscitation are critical in prevention of serious morbidity and mortality from obstetric hemorrhage in the third trimester.

II. PLACENTAL ABRUPTION
   A. Refers to the state in which all (complete abruption) or part (partial abruption) of the placenta separates from the uterus after 20 weeks' gestation but prior to delivery.
   B. Incidence is 0.4% to 1% of pregnancies, with 80% occurring prior to the onset of labor.

C. Fetal and neonatal morbidity and mortality associated with placental abruption are linked with preterm birth, low birth weight, and fetal distress

D. Risk factors include trauma, hypertension, cocaine use, thrombophilias, preterm premature rupture of membranes, rapid decompression of amniotic fluid, and cigarette smoking.

E. Results from disruption of maternal vessels in the decidua basalis where they interface with the villi of the placental cytotrophoblast. May result from trauma or a chronic pathologic vascular process.

F. Most common presentation is vaginal bleeding, although 20% of patients will not exhibit bleeding. Half of patients will present with abdominal pain and uterine contractions.

G. Physical examination may reveal a rigid, firm uterine fundus.

H. The fetal heart tracing may have signs of fetal distress.

I. Ultrasound may show a retroplacental hematoma, but the sensitivity of ultrasound in detection of placental abruption is poor.

J. If massive bleeding is present, clinical and laboratory evidence of disseminated intravascular coagulation may be associated.

III. PLACENTA PREVIA

A. *Placenta previa* refers to the implantation of the placenta over the cervical os. This may be complete (entirely covering the cervical os), partial (only a portion of the placental covers the cervical os), or marginal (the placenta approaches but does not cover the cervical os).

B. Placenta previa complicates 1 in 200 pregnancies.

C. Risk factors include placenta previa in a prior pregnancy, previous cesarean delivery or other uterine incision, and advanced maternal age. Previous cesarean section remains the most important risk factor for development of placenta previa, with the risk increasing with the number of previous cesarean sections.

D. The classic presentation of placenta previa is painless vaginal bleeding. All patients presenting with vaginal bleeding in pregnancy should have ultrasound imaging to determine the location of the placenta.

E. **DO NOT** perform digital examination of the cervix in patients with placenta previa—this could precipitate hemorrhage.

IV. MANAGEMENT OF THIRD TRIMESTER BLEEDING

A. Third trimester bleeding is an obstetric emergency. Maternal hemodynamic status should be monitored closely and fetal status should be assessed with continuous fetal heart rate monitoring.

B. Two large-bore intravenous lines should be placed to allow rapid replacement of any lost intravascular volume.

C. If blood loss is large, ongoing, or associated with hypotension, transfuse early with packed red blood cells.

D. In addition to measurement of hemoglobin, platelet count and blood type assess coagulation status with measurements of the prothrombin time, activated partial thromboplastin time, and fibrinogen. Coagulopathy should be corrected with fresh frozen plasma or cryoprecipitate as necessary.

E. When maternal hypovolemia, coagulopathy, or nonreassuring fetal heart rate status exist, expedite delivery to prevent maternal and fetal morbidity. Delivery is always by cesarean section for placenta previa and abruption.

LABOR AND DELIVERY

I. INTRODUCTION. Not infrequently, women present in the advanced stages of labor, and movement to the labor and delivery suite for delivery may not be possible. Basic aspects of labor and delivery are reviewed in the following.

II. NORMAL LABOR

A. Normal labor is divided into three stages:

1. The first stage of labor starts with the onset of contractions until the cervix is completely dilated. The first stage of labor is further divided into the:
   a. Latent phase—The period from a closed cervix to 4 cm of dilation.
   b. Active phase—The period from 4 cm of dilation to complete cervical dilation. The active phase progresses at a minimum of 1.2 cm/h in primigravida women, but is usually faster in multiparous patients.
2. The second stage of labor is time from complete cervical dilation until delivery of the fetus.
3. The third stage of labor is the time from delivery of the fetus until delivery of the placenta. This should last less than 30 minutes.

B. Labor progresses in an orderly fashion
1. The head becomes engaged in the maternal pelvis.
2. The head of the fetus flexes, minimizing the diameter passing through the pelvic inlet.
3. The head descends through the pelvis.
4. The fetal head rotates internally.
5. The fetal head extends and passes through the budging introitus.
6. The fetal head rotates externally.
7. The shoulders pass below the pubic symphysis and the remainder of the fetus is delivered.

C. The role of the delivering clinician is as follows:
1. As the fetal head extends and delivers through the introitus, the delivering clinician should place his or her hands on the fetal head and support the perineum to ensure that the head delivers in a controlled fashion. Rapid extension and delivery can result in increased perineal trauma and greater damage to the anal sphincter.
2. After delivery of the head, a bulb suction device is used to clear amniotic fluid and blood from the mouth and nares of the infant.
3. The finger should be swept over the neck to assess for the presence of a nuchal umbilical cord. The cord usually sweeps easily over the fetal head. If the cord is too tight to move over the fetal head easily, it may be doubly clamped and ligated to facilitate delivery.
4. After delivery of the head and restitution (external rotation), the fetal shoulders should be gently guided below the pubic symphysis. It is important to avoid excessive traction at this point as doing so may result in brachial plexus injury. The posterior shoulder is then delivered.
5. Perineal lacerations are common following delivery. Consultation with an obstetrician should be made in the emergency department setting for repair of perineal lacerations.

D. *Shoulder dystocia* refers to a delay in delivery of the fetal shoulder after delivery of the fetal head. It is an obstetric emergency; do the following:
1. Call for assistance and immediate backup by an obstetrician.
2. Hyperflex the maternal legs toward the maternal abdomen, thus widening the pelvic outlet (McRobert's maneuver).
3. Apply suprapubic pressure to attempt to displace the fetal shoulder below the pubic symphysis.
4. Try to deliver the posterior arm. Cutting an episiotomy may facilitate performance of this and other maneuvers.
5. If these maneuvers are not successful, two fingers are placed against the posterior shoulder and pressure is applied toward the fetal back. This should rotate the shoulders into the wider diameter of the pelvis (Wood's Screw Maneuver).
6. The posterior arm is delivered.
7. With failure of these maneuvers, deliberate fracture of the fetal clavicle may facilitate delivery.

ACUTE PELVIC INFLAMMATORY DISEASE

I. INTRODUCTION. PID is an inflammatory condition of the upper genital tract caused by upward ascension of microorganisms from the lower genital tract. This disease may include any combination of infection of the endometrium (endometritis), fallopian tubes (salpingitis), or peritoneal cavity. The disease may also include the development of tubo-ovarian abscess. Prompt diagnosis and treatment of PID is important to prevent both short- and long-term morbidities in women with the diagnosis. The consequences of PID include infertility, increased risk of ectopic pregnancy, and chronic pelvic pain.

II. EPIDEMIOLOGY AND PATHOPHYSIOLOGY

  A. The Center for Disease Control (CDC) estimates approximately 780,000 new cases of PID diagnosed annually in the United States.
  B. Many cases of PID go unrecognized and undiagnosed (silent PID).
  C. Risk factors for development of PID include:
   1. Young age
   2. Multiple sex partners
   3. Young age of sexual debut
   4. Lack of use of barrier contraception
  D. Occurs as a result of the ascension of microorganisms from the vagina and endocervix into the endometrium, fallopian tubes, and pelvic peritoneum.
  E. Most cases are caused by *Neisseria gonorrhea* (43%), 10% caused by *Chlamydia trachomatis* alone, and 12% caused by coinfection with both organisms.
  F. The remaining cases of PID is caused by infection with anaerobic bacteria, *Mycoplasma*, and *Ureaplasma*.

III. DIAGNOSIS

  A. Bedside clinical diagnosis is challenging and often inaccurate secondary to wide variation in severity of symptoms.
  B. Gold standard for diagnosis is laparoscopy with directed biopsy and culture, although this is not practical or necessary for most patients.
  C. Treatment for PID should be initiated in women with abdominal or pelvic pain (assuming no other identifiable cause) if one or more of the following is noted:
   1. Cervical motion tenderness
   2. Uterine tenderness
   3. Adnexal tenderness
  D. Each of the following further supports the diagnosis:
   1. Temperature greater than 101°F
   2. Mucopurulent cervical discharge
   3. White blood cells on wet mount
   4. Elevated sedimentation rate
   5. Elevated C-reactive protein
   6. Positive testing for *N. gonorrhea* or *C. trachomatis*.

IV. MANAGEMENT

  A. The goal of management is to treat the immediate symptoms of pain and to prevent later consequences including infertility, ectopic pregnancy, and chronic pelvic pain.
  B. Tables 57-1 to 57-3 show the CDC criteria for hospitalization and antibiotic treatment of patients with PID.

TABLE 57-1	Criteria for Hospitalization of Patients with Acute PID

Surgical emergencies such as appendicitis cannot be excluded
The patient is pregnant
The patient does not respond clinically to oral antibiotic therapy
The patient is unable to tolerate or follow an outpatient treatment regimen
The patient has severe illness with nausea, vomiting, or high fever
The patient has a tubo-ovarian abscess
Immunodeficiency

TABLE 57-2   **CDC Recommended Treatment Schedules for Parenteral Treatment of Acute PID**

Regimen A
  Cefotetan 2 g IV every 12 h
  Or
  Cefoxitin 2 g IV every 6 h
  Plus
  Doxycycline 100 mg PO or IV every 12 h
The regimen is given for at least 24 h after patient clinically improves. After discharge from the
  hospital, continue doxycycline 100 mg PO bid to complete a 14-d course
Regimen B
  Clindamycin 900 mg IV every 8 h
  Plus
  Gentamicin loading dose IV or IM (2 mg/kg) followed by a maintenance dose (1.5 mg/kg) every
    8 h. Single daily dosing (3–5 mg/kg) can be substituted
The regimen is given for at least 24 h after patient clinically improves. After discharge from the
  hospital, continue doxycycline 100 mg PO bid or clindamycin 450 mg PO qid to complete 14 d
  of therapy.

V. TUBO-OVARIAN ABSCESS

  A. This is a common complication of PID (up to one-third of hospitalized patients).
  B. Suspected when abdominal pain is lateralized. On physical examination there is
     usually a tender palpable adnexal mass. Ultrasound confirms the diagnosis.
  C. Patients with tubo-ovarian abscess should initially have a trial of medical therapy
     with a CDC recommended treatment regimen. All patients should be admitted.
  D. If patients do not have a clinical response in 2 to 4 days or if the abscess is large,
     the abscess should be surgically managed. One option is ultrasound guided drainage,
     although recurrences are common.

ABNORMAL UTERINE BLEEDING

  I. INTRODUCTION. Abnormal uterine bleeding can be caused by anatomic abnormalities
  or abnormalities of the menstrual cycle. The term "dysfunctional uterine bleeding"
  describes bleeding that is unrelated to anatomic abnormalities. *Menorrhagia* refers to

TABLE 57-3   **CDC Treatment Schedule for Oral Treatment of Acute PID**

Ceftriaxone 250 mg IM in a single dose
Plus
Doxycycline 100 mg PO every 12 h for 14 d with or without metronidazole 500 mg PO every 12 h
  for 14 d
Or
Cefoxitin 2 g IM in a single dose and Probenecid 1 g orally administered concurrently in a single
  dose
Plus
Doxycycline 100 mg PO every 12 h for 14 d with or without 500 mg PO every 12 h for 14 d
Or
Other parenteral third-generation cephalosporin
Plus
Doxycycline 100 mg PO every 12 h for 14 d with or without Metronidazole 500 mg PO every 12 h
  for 14 d

heavy uterine bleeding at the expected time of menses. The normal menses usually results in the approximately 80 mL of blood loss and lasts for less than 7 days. Bleeding in excess of this amount or lasting longer than 7 days constitutes menorrhagia. As a practical matter, it is difficult to quantify the volume of blood loss with each menses. The number of pads or tampons used during menses serves as a surrogate measure of blood loss, although even pad counts may not accurately estimate blood loss. *Metrorrhagia* is the term used to describe bleeding that occurs between menses. *Menometrorrhagia* refers to heavy menses in addition to bleeding between menses.

II. PATHOPHYSIOLOGY

    A. Anatomic causes of abnormal uterine bleeding include:
        1. Leiomyomas (fibroids) are a common cause
        2. Endometrial polyps
        3. Endometritis
        4. Endometrial hyperplasia
        5. Endometrial cancer
    B. The most common cause of dysfunctional uterine bleeding is anovulation. Risk factors for dysfunctional uterine bleeding include obesity, thyroid dysfunction, endometrial atrophy, and bleeding dyscrasias.

III. EVALUATION

    A. The initial approach is based on a directed history and physical examination, including vital signs and including orthostatic testing plus a pelvic examination including a speculum examination. Look for lower genital tract causes of vaginal bleeding. In addition, assess the size, texture, and mobility of the uterus.
    B. Order a urine hCG to assess for potential pregnancy. Also, a complete blood count can be obtained to assess for anemia and to assess red blood cell indices. In select cases of heavy, recurrent or bleeding in more than one site, assess coagulation with a prothrombin time, activated partial thromboplastin time, and fibrinogen level.
    C. Pelvic imaging with ultrasound is sometimes helpful, although the history and above examination alone is usually sufficient for the initial evaluation.

IV. MANAGEMENT

    A. Patients presenting with profuse vaginal hemorrhage should receive the same care as any patient presenting with life-threatening bleeding. Intravenous volume replacement is initiated with crystalloids, adding packed red blood cells if necessary. Consult a gynecologist while resuscitating the patient, since the quickest and most effective way to relieve profuse hemorrhage often is dilation and curettage.
    B. Medical therapy for heavy bleeding in the absence of life-threatening hemorrhage includes:
        1. Intravenous estrogen administered as conjugated equine estrogens, 25 mg every 6 hours.
        2. Oral estrogen administered as conjugated equine estrogens, 2.5 mg every 6 hours.
        3. Oral contraceptives.
        4. Medroxyprogesterone acetate.
        5. If anemic, give iron supplementation.
        6. Arrange follow-up with a women's health provider as endometrial biopsy may be necessary in patients at risk of endometrial hyperplasia or malignancy.

V. GYNECOLOGIC CAUSES OF ABDOMINAL PAIN

    A. Ovarian cysts
        1. Commonly cause pelvic pain and are classified as either functional (arise as a result of the normal menstrual cycle) or neoplastic (a true cyst that arises from the epithelium).
        2. Rupture, hemorrhage, or torsion may cause pain.
        3. Diagnosis is made by history and physical examination. Pelvic ultrasound will confirm the diagnosis and define the type of cyst.

4. Management is supportive, including appropriate pain therapy. Non-steroidal agents are first line choices, with opioids for more severe discomfort (this much pain should prompt a search for ovarian torsion).
5. Hemorrhagic cysts may require surgical management if severe or evolving anemia. Oral contraceptives do not cause regression of existing ovarian cysts but may prevent formation of new functional cysts.

B. Ovarian torsion

1. Ovarian torsion occurs when the ovary (and most often the fallopian tube) twists on its ligamentous support, compromising blood flow to the adnexa. As the ovarian veins and lymphatic system are obstructed, the adnexa become increasingly edematous.
2. Patients often present with unilateral exquisite abdominal pain that is sudden and severe, but pain is occasionally just moderate or intermittent.
3. Pain may be accompanied by nausea and vomiting, mimicking appendicitis.
4. An adnexal mass is sometimes palpable and examination may reveal lateralized severe lower abdominal tenderness.
5. Pelvic ultrasound may aid in diagnosis by demonstrating an adnexal mass. Color Doppler to detect obstructed flow may aid in the diagnosis of ovarian torsion but should not be relied upon to exclude the diagnosis.
6. Gynecologic consultation is necessary to provide relief of pain and possible preservation of ovarian function using surgical intervention. The adnexa may be "untwisted" with removal of the causative mass. If there is evidence of tissue necrosis (failure of return of pink color 30 minutes after untwisting) the adnexa should be removed.

C. Endometritis

1. Defined as infection of the endometrium. Infection may also extend to the myometrium (endomyometritis).
2. Endometritis may be diagnosed following vaginal or cesarean delivery. Additionally, endometritis may occur following therapeutic or spontaneous abortion. Endometritis can also occur in the non-pregnant patient.
3. Pathophysiology and management depends on whether the endometritis is related to pregnancy and whether this pregnancy ended in abortion or delivery.
4. Infections are often polymicrobial and may involve aerobic and anaerobic species. Other pathogens include group B beta streptococcus, *Staphylococcus aureus*, *Bacteroides* species, *N. gonorrhea*, and *C. trachomatis*. *Clostridium sordellii* is an uncommon but lethal (toxic shock producing trigger) pathogen.
5. Commonly presents within 5 days after procedure or delivery.
6. Symptoms include abdominopelvic pain, fever, and a foul smelling discharge.
7. Physical examination reveals uterine tenderness.
8. In most cases, treatment requires admission to the hospital and broad spectrum parenteral antibiotics, although select patients may be suitable for outpatient management.
9. Ultrasound to search for retained products of conception is helpful in patients not responding to antibiotic therapy. Dilation and curettage is necessary in patients with endometritis and retained products of conception.

D. Endometriosis

1. Condition in which hormonally responsive implants of endometrial tissue are present in the abdominopelvic cavity on areas such as the peritoneum, bladder, and bowel.
2. Present in up to 15% of premenopausal women.
3. The etiology of endometriosis is uncertain but may be related to retrograde menstruation through the fallopian tube.
4. The most common complaint is cyclic abdominal pain and painful menses (dysmenorrhea).
5. Physical examination reveals abdominal and pelvic tenderness. An ovarian mass may be palpated and may represent an endometrioma, or the so-called "chocolate cyst." Recto-vaginal examination may reveal nodularity in the recto-vaginal septum or utero-sacral ligaments.

6. Similar to simple ovarian cysts, acute management centers on pain control. Patients with endometriosis will need outpatient gynecologic management to determine what medical or surgical treatment plan is most appropriate.

E. Adenomyosis

1. Adenomyosis is the proliferation of endometrial glands within the myometrial walls.
2. Patients present with abnormal uterine bleeding and dysmenorrhea.
3. Physical examination reveals an enlarged, globular, tender uterus.
4. The diagnosis of adenomyosis is clinical, with pelvic ultrasound most often being of limited value. MRI may confirm the diagnosis.
5. Acute management of adenomyosis includes pain control. Patients with adenomyosis will need outpatient gynecologic management to determine what medical or surgical treatment plan is most appropriate.

F. Intra-abdominal adhesions

1. May be a cause of abdominal pain and may be associated with bowel obstruction.
2. Risk factors include prior pelvic surgery, endometriosis, a history of PID, and radiation therapy.
3. Initial management of patients suspected of having pain secondary to adhesions is with supportive analgesia. Surgical lysis is reserved for refractory cases or cases of suspected bowel obstruction.

BARTHOLIN'S ABSCESS

I. INTRODUCTION. Bartholin's glands are mucous secreting structures located at 4 and 8 o'clock in the posterior introitus. These normally small glands drain through duct openings in the vulvar vestibule. Bartholin's glands can become obstructed resulting in a cyst formation or, if infected, an abscess.

II. EPIDEMIOLOGY AND PATHOPHYSIOLOGY

A. Most commonly affects women in the third decade of life, and 2% of women develop a Bartholin's cyst or abscess during their lifetime.
B. Infections are generally polymicrobial and caused by a wide variety of organisms. Anaerobes are the most commonly isolates, and *E.coli* is the most common aerobic species isolated. *N. gonorrhea and C. trachomatis* are uncommonly isolated.

III. DIAGNOSIS

A. Patients with Bartholin's gland abscess usually present with the complaint of a painful mass in the posterior vulva.
B. Physical examination reveals a tender, indurated, erythematous mass at the posterior vulvar vestibule. Occasionally, spontaneous drainage of purulent material occurs.
C. Induration and swelling that is more anterior is likely not a Bartholin's abscess but rather a labial abscess.

IV. MANAGEMENT

A. Simple incision and drainage of Bartholin's abscesses **should not** be performed as the recurrence rate is unacceptably high.
B. A preferred option is use of a Word catheter
    1. The vulva is prepared with betadine and anesthetized with 1% lidocaine.
    2. A 5 mm incision is made distal to the hymeneal ring, but proximal to the labia minora in the vulvar vestibule at the location of the abscess.
    3. The abscess is drained completely and an instrument is used to break up loculations. Cultures can be sent at this time. The abscess is then irrigated copiously.
    4. The Word catheter is placed and filled with 3 cc of saline. The end of the catheter should be tucked into the vagina.
    5. The catheter should be left in place for at least 4 weeks to allow epithelialization.
    6. Unless there is surrounding cellulitis or the patient is diabetic, antibiotics are not necessary.
C. Another option is marsupialization of a Bartholin's cyst.

1. The vulva is prepared with betadine and anesthetized with 1% lidocaine.
2. A 3 cm incision is made distal to the hymeneal ring, but proximal to the labia minora in the vulvar vestibule. The incision is carried through to the underlying cyst or abscess wall.
3. The abscess is drained completely and an instrument is used to break up loculations. Cultures can be sent at this time. The abscess is then irrigated copiously.
4. The cyst wall is then everted and sutured with absorbable suture to the skin of the introitus laterally and the vaginal mucosa medially.

D. Excision of Bartholin's gland is performed for recurrent abscesses. This procedure should only be performed in the operating room setting by an experienced gynecologist.

MASTITIS

I. INTRODUCTION. Mastitis is infection of the breast tissue.

II. EPIDEMIOLOGY AND PATHOPHYSIOLOGY
A. Occurs in 1.4% to 8.9% of lactating women.
B. Most common during the first 3 weeks after delivery.
C. Cracks in the skin of the nipple or breast allow the entry of bacteria. The most common pathogens are *Staphylococcus* species, *E. coli*, and *Streptococcus*.

III. DIAGNOSIS
A. Patients present with the complaint of breast pain (usually unilateral). In addition, they may complain of fever, chills, malaise, and body aches
B. Physical examination reveals erythema, tenderness, induration, and warmth to the touch. Careful palpation should be performed to exclude the presence of a breast abscess.

IV. MANAGEMENT
A. Treatment consists of antibiotic therapy, usually with an extended penicillin (such as dicloxacillin or nafcillin) or a first generation cephalosporin (cephalexin) for 10 to 14 days.
B. Lactating mothers should continue to breast feed or pump on the affected breast, although this may be painful.
C. Warm compresses should be encouraged.
D. Patients should wear a supporting bra even while sleeping.
E. Follow-up should be arranged within several days to ensure that the mastitis is resolving.
F. Breast abscess develops in 10% of women with mastitis. Findings include a tender, fluctuant mass in the breast and can be confirmed by ultrasound. The breast abscess should be incised and drained. Obtain cultures and antibiotic sensitivities from the abscess material.

SEXUAL ASSAULT

I. INTRODUCTION. Sexual assault is a common and increasingly prevalent problem in the United States. Although many sexual assaults are never reported, providers must be prepared to care for victims of sexual assault.

II. INCIDENCE AND EPIDEMIOLOGY
A. The true population incidence is unknown.
B. Women between the ages of 17 and 25 are the most common victims of rape, and nearly three quarters of these women know the assailant.
C. One-third of rapes involve oral or anal penetration.

III. MANAGEMENT
A. The victim should be immediately taken to a private room in the emergency department or care site. With the permission of the victim, and not to impede evaluation

and treatment of medical/traumatic needs, law enforcement personnel should be contacted early to aid with the combined medical–legal needs. Also, a sexual assault team or an experienced clinician is preferred to provide the best possible evaluation and care.

B. Try to detail all of the specifics of the assault that the patient can remember.

C. Gather all clothes and label with the patient's name, date, and time of collection. Evidence should never be left unattended and should be stored in designated collection bags to maintain the chain of evidence for law enforcement.

D. After an appropriate general examination, search for any moist or dried secretions, stains, hair, or foreign material and collect these. A Wood's lamp may make collection easier. Perform a complete pelvic examination, again with attention to the presence of any secretions, stains, hair, or foreign material. Comb the pubic hair and send the material with the comb to the laboratory. With the speculum examination, look carefully to find any trauma to the vaginal walls. Also, collect vaginal fluid to be examined for the presence of sperm. If intercourse was greater than 72 hours prior to presentation, swabs of the cervix may yield sperm. Obtain swabs to examine for gonorrhea, chlamydia, and trichomonas. Perform a bimanual examination to assess for pelvic trauma. Include a rectal examination as necessary with the collection of appropriate specimens. Finally, obtain blood to test for HIV, hepatitis B, and syphilis. In select cases, directed toxicology screening may be needed.

E. Emergency contraception should be offered to all victims of sexual assault as indicated. Immediate counseling should be available, along with structured follow-up for medical and psychological assessment after the initial evaluation.

F. Depending on state and local regulations, other specimens may be collected such as blood, saliva, and fingernail debris. It is important to be familiar with local regulations and hospital policy when gathering evidence and caring for the victim of sexual assault—this is another reason for creating trained sexual assault teams or clinicians.

LOWER GENITAL TRACT TRAUMA

I. INTRODUCTION. Vulvar and vaginal trauma may occur in both the obstetric and non-obstetric setting, and may be penetrating or non-penetrating.

II. VULVAR AND VAGINAL HEMATOMA

A. Most commonly encountered trauma in the vulva is the straddle injury.

B. Because of the dense vascularity of the vulva and vagina, bleeding is often profuse. Contained bleeding may result in a vulvar or vaginal hematoma.

C. Nonexpanding hematomas should be observed. The pressure of the hematoma may be sufficient to tamponade bleeding. Insert a urinary catheter if outflow is obstructed.

D. If the hematoma is expanding or hemodynamic compensation is lost, the hematoma should be opened and explored in the operating room to identify and stop the bleeding site.

III. VULVAR AND VAGINAL LACERATIONS

A. If the laceration is superficial and hemostatic, it is not necessary to suture the injury. If bleeding is light, use a hemostatic agent (such as silver nitrate or Monsel's solution).

B. Deep lacerations are best repaired in the operating room.

C. Deep lacerations should be repaired in layers with absorbable suture after copious irrigation. Avoid placement of sutures in the bladder anteriorly and the rectum posteriorly.

D. If there is evidence of infection, leave the wound open for later repair or allow healing by secondary intention.

AXIOMS

- Ectopic pregnancy can result in maternal death; prompt diagnosis and treatment is critical.
- Third trimester bleeding is an obstetric emergency.
- Prompt diagnosis and treatment of PID is important to prevent both short- and long-term morbidity.

■ Simple incision and drainage of Bartholin's abscesses **should not** be performed; recurrence rate is unacceptably high.

Suggested Readings

Bangsgaard N, Lund CO, Ottesen B, et al. Improved fertility following conservative surgical treatment of ectopic pregnancy. *BJOG* 2003;110(8):765–770.

Barnhart KT, Sammel MD, Rinaudo PF, et al. Symptomatic patients with an early viable intrauterine pregnancy: HCG curves redefined. *Obstet Gynecol* 2004;105(1):50–55.

Center for Disease Control and Prevention. Sexually transmitted disease treatment guidelines 2010. *MMWR Recomm Rep* 2010;59(RR-12):1–110.

Nelson AL, Sinow RM, Renslo R, et al. Endovaginal ultrasonographically guided transvaginal drainage for treatment of pelvic abscesses. *Am J Obstet Gynecol* 1995;172(6):1926–1932; discussion 1932–1935.

Zweizig S, Perron J, Grubb F, et al. Conservative management of adnexal torsion. *Am J Obstet Gynecol* 1993;168(6 Pt 1):1791–1795.

58 Laparoscopic Treatment of the Acute Abdomen

Abe Fingerhut and Mousa Khoursheed

I. INTRODUCTION. Minimal access techniques (including percutaneous, interventional radiology techniques) are used often in the emergency situation. Employed for emergency diagnostic and therapeutic procedures as early as 1991, laparoscopy now has gained a well-defined and often validated position in the armamentarium of management of acute abdominal diseases.

As the accuracy of imaging techniques has improved over the last few years, the need for laparoscopy as an isolated diagnostic tool without any indication for laparoscopic therapy has diminished. A wide array of laparoscopic therapeutic options is available; many well adapted to emergency surgery.

II. DEFINITIONS. Definitions vary for "acute abdomen," "acute abdominal pain," "acute care surgery," "emergency," or "urgent surgery."

- **A.** The *acute abdomen* is defined as any acute intra-abdominal condition of abrupt onset, usually associated with pain due to inflammation, perforation, obstruction, infarction, or rupture of abdominal organs, and usually requiring emergency surgical intervention.
- **B.** *Acute abdominal pain* is defined as any medium or severe abdominal pain of less than 7 days duration.
- **C.** *Acute care* can be defined as:
    - **1.** Medical treatment for individuals with short-term illnesses or health problems (National Caregivers Library)
    - **2.** Comprehensive patient management from emergency room arrival to hospital discharge and seamless 24/7 services
- **D.** The distinction between **emergency surgery** (immediate life-saving operation, usually within 1 hour, with simultaneous resuscitation) and **urgent surgery** (operation performed as soon as possible after resuscitation, usually within 24 hours) is semantic as best, as the two terms have been used interchangeably in the literature. Most of the literature speaks of emergency surgery as any operation taking place during the acute phase of disease; ideally, as quickly as possible after stabilization.
- **E.** *Emergency admission*, defined as an "unpredictable admission at short notice because of clinical need" by the NHS Data Model and Dictionary, accounts for 35% of total admissions on general surgical units; 9.7% of all emergency surgical admissions were for abdominal pain.

III. OPERATION ROOM AND ERGONOMIC CONSIDERATIONS

- **A.** As for any laparoscopic procedure, the ergonomic and technical aspects of minimal access surgery in emergency surgery are important issues and directly affect outcomes.
    - **1.** Patient
        - **a.** Positioned supine (dorsal decubitus) for most operations
            - **i.** One arm in abduction if need be for anesthesiology purposes
            - **ii.** If not, both arms tucked alongside patient
            - **iii.** Legs spread apart
        - **b.** Prepped and draped so that any unexpected findings or the need to convert to open surgery can be managed without delay
        - **c.** Insertion of a bladder catheter is a wise precaution

2. Surgeon position
   a. Stands between the legs ("French position")
   b. Or on the side opposite the target organ
   c. With possibility of moving around to gain access to all four quadrants of the abdomen as required
3. Operating room
   a. The surgeon, scrub, and circulating nurses share the responsibility of:
      i. Appropriate laparoscopic instruments and equipment setup, adapted to the envisioned procedure
      ii. Laparotomy instruments and equipment ready for use
      iii. Vascular surgery instruments and equipment within easy and rapid reach in case of bleeding
   b. Monitor and screen position
      i. Flat screen placed at 15 degrees below the eye level
      ii. Or at the gaze-down level (height at the level of the surgeon's elbows)
      iii. Monitors should be mobile and moved according to the site of the pathology to keep the alignment necessary for optimal ergonomic conditions
4. Trocar setup
   a. Should allow full and unrestricted exploration of the abdominal cavity, irrespective of the location of the underlying pathology
   b. Initial trocar layout depends on preoperative clinical findings and diagnostic probabilities:
      i. for acute abdominal pain predominating in the right lower quadrant, plan complete exploration of the pelvis and the genital organs as well as the appendix
      ii. In case of intestinal dilation (intestinal obstruction or ileus secondary to peritonitis or abscess), stay lateral to view the middle of the abdomen
      iii. Avoid previous scars (incisions or drainage sites)
      iv. Additional trocars can be added as needed
      v. Unless prior abdominal surgery suggests otherwise, the first trocar can be inserted near the umbilicus
      vi. At least one trocar is necessary to manipulate, palpate, or move viscera for exploration
5. Insertion
   a. We recommend the open approach for creation of pneumoperitoneum and insertion of the first trocar
   b. If incidental enterotomy occurs, repair immediately
6. Laparoscope
   a. The choice between the smaller 5 mm laparoscope should be weighed against the better lighting and view associated with the 10 mm scope
   b. Both a 0-degree and a 30-degree (or greater) scope should be available
7. Essential instrumentation
   a. Several 5, 10, and 12 mm ports
   b. Atraumatic grasping forceps and clamps
   c. Right-angle forceps
   d. Titanium and absorbable clips
   e. Two or more needle holders
   f. An energy-driven (ultrasonic or bipolar) coagulation device
   g. Traditional laparoscopic scissors
   h. Powerful suction–irrigation device
   i. Swabs
   j. Umbilical tapes, rubber drains, tourniquets
   k. Clamps and bulldog vascular clamps
   l. Plastic bags for specimen extraction
8. As appropriate, never hesitate to change the optical device and manipulation instruments from one port to another, or to insert another trocar, to be able to view the entire field and maintain optimal ergonomic conditions

B. The peritoneal cavity is entered and explored in its entirety.

    1. The cause of the acute abdomen is obvious (perforated appendix, ulcer, or sigmoid diverticulitis): Treat (see later, as appropriate).

    2. The cause is not obvious.

        a. Note the area of maximal inflammation, concentration of pus, or blood, as in the case of ruptured ectopic pregnancy.

        b. Routine, systematic, and complete exploration is mandatory (check list highly recommended)

IV. INDICATIONS ACCORDING TO DISEASE

A. Peritonitis

    1. Classical goals include source control, reduction of bacterial contamination, and prevention of persistent or recurrent infection

        a. Source control can be accomplished laparoscopically in most cases (closure, resection)

        b. Reduction of bacterial contamination

            i. Use high pressure irrigation and suction devices.

            ii. Although lavage with saline has never been formally demonstrated in patients receiving adequate, systemic antibacterial therapy, adequate peritoneal irrigation is probably more important than the method of closure.

            iii. All gross purulent exudates, fecal debris, food particles as well as intraperitoneal lavage must be aspirated.

            iv. Addition of:

                a) Antibiotics to the lavage solution of little benefit

                b) Antiseptics, same remark and may even be detrimental

            v. Ideal volume for lavage in peritonitis is not known:

                a) Between 4 and 30 L recommended in the literature

            vi. Abdominal drainage as needed

        c. Prevention of recurrence depends on the cause

            i. Does not always require a radical solution (e.g., perforated diverticular disease)

    2. The advantages of laparoscopic treatment of peritonitis, irrespective of the origin, include:

        a. The possibility of full exploration of the abdominal cavity with minimal parietal insult, avoiding long incisions which carry a high rate of surgical site postoperative infection and incisional hernia

        b. Most causes of peritonitis (perforated duodenal ulcer, perforated appendicitis, perforation in diverticular disease, postoperative leakage after index laparoscopic operations) can also be treated laparoscopically

        c. If needed, stoma formation may be accomplished laparoscopically

    3. Precaution: Maintain pneumoperitoneum pressures between 8 and 12 mm Hg, not higher

B. Acute appendicitis

    1. Still a topic of much debate

        a. Although readily feasible

        b. Routine laparoscopic appendectomy costs are disproportionate to advantages

    2. Main indication: Acute appendicitis (including perforated appendicitis, abscess, and peritonitis) that would normally require large incisions

    3. Prevention of residual post-laparoscopic appendectomy abscess, reported to be higher in the literature for laparoscopic appendectomy, must be avoided

        a. Complete abdominal exploration

        b. Adequate lavage

        c. Complete aspiration

        d. Drains generally not required

    4. Major advantages of the laparoscopic approach:

        a. In the overweight or obese patient

        b. In ectopic location of appendix

        c. In fertile female when all other diagnostic methods are inconclusive

5. Debate as to how to best close the appendicular stump during laparoscopic appendectomy
   a. Loop closure best
   b. Staples
      i. May reduce operative time and superficial wound (but not deep organ space surgical site) infections in difficult stump closure (when loop closure seems difficult or inappropriate [stump necrosis] or need for speed)
      ii. But should not be used routinely because of higher costs
6. Reversed conversion advocated by some (including this author):
   a. Start with 10 to 12 mm horizontal incision in right iliac fossa (to perform appendectomy with classical laparotomy instruments)
   b. Convert to laparoscopy through the 10 to 12 mm incision (called "reversed conversion") if difficulty arises (ectopic appendix or perforated appendicitis with localized or generalized peritonitis) rather than to extend the incision or revert to a midline incision

C. Acute pelvic problems in the female
1. Ectopic pregnancy
   a. Ideal setting for emergency laparoscopic surgery
   b. Possible in the hemodynamically stable patient
   c. Heparinized saline may be used in cases of large hematoma
   d. Requires clinical experience and skills (intracorporeal suturing and knotting techniques), as well as specific equipment (vacuum, special suction probe) if the tubes are to be spared
2. Adnexal torsion
   a. Readily treated laparoscopically

D. Perforated gastroduodenal ulcer
1. Particularly amenable to laparoscopic repair in the hemodynamically normal patient
   a. Especially in patients without Boey risk factors (see Chapter 51)
2. Main advantages
   a. Less postoperative pain
   b. Less surgical site morbidity (no need for long incisions, or to extend the initial incision)
3. Treatment of choice: Closure of the perforation (more extensive operations are uncommonly needed in the era of adequate and effective medical treatment of *Helicobacter pylori* infection)
   a. Definite need for adequate surgical skills and especially intracorporeal suturing techniques for closure, may be reinforced with fibrin glue, absorbable mesh, or omentoplasty
   b. Closure may be accomplished with fibrin glue, omentum alone
      i. A hybrid NOTES procedure consists of drawing the omentum through the perforation by means of an endoluminal endoscope
   c. Two possible exceptions to simple closure
      i. Those rare patients who are *H. pylori* negative
      ii. Or who cannot stop taking NSAID
   d. Particular attention should be paid to the quality of closure to keep the reoperation rate low (reported to be higher with laparoscopic closure than with open repair when results of the controlled trials comparing the two approaches were analyzed together)
   e. Laparoscopic treatment may be difficult/dangerous in patients:
      i. With Boey risk factors
      ii. Ulcer diameter greater than
         a) 10 mm (risk factor for conversion)
         b) Larger than 20 mm perforation (12% failure rate if simple suture techniques are employed)
4. The same therapeutic principles apply for gastric ulcer perforation: In this setting, however, a biopsy must be obtained to exclude carcinoma

E. Acute cholecystitis
   1. Operative treatment of acute cholecystitis is cholecystectomy
   2. However, cholecystectomy for acute cholecystitis can be challenging
       a. Inflamed, thickened but fragile gallbladder wall
       b. Adhesions of adjacent organs
       c. Distorted anatomy
           i. Main biliary ducts are at risk
               a) Risk of common bile duct injury increased two- to five-fold
           ii. Critical view of safety may be difficult
       d. Safety measures include:
           i. Stay anterior to Rouvières sulcus
           ii. Anterograde dissection of gallbladder
           iii. Intraoperative cholangiogram strongly indicated
               a) Goal of IOC
                   1) More importantly than to detect common bile duct stones
                   2) Above all, to delineate the biliary tree after dissection but before division of structures thought to belong to the biliary system
                   3) While not always capable of preventing bile duct injuries, reduces the overall rate of bile duct injury, allows the early detection and repair (well-recognized and all-important prognostic factor)
   3. Timing of operation
       a. Early cholecystectomy (within 48 hours from onset) is preferred
       b. If not, within the first week
       c. If not, only after 6 to 8 weeks
   4. Indications according to the Tokyo consensus (2007) classification of acute cholecystitis
       a. Grade I (mild acute cholecystitis), that is, acute cholecystitis with no organ dysfunction and disease limited to the gallbladder
           i. Ideal indication for laparoscopic cholecystectomy
           ii. Observation under medical treatment or transhepatic drainage (cholecystostomy) are other alternatives
       b. Grade II (moderate acute cholecystitis): Extensive disease in the gallbladder
           i. No organ dysfunction, but severe signs of infection (elevated white blood cell, palpable tender mass [gallbladder], symptoms persisting for more than 72 hours, significant inflammatory changes in the gallbladder seen on imaging studies)
           ii. Can also be treated with laparoscopic cholecystectomy although transhepatic drainage may be considered an acceptable indication
       c. Grade III (severe acute cholecystitis including gangrenous cholecystitis or empyema) corresponds to acute cholecystitis with organ dysfunction
           i. Laparoscopic cholecystectomy is possible after stabilization.
           ii. Conversion rate to open cholecystectomy is increased three-fold.
           iii. Overall postoperative complications occur more often.
           iv. Subtotal cholecystectomy has its proponents (but has not been proven to provide better outcomes than laparoscopic cholecystectomy, even in the elderly or the surgically unfit).
F. Complicated diverticular disease
   1. In Hinchey I and IIa stages, medical treatment, combined or without percutaneous drainage, is usually effective in controlling symptoms (see Chapter 52).
   2. However, in patients with persistent septic signs after drainage and in patients with Hinchey IIb and Hinchey III disease, surgical treatment is indicated (one register-based and two randomized controlled studies have shown that laparoscopic treatment is safe and as effective as open treatment).
   3. The general approach for decades has been Hartman Resection for perforated diverticulitis. Hartman Resection is still the safest approach for feculent peritonitis (Hinchey IV). A more recent approach (which needs further validation) for Hinchey IIb and III involves simple laparoscopic lavage, associated or not with

suture and/or drainage, with the aim of sparing the patient from both a major bowel resection and stoma creation. (Hartman resection is still recommended for the hemodynamically unstable patient or the immunosuppressed patient with Hinchey IIb or III disease.)

a. Laparoscopic lavage with 4 L of saline followed by drainage plus antibiotic therapy has been reported to be successful in more than 90% of cases and decreases mortality and morbidity (particularly surgical site complications such as dehiscence, wound infection, and incisional hernia and the need for a stoma).

b. If the perforation is found, a suture or fibrin glue closure can be attempted, eventually reinforced with an omental patch. However, do not persevere in finding the perforation at all costs.

c. Some authors propose elective colonic resection within 3 to 6 months, but others limit treatment to simple peritoneal lavage and do not propose any further treatment.

d. Conversion should be considered:
  i. When exploration of the abdomen is difficult because of adhesions, intestinal dilatation, or suspicion of other cause (e.g., malignant disease) of symptoms
  ii. When severe peritonitis with abundant false membranes is found and cannot be treated satisfactorily laparoscopically

e. Emergency colonic resection should be performed laparoscopically only if local expertise is available.

G. Intestinal obstruction

1. No longer considered a contraindication to laparoscopy

2. Excellent indication for laparoscopic exploration and treatment when the obstruction is caused by localized (e.g., post-appendectomy) adhesions or bands

3. Challenges
  a. Adhesions frequently prevent easy access to the peritoneal cavity
  b. Intestinal distension is:
    i. not only an obstacle to clear visibility, complete exploration
    ii. but also associated with specific intraoperative difficulties (fragile intestinal serosa), rendering grasping and retraction somewhat difficult and dangerous
  c. All possible precautions should be taken to stay away from abdominal scars for the creation of pneumoperitoneum or initial trocar insertion.
    i. Blind (closed) insertion of the Veress needle or first trocar (direct) is ill advised.
    ii. First trocar insertion should be performed "open," at a location at a distance from any scars, usually the left hypochondrium.
    iii. The sonographic visceral slide sign and the use of optical trocars may be particularly interesting options in this setting.
  d. Special instruments may be necessary including
    i. Dissectors (Maryland) and retractors
    ii. Angled scopes are ideal for viewing behind and lateral to adhesions, especially when it is difficult to mobilize the bowel
    iii. Specially designed decompression tubes
  e. In case of vascular compromise or necrotic bowel, intestinal handling may become the major issue, and it is preferable to convert to open laparotomy rather than to provoke a rupture with inundation of the peritoneal cavity with septic contents.
  f. Intestinal resection may be accomplished laparoscopically, but every precaution must be taken to avoid spillage of septic intestinal contents. Thus, open resection may be a safer option with high risk of spillage of intestinal contents.

H. Incarcerated/strangulated hernias

1. No studies are available comparing the laparoscopic to the open approach in emergency adult cases of incarcerated/strangulated inguinal or incisional hernia.

2. Either TEP or TAPP can be proposed to repair incarcerated inguinal hernia, to resect bowel, whenever needed, or to repair an occult contralateral hernia with overall rates of complications, recurrences, and hospital stay very similar to the rates documented in open repair for strangulated/incarcerated hernias.

3. "Hernioscopy," a mixed laparoscopic open technique for incarcerated hernias, has been found to be effective in one randomized controlled study.

4. Laparoscopy is feasible, if the expertise is available, to repair complicated and/or non-reducible retro-xiphoid or diaphragmatic hernias, para-esophageal hernias, rare abdominal wall acute hernias, such as supra-vesical and Spigelian, or obturator hernias, and internal hernias.

5. Aside from problems common to all obstruction (marked abdominal distention, distended bowel, difficulty in assessment of ischemia, need for bowel resection or need to handle a highly inflamed or fragile bowel segment), two aspects are specific to laparoscopic management of incarcerated hernia, irrespective of its type:

a. Obtain adequate overlap (5 cm recommended by most) of the mesh in major wall defects with loss of domain.

b. Use of mesh when either an inadvertent enterotomy occurs or when the bowel contents are ischemic/necrotic/perforated. In this setting most authors refrain from inserting a synthetic mesh, or prefer biologic meshes.

I. Mesenteric ischemia

1. Occurs most often in the elderly, frequently with comorbidity

2. As (especially unnecessary) laparotomy is poorly tolerated, laparoscopy in this setting may be performed at the bedside, if the patient cannot be transported to the operating suite

3. Of particular concern in this setting: Potential adverse effect of pneumoperitoneum on mesenteric blood flow

a. Recommendation: Work with low intra-abdominal pressure

b. In case of doubtful intestinal vitality: Use of intraoperative Doppler, fluorescein injection, or specific tissue oxygen saturation probes may help to determine small bowel viability

4. When a second-look procedure is indicated, some authors have recommended the following approach:

a. Leave trocars (used for the initial procedure) in place within the abdominal wall

b. Ensure access site sterility with occlusive dressings

c. Use same trocars for second look

J. Immediate laparoscopy for postoperative complications after initial laparotomy/laparoscopy/endoscopic procedures

1. Postoperative complications such as hemorrhage, intra-abdominal abscess, small bowel obstruction, bile leak, ischemic bowel disease, retrieval of retained foreign bodies, and anastomotic leakage may, at one time or another, warrant early postoperative re-exploration

2. Advantages of laparoscopy early in the postoperative period:

a. avoidance of risks of a negative laparotomy

b. decreased risk of surgical site complications

c. ensuring rapid diagnosis of intra-abdominal complications

d. thus decreasing the overall morbidity related to these complications

3. Second-look laparoscopy may be used in a variety of pathologies including mesenteric ischemia, abdominal trauma or in the postoperative patient, irrespective of the type (laparoscopy or laparotomy) of initial operation

a. Precautions:

i. Beware of early adhesions

ii. Caution if abdominal distension

iii. Check bowel vitality

b. Particularly interesting is early laparoscopic exploration for same-hospital stay postoperative obstruction in laparoscopic operations such as bariatric surgery

       i. Of importance, the surgeon must identify all limbs (best achieved by starting at the terminal ileum and working retrograde to the jejunojejunostomy and proximally to the Roux and biliopancreatic limbs)

       ii. Particular attention should be paid to mesenteric defects that should be closed with non-absorbable sutures

4. Iatrogenic perforations

   a. After colonoscopy (the most frequent)

       i. Early (<24 hours) laparoscopic management of colonoscopy perforation is safe.

          a) Reduced surgical and psychological stress for the patient because of its low morbidity and mortality

          b) Laparoscopic perforation suture, peritoneal lavage and drainage may be accomplished if performed within 24 hours of onset without the need for protective stoma

       ii. Conversion after a loyal attempt at laparoscopic repair is not a failure: Patient safety is the priority.

       iii. Endoscopic closure or clipping is possible by experienced gastroenterologists.

   b. After ERCP perforation

       i. When indicated, simple drainage performed laparoscopically seems feasible.

K. Laparoscopy in the critically ill in the intensive care unit

  1. Rationale

   a. Clinical diagnosis is unreliable in patients with pharmacologic and metabolic obtundation, prior intubation, compounding comorbidities, unexplained sepsis, acidosis, or multisystem organ failure

   b. Investigational procedures, transportation to the radiology suite or the operation room are problematic in these patients

   c. Diagnosis and concomitant or two-stage laparoscopic treatment are possible in the most frequent diagnoses

       i. Acalculous cholecystitis, gastrointestinal tract perforation, intestinal ischemia, pancreatitis, bowel obstruction, and intra-abdominal hemorrhage

V. LAPAROSCOPY IN THE PREGNANT WOMAN

A. Although highly debated, laparoscopy can be performed safely in the pregnant woman in all trimesters (SAGES recommendations)

  1. The advantages of laparoscopy in the emergency surgery setting may, however, be offset by the increased fetal mortality rate when performed during the first trimester

B. Precautions

  1. Mandatory open approach (no Veress needle) and more cephalad trocar insertion, adapted to the volume of the uterus, for creation of pneumoperitoneum

VI. DOES CONVERSION HAVE AN ADVERSE EFFECT ON EMERGENCY SURGERY?

A. Conversion rates range (proportionally to the complexity of the procedure) from

  1. 11.7% to 25% in peritonitis

  2. 9.7% to 21.2% in acute appendicitis

  3. 0% to 29% in peptic ulcer perforation

  4. 5.3% to 30% in acute cholecystitis

  5. 0% to 83% in colonic perforation (mostly complicated diverticular disease)

  6. 16% to 45% in intestinal occlusion

B. No adverse effects per se, but these patients may have:

  1. More surgical site and overall morbidity

  2. Longer convalescence

C. Conversion from laparoscopic to open surgery should never be considered a failure; but rather a wise decision to ensure patient safety and complete the emergency surgery as needed. Pre-emptive conversion (i.e., before an intraoperative event makes it mandatory) is associated with better outcome than reactive conversion (after the event occurs).

Suggested Readings

Agresta F, Ciardo LF, Mazzarolo G, et al. Peritonitis: laparoscopic approach. *World J Emerg Surg* 2006;1:9. doi:10.1186/1749-7922-1-9.

Alamili M, Gögenur I, Rosenberg J. Acute complicated diverticulitis managed by laparoscopic lavage. *Dis Colon Rectum* 2009;52:1345–1349.

Arnell TD. Minimally Invasive Reoperation following Laparotomy. *Clin Colon Rectal Surg* 2006;19:223–227.

Berci G, Sackier JM, Paz-Partlow M. Emergency laparoscopy. *Am J Surg* 1991;161:332–335.

Bertleff MJOE, Lange JF. Perforated Peptic Ulcer Disease: a review of history and treatment. *Dig Surg* 2010;27:161–169.

Boey J, Choi SK, Poon A, et al. Risk stratification in perforated duodenal ulcer: a prospective validation of predictive factors. *Ann Surg* 1987;205:22–26.

Bosscha K, van Vroonhoven THMV, et al. Surgical management of severe secondary peritonitis. *Br J Surg* 1999;86:1371–1372.

Brandt D, Gervaz P, Durmishi Y, et al. Percutaneous CT scan-guided drainage vs. antibiotherapy alone for Hinchey II diverticulitis: a case-control study. *Dis Colon Rectum* 2006;49:1533–1538.

Campanelli G, Catena F, Ansaloni L. Prosthetic abdominal wall hernia repair in emergency surgery: from polypropylene to biological meshes. *World J Emergency Surg* 2008;3:33. doi:10.1186/1749-7922-3-33.

Chu T, Chandhoke RA, Smith PC, et al. The impact of surgeon choice on the cost of performing laparoscopic appendectomy. *Surg Endosc* 2011;25:1187–1191. doi:10.1007/s00464-010-1342-1.

Coimbra C, Bouffioux L, Kohnen L, et al. Laparoscopic repair of colonoscopic perforation: a new standard. *Surg Endosc* 2011;25:1514–1517.

De Bakker JK, Dijksmann LM, Donkervoort SD. Safety and outcome of general surgical open and laparoscopic procedures during pregnancy. *Surg Endosc* 2011;25:1574–1578.

De Visser H, Heijnsdijk EAM, Herder JL, et al. Forces and displacements in colon surgery. *Surg Endosc* 2002;16:1426–1430.

Dedemadi G, Sgourakis G, Radtke A, et al. Laparoscopic versus open mesh repair for recurrent inguinal hernia: a meta-analysis of outcomes. *Am J Surg* 2010;200:291–297.

Deeba S, Purkayastha S, Paraskevas P, et al. Laparoscopic approach to incarcerated and strangulated inguinal hernias. *JSLS* 2009;13:327–331.

Durmishi Y, Gervaz P, Brandt D, et al. Results from percutaneous drainage of Hinchey stage II diverticulitis guided by computed tomography scan. *Surg Endosc* 2006;20:1129–1133.

Enochsson L, Hellberg A, Rudberg C, et al. Laparoscopic vs open appendectomy in overweight patients. *Surg Endosc* 2001;15:387–392. doi:10.1007/s004640000334.

Eypasch E, Troidl H, Mennigen R, et al. Laparoscopy via an indwelling cannula: an alternative to planned relaparotomy. *Br J Surg* 1992;79:1395.

Fingerhut A, Millat B, Borie F. Prevention of complications in laparoscopic surgery. In: Eubanks S, Swanstrom L, Soper N (eds). *Mastery of endoscopic and laparoscopic surgery.* Philadephia, PA: Lippincott; 2004.

Fingerhut A. Reversed conversion revisited. *Surg Innov* 2011;18:5–7.

Fingerhut A, Millat B, Borrie F. Laparoscopic versus open appendectomy: time to decide. *World J Surg* 1999;23:835–845.

Fletcher DR, Hobbs MST, Tan P, et al. Complications of cholecystectomy: risks of the laparoscopic approach and protective effects of operative cholangiography. A population-based study. *Ann Surg* 1999;229:449–457.

Flum DR, Dellinger EP, Cheadle A, et al. Intraoperative cholangiography and risk of common bile duct injury during cholecystectomy. *JAMA* 2003;289:1639–1644.

Gervaz P, Inan I, Perneger T, et al. A prospective, randomized, single-blind comparison of laparoscopic versus open sigmoid colectomy for diverticulitis. *Ann Surg* 2010;252:3–8.

Gervaz P, Mugnier-Konrad B, Morel P, et al. Laparoscopic versus open sigmoid resection for diverticulitis: Long-term results of a prospective, randomized trial. *Surg Endosc* 2011;25:3373–3378.

Greenwald JA, McMullen HF, Coppa GF, et al. Standardization of surgeon-controlled variables: impact on outcome in patients with acute cholecystitis. *Ann Surg* 2000;231:339–344.

Guller U, Rosella L, Karanicolas PJ, et al. Population-based trend analysis of 2813 patients undergoing laparoscopic sigmoid resection. *Arch Surg* 2003;138:1179–1186.

Gurusamy K, Samraj K, Gluud C, et al. Meta-analysis of randomized controlled trials on the safety and effectiveness of early versus delayed laparoscopic cholecystectomy for acute cholecystitis. *Br J Surg* 2010;97:141–150.

Gurusamy KS, Samraj K. Early versus delayed laparoscopic cholecystectomy for acute cholecystitis. *Cochrane Database Syst Rev* 2006;4:CD005440.

Hamdan K, Somers S, Chand M. Management of late postoperative complications of bariatric surgery. *Br J Surg* 2011;98:1345–1355.

Hanna GB, Shimi SM, Cuschieri A. Task performance in endoscopic surgery is influenced by location of the image display. *Ann Surg* 1998;227:481–484.

Hellberg A, Rudberg C, Enochsson L, et al. Conversion from laparoscopic to open appendicectomy: a possible drawback of the laparoscopic technique? *Eur J Surg* 2001;167:209–213.

Hemmila MR, Birkmeyer NJ, Arbabi S, et al. Introduction to propensity scores: a case study on the comparative effectiveness of laparoscopic vs open appendectomy. *Arch Surg* 2010;145:939–945.

Hirota M, Takada T, Kawarada Y, et al. Diagnostic criteria and severity assessment of acute cholecystitis: Tokyo Guidelines. *J Hepatobiliary Pancreat Surg* 2007;14:78–82.

Kenyon TA, Urbach DR, Speer JB, et al. Dedicated minimally invasive surgery suites increase operating room efficiency. *Surg Endosc* 2001;15:1140–1143.

Klarenbeek BR, Veenhof AA, Bergamaschi R, et al. Laparoscopic sigmoid resection for diverticulitis decreases major morbidity rates: a randomized control trial: short-term results of the Sigma Trial. *Ann Surg* 2009;249:39–44.

Krahenbuhl L, Sclabas G, Wente MN, et al. Incidence, risk factors, and prevention of biliary tract injuries during laparoscopic cholecystectomy in Switzerland. *World J Surg* 2001;25:1325–1330.

Larobina M, Nottle P. Complete evidence regarding major vascular injuries during laparoscopic access *Surg Laparosc Endosc Percutan Tech* 2005;15:119–123.

Lau H, Lo Y, Patil NG, et al. Early versus delayed-interval laparoscopic cholecystectomy for acute cholecystitis. A metaanalysis. *Surg Endosc* 2006;20:82–87.

Lau H. Laparoscopic repair of perforated peptic ulcer: a meta-analysis. *Surg Endosc* 2004;18:1013–1021.

Lee CW, Sarosi GA. Emergency ulcer surgery. *Surg Clin N Am* 2011;91:1001–1013.

Levard H, Boudet MJ, Msika S, et al. Laparoscopic treatment of acute small bowel obstruction: a multicentre retrospective study. *ANZ J Surg* 2001;71:641–646.

McCormack K, Scott NW, Go PM, et al. Laparoscopic techniques versus open techniques for inguinal hernia repair. *Cochrane Database Syst Rev* 2003:CD001785.

Merlin TL, Hiller JE, Maddern GJ, et al. Systematic review of the safety and effectiveness of methods used to establish pneumoperitoneum in laparoscopic surgery. *Br J Surg* 2003;90:668–679.

Myers E, Hurley M, O'Sullivan GCO, et al. Laparoscopic peritoneal lavage for generalized peritonitis due to perforated diverticulitis. *Br J Surg* 2008;95:97–101.

Navez B, Delgadillo X, Cambier E, et al. Laparoscopic approach for acute appendicular peritonitis: efficacy and safety: a report of 96 consecutive cases. *Surg Laparosc Endosc Percutan Tech* 2001;11:313–316.

Navez B, Tassetti V, Scohy JJ, et al. Laparoscopic management of acute peritonitis. *Br J Surg* 1998;85:32–36.

Neudecker J, Sauerland S, Neugebauer E, et al. The European Association for Endoscopic Surgery clinical practice guideline on the pneumoperitoneum for laparoscopic surgery. *Surg Endosc* 2002;16:1121–1143.

Papi C, Catarci M, D'Ambrosjo L, et al. Timing of cholecystectomy for acute calculous cholecystitis: a meta-analysis. *Am J Gastroenterol* 2003;99:147–155.

Platell C, Papadimitriou JM, Hall JC. The influence of lavage on peritonitis. *J Am Coll Surg* 2000;191:672–680.

Rosin D, Zmora O, Khaikin M, et al. Laparoscopic management of surgical complications after a recent laparotomy. *Surg Endosc* 2004;18:994–996.

Sajid MS, Rimple J, Cheek E, et al. Use of endo-GIA versus endo-loop for securing the appendicular stump in laparoscopic appendicectomy: a systematic review. *Surg Laparosc Endosc Percutan Tech* 2009;19:11–15.

Sauerland S, Jaschinski T, Neugebauer EA. Laparoscopic versus open surgery for suspected appendicitis. *Cochrane Database Syst Rev* 2010;(10):CD001546.

Sgourakis G, Radtke A, Sotiropoulos GC, et al. Assessment of strangulated content of the spontaneously reduced inguinal hernia via hernia sac laparoscopy: preliminary results of a prospective randomized study. *Surg Laparosc Endosc Percutan Tech* 2009;19:133–137.

Shah RH, Sharma A, Khullar R, et al. Laparoscopic repair incarcerated ventral abdominal wall hernia. *Hernia* 2008;12:457–463.

Shikata S, Noguchi Y, Fukui T. Early versus delayed cholecystectomy for acute cholecystitis: a meta-analysis of randomized controlled trials. *Surg Today* 2005;35:553–560.

Shukla PJ, Maharaj R, Fingerhut A. Ergonomics and technical aspects of minimal access surgery in acute surgery. *Eur J Trauma Emerg Surg* 2010;36:3–9.

Siddiqui T, MacDonald A, Chong PS, et al. Early versus delayed laparoscopic cholecystectomy for acute cholecystitis: a meta-analysis of randomized clinical trials. *Am J Surg* 2008;195:40–47.

Singhal T, Balakrishnan S, Hussain A, et al. Laparoscopic subtotal cholecystectomy: initial experience with laparoscopic management of difficult cholecystitis. *Surgeon* 2009;7:263–268.

Stocchi L. Current indications and role of surgery in the management of sigmoid diverticulitis. *World J Gastroenterol* 2010;16:804–817.

Sugimoto K, Hirata M, Kikuno T, et al. Large-volume intraoperative peritoneal lavage with an assistant device for treatment of peritonitis caused by blunt traumatic rupture of the small bowel. *J Trauma* 1995;39:689–692.

Sugimoto K, Hirata M, Takishima T, et al. Mechanically assisted intraoperative peritoneal lavage for generalized peritonitis as a result of perforation of the upper part of the gastrointestinal tract. *J Am Coll Surg* 1994;179:443–448.

Swank HA, Eshuis EJ, van Berge Henegouwen, et al. Short and long-term results of open versus laparoscopic appendectomy. *World J Surg* 2011;35:1221–1226.

Tan HL, Shankar KR, Ade-Ajayi N, et al. Reduction in visceral slide is a good sign of underlying postoperative viscero-parietal adhesions in children. *J Pediatr Surg* 2003;38:714–716.

Taylor CJ, Layani L, Ghusn MA, et al. Perforated diverticulitis managed by laparoscopic lavage. *ANZ J Surg* 2006;76:962–965.

Winbladh A, Gullstrand P, Svanvik J, et al. Systematic review of cholecystostomy as a treatment option in acute cholecystitis. *HPB (Oxford)* 2009;11:183–193.

Zamir G, Reissman P. Diagnostic laparoscopy in mesenteric ischemia. *Surg Endosc* 1998;12:390–393.

Miscellaneous Procedures

Glen Tinkoff and Frederick Giberson

INTRODUCTION

Many procedures are performed as adjuncts to the resuscitation of the trauma patient in the emergency department or at the bedside in the ICU. We describe approaches and where available, the internet URL addresses of images and video clips of these procedures in the public domain have also been cited.

I. ADJUNCTIVE PROCEDURES TO RESUSCITATON
A. Naso/orogastric tube intubation
1. Indications
a. Gastric decompression
b. Gastric lavage
2. Contraindications
a. Mid-face or basilar skull fracture (use an orogastric route)
b. Obstruction of the naso/oropharynx, or esophagus
3. Technique
a. In the conscious patient, nasal insertion is preferred if not contraindicated; in patients who are unconscious or have been intubated, the oral route is preferred.
b. Lubricate tube with a water soluble lubricant.
c. Elevate head of bed, if possible.
d. If inserting nasally, introduce the tube gently into the nostril; slowly direct the tube posteriorly and caudad into the posterior oropharynx by inserting short increments (*do not advance upward*—a common error, usually done when external nasal slope is followed instead of passage directly posterior). If inserting orally, advance tube to the posterior oropharynx over the tongue in a similar fashion.
e. Do not advance the tube while the patient is talking or inhaling.
f. If possible, the tube should be inserted by gently advancing as the patient swallows.
g. Once in the esophagus, the tube should advance easily into the stomach. Gagging is common during insertion; if the patient loses their voice, becomes hoarse, or has violent coughing, withdraw the tube as it is likely to be in the trachea.
h. Inject air into the tube via a large syringe and auscultate over the left upper quadrant of the abdomen for a "rush" of air.
i. If gastric location is confirmed with air injection, irrigate the tube with normal saline and aspirate to remove particulate gastric contents.
j. Secure the tube with adhesive tape.
k. Attach to low continuous suction (if a sump tube).
4. Complications
a. Epistaxis (nasal placement)
b. Sinusitis (nasal placement greater than 24 hours)
c. Pneumothorax
d. Aspiration
e. Intracranial insertion (nasal placement)

5. Available internet video
   a. http://emedicine.medscape.com/article/80925-overview#a15
   b. http://www.nejm.org/doi/full/10.1056/NEJMvcm050183#figure=preview.gif

B. Optical tonometry/lateral canthotomy

1. Indications
   a. Traumatic retrobulbar hematoma with intraocular pressure (IOP) >30 mm Hg
   b. Proptosis
   c. Decreased visual acuity
   d. Presence of retrobulbar hematoma

2. Contraindications
   a. Globe rupture

3. Technique of optical tonometry (e.g., Tono-Pen®)
   a. Clear debris, cleanse and prep affected periorbital area
   b. Apply topical ocular anesthetic (e.g., tetracaine, proparacaine) to cornea
   c. Place cover over probe tip
   d. Activate and calibrate device
   e. Take measurement of affected eye by lightly touching the cornea and listening for the "click"; take at least four separate readings or until instrument signals and provides an average reading
   f. If IOP >30 mm Hg, perform a lateral canthotomy

4. Technique of lateral canthotomy
   a. Infiltrate dermis above lateral canthus with 1 to 2 cc of 1% to 2% lidocaine with epinephrine
   b. Apply straight hemostat from lateral canthus toward bony orbit for 30 to 90 seconds
   c. Incise demarcated area 1 to 2 cm
   d. With forceps, pull caudad on lower led to visualize inferior lateral canthal tendon
   e. Incise inferior canthal tendon with iris scissors
   f. Reassess IOP—if increased, lift upper eyelid and incise superior lateral canthal tendon

5. Complications
   a. Infection
   b. Hemorrhage
   c. Injury to globe

6. Available internet video
   a. Optical tonometry
      i. http://www.youtube.com/watch?v=-l2fS4ykYsc...feature=related
      ii. http://www.youtube.com/watch?v=-Y3KtAnbuFo...feature=related
   b. Lateral canthotomy
      i. http://emedicine.medscape.com/article/82812-overview#a15

C. Reduction of common dislocations

1. General considerations
   a. Manage life-threatening injuries first.
   b. Perform a thorough neurovascular examination of the affected extremity.
   c. Confirm clinical findings with appropriate radiologic assessment.
   d. Know the joint anatomy well.
   e. If an associated fracture is evident, consult an orthopedic surgeon early.
   f. Administer adequate IV analgesia and sedation with appropriate hemodynamic monitoring before proceeding.
   g. If unable to reduce the dislocation or reduction is lost, splint the extremity in position and obtain orthopedic consultation.

2. Reduction of a shoulder dislocation
   a. Anterior dislocation (most common)
      i. Place patient supine with the affected arm adducted with elbow flexed at 90 degrees.
      ii. Hold the patient's wrist and slowly externally rotate.

    iii. Continue the external rotation until the forearm is near the coronal plane.

    iv. If this maneuver is unsuccessful, lift the arm perpendicular to the patient's torso while applying axial traction and rotate the arm externally.

    v. If the shoulder still remains dislocated, consider utilizing traction–countertraction.

    vi. Flex the patient's elbow on the affected side to 90 degrees and wrap a sheet or strap around the proximal forearm.

    vii. Wrap a sheet or strap around the upper chest under the axilla of the affected shoulder to provide countertraction.

    viii. Apply traction to the arm while an assistant applies countertraction.

    ix. Also gently rotate the arm externally to facilitate reduction.

b. Posterior dislocation

    i. Posterior dislocation is usually amenable to closed reduction only if there is minimal displacement and recent onset.

    ii. Use traction–countertraction method as described previously.

    iii. Abduct and internally rotate the affected arm.

    iv. Apply anteriorly directed pressure on the humeral head.

c. Post-procedure care

    i. Reassess neurovascular status (notably sensation on shoulder area).

    ii. Confirm reduction of the dislocation with post-reduction radiographs that include a lateral view.

    iii. Immobilize the reduced shoulder with sling.

d. Complications

    i. Displacement of fractures of the humeral neck

    ii. Avascular necrosis of the humeral head

    iii. Neurovascular injury

    iv. Joint instability leading to recurrent dislocation

3. Reduction of a hip dislocation

a. Posterior dislocation (most common)

    i. Confirm diagnosis based on the presence of a shortened, internally rotated lower extremity on physical examination and on radiologic examination, the femoral head located posterior to the acetabulum.

    ii. Have an assistant apply countertraction by pushing on the anterior superior iliac spines

    iii. Hold affected leg in adduction with the knee flexed.

    iv. Apply axial traction, in line with the deformity while gently flexing the hip to 90 degrees or until reduction is achieved.

b. Anterior dislocation

    i. In anterior hip dislocations, the femoral head is displaced anterior to the acetabulum causing the lower extremity to be shortened and externally rotated. On radiologic assessment, the femoral head should lie over the obturator foramen.

    ii. Have an assistant apply countertraction by pushing on the anterior superior iliac spines.

    iii. Hold affected leg in abduction, with the knee slightly flexed.

    iv. Apply axial traction, in line with the deformity, and gently adduct and internally rotate until reduction is achieved.

c. Post-reduction care

    i. Reexamine the hip range of motion to assess stability.

    ii. Repeat the neurovascular examination.

    iii. Immobilize; use a knee immobilizer for posterior and an abduction pillow for anterior dislocations.

    iv. Obtain appropriate post-reduction imaging studies.

    v. If the hip is unstable, a traction pin may be needed.

d. Complications

    i. Nerve or vascular injury

    ii. Avascular necrosis of the femoral head

      iii. Osteoarthritis

      iv. Heterotopic ossification

4. Reduction of an ankle dislocation

  a. Posterior dislocation (most common)

      i. Grasp the foot by the heel and forefoot while an assistant holds the leg at the knee in flexion.

      ii. Plantar flex the foot slightly and apply axial traction.

      iii. Slowly push the heel anteriorly against downward countertraction on the tibia until reduction is achieved.

      iv. Keep the foot in dorsiflexion until splinted.

  b. Anterior dislocation

      i. Grasp the foot by the heel and forefoot while an assistant holds the leg at the knee in flexion.

      ii. Dorsiflex the foot and apply axial traction.

      iii. Slowly push the forefoot posteriorly against upward countertraction on the tibia until reduction is achieved.

      iv. Keep the foot in plantar flexion until splinted.

  c. Lateral dislocation

      i. Associated with malleoli fractures often managed with open reduction and internal fixation.

      ii. Closed reduction achieved in a similar manner to posterior dislocation except foot should be manipulated medially or laterally as needed to achieve reduction.

  d. Post-procedure care

      i. Splint the ankle at 90 degrees with a posterior short leg splint.

      ii. Reassess neurovascular status.

      iii. Repeat radiologic assessment to confirm reduction.

  e. Complications

      i. Neurovascular injury, uncommon

      ii. Loss of range of motion

      iii. Joint instability

      iv. Chronic pain

5. Available internet video

  a. Shoulder (anterior)—http://emedicine.medscape.com/article/109130-overview #a15

  b. http://www.youtube.com/watch?v=CGvy6sA2OD4...feature=youtube_gdata_player

  c. Hip (posterior)—http://www.medicalvideos.us/videos/1598/

  d. Ankle (posterior)—http://emedicine.medscape.com/article/109244-overview #a15

D. Ring removal from a compromised digit

1. Indications

  a. Removal of ring or other constricting object from a compromised or potentially compromised digit.

  b. If neurovascular compromise, ring cutter or other metal cutting instrument should be employed.

2. Technique

  a. Elevate finger relative to others above head and/or torso and compress it manually.

  b. Pass tape/suture under ring (may be facilitated with a hemostat) then wrap proximal to distal with umbilical tape or heavy silk in spiral fashion from tip to base.

  c. Lubricate ring generously.

  d. Apply gentle pull traction on ring and toward tip and unwrap the tape/suture from under ring while pushing ring toward tip of the finger.

  e. The finger portion from a powder-free latex glove can be used in similar manner with cut edge pulled under the ring.

  f. If this fails, the ring must be cut to relieve neurovascular compromise.

3. Complications
   a. Injury to underlying skin and soft tissue structures
   b. Fracture/dislocation of the proximal phalanx
4. Available internet images
   a. http://www.knowabouthealth.com/quick-tips-to-remove-stuck-ring-from-swollen-finger/3510/

E. Skeletal traction pin insertion
1. Indications
   a. Femur fracture which cannot undergo early definitive treatment (i.e., severe TBI)
2. Contraindications
   a. Unstable knee injury
   b. Open distal femur or proximal fibula fracture
3. Technique
   a. For short duration (i.e., 2 to 3 days), insert 1 cm distal to anterior tibial tubercle.
   b. For more prolonged traction (i.e., ≈1 week) insert into distal femur.
   c. Align leg from the great toe, through the patella to the anterior iliac spine.
   d. Elevate the leg to allow the drill handle to turn without striking the bed.
   e. Prepare and drape the knee and proximal tibia.
   f. Infiltrate entry and exit sites with local anesthetic.
   g. Use a non-threaded Steinman pin or Kirschner wire for tibial insertion (a threaded pin should be used with femoral insertion).
   h. Make a small skin incision laterally, 2 cm distal and posterior to the anterior tibial tubercle or 2 cm above the femoral condyles.
   i. Engage the pin/wire against the bone and stay parallel to the ground.
   j. Drill through both cornices. When the pin pushes against the medial skin, the skin is incised with the scalpel. The pin/wire should extend beyond the skin 1 to 2 in.
   k. Cut the pin/wire to length and cap the ends with corks or rubber stoppers.
   l. Attach the pin/ wire into the appropriate bow and traction.
   m. Dress the pin sites with povidone-iodine and 2 × 2 gauze.
4. Complications
   a. Failure to obtain purchase into bone
   b. Bleeding
   c. Pin site infection
5. Available internet video
   a. http://www.youtube.com/watch?v=WXN9RMjyn4M...feature=email

II. SPLINT APPLICATION
A. Indications
   1. Temporary immobilization of an injured extremity (esp. fractures)
B. Contraindications
   1. Destructive soft tissue injury
   2. Vascular compromise of the distal extremity
   3. Presence of a compartment syndrome
   4. Neuropathic extremity
C. General splinting technique
1. Pre-procedure
   a. Examine extremity including a detailed neurovascular examination.
   b. Reduce fracture, if necessary.
   c. Irrigate, debride, and dress any open wounds.
   d. Complete any radiologic assessment necessary.
2. General splinting procedure
   a. Apply stockinette (optional); avoid wrinkles
   b. Measure length of splinting material (plaster sheets or pre-fabricated fiberglass of appropriate width to span above and below the fracture site and associated joints.

    c. If using plaster (eight layers for upper extremity and 12 layers for lower extremity splints), add several layers of cotton padding (Webril®) on extremity and to surface of the splinting material that will be next to patient's skin; provide length of padding to extend over the edges of the splint.

    d. Soak plaster splint material in tepid temperature water and allow excess to drain. If using fiberglass, do not soak—a light spray/short rinse under water is plenty to begin the setting process (too much water interferes).

    e. Place splint with padding facing the skin, roll the ends of the stockinette over the splint and secure in place with rolled gauze (Kerlix®) and elastic bandage (Ace®) from the distal to proximal extent of the splint being fashioned.

    f. Gently mold the splint to the contour of the extremity and allow to set until firm—this is much faster for fiberglass (5 to 10 minutes) than plaster.

3. Post-procedure

    a. Post splinting x-rays are key if any manipulation occurred.

    b. Reassess neurovascular status of the splinted extremity. If there are signs of neurovascular compromise, loosen or remove then reapply the splint.

D. Splint types

1. Upper extremity

    a. Coaptation

        i. Extends along upper arm beginning in axilla wrapping around elbow and then along lateral aspect of upper extremity.

        ii. Elbow should remain at 90 degrees of flexion.

        iii. Immobilizes fractures of proximal and mid-shaft humerus.

    b. Long arm

        i. Extends along dorsal surface of arm from proximal humerus to wrist with elbow at 90 degrees flexion and neutral position of wrist.

        ii. Immobilizes fractures of proximal forearm, elbow, distal humerus.

    c. Sugar tong

        i. Extends from the metacarpophalangeal joints on the dorsum of the hand, around the elbow, along the volar aspect of the mid-palmar crease. Elbow is maintained at 90 degrees flexion with neutral position of wrist.

        ii. Immobilizes wrist and forearm while preventing supination/pronation.

        iii. Utilized for fractures of distal forearm and wrist.

    d. Short arm

        i. Extends along dorsal aspect of forearm from metacarpal heads to mid-forearm.

        ii. Allows unencumbered flexion of the elbow.

        iii. Forearm should remain in neutral position with wrist at 20 degrees of extension.

        iv. Utilized for second to fifth metacarpal fractures, carpal bone fractures (excluding scaphoid fractures), and wrist sprains.

    e. Thumb spica

        i. Extends along radial aspect of the forearm from tip of thumb to proximal forearm with the forearm in neutral position with the wrist at 20 degrees of extension and thumb slightly flexed.

        ii. Splint material is molded around the thumb, thereby immobilizing the thumb and preventing flexion or extension of the wrist.

        iii. Utilized for fractures of scaphoid and lunate bones, first metacarpal and thumb.

    f. Ulnar gutter

        i. Extends along the ulnar aspect of the forearm from the distal interphalangeal joint of the fifth digit to the proximal forearm.

        ii. Forearm is kept in neutral position with the wrist at 20 degrees of extension.

        iii. The metacarpal/phalangeal joints are flexed at 50 degrees with the proximal and distal interphalangeal joints in slight flexion.

        iv. Immobilizes fractures of the fourth and fifth phalanges and metacarpals and ulnar styloid fractures.

2. Lower extremity
a. Posterior long leg
- **i.** Extends from mid to proximal thigh to approximately 5 cm proximal to the malleoli along the posterior leg.
- **ii.** Knee joint should remain flexed at 10 to 20 degrees.
- **iii.** Utilized for immobilization of fractures of distal femur, proximal to the tibia/fibula, and acute dislocation of knee.
- **iv.** A pre-fabricated knee immobilizer can also be utilized.

b. Posterior short leg
- **i.** Extends posteriorly from metatarsal heads to just below fibular head.
- **ii.** Maintain 90 degrees at the ankle and keep the fibular head clear to avoid compression of peroneal nerve.
- **iii.** Commonly used for severe ankle sprains, fractures of the ankle or foot.

E. Complications
1. Vascular compromise
2. Neuropathy
3. Dermatitis
4. Pressure sores

F. Available internet images/video
1. General principles http://www.nejm.org/doi/full/10.1056/NEJMvcm0801942#figure=preview.gif
2. Coaptation—http://www.steinergraphics.com/surgical/006_17.2.html
3. Posterior long arm—http://emedicine.medscape.com/article/1355110-overview#a15
4. Sugar Tong—http://emedicine.medscape.com/article/80127-overview#a15
5. Short arm—http://emedicine.medscape.com/article/109769-overview#a15
6. Thumb spica—http://emedicine.medscape.com/article/80127-overview#a15
7. Ulnar gutter—http://emedicine.medscape.com/article/80165-overview#a15
8. Posterior long leg—http://emedicine.medscape.com/article/1355131-overview#a15
9. Posterior short leg—http://emedicine.medscape.com/article/80070-overview#aw2aab6b4aa

G. Pelvic sling/binder application
1. Indications
a. Mechanically unstable pelvis
- **i.** Unstable fracture patterns:
  - **a)** >2.5 cm symphysis diastasis
  - **b)** Displaced pubic rami fractures
  - **c)** >1 cm SI joint widening or displacement of a sacral fracture
  - **d)** Fracture/dislocation of the SI joint complex
  - **e)** Displacement of a hemi-pelvis

b. Suspected pelvic hemorrhage in a patient with a pelvic ring fracture

2. Contraindications
a. Stable pelvic fractures
- **i.** Minimally displaced pubic rami fracture
- **ii.** Non or minimally displaced sacral ala fracture
- **iii.** Isolated iliac wing fractures
- **iv.** Avulsion fractures at muscle insertions

b. Penetrating pelvic trauma

3. Technique
a. During a log roll, place binder or folded sheeting behind patient with the bottom edge at the level of the greater trochanters.
b. Manually reduce and hold pelvic reduction in place.
c. Wrap binder or folded sheeting around patient.
d. For sheeting, overlap ends and tie in place (pelvic sling).
e. For binder, secure over anterior pelvis applying pressure to lateral pelvis. Most pre-fabricated binders utilize a belt or Velcro® apparatus.
f. In male patients, make certain that the genitalia are elevated out of the groin.

    g. Remove only after resuscitation completed, hemodynamically stable, and definitive fixation of the pelvis is imminent. Monitor vital signs including pain scale during removal and replace if they deteriorate.

  4. Complications
    a. Failure to stop pelvic hemorrhage
    b. Compartment syndrome

  5. Available internet video
    a. http://video.google.com/videoplay?docid=-3053627367877537352#

H. Traction splint application

  1. Indications
    a. Femur fracture—diaphyseal

  2. Contraindications
    a. Pelvic fracture
    b. Significant foot/ankle fracture
    c. Associated destructive soft tissue injury

  3. Technique
    a. Minimum, two-person procedure
    b. Prepare the splint (e.g., Hare®, Sager®) before application (i.e., measure limb length and obtain straps)
    c. Administer intravenous (IV) analgesia.
    d. Assess the distal pulses before applying the splint.
    e. Apply manual traction via the foot strap while raising the leg.
    f. In a coordinated and precise effort, position the splint under the leg with the proximal covered rim of the splint against the ischial tuberosity.
    g. Slowly apply traction to the foot strap after affixing the traction hook to the foot strap sling.
    h. Apply leg straps (usually Velcro) to secure the leg in the splint; the straps do not need to be tight.
    i. Reassess distal pulses after the splint is applied.

  4. Complications
    a. Sloughing of skin at the ankle
    b. Loss of pulses/ischemia

  5. Available internet video
    a. http://www.youtube.com/watch?v=qs6RciOHM4U...feature=youtube_gdata_player
    b. http://www.youtube.com/watch?v=VjmFVHsH95o...feature=youtube_gdata_player

III. URINARY CATHETER/SUPRAPUBIC CATHETER INSERTION

A. Urinary catheter insertion

  1. Indications
    a. Hemodynamic instability
    b. Distended abdomen
    c. Obvious indication for operative intervention (i.e., open fracture)
    d. External signs of major torso trauma
    e. Spinal fractures/spinal cord injury

  2. Contraindications
    a. Stable patient with minimal evidence of trauma
    b. High suspicion of urethral injury in the male
    c. Blood in urethral meatus (concerning for urethral injury and may convert to complete disruption)
    d. Scrotal ecchymosis
    e. Boggy or high-riding prostate on rectal examination

  3. Technique
    a. Insertion in the male patient
      i. Prepare the glans of the penis with antiseptic solution
      ii. With the non-dominant hand, gently stretch the shaft of the penis and extend upward.

    iii. Hold the catheter close to the meatus and with the dominant hand; gently insert the catheter in short increments.

    iv. Resistance should be met at the posterior urethral sphincter. Apply gentle, forward pressure on the catheter until the sphincter relaxes.

    v. When urine is obtained, advance the catheter its full length to avoid inflation of the balloon in the urethra.

    vi. Inflate the balloon, and then gently withdraw the catheter until stopped by the balloon.

    vii. If urine is not observed, apply suprapubic pressure. If urine is still not obtained, irrigate the catheter. If no urine still, abort the insertion attempt and do either sonographic assessment of the bladder or an urethrocystogram.

  b. Insertion in the female patient

    i. The technique is similar to male but the female urethra is shorter, and the location of the urethral meatus can be difficult to visualize. Vaginal insertion is common.

    ii. If possible, use supplemental lighting and assistance.

    iii. Place the patient in a frogleg position and have an assistant spread labial folds.

  c. Insertion in the pediatric patient

    i. Use an appropriately sized catheter (a small polyethylene feeding tube can be also be used).

    ii. Gentle insertion is essential.

    iii. During insertion, spontaneous voiding is common.

4. Complications

  a. Urethral injury/stricture

  b. Urinary tract infection

5. Available internet video

  a. http://www.nejm.org/doi/full/10.1056/NEJMvcm054648#figure=preview.gif

  b. http://www.nejm.org/doi/full/10.1056/NEJMvcm0706671#figure=preview.gif

B. Suprapubic catheter insertion

1. Indications

  a. Urethral injury

  b. Urethral obstruction

  c. Benign prosthetic hypertrophy (BPH)

2. Contraindications

  a. Absence of a palpable bladder or sonographically localized distended urinary bladder

  b. Coagulopathy (relative, and until the abnormality is corrected)

  c. Prior lower abdominal or pelvic surgery

3. Technique

  a. Palpate the distended bladder and perform ultrasonography to verify its location.

  b. Mark the insertion site at the midline and two fingers (4 to 5 cm) above the pubic symphysis.

  c. Prep and drape from the pubis to the umbilicus.

  d. Anesthetize the dermis and rectus fascia at the insertion site mark and make a small incision with an 11 scalpel.

  e. Advance a "finder" needle with syringe (preferably with sonographic guidance) until urine is obtained; note the direction and depth of the needle.

  f. One of two basic approaches can utilized: (1) Trocar approach or (2) an approach utilizing a modified Seldinger technique with "peel-away" catheter (both are available in pre-fabricated kits).

  g. Trocar approach

    i. Insert and secure a trocar into a Malecot catheter so that the trocar tip projects 2.5 mm from the distal end of the catheter. Connect the 60 mL syringe.

      ii. Place the tip of the catheter/trocar unit into the skin incision and direct it caudally at a 20-degree angle and advance until urine enters the syringe.

      iii. Once urine enters the syringe, advance catheter/trocar unit 3 to 4 additional centimeters.

      iv. Advance the catheter over the trocar and then, withdraw the trocar.

    h. Modified Seldinger technique with "peel-away" catheter

      i. Introduce a guidewire through the finder needle

      ii. Slide the needle out and insert the "peel away" catheter with dilator over the guidewire

      iii. Remove dilator and guidewire

      iv. Insert 14 Fr Foley catheter and inflate balloon

      v. Remove the "peel away" catheter

    i. Connect to a urinary bag and secure the catheter to the skin and dress.

  4. Complications

    a. Intraperitoneal visceral injury

    b. Gross hematuria (common)

    c. Post-obstructive diuresis

    d. Cellulitis

    e. Malposition/dislodgement/ obstruction of tube

  5. Available internet video

    a. http://emedicine.medscape.com/article/145909-overview#a15

    b. http://www.medicalvideos.us/play.php?vid=1651

IV. ICU BEDSIDE PROCEDURE

A. Fiberoptic bronchoscopy (fob)

  1. Indications

    a. Adjunct to endotracheal intubation

    b. Evaluation of posttraumatic hemoptysis, acute inhalation injury, suspected bronchial injury, or injury caused by prolonged intubation.

    c. Extraction of foreign bodies

    d. Clearance of secretions and mucous plugs

    e. Diagnosis of nosocomial pneumonia

  2. Contraindications

    a. Uncooperative patient

    b. Persistent, marked hypoxemia or hypercarbia (relative, since this is sometimes an indication)

    c. Severe bronchospasm

    d. Severe pulmonary hypertension

    e. Cardiac ischemia

    f. Coagulopathy

  3. Procedure

    a. Most trauma patients needing FOB will have an endotracheal tube in place.

    b. For patients not intubated, the most skilled person performs FOB.

    c. Have cardiac and pulse oximetry monitoring and skilled assistance at the bedside.

    d. Generally, ≥ 8 mm internal diameter endotracheal or tracheostomy tube is preferred for FOB.

    e. Maintain 100% FiO_2 throughout the procedure and minimize airway suctioning to avoid reduced tidal volumes.

    f. Make adjustments to mechanical ventilation before the procedure to maintain adequate minute ventilation and avoid increased inflation pressures.

    g. Use local anesthetics judiciously—e.g., 200 to 300 mg of topical lidocaine (20 to 30 mL of 1% lidocaine solution).

    h. Premedication with IV analgesics and sedatives as indicated.

    i. Use silicone spray rather than wet lubricant.

    j. Consider use of a swivel adaptor, which minimizes air leak.

4. Diagnosis of nosocomial pneumonia
   a. Cultures of sputum aspirates or traditional FOB specimens are unreliable because of contamination by upper airway secretions.
   b. Protected brush catheter (PBC)
      i. A PBC is a telescoping double catheter with a recessed sterile brush.
      ii. The inner catheter with brush can be advanced into subsegmental bronchi for sampling of focal infiltrates.
      iii. Avoid proximal lidocaine administration and suctioning during the procedure.
      iv. Post stamping. Retract the inner catheter and brush and remove from the bronchoscope. The brush is severed from the catheter for quantitative cultures ($>10^3$ colonies per milliliter).
   c. Bronchoalveolar lavage (BAL)
      i. Bronchoscopic tip is wedged into a subsegmental bronchi.
      ii. Instill sterile normal saline solution (NSS: 50 to 100 mL) and remove via suction.
      iii. Take quantitative cultures of the sample ($>10^4$ colonies per milliliter).
5. Available internet videos
   a. http://www.youtube.com/watch?v=VLsXe5oB2W0...feature=related
   b. http://www.youtube.com/watch?v=kQCFp_819CU...feature=related
B. Inferior vena cava filter insertion
1. Indications
   a. Recurrent pulmonary embolism despite anticoagulation
   b. Venous thromboembolism disease with contraindication to systemic anticoagulation
   c. Progression of ileofemoral clot despite anticoagulation
   d. Large, free-floating thrombus in the iliac vein or IVC
   e. Massive pulmonary embolism (PE) in which recurrent emboli would prove fatal
   f. During or after surgical embolectomy
   g. Prophylaxis in patients who cannot receive anticoagulation because of bleeding risk and with high risk injury pattern (e.g., severe closed head injury, spinal cord injury, complex pelvic fractures with associated long bone fracture, or multiple long bone fractures).
   h. Bedside insertion of IVC filters can be performed with minimal complications and eliminate the risk associated with intrahospital transport.
2. Contraindications
   a. Thrombus between access site and site of deployment (choose alternate site)
3. Technique
   a. Equipment
      i. Fluoroscopic image intensifier and monitor (Cine-loop and subtraction capabilities preferred) and fluoroscopic-ready bed
      ii. Lead aprons, sterile barriers, gowns, masks, caps
      iii. Introducer kits with guidewire
      iv. Intravenous contrast material
      v. Heparinized saline (10 U/mL NSS)
      vi. Radiopaque markers for measurements
      vii. Note: Be familiar with introducer system and size restrictions of individual vena cava filters
   b. Procedure
      i. Right internal jugular or femoral venous access approach is preferred.
      ii. Prepare access site with povidone-iodine solution or chlorhexidine gluconate.
      iii. Identify T-12 and all lumbar vertebrae under fluoroscopic guidance.
      iv. Gain venous access and advance guidewire under fluoroscopic guidance.
      v. Insert introducer with dilator previously flushed with heparin solution.
      vi. Perform venogram (hand-injected or power-injected, if available) to assess for anomalies, venal caval size, and location of renal veins.

      vii. Flush introducer with heparinized saline and solution and advance filter into infrarenal position. Deploy filter under fluoroscopic guidance.

    viii. Remove introducer and hold pressure at site for 10 minutes or until bleeding stops.

      ix. Confirm placement of IVC filter with abdominal x-ray.

  4. Complications

    a. Filter tilting, malposition, or migration

    b. IVC erosion or obstruction

    c. IVC thrombosis

    d. Insertion site thrombosis

    e. Bleeding

    f. Pulmonary contusion

  5. Available Internet Videos

    a. http://www.cookmedical.com/di/educationMedia.do?mediaId=527

    b. http://www.cookmedical.com/di/datasheetMedia.do?mediaId=582...id=4354

C. Nasoenteric post-pyloric feeding tube insertion

  1. See section IIA for Naso/orogastric insertion technique.

  2. Use an 8, 10, or 12 Fr enteric feeding tube (length >100 cm) with Y adapter and stylet.

  3. A prokinetic agent (e.g., Metoclopramide) can be administered prior to insertion to aide in pyloric passage.

  4. Once the tube is confirmed in intragastric position, roll the patient to the right lateral decubitus position, if possible.

  5. With the stylet still in place, rapidly insufflate the stomach with 500 to 1,000 mL of air, using the 60 mL regular tip syringe.

  6. Advance the feeding tube to a point such that only 10 cm of tubing remains externally.

  7. Return the patient to the supine position with stylet in place and secure the tube with tape.

  8. Assess tube position with chest or abdominal x-ray study.

    a. If the tube is transpyloric, flush with 10 mL of sterile water and remove stylet before initiating tube feeds.

    b. If the tube is at the pylorus, wait 24 to 48 hours and reassess.

    c. If the tube is looped around the stomach with the tip away from a pylorus, retract it to the centimeter mark estimating gastric placement. Consider administering a dose of a prokinetic agent and reattempt tube insertion.

  9. When properly positioned, secure tube to patient's nose and cheek and note centimeter marking on the tube at the tip of the patient's nose.

 10. If unsuccessful in transpyloric passage, arrange for a fluoroscopic or endoscopic manipulation.

D. Percutaneous endoscopic gastrostomy (PEG)

  1. Indication

    a. Long-term gastric access for either decompression or feeding. In general, if a patient is not expected to survive >30 days or will likely be eating within 14 days, a PEG is not indicated.

  2. Technical points (a detailed technical review of this procedure is beyond the scope of this manual)

    a. In general, plan the procedure for periods of optimal staffing and if possible include the use of gastrointestinal endoscopy nurses.

    b. Be prepared and equipped to safely give moderate sedation, including appropriate agents, an airway skilled physician, and continuous blood pressure, electrocardiography (ECG), and pulse oximetry monitoring.

    c. If a PEG and tracheostomy are both planned, the PEG should follow because the endotracheal tube will have been removed, facilitating endoscopy.

    d. A PEG is a three-person procedure, including the airway/monitoring physician or practitioner.

    e. Endoscopically inspect the esophagus, stomach, and duodenum before beginning placement of the PEG tube.

f. Gastric insufflation, transabdominal illumination, and endoscopic visualization of finger depression of the abdominal wall are essential for proper placement.

g. Most endoscopists do not routinely reintroduce the endoscope to inspect the stomach after placement.

h. Feeding can usually be started immediately after insertion.

3. Complications
a. Pneumoperitoneum (common)
b. Misplacement and inadvertent organ injury
c. Early tube removal with gastric perforation
d. Tube site cellulitis or hemorrhage
e. Gastrocutaneous fistula
f. Tube related mechanical problems (e.g., clogging, breakage)

4. Available internet video
a. http://www.youtube.com/watch?v=HmvFv1jswzg

E. Percutaneous tracheostomy

1. Indications
a. Airway protection
b. Pulmonary toilet
c. Prolonged ventilatory support
d. Decontamination of oropharynx
e. Extensive orofacial trauma

2. Contraindications
a. If an urgent airway is needed, cricothyrotomy, not a tracheostomy, is used

3. Technique (A detailed description of open and percutaneous tracheostomy is beyond the scope of this manual.)
a. Utilizing bronchoscopic guidance is the preferred method.
b. Plan and time procedure for periods of optimal staffing. Similar to the PEG, this bedside procedure is a three-person procedure including the person dedicated to airway and overall monitoring.
c. Have a checklist of supplies and all available before the procedure. An appropriate sized tracheostomy tube fitted to the dilators should be opened, tested, and prepared for insertion before beginning the procedure. Have an instrument tray for open tracheostomy available.
d. Ensure adequate lighting over the patient's neck and anterior chest region.
e. Use full sterile barriers, and place equipment open and on tables, not directly on the bed.
f. Have resources for moderate or deep sedation available, including appropriate agents, continuous blood pressure, ECG, and pulse oximetry monitoring.
g. Position the patient to extend the neck if possible. The anterior neck skin is prepared, draped, and anesthetized with local anesthesia.
h. If a PEG is planned at the same time, it should usually follow the tracheostomy because the endotracheal tube will have been removed, facilitating endoscopy.

4. Complications
a. The most serious complication is loss of the airway during the procedure; usually associated with hypoxia and bradycardia. If uncertain about position of the endotracheal tube or tracheostomy tube—reintubate from above *immediately.*
b. Other complications
   i. Tube misplacement (e.g., pre-tracheal) or dislodgement
   ii. Tracheal laceration, stenosis
   iii. Bleeding
   iv. Pneumothorax
   v. Laryngeal nerve injury
   vi. Tracheoinnominate fistula

5. Available internet video
a. http://www.youtube.com/watch?v=6TVOSb6sqL8

AXIOMS

- Always remember—no procedure is "minor"!
- In ocular trauma with any new vision loss, an intraocular pressure >30 mm Hg warrants consideration of lateral canthotomy.
- Avoid nasal insertion of a gastric tube in patients with mid-face or basilar skull fracture.
- Reduction of a dislocation utilizes traction opposite to the distracting force which originally caused it.
- Always assess and reassess neurovascular status and fracture alignment before and after placement of splint or traction pin.
- For bedside procedures such as tracheostomy, PEG, FOB, and IVC filter insertion, have resources and monitoring available to safely provide systemic analgesia and sedation and to secure an airway if needed.

Suggested Readings

Brohl K. *The Ideal Pelvic Binder: What's important in a pelvic binder?* Available at: http://www.trauma.org/index.php/main/article/657/. Accessed August 2011.

Buttaravoli PM, Stair TO, eds. *Common Simple Emergencies.* Available at: http://www.ncemi.org/cse/cse1005.htm. Accessed August 2011.

Davenport MD, Schraga ED, eds. *Ankle Dislocation Reduction.* Available at: http://emedicine.medscape.com/article/109244-overview#a15. Accessed August 2011.

Dellinger PR. Fiberoptic bronchoscopy in critical care medicine. In: Shoemaker WC, Ayers SH, Grenvig A, Holbrook PR, eds. *Textbook of Critical Care.* Philadelphia, PA: WB Saunders; 1995:761–769.

Elisa A, Shraga E, eds. *Joint Reduction, Shoulder Dislocation, Anterior.* Available at: http://emedicine.medscape.com/article/109130-overview#a01. Accessed August 2011.

Fitch MT, Nicks BA, Pariyadath M, et.al. Basic splinting techniques. *NEJM* 2008;359:e32.

Kaushal HS, Chilembwe M, eds. *Essential Emergency Procedures.* Philadelphia, PA: Lippincott Williams & Wilkins; 2007.

Liu LG, Kulkarni R, eds. *Lateral Orbital Canthotomy.* Available at: http://emedicine.medscape.com/article/82812-overview#a15. Accessed August 2011.

Mayeaux EJ. *The Essential Guide to Primary Care Procedures.* Philadelphia, PA: Lippincott Williams & Wilkins; 2009.

Milligan BT, Schraga ED, eds. *Joint Reduction, Shoulder Dislocation, Posterior.* Available at: http://emedicine.medscape.com/article/109149-overview. Accessed August 2011.

Rogers, FB, Cipolle MD, et al. Practice management guidelines for the management of venous thromboembolism in trauma patients. Available at http://www.east.org.

Schultz MD, Santatello SA, Monk J, et al. An improved method for transpyloric placement of nasoenteric feeding tubes. *Int Surg* 1993;78:79–82.

Shlamovitz GZ, Kim ED, eds. *Suprapubic Catheterization.* Available at: http://emedicine.medscape.com/article/145909-overview. Accessed August 2011.

Shlamovitz GZ, Kulkarni R, eds. *Gastric Intubation.* Available at: http://emedicine.medscape.com/article/80925-overview#a01. Accessed August 2011.

Wheeless GR, ed. Femoral and Tibial Traction Pins in Wheeless' Textbook of Orthopaedics. http://www.wheelessonline.com/ortho/femoral_and_tibial_traction_pins. Accessed August 2011.

60 Scoring for Injury and Emergency Surgery

Edward Kwon and John Fildes

I. **INTRODUCTION.** Injury severity scoring in trauma plays many important roles in the management of the injured patient, beginning with quantifying injuries. This allows the stratification of patients based on the types of injuries and predicts the probability of survival based on severity of injury. These two main functions play a particularly important role in field triage, identification of patients who may require higher levels of care, and allocation of resources.

A. In addition, scoring systems play a valuable role in research allowing similarly injured patient populations to be compared. Scoring systems in trauma surgery are widely used in research and measurement of outcomes of the injured patient.

B. Scoring systems in emergency general surgery are not as well established as for trauma.

C. **Types of scoring systems.** Three major types of scoring systems are used to assess the severity of injury: Anatomic, physiologic, and combined. Anatomic scoring systems as suggested by the name, consider solely the anatomic characteristics of injuries for stratification, the best known of which include the Abbreviated Injury Scale (AIS), Injury Severity Score (ISS) and the individual organ injury scales. Physiologic scoring systems utilize various physiologic markers such as blood pressure, heart rate, and similar variables to assess severity including the Glasgow Coma Scale (GCS), Revised Trauma Score (RTS) and the Acute Physiology and Chronic Health Evaluation II Score (APACHE II). Combined scoring systems are a composite of anatomic and physiologic scoring systems utilized mainly to predict outcomes. Examples of combined systems include the Trauma and Injury Severity Score (TRISS) and "A Severity Characterization of Trauma (ASCOT)."

II. SCORING SYSTEMS IN INJURY AND TRAUMA

A. Anatomic scoring

1. **Abbreviated Injury Scale (AIS).** The AIS was developed in 1969 by a Joint Committee of the American Medical Association called the Society of Automotive Engineers and the Association for the Advancement of Automotive Medicine and has undergone several revisions, most recently in 2008. AIS is a consensus derived scale rather than a scoring system, which classifies injuries into six separate body regions including head/neck, face, thorax, abdomen/pelvis, extremities, and external structures. Injuries are then further stratified into types of injuries and assigned a score of 1 to 6 with 1 representing minimal injury and 6 a fatal injury (Table 60-1). The AIS is a useful descriptive tool to catalogue similar injuries rather than a predictive model, as there is no linear correlation between classified injuries and outcomes, and does not account for multiple injuries in a given patient.

2. **Injury Severity Score (ISS).** The ISS was proposed in 1974 to more accurately assess severity of injury by recognizing that patients who did not have similar injuries may still have similar overall injury severity based on multiple injuries. ISS is based on the AIS and calculated by the squaring of the highest AIS scores in the three most severely injured areas and adding the scores. An AIS score in any anatomical region of 6 automatically equates to an ISS of 75 and is considered fatal. A higher ISS score correlates with severity of injury and mortality. An ISS score between 1 and 8 (minor) is associated with a mortality of 1%; ISS 9 to 15 (moderate), a mortality of 2%; ISS 16 to 24 (severe), a mortality of 7%; and ISS

TABLE 60-1	General Categories of the Abbreviated Injury Scale

Abbreviated injury scale

Injury	Score
Minor	1
Moderate	2
Serious	3
Severe	4
Critical	5
Unsurvivable	6

>24 (very severe) a mortality of >30% (Table 60-2). The major limitations of the ISS are because it is based on the AIS; ISS does not account for multiple injuries in a given body region, underestimates severity and weighs all body regions equally. For example, an AIS injury of 5 in an extremity is equal to an AIS injury of 5 in the head although an extremity AIS of 5 is associated with a much lower mortality. Despite these limitations, the ISS is the most popular scoring system.

3. **New Injury Severity Score (NISS).** The NISS was created in 1997 to address the limitation of the ISS in its inability to account for more than one injury in a given anatomic region. NISS is calculated in the same manner to the ISS but uses the three highest AIS scores regardless of anatomic region, thus allowing for multiple injuries in a single anatomic region. The NISS has been found to have increased correlation with mortality compared to ISS. However, ISS remains the standard anatomic ISS.

4. **American Association for the Surgery of Trauma (AAST) Organ Injury Scale (OIS).** The OIS was developed in 1987 by a committee appointed by the AAST as a method to accurately describe and stratify the severity of injuries to individual organs (see the Injury Scales Appendix). The individual organ scales

TABLE 60-2	Case Fatality Rates by Injury Severity Score from the 2010 National Trauma Data Base

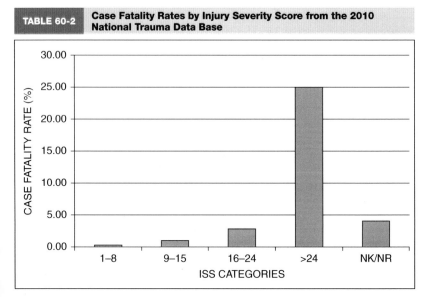

| TABLE 60-3 | Example of AAST OIS Score for Splenic Injury |

Grade[a]	Injury type	Description of injury	ICD-9	AIS-90
I	Hematoma	Subcapsular, <10% surface area	865.01 865.11	2
	Laceration	Capsular tear, <1 cm parenchymal depth	865.02 865.12	2
II	Hematoma	Subcapsular, 10–50% surface area Intraparenchymal, <5 cm in diameter	865.01 865.11	2
	Laceration	Capsular tear, 1–3 cm parenchymal depth that does not involve a trabecular vessel	865.02 865.12	2
III	Hematoma	Subcapsular, >50% surface area or expanding; ruptured subcapsular or parenchymal hematoma; intraparenchymal hematoma ≥5 cm or expanding		3
	Laceration	>3 cm parenchymal depth or involving trabecular vessels	865.03 865.13	3
IV	Laceration	Laceration involving segmental or hilar vessels producing major devascularization (>25% of spleen)		4
V	Laceration	Completely shattered spleen	865.04	5
	Vascular	Hilar vascular injury which devascularizes spleen	865.14	5

[a]Advance one grade for multiple injuries up to grade III.

were developed by literature examination and expert consensus. Individual organ injuries are given a score from 1 to 6 based on specified parameters; such as anatomic location within an organ, size of injury, laceration versus hematoma, and blunt versus penetrating, thereby reflecting severity (Table 60-3). The OIS score provides a common descriptive terminology for individual organ injuries based on severity making it particularly useful for clinical research, prognostication, and therapeutic planning as well as its wide acceptance.

5. **Anatomic profile (AP).** The AP was developed in 1990 to address the limitations of the ISS counting only injury to the single most severe injury in a given body region and the assignment of equal weights to injuries regardless of body region. The AP divides injuries into three different body regions including head/spine, neck/thorax, and other. All injuries within a given body region with an AIS >2 are then modified and weighted and used in an equation to calculate the AP score. Despite the increased sensitivity of the AP in comparison to the ISS in predicting mortality, it has not gained wide acceptance.

6. **International classification of diseases injury severity score (ICISS).** Proposed in 1996, the ICISS is a scoring system, which is based on ICD-9 codes rather than AIS scores. Survival risk ratios (SRR) are determined for each ICD-9 code utilizing trauma databases to identify the number of patients who survive each coded injury and dividing that number by the total number of patients with that particular injury. The product of all of the SRR for a given patient is then calculated to give the ICISS. The ICISS more accurately predicts survival and mortality compared to ISS and also has the advantage of requiring only the ICD-9 codes to calculate which is readily available as all hospitals utilize ICD-9 coding for reimbursement.

B. **Physiologic scoring**

1. **Glasgow Coma Scale (GCS).** Introduced in 1974, the GCS scoring system is one of the most widely used and accepted trauma scoring systems. The GCS score is used to stratify neurologic injury based on three clinical findings: Eye opening,

TABLE 60-4 **Glasgow Coma Scale**

Eye opening (4)	Spontaneous	4
	To voice	3
	To pain	2
	None	1
Verbal response (5)	Oriented	5
	Confused	4
	Inappropriate	3
	Incomprehensible	2
	None	1
Motor response (6)	Follows commands	6
	Localizes to pain	5
	Withdraws to pain	4
	Flexion (decorticate posturing)	3
	Extension (decerebrate posturing)	2
	None	1
Total GCS		3–15

verbal expression, and motor response. Each component is given a score based on the best response with a range of 1 to 4 for eye opening, 1 to 5 for verbal, and 1 to 6 for motor response to yield the sum overall GCS of 3 to 15 (Table 60-4). The GCS score allows the stratification of neurologic injury in a rapid and simple manner making it particularly useful for field and hospital triage, management decisions (intubation, intracranial pressure monitoring, and surgical decompression), as well as prognostication and research. While used outside neurotrauma, the GCS is not designed for other conditions and has an uneven utility in those settings.

2. **Trauma Score (TS) and Revised Trauma Score (RTS).** The trauma score was developed in 1981 in an effort to utilize physiologic parameters in the assessment of injury severity including respiratory rate, respiratory effort, systolic blood pressure, capillary refill, and GCS as its variables. The TS was then revised in 1989 to address the subjective components of the TS namely respiratory effort and capillary refill. The RTS is calculated utilizing the GCS, systolic blood pressure, and respiratory rate. Depending on the findings within each of these categories, a coded value is assigned to each category. The coded values are then assigned a weighted constant and summated to yield the RTS (Table 60-5). Notably, the RTS is heavily weighted with respect to the GCS score to account for neurologic injuries without multisystem injuries. Given the simplicity of calculation and good

TABLE 60-5 **Revised Trauma Score**

Glasgow coma scale (GCS)	Systolic blood pressure mm Hg (SBP)	Respiratory rate per minute (RR)	Coded value
13–15	>89	10–29	4
9–12	76–89	>29	3
6–8	50–75	6–9	2
4–5	1–49	1–5	1
3	0	0	0

RTS = 0.9368 GCS + 0.7326 SBP + 0.2908 RR.

correlation with probability for survival, the RTS is often used for triage decisions and is the most widely accepted of physiologic trauma scoring systems.

3. **Pediatric Trauma Score (PTS).** The PTS was proposed in 1981 as an RTS designed for the pediatric population. It utilizes six components: Weight, airway, systolic blood pressure, central nervous system, open wound, and skeletal injury. Each component is given a score with a range from -1 to $+2$ and all of the components are summated to give a final score range of -6 to $+12$. There is good correlation of decreasing PTS with increased mortality; PTS is useful for triage decisions.

C. **Combined scores**

1. **Trauma and Injury Severity Score (TRISS).** The TRISS was introduced in 1988 and combines elements of the ISS, RTS, patient age, and injury mechanism to calculate probability of survival. Calculation of the TRISS is complicated, as it relies on both the ISS and RTS, which are then multiplied by a coefficient determined from the Major Trauma Outcome Study and then finally derived by use of an equation accounting for age and mechanism. The complexity of its determination yields a high predictive value for survival. However, the cumbersome nature of it calculation limits it applicability to research and outcomes analysis. The TRISS may be particularly useful in quality improvement initiatives of trauma centers as it may be used to identify patients for peer review analysis based on deaths, which fall out of the predictive model.

2. **A Severity Characterization of Trauma (ASCOT).** ASCOT was created in 1990 to improve on the TRISS methodology by replacing the ISS with an anatomical profile similar to the AP, thereby removing the limitations of the ISS. The components of ASCOT include age, RTS, and an anatomic profile. Calculation of ASCOT is more complex than TRISS and most studies have attributed equivalent or minimal improvements to predictive value compared to TRISS leading to mixed acceptance of ASCOT.

III. **SCORING SYSTEMS IN EMERGENCY GENERAL SURGERY.** As mentioned previously, scoring systems for emergency general surgery have not been as well established as they have been for the field of trauma surgery. Ideally, a scoring system in emergency general surgery would accurately describe the severity of a surgical emergency with respect to anatomic location and the overall physiology of the patient. In considering emergency general surgery scoring systems as in trauma scoring, there appears to be two major categories: The anatomic or pathology specific and the physiologic systems. Listed below are some of the examples of such scoring systems useful in the field of emergency general surgery.

A. **Anatomic/pathology specific scores**

1. **Diverticulitis**

a. **Hinchey classification.** The Hinchey classification was proposed in 1978 and is the most commonly used system to describe the severity of diverticulitis. Initially used to describe findings at time of laparotomy and guide surgical management, it is currently used to classify diverticulitis based on CT scan findings. The classification ranges from stage 1 to stage 4 with increasing severity (Table 60-6). Although there is some controversy concerning the optimal

TABLE 60-6	Hinchey Classification for Diverticulitis

Stage	Description
I	Pericolic or mesenteric abscess
II	Walled off pelvic abscess
III	Generalized purulent peritonitis
IV	Generalized fecal peritonitis

TABLE 60-7	Pediatric Appendicitis Score (PAS)

Variable	Points
Cough/percussion/hopping tenderness in right lower quadrant of abdomen	2
Anorexia	1
Pyrexia	1
Nausea/emesis	1
Tenderness over right iliac fossa	2
Leukocytosis	1
Polymorphonuclear neutrophilia	1
Migration of pain	1
Total score	10

management of acute diverticulitis, the Hinchey stage is a useful guideline for management and is also predictive of perioperative complication.

2. **Appendicitis**

   a. **Alvarado score.** The Alvarado score was developed in 1988 to stratify patients in need of surgical intervention for acute appendicitis and decrease delays in treatment and negative appendectomy rates. The Alvarado score is calculated based on 6 history and clinical examination findings and 2 laboratory values with an emphasis on right lower quadrant tenderness and leukocytosis for a total of 10 points. The Alvarado score is not widely used.

   b. **Pediatric Appendicitis Score (PAS).** The PAS is a diagnostic scoring system similar to the Alvarado scoring system. It was developed in 2002 specifically for assessment of appendicitis in the pediatric population (age 4 to 15 years) to increase the accuracy of diagnosis of appendicitis and decrease the rates of non-therapeutic surgical interventions. The PAS is based on eight variables including history and physical examination findings and laboratory findings. Each variable is assigned a point based on correlation coefficients with acute appendicitis and the overall score is determined by the sum for a total possible of 10 (Table 60-7). A recent prospective validation of the PAS suggests that a score of ≤4 is highly unlikely to be acute appendicitis, a score of ≥8 is highly likely to be acute appendicitis, and score of 5 to 7 would benefit from additional studies and imaging.

3. **Cholecystitis**

   a. **Tokyo guidelines.** The Tokyo guidelines for severity assessment of acute cholecystitis were proposed in 2006 based on systematic review of the available literature and expert consensus opinion. The Tokyo guidelines were created as method to stratify the severity of disease and as a guide for optimal management. There are three grades in the Tokyo classification: Grade I—mild, grade II—moderate, and grade III—severe (Table 60-8). Grade I acute cholecystitis refers to the patient in whom cholecystectomy is a safe and low risk operative procedure in the acute phase. Grade II describes those patients in whom cholecystectomy may not be optimal in the acute phase, secondary to likely increased operative difficulty and who may benefit from a period of nonoperative management followed by interval cholecystectomy. Grade III describes the patient who will require intensive care and urgent treatment (operation or drainage) despite operative risks. The Tokyo severity assessment of acute cholecystitis serves as a useful guideline for the optimal timing of management of acute cholecystitis, however awaits further study for validation.

4. **Pancreatitis**

   a. **Ranson's criteria.** Ranson's score or Ranson's criteria proposed in 1974 is the best known scoring system for acute pancreatitis. Initially designed to stratify the severity of acute pancreatitis mainly in alcohol-induced pancreatitis, the

TABLE 60-8	Tokyo Classification for Severity Assessment of Acute Cholecystitis

Grade	Criteria
I—mild	Acute cholecystitis that does not meet criteria for grade II or III. Acute cholecystitis in the otherwise healthy patient with no organ dysfunction and only mild inflammatory changes in the gallbladder.
II—moderate	The presence of any one of the following criteria: **1.** Elevated WBC ($>18,000/mm^3$) **2.** Palpable tender mass in the right upper quadrant **3.** Duration of complaints >72 h **4.** Marked local inflammation (biliary peritonitis, pericholecystic abscess, hepatic abscess, gangrenous cholecystitis, emphysematous cholecystitis)
III—severe	The presence of any one of the following criteria: **1.** Cardiovascular dysfunction (hypotension requiring treatment with dopamine ≥ 5 μg/kg/min, or any dose of dobutamine) **2.** Neurologic dysfunction (decreased level of consciousness) **3.** Respiratory dysfunction (PaO_2/FiO_2 ratio <300) **4.** Renal dysfunction (oliguria, creatinine >2.0 mg/dL) **5.** Hepatic dysfunction (INR >1.5) **6.** Hematologic dysfunction (platelet count $<100,000/mm^3$)

criteria were modified 8 years later to include gallstone pancreatitis. Ranson's score remains in wide use today for the assessment of acute pancreatitis regardless of etiology. Ranson's criteria consist of 11 signs within the initial 48 hours of presentation which have prognostic significance (Table 60-9). Each of the 11 signs is assigned 0 or 1 point for a total possible score of 11. A score <3 implies less severe acute pancreatitis and corresponds to a mortality of $\sim 1\%$ while a score >3 implies severe pancreatitis and corresponds to a mortality of $\sim 15\%$ for a score of 3 to 4, 50% for 5 to 6, and 100% for >6. There are limitations to Ranson's criteria including a requisite 48 hours for completion of scoring and a relatively modest positive predictive value. However, it remains

TABLE 60-9	Ranson's Criteria for Acute Pancreatitis

	Non gallstone pancreatitis	Gallstone pancreatitis
Admission	Age >55 y WBC $>16,000/mm^3$ Blood glucose >200 mg/dL Serum lactate dehydrogenase >350 IU/L Serum aspartate aminotransferase >250 IU/L	Age >70 y WBC $>18,000/mm^3$ Blood glucose >220 mg/dL Serum lactate dehydrogenase >400 IU/L Serum aspartate aminotransferase >250 IU/L
Initial 48 h	Hematocrit decrease $>10\%$ Blood urea nitrogen increase >5 mg/dL Serum calcium <8 mg/dL $PaO_2 <60$ mm Hg Serum base deficit >4 mEq/L Fluid sequestration >6 L	Hematocrit decrease $>10\%$ Blood urea nitrogen increase >2 mg/dL Serum calcium <8 mg/dL NA Serum base deficit >5 mEq/L Fluid sequestration >4 L

TABLE 60-10 CT Severity Index for Acute Pancreatitis (Balthazar Score)

Balthazar grade	CT findings	Point(s)
A	Normal CT	0
B	Focal or diffuse enlargement of pancreas	1
C	Pancreatic gland abnormalities and peripancreatic inflammation	2
D	Single ill-defined fluid collection or phlegmon	3
E	$\geq$2 poorly defined collections or presence of gas in or adjacent to pancreas	4
Degree of necrosis		Additional points
0		0
$\leq$30%		2
30–50%		4
>50%		6

a widely used tool for both triage and prognostication of the patient with acute pancreatitis.

  b. **CT severity index for pancreatitis (Balthazar score).** The Balthazar score for acute pancreatitis was proposed in 1985 as a severity index for acute pancreatitis based on initial CT findings. The CT severity index or Balthazar score is based on a point system assigned from the Balthazar grade of pancreatitis and the degree of necrosis (Table 60-10). An increasing CT severity index has been shown to be associated with increasing morbidity and mortality in acute pancreatitis: CT severity index of 0 to 1 is associated with 0% morbidity and mortality, 2 is associated with 0% mortality and 4% morbidity, and 7 to 10 is associated with 17% mortality and 92% morbidity. The CT severity index has been suggested to be a more accurate prognostic tool than Ranson's criteria in acute pancreatitis. However, as it requires CT scan with intravenous contrast, its utility may be best limited to those cases with a high suspicion for severe acute pancreatitis.

5. **Necrotizing soft tissue infections**
    a. **Necrotizing soft tissue infection (NSTI) clinical score.** The NSTI clinical score was proposed in 2009 as a method to categorize the severity of necrotizing soft tissue infections and identify patients at high risk for mortality at the time of presentation. The NTSI score consists of 3 major and 3 minor variables which were found to be independent predictors of mortality. Each of the minor variables is assigned a single point and the major variables 3 points (Table 60-11). Based on the total score, the severity of the NSTI is assigned to a group which is stratified according to risk of mortality: Group 1 consists of 0 to 2 points and is associated with ~6% mortality, group 2 consists of

TABLE 60-11 Necrotizing Soft Tissue Infection Clinical Score (NSTI Score)

Variable (on admission)	Points
Heart rate >110/min	1
Temperature <36°C	1
Serum creatinine >1.5 mg/dL	1
Age >50 y	3
WBC >40,000/mm^3	3
Hematocrit >50%	3

3 to 5 points and is associated with ~24% mortality and group 3 consists of ≥6 points and is associated with ~88% mortality. The NTSI clinical scoring system is a useful method of severity assessment based on readily available physiologic parameters at admission which can be used to guide triage, management options, as well as for comparison across institutions for research purposes.

B. **Physiologic scores.** Unlike scoring systems in the field of trauma, there are no specific physiologic scoring systems for emergency general surgery. The most often used physiologic scores for emergency general surgery utilize general physiologic scores such as the Acute Physiology and Chronic Health Evaluation (APACHE) and Systemic Inflammatory Response Syndrome Score (SIRS Score). Listed below are brief descriptions of some of these two common physiologic scoring systems.

1. **Acute Physiology and Chronic Health Evaluation II (APACHE II).** The APACHE II score was proposed in 1985 as a severity of disease measure for adult patients admitted to the intensive care unit. The APACHE II scoring system is a modification of the original APACHE score, which assessed severity of disease based on 34 physiologic variables, whereas APACHE II utilizes 12 variables and also considers age and chronic health problems. The variables included in the calculation of the APACHE II score include: Temperature, mean arterial blood pressure, heart rate, respiratory rate, oxygenation (PaO_2), arterial pH, serum sodium, serum potassium, serum creatinine, hematocrit, white blood cell (WBC) count, and GCS. Depending on the value of each variable, a point of 1 to 4 is assigned. Additional points are given for increasing age, chronic health problems, and emergency versus elective postoperative patients. The points are then summed to yield the APACHE II score, which correlates with an increase in mortality as the score increases. There are numerous websites that contain convenient calculators for the computation of the APACHE II score and predicted mortality. Although the APACHE II score was initially designed for patients on admission to the ICU, it has been found to be a useful marker of overall physiologic impairment. In the realm of emergency general surgery, the APACHE II score is validated as a tool for risk stratification of patients undergoing emergency surgery, when the APACHE II score is calculated prior to surgical intervention. APACHE II has also been found useful as a guide for emergent surgical treatment such as pancreatitis and perforated peptic ulcer. There has been an additional modification to the APACHE scoring system in APACHE III; however, APACHE II appears to be favored at the current time despite various criticisms of, underestimation or overestimation of mortality.

2. **Systemic Inflammatory Response Syndrome score (SIRS score).** The SIRS score proposed in 1992 with the definition of a systemic inflammatory response syndrome at the American College of Chest Physicians/Society of Critical Care Medicine consensus conference is a method to assess the overall physiologic derangement of a given patient. The SIRS score utilizes four parameters: Temperature, heart rate, respiratory rate, and white blood cell count. Each parameter is assigned 1 point for a total possible score of 4 (Table 60-12). The presence of SIRS, defined as the presence of ≥2 of the parameters included in the SIRS

TABLE 60-12	Systemic Inflammatory Response Syndrome Score (SIRS Score)
Variable	**Points**
Temperature >38°C or <36°C	1
Heart rate >90 beats/min	1
Respiratory rate >20 breaths/min, $PaCO_2$ <32 mm Hg	1
White blood cell count >12,000/mm³, <4000/mm³, or ≥10% bands	1
Total score	0–4

score has been shown to be a predictor of increased mortality in the acutely ill patient. In critical surgical patients including trauma patients, the SIRS score has also been demonstrated to be a useful predictor of outcome. Within the initial 24 hours of surgery, the SIRS score has been shown to overestimate the inflammatory response secondary to the various physiologic insults of surgery. After the initial 24 hours of ICU resuscitation, the SIRS score decreases and a persistently elevated SIRS score after 24 hours correlates with increased mortality and multiple organ dysfunction. The SIRS score is a convenient method to identify patients at high risk for multiple organ dysfunction and a poor outcome. The limitation is that some patient have systemic inflammation or infection but only one – albeit often marked – SIRS criterion.

AXIOMS

- Scoring systems in trauma and emergency general surgery allow comparisons of patients with similar injuries/pathology across systems and institutions, making it particularly useful for measuring outcomes and quality improvement.
- Clinically severity scoring can be useful for triage, the allocation of resources, and as a guide for therapeutic intervention.
- There are numerous scoring systems available in the field of trauma surgery designed for different purposes and selection of an individual scoring system is dependent upon the information sought.
- Emergency general surgery is an evolving specialty and the development of scoring systems specific to this specialty is a useful and important endeavor to provide standardized and uniform care.

Suggested Readings

Anaya DA, Bulger EM, Kwon YS, et al. Predicting death in necrotizing soft tissue infections: a clinical score. *Surg Infect (Larchmt)* 2009;10(6):517–522.

Baker SP, O'Neill B, Haddon W, et al. The injury severity score: a method for describing patients with multiple injuries and evaluating emergency care. *J Trauma* 1974;14(3):187–196.

Balthazar EJ, Robinson DL, Megibow AJ, et al. Acute pancreatitis: value of CT in establishing prognosis. *Radiology* 1990;174:331–336.

Bhatt M, Joseph L, Ducharme F, et al. Prospective validation of the pediatric appendicitis score in a Canadian pediatric emergency department. *Acad Emerg Med* 2009;16(7):591–596.

Bone RC, Balk RA, Cerra FB, et al. Definitions for sepsis and organ failure, and guidelines for the use of innovative therapies in sepsis. The ACCP/SCCM Consensus Conference Committee. American College of Chest Physicians/Society of Critical Care Medicine. *Chest* 1992;136(5 Suppl):e28.

Boyd CR, Tolson MA, Copes WS. Evaluating trauma care: the TRISS method. Trauma Score and the Injury Severity Score. *J Trauma* 1987;27:370–378.

Champion HR, Copes WS, Sacco WJ, et al. Improved predictions from a severity characterization of trauma (ASCOT) over trauma and injury severity score (TRISS): results of an independent evaluation. *J Trauma* 1996;40(1):42–48; discussion 48–49.

Champion HR, Sacco WJ, Carnazzo AJ, et al. Trauma score. *Crit Care Med* 1981;9(9):672–676.

Champion HR, Sacco WJ, Copes WS, et al. A revision of the trauma score. *J Trauma* 1989;29(5):623–629.

Dierking BH, Ramenofsky ML. The pediatric trauma score: an effective method of field triage. *JEMS* 1988;13(5):70–72.

Hinchey EJ, Schaal PG, Richards GK. Treatment of perforated diverticular disease of the colon. *Adv Surg* 1978;12:85–109.

Hirota M, Takada T, Kawarada Y, et al. Diagnostic criteria and severity assessment of acute cholecystitis: Tokyo Guidelines. *J Hepatobiliary Pancreat Surg* 2007;14(1):78–82.

Knaus WA, Draper EA, Wagner DP, et al. Apache II: A severity of disease classification system. *Crit Care Med* 1985;13(10):818–829.

Osler T, Rutledge R, Deis J, et al. ICISS: an international classification of disease-9 based injury severity score. *J Trauma* 1996;41(3):380–386; discussion 286–288.

Ranson JH, Rifkind RM, Roses DF. Prognostic signs and the role of operative management in acute pancreatitis. *Surg Gynecol Obstet* 1974;139(1):69–81.

Sasser SM, Hunt RC, Sullivent EE, et al. Guidelines for Field Triage of Injured Patients: Recommendations of the National Expert Panel on Field Triage. *MMWR Recomm Rep.* 2009;58(RR-1):1–35.

Teasdale G, Jennett B. Assessment of coma and impaired consciousness: a practical scale. *Lancet* 1974;2(7872):81–84.

APPENDIX A

Injury Scales

TABLE A-1 Cervical Vascular Organ Injury Scale

Grade	Description of injury	AIS-90
I	Thyroid vein	1–3
	Common facial vein	1–3
	External jugular vein	1–3
	Non-named arterial/venous branches	1–3
II	External carotid arterial branches (ascending pharyngeal, superior thyroid, lingual, facial maxillary, occipital, posterior auricular)	1–3
	Thyrocervical trunk or primary branches	1–3
	Internal jugular vein	1–3
III	External carotid artery	2–3
	Subclavian vein	3–4
	Vertebral artery	2–4
IV	Common carotid artery	3–5
	Subclavian artery	3–4
V	Internal carotid artery (extracranial)	3–5

[a]Increase one grade for multiple grade III or IV injuries involving more than 50% vessel circumference. Decrease one grade for less than 25% vessel circumference disruption for grade IV or V.

TABLE A-2 Chest Wall Injury Scale[a]

Grade	Injury type	Description of injury	AIS-90
I	Contusion	Any size	1
	Laceration	Skin and subcutaneous	1
	Fracture	<3 ribs, closed; non-displaced clavicle closed	1–2
II	Laceration	Skin, subcutaneous and muscle	1
	Fracture	≥3 adjacent ribs, closed	2–3
		Open or displaced clavicle	2
		Non-displaced sternum, closed	2
		Scapular body, open or closed	2
III	Laceration	Full thickness including pleural penetration	2
	Fracture	Open or displaced sternum	2
		Flail sternum	2
		Unilateral flail segment (<3 ribs)	3–4
IV	Laceration	Avulsion of chest wall tissues with underlying rib fractures	4
	Fracture	Unilateral flail chest (≥3 ribs)	3–4
V	Fracture	Bilateral flail chest (≥3 ribs on both sides)	5

[a]This scale is confined to the chest wall alone and does not reflect associated internal or abdominal injuries. Therefore, further delineation of upper versus lower or anterior versus posterior chest wall was not considered, and a grade VI was not warranted. Specifically, thoracic crush was not used as a descriptive term; instead, the geography and extent of fractures and soft tissue injury were used to define the grade.

TABLE A-3   Heart Injury Scale

Grade	Description of injury	AIS-90
I	Blunt cardiac injury with minor ECG abnormality (nonspecific ST or T wave changes, premature atrial or ventricular contraction or persistent sinus tachycardia)	3
	Blunt or penetrating pericardial wound without cardiac injury, cardiac tamponade, or cardiac herniation	
II	Blunt cardiac injury with heart block (right or left bundle branch, left anterior fascicular, or atrioventricular) or ischemic changes (ST depression or T wave inversion) without cardiac failure	3
	Penetrating tangential myocardial wound up to, but not extending through, endocardium, without tamponade	3
III	Blunt cardiac injury with sustained ($\geq$6 beats/min) or multifocal ventricular contractions	3–4
	Blunt or penetrating cardiac injury with septal rupture, pulmonary or tricuspid valvular incompetence, papillary muscle dysfunction, or distal coronary arterial occlusion without cardiac failure	3–4
	Blunt pericardial laceration with cardiac herniation	
	Blunt cardiac injury with cardiac failure	3–4
IV	Penetrating tangential myocardial wound up to, but extending through, endocardium, with tamponade	3
	Blunt or penetrating cardiac injury with septal rupture, pulmonary or tricuspid valvular incompetence, papillary muscle dysfunction, or distal coronary arterial occlusion producing cardiac failure	3
	Blunt or penetrating cardiac injury with aortic, mitral valve incompetence	
	Blunt or penetrating cardiac injury of the right ventricle, right atrium, or left atrium	5
	Blunt or penetrating cardiac injury with proximal coronary arterial occlusion	5
	Blunt or penetrating left ventricular perforation	5
	Stellate wound with <50% tissue loss of the right ventricle, right atrium, or of left atrium	5
V	Blunt avulsion of the heart; penetrating wound producing >50% tissue loss of a chamber	6

[a]Advance one grade for multiple wounds to a single chamber or multiple chamber involvement.

TABLE A-4   Lung Injury Scale

Grade[a]	Injury type	Description of injury	AIS-90
I	Contusion	Unilateral, <1 lobe	3
II	Contusion	Unilateral, single lobe	3
	Laceration	Simple pneumothorax	3
III	Contusion	Unilateral, >1 lobe	3
	Laceration	Persistent (>72 h) air leak from distal airway	3–4
	Hematoma	Nonexpanding intraparenchymal	
IV	Laceration	Major (segmental or lobar) air leak	4–5
	Hematoma	Expanding intraparenchymal	
	Vascular	Primary branch intrapulmonary vessel disruption	3–5
V	Vascular	Hilar vessel disruption	4
VI	Vascular	Total uncontained transection of pulmonary hilum	4

[a]Advance one grade for bilateral injuries up to grade III. Hemothorax is scored under thoracic vascular injury scale.

TABLE A-5	**Thoracic Vascular Injury Scale**

Grade[a]	Description of injury	AIS-90
I	Intercostal artery/vein	2–3
	Internal mammary artery/vein	2–3
	Bronchial artery/vein	2–3
	Esophageal artery/vein	2–3
	Hemizygous vein	2–3
	Unnamed artery/vein	2–3
II	Azygos vein	2–3
	Internal jugular vein	2–3
	Subclavian vein	3–4
	Innominate vein	3–4
III	Carotid artery	3–5
	Innominate artery	3–4
	Subclavian artery	3–4
IV	Thoracic aorta, descending	4–5
	Inferior vena cava (intrathoracic)	3–4
	Pulmonary artery, primary intraparenchymal branch	3
	Pulmonary vein, primary intraparenchymal branch	3
V	Thoracic aorta, ascending and arch	5
	Superior vena cava	3–4
	Pulmonary artery, main trunk	4
	Pulmonary vein, main trunk	4
VI	Uncontained total transection of thoracic aorta or pulmonary hilum	5

[a]Increase one grade for multiple grade III or IV injuries if more than 50% circumference; decrease one grade for grade IV injuries if less than 25% circumference.

TABLE A-6	**Diaphragm Injury Scale**

Grade[a]	Description of injury	AIS-90
I	Contusion	2
II	Laceration <2 cm	3
III	Laceration 2–10 cm	3
IV	Laceration >10 cm with tissue loss ≤25 cm^2	3
V	Laceration with tissue loss >25 cm^2	3

[a]Advance one grade for bilateral injuries up to grade III.

TABLE A-7   Spleen Injury Scale (1994 revision)

Grade[a]	Injury type	Description of injury	AIS-90
I	Hematoma	Subcapsular, <10% surface area	2
	Laceration	Capsular tear, <1 cm parenchymal depth	2
II	Hematoma	Subcapsular, 10%–50% surface area intraparenchymal, <5 cm in diameter	2
	Laceration	Capsular tear, 1–3 cm parenchymal depth that does not involve a trabecular vessel	2
III	Hematoma	Subcapsular, >50% surface area or expanding; ruptured subcapsular or parenchymal hematoma; intraparenchymal hematoma ≥5 cm or expanding	3
	Laceration	>3 cm parenchymal depth or involving trabecular vessels	3
IV	Laceration	Laceration involving segmental or hilar vessels producing major devascularization (>25% of spleen)	4
V	Laceration	Completely shattered spleen	5
	Vascular	Hilar vascular injury with devascularized spleen	5

[a]Advance one grade for multiple injuries up to grade III.

TABLE A-8   Liver Injury Scale (1994 revision)

Grade[a]	Type of injury	Description of injury	AIS-90
I	Hematoma	Subcapsular, <10% surface area	2
	Laceration	Capsular tear, <1 cm parenchymal depth	2
II	Hematoma	Subcapsular, 10%–50% surface area intraparenchymal <10 cm in diameter	2
	Laceration	Capsular tear 1–3 cm parenchymal depth, <10 cm in length	2
III	Hematoma	Subcapsular, >50% surface area of ruptured subcapsular of parenchymal hematoma; intraparenchymal hematoma >10 cm or expanding	3
	Laceration	>3 cm parenchymal depth	3
IV	Laceration	Parenchymal disruption involving 25%–75% hepatic lobe or 1–3 Couinaud's segments	4
V	Laceration	Parenchymal disruption involving >75% of hepatic lobe or >3 Couinaud's segments within a single lobe	5
	Vascular	Juxtahepatic venous injuries; i.e., retrohepatic vena cava/central major hepatic veins	5
VI	Vascular	Hepatic avulsion	6

[a]Advance one grade for multiple injuries up to grade III.

TABLE A-9   Extrahepatic Biliary Tree Injury Scale

Grade[a]	Description of injury	AIS-90
I	Gallbladder contusion/hematoma	2
	Portal triad contusion	2
II	Partial gallbladder avulsion from liver bed; cystic duct intact	2
	Laceration or perforation of the gallbladder	2
III	Complete gallbladder avulsion from liver bed	3
	Cystic duct laceration	3
IV	Partial or complete right hepatic duct laceration	3
	Partial or complete left hepatic duct laceration	3
	Partial common hepatic duct laceration (<50%)	3
	Partial common bile duct laceration (<50%)	3
V	>50% transection of common hepatic duct	3–4
	>50% transection of common bile duct	3–4
	Combined right and left hepatic duct injuries	3–4
	Intraduodenal or intrapancreatic bile duct injuries	3–4

[a]Advance one grade for multiple injuries up to grade III.

TABLE A-10   Pancreas Injury Scale

Grade[a]	Type of injury	Description of injury	AIS-90
I	Hematoma	Minor contusion without duct injury	2
	Laceration	Superficial laceration without duct injury	2
II	Hematoma	Major contusion without duct injury or tissue loss	2
	Laceration	Major laceration without duct injury or tissue loss	3
III	Laceration	Distal transection or parenchymal injury with duct injury	3
IV	Laceration	Proximal transection or parenchymal injury involving ampulla[b]	4
V	Laceration	Massive disruption of pancreatic head	5

[a]Advance one grade for multiple injuries up to grade III.
[b]—head; —body; —tail. Proximal pancreas is to the patients' right of the superior mesenteric vein.

TABLE A-11   Esophagus Injury Scale

Grade[a]	Description of injury	AIS-90
I	Contusion/hematoma	2
	Partial thickness laceration	3
II	Laceration <50% circumference	4
III	Laceration >50% circumference	4
IV	Segmental loss or devascularization <2 cm	5
V	Segmental loss or devascularization >2 cm	5

[a]Advance one grade for multiple lesions up to grade III.

TABLE A-12 Stomach Injury Scale

Grade[a]	Description of injury	AIS-90
I	Contusion/hematoma	2
	Partial thickness laceration	2
II	Laceration <2 cm in GE junction or pylorus	3
	<5 cm in proximal 1/3 stomach	3
	<10 cm in distal 2/3 stomach	3
III	Laceration >2 cm in GE junction or pylorus	3
	>5 cm in proximal 1/3 stomach	3
	>10 cm in distal 2/3 stomach	3
IV	Tissue loss or devascularization <2/3 stomach	4
V	Tissue loss or devascularization >2/3 stomach	4

[a]Advance one grade for multiple lesions up to grade III.
GE, gastroesophageal.

TABLE A-13 Duodenum Injury Scale

Grade[a]	Type of injury	Description of injury	AIS-90
I	Hematoma	Involving single portion of duodenum	2
	Laceration	Partial thickness, no perforation	3
II	Hematoma	Involving more than one portion	2
	Laceration	Disruption <50% of circumference	4
III	Laceration	Disruption 50%–75% of circumference of D2	4
		Disruption 50%–100% of circumference of D1, D3, D4	4
IV	Laceration	Disruption >75% of circumference of D2	5
		Involving ampulla or distal common bile duct	5
V	Laceration	Massive disruption of duodenopancreatic complex	5
	Vascular	Devascularization of duodenum	5

[a]Advance one grade for multiple injuries up to grade III.
D1, first portion of duodenum; D2, second portion of duodenum; D3, third portion of duodenum; D4, fourth portion of duodenum.

TABLE A-14 Small Bowel Injury Scale

Grade[a]	Type of injury	Description of injury	AIS-90
I	Hematoma	Contusion or hematoma without devascularization	2
	Laceration	Partial thickness, no perforation	2
II	Laceration	Laceration <50% of circumference	3
III	Laceration	Laceration ≥50% of circumference without transection	3
IV	Laceration	Transection of the small bowel	4
V	Laceration	Transection of the small bowel with segmental tissue loss	4
	Vascular	Devascularized segment	4

[a]Advance one grade for multiple injuries up to grade III.

TABLE A-15	Colon Injury Scale

Grade[a]	Type of injury	Description of injury	AIS-90
I	Hematoma	Contusion or hematoma without devascularization	2
	Laceration	Partial thickness, no perforation	2
II	Laceration	Laceration <50% of circumference	3
III	Laceration	Laceration ≥50% of circumference without transection	3
IV	Laceration	Transection of the colon	4
V	Laceration	Transection of the colon with segmental tissue loss	4
	Vascular	Devascularized segment	4

[a]Advance one grade for multiple injuries up to grade III.

TABLE A-16	Rectum Injury Scale

Grade[a]	Type of injury	Description of injury	AIS-90
I	Hematoma	Contusion or hematoma without devascularization	2
	Laceration	Partial-thickness laceration	2
II	Laceration	Laceration <50% of circumference	3
III	Laceration	Laceration ≥50% of circumference	4
IV	Laceration	Full-thickness laceration with extension into the perineum	5
V	Vascular	Devascularized segment	5

[a]Advance one grade for multiple injuries up to grade III.

TABLE A-17	Abdominal Vascular Injury Scale

Grade[a]	Description of injury	AIS-90
I	Non-named superior mesenteric artery or superior mesenteric vein branches	NS
	Non-named inferior mesenteric artery or inferior mesenteric vein branches	NS
	Phrenic artery or vein	NS
	Lumbar artery or vein	NS
	Gonadal artery or vein	NS
	Ovarian artery or vein	NS
	Other non-named small arterial or venous structures requiring ligation	NS
II	Right, left, or common hepatic artery	3
	Splenic artery or vein	3
	Right or left gastric arteries	3
	Gastroduodenal artery	3
	Inferior mesenteric artery, or inferior mesenteric vein, trunk	3
	Primary named branches of mesenteric artery (e.g., ileocolic artery) or mesenteric vein	3
	Other named abdominal vessels requiring ligation or repair	3

(continued)

Abdominal Vascular Injury Scale (*Continued*)

Grade[a]	Description of injury	AIS-90
III	Superior mesenteric vein, trunk	3
	Renal artery or vein	3
	Iliac artery or vein	3
	Hypogastric artery or vein	3
	Vena cava, infrarenal	3
IV	Superior mesenteric artery, trunk	3
	Celiac axis proper	3
	Vena cava, suprarenal and infrahepatic	3
	Aorta, infrarenal	4
V	Portal vein	3
	Extraparenchymal hepatic vein	3 (hepatic vein) 5 (liver + veins)
	Vena cava, retrohepatic or suprahepatic	5
	Aorta suprarenal, subdiaphragmatic	4

[a]This classification system is applicable to extraparenchymal vascular injuries. If the vessel injury is within 2 cm of the organ parenchyma, refer to specific organ injury scale. Increase one grade for multiple grade III or IV injuries involving >50% vessel circumference. Downgrade one grade if <25% vessel circumference laceration for grades IV or V.
NS, not scored.

TABLE A-18 **Adrenal Organ Injury Scale**

Grade[a]	Description of injury	AIS-90
I	Contusion	1
II	Laceration involving only cortex (<2 cm)	1
III	Laceration extending into medulla (≥2 cm)	2
IV	>50% parenchymal destruction	2
V	Total parenchymal destruction (including massive intraparenchymal hemorrhage)	3
	Avulsion from blood supply	3

[a]Advance one grade for bilateral lesions up to grade V.

TABLE A-19 **Kidney Injury Scale**

Grade[a]	Type of injury	Description of injury	AIS-90
I	Contusion	Microscopic or gross hematuria, urologic studies normal	2
	Hematoma	Subcapsular, nonexpanding without parenchymal laceration	2
II	Hematoma	Non-expanding perirenal hematoma confined to renal retroperitoneum	2
	Laceration	<1 cm parenchymal depth of renal cortex without urinary extravasation	2
III	Laceration	>1 cm parenchymal depth of renal cortex without collecting system rupture or urinary extravasation	3
IV	Laceration	Parenchymal laceration extending through renal cortex, medulla, and collecting system	4
	Vascular	Main renal artery or vein injury with contained hemorrhage	4
V	Laceration	Completely shattered kidney	5
	Vascular	Avulsion of renal hilum which devascularizes kidney	5

[a]Advance one grade for bilateral injuries up to grade III.

TABLE A-20   Ureter Injury Scale

Grade[a]	Type of injury	Description of injury	AIS-90
I	Hematoma	Contusion or hematoma without devascularization	2
II	Laceration	<50% transection	2
III	Laceration	≥50% transection	3
IV	Laceration	Complete transection with <2 cm devascularization	3
V	Laceration	Avulsion with >2 cm of devascularization	3

[a]Advance one grade for bilateral up to grade III.

TABLE A-21   Bladder Injury Scale

Grade[a]	Injury type	Description of injury	AIS-90
I	Hematoma	Contusion, intramural hematoma	2
	Laceration	Partial thickness	3
II	Laceration	Extraperitoneal bladder wall laceration <2 cm	4
III	Laceration	Extraperitoneal (≥2 cm) or intraperitoneal (<2 cm) bladder wall laceration	4
IV	Laceration	Intraperitoneal bladder wall laceration ≥2 cm	4
V	Laceration	Intraperitoneal or extraperitoneal bladder wall laceration extending into the bladder neck or ureteral orifice (trigone)	4

[a]Advance one grade for multiple lesions up to grade III.

TABLE A-22   Urethra Injury Scale

Grade[a]	Injury type	Description of injury	AIS-90
I	Contusion	Blood at urethral meatus; urethrography normal	2
II	Stretch injury	Elongation of urethra without extravasation on urethrography	2
III	Partial disruption	Extravasation of urethrography contrast at injury site with visualization in the bladder	2
IV	Complete disruption	Extravasation of urethrography contrast at injury site without visualization in the bladder; <2 cm of urethra separation	3
V	Complete disruption	Complete transection with ≥2 cm urethral separation, or extension into the prostate or vagina	4

[a]Advance one grade for bilateral injuries up to grade III.

TABLE A-23	Uterus (nonpregnant) Injury Scale

Grade[a]	Description of injury	AIS-90
I	Contusion/hematoma	2
II	Superficial laceration (<1 cm)	2
III	Deep laceration (≥1 cm)	3
IV	Laceration involving uterine artery	3
V	Avulsion/devascularization	3

[a]Advance one grade for multiple injuries up to grade III.

TABLE A-24	Uterus (pregnant) Injury Scale

Grade[a]	Description of injury	AIS-90
I	Contusion or hematoma (without placental abruption)	2
II	Superficial laceration (<1 cm) or partial placental abruption <25%	3
III	Deep laceration (≥1 cm) occurring in second trimester or placental abruption >25% but <50%	3
	Deep laceration (≥1 cm) in third trimester	4
IV	Laceration involving uterine artery	4
	Deep laceration (≥1 cm) with >50% placental abruption	4
V	Uterine rupture	
	Second trimester	4
	Third trimester	5
	Complete placental abruption	4–5

[a]Advance one grade for multiple injuries up to grade III.

TABLE A-25	Fallopian Tube Injury Scale

Grade[a]	Description of injury	AIS-90
I	Hematoma or contusion	2
II	Laceration <50% circumference	2
III	Laceration ≥50% circumference	2
IV	Transection	2
V	Vascular injury; devascularized segment	2

[a]Advance one grade for bilateral injuries up to grade III.

TABLE A-26	Ovary Injury Scale	
Grade[a]	Description of injury	AIS-90
I	Contusion or hematoma	1
II	Superficial laceration (depth <0.5 cm)	2
III	Deep laceration (depth ≥0.5 cm)	3
IV	Partial disruption of blood supply	3
V	Avulsion or complete parenchymal destruction	3
[a]Advance one grade for bilateral injuries up to grade III.		

TABLE A-27	Vagina Injury Scale	
Grade[a]	Description of injury	AIS-90
I	Contusion or hematoma	1
II	Laceration, superficial (mucosa only)	1
III	Laceration, deep into fat or muscle	2
IV	Laceration, complex, into cervix or peritoneum	3
V	Injury into adjacent organs (anus, rectum, urethra, bladder)	3
[a]Advance one grade for multiple injuries up to grade III.		

TABLE A-28	Vulva Injury Scale	
Grade[a]	Description of injury	AIS-90
I	Contusion or hematoma	1
II	Laceration, superficial (skin only)	1
III	Laceration, deep (into fat or muscle)	2
IV	Avulsion; skin, fat or muscle	3
V	Injury into adjacent organs (anus, rectum, urethra, bladder)	3
[a]Advance one grade for multiple injuries up to grade III.		

TABLE A-29	Testis Injury Scale	
Grade[a]	Description of injury	AIS-90
I	Contusion/hematoma	1
II	Subclinical laceration of tunica albuginea	1
III	Laceration of tunica albuginea with <50% parenchymal loss	2
IV	Major laceration of tunica albuginea with ≥50% parenchymal loss	2
V	Total testicular destruction or avulsion	2
[a]Advance one grade for bilateral lesions up to grade V.		

TABLE A-30   Scrotum Injury Scale

Grade	Description of injury	AIS-90
I	Contusion	1
II	Laceration <25% of scrotal diameter	1
III	Laceration ≥25% of scrotal diameter	2
IV	Avulsion <50%	2
V	Avulsion ≥50%	2

TABLE A-31   Penis Injury Scale

Grade[a]	Description of injury	AIS-90
I	Cutaneous laceration/contusion	1
II	Buck's fascia (cavernosum) laceration without tissue loss	1
III	Cutaneous avulsion	3
	Laceration through glans/meatus	3
	Cavernosal or urethral defect <2 cm	3
IV	Partial penectomy	3
	Cavernosal or urethral defect ≥2 cm	3
V	Total penectomy	3

[a]Advance one grade for multiple injuries up to grade III.

TABLE A-32   Peripheral Vascular Organ Injury Scale

Grade[a]	Description of injury	AIS-90
I	Digital artery/vein	1–3
	Palmar artery/vein	1–3
	Deep palmar artery/vein	1–3
	Dorsalis pedis artery	1–3
	Plantar artery/vein	1–3
	Non-named arterial/venous branches	1–3
II	Basilic/cephalic vein	1–3
	Saphenous vein	1–3
	Radial artery	1–3
	Ulnar artery	1–3
III	Axillary vein	2–3
	Superficial/deep femoral vein	2–3
	Popliteal vein	2–3
	Brachial artery	2–3
	Anterior tibial artery	1–3
	Posterior tibial artery	1–3
	Peroneal artery	1–3
	Tibioperoneal trunk	2–3
IV	Superficial/deep femoral artery	3–4
	Popliteal artery	2–3
V	Axillary artery	2–3
	Common femoral artery	3–4

[a]Increase one grade for multiple grade III or IV injuries involving >50% vessel circumference. Decrease one grade for <25% vessel circumference disruption for grades IV or V.

Suggested Readings

Moore EE, Cogbill TH, Jurkovich GJ, et al. Organ injury scaling III: Chest wall, abdominal vascular, ureter, bladder, and urethra. *J Trauma* 1992;33:337.

Moore EE, Cogbill TH, Jurkovich GJ, et al. Organ injury scaling V: Spleen and liver (1994 revision). *J Trauma* 1995;38:323.

Moore EE, Cogbill TH, Malangoni MA, et al. Organ injury scaling II: Pancreas, duodenum, small bowel, colon, and rectum. *J Trauma* 1990;30:1427.

Moore EE, Cogbill TH, Malangoni MA, et al. Organ injury scaling. *Surg Clin North Am* 1995;75:293–303.

Moore EE, Dunn EL, Moore JB, et al. Penetrating abdominal trauma index. *J Trauma* 1981;21:439.

Moore EE, Jurkovich GJ, Knudson MM, et al. Organ injury scaling VI: Extrahepatic biliary, esophagus, stomach, vulva, vagina, uterus (nonpregnant), uterus (pregnant), fallopian tube, and ovary. *J Trauma* 1995;39:1069–1070.

Moore EE, Malangoni MA, Cogbill TH, et al. Organ injury scaling IV: Thoracic vascular, lung, cardiac, and diaphragm. *J Trauma* 1994;36:299.

Moore EE, Malangoni MA, Cogbill TH, et al. Organ injury scaling VII: Cervical vascular, peripheral vascular, adrenal, penis, testis, and scrotum. *J Trauma* 1996;41:523–524.

Moore EE, Shackleford SR, Pachter HL, et al. Organ injury scaling: Spleen, liver, and kidney. *J Trauma* 1989;29:1664.

Tinkoff G, Esposito TJ, Reed J, et al. American association for the surgery of trauma organ injury scale I: spleen, liver, and kidney, validation based on the national trauma data bank. *J Am Coll Surg* 2008;207:646.

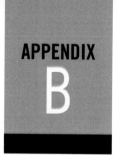

APPENDIX

B

Frequently Used Forms

PHYSICIAN ORDER SET

AUTHORIZATION IS GIVEN TO THE PHARMACY TO DISPENSE AND TO THE
NURSE TO ADMINISTER THE GENERIC OR CHEMICAL EQUIVALENT WHEN
THE DRUG IS FILLED BY THE PHARMACY OF THE UPMC HEALTH SYSTEM
HOSPITAL-UNLESS THE PRODUCT NAME IS CIRCLED.

IMPRINT PATIENT IDENTIFICATION HERE

Trauma Surgery: Admission: Non-ICU—Physician Order Set

Nursing Unit: ☐ Regular _____ ☐ Telemetry _____ Attending Physician: _____

Diagnosis: _____ Condition: _____

Allergies: _____

Check All Orders That Apply with a ☒ *& All Handwritten Orders Should Be BLOCK PRINTED for Clarity*

Communication Orders

☐ 23-Hour observation status

☐ Thoraco-lumbar spine (TLS) precautions

☐ C-spine precautions (NO pillow)

☐ Reverse Trendelenberg 30 degrees

☐ Head of bed elevated 30 degrees

☒ Notify house officer of patient arrival to nursing unit

☒ Call physician if any of the following occur:

☐ Restraints: Refer to Rastraints Orders Form

- Temperature >38.5° or <36°
- Heart rate >120 or <50 beats per minute
- Systolic blood pressure <90 or >150 mmHg
- Diastolic blood pressure >100 or <60 mmHg

- SaO$_2$ <92%
- Urine output <250 mL/8 hours
- New onset of lethargy, difficulty waking agitation delirium
- Other: _____

- Respiratory rate >30 or <10 breaths/min
- Accucheck glucose <70 or >350 mg%

Vital Signs

☐ Cardiac telemetry (only in monitored bed)

☐ Vital sign checks: ☐ q 4 hours ☐ q 2 hours

☐ Neurological checks: ☐ q 8 hours ☐ q 6 hours ☐ q 4 hours ☐ q 2 hours

☐ Neurovascular checks: ☐ q 8 hours ☐ q 6 hours ☐ q 4 hours ☐ q 2 hours

☐ Pulse Oximetry: ⇨ ☐ with vitals signs ☐ Continuous

Activity

☐ Bed rest ☐ Logroll q 2 hours ☐ Out of bed ad lib ☐ Out of bed to chair with assistance (select one): ☐ bid ☐ tid

☐ Overhead Trapeze

☐ Ambulate as tolerated (select all that are appropriate): **May order only if patient does NOT have C-spine precautions.**

☐ No weightbearing limitations

☐ RUE ⇨ ☐ WBAT ☐ NWB ☐ Touch down WB

☐ LUE ⇨ ☐ WBAT ☐ NWB ☐ Touch down WB

☐ RLE ⇨ ☐ WBAT ☐ NWB ☐ Touch down WB ☐ Pivot-transfer only

☐ LLE ⇨ ☐ WBAT ☐ NWB ☐ Touch down WB ☐ Pivot-transfer only

_____   _____

(BLOCK Print Name)   (Signature)

Date/Time: _____   Pager # _____

Additional Handwritten Orders Should Be Placed at the **End** of This Order Set.

☐ **Order Set Faxed to Pharmacy By:**

(name/time) _____ Unit: _____

0031-01-U   Form ID: PUH-1164   Last Revision Date: 02/17/2007   Page 1 of 5

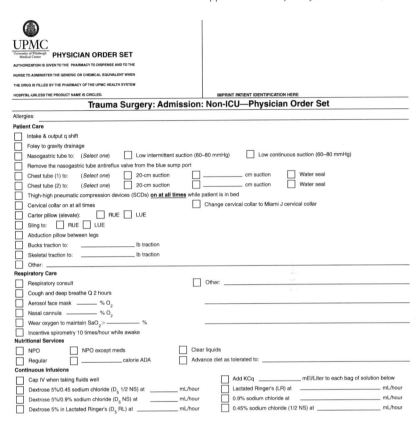

UPMC
University of Pittsburgh
Medical Center **PHYSICIAN ORDER SET**

AUTHORIZATION IS GIVEN TO THE PHARMACY TO DISPENSE AND TO THE

NURSE TO ADMINISTER THE GENERIC OR CHEMICAL EQUIVALENT WHEN

THE DRUG IS FILLED BY THE PHARMACY OF THE UPMC HEALTH SYSTEM

HOSPITAL-UNLESS THE PRODUCT NAME IS CIRCLED.

IMPRINT PATIENT IDENTIFICATION HERE

Trauma Surgery: Admission: Non-ICU—Physician Order Set

Allergies:

Patient Care

☐ Intake & output q shift

☐ Foley to gravity drainage

☐ Nasogastric tube to: (Select one) ☐ Low intermittent suction (60–80 mmHg) ☐ Low continuous suction (60–80 mmHg)

☐ Remove the nasogastric tube antireflux valve from the blue sump port

☐ Chest tube (1) to: (Select one) ☐ 20-cm suction ☐ _____ cm suction ☐ Water seal

☐ Chest tube (2) to: (Select one) ☐ 20-cm suction ☐ _____ cm suction ☐ Water seal

☐ Thigh-high pneumatic compression devices (SCDs) **on at all times** while patient is in bed

☐ Cervical collar on at all times   ☐ Change cervical collar to Miami J cervical collar

☐ Carter pillow (elevate): ☐ RUE ☐ LUE

☐ Sling to: ☐ RUE ☐ LUE

☐ Abduction pillow between legs

☐ Bucks traction to: _____ lb traction

☐ Skeletal traction to: _____ lb traction

☐ Other: _____

Respiratory Care

☐ Respiratory consult   ☐ Other: _____

☐ Cough and deep breathe Q 2 hours

☐ Aerosol face mask _____ % O_2

☐ Nasal cannula _____ % O_2

☐ Wear oxygen to maintain SaO_2 > _____ %

☐ Incentive spirometry 10 times/hour while awake

Nutritional Services

☐ NPO   ☐ NPO except meds   ☐ Clear liquids

☐ Regular   ☐ _____ calorie ADA ☐ Advance diet as tolerated to: _____

Continuous Infusions

☐ Cap IV when taking fluids well   ☐ Add KCq _____ mEl/Liter to each bag of solution below

☐ Dextrose 5%/0.45 sodium chloride (D_5 1/2 NS) at _____ mL/hour   ☐ Lactated Ringer's (LR) at _____ mL/hour

☐ Dextrose 5%/0.9% sodium chloride (D_5 NS) at _____ mL/hour   ☐ 0.9% sodium chloride at _____ mL/hour

☐ Dextrose 5% in Lactated Ringer's (D_5 RL) at _____ mL/hour   ☐ 0.45% sodium chloride (1/2 NS) at _____ mL/hour

_____   _____

(BLOCK Print Name)   (Signature)

Date/Time: _____   Pager # _____

Additional Handwritten Orders Should Be Placed at the **End** of This Order Set.

☐ **Order Set Faxed to Pharmacy By:**
(name/time)   **Unit:**

0031-01-U   Form ID: PUH-1164   Last Revision Date: 02/17/2007   Page 2 of 5

PHYSICIAN ORDER SET

AUTHORIZATION IS GIVEN TO THE PHARMACY TO DISPENSE AND TO THE

NURSE TO ADMINISTER THE GENERIC OR CHEMICAL EQUIVALENT WHEN

THE DRUG IS FILLED BY THE PHARMACY OF THE UPMC HEALTH SYSTEM

HOSPITAL-UNLESS THE PRODUCT NAME IS CIRCLED.

IMPRINT PATIENT IDENTIFICATION HERE

Trauma Surgery: Admission: Non-ICU—Physician Order Set

Allergies: _____

Medications   Do **NOT** exceed a total of 4,000 mg of acetaminophen in a 24-hour period.

- ☐ Docusate 100 mg po bid   ☐ Senokot S two tabs po q Hs prn constipation
- ☐ Enoxaparin (**Lovenox**) 30 mg subcutaneous bid (*DVT Prophylaxis*) <u>Do **NOT** substitute.</u>
- ☐ Famotidine (**Pepcid**) 20-mg IV bid until patient is taking po, then discontinue and start Famotidine 20 mg po bid
- ☐ For patients <65 years of age: Prochlorperazine (**Compazine**) 10-mg IV q 6 hours prn for nausea
- ☐ For patients >65 years of age: Ondansetron (**Zofran**) 4-mg IV Q 6 hours PRN nausea
- ☐ Antibiotic for treatment: Dose: _____   Route: _____   Freq: _____   _____   _____   _____
- ☐ See separate PCA order sheet
- ☐ Ibuprofen 600 mg po q 6 hours around the clock for pain   ☐ Acetaminophen 650 mg po/PR q 4 hours prn for fever/mild pain (1–3)
- ☐ Acetaminophen 325 mg/Oxycodone hydrochloride 5 mg (**Percocet**) <u>1</u> tablet po q 4 hours prn for moderate pain (4–6)
- ☐ Acetaminophen 325 mg/Oxycodone hydrochloride 5 mg (**Percocet**) <u>2</u> tables po q 4 hours prn for severe pain (7–10)
- ☐ Acetaminophen 325 mg/Hydrocodone bitattrate 5 mg (**Vicodin**) <u>1</u> tablet po q 4 hours prn for moderate pain (4–6)
- ☐ Acetaminophen 325 mg/Hydrocodone bitattrate 5 mg (**Vicodin**) <u>2</u> tables po q 4 hours prn for severe pain (7–10)
- ☐ Acetaminophen 325 mg/Oxycodone 5 mg (**Roxiect**) <u>5</u> mL po q 4 hours prn for moderate pain (4–6)
- ☐ Acetaminophen 325 mg/Oxycodone 5 mg (**Roxiect**) <u>10</u> mL po q 4 hours prn for severe pain (7–10)
- ☐ Morphine 1-mg IV q one hour prn mild to moderate pain (4–6)
- ☐ Morphine 2-mg IV q one hour prn severe pain (7–10)

Labs

Now
_____

☐ Lytes	☐ Lytes	☐ PT
☐ BUN/Creatinine	☐ BUN/Creatinine	☐ PTT
☐ Glucose	☐ Glucose	☐ Sodium
☐ CBC. Diff	☐ CBC, Diff	☐ Potassium
☐ Platelet count	☐ Platelet count	☐ Magnesium
☐ CPK/MB q _____ hours x _____		☐ Phosphorus

☐ Calcium
☐ Hct
☐ _____
☐ _____
☐ _____
☐ _____

- ☐ CPK/MB q _____ hours x _____
- ☐ CPK q _____ hours x _____
- ☐ Troponin I q _____ hours x _____
- ☐ Accucheck glucose q _____ hours x _____
- ☐ Hct q _____ hours x _____
- ☐ Urinalysis

_____   _____
(**BLOCK** Print Name)   (Signature)

Date/Time _____   Pager# _____

Additional Handwritten Orders Should Be Placed at the <u>End</u> of This Order Set.

☐ **Order Set Faxed to Pharmacy By:**
(name/time)   Unit: _____

UPMC
University of Pittsburgh
Medical Center **PHYSICIAN ORDER SET**

AUTHORIZATION IS GIVEN TO THE PHARMACY TO DISPENSE AND TO THE

NURSE TO ADMINISTER THE GENERIC OR CHEMICAL EQUIVALENT WHEN

THE DRUG IS FILLED BY THE PHARMACY OF THE UPMC HEALTH SYSTEM

HOSPITAL-UNLESS THE PRODUCT NAME IS CIRCLED.

IMPRINT PATIENT IDENTIFICATION HERE

Trauma Surgery: Admission: Non-ICU—Physician Order Set

Allergies:

Diagnostic Tests

☐ 12-lead EKG

Radiology

☐ CXR ☐ In the department ☐ Portable ☐ In am (_____/_____/_____) re: _____

☐ CT chest   Clinical indication: _____

☐ Ct head ☐ In am (_____/_____/_____)   Clinical indication: _____

☐ CT abdomen/pelvis   Clinical indication: _____

☐ MRI:_____ Clinical indication: _____

☐ Other:_____ Clinical indication: _____

Consults

☐ Orthopaedic consult, clinical indication: _____

☐ Spine trauma consult, clinical indication: _____

☐ Neurosurgery consult, clinical indication: _____

☐ Facial service consult, clinical indication: _____

☐ Hand surgery consult, clinical indication: _____

☐ Ophthalmology consult, clinical indication: _____

☐ PMR consult, clinical indication: Status: Postrauma

☐ Psychiatry consult, clinical indication: _____

☐ PT consult, reason: _____

☐ OT consult, reason: _____

☐ Social work consult, reason: _____

☐ Substance abuse treatment referral

(**BLOCK** Print Name) _____   (Signature) _____

Date/Time: _____   Pager # _____

Additional Handwritten Orders Should Be Placed at the <u>End</u> of This Order Set.

☐ **Order Set Faxed to Pharmacy By:**
(name/time) _____   **Unit:** _____

0031-01-U   Form ID: PUH-1164   Last Revision Date: 02/17/2007   Page 4 of 5

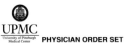

PHYSICIAN ORDER SET

AUTHORIZATION IS GIVEN TO THE PHARMACY TO DISPENSE AND TO THE

NURSE TO ADMINISTER THE GENERIC OR CHEMICAL EQUIVALENT WHEN

THE DRUG IS FILLED BY THE PHARMACY OF THE UPMC HEALTH SYSTEM

HOSPITAL-UNLESS THE PRODUCT NAME IS CIRCLED.

IMPRINT PATIENT IDENTIFICATION HERE

Trauma Surgery: Admission: Non-ICU—Physician Order Set

Allergies:

Additional Orders Should Be BLOCK PRINTED for Clarity	
The following abbreviations are disallowed: u (unit), MS and MSO4 (morphine), MgSO4 (magnesium sulfate),	
QD (daily), QOD (every other day), IU (international units)	
Other Orders	**Medication Orders**
Safe Prescribing Practices: Verify all orders by reading the order back to the prescriber. Do not use zeros following a decimal point. Use a zero before a decimal point. Order IV medications by dose per time (e.g., mg/h). Order levothyroxine in micrograms (µg), not mg doses	

(BLOCK Print Name)

(Signature)

Date/Time:

Pager #

☐ **Order Set Faxed to Pharmacy By:**
   (name/time)   **Unit:**

0031-01-U   Form ID: PUH-1164   Last Revision Date: 02/17/2007   Page 5 of 5

UPMC
University of Pittsburgh
Medical Center

Admission Orders: Trauma ICU

AUTHORIZATION IS GIVEN TO THE PHARMACY TO DISPENSE AND TO THE
NURSE TO ADMINISTER THE GENERIC OR CHEMICAL EQUIVALENT WHEN
THE DRUG IS FILLED BY THE PHARMACY OF UPMC-UNLESS THE PRODUCT
NAME IS CIRCLED.

IMPRINT PATIENT IDENTIFICATION HERE

Admit Unit	
Service	
Diagnosis	
Allergies	
Condition	☐ Critical ☐ Serious ☐ Fair ☐ Good
Vital Signs	☐ Vital signs, I and O, monitoring and turning per ICU standards
Activity	☐ Bed rest ☐ Mobilize to chain
Precautions	☐ None ☐ C-spine ☐ TLS
	☐ Logroll only
Position	☒ Elevate HOB 30° per ICU standards
Nutrition	☐ NPO ☐ Ice chips ☐ Sips ☐ TPN
Enteral	Product _____ mL/h
Devices	☐ Pneumatic compression devices
NG tube	☐ Intermittent suction ☐ Continuous ☐ Gravity
Chest tubes	☐ Suction _____ cm H$_2$O ☐ Water seal
Drains	
Traction	
Other	
Dressings	

IV Fluids	**Maintenance Infusion Rate:** _____ mL/h
Type	☐ D5W ☐ D5W with KCL _____ mEq/L
	☐ LR ☐ LR with KCL _____ mEq/L
	☐ 0.9% NaCl ☐ 0.9% NaCl with KCL ___ mEq/L
	☐ 0.45% NaCl ☐ 0.45% NaCl with KCL ___ mEq/L
Phamacy additive	☐ MVI 10 mL/L in IV above
Other	
Blood	☐ Type and screen ☐ Hold _____ Units PRBC
Transfuse	_____ Units PRBC _____ Units FFP _____ Units Plts

Medications	Dose	Route	Frequency/Indication
☐ Famotidine	20 mg	IV	Q 12 hours
☐ Enoxaparin	30 mg	Subq	Q 12 hours Do NOT Substitute
☐ Dalteparin	5,000 u	Subq	Q 24 hours
☐ Heparin	5,000 u	Subq	Q 12 hours
☐ Propofol	mg/kg/m	IV	
☐ Lorazepam	mg	IV	
☐ Haloperidol	mg	IV	
☐ Morphine	mg	IV	
☐ Fentanyl	mg	IV	
☐ Phenytoin	mg	IV	
☐ Labeltalol	mg	IV	
☐ Hydralazine	mg	IV	
☐ Metoprolol	mg		
☐ Ondansetron	mg	IV	
☐ Cefazolin	g	IV	
☐ Acetaminophen	mg		
☐ Regular insulin sliding scale		12 units	☐ 20 units ☐ 28 units
☐ Insulin infusion per unit protocol			
☐ PCA per order form			
☐ Chlorhexidine (0.12%) mouth rinse per unit protocol			
☐ Titrate propofol to Ramsay sedation scale		☐ 2 ☐ 3 ☐ 4	
☐ BP Rx Threshold ☐ SBP > ☐ MAP > _____ mmHg			
☐ Hold Metoproll or HR <60 bpm or SBP <100 mmHg			

Electrolytes			
KCL	☐ Per protocol Target ☐ 3.5 mEq/L ☐ 4.2 mEq/L		
Magnesium Sulf	☐ 4-g IV over 4 hours prn Mg^{+2} < 2 mEq/L		
Phosphate	☐ Phos. <1.0 mg/dL 30 mmol over 6 hours—IV		
	☐ Phos. 1.0–2.0 mg/dL 15 mmol over 4 hours—IV		
Phosphate given as KPO$_4$ unless K >4.0 mEq/L NaPO$_4$ when K >4.0 mEq/L.			

Physician Name (Print) _____

Pager # _____

Physician (Signature) _____

Date: _____   Time: _____

☐ **Order Set Faxed to Pharmacy By:**
(name/time) _____

0031-01-U   Form ID: PUH-1402   Last Revision Date: 08/15/2006

Page 1 of 2

UPMC
University of Pittsburgh
Medical Center

Admission Orders: Trauma ICU

AUTHORIZATION IS GIVEN TO THE PHARMACY TO DISPENSE AND TO THE
NURSE TO ADMINISTER THE GENERIC OR CHEMICAL EQUIVALENT WHEN
THE DRUG IS FILLED BY THE PHARMACY OF THE UPMC-HOSPITAL-UNLESS
THE PRODUCT NAME IS CIRCLED.

IMPRINT PATIENT IDENTIFICATION HERE

Ventilator	☐ AC ☐ IMV ☐ PSV	cm H_2O	**Diagnostics**	☐ Portable CXR ☐ STAT ☐ In AM
Settings	RR / Tidal volume / FiO$_2$ / PEEP			☐ 12-lead EKG ☐ STAT ☐ In AM
	Bpm / mL / cm H_2O		CT scan	
Other			MRI	
BiPap	Mode / IPAP / EPAP		X-rays	

Weaning	☒ Wean ventilator per protocol ☐ Extubate

Oxygen Rx	☐ AFM % ☐ Nasal cannula L/min

Consults

Toilet	☐ Per respiratory care protocol/pathway
Directed	☐ Incentive spirometry ☐ PEP ☐ Flutter valve
	☐ IPPB ☐ CPAP ☐ NT suction
	Administer directed pulmonary toilet every ___ hours

☐ Orthopaedics	☐ Neurosurgery	☐ Plastic Surgery
☐ Maxillofacial Surgery	☐ ENT	☐ Ophthalmology
☐ Rehabilitation Medicine	☐ Physical Therapy	☐ Occupational Therapy
☐ Social Service		

Bronchodilator	Administer bronchodilators every ___ hours
Method	☐ MDI ☐ Nebulizer ☐ IPPB
Drug	

ICU Physician or Primary Service Notifications

☒ Temperature >38.5° or <36°C
☒ Systolic blood pressure <90 mmHg or >160 mmHg
☒ Mean arterial pressure <60 mmHg or >110 mmHg

Labs	
STAT	☐ ABG ☐ HCT ☐ Glu ☐ K$^+$ ☐ Na$^+$
	☐ Ca^{+2} ☐ Lytes ☐ Lactate ☐ BUN/Creatinine
	☐ Ca/Mg/Phos ☐ LFTs ☐ Bili ☐ Urinalysis
	☐ Troponin I ☐ CPK/MB
	☐ CBC ☐ Diff ☐ Platelets ☐ PT/PTT
Cultures	☐ Blood x 2 ☐ Urine ☐ Blind BAL ☐ Sputum

☒ Urine output <25 mL/h or >300 mL/h
☒ Respiratory rate <10 or >30 breaths/min
☒ Pulse <50 or >120 bpm
☒ Pulse oximetry saturation <90%
☒ Pain score >5 or pain interfering with therapy
☒ Intracranial pressure sustained >30 mmHg

Morning Labs	☐ Lytes/BUN/Creatinine ☐ Ca/Mg/Phos
	☐ Glucose ☐ ABG ☐ CBC
	☐ CBC ☐ WBC diff ☐ Platelets ☐ PT/PTT

CCM Fellow/Attending Notification

☒ Oliguria unresponsive to fluid challenge within 1 hour
☒ Hypotension unresponsive to fluid challenge within 15 minutes
☒ Hypotension necessitating >20% escalation in vasopressor dosage

Monitoring	Frequency		Duration
Glucose every:	hours	x	hours
Hematocrit every:	hours	x	hours
ABG every:	hours	x	hours
Troponin I every:	hours	x	hours
every:	hours	x	hours

☒ CI <2.0 L/min/M^2 unresponsive to fluid challenge within 15 minutes
☒ Worsening oxygenation requiring >10% escalation in FiO$_2$
☒ New or worsening bleeding
☒ New seizures, anisocoria, focal weakness, or unresponsiveness

---

Physician Name (Print) _____

Pager # _____

Physician (Signature) _____

Date: _____ Time: _____

☐ **Order Set Faxed to Pharmacy By:**
(name/time) _____

0031-01-U   Form ID: PUH-1402 Last Revision Date: 08/15/2006

UPMC
University of Pittsburgh
Medical Center

**TRAUMA ADMISSION
HISTORY AND PHYSICAL**

999900

Date : 2007   ED Arrival Time: _____

History (Mechanism of Injury): ☐ N/A

1. Blunt: ☐ MVC: Driver/Passenger   Restrained/Unrestrained

☐ MCC: Driver/Passenger   Helmet/Unhelmeted   ☐ ATV   ☐ Assault   ☐ Fall _____(ht)   ☐ Ped struck   ☐ Other: _____

2. Penetrating: ☒ Firearm   ☐ Stab wound   ☐ Other: _____

IMPRINT PATIENT IDENTIFICATION HERE   Page 1 of 4

Description of Injury (location, duration, quality, severity, timing, context, signs and symptoms, modifying factors):   ☐ Scene run
27 y/o male gunshot wound to the chest, rt arm, hip with a pneumothorax.

Prehospital care: _____   Location of care: _____

Past Medical History: ☐ Coronary artery disease   ☐ COPD   ☐ Stroke   ☐ DM   ☐ Obesity   ☐ Hypertension   ☐ Asthma   ☐ MI   ☐ Afib

☐ Cancer: _____   ☐ Other: _____

Home medications: _____

Past Surgical History: _____

Medications: ☐ ASA ☐ Plavix ☐ Coumadin | **Allergies:** ☐ NKDA

☒ Unable to obtain because of the emergent nature of the patient ☐ Unable to obtain because: ☐ No reported medical history

Past Family History: ☐ Coronary artery disease   ☐ COPD   ☐ Stroke   ☐ DM   ☐ Obesity   ☐ Hypertension   ☐ Asthma   ☐ MI   ☐ Afib

☐ Cancer: _____   ☐ Other: _____   **Relation to patient:** _____

☒ Unable to obtain because of the emergent nature of patient ☐ Unable to obtain because: ☐ No significant family history

Past Social History: ☐ Tobacco _____ ppd   ☐ EtOH _____ per day/week   ☐ Drugs   Occupation: _____

☒ Unable to obtain because of the emergent nature of patient   ☐ Unable to obtain because:

REIVIEW OF SYSTEMS

Constitutional	Neg/Pos	Findings:		Musculoskeletal	Neg/Pos	Findings:
Eyes	Neg/Pos	Findings:		Neurological	Neg/Pos	Findings:
Ears, Nose Mouth/Throat	Neg/Pos	Findings:		Psychiatric	Neg/Pos	Findings:
Cardiovascular	Neg/Pos	Findings:		Endocrine	Neg/Pos	Findings:
Respiratory	Neg/Pos	Findings:		Hematologic/ Lymphatic	Neg/Pos	Findings:
Gastrointestinal	Neg/Pos	Findings:		Skin	Neg/Pos	Findings:
Genitourinary	Neg/Pos	Findings:		Allergic/ Immunologic	Neg/Pos	Findings:

☐ All other systems have been reviewed and are negative   ☒ Unable to obtain because:

Initial Trauma Room VS: P: 114   BP: RESP: O$_2$ Saturation: T: Height: Weight:

Primary Survey

Airway: Patent (Yes) No   intubation | Breathing: intubation

Circulation: Pulse/Strength   0   1+   2+   Site:

Interventions on the primary survey:

9655-01-U   Form ID: PUH-2233-3670   Last Revision Date: 5/19/2006

Name: _____   Page 1 of 4

NAME:_____ D.O.B:_____ MEDICAL RECORD#: _____ DATE: _____

Glasgow Coma Scale (GCS):

| Eye Opening: None 1 | Verbal Response: None 1 | Motor Response: None 1 | GCS Total: 3 |

Pupils: R: _2_ L: _2_ [X] Equal and reactive to light ☐ Unequal ☐Reactive R Yes/No ☐Reactive L Yes/No

☐ Unable to assess: _____ Cranial pairs:_____

Neurological Exam

Peripheral Function (sensory/motor):
UE R: S_____ M____ L: S_____ M____
LE R: S_____ M____ L: S_____ M____

Psych: ☐ Combative ☐ Agitated [X] Somnolent ☐ Cooperative

Other:

Head:

Face:

ENT:
TM's: R/L _____

Neck
Pain on palpation: Yes/No
Deformities: Yes/No
Distracting injuries: Yes/No   Peripheral neurological deficits Yes/No
Altered mental status (includes alcohol) Yes/No
Cervical collar in place (Yes)/No Carotid pulse: R: 0 1+ (2+) L: 0 1+ (2+)

Chest
Breath sounds: rhonci on breath sounds
[X] Present   (R)(L)
☐ Diminished   R / L
☐ Absent   R / L
☐ Presence of subcutaneous emphysema: R Yes/No   L Yes/No

Cardiac:

Abdomen
Pain on palpation: Yes/No If yes, where: _____
[X] F.A.S.T. Free fluid: Yes/(No) If yes, where: _____
☐ Indeterminate

Vascular Exam
Carotid	**R:** 0 1+ (2+) **L:** 0 1+ (2+)	Femoral	**R:** 0 1+ (2+) **L:** 0 1+ 2+
Axillary	**R:** 0 1+ 2+ **L:** 0 1+ 2+	Popliteal	**R:** 0 1+ 2+ **L:** 0 1+ 2+
Brachial	**R:** 0 1+ 2+ **L:** 0 1+ 2+	Dorsalis pedis	**R:** 0 1+ 2+ **L:** 0 1+ 2+
Brachial	**R:** 0 1+ 2+ **L:** 0 1+ 2+	Posterior tibial	**R:** 0 1+ 2+ **L:** 0 1+ 2+

Pelvis
Stable: Yes/No

GU/Perineum:
☐ Hemocult +   ☐ Gross blood +

Skin:

Rectal: no gross blood, good tone

Pelvic Exam:
☐ Deferred

Thoracic Lumbar, Sacral Spine:
Spontaneous pain: Yes/No If yes, where? _____
Pain on palpation: Yes/No If yes, where? _____
Deformities: Yes/No If yes, where? _____

Secondary Survey

Cranial pairs:_____
Add Physical Exam Findings:

Gunshot Wound
Gunshot Wound
Gunshot Wound

Legend: A—Abrasion L—Laceration S—Stab Wound
C—Contusion GSW—Gunshot Wound UW—Unspecified
CF—Closed Fracture OF—Open Fracture

Additional Descriptions:

Secondary Survey

Name:

NAME: _____ D.O.B.: _____ MEDICAL RECORD #: _____ DATE: _____

Preliminary Imaging Performed/Reviewed:	Date:	For acute trauma (circle):	Findings:
☒ CXR	2007/01/27	☒ Pending Neg/Pos	
☐ Pelvis	_____	☐ Pending Neg/Pos	
☐ Neck (simple films)	_____	☐ Pending Neg/Pos	
☐ Extremity films	_____	☐ Pending Neg/Pos	
☐ CT head	_____	☐ Pending Neg/Pos	
☐ CT neck	_____	☐ Pending Neg/Pos	
☐ CT chest	_____	☐ Pending Neg/Pos	
☐ CT abdomen/pelvis	_____	☐ Pending Neg/Pos	
☐ Other: _____	_____	☐ Pending Neg/Pos	
☐ Other: _____	_____	☐ Pending Neg/Pos	

Name:

9655-01-U

NAME: _____ D.O.B.: _____ MEDICAL RECORD . _____ DATE: _____

A. Injuries and Problems Identified:

Date of Diagnosis:

		Error
_____	1. 879.8 GUNSHOT WOUNDS, MULTIPLE	☐
_____	2.	☐
_____	3.	☐
_____	4.	☐
_____	5.	☐
_____	6.	☐

B. Injuries and Problems to Rule Out:

C. Plan:

1.

2.

3.

D. Attending Note and Attestation: ☐ Patient to follow up in clinic. Discharge to home.

I saw the patient. I personally examined the patient. I agree with the notes written by the resident.

☐ With the exception of:

☐ With the addition of:

Procedures: ☐ Chest tube 32020 ☐ Intubation 31500 ☐ DPL 49080 ☐ Cricothyroidotomy 31605 ☐ CPR 92950 ☐ Cystogram 51605

☐ Urethrogram 74450 ☐ Thoracotomy 32160 ☐ Arterial line 36620 ☐ Percutan. cent. line 36556 ☐ Cutdown cent. line 36558

☐ Other: _____ ☐ Other: _____ ☐ Other: _____

| Critical Care: | 30–74 min. (99291) | 75–104 min. (99291, 99292×2) | 105–134 min. (99291, 99292×2) | 135–164 min. (99291, 99292×2) | 165–194 min. (99291, 99292×2) | _____ (min.) |

Initial IP: _____ Subsequent Care: _____ 23 H. Admit to Obs: _____ ☐ 99217 Discharge from Obs

☒ 99499 (resus) Admit, discharge same calendar day. _____ ☐ 99238 discharge (<30 min.) _____ (min.) ☐ 99239 discharge (<30 min.) _____ (min.)

☐ No charge **Modifiers:** ☐ –24 E/M unrelated to recent surgery ☐ 25 separate E/M encounter with minor procedure ☐ 57 Decision for surgery within 24 hours

Signature attests that all four pages have been reviewed and completed.

Housestaff Physician/Other Signature: _____

Title: _____ Pager: _____ Date/Time: _____

Attending Physician Signature: _____

Title: _____ Pager: _____ Date/Time: _____

Name:

Assessment and Plan

Visit

UPMC | University of Pittsburgh Medical Center
200 Lothrop Street
Pittsburgh, PA 15213-2582

TRAUMA CARE FLOW RECORD

IMPRINT PATIENT IDENTIFICATION HERE

Date: _____ Treatment room: _____

Mechanism of injury:
- ☐ MVC
- ☐ ATV
- ☐ GSW
- ☐ Stab
- ☐ Assault
- ☐ Motorcycle
- ☐ Fall _____ ft.
- ☐ Other

Arrived by:
- ☐ Self
- ☐ Air
- ☐ Ambulance

Transferred from:
- ☐ Home
- ☐ Scene
- ☐ Hospital

Details of injury/prehospital report: _____

V.S. at scene: _____

Loss of consciousness: ☐ Yes ☐ No ☐ Unknown

Prehospital interventions:
- ☐ CPR ☐ In progress
- ☐ Intubation
- ☐ O₂
- ☐ Cervical collar
- ☐ CID
- ☐ Blackboard
- ☐ Splint
- ☐ Chest tube
- ☐ Ng ☐ Og
- ☐ Foley
- ☐ Medication PTA

Total Intake	Output
Crystalloid: _____	
Colloid: _____	

Trauma team activated:
☐ Yes ☐ No

Level I Time: _____
Level II Time: _____

PERSONNEL RESPONSE

	NAME	ARRIVAL TIME
Triage Nurse		
Nurse Recorder		
Primary Trauma Nurse		
Secondary Trauma Nurse		
ED Attending		
Trauma Attending		
Chief Resident		
Team Leader		
CCM/Anesthesia		
Social Service		
Relief Nurse		

Consults	Name	Time called	Returned Call	Time Arrived
Orthopedics				
Neurosurgery				
Eye				
Hand				
Face				

Medical History: _____

Medications: _____

Allergies: _____

Pregnant: ☐ Yes ☐ No   LMP _____
Tetanus: _____

PATIENT ARRIVAL TIME: _____

3272-01-U   FORM 1064-2400-0207A

NAME _____ MEDICAL RECORD _____ DATE _____

TIME	S/P CUFF	S/P DINAMAP	PULSE	RESP/ SPONT ASSIST	EKG	SAO₂	O₂/l	GCS TOTAL	PAIN SCALE	NURSING OBSERVATIONS PATIENT RESPONSE TO TREATMENTS	INITIALS

Disposition _____ Intake _____ Time _____

I&O _____ Output _____

Total _____

C-spine precaution ☐

T/L/S precaution ☐

Airway patent ☐ O₂ _____
Intubated ☐
IV's Patient ☐
Fluid _____ Patient ☐

Physician MD Signature: _____

Accompanied by: ☐ Rn ☐ PCT ☐ Escort
GCS _____

Last Set V/S _____
Monitor Rhythm _____
- Lacerations Sutured ☐ Done ☐ N/A
- Splints in Place ☐ Done ☐ N/A Not Done _____

Transferring Rn _____

LIST BELONGINGS: _____

VALUABLES
(List above)
- ☐ With Patient
- ☐ To Family
- ☐ Security
- ☐ Other

CLOTHING
- ☐ Cut Off
- ☐ With Patient
- ☐ To Family
- ☐ Security
- ☐ Other

FINAL DISPOSITION _____ TIME _____

767

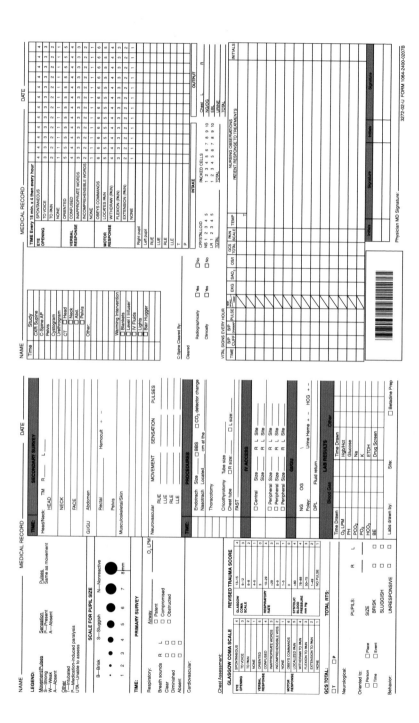

3272-02-U FORM 1064-2400-0207B

UPMC
University of Pittsburgh
Medical Center

PHYSICIAN ORDER SET

AUTHORIZATION IS GIVEN TO THE PHARMACY TO DISPENSE AND TO THE
NURSE TO ADMINISTER THE GENERIC OR CHEMICAL EQUIVALENT WHEN
THE DRUG IS FILLED BY THE PHARMACY OF THE UPMC HEALTH SYSTEM
HOSPITAL–UNLESS THE PRODUCT NAME IS CIRCLED.

IMPRINT PATIENT IDENTIFICATION HERE

TRAUMA PATIENT: DISCHARGE ORDERS AND INSTRUCTIONS

Attending physician:

Allergies:

[X] Discharge to:

Injuries:

1		5	
2		6	
3		7	
4		8	

Check All Orders That Apply with an [X] . *All Handwritten Orders Should Be* <u>BLOCK PRINTED</u> *for Clarity*

[X] Call **(412) 647-2002** if you experience any of the following or if you have any questions that are not listed below:

- Persistent headache
- Nausea/vomiting
- Dizziness
- Ringing in the ears
- Numbness/tingling

- Abdominal pain
- Warmth at wound site
- Night sweats
- Chest pain
- Fever/chills

- Shortness of breath
- Visual changes
- Pain not relived with prescribed medicine
- Increased redness or wound drainage
- Significant new problems not specified above

IF YOU BELIEVE YOU HAVE A LIFE-THREATENING EMERGENCY,
PLEASE CALL <u>911</u> OR YOUR LOCAL EMERGENCY MEDICAL SERVICE (EMS)

CLINIC	ATTENDING PHYSICIAN	WHEN	PLACE	PHONE #
Trauma	TraumaClinic		Falk Clinic 6B	(412) 648-3164 or (412) 648-3167
Orthopaedics				
Neurosurgery				
Other Services				
Other Services				
Services	**Name**		**Phone #**	
Home Care				
Equipment Company				

(BLOCK Print Name)

Date/Time:

(Signature)

Pager #:

[ ] Order Set Faxed to Pharmacy By:
(name/time)

Unit:

0031-01-U   Form ID: PUH-1495   Last Revision Date: 10/01/2006

Page 1 of 3

UPMC
University of Pittsburgh
Medical Center

PHYSICIAN ORDER SET

AUTHORIZATION IS GIVEN TO THE PHARMACY TO DISPENSE AND TO THE
NURSE TO ADMINISTER THE GENERIC OR CHEMICAL EQUIVALENT WHEN
THE DRUG IS FILLED BY THE PHARMACY OF THE UPMC HEALTH SYSTEM
HOSPITAL-UNLESS THE PRODUCT NAME IS CIRCLED.

IMPRINT PATIENT IDENTIFICATION HERE

TRAUMA PATIENT: DISCHARGE ORDERS AND INSTRUCTIONS

Do you have a primary care physician? ☐ No ☐ Yes   Name: _____

If yes, notify your primary care physician of your admission to the hospital

Ask if a follow-up appointment in the office of your primary care physician is needed.

Diet: _____

Activity

Walking: ☐ No restrictions   ☐ Weightbearing restrictions (check all that are applicable)

☐ Pivot transfer   ☐ Touchdown   ☐ Nonweightbearing

☐ LLE   ☐ RLE   ☐ LUE   ☐ RUE

Sitting:	☐ No Restrictions	☐ Hip flexion precautions no greater than 30/60/90° Other: _____
Lifting:	☐ No Restrictions	☐ No lifting greater than (5–10) lb
Stairs:	☐ No Restrictions	☐ Limit use
Driving:	☐ No Restrictions	☐ No driving until seen for follow-up ☐ No driving while taking pain medications
Work:	☐ No Restrictions	☐ No work until seen for follow-up ☐ Light duty
School:	☐ No Restrictions	☐ No school until seen for follow-up ☐ May attend, but no physical activity
Bathing:	☐ No Restrictions	☐ May shower ☐ No tub baths ☐ Sponge bathe ONLY
Sexual Activity:	☐ No Restrictions	☐ Restrictions: _____

Special Care In Instructions (when applicable)

☐ Wound Care/Dressing Changes: _____

☐ Incentive Spirometry (send home with patient) _____

☐ Pin Care _____

☐ Ostomy Care: _____

☐ Drain Care (i.e., flushing drains, recording outputs, bring output #s to clinic): _____

☐ Braces/Slings/Splings: _____

☐ Laboratory Studies: Date and Place to be drawn: _____

PA Trauma Outcome Functional Status

Feeding _____ Expression _____ Locomotion _____ Social interaction _____ Transportation/mobility _____

(**BLOCK** Print Name) _____   (Signature) _____

Date/Time: _____   Pager #: _____

☐ **Order Set Faxed to Pharmacy By:**
(name/time) _____   **Unit:** _____

0031-01-U   Form ID: PUH-1304   Last Revision Date: 10/01/2006   Page 2 of 3

UPMC
University of Pittsburgh
Medical Center

PHYSICIAN ORDER SET

AUTHORIZATION IS GIVEN TO THE PHARMACY TO DISPENSE AND TO THE
NURSE TO ADMINISTER THE GENERIC OR CHEMICAL EQUIVALENT WHEN
THE DRUG IS FILLED BY THE PHARMACY OF THE UPMC HEALTH SYSTEM
HOSPITAL-UNLESS THE PRODUCT NAME IS CIRCLED.

IMPRINT PATIENT IDENTIFICATION HERE

TRAUMA PATIENT: DISCHARGE ORDERS AND INSTRUCTIONS

Medications   *Do **NOT** drive or consume alcoholic beverages while taking pain medications.*
*This **DOES NOT** include Tylenol™ or other antiinflammatory medications.*

Drug _____ Dose _____ Route _____ Frequency _____ Amount Dispenensed _____

Drug _____ Dose _____ Route _____ Frequency _____ Amount Dispenensed _____

Drug _____ Dose _____ Route _____ Frequency _____ Amount Dispenensed _____

Drug _____ Dose _____ Route _____ Frequency _____ Amount Dispenensed _____

Drug _____ Dose _____ Route _____ Frequency _____ Amount Dispenensed _____

Drug _____ Dose _____ Route _____ Frequency _____ Amount Dispenensed _____

Medication Reconciliation

☐ I have reviewed the current list of medications, the new medications ordered, and compared them to the home medication list.

_____   _____
(**BLOCK** Print Name)   (Signature)

Date/Time: _____   Pager #: _____

Discharge instructions given by: _____ / _____
                Registered Nurse (Print Name)   /   Registered Nurse (Signature)   Date

I have received Healthy Lifestyle information material. The information covers the benefits of healthy eating, regular exercise,
and health care tips related to diabetes, stroke, and key points of heart failure management including signs and symptoms
to report to physician, daily weight instruction, daily activity review, and dietary choices. Additional information addresses
smoking cessation, warning signs of cancer, and steps to control and prevent the spread of infection.
Patient verifies understanding of Discharge Instructions and is leaving with all valuables/belongings.

_____   _____
Patient/Significant Other Signature   Date/Time

Give photocopy of Orders/Instructions to patient.

☐ **Order Set Faxed to Pharmacy By:**
   (name/time)   **Unit:** _____

0031-01-U   Form ID: PUH-1495   Last Revision Date: 10/01/2006   Page 3 of 3

Index

Note: Page number followed by f and t indicates figure and table respectively.